Diagnostic Testing and Nursing Implications

A Case Study Approach

Diagnostic Testing and Nursing Implications

A Case Study Approach

Kathleen Deska Pagana, Ph.D., R.N.

Professor
Department of Nursing, Lycoming College
Williamsport, Pennsylvania

Timothy James Pagana, M.D., F.A.C.S.

Surgical Oncologist
Williamsport, Pennsylvania

Fifth Edition

With 112 illustrations

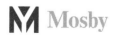 Mosby

St. Louis Baltimore Boston Carlsbad Chicago Minneapolis New York Philadelphia Portland
London Milan Sydney Tokyo Toronto

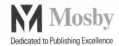

Editor: Loren S. Wilson
Developmental Editor: Brian Dennison
Project Manager: Mark Spann
Production Editor: Monica Groth Farrar
Designer: Bill Drone
Manufacturing Manager: Don Carlisle
Background Cover Image: Gary Chapman/Image Bank
Cover Photos: PhotoDisc

FIFTH EDITION

Composition by The Clarinda Company
Lithography/color film by The Clarinda Company
Printing/binding by R.R. Donnelley & Sons Company

Mosby, Inc.
11830 Westline Industrial Drive
St. Louis, Missouri 63146

Library of Congress Cataloging in Publication Data

Pagana, Kathleen Deska
    Diagnostic testing & nursing implications : a case study approach
 / Kathleen Deska Pagana, Timothy James Pagana. —5th ed.
    p. cm.
    Includes bibliographical references and index.
    ISBN 0-323-00289-7
    1. Diagnosis. 2. Nursing.   3. Diagnosis—Case studies.
  4. Nursing—Case studies.   I. Pagana, Timothy James
  II. Title.
    [DNLM: 1. Laboratory Techniques and Procedures nurses'
instruction. 2. Nursing Assessment. QY 4P128d 1998]
  RT48.5.P32 1998
  616.07′5′024613—dc21
  DNLM/DLC
  for Library of Congress   98-34086
                                              CIP

99 00 01 02 03 / 9 8 7 6 5 4 3 2 1

We lovingly dedicate this book to our three daughters:

Jocelyn Marie Pagana

Denise Kathleen Pagana

Theresa Noel Pagana

Preface

With the ever-increasing advances in technology, it remains a major challenge to stay current in the exciting field of diagnostic and laboratory testing. Although this fifth edition represents a major revision of this widely used textbook, its purpose remains the same: to make the study of diagnostic and laboratory testing interesting and enjoyable.

NEW TO THIS EDITION

Three of the major changes of this edition include a more contemporary design in which color has been added, the alphabetical listing of tests within each body system chapter, and the complete reorganization of the introductory chapter. Chapter 1 (General Guidelines for Diagnostic and Laboratory Testing) provides an overview of the major types of laboratory tests and diagnostic procedures to ensure patient safety and clinical accuracy.

All of the studies have been updated, and many sections have been completely rewritten. Many new studies, such as bone densitometry, fetal biophysical profile, breast scintigraphy, breast cancer genetic screening, white blood cell scan, and sleep apnea studies, are included in this edition. New case studies address topics such as inflammatory bowel disease, sleep apnea, testicular torsion, and cervical cancer.

ORGANIZATION

This book is unique in the field of diagnostic testing because of the organization of information, application of the case study approach, inclusion of review questions and answers, and the extensive use of illustrations. Nursing implications are comprehensive and clearly stated. The format of this book invites the reader to a full and logical understanding of diagnostic tests and abnormal findings through interesting case studies. This book supplies the diagnostic testing information needed to provide thorough and accurate patient teaching and patient preparation so that tests can be performed accurately and safely.

Chapters are arranged according to body systems (e.g., cardiovascular, reproductive, and nervous systems). The advantage of this feature is that tests relating to a certain system (e.g., EKG, cardiac catheterization, cardiac enzymes) are all discussed in the same chapter. This body system approach has been beneficial to nurse educators who have selected chapters of this book as required or recommended reading in their courses. For ease in locating material, studies are presented alphabetically within each chapter.

A special feature of this book is a concise, yet complete, discussion of anatomy and physiology, which introduces each chapter. Although we assume that the reader has a basic knowledge of anatomy and physiology, this information is included to provide a general overview of the system to be discussed. The inclusion of this material ensures a better understanding of the related diagnostic procedures.

Case studies enhance the understanding of tests and include the following information: the presentation of a commonly seen patient problem, the results (including normal values) of diagnostic studies performed, and a diagnostic analysis, which explains the interpretation of these studies and patient treatment. Additionally, critical thinking questions related to each case have been added in this edition to challenge the reader to make sound clinical decisions using the information gained in the case presentation. The purpose of the case study is to stimulate the reader's interest by providing an actual patient problem and treatment of the problem based on accurate diagnostic testing. Case studies are distributed throughout each chapter and provide application for key diagnostic and laboratory tests.

TEST FORMAT

A major feature of the text is its consistent format. Test name, test type, normal values, possible critical values, rationale, potential complications, interfering factors, procedure, contraindications, and nursing implications are discussed for each test. The *test name* includes the complete name of the study followed by a complete list of abbreviations and alternative test names. The *test type* identifies whether the test is, for example, a radiographic procedure, ultrasound test, blood test, sputum test, or microscopic examination. This section helps the reader to identify the source of the laboratory specimen or the location of the diagnostic procedure. *Normal values* are listed, when appropriate, for the infant, child, adult, and elderly person. Also, when appropriate, values

are listed according to gender. Because many laboratories are now using the System of International Units (SI units), most common laboratory values are expressed both in conventional and SI units. Normal values may vary because of different laboratory methods. We encourage the reader to check the normal values at the institution where the test is performed. *Possible critical values* indicate results that are well outside the range of normal. These results generally require immediate interventions.

The *rationale* for a study includes a discussion of the relevant anatomy and physiology and indications for the test. *Potential complications* also are listed. Factors that can invalidate the test or make the test results unreliable are listed in *interfering factors*. The *procedure* describes how the study is performed; who performs the study; where the study is performed; the patient's position during the study; the need for anesthesia or sedation; patient sensation; and the duration of the procedure. (The procedure may vary somewhat in different institutions and in different areas of the country.) *Contraindications* are crucial because they alert the nurse to patients who should not undergo the test. Patients frequently highlighted in this section include those who are pregnant, who are allergic to iodinated or contrast dyes, or who have bleeding disorders.

Nursing implications are comprehensive and address the patient's psychologic, as well as physiologic, needs. Included in this section are nursing interventions (with rationales) that should be performed before, during, and after the study to ensure the accuracy of the procedure and the safety of the patient. Potential problems are identified, and key areas of nursing assessment and intervention are described. Patient teaching priorities are noted with a special icon to highlight information that the nurse communicates to the patient.

SPECIAL FEATURES

Review questions and answers are included at the end of each chapter to describe common nursing problems associated with patients undergoing diagnostic tests and to ensure comprehension of the diagnostic studies. The review questions challenge the reader to correlate previously presented material with problematic circumstances that frequently occur in nursing practice. Answers are provided after each question. *A Comprehensive Practice Test* in National Council Licensure Examination (NCLEX) format is located at the end of the book. Answers with rationales are included to help readers measure their understanding of diagnostic testing. A bibliography is provided at the end of each chapter for the reader who wishes to find additional information on a particular diagnostic procedure.

The two-color design highlights important information and enhances the visual appeal of this new edition. Many new, two-color illustrations and tables clarify and simplify content. In addition to being interesting and helpful to nurses and nursing students, these illustrations have proved to be advantageous in patient education.

The concise table of contents directs the reader to the appropriate chapter outline, which includes page references to each test in the chapter for quick location of test information. This edition's user-friendly organization is exemplified by extensive cross-referencing. Appendix A provides an alphabetical list of all the tests discussed in the book. Appendix B features a list of the studies according to test type. This listing helps the reader to learn about similarly performed tests and procedures (e.g., nuclear scans of the brain, bone, and gallbladder). Appendix C lists the abbreviations for diagnostic and laboratory tests. This should be extremely useful for those puzzled by abbreviations such as DSA, EGD, ERCP, KUB, and AST. Typical abbreviations and units of measurement can be found inside the book's front cover. Appendix D provides a brief list of normal values for commonly performed blood tests.

ACKNOWLEDGMENTS

We wish to sincerely thank the many people throughout the country who sent in comment cards with recommendations for improving this book. All evaluations and reviews were most helpful in planning for this fifth edition. We sincerely appreciate the efforts of our editors, Loren Wilson and Brian Dennison, for their help in ensuring the high quality of the book.

Kathleen Deska Pagana
Timothy James Pagana

Contents

Chapter 1

General Guidelines for Diagnostic and Laboratory Testing

The complete evaluation of a patient usually requires a thorough health history and physical examination along with efficient diagnostic testing. The correct use of diagnostic testing can confirm or eliminate the presence of disease and improve the cost efficiency of screening tests. Finally, appropriate and thoughtfully timed diagnostic testing allows monitoring of both the disease and effectiveness of treatment.

Health care economics demands that laboratory and diagnostic testing be performed accurately and in a timely manner. Tests should not have to be repeated because of problems with patient preparation, test procedure, and/or specimen collection technique. The interpretation of diagnostic testing is no longer left to the physician alone. In today's complex environment of highly technical testing and economic restrictions, nurses must be able to interpret diagnostic testing to develop timely and effective treatment.

The following guidelines will describe the responsibilities of nurses and other health care providers to ensure safety and accuracy in diagnostic testing. A brief overview of the major types of studies (hematologic, endoscopic, microscopic, nuclear scan, stool, ultrasonographic, urine, and x-ray) is included to provide a basic foundation for understanding laboratory and diagnostic testing.

UNIVERSAL PRECAUTIONS

The Centers for Disease Control and Prevention's guidelines for Universal Precautions have been established to protect health care workers from infectious agents (Box 1-1). This policy recommends that blood and body fluids be considered as potentially infectious.

SEQUENCING AND SCHEDULING OF TESTS

Because of the cost and complexity of laboratory and diagnostic testing, it is important that tests be scheduled in the most efficient, sequential manner. Guidelines apply when multiple tests must be performed in a limited period because one type of test can interfere with another. For example, radiographic examinations that do not require the administration of contrast material should precede examinations that do. Radiographic studies that use barium should be scheduled after ultrasonography studies. An essential component of this scheduling process involves communication and collaboration with health care workers in other departments.

Box 1-1	*Universal Precautions*

Universal Precautions have been mandated by the Occupational Safety and Health Administration (OSHA). Their purpose is to protect health care workers from contracting illnesses from specimens, patients, and the work environment. They can be summarized as follows:

Wear gowns, gloves, face masks, protective eyewear and clothing (including laboratory coat) whenever exposed to blood or other body fluids.

If the health care worker's skin is open, gloves should be worn during direct patient care.

Mouth-to-mouth emergency resuscitation equipment should be available in strategic locations. The mouthpieces should be individualized for each health care worker. Ambu bags are preferable. Saliva is considered to be an infectious fluid.

Dispose of all sharp items into puncture-resistant containers.

Do not recap, bend, break, or remove needles from syringes.

Immediately remove gloves that have either a hole or tear.

Before disposal, all patient-related wastes must be labeled as a biohazard.

All specimens must be transported in leak-proof containers.

Eating, drinking, applying cosmetics, or handling contact lenses is prohibited in patient care areas.

Presume all patients have hepatitis B and human immunodeficiency virus (HIV).

If a health care worker has been exposed to blood or other body fluids (e.g., needle stick), test the health care worker and patient for hepatitis and HIV.

BEFORE THE TEST

Patient preparation is vital to the success of diagnostic testing. Development of and adherence to guidelines for patient preparation require an understanding of the procedure. It is vital to obtain a thorough patient health history to identify contraindications to a specific test. Recognizing and counseling patients at risk for potential complications are important. Fears and concerns of the patient must be addressed before testing. To avoid misinterpretation of diagnostic testing, documentation and a thorough understanding of factors (e.g., medications, previous test) that could interfere with the test results are essential.

Pretest preparation procedures must be closely followed. Dietary restrictions are an important consideration. Because many blood tests and procedures require fasting, they should be performed as early in the morning as possible to diminish patient discomfort. Studies such as the barium enema, colonoscopy, upper gastrointestinal (GI) endoscopy, and intravenous pyelogram (IVP) are more accurate if the patient has had nothing by mouth (NPO, *nil per os*) for several hours before the test. Dietary restrictions also may be important for reasons of safety. For example, upper GI endoscopy requires that the patient be NPO for 8 to 12 hours before the test to prevent gagging, vomiting, and aspiration. Bowel preparation is an important part of many procedures that evaluate the mucosa of the gastrointestinal tract.

Patient Identification

Proper identification of the patient is a key safety factor. The patient's name should be verified by checking the patient identification band and test requisition slip. No specimens should be collected or procedures performed until the patient is properly identified. All specimens should be labeled with the correct patient name. Test results are useless and costly if they are reported for the wrong patient.

Patient Education

Patient education is the most important factor in obtaining accurate and useful test results. All phases of the testing process (before, during, and after) must be thoroughly explained to the patient. Complete understanding of these phases is essential to the development of nursing priorities

and clinical pathways related to diagnostic testing. Patients want to know what tests they will have and why they are needed. Patient education decreases apprehension and increases cooperation. It further ensures that the test will not need to be repeated because of improper preparation. Fasting requirements and bowel preparations must be explained clearly to the patient. Written instructions are essential. Medications sometimes may need to be discontinued for a period before certain tests. This information should be determined in consultation with the physician. Medications that are not discontinued are often listed on the test requisition slip to aid in interpretation of test results.

Variables That Affect Test Results

Many laboratory tests are affected by variables that must be considered when interpreting results. A discussion of some of these key variables follows:

- Age: Pediatric reference values differ from adult values. Likewise, geriatric patients may have a range of normalcy that varies from that of middle-aged patients.
- Gender: Values differ between the sexes, usually because of increased muscle mass in men and differences in hormonal secretion.
- Race: The patient's race generally has little effect on laboratory values. Race or origin is more important with regard to genetic diseases.
- Pregnancy: Many endocrinologic, hematologic, and biochemical changes occur during pregnancy. These changes significantly affect test results.
- Food ingestion: Several serum values are affected markedly by food. To avoid the effects of diet on laboratory tests, many tests are obtained after the patient has fasted.
- Posture: Changes in body position affect the concentration of several components in the peripheral bloodstream. Therefore, it is often important to note on the test requisition slip

whether the patient was in the supine, sitting, or standing position when the blood was drawn.

DURING THE TEST

The extent to which a health care provider is knowledgeable about a procedure can be a determinant of its successful outcome. Furthermore, the presence of a knowledgeable and supportive health care provider during a procedure is invaluable to the patient.

Transport and Processing of Specimens

Delivering specimens to the laboratory in an acceptable state for examination is important. The specimen generally should be transported to the laboratory as soon as possible after collection. Delays may result in rejection of the specimen. Some specimens must be fixed or treated immediately before arrival in the laboratory.

System of International Units

The System of International Units (SI units) is a method of reporting laboratory values in terms of standardized international measurements. This system currently is used in many countries, with an expectation that it will be adopted worldwide. Throughout this book, results are given in conventional units and SI units whenever possible.

AFTER THE TEST

Posttest care is an important part of total patient care. Attention should be directed to the patient's concerns about possible results or difficulties of the procedure. Patient treatment subsequent to testing must be appropriately provided. For example, after a barium test, a bowel cathartic is usually indicated. However, if a bowel obstruction has been identified, catharsis would be contrain-

dicated. Recognition and rapid institution of treatment for complications, such as bleeding, shock, or bowel perforation, are vital.

Reporting of Test Results

To be clinically useful, results must be reported promptly. The data must be documented in the appropriate medical record and presented in a clear manner that is easily interpreted. As in all phases of testing, communication among health care professionals is important.

MAJOR TYPES OF STUDIES
Blood Studies

Blood studies are used to assess a multitude of body processes and disorders. Common studies assess the quantity of red and white blood cells, as well as the levels of enzymes, lipids, clotting factors, hormones, and metabolic waste products, such as urea nitrogen.

Blood samples may be obtained using the following three methods: venous, arterial, and skin puncture. The ease of obtaining venous blood makes it the primary source of blood collection. It is relatively free of complications. *Venipuncture* is usually obtained by drawing a blood specimen from a superficial vein. The site most often used is the antecubital fossa of the arm because several large superficial veins are available there (Figure 1-1).

Arterial blood is used to measure oxygen, carbon dioxide (CO_2), and pH, which are often referred to as arterial blood gases (ABGs). They are described on p. 145. *Arterial punctures* are more difficult to perform than venipuncture. They also cause a significant amount of patient discomfort. The brachial and radial arteries are most often used for arterial puncture (Figure 1-2).

Skin puncture (sometimes called *capillary puncture*) is the method of choice for obtaining blood from pediatric patients, especially infants, because large amounts of blood required for repeated venipuncture could result in anemia. However, skin punctures are also used in adult

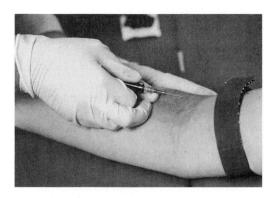

Figure 1-1 Performing venipuncture.

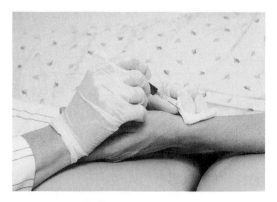

Figure 1-2 Drawing arterial blood. Note that the needle is at a 45-degree angle.

patients. Common puncture sites include the fingertips, earlobes, and heels.

Multiphasic screening machines can perform many blood tests quickly and simultaneously, using only a small blood sample. An example of this type of instrument is the *sequential multiple analyzer (SMA)*. An SMA-12 performs 12 tests, whereas an SMA-6 performs 6 tests. Advantages of these machines are that results are available more quickly and costs are lowered because performing a panel of tests is less expensive than performing each test individually.

Endoscopic Studies

Endoscopy refers to the inspection of body cavities with an endoscope. Endoscopic procedures are named for the organ or body area to be visualized and/or treated. See Table 1-1 for an overview of body areas that can be viewed endoscopically.

In addition to direct observation, endoscopy permits the biopsy of suspicious pathology, removal of polyps, injection of variceal blood vessels, and performance of many surgical procedures. Laser beams can be used to remove tissue or for coagulation. Furthermore, strictures within a lumen of a hollow viscus can be dilated and stented during endoscopy.

Endoscopes can be inserted through a body orifice (e.g., rectum) or small incision (e.g., arthroscopy). Endoscopes are available in two basic

types: flexible and rigid. *Flexible fiberoptic endoscopes* are used most often in pulmonary and gastrointestinal endoscopy. These scopes allow the transmission of images over flexible, light-carrying bundles of glass wires. These scopes contain accessory lumens for the insertion of instruments, water, and medication or the aspiration of debris.

Rigid endoscopes are used for operative endoscopy (e.g., laparoscopy) or endourology and are lighted by fiberoptic cords that transmit a bright beam through the scope.

Most endoscopic procedures now performed are able to be viewed by others, who then can actively assist the surgeon. This is possible because a camera containing a video chip in its tip is placed over the viewing lens and the image is then transmitted to a nearby television monitor. In many situations, endoscopy eliminates the need for open surgery.

Microscopic Studies

Microscopic examinations are essential for the diagnosis and treatment of numerous diseases and infectious processes. Microbiologic specimens can be collected from many sources, such as tissue and organ biopsy samples, blood, urine, wound drainage, cervical secretions, and sputum.

Microscopic examinations are used to evaluate histology and cytology and to identify bacteria and other infecting organisms. Included in micro-

TABLE 1-1   Endoscopic Procedures and Areas of Visualization

Procedure	Area of Visualization
Arthroscopy	Joints
Bronchoscopy	Larynx, trachea, bronchi, and alveoli
Colonoscopy	Rectum and colon
Colposcopy	Vagina and cervix
Cystoscopy	Urethra, bladder, ureters, and prostate
Enteroscopy	Upper colon and small intestine
Endourology	Bladder and urethra
Endoscopic retrograde cholangiopancreatography (ERCP)	Pancreatic and biliary ducts
Esophagogastroduodenoscopy (EGD)	Esophagus, stomach, duodenum
Fetoscopy	Fetus
Gastroscopy (part of EGD)	Stomach
Hysteroscopy	Uterus
Laparoscopy	Abdominal cavity
Mediastinoscopy	Mediastinal lymph nodes
Sigmoidoscopy	Anus, rectum, sigmoid colon
Sinus endoscopy	Sinus cavities
Thoracoscopy	Pleura and lungs
Transesophageal echocardiography (TEE)	Heart

scopic studies are culture and sensitivity testing (see p. 173), which are important for identifying and treating an infectious organism. A Gram stain is just one of the microscopic examinations performed with microbiologic testing.

Nuclear Medicine Studies

Anatomic and functional abnormalities of various organs can be identified through nuclear medicine studies. To do so, a *radiopharmaceutical,* which is a combination of a radionuclide and transport molecule, is administered and photons emitted from an organ subsequently are detected. Nuclear medicine studies do not identify the specific cause of the abnormality. Instead, they provide supportive information to be used in conjunction with other diagnostic modalities.

The radionuclides used in nuclear scanning have short half-lives, which is the time required for 50% of the radioactive atom to decay. Technetium (Tc)-99m is used extensively in nuclear scanning because its half-life is 6 hours and emits low levels of gamma rays. Other commonly used radionuclides include gallium, thallium, and iodine.

For most nuclear scans, radiopharmaceuticals are given intravenously. Less commonly used methods of administration include the oral and inhalation routes. After the radioisotope concentrates in the desired area, it emits gamma rays. The area is scanned with a gamma camera (scintillation scanner), which detects and records the emission of gamma rays. For each gamma ray detected, a light particle is emitted from the scintillator. A computer translates these light readings into a two-dimensional image or scan (scintigram), which is printed in various shades of color. Scanning usually takes place in the nuclear medicine department.

During nuclear scanning, the patient is exposed to a small amount of radiation. The short half-lives of the radioisotopes result in minimal radiation contamination of fecal and urine wastes. Nuclear scans are contraindicated in pregnant women and nursing mothers because of the potential risk of injury to the fetus or infant.

Stool Studies

Stool represents the waste products of digested food. It also includes bile, mucus, shed epithelial cells, bacteria, and inorganic salts. Normally, food is passed through the stomach, into the duodenum, and into the small bowel, where most of the nutrient and electrolyte absorption occurs. The liquid stool is then passed into the colon, where most of the water is reabsorbed.

Stool studies are utilized to evaluate the function and integrity of the bowel. These studies are performed to evaluate patients with intestinal bleeding, infections, infestations, inflammation, malabsorption, and diarrhea.

Ultrasound Studies

Ultrasonography, or ultrasound, sends harmless, high-frequency sound waves into the body and records the pattern of the echo as the sound waves bounce back or "echo off" body areas and return to the transducer. The transducer converts the echoes to electrical impulses and then transforms these to visual images or audible signals. Photographs and videotapes are made for study and evaluation.

The key advantages of ultrasonography are that it is noninvasive and requires no ionizing radiation for imaging. Because multiple images and repeat studies can be obtained with no risk of radiation exposure, this test can be performed in an office, laboratory, or at the bedside. Ultrasonography is less expensive than a computed tomography (CT) or magnetic resonance imaging (MRI) scan. No contrast is required for testing because the image occurs as a natural result of the way various tissues reflect the ultrasound wave.

Urine Studies

Urine is derived from filtration of the blood by the nephrons in the kidneys. Urine is nearly all water, with a small percentage of solutes. All end products of metabolism and all potentially harmful materials are excreted in the urine to maintain normal acid/base ratio, fluid and electrolyte balance, and homeostasis.

Urine generally reflects the blood level for any analyte. If the blood level is elevated and the kidneys are working well, the urine level for that same product can be expected to be high. If the urine level is not high, the kidneys may be diseased, resulting in high levels of the analyte in the blood. In some instances, certain blood solute products (e.g., glucose) are not filtered from the blood unless threshold levels of the solute are exceeded.

Urine specimens are usually painlessly obtained and provide much information quickly and economically. Although blood tests provide valuable information about the body, urinalysis may be preferred for several reasons:

1. A 24-hour urine collection will reflect homeostasis and disease better than a blood specimen obtained randomly.
2. Some products to be tested for are rapidly cleared by the kidneys and may not be apparent in the blood (e.g., Bence Jones protein). Results of a blood test therefore may be normal, whereas urinalysis indicates the presence of these products.
3. The serum product being tested may be affected by renal clearance (e.g., sodium). Therefore, a urine specimen to measure the sodium concentration will add significant additional information to a serum sodium level.
4. Urine testing is performed easily and does not require an invasive skin puncture.
5. Many urine tests are less expensive to perform than blood tests. The urine test may be less accurate or only qualitative, but it may be all that is needed.

The urine reagent strip has replaced many complicated individual chemical analyses for determining various components in the urine. For example, estimation of glucose, albumin, hemoglobin, and bile concentrations, as well as urinary pH, specific gravity, protein, ketone bodies, nitrates, and leukocyte esterase, can be determined easily by using a dipstick. Dipsticks are small strips of paper impregnated with a chemical that reacts to products in the urine by changing color.

The color correlates with concentrations of the analyte in the urine. Many tests can be performed with one dipstick.

X-ray Studies

Because of the ability of x-rays to penetrate human tissue, radiographic studies provide a valuable picture of bodily structures. X-ray studies can be as simple as a routine chest x-ray or as complex as a dye-enhanced cardiac catheterization. With increasing concern about radiation exposure, it is important to realize that the patient may want to know if the proposed benefit outweighs the risk involved.

X-rays are radiographs of body structures that appear like negatives of photographs. Radiography is based on the ability of x-rays to penetrate tissues and organs differently according to tissue density. X-rays are generated by a machine that passes a high-voltage electrical current through a tungsten filter within a vacuum tube (x-ray tube). As the x-ray passes through body tissues, images are formed on photographic film positioned on the other side of the body. Images are produced in varying degrees of dark and light according to the amount of x-ray absorbed by the tissues. The greater the amount of energy absorbed, the less x-ray reaches the film, and the whiter the image appears on the film. For example, bones are white because the x-rays cannot penetrate bone to reach the film. When bones are fractured, the break is visible as a radiolucent (black) line. Because patients with osteoporosis have less calcium in their bones, their films are gray and porous. X-rays can easily penetrate air. Therefore, areas filled with air or gas (e.g., lungs or bowel) appear black or dark on the film. Muscles, blood, organs, and other tissues appear as various shades of gray because they are denser than air but not as dense as bone.

By filming the body from front to back, as well as from the side, a three-dimensional examination can be obtained. These views are called *anteroposterior (AP)* and *lateral.* They are the basic views of most x-rays. *Posteroanterior (PA)* refers to filming the body from back to front. *Oblique* views can obtain an image of a body area not visible from the AP, PA, and lateral views.

Because of radiation exposure risks, x-ray studies should not be performed more often than necessary. For this reason, patients should be adequately prepared for the test to reduce the need for repeated films. Patients should be shielded from unnecessary exposure with lead aprons and gloves. Women who are having menses or are within 10 to 12 days after normal menses can have a diagnostic x-ray safely. Otherwise, no women in their childbearing years should have x-ray examinations unless a pregnancy test is performed and is negative. These restrictions exist to avoid exposure and possible harm to a fetus in the event a woman is unknowingly pregnant.

● ● ●

Knowledgeable interpretation of diagnostic testing is key for effective collaboration among health care providers to provide the most efficient patient care. The safety and success of diagnostic testing often depend on the nurse and other health care professionals. The safety of the patient and health care professionals depends on the creation of practice guidelines and standards of care. These can be developed effectively only with a thorough understanding of laboratory and diagnostic testing.

Chapter 2

Diagnostic Studies Used in the Assessment of the
Cardiovascular System

ANATOMY AND PHYSIOLOGY

The heart is located within the mediastinum (the midline cavity between the lungs) and is divided by a septum into the right and left sides. The right side contains unoxygenated (i.e., "prepulmonary") blood, and the left side contains the oxy-

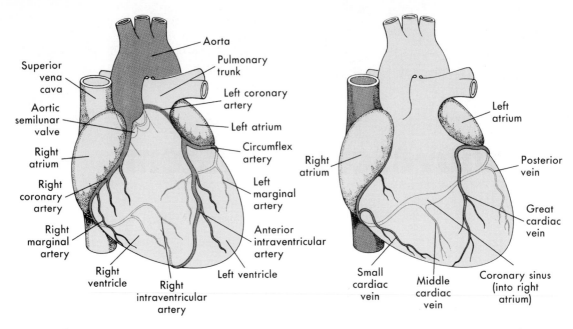

Figure 2-1   Anterior and posterior surfaces of heart, illustrating location and distribution of principle coronary vessels.

genated (i.e., "postpulmonary") blood. Each side is composed of an atrium and a ventricle (Figure 2-1). Unoxygenated venous blood from the venae cavae enters the right atrium and flows into the right ventricle. This ventricle pumps the blood forward into the pulmonary artery leading to the lungs, where it is oxygenated. The oxygenated blood then enters the left atrium, which pumps it into the left ventricle. The left ventricle then pumps the blood into the aorta and through the arteries. The pumping force of the left ventricle pushes the blood through the arterial and venous systems to provide the return of blood to the heart.

The flow of blood must be constantly "forward." Valves exist between all chambers of the heart to prevent any backward flow of blood. The tricuspid and mitral (atrioventricular) valves are located between the atria and ventricles on the right and left sides of the heart, respectively. These valves prevent potentially harmful backflow of blood from the ventricles into the atria. The pulmonary valve is located between the right

ventricle and the pulmonary artery, and the aortic valve is located between the left ventricle and the aorta. These semilunar valves prevent potentially harmful backflow of the blood from the aorta and pulmonary artery to the ventricles.

The heart wall is made up of three distinct tissue layers in both the atria and the ventricles. The bulk of the heart wall is called the *myocardium.* The inner lining surface, which comes in contact with the blood, is called the *endocardium.* The outer lining of the heart wall is called the *epicardium.* The heart is surrounded by a saclike tissue called the *pericardium.* The myocardial cells receive their blood supply from the right and left coronary arteries, which arise from the aorta near its origin (see Figure 2-1).

Specialized cells, located in the superior portion of the atrial wall, form the sinoatrial (SA) node. Here the electrical impulse, which normally stimulates myocardial contraction, begins. The SA node generates about 60 to 100 impulses/minute in the resting state. These impulses are conducted through the atrial muscle cells to the atrioventric-

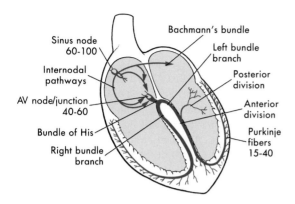

Figure 2-2 Electrical conduction system with the rates of the potential pacemakers.

ular (AV) node, located in the lower part of the right atrium. The AV node then relays the electrical impulses by way of specialized nerve fibers known as the *bundle of His,* which is located in the septum between the right and the left ventricles. Purkinje fibers then carry the impulses throughout the ventricular walls, stimulating the myocardium to contract (Figure 2-2).

If the SA node fails to generate an electrical impulse, the AV node (with an intrinsic rate of 40 to 60 impulses/minute) takes over as impulse generator. If both the SA node and the AV node malfunction, the myocardium will beat at its own ventricular intrinsic rate of 20 to 40 beats/minute.

Apolipoproteins (Apolipoprotein A-I [Apo A-I], Apolipoprotein B [Apo B], Lipoprotein (a) [Lp (a)])

Test type Blood

Normal values
Apo A-I
Adult/elderly
  Male: 75-160 mg/dl
  Female: 80-175 mg/dl
Child
  Newborn
    Male: 41-93 mg/dl
    Female: 38-106 mg/dl

6 months-4 years
  Male: 67-167 mg/dl
  Female: 60-148 mg/dl
5-17 years: 83-151 mg/dl

Apo B
Adult/elderly
  Male: 50-125 mg/dl
  Female: 45-120 mg/dl
Child
  Newborn: 11-31 mg/dl
  6 months-3 years: 23-75 mg/dl
  5-17 years:
    Male: 47-139 mg/dl
    Female: 41-132 mg/dl

Apo A-I/apo B ratio
Male: 0.85-2.24
Female: 0.76-3.23

Lipoprotein (a)
Caucasian (5th-95th percentile)
  Male: 2.2-49.4 mg/dl
  Female: 2.1-57.3 mg/dl
African-American (5th-95th percentile)
  Male: 4.6-71.8 mg/dl
  Female: 4.4-75.0 mg/dl

Rationale
This test is used to evaluate the risks of atherogenic heart and peripheral vascular diseases. The protein component of lipoproteins, which plays an important role in lipid transport, is composed of several specific polypeptides called *apolipoproteins.* Apolipoproteins are also involved in binding lipoproteins to lipoprotein receptors at the cell surface, thus facilitating lipid uptake by cells.

Apolipoprotein A-I (apo A-I) is the major polypeptide component of high-density lipoprotein (HDL [see p. 43]). In general, as HDL levels increase, apo A-I values increase. Apo A-I has been proposed to be a better index of atherogenic risk than is the HDL assay.

Apolipoprotein B (apo B) is the major polypeptide component of low-density lipoprotein (LDL) and very low-density lipoprotein (VLDL [see p. 43]). Apo B has been shown to exist in two forms: apo B-100 and apo B-48. Apo B-100 is the principle transport mechanism for endogenous cholesterol. Some believe that apo B-100 may be a better indicator of atherosclerotic heart disease than is LDL. Apo B-48, which is of intestinal origin and found mainly in chylomicrons, serves to transport ingested lipids through the intestines and into the bloodstream.

Lipoprotein (a) [Lp(a)] (referred to as *lipoprotein little a*) is a recently discovered lipoprotein. The two polypeptide components of Lp(a) are apo (a) and an LDL-like protein containing apo B-100. Recent research has suggested that increased levels of Lp(a) may be an independent risk factor for atherosclerosis. It is suggested that, following endothelial damage, Lp(a) may insinuate itself into the arterial wall, inhibiting the cleavage of fibrin in microthrombi by competing with plasminogen for access to fibrin. Atherosclerotic damage of the arterial wall soon follows, leading to occlusive disease or aneurysm.

Decreased levels of apo A-I and increased levels of apo B-100 are associated with increased risk of coronary heart disease. Reports also indicate that a low ratio of apo A-I to apo B may be a good predictor of coronary heart disease. Individuals with increased concentrations of Lp(a) appear to have a significantly higher risk for coronary heart disease.

These and other apolipoproteins are associated with the identification of other maladies. For example, the apo E4 (APOE4) gene has been proposed as a risk factor for Alzheimer's disease.

Interfering factors

Factors that interfere with determining apolipoprotein levels include the following:

- Physical exercise, because it may *increase* apo A-I levels
- Smoking, because it may *decrease* levels of apo A-I
- Diets high in carbohydrates or polyunsaturated fats, because they may *decrease* apo A-I levels

- Diets high in saturated fats and cholesterol, because they may *increase* apo B levels

Procedure

The patient must fast 12 to 14 hours after eating a low-fat meal before testing. Only water is permitted. Apolipoproteins are affected by a previous meal. Alcohol should not be taken 24 hours before the test. A peripheral venipuncture is performed, and 5 to 10 ml of blood is collected in a red-top tube.

Nursing implications with rationale

Before

☞ Instruct the patient to fast 12 to 14 hours before the test. Only water is permitted. Tell the patient that smoking is prohibited because it may decrease levels of apo A-1.

During

- Indicate on the laboratory slip any drugs that may affect test results.

After

- After the venipuncture, apply pressure or a pressure dressing to the site to prevent further bleeding. Observe the site for bleeding.

Arteriography of the Lower Extremities (Femoral Angiogram)

Test type X-ray with contrast dye

Normal values

Normal arterial vasculature anatomy without evidence of occlusion or aneurysm

Rationale

Femoral arteriography allows for accurate identification and location of occlusions within the femoral arterial system. After a catheter is placed in the femoral artery, radiopaque dye is injected. Radiographic films are taken immediately in a timed sequence to allow radiographic visualization of the arterial system of the lower extremity. Total or near-total occlusion of the flow of dye is seen in arteriosclerotic vascular occlusive disease.

Arterial emboli or acute thrombosis will be seen as total occlusions of the femoral artery or its branches. Arterial trauma, such as lacerations or intimal tears (lacerations of the inner vessel lining), are likewise seen as total or near-total obstructions to the flow. Fusiform dilation of the femoral artery or its branches is indicative of aneurysm. Unusual arterial disorders, such as Buerger's disease and fibromuscular dysplasia, have pathognomonic arteriographic findings.

Arterial vascular balloon dilation can be performed if a short segment arterial stenosis is identified. In this instance, the guide wire is left in place, and a balloon catheter is inserted over it. The dilating balloon is inflated, and the arteriosclerotic plaque is dilated gently and persistently.

Femoral arteriography is usually done electively on patients who have symptoms and signs of peripheral vascular disease. However, emergency arteriography is needed when blood flow to an extremity has ceased suddenly. Immediate surgical therapy is needed, and that surgery is most effective when the surgeon has knowledge of the etiology and location of the sudden occlusion. This knowledge can be obtained only by arteriography.

Potential complications

Potential complications associated with femoral arteriography are as follows:

- Hemorrhage at the site of the arterial puncture
- Pseudoaneurysm formation
- Catheter dissection of the intimal lining of the artery from the remaining wall
- Arterial thrombosis, embolism, or pseudoaneurysm in the peripheral artery used for catheter access
- Allergic reactions to iodinated dye
  These vary from flushing, itching, and urticaria to severe, life-threatening anaphylaxis (evidenced by respiratory distress, drop in blood pressure, shock). In the event of anaphylaxis, the patient is treated with diphenhydramine (Benadryl), steroids, and epinephrine. Oxygen and endotracheal equipment should be on hand for immediate use.

- Dye-induced renal failure in the elderly patient who is chronically dehydrated or who has mild renal failure.

Procedure

Preferably, the patient is kept fasting for 8 hours, although this is not necessary. Usually, sedation (meperidine) is ordered, if needed, for arteriography. The patient is taken to the "special studies" arteriography laboratory (usually in the radiology department) and placed on a special movable table. He or she is asked to lie still and in the supine position. To decrease the possibility of spasm or emboli, the femoral artery on the side opposite the involved extremity is catheterized after the groin is prepared and draped in a sterile manner. A radiopaque catheter is guided under radiographic visualization into the proximal iliac artery, through the aorta, and down the leg to be studied. Once the catheter is positioned in the involved femoral vessel, radiopaque dye is injected, and radiographic films of the thigh, calf, and ankle are taken immediately in a timed sequence. This allows visualization of the femoral artery and its branches. After the films are taken, the catheter is removed, and a pressure dressing is applied to the puncture site.

As with all arteriograms, when the dye is injected, the patient will feel an uncomfortable and sometimes painful heat flash, which usually lasts less than 10 seconds. This, along with the initial arterial puncture, is the only discomfort the patient will feel. A radiologist performs this study in approximately 40 minutes.

Contraindications

Contraindications for femoral arteriography are as follows:

- Patients who are unable to cooperate during the test
- Patients with an iodine dye allergy who have not received preventive medication for allergy
- Patients who are pregnant, because of radiation exposure to the fetus

- Patients with renal disorders, because iodinated contrast is nephrotoxic
- Patients with a bleeding propensity, because of potential difficulties in sealing the arterial or venous puncture site

Nursing implications with rationale

Before

- Explain the procedure to the patient. Tell the patient where the catheter will be inserted. Inform the patient that he or she will feel a warm flush when the dye is injected. Provide emotional support.
- Assess the patient for allergies to iodine dye.
- Keep the patient NPO from midnight on the day of the study.
- Ensure that informed, written consent for this procedure is obtained before administering the preprocedure medications.
- Mark the patient's peripheral pulses with a pen before arterial catheterization to permit assessment of pulses after the procedure.
- Instruct the patient to void before the study, because iodinated dye can act as an osmotic diuretic.
- Be certain that coagulation studies (prothrombin time [PT], partial thromboplastin time [PTT], bleeding time) are normal because of the risk of bleeding.

After

- Keep the patient on bed rest for about 8 hours after the procedure to allow complete sealing of the puncture site.
- Observe the catheter insertion site for inflammation, hemorrhage, hematoma, or the absence of peripheral pulses. Usually, apply a pressure dressing and sandbag to the catheter site. Assess the involved extremity for numbness, tingling, pain, or loss of function. The color and temperature of the involved extremity are compared with the color and temperature of the uninvolved extremity.
- Assess the vital signs for evidence of bleeding (decreased blood pressure and increased pulse). Vital sign measurements are usually ordered every 15 minutes for four times, then every 30 minutes for four times, then every hour for four times, and then every 4 hours. Of course, one may take these more frequently.
- Apply cold compresses to the puncture site, if needed, to reduce discomfort and swelling.
- Administer mild analgesics, if these have been ordered. If the patient is having continuous, severe pain, the physician should check the site because a hematoma may be forming.

Case Study

Peripheral Vascular Disease

Mr. R. was a 52-year-old man who complained of pain and cramping in his right calf while walking two blocks. The pain was relieved with cessation of activity. The pain had been increasing in frequency and intensity. Physical examination findings were essentially normal except for decreased hair on the right leg. The patient's popliteal, dorsalis pedis, and posterior tibial pulses were markedly decreased compared with those of his left leg.

Studies

Routine laboratory work
Doppler ultrasound systolic pressures, p. 52

Results

Within normal limits (WNL)
Femoral: 130 mm Hg; popliteal: 90 mm Hg; posterior tibial: 88 mm Hg; dorsalis pedis: 88 mm Hg (normal: same as brachial systolic blood pressure)

Arterial plethysmography	Decreased amplitude of distal femoral, popliteal, dorsalis pedis, and posterior tibial pulse waves;
Femoral arteriography of right leg, p. 12	Obstruction of the femoral artery at the midthigh level

Diagnostic Analysis

With the clinical picture of classic intermittent claudication, the noninvasive Doppler and plethysmographic arterial vascular study merely documented the presence and location of the arterial occlusion in the proximal femoral artery. Most vascular surgeons then require arteriography to document the location of the vascular occlusion. Mr. R. underwent a bypass from the proximal femoral artery to the popliteal artery. After surgery he was asymptomatic.

Critical Thinking Questions

1. What was the cause of Mr. R.'s pain and cramping?
2. Why was there decreased hair on Mr. R.'s right leg?
3. What would be the key nursing assessments after surgery to determine the adequacy of Mr. R.'s circulation?

Aspartate Aminotransferase (AST; Formerly Called Serum Glutamic-Oxaloacetic Transaminase [SGOT])

Test type Blood

Normal values

Age	Normal Value (U/L)
0-5 days	35-140
<3 yr	15-60
3-6 yr	15-50
6-12 yr	10-50
12-18 yr	10-40
Adult	8-20
Females	Slightly higher than males
Elderly	Slightly higher than adults

Rationale

AST is an enzyme found in very high concentrations within highly metabolic tissue such as the heart muscle, liver cells, skeletal muscle cells, and, to a lesser degree, in the kidneys, pancreas and red blood cells (RBCs). When disease or injury affects the cells of these tissues, the cells lyse.

Then AST is released, picked up by the blood, and the serum level rises. The amount of AST elevation is directly related to the number of cells affected by the disease or injury. Further, the elevation is dependent on the time after the injury that the blood is drawn. AST is cleared from the blood in a few days. Serum AST levels become elevated 8 hours after cell injury, peak at 24 to 36 hours, and return to normal in 3 to 7 days. If the cellular injury is chronic, levels will be elevated persistently.

The AST enzyme is included among others in the cardiac enzyme series. Although not specific for myocardial injury, when it is observed with the enzymes creatine phosphokinase (CPK) (see p. 28) and lactic dehydrogenase (see p. 42), it is useful in diagnosis of a myocardial infarction (MI). It aids in determining the timing of a recent MI and the extent of the MI. In the case of an acute MI, the AST level rises within 6 to 10 hours after MI, peaks at 12 to 48 hours, and returns to normal in 3 to 4 days, assuming further cardiac injury does not occur (Table 2-1). A second rise in AST would indicate extension or progression of myocardial injury despite therapy. Myocardial injuries, such as an-

TABLE 2-1	Timing of Appearance and Disappearance of Commonly Used Cardiac Enzymes		

	Hours		**Days**
Enzyme	**Starts to Rise**	**Peaks**	**Returns to Normal**
Total CPK	4-6	18	2-3
CPK-MB	4	18	2
AST	8	12-48	4
LDH	24	72	8-9
Troponin T	4-6	10-24	10
Troponin I	4-6	10-24	4

CPK, Creatine phosphokinase; *AST,* aspartate aminotransferase; *LDH,* lactic dehydrogenase.

gina, pericarditis, or rheumatic carditis, do not increase the AST level.

As with CPK, serial determinations of AST are necessary in determining the timing, initiation, and resolution of an MI. Unlike the isoenzyme CPK-MB, however, AST is much less specific for infarction of myocardial muscle cells.

Because AST also exists within liver cells, diseases that affect hepatocytes will cause elevated levels of this enzyme. In acute hepatitis, AST levels can rise 20 times the normal value. In acute extrahepatic obstruction (e.g., gallstone), AST levels quickly rise to 10 times the normal and swiftly fall. In patients with cirrhosis, the level of AST depends on the amount of active inflammation.

Serum AST levels are often compared with alanine aminotransferase (ALT, see p. 15) levels. The AST/ALT ratio is usually greater than 1.0 in patients with alcoholic cirrhosis, liver congestion, and metastatic tumor of the liver. Ratios less than 1.0 may be seen in patients with acute hepatitis, viral hepatitis, or infectious mononucleosis.

Patients with acute pancreatitis, acute renal diseases, musculoskeletal diseases, or trauma may have a transient rise in serum AST. Patients with RBC abnormalities, such as acute hemolytic anemia and severe burns, also can have elevations of this enzyme.

Interfering factor
A factor that interferes with determining AST levels is exercise, which may cause *increased* levels.

Procedure
No fasting is required. A venous blood sample is collected in a red-top tube.

Nursing implications with rationale
During
☞ Explain the need for this procedure to the patient.
After
■ After venipuncture, apply pressure or a pressure dressing to the site to prevent further bleeding. Observe the site for bleeding.

Cardiac Catheterization (Coronary Angiography, Angiocardiography, Ventriculography)

Test type X-ray with contrast dye

Normal values
Normal heart-muscle motion, normal and patent coronary arteries, normal great vessels, and normal intracardiac pressures and volumes

Rationale
Cardiac catheterization is a procedure that allows the heart, great blood vessels (i.e., aorta, inferior vena cava, pulmonary artery and vein) and coronary arteries to be studied. A catheter is passed into the heart through a peripheral vein (for right-heart catheterization) or artery (for left-heart catheterization). Through the catheter, pressures are recorded, and radiographic dyes are injected. With the assistance of computer calculations, cardiac output and other measures of cardiac functions can be determined. Cardiac catheterization is indicated for the following reasons:

1. To identify, locate, and quantify the severity of atherosclerotic, occlusive coronary artery disease

TABLE 2-2 Pressures and Volumes Used in Cardiac Monitoring

	Description	Normal Value
Pressures		
Routine blood pressure	Routine brachial artery pressure	90-140/60-90 mm Hg
Systolic left ventricular pressure	Peak pressure in the left ventricle during systole	90-140 mm Hg
End-diastolic left ventricular pressure	Pressure in the left ventricle at the end of diastole	4-12 mm Hg
Central venous pressure	Pressure in the superior vena cava	2-14 cm H_2O
Pulmonary wedge pressure	Pressure in the pulmonary venules, an indirect measurement of left atrial pressure and left ventricular end-diastolic pressure	Left atrial: 6-15 mm Hg
Pulmonary artery pressure	Pressure in the pulmonary artery	15-28/5-16 mm Hg
Aortic artery pressure	Same as routine blood pressure	
Volumes		
End-diastolic volume (EDV)	Amount of blood present in the left ventricle at the end of diastole	50-90 ml/m^2
End-systolic volume (ESV)	Amount of blood present in the left ventricle at the end of systole	25 ml/m^2
Stroke volume (SV)	Amount of blood ejected from the heart in one contraction (SV = EDV − ESV)	45 ± 12 ml/m^2
Ejection fraction (EF)	Proportion (fraction) of EDV ejected from the left ventricle during systole (EF = SV/EDV)	0.67 ± 0.07
Cardiac output (CO)	Amount of blood ejected by the heart in 1 min	3-6 L/min
Cardiac index (CI)	Amount of blood ejected by the heart in 1 min per square meter of body surface area (CI = CO/body surface area)	2.8-4.2 L/min/m^2 in a patient with 1.5 m^2 of body surface area

2. To evaluate the severity of acquired and congenital cardiac valvular or septal defects
3. To determine the presence and degree of congenital cardiac abnormalities, such as transposition of great vessels, patent ductus arteriosus, and anomalous venous blood return to the heart
4. To evaluate the success of previous cardiac surgery or balloon angioplasty
5. To evaluate cardiac muscle function
6. To identify and quantify ventricular aneurysms
7. To identify and locate acquired disease of the great vessels, such as atherosclerotic occlusion or aneurysms within the aortic arch
8. To evaluate patients with acute myocardial infarction and facilitate infusion of thrombolytic agents into the occluded coronary arteries
9. To insert a catheter to monitor right-sided heart pressures, such as pulmonary artery and pulmonary wedge pressures, and measure cardiac output. Cardiac output can be measured only during right-sided heart catheterization. Table 2-2 provides pressures and volumes used in cardiac monitoring.

10. To perform dilation of stenotic coronary arteries (angioplasty), place coronary artery stents, or perform laser atherectomy

Cardiac catheterization is performed under sterile conditions. In right-sided heart catheterization, usually the subclavian, brachial, or femoral vein is used for vascular access (Figure 2-3).

In left-sided heart catheterization, usually the right femoral artery is cannulated. Alternatively, however, the brachial or radial artery may be chosen. As the catheter is placed into the great vessels of the heart chamber, pressures are monitored and recorded. Blood samples for analysis of oxygen (O_2) content are also obtained. The catheter is advanced with appropriate guidance into the desired position. After pressures are obtained, angiographic visualization of the heart chambers, valves, and coronary arteries is achieved with the injection of radiographic dye.

Transluminal coronary angioplasty is a therapeutic procedure that can be performed during coronary angiography in medical centers where open heart surgery is available. During this procedure, a specific, specially designed balloon catheter is introduced into the coronary arteries and placed across the stenotic area of the coronary artery. This area can then be dilated by controlled inflation of the balloon. The coronary arteriogram is then repeated to document the effects of the forceful dilation of the stenotic area. Coronary arterial *stents* can be placed at the site of previous stenosis after angioplasty to maintain patency for longer periods. Likewise, *laser atherectomy* of coronary arterial plaques can be performed to more permanently open hard, atheromatous plaques.

Potential complications

Potential complications associated with cardiac complications are as follows:

- Cardiac arrhythmias (dysrhythmias)
  These can be induced by placement of the catheter within the heart.
- Perforation of the heart myocardium
  This can occur as a result of increased pressure placed on the catheter.
- Embolic stroke (cerebrovascular accident) or myocardial infarction
  These problems may occur if the catheter were to dislodge an atheromatous plaque.
- Arterial thrombosis, embolism, or pseudoaneurysm in the peripheral artery used for access
- Allergic reactions to iodinated dye
  Allergic reactions vary from flushing, itching, and urticaria to severe, life-threatening anaphylaxis (evidenced by respiratory distress, drop in blood pressure, and shock). In the event of anaphylaxis, the patient is treated with diphenhydramine, steroids, and epinephrine. O_2 and endotracheal equipment should be on hand for immediate use.
- Infection at the catheter insertion site
- Pneumothorax following misplaced subclavian vein catheterization of the right side of the heart
- Dye-induced renal failure in the elderly patient who is chronically dehydrated or has mild renal failure

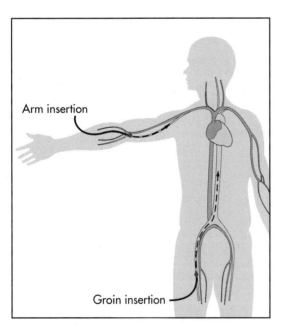

Arm insertion

Groin insertion

Figure 2-3 Insertion sites for cardiac catheterization.

Procedure

The patient is kept fasting from solid food for 6 to 8 hours before catheterization. Fluids are often permitted until 3 hours before the study. The patient is often sedated with midazolam (Versed) and either meperidine (Demerol) or morphine 30 to 60 minutes before the study. Young children require general anesthesia.

Electrocardiograph (EKG) leads are placed on the four extremities. A peripheral intravenous (IV) needle is inserted to allow venous access in the event that antiarrhythmic drugs are needed. Cardiac catheterization is performed under sterile conditions. The catheter insertion site is prepared and anesthetized with a local anesthetic, such as lidocaine (Xylocaine).

To study the *right side* of the heart, a sterile radiopaque catheter is inserted into the antecubital, femoral, or subclavian vein and then into the superior or inferior vena cava. The catheter is then advanced through the right atrium and ventricle and, later, into the pulmonary artery. The course of the catheter is followed by fluoroscopy. Pressures are recorded, and radiopaque dye may be injected. Radiographic films may be taken at any time. The heart is constantly monitored during the procedure. Premature ventricular contractions (PVCs) may occur as the catheter is passed into the ventricle. An increase in PVCs may necessitate the IV administration of lidocaine or the withdrawal of the catheter. Routine blood pressures are checked regularly during the procedure. As the catheter is passed through the heart, pressures within the superior vena cava, right atrium, right ventricle, and pulmonary artery are recorded. Blood samples are drawn for analyses of O_2 content. Radiopaque dye may be injected at selected sites to permit opacification of the right-heart chambers with cinegraphic recording. Catheterization of the right side of the heart is usually performed in the cardiac catheterization laboratory, but it may also be performed at the bedside in the coronary care unit (CCU) or intensive care unit (ICU).

For *left-sided* heart catheterization, the catheter is usually passed in retrograde fashion from the femoral or brachial artery into the aorta and then into the left ventricle. Monitoring is similar to right-sided catheterization. Once the catheter is correctly positioned by fluoroscopy, pressure readings are measured, and blood samples are drawn for O_2 content. Radiopaque dye is injected into the left ventricle and "movie-type" radiographic films (cineventriculography) are taken. Angiographic visualization of the coronary arteries is one of the most commonly applied diagnostic procedures performed during cardiac catheterization. For the visualization of the coronary arteries, special catheters are placed at the orifice of the arteries, dye is then injected, and the arteries are visualized (coronary cineangiography [Figure 2-4]). During the injection of dye into the coronary arteries, the table is moved from side to side or tilted. The patient may feel as if he or she is falling. Left-sided catheterization is usually performed in the cardiac catheterization laboratory.

For *transluminal coronary angioplasty*, a specially designed balloon catheter is introduced via the coronary catheter and placed across a stenotic area of the coronary artery. This area can then be dilated by controlled inflation of the balloon catheter. The coronary arteriogram is repeated to document the effect of the forceful dilation of the stenotic area of the coronary artery.

After the study of either side of the heart, the cardiac catheter is removed. The insertion site is immobilized for several hours. Pressure is applied to the site. Vital signs are monitored frequently over the next 4 to 6 hours. The puncture site is assessed for signs of bleeding. Peripheral pulses, color, temperature, and neurologic status are evaluated in the involved extremity every hour.

For most patients, cardiac catheterization is an anxiety-producing experience. The patient must lie still on a hard examination table that may rotate in several positions. The room is usually darkened to allow for visualization of the fluoroscopic screen. The patient's arm may feel as though it is "going to sleep" if the brachial artery is used for access. As the catheter touches the ventricles, the patient may feel palpitations (i.e., the heart skipping a beat) because of PVCs. When the radiopaque dye is injected, the patient may feel a warm flush. This feeling of warmth fre-

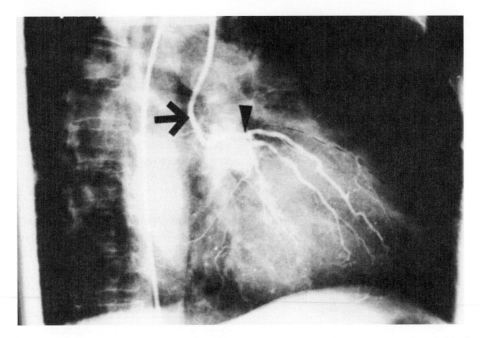

Figure 2-4 Coronary angiogram, lateral view. Black arrow indicates angiocatheter; black pointer indicates narrowing of the left coronary artery. Dotted line indicates what would have been the normal course of the anterior descending artery had proximal narrowing not occurred. Dye-filled vessels represent collateralization.

quently is so strong that it simulates being thrown into a fire. Although transient (4 to 10 seconds), it is very uncomfortable. Some patients have a tendency to cough as the catheter is passed into the pulmonary artery. Cardiologists perform catheterization in approximately 1 to 3 hours. Because of tremendous improvements in safety, cardiac catheterization can now be performed on either an inpatient or outpatient basis.

Contraindications

Contraindications for cardiac catheterization are as follows:

- Patients who are unable to cooperate during the test
- Patients who would refuse intervention if a surgically amenable lesion were found
- Patients with an iodine dye allergy who have not received preventive medication for allergy

- Patients who are pregnant, because of radiation exposure to the fetus
- Patients with renal disorders, because iodinated contrast is nephrotoxic
- Patients with a bleeding propensity, because the arterial or venous puncture site may not seal

Nursing implications with rationale

Before

- Explain the procedure to the patient. Ask the patient to verbalize his or her understanding of the procedure. Describe the sensations that the patient is likely to have (see the previous discussion under Procedure). Allow the patient ample time to verbalize apprehensions or fears regarding this test.
- Locate the catheter insertion site for the patient and explain that a local anesthetic will be used.

✏ Inform the patient that the insertion site will be shaved and prepared with an antiseptic scrub to avoid infection.

■ Withhold food and fluid for 6 to 8 hours before the procedure to prevent vomiting and aspiration during the study.

■ Determine whether the patient has any dye allergies. If so, he or she should be given a medication regimen to prevent allergic reaction. A commonly used regimen is prednisone, 5 mg four times daily, and diphenhydramine, 25 mg four times daily, for 3 days before and after the test.

■ Mark the patient's peripheral pulses with a pen before catheterization. This will permit quicker assessment of the pulses after the procedure. Note and record the quality of the pulses as baseline data.

✏ Tell the patient that he or she will be lying still on a hard table for the duration of this procedure and that the room will be darkened at intervals.

■ Administer the preprocedure drugs as ordered before catheterization.

After

■ Most patients are very tired after this procedure, and the physician often orders bed rest for several hours to allow the arterial puncture site to completely seal. Enforce safety measures, such as elevated side rails, until the effect of the preprocedure medications has worn off.

■ Keep the extremity in which the catheter was placed straight and immobilized for several hours after catheterization to prevent bleeding and discomfort. Apply ice to the site, if ordered. The physician may order a sandbag for femoral arterial access sites.

■ Monitor the patient's vital signs at frequent intervals (usually every 15 minutes for four times, then every 30 minutes for four times, then every hour for four times, and then every 4 hours) for arrhythmias and hypotension. Report abnormalities to the physician.

■ After the procedure, observe the arterial puncture site for hemorrhage, inflammation, hematoma, or absence of pulse. Check the peripheral pulses and compare the quality of the pulses

with the preprocedure baseline values. Assess the extremity for signs of ischemia (i.e., numbness, tingling, pain, absence of peripheral pulses, and loss of function). The color and temperature of the extremity are compared with the color and temperature of the uninvolved extremities.

■ Encourage fluids after the procedure to aid in eliminating the contrast medium.

■ Encourage the patient to verbalize his or her experience with cardiac catheterization.

Cardiac Radionuclear Scanning
(Myocardial Scan, Cardiac Scan, Nuclear Cardiac Scanning, Heart Scan, Thallium Scan, Multiple Gated Acquisition [MUGA] Scan, Isonitrile Scan, Sestamibi Scan)

Test type Nuclear scan

Normal values
Normal myocardial ejection fraction and coronary perfusion

Rationale
Cardiac radionuclear scanning is a noninvasive and safe method of recognizing alterations of left ventricular muscle function and coronary artery blood distribution. Many different radiocompound materials can be used, most often technetium-99m (Tc 99m) pertechnetate, thallium (Tl) 201, or Tc 99m pyrophosphate. When these compounds are injected intravenously and a radiation detector is placed over the heart, an image of the heart can be recorded and photographed.

In evaluating the patency of the coronary arteries, the characteristic abnormality varies according to the type of radiocompound used. When Tl is used, all normal myocardial cells take up the substance and appear on the photoscan. Ischemic or infarcted cells do not take up the substance and appear as "cold spots," devoid of nuclear material and surrounded by normal cells. Tc 99m sestamibi (isonitrile) presents a similar picture. It is an even better cardiac imaging agent. Higher quality images can be obtained on the first pass, providing information similar to that of angiocardiography. Perfusion images, ventricular function, and gated-pool ejection fractions (GPEFs) can all be obtained with a single injection. This is often called a *myocardial perfusion scan.* Furthermore, with the use of isonitrile, an ischemic area will be visible several hours after an ischemic event.

Tc 99m pyrophosphate is a radionuclide that binds with calcium. When ischemia or early infarction has occurred, intracellular calcium leaks out of the cardiac muscle cells. The level of calcium in the area of injury is high. The Tc 99m pyrophosphate binds to that calcium and creates an area of increased radionuclide uptake ("hot spot"). This is often called a *myocardial infarction scan.* Cardiac scanning with Tc 99m pyrophosphate is particularly useful in cases in which ischemia is difficult to diagnose. For example, in a patient with ventricular hypertrophy or left bundle branch block, the EKG is unreliable. If such a patient has chest pain and the pyrophosphate scan is positive, muscle injury can be said to have occurred. This type of scan is also especially helpful if the patient has had chest pain 5 to 10 days before seeing a physician. Because the pyrophosphate scan stays positive for that long a period, the delayed diagnosis of MI can be made.

Using the radionuclides just mentioned, cardiac nuclear scanning is used to indicate myocardium ischemia or infarction. It can be used in acute events of chest pain. Ischemia/infarction would be evident as just described. Cardiac scanning also can be used to assess myocardial ischemia during stress testing (see p. 23). In some cases, no evidence of diminished blood supply to the myocardium is evident during the resting state. When the heart is under stress, however, evidence of myocardial ischemia can become obvious and is easily detected by nuclear stress testing. In this form of nuclear cardiac scanning, the radionuclide is injected intravenously at the point of maximal cardiac stress. The radionuclide accumulates in the myocardium in direct proportion to the regional myocardial blood flow. The normal myocardium will have much greater radionuclide activity than the ischemic myocardium. In comparing this stress testing with a resting cardiac nuclear scan, one can see exercise-induced ischemia. This is known as *stress testing utilizing cardiac nuclear scanning* as the method of cardiac imaging or monitoring. This test not only is beneficial in detecting coronary occlusive disease but also is successful in assessing postoperative patency of a coronary bypass graft.

For an evaluation of myocardial function, Tc 99m pertechnetate or Tc 99m albumin is used to measure the portion of blood ejected from the ventricle during one cardiac cycle, known as the *ejection fraction.* Normally, more than 65% of the blood is ejected from the ventricle during systole. Values less than that indicate decreased contractility of the heart caused by ischemia or infarction or by cardiomyopathy. Computers can be synchronized with the EKG during scanning. This form of determination of ventricular function is called *gated pool imaging* or the *gated pool ejection fraction. Multiple gated acquisition (MUGA) scan* is another name for this test, based on the name of the computer machinery originally required for this determination.

This computer-assisted gated (synchronized) cardiac scan can also allow the myocardial wall to be photographed while in motion. This allows visualization of the myocardium during several cardiac cycles, and contractility of the myocardium can be determined. This imaging technique is called *nuclear ventriculography* and can provide the same information as radiographic ventriculography, which is performed during cardiac catheterization (see p. 16). However, the nuclear scans are noninvasive and much safer. Ischemic areas are seen to be hypokinetic on scan. Infarcted areas are akinetic on scan. This is also evident after stress during a cardiac stress test.

Single-photon emission (the radionuclear materials just discussed emit single photons) computed tomography (SPECT) has been used to visualize the heart from many different angles. These images are then reconstructed using techniques similar to computed tomography (CT) scanning, and three-dimensional images of the physiologic cardiac processes are obtained. Areas of myocardial ischemia can be seen with far greater resolution and can be more accurately quantified.

Procedure

The unsedated patient is given an IV injection of the appropriate radionuclide. Most injections are given in a peripheral vein. Fasting requirements vary with the type of procedure indicated. Shortly thereafter (but in less than 4 hours) a gamma-ray detector is placed over the precordium. The patient is first placed in the supine position, then in the lateral position, and then in both oblique positions. The detector records the image of the heart, and an image is taken. The only part of the test that is at all uncomfortable is the venous puncture required for the injection. A nuclear medicine technician performs the myocardial scan in fewer than 30 minutes.

Contraindications

Contraindications for cardiac radionuclear scanning are as follows:

- Patients who are uncooperative, because they must lie still for a short period
- Patients who are pregnant, because of fetal exposure to radionuclide material

Nursing implications with rationale

Before

☞ Explain the procedure to the patient. Encourage verbalization of patient's fears.

☞ Inform the patient that smoking is prohibited for several hours before the test. Nicotine causes transient coronary artery spasm, which may last up to 12 hours.

☞ Provide the patient with specific instructions regarding fasting and taking medications before the test. Instructions will vary according to the different types of cardiac scans.

After

☞ Reassure the patient that this procedure is safe because only trace doses of radioisotopes are used. No precautions need to be taken against radioactive exposure to personnel and family.

- If stress testing was performed, evaluate the patient's vital signs at frequent intervals.

Cardiac Stress Testing (Stress Testing, Exercise Testing, Electrocardiograph [EKG] Stress Testing, Exercise Testing, Nuclear Stress Testing, Echo Stress Testing)

Test type Electrodiagnostic

Normal values

The patient is able to obtain and maintain maximal heart rate of 85% for predicted age and gender with no cardiac symptoms or EKG change. No cardiac muscle wall dysfunction

Rationale

Stress testing is a noninvasive study that provides information about the patient's cardiac function. In this test, the heart is evaluated while it undergoes stress in some way. Changes indicating ischemia indicate coronary occlusive disease. Stress testing is used in the following situations:

1. To evaluate chest pain in a patient suspected of having coronary disease. Occasionally a person may have significant coronary stenosis that is not apparent during normal physical activity. If, however, the pain can be reproduced with exercise, one may infer that coronary occlusion is present.
2. To determine the limits of safe exercise during a cardiac rehabilitation program or to assist patients with cardiac disease in maintaining good physical fitness
3. To detect labile or exercise-related hypertension
4. To detect intermittent claudication in patients with suspected vascular occlusive disease in the extremities. In this situation, the patient may experience leg muscle cramping while performing the exercise.
5. To evaluate the effectiveness of treatment in patients who take antianginal or antiarrhythmic medications
6. To evaluate the effectiveness of cardiac intervention, such as bypass grafting or angioplasty

The most commonly used method of stress is exercise (bike or treadmill). Chemical stress methods are becoming more commonly used because of their safety and increased accuracy.

During *exercise stress testing*, the EKG, heart rate, and blood pressure are monitored while the patient experiences cardiac stress. The treadmill test is the most frequently used, because it is the most easily standardized and reproducible (Figure 2-5).

Exercise stress testing is based on the principle that occluded arteries will be unable to meet the heart's increased demand for blood during the testing. This may become obvious with symptoms (e.g., chest pain, fatigue, dyspnea, tachycardia, cardiac arrhythmias, fall in blood pressure) or EKG changes (e.g., ST-segment variance of 1 mm, increasing PVCs, or other rhythm disturbances). An advantage of stress testing is that these symptoms can be stimulated and identified in a safe environment. Besides the electro-diagnostic method of cardiac evaluation, the stressed heart can also be evaluated by nuclear scanning or echocardiography. Findings of ischemia are discussed below.

When exercise testing is not advisable or the patient is unable to exercise to a level adequate to stress the heart (e.g., patients with an orthopedic, arthritic, neurologic, or pulmonary limitation), *chemical stress testing* is recommended. Chemical stress testing is increasing because of its accuracy and ease of performance. Although chemical stress testing is less physiologic than exercise testing, it is safer and more controllable. Dipyridamole (Persantine) is a coronary vasodilator. If one coronary artery is significantly occluded, the coronary blood flow is diverted to the opened vessels. This causes a "steal syndrome" away from the stenotic or occluded coronary vessel, that is, the dipyridamole-induced vascular dilation "steals" the blood from the ischemic areas and diverts it to the open, dilated coronary vessels. Caution must be taken, however, because this can precipitate angina or myocardial infarction. This test should be performed only with a cardiologist in attendance. IV aminophylline can reverse the effect of dipyridamole. Adenosine works similarly to dipyridamole.

Dobutamine is another chemical that can stress the heart. Dobutamine stimulates the heart function. This entails administration of progressively greater amounts of dobutamine at 3-minute intervals. The normal heart muscle increases (augments) its contractility (wall motion). Ischemic muscle has no augmentation. In fact, in time the ischemic area becomes hypokinetic. Infarcted tissue is akinetic. In chemical stress testing, the stressed heart is evaluated by nuclear scanning or echocardiography.

Pacing is another method of stress testing. In patients with permanent pacemakers, the rate of capture can be increased to a level that would be considered a cardiac stress. The heart is then evaluated electrodiagnostically or with nuclear scanning or echocardiography.

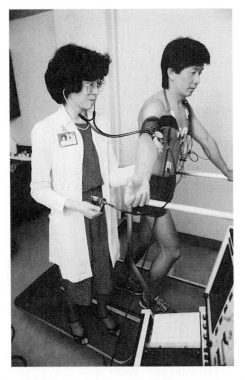

Figure 2-5 Exercise stress testing. Patient is walking on a treadmill while blood pressure, EKG, and other parameters are being monitored.

Methods of evaluation of the heart include electrophysiologic (e.g., EKG), nuclear scanning, and echocardiography. Echocardiography is fast becoming the method of choice for urgent and elective cardiac evaluation, with or without stress testing.

Potential complications

Potential complications associated with cardiac stress testing are as follows:

- Fatal cardiac arrhythmias induced by stress testing
- Severe angina or MI during stress testing
- Fainting

Interfering factors

Factors that interfere with cardiac stress testing include the following:

- Heavy meal before testing
  This can divert blood to the gastrointestinal (GI) tract.
- Smoking
  This can cause coronary artery spasm.
- Medical problems, such as hypertension, valvular heart disease (especially of the aortic valve), severe anemia, hypoxemia, and chronic pulmonary disease
  These problems can diminish the patient's tolerance to cardiac stress.
- Left bundle branch block
  The EKG is not a reliable indicator of ischemia in these patients.

Procedure

The patient reports to the cardiology clinic, usually after 4 hours of abstinence from eating, drinking, and smoking. Two methods of exercise stress testing include pedaling a stationary bicycle and walking on a treadmill. With the stationary bicycle, the pedaling tension is slowly increased to elevate the heart rate. With the treadmill test, the speed and grade of incline are increased. The various grades of exercise are determined by the cardiologist in attendance based on estimation of cardiac function capabilities. The usual goal of the exercise stress testing is to increase the heart rate to just below maximal levels or to the target heart rate. Usually, the target heart rate is 80% to 90% of the maximal heart rate. The test is usually discontinued if the patient reaches that target heart rate or develops symptoms or EKG changes. The maximal heart rate is determined by a chart that takes into account the patient's age (about 230 minus the patient's age) and gender.

For exercise stress testing evaluated by the EKG, electrodes are placed on the patient and attached to a monitor. A prestress test EKG is recorded. Vital signs are taken to obtain baseline values. During stress testing the EKG, heart rate, and blood pressure are recorded continuously. After the stress test, EKGs and vital signs are recorded at intervals during a 5- to 10-minute recovery period. A cardiologist performs a stress test in approximately 30 to 45 minutes.

With increasing frequency, echocardiography is used to evaluate the heart muscle wall function during stress testing. In this circumstance, a cardiac echogram is performed immediately after the cardiac stress has been applied.

Cardiac nuclear scanning is also used in stress testing. In this circumstance, a baseline nuclear scan is performed. Usually a chemical stress agent is administered, and the cardiac scan is repeated. This test is performed in the nuclear medicine department.

Contraindications

Contraindications for cardiac stress testing are as follows:

- Patients with unstable angina, because stress may induce an infarction
- Patients with severe aortic valvular heart disease, because of their low stress tolerance
- Patients who have recently had an MI
  In this case, however, limited stress testing can be done.
- Patients with severe congestive heart failure
- Patients who have severe claudication
  These patients cannot walk adequately to stress their hearts. However, they can be stressed chemically.

Nursing implications with rationale

Before

☑ Explain the procedure to the patient. Describe the type of exercise testing that will be used. Many patients are anxious and require considerable emotional support.

■ Ensure that the physician has obtained written and informed consent for this procedure.

☑ Instruct the patient to eat a light meal, without coffee or tea (stimulants) or alcohol (a depressant), 4 hours before the test. Heavy meals divert blood to the gastrointestinal tract, and, when exercise is begun, a large portion of the remaining blood goes to skeletal muscle. A heavy meal before stress testing may cause signs of ischemia much earlier than if no meal had been eaten.

☑ Instruct the patient that smoking is not permitted for at least 4 hours before the test. Nicotine causes transient coronary artery spasm, which may last up to 12 hours.

☑ Instruct the patient to get adequate sleep the night before the test.

☑ Instruct the patient to wear loose-fitting clothes with a shirt that buttons down the front. This facilitates application of monitoring devices. Women should wear a bra.

☑ Inform the patient that he or she will need to wear comfortable, well-fitting shoes with rubber soles. This will ensure safety and stability on the inclined treadmill or stairs. Slippers are not permitted.

■ Some physicians may want their patients to discontinue certain drugs (e.g., beta-blockers such as propranolol [Inderal], which limit the heart rate) before the stress test. Some patients who are taking digoxin may have drug-induced ST segment changes that are related to exercise.

■ Patients taking coronary vasodilators, such as nitroglycerine, may perform at a higher level of exercise and may have fewer arrhythmias, thus masking an ischemic response.

During

☑ Instruct the patient to report any signs of chest pain, exhaustion, shortness of breath, or generalized fatigue during the test.

After

☑ Advise the patient to rest for several hours and avoid stimulants or extreme temperature changes.

☑ Instruct the patient not to take a hot shower for at least 2 hours. A hot shower may cause an increase in cutaneous vasodilation and lead to orthostatic hypotension. This is especially hazardous for patients whose blood pressure dropped during the stress test.

■ If the stress test's results are positive, encourage the patient to verbalize his or her feelings, and provide emotional support.

Carotid Duplex Scanning (Carotid Doppler Ultrasound)

Test type Ultrasound

Normal values

Carotid artery free of plaques and stenosis

Rationale

This Doppler ultrasound test is performed to identify occlusive disease in the carotid artery or its branches. It is recommended for patients with headaches and with neurologic symptoms, such as transient ischemic attacks (TIAs), hemiparesis, paresthesia, and acute speech or visual deficits.

Carotid duplex scanning is a noninvasive ultrasound test used on the extracranial carotid artery to detect occlusive disease directly. The duplex concept is based on the ability to define the carotid artery walls within a two-dimensional image and uses a pulse Doppler probe to evaluate flow velocities and direction within the artery. This technique can measure the amplitude and waveform of the carotid arterial pulse. Furthermore, a two-dimensional image of the carotid artery can be produced. As a result, one can directly visualize possibly stenotic or occluded arteries and the arterial flow disruption.

Procedure

No special preparation is required. The patient is placed in the supine position, with the head supported to prevent lateral motion. A water-soluble gel is used to couple the sound from the transducer to the skin surface. Images of the carotid artery and pulse wave form are obtained. This test is performed by an ultrasound technologist in the ultrasound or radiology department in approximately 15 to 30 minutes. It is interpreted by the radiologist, usually that same day. No discomfort is associated with this test.

Nursing implications with rationale

Before

☞ Explain the procedure to the patient. Assure him or her that this is a painless study.

☞ Explain to the patient that a gel will be applied to the skin over the area to enhance transmission of sound waves.

After

■ Remove the gel from the patient's neck area.

Cholesterol

Test type Blood

Normal values

Adult/elderly: <200 mg/dl or 5.20 mmol/L (SI units)

Child: 120-200 mg/dl

Infant: 70-175 mg/dl

Newborn: 53-135 mg/dl

Rationale

Cholesterol is the main lipid associated with arteriosclerotic vascular disease. Cholesterol, however, is required for the production of steroids, sex hormones, bile acids, and cellular membranes. Most of the cholesterol we eat comes from foods of animal origin. The liver metabolizes the cholesterol to its free form, and cholesterol is transported in the bloodstream by lipoproteins. Nearly 75% of the cholesterol is bound to low-density lipoproteins (LDLs [see p. 43]), and 25% is bound to high-density lipoproteins (HDLs [see p. 43]). It is the LDL that is most directly associated with increased coronary heart disease (CHD) risk.

The purpose of cholesterol testing is to identify patients at risk for arteriosclerotic heart disease. Cholesterol testing is usually done as a part of lipid profile testing, which also evaluates lipoproteins (see p. 43) and triglycerides (see p. 51). By itself, cholesterol is not a totally accurate predictor of heart disease since there is considerable overlap in what are considered normal and high-risk levels. Because of considerable variation in cholesterol levels, elevated results should be corroborated by repeating the study. The two results should be averaged to obtain an accurate cholesterol-for-risk assessment. See Table 2-3 for an evaluation of coronary heart disease risk according to cholesterol levels.

Because the liver is required to metabolize ingested cholesterol products, subnormal cholesterol levels are indicative of severe liver diseases. Further, because the main source of cholesterol is diet, malnutrition is also associated with low cholesterol levels. Certain illnesses can affect cholesterol levels. For example, patients with an acute MI may have as much as a 50% reduction in cholesterol level for as long as 6 to 8 weeks. Familial hyperlipidemias and hyperlipoproteinemias are often associated with high cholesterol.

TABLE 2-3	Total Cholesterol as an Indicator of Coronary Heart Disease in mg/100 ml (SI Units: mmol/L)*		
Age (yr)	Low Risk	Moderate Risk	High Risk
2-19	<170 (4.4)	171-185	>185 (4.8)
20-29	<200 (5.5)	201-220	>220 (5.7)
30-39	<220 (5.7)	221-240	>240 (6.2)
>40	<240 (6.2)	241-260	>260 (6.8)

*When cholesterol testing is combined with measurement of lipoproteins, risk of coronary heart disease can be more accurately calculated.

Interfering factors
Factors that can interfere with cholesterol testing include the following:

- Pregnancy, because it is usually associated with *elevated* cholesterol levels
- Oophorectomy and postmenopausal status, because of the association with *increased* levels

Procedure
The patient must fast 12 to 14 hours after eating a low-fat meal before testing. Only water is permitted. Although cholesterol levels rise only minimally after a meal, early-morning fasting cholesterols are more easily compared when performed serially. In addition, lipoproteins, which are often ordered simultaneously, are affected by a previous meal. Therefore, fasting is usually requested. Alcohol should not be taken 24 hours before the test. A peripheral venipuncture is performed, and 5 to 10 ml of blood is collected in a red-top tube. A fingerstick method often is used in mass screenings. Less than a 5% difference in cholesterol exists between these two methods.

Nursing implications with rationale
Before
- Instruct the patient to fast 12 to 14 hours after eating a low-fat meal. Tell the patient that dietary intake for 2 weeks before testing will affect results. Therefore, it is suggested that the patient eat a normal diet for at least 1 week before testing.

During
- Indicate any drugs that may affect cholesterol levels on the laboratory requisition slip.

After
- After the venipuncture, apply pressure or a pressure dressing to the site to prevent further bleeding. Observe the site for bleeding.
- Instruct patients with high cholesterol levels about (1) appropriate body weight, (2) exercise, and (3) following a low-cholesterol diet (i.e., avoid animal fats, replace saturated fats with polyunsaturated fats, and increase ingestion of fruits and vegetables).

Creatine Phosphokinase (CPK, CP, Creatine Kinase [CK])

Test type Blood

Normal values
Total CPK:
Adult/elderly
    Male: 12-70 U/ml or 55-170 U/L (SI units)
    Female: 10-55 U/ml or 30-135 U/L (SI units)
Values are higher after exercise
Newborn: 68-580 U/L (SI units)
Isoenzymes
    CPK-MM: 100%
    CPK-MB: 0% (0-3.0 ng/ml)
    CPK-BB: 0%

Rationale
Creatine phosphokinase (CPK) is found predominantly in the heart muscle, skeletal muscle, and brain. Serum CPK levels are elevated whenever injury occurs to these muscle or nerve cells. CPK levels can rise within 6 hours after damage. If damage is not persistent, the levels peak at 18 hours after injury and return to normal in 2 to 3 days. (See Table 2-1, p. 16.)

To test specifically for myocardial muscle injury, electrophoresis is performed to detect the three CPK isoenzymes: CPK-BB (CPK1), CPK-MB (CPK2), and CPK-MM (CPK3). The CPK-MB isoenzyme portion appears to be specific for myocardial cells. CPK-MB levels rise 3 to 6 hours after infarction occurs. If there is no further myocardial damage, the level peaks at 12 to 24 hours and returns to normal 12 to 48 hours after infarction. CPK-MB levels usually do not rise with transient chest pain caused by angina, pulmonary embolism, or congestive heart failure. One can expect to see a rise in CPK-MB in patients with unstable angina, shock, malignant hyperthermia, myopathies, or myocarditis.

Besides in MI, CPK-MB levels are elevated in patients with myocarditis and Reye's syndrome. Very small amounts of CPK-MB also exist in skeletal muscle. Severe injury to skeletal muscle can be significant enough to raise the CPK-MB isoenzyme above normal. To avoid the misdiagnosis of myocardial injury, a *relative index* is calculated to determine whether myocardial injury has occurred. This relative index is a mathematic calculation of the ratio of CPK-MB to total CPK. A relative index of >2.5 is highly suggestive of myocardial injury.

The CPK-MB isoenzyme level is helpful in both quantifying the degree of MI and timing the onset of infarction. With the more frequent use of thrombolytic therapy for MI, the CPK-MB isoenzyme is often used to determine appropriateness of thrombolytic therapy. High CPK-MB levels would suggest that significant infarction has already occurred, thereby precluding the benefit of thrombolytic therapy.

Because the CPK-BB isoenzyme is predominantly found in the brain and lung, injury to either of these organs (e.g., cerebrovascular accident, pulmonary infarction) will be associated with elevated levels of this isoenzyme.

The CPK-MM isoenzyme normally comprises almost all of the circulatory total CPK enzymes in healthy people. When the total CPK level is elevated as a result of increases in CPK-MM, injury to or disease of the skeletal muscle is present. Examples of this include: myopathies, vigorous exercise, multiple intramuscular (IM) injections, electroconvulsive therapy, cardioversion, chronic alcoholism, or surgery. Because CPK is made only in the skeletal muscle, the normal value of total CPK (and therefore CPK-MM) varies according to a person's muscle mass. Large, muscular people normally may have a CPK level in the high range of normal.

Creatine phosphokinase is the chief cardiac enzyme studied in patients with heart disease. Because its blood clearance and metabolism are well known, its frequent determination (on admission, at 12 and 24 hours) can accurately reflect the timing, quantity, and resolution of an MI. Lactic dehydrogenase (see p. 42) and aspartate amino- transferase (see p. 15) are other cardiac enzymes used to confirm an MI.

New blood assays for cardiac markers have promised to detect acute MI rapidly and accurately in the emergency room. One of these new assays is troponin. *Troponin* is a protein complex consisting of three isotypes (T, I, and C). Troponin T and troponin I have the potential to become better diagnostic markers for acute MI than existing enzymes. The normal value for troponin I should be <0.4 ng/ml.

Interfering factors

Factors that interfere with creatine phosphokinase testing include the following:

- IM injections, which may cause *elevated* CPK levels
- Strenuous exercise and recent surgery, which may cause *increased* levels
- Early pregnancy, because it may produce *decreased* levels
- Muscle mass, because it is directly related to one's normal CPK level

Procedure

A venous blood sample is collected in a red-top tube. This is usually done initially on admission and 12 hours later, followed by daily testing for 3 days and then 1 week later. The venipuncture sites are rotated to save veins. It is important to avoid hemolysis during phebotomy. The exact time and date of venipuncture should be recorded on each laboratory slip. This aids in the interpretation of the temporal pattern of enzyme elevations.

Nursing implications with rationale

Before

☞ Explain the procedure to the patient. Discuss the need and reason for frequent venipuncture in diagnosing an MI.

After

- After venipuncture, apply pressure or a pressure dressing to the site to prevent further bleeding. Observe the site for bleeding.

Case Study

Angina

Mr. J.P. was a 48-year-old man admitted to the coronary care unit complaining of substernal chest pain. During the 4 months preceding admission, he noted chest pain radiating to his neck and jaw during exercise or emotional upsets. The pain dissipated when he discontinued the activity or relaxed. The results of his physical examination were essentially normal except for a systolic murmur heard best at the apex of the precordium and radiating into the left axilla.

Studies	Results
Routine laboratory work	Within normal limits (WNL)
Cardiac enzyme studies	
Creatine phosphokinase (CPK), p. 28	20 mU/ml (normal: 5-75 mU/ml)
CPK-MB	2 ng/ml (normal: 0-3 ng/ml)
Lactic dehydrogenase (LDH), p. 42	120 ImU/ml (normal: 90-200 ImU/ml)
Serum aspartate aminotransferase (AST; formerly serum glutamic oxaloacetic transaminase, SGOT), p. 15	24 IU/L (normal: 5-40 IU/L)
Electrocardiography (EKG), p. 34	Evidence of left ventricular hypertrophy
Chest x-ray study, p. 155	WNL
Exercise stress test, p. 23	Positive: pain reproduced, ST segment depression noted on EKG (normal: negative)
Echocardiography, p. 32	Normal ventricular wall motion
Transesophageal echocardiography (TEE), p. 49	Mitral regurgitation, dilated left atrium
Lipoproteins, p. 43	
HDL	20 mg/dl (normal: >45 mg/dl)
LDL	280 mg/dl (normal: 60-180 mg/dl)
VLDL	30% (normal: 25%-50%)
Cardiac catheterization, p. 16	*Pressures* All WNL except: Left ventricular systolic pressure: 140 mm Hg (normal: 90-140 mm Hg) Aortic systolic pressure: 130 mm Hg (normal: 90-140 mm Hg) Ventricular-aortic pressure gradient: 5 mm Hg (normal: 0)
	Left ventricular function Cardiac output: 3.5 L/min (normal: 3-6 L/min)

End diastolic volume (EDV): 60 ml/m^2
(normal: 50-90 ml/m^2)
End systolic volume (ESV): 22 ml/m^2
(normal: 25 ml/m^2)
Stroke volume (SV): 38 ml/m^2
(SV = EDV − ESV)
Ejection fraction: 0.63
(normal: 0.67 ± 0.07)

Cineventriculography
Mitral regurgitation present, normal
muscle function
(normal: normal ventricle)

Analysis of O$_2$ gas content
No shunting (normal: no shunting)

Coronary angiography (coronary cineangiography)
90% narrowing of left coronary artery
(see Figure 2-4, p. 20)
(normal: no narrowing)

Cardiac radionuclear scanning, p. 21 — Scans normal except for thallium scan, which showed localized area of decreased uptake in the myocardium during exercise

Cholesterol, p. 27 — 502 mg/dl
(normal: <200 mg/dl)

Triglycerides, p. 51 — 198 mg/dl
(normal: 40-150 mg/dl)

Diagnostic Analysis

Cardiac radionuclear scanning, EKG, and serial cardiac enzyme studies ruled out the possibility of MI. Stress testing and a thallium nucleotide scan indicated that the patient was having exercise-related myocardial ischemia (angina). Echocardiography indicated the heart muscle was functioning well. Transesophageal echocardiography indicated that the patient had significant mitral regurgitation. Cardiac catheterization with cineventriculography demonstrated near-normal ventricular function, and coronary angiography indicated significant narrowing of the left coronary artery. Mitral regurgitation was also seen. The patient's angina was then thought to be caused by the coronary artery disease. Open-heart surgery was performed. Mr. J.P.'s mitral valve was replaced with a prosthesis, and an aortocoronary artery bypass graft was performed. Postoperatively, Mr. J.P. had a large pleural effusion. This diminished his heart function. He underwent pericardiocentesis, and his function improved. Because his serum lipids study showed type IIa hyperlipidemia, a low-cholesterol diet and cholesterol-lowering agents were prescribed. Six months later he was asymptomatic and jogging 5 miles per day.

Continued

Case Study—cont'd

Angina

Critical Thinking Questions

1. Based on the ratio of cholesterol to HDL, what is the patient's risk for coronary heart disease?
2. If these blood tests were drawn 1 year ago, what treatment would have been indicated?
3. Could surgery have been avoided?

Echocardiography (Cardiac Echo, Heart Sonogram, Transthoracic Echocardiography [TTE])

Test type Ultrasound

Normal values

Normal position, size, and movement of the cardiac valves and heart muscle wall

Normal directional flow of blood within the heart chambers

Rationale

Echocardiography is a noninvasive ultrasound procedure used to evaluate the structure and function of the heart. This study is done most commonly to evaluate heart wall motion, which is a measure of heart wall function. In diagnostic ultrasonography, a harmless, high-frequency sound wave emitted from a transducer penetrates the heart. Sound waves are bounced off the heart structures and reflected back to the transducer and then electronically converted into a pictorial image that is recorded on graph paper or film.

M-mode echocardiography is a linear tracing of the motion of the heart structures over time. This allows the various cardiac structures to be located and studied regarding their movement during a cardiac cycle.

Two-dimensional (2D) echocardiography angles a beam within one sector of the heart. This produces a picture of the spatial anatomic relationships within the heart.

Color Doppler echocardiography demonstrates the direction of the blood flow and measures changes in velocity of blood flow within the heart and great vessels. Turbulent blood or altered velocity and direction of blood flow can then be identified by changes in color. In most Doppler ultrasound color-flow imaging, blue and red represent the direction of a given stream of blood; the various hues from dull to bright represent varying blood velocities. The most useful application of color-flow imaging is determining the direction and turbulence of blood flow across regurgitant or narrowed valves. Doppler color-flow imaging also may be helpful in assessing proper functioning of prosthetic valves.

Echocardiography generally is used in the diagnosis of a pericardial effusion, valvular heart disease (e.g., mitral valve prolapse, stenosis, regurgitation), subaortic stenosis, myocardial wall abnormalities (e.g., cardiomyopathy), infarction, and aneurysm. Cardiac tumors (e.g., myxomas) are easily diagnosed with ultrasound. Atrial and ventricular septal defects and other congenital heart diseases are also recognized by ultrasound. Finally, postinfarction mural thrombi are readily apparent with this testing.

Echocardiography is also used in *cardiac stress testing*. It is fast becoming the method of choice in heart imaging for stress testing. During an exercise or chemical cardiac stress test, ischemic muscle areas are evident as hypokinetic areas within the myocardium. Echocardiography is being used with increased frequency in emergent and urgent evaluations of patients with chest pain. If the myocardium is normal and without areas of hypokinesia, no coronary artery occlusive disease is suspected. If, however, a hypokinetic or akinetic area is noted, ischemia or infarction has occurred, and the chest pain is cardiac in origin.

It is now possible to perform echocardiography via the esophagus using a probe mounted on an endoscope. This is referred to as transesophageal echocardiography (TEE [see p. 49]). Fetal echocardiograms can now identify significant congenital heart disease before birth.

Interfering factors

Factors that interfere with echocardiography include the following:

- Patients who have severe chronic obstructive pulmonary disease (COPD)
  These patients have a significant amount of air and space between the heart and chest cavity. Air space does not conduct ultrasound waves well.
- Patients who are obese
  In these patients the space between the heart and the transducer is greatly enlarged; therefore, accuracy of the test is decreased.

Procedure

No patient sedation or fasting is required. The patient must undress to the waist. The patient lies on a bed, first in the supine position and then in the left lateral decubitus position. The ultrasonographer (a trained technician or cardiologist) applies mineral oil or glycerine to the skin over the fourth left intercostal space. This paste is used to enhance transmission and reception of sound waves. The technician places a pencil-like probe (transducer) on the skin and then tilts or rocks it into various positions (Figure 2-6) to inscribe an arc that will demonstrate several areas of the heart sequentially. An EKG is recorded simultaneously during echocardiography to time the events demonstrated by ultrasound with the cardiac cycle. During this study, drugs such as amyl nitrate may be administered to increase the contractility of the heart and provide additional information about the valves.

Echocardiography is usually performed in a darkened room in a cardiology clinic or in the cardiologist's office. It can be performed at the bedside or in the emergency room in an emergency situation (e.g., if needed to rule out pericardial effusion or evaluate a patient who is having an MI). The duration of this study is approximately 15 to 45 minutes. Most patients will not feel any discomfort during this procedure, although some may complain of pressure from the probe pressing

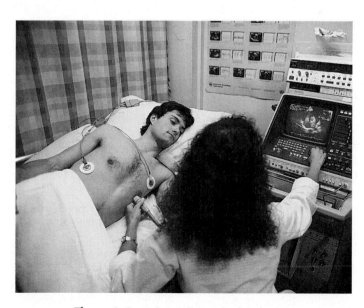

Figure 2-6 Echocardiography laboratory.

against the chest or the cool temperature of the transmission gel.

Nursing implications with rationale

Before

☞ Explain the procedure to the patient. Assure him or her that this is a painless study. Provide as much privacy and draping as possible.

☞ Explain to the patient that a gel will be applied to the skin over the heart to enhance the transmission of sound waves. Tell the patient that an EKG is normally run continuously during the study. Limb EKG leads will be applied (see EKG study, p. 34).

■ Make sure that the request form for echocardiography includes the patient history and the specific problem that the referring physician suspects.

After

■ Remove the gel from the patient's chest.

Electrocardiography
(Electrocardiogram [EKG, ECG])

Test type Electrodiagnostic

Normal values

Normal heart rate (60 to 100 beats/minute), rhythm, and wave deflections

Rationale

Electrocardiography is a graphic representation of the electrical impulses that the heart generates during the cardiac cycle. These electrical impulses are conducted to the body's surface, where they are detected by electrodes placed on the patient's limbs and chest. The monitoring electrodes detect the electrical activity of the heart from various spatial perspectives. This test is used in evaluating arrhythmias, conduction defects, myocardial injury and damage, hypertrophy (both left and right), and pericardial diseases. It also is used to assist in the diagnosis of other noncardiac diseases, such as electrolyte abnormalities, drug level abnormalities, and pulmonary diseases.

The EKG lead system is composed of several electrodes that are placed on each of the four extremities and at varying sites on the chest. Each combination of electrodes is called a *lead*. There are six limb leads (combination of electrodes on the extremities) and six chest leads (corresponding to six sites on the chest). Leads I, II, and III are considered the *standard limb leads*. Lead I records the difference in electrical potential between the left arm (LA) and the right arm (RA). Lead II records the electrical potential between the RA and the left leg (LL). Lead III reflects the difference between the LA and the LL. The right leg (RL) electrode is an inactive ground in all leads. There are three *augmented limb leads:* aV_R, aV_L, and aV_F (a, augmented; V, vector [unipolar]; R, right arm; L, left arm; F, left foot or leg). The augmented leads measure the electrical potential between the center of the heart and the right arm (aV_R), the left arm (aV_L), and the left leg (aV_F). The six standard *chest*, or *precordial, leads* (V_1, V_2, V_3, V_4, V_5, V_6) are recorded by placing electrodes at six different positions on the chest, surrounding the heart (see the discussion later in this chapter for exact locations).

In general, it is said that leads II, III, and aV_F look at the inferior portion of the heart. Leads aV_L and I look at the lateral portion of the heart. Leads V_2 to V_4 look at the anterior portion of the heart.

The EKG is recorded on special paper with a graphic background of horizontal and vertical lines for rapid measurement of time intervals (X coordinate) and voltages (Y coordinate). Time duration is measured by vertical lines 1 mm apart, each representing 0.04 second. Voltage is measured by horizontal lines 1 mm apart. Five 1-mm squares equal 0.5 mV.

The normal EKG pattern is composed of waves arbitrarily designated by the letters P, Q, R, S, and T. The Q, R, and S waves are grouped together and described as the QRS complex. The significance of the waves and time intervals is as follows (Figure 2-7):

P wave. This represents atrial electrical depolarization associated with atrial contraction. It represents electrical activity associated with the spread of the original impulse from the SA node through the atria. If the P waves are absent or al-

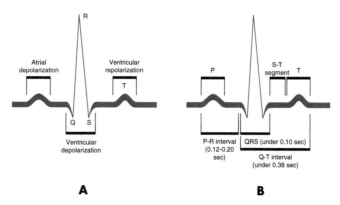

Figure 2-7 **A,** Normal EKG deflections during depolarization and repolarization of the atria and ventricles. **B,** Principle EKG intervals between P, QRS, and T waves.

tered, the cardiac impulse originates outside the SA node.

PR interval. This represents the time required for the impulse to travel from the SA node to the AV node. If this interval is prolonged, a conduction delay exists in the AV node (e.g., a first-degree heart block). If the PR interval is shortened, the impulse must have reached the ventricle through a shortcut (as in Wolff-Parkinson-White syndrome).

QRS complex. This represents ventricular electrical depolarization associated with ventricular contraction. This complex consists of an initial downward (negative) deflection (Q wave), a large upward (positive) deflection (R wave), and a small downward deflection (S wave). A widened QRS complex indicates abnormal or prolonged ventricular depolarization time (as in a bundle-branch block).

ST segment. This represents the period between the completion of depolarization and the beginning of repolarization of the ventricular muscle. This segment may be elevated or depressed in transient muscle ischemia (e.g., angina) or in muscle injury (as in the early stages of MI).

T wave. This represents ventricular repolarization (i.e., return to neutral electrical activity).

U wave. This deflection follows the T wave and is usually small. It represents repolarization of the Purkinje nerve fibers within the ventricles.

Through the analysis of these waveforms and time intervals, valuable information about the heart may be obtained. It is important to note that the EKG may be normal, even in the presence of heart disease, if the disorder does not affect the electrical activity of the heart.

For some patients at high risk for malignant ventricular arrhythmias, a *signal-averaged EKG (SAEKG)* can be performed. This test averages several hundred QRS waveforms to detect late potentials that are likely to lead to ventricular arrhythmias. SAEKGs have been a useful precursor to electrophysiologic studies (see p. 38) because they can identify ventricular tachycardia in patients with unexplained syncope.

The EKG should be studied in an orderly manner. The five basic steps to the identification of cardiac arrhythmias are as follows:

1. Calculate the heart rate. This can be done easily by counting the number of complete cycles (R wave to R wave is one cycle) in a 6-inch strip (6 seconds) of EKG paper and multiplying this number by 10 to get the rate/minute. The normal rate should be 60 to 100 beats/minute. *Bradycardia* describes a rate below 60, and *tachycardia* describes a rate over 100 (Figure 2-8). Several other methods are also used to calculate heart rate.

2. Measure the rhythm of the R waves. R waves that occur at regular intervals con-

EKG

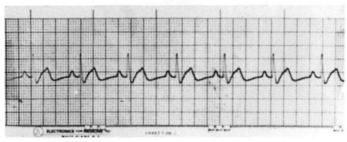

Normal sinus rhythm

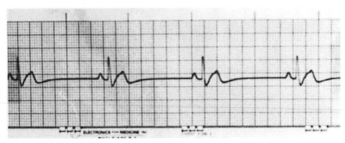

Sinus bradycardia

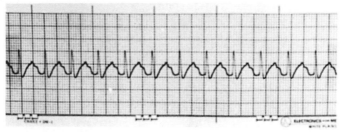

Sinus tachycardia

Figure 2-8 Common EKG rhythm strips. *Top,* Normal sinus rhythm (NSR) (rate, 80 beats/minute); *middle,* sinus bradycardia (rate, 40 beats/minute); *bottom,* sinus tachycardia (rate, 140 beats/minute).

stitute regular rhythm. When the difference between two R waves is greater than 0.12 second, the ventricular rhythm is irregular.

3. Examine the P wave. A normally positioned P wave (see Figure 2-7) preceding each QRS complex indicates a sinus rhythm. If P waves are absent or abnormally shaped, the

cardiac impulse is originating outside of the SA node (ectopic pacemaker).

4. Measure the PR interval. An increase or decrease in this interval is an indication of a defect in the conduction system between the atria and ventricles (see Figure 2-7).

5. Measure the QRS complex. A widened QRS complex indicates an intraventricular con-

EKG

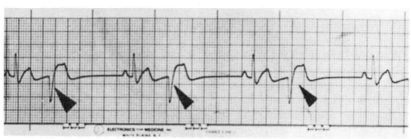

PVCs

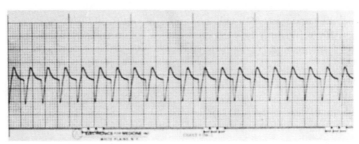

Ventricular tachycardia

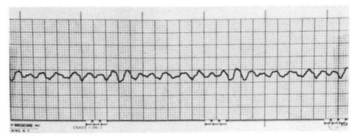

Ventricular fibrillation

Figure 2-9 Serious dysrhythmias. *Top,* Multiple premature ventricular contractions (PVCs) (black pointers indicate PVCs); *middle,* ventricular tachycardia; *bottom,* ventricular fibrillation.

duction defect (such as PVCs). See Figures 2-8 and 2-9 for a sample of normal sinus rhythm and some of the more common arrhythmias. A more thorough and comprehensive discussion of EKG interpretation may be found elsewhere and is beyond the scope of this chapter.

Interfering factors

Factors that interfere with EKG include the following:

- Inaccurate placement of the electrodes
- Electrolyte imbalances
- Poor contact between the skin and electrodes

- Movement or muscle tremors (twitching) during the test

Procedure

The patient is placed in the supine position on a table or bed. The machine is turned on so that it will be ready to use after the electrodes are applied. The skin areas designated for electrode placement are prepared by using alcohol swabs or sandpaper to remove skin oil or debris. Sometimes the skin is shaved if the patient has a large amount of hair. Electrode paste is applied to ensure electrical conduction between the skin and electrodes. The four limb leads are usually held in place by straps that encircle the extremity. Newer machines have clamps (much like a clothespin) that can easily be opened and applied. Many cardiologists recommend that arm electrodes be placed on the upper arm because fewer muscle tremors are detected there. The chest leads (suction cups) are applied either one at a time, three at a time, or all six at once, depending on the type of EKG machine. These leads are positioned as follows:

V$_1$: In the fourth intercostal space (4ICS) at the right sternal border
V$_2$: In 4ICS at the left sternal border
V$_3$: Midway between V$_2$ and V$_4$
V$_4$: In the fifth intercostal space (5ICS) at the midclavicular line
V$_5$: At the left anterior axillary line at the level of V$_4$ horizontally
V$_6$: At the left midaxillary line on the level of V$_4$ horizontally

Although this procedure entails no discomfort for the patient, he or she must lie still and not talk while the EKG is recorded. Cardiac technicians and nurses perform the procedure in less than 5 minutes in the "heart station" or at the bedside.

Nursing implications with rationale

Before
- Explain the procedure to the patient. Assure him or her that the flow of electrical current is *from* the patient. He or she will feel nothing during this procedure.

- Expose only the patient's chest and arms. Keep the abdomen and thighs adequately covered.
- Prepare the patient's skin and apply only a small amount of electrode gel. A large amount may produce a wandering baseline by allowing movement of the electrode. The gel will usually feel cold.
- Apply the electrodes and wires so that tension on the electrodes is avoided.

After
- After the EKG is recorded, remove the electrodes from the patient's skin and wipe off the electrode gel.
- If Holter monitoring (see p. 40) is being used, explain the procedure carefully to the patient.

Electrophysiologic Study (EPS, Cardiac Mapping)

Test type Electrodiagnostic

Normal values

Normal conduction intervals, refractive periods, and recovery times

Rationale

EPS is a method of studying evoked potentials within the heart. It is used to evaluate patients with syncope, palpitations, or arrhythmias; identify the location of conduction defects that cause abnormal electroconduction and arrhythmias; and monitor antiarrhythmic therapy.

In this invasive procedure, multiple electrode catheters are fluoroscopically placed through a peripheral vein and into the right atrium and/or ventricle or, less often, through an artery into the left atrium and/or ventricle. With close cardiac monitoring, the electrode catheters are used to pace the heart and potentially induce arrhythmias. Defects in the heart conduction system can then be identified; arrhythmias that are otherwise unapparent also can be induced, identified, and treated. The effectiveness of the antiarrhythmic drugs (e.g., lidocaine, phenytoin, quinidine) can be assessed by determining the electrical threshold required to induce arrhythmias.

EPS also can be therapeutic. With the use of radiofrequency, sites with documented low thresholds for inducing arrhythmias can be obliterated to stop the arrhythmias.

Potential complications

Potential complications associated with electrophysiologic studies are as follows:

- Cardiac arrhythmias leading to ventricular tachycardia or fibrillation
  These can be induced during the procedure.
- Perforation of the myocardium from the catheter
- Catheter-induced embolic cerebrovascular accident (CVA) (stroke) or MI
- Peripheral vascular emboli at the site of catheter placement
- Hemorrhage from failure to seal the arterial puncture site
- Phlebitis at the venipuncture site

Procedure

The patient is usually kept fasting for 6 to 8 hours before the EPS, although fluids are often permitted until 3 hours before the test. EKG leads are placed. A peripheral IV line is inserted for administration of medications. The EPS catheter insertion site is prepared and anesthetized with a local anesthetic, such as lidocaine. Catheters are inserted into a vein or artery (usually femoral) and threaded via fluoroscopy to the right and left sides of the heart, respectively. Baseline surface and intracardiac EKGs are recorded. Various parts of the conduction system are stimulated by atrial or ventricular pacing. Mapping, or locating the site of origin of a recurrent ventricular tachycardia, can be done. Drugs are administered via the IV line to assess the efficacy of certain drugs for arrhythmias.

For most patients, this is an anxiety-producing experience. The patient must lie still on a hard x-ray table in a darkened room. He or she may have sensations of palpitations and lightheadedness or dizziness. These sensations should be reported to the physician. After completion of the test, the catheters are removed and direct pressure is applied to the insertion site. Occasionally a catheter may be left in place for follow-up studies the next day. A cardiologist performs this procedure in 1 to 4 hours.

Contraindications

Contraindications for electrophysiologic studies are as follows:

- Patients who are uncooperative
- Patients with acute MI
  These patients may extend their infarction with rapid pacing.

Nursing implications with rationale

Before

- ☞ Explain the procedure to the patient. Ask the patient to verbalize his or her understanding of the test and then reinforce the patient's understanding.
- ☞ Describe the sensations that the patient is likely to have (see the previous discussion under Procedure). Allow the patient ample time to verbalize apprehensions or fears regarding this test.
- ☞ Locate the catheter insertion site for the patient and explain that a local anesthetic will be used. Inform the patient that the insertion site will be shaved and prepped with an antiseptic scrub to avoid infection.
- Withhold food or fluid for 6 to 8 hours before the procedure to prevent vomiting and aspiration during the study.
- Mark the patient's peripheral pulses with a pen before catheterization. This will permit quick assessment of the pulses after the procedure. Note and record the quality of the pulses as baseline data.
- ☞ Tell the patient that he or she will be lying still on a hard table for the duration of this procedure and that the room will be darkened at intervals.

After

- The patient is usually kept on bed rest for several hours to allow complete sealing of the puncture site.
- ☞ Instruct the patient to keep the extremity in which the catheter was placed straight and im-

mobilized for several hours to prevent bleeding and discomfort. Apply ice to the site, if ordered.

- Monitor the patient's vital signs at frequent intervals (usually every 15 minutes for four times, then every 30 minutes for four times, then every hour for four times, then every 4 hours) for dysrhythmias and hypotension. Any abnormalities should be reported to the physician.

- Observe the puncture site for hemorrhage, inflammation, hematoma, or absence of pulse. Check the peripheral pulses and compare the quality of the pulses with the preprocedure baseline values. Assess the extremity for signs of ischemia (numbness, tingling, pain, absence of peripheral pulses, and loss of function). Compare the color and temperature of the extremity with the uninvolved extremity.

- Additional monitoring may be needed for any medications that the patient received during the procedure. For example, a patient receiving quinidine should be monitored for hypotension and abdominal cramping.

- If an electrocatheter is left in place for subsequent studies, it is sutured in place and covered with a sterile dressing.

- If the patient has an adverse reaction to a drug administered during EPS, the EKG should be carefully monitored until the drug is eliminated from the body.

Holter Monitoring (Ambulatory Monitoring, Ambulatory Electrocardiography, Event Recorder)

Test type Electrodiagnostic

Normal values
Normal sinus rhythm

Rationale
Holter monitoring is a continuous recording of the electrical activity of the heart. Holter monitoring is used to record a patient's heart rate and rhythm for one or more days. With this technique, an EKG is recorded continuously during unrestricted activity, rest, and sleep. The Holter monitor is equipped with a clock that permits accurate time monitoring on the EKG tape. The patient is asked to carry a diary and record daily activities, as well as any cardiac symptoms that may develop during monitoring. Symptoms such as chest pain, syncope, or palpitations can be noted and recorded when the patient pushes a button on the event recorder.

The Holter monitor is used primarily to identify suspected cardiac rhythm disturbances and to correlate these disturbances with symptoms such as dizziness, syncope, palpitations, or chest pain. The monitor is also used to assess pacemaker function and the effectiveness of antiarrhythmic medications.

Interfering factors
Interruption in the electrode contact with the skin interferes with Holter monitoring.

Procedure
A small, portable monitor is attached to EKG leads (see p. 34) and carried by the patient in a sling around the chest or abdomen for up to several weeks (Figure 2-10). The patient records daily activities in a diary to see if there is a correlation between the symptoms and EKG findings. At the completion of the test, the tape is scanned for abnormalities.

Event recorders are now being used to follow patients with periodic fainting or near-syncope. Patients may attach these small devices to themselves if they feel symptoms or arrhythmias. The recorders have electrodes that the patients simply hold to their chests to record the EKG. Some recorders store the information, which can later be relayed by telephone to the physician's office. (This feature is convenient if patients have brief periods of symptoms or arrhythmias while driving, for instance.) Other recorders require patients to call the physician's office during the symptomatic event so the EKG is directly transmitted by telephone.

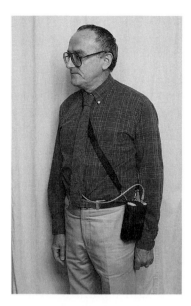

Figure 2-10 Patient wearing Holter monitor.

After completion of the test period, usually 24 to 72 hours, the Holter monitor is removed, and the tape is played back at high speeds. The EKG tracing usually is interpreted by a computer, which can detect abnormal wave patterns that occurred during the testing. The cardiologist then reviews any abnormalities.

Contraindications
Contraindications for Holter monitoring are as follows:

- Patients who cannot maintain the lead placement
- Patients who cannot record in a diary significant activities or symptomatic events

Nursing implications with rationale
Before
- ☞ Explain the procedure to the patient. Inform the patient about the care of the monitor. Tell the patient that the monitor cannot get wet; therefore, bathing, swimming, and showering must be avoided.

- ☞ Tell the patient that electrical gadgets, such as electrical toothbrushes, can cause artifacts on the EKG tape. Therefore, their use should be noted in the diary.
- ☞ Assure the patient that the electrical flow is coming from him or her and not from the machine.

During
- ■ Use a tight undershirt or netlike dressing to hold the leads in place.

After
- ■ Gently remove the tape and other materials securing the electrodes.
- ■ Wipe off the electrode gel.
- ☞ Tell the patient that the test interpretation will not be available for several days.

Lactic Acid (Lactate)

Test type Blood

Normal values
Venous blood: 0.5 to 2.2 mmol/L
Arterial blood: 0.9 to 1.7 mmol/L

Rationale
Normally, glucose is metabolized to carbon dioxide (CO_2) and water (H_2O) for energy. When oxygen to the tissues is diminished, anaerobic metabolism of glucose occurs and lactate (lactic acid) is formed instead of CO_2 and H_2O. The liver, when hypoxic, fails to clear the lactic acid; therefore, lactic acid levels accumulate and cause lactic acidosis (LA). Lactate therefore is a sensitive and reliable indicator of tissue hypoxia. The hypoxia may be local (e.g., mesenteric ischemia, extremity ischemia) or general (e.g., shock). Lactic acid levels are used to document the presence of tissue hypoxia, determine the degree of hypoxia, and monitor the effect of therapy. Lactic acidosis not caused by hypoxia is classified as type I LA and is caused by diseases such as glycogen storage or liver diseases, or by drugs. Lactic acidosis caused by hypoxia is classified as type II LA, with shock, convulsions, and extremity ischemia among the

most common causes. Type III LA is idiopathic and most commonly seen in patients with nonketotic diabetes. The pathophysiology of lactic acid accumulation in type III is not known.

Interfering factors

Factors that interfere with lactic acid testing include the following:

- Prolonged use of a tourniquet or hand clenching, both of which may *increase* lactate levels

Procedure

No fasting is required. The patient should avoid making a fist before and during blood withdrawal. If possible, avoid the use of a tourniquet. Approximately 7 ml of venous blood or 4 to 7 ml of arterial blood is collected in a red-top tube.

Nursing implications with rationale

Before

- Explain the reason for this test. Tell the patient that no fasting is required.

After

- After venipuncture, apply pressure or a pressure dressing to the site to prevent further bleeding. Observe the site for bleeding.
- After an arterial puncture, apply pressure for 3 to 5 minutes to avoid hematoma formation. Observe the site for bleeding.

Lactic Dehydrogenase (LDH)

Test type Blood

Normal values

Adult/elderly: 45-90 U/L (30° C), 115-225 IU/L, or 0.4-1.7 mmol/L (SI units)
Isoenzymes in adult/elderly values
   LDH-1: 17% to 27%
   LDH-2: 27% to 37%
   LDH-3: 18% to 25%
   LDH-4: 3% to 8%
   LDH-5: 0% to 5%

Child: 60-170 U/L (30° C)
Infant: 100-250 U/L (30° C)
Newborn: 160-450 U/L (30° C)

Rationale

LDH is an enzyme found in many body tissues, especially the heart, liver, RBCs, kidneys, skeletal muscle, brain, and lungs. Because LDH is widely distributed throughout the body, the total LDH level is not a specific indicator of any one disease or indicative of injury to any one organ. When disease or injury affects cells containing LDH, these cells lyse and LDH is spilled into the bloodstream, where it is identified in higher than normal levels. The LDH value is a measure of total LDH; five separate fractions (isoenzymes) make up the total LDH. Each tissue contains a predominance of one or more LDH enzymes.

Isoenzyme LDH-1 generally comes from the heart; LDH-2 originates primarily from the reticuloendothelial system; LDH-3 comes from the lungs and other tissues; LDH-4 originates from the kidney, placenta, and pancreas; and LDH-5 comes from the liver and striated muscle. Normally, LDH-2 makes up the greatest percentage of total LDH.

The following patterns of LDH isoenzymes are specific for certain diseases:

1. Isolated elevation of LDH-1 (above LDH-2) indicates myocardial injury.
2. Isolated elevation of LDH-5 indicates hepatocellular injury or disease.
3. Elevations of LDH-2 and 3 indicate pulmonary injury or disease.
4. Elevations of all LDH isoenzymes indicate multiorgan injury (e.g., MI with congestive heart failure causing pulmonary and hepatic congestion along with decreased renal perfusion). This pattern can also indicate advanced malignancy or diffuse autoimmune inflammatory diseases, such as systemic lupus erythematosus.

With myocardial injury, the serum LDH level rises within 24 to 48 hours after an MI, peaks in 2 to 3 days, and returns to normal in approximately

5 to 10 days. This makes the serum LDH level especially useful for a delayed diagnosis of patients with MI (i.e., the patient reports having had severe chest pain 4 days earlier). In patients with MI, the LDH-1 level is a more sensitive and specific indicator of MI than the total LDH level. Its sensitivity alone is greater than 95%. Normally, the LDH-2 fraction is greater than the LDH-1 fraction. Therefore, the normal LDH-1/LDH-2 ratio is less than 1. When the LDH-1 level is greater than LDH-2, myocardial injury is strongly suspected. The reversal of the normal ratio is referred to as a *flipped LDH* (i.e., the LDH-1/LDH-2 ratio of less than 1 is reversed). In an acute MI, the flipped LDH ratio usually appears in 12 to 24 hours and is present within 48 hours in approximately 80% of patients. When LDH-2 is greater than LDH-1 (a normal LDH-1/LDH-2 ratio), it is considered reliable evidence against MI. In the patient with chest pain caused by angina only, the LDH will probably not be elevated.

It is important to note that two diseases causing elevated LDH may coexist and obscure each other. For example, a patient who has liver disease may also be having an acute MI. The elevation in LDH-1 may be obscured by the elevation of LDH-5. An elevated LDH level with greater than 40% of LDH-1 is diagnostic of myocardial damage.

LDH is also measured in other body fluids. Elevated urine levels of total LDH indicate neoplasm or injury to the urologic system. When the LDH in an effusion (pleural, cardiac, or peritoneal) is greater than 60% of the serum total LDH (i.e., effusion LDH/serum LDH ratio is greater than 0.6), the effusion is said to be an *exudate* and not a *transudate*.

Interfering factors

Factors that interfere with LDH testing include the following:

■ Hemolysis of blood
This will cause false-positive LDH levels because LDH exists in the RBCs. Lysis of these cells causes the LDH to be released into the

blood specimen and falsely *elevates* the LDH level.
■ Strenuous exercise
This may cause *elevation* of total LDH and specifically LDH-1, 2, and 5.

Procedure

No fasting is required. A venous blood sample is collected in a red-top tube.

Nursing implications with rationale

Before

☞ Explain the need for this test to the patient. Inform the patient if he or she will be receiving frequent venipunctures for evaluation of an MI.

After

■ After venipuncture, apply pressure or a pressure dressing to the site to prevent further bleeding. Observe the site for bleeding.

Lipoproteins (High-Density Lipoprotein [HDL], Low-Density Lipoprotein [LDL], Very Low-Density Lipoprotein [VLDL])

Test type Blood

Normal values

HDL:
Male: >45 mg/dl or >0.75 mmol/L (SI units)
Female: >55 mg/dl or >0.91 mmol/L (SI units)
LDL: 60-180 mg/dl or <3.37 mmol/L (SI units)
VLDL: 25% to 50%

Rationale

Lipoproteins are proteins in the blood whose main purpose is to transport cholesterol, triglycerides, and other insoluble fats. They are used as markers indicating the levels of lipids in the bloodstream. With the use of electrophoresis, these lipoproteins can be grouped into the following types:

1. Chylomicrons, which are primarily triglycerides

2. LDLs (beta lipoproteins), which are primarily cholesterol
3. VLDLs (pre-beta lipoproteins), which are mainly triglycerides
4. HDLs (alpha lipoproteins), which are predominantly protein with a small amount of cholesterol

Lipids and cholesterol are used in the synthesis of sterol hormones (adrenals and gonadals). They are important in the structure of cellular membranes. Cholesterol is an integral part of bile. The lipid profile usually measures total cholesterol, triglycerides, HDL, LDL, and VLDL.

HDLs are carriers of cholesterol. They are produced in the liver and, to a smaller degree, in the intestines. It is suspected that the purpose of HDLs is to remove cholesterol from the peripheral tissues and transport it to the liver for excretion. Also, HDLs may have a protective effect by preventing cellular uptake of cholesterol and lipids. These potential actions may be the source of the protective cardiovascular characteristics associated with HDLs (good cholesterol) within the blood. Both HDL and total cholesterol are independent variables of CHD risk (Table 2-4). When they are combined in a ratio, the accuracy of prediction is increased. The total cholesterol/HDL ratio should be at least 5:1; 3:1 is ideal (Table 2-5).

LDLs are also cholesterol-rich. Cholesterol carried by LDLs can be deposited into the peripheral tissues and is associated with an increased risk of arteriosclerotic heart and peripheral vascular disease. Therefore, high levels of LDL (bad cholesterol) are atherogenic. The LDL level should be less than 160 mg/dl in persons with coronary artery disease and less than 180 mg/dl in those without disease. LDL is usually derived by the Friedwald formula by subtracting the HDL plus one fifth of the triglycerides from the total cholesterol:

$$LDL = \text{Total cholesterol}$$
$$- (HDL + \text{Triglycerides}/5)$$

Other formulas for deriving LDL account for different sets of normal values.

Although VLDLs carry a small amount of cholesterol, they are the predominant carriers of blood triglycerides. To a lesser degree, VLDLs also are associated with an increased risk of arteriosclerotic occlusive disease. The VLDL value is usually expressed as a percentage of total cholesterol. Levels in excess of 25% to 50% are associated with increased risk of coronary disease.

The HDL, LDL, and VLDL levels are part of a lipid profile test that also evaluates cholesterol (see p. 27) and triglycerides (see p. 51). The lipoprotein test is used to assess the risk of coronary artery disease. High levels of the protective HDL are associated with a decreased risk of coro-

TABLE 2-4 HDL as an Indication of Risk for Coronary Heart Disease

	HDL mg/dl (SI Units)	
Risk Level	Male	Female
Low	60 (1.55)	70 (1.81)
Moderate	45 (1.17)	55 (1.42)
High	25 (0.65)	35 (0.90)

TABLE 2-5 Cholesterol-to-HDL Ratio as an Indicator of Risk of Coronary Heart Disease*

	Ratio	
Risk	Male	Female
Half average	3.4	3.3
Average	5.0	4.4
2 × average	10.0	7.0
3 × average	24.0	11.0

*When cholesterol testing is combined with measurement of lipoproteins, risk of coronary heart disease can be more accurately calculated.

nary disease, whereas high levels of LDL and VLDL are associated with an increased risk of coronary occlusive disease.

Genetic makeup is probably the most important determinant of lipoprotein level. However, frequent physical activity and moderate alcohol intake may increase HLD levels. Poor dietary habits associated with an increased intake of animal fats and snack foods also are known to increase LDL and VLDL levels.

Interfering factors

Factors that interfere with lipoprotein testing include the following:

- Smoking and alcohol ingestion, because they *decrease* HDL levels
- Binge eating, because it can alter lipoprotein values
- Age and gender, because they affect HDL levels
- Postmyocardial infarction
  HDL values, like cholesterol, tend to *decrease* significantly for as long as 3 months following MI

Procedure

After eating a low-fat meal, the patient must fast 12 to 14 hours before testing. Only water is permitted. Lipoproteins are affected by a previous meal. Alcohol should not be taken 24 hours before the test. A peripheral venipuncture is performed, and 5 to 10 ml of blood is collected in a red-top tube.

Nursing implications with rationale

Before
☞ Instruct the patient to fast for 12 to 14 hours before testing. Only water is permitted. Inform the patient that dietary indiscretion within the previous few weeks may influence results.

During
- Indicate on the laboratory requisition slip any drugs that may affect test results.

After
- After the venipuncture, apply pressure or a pressure dressing to the site to prevent further bleeding. Observe the site for bleeding.

☞ Instruct patients with high lipoprotein levels about diet, exercise, and appropriate body weight.

Pericardiocentesis

Test type Fluid analysis

Normal values

Minimal amount of clear, straw-colored fluid without evidence of bacteria, blood, or malignant cells

Rationale

Pericardiocentesis, the aspiration of fluid from the pericardial sac with a needle, may be performed for therapeutic and diagnostic purposes. Therapeutically, the test is performed to relieve cardiac tamponade by removing blood or fluid to improve diastolic filling. Diagnostically, pericardiocentesis is performed to remove a sample of pericardial fluid for laboratory examination to determine the cause of the fluid accumulation. This is similar to the evaluation described for pleural fluid on p. 174.

Potential complications

Potential complications associated with pericardiocentesis are as follows:

- Laceration of the coronary artery or myocardium by the aspirating needle
- Ventricular arrhythmias induced by the aspirating needle
- MI, if the needle were to injure the myocardium
- Pneumothorax caused by inadvertent puncture of the lung
- Hepatic laceration caused by inadvertent puncture of the liver
- Pleural/pericardial infection caused by the aspirating needle

Procedure

No fluid or food restrictions are necessary before this procedure. (However, for an elective procedure the patient is often kept fasting for 4 to 6

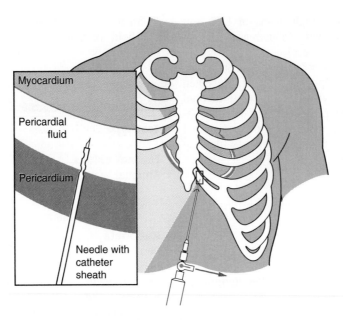

Figure 2-11 Pericardiocentesis procedure and aspiration of pericardial fluid. For recurrent cardiac tamponade and large pericardial effusion, the indwelling catheter may remain.

hours.) Pericardiocentesis is usually performed with the patient in a supine position with the head of the bed elevated 60 degrees. A peripheral IV is obtained. An area in the fifth to sixth intercostal space at the left sternal margin (or subxyphoid) is antiseptically prepared with povidone-iodine solution and injected with a local anesthetic. A large-bore, short-beveled pericardiocentesis needle attached to a three-way stopcock with a 50-ml syringe is introduced at a 20- to 30-degree angle to the frontal plane. An EKG lead wire is attached to the needle. As the needle is inserted through the chest wall into the pericardial sac (Figure 2-11), the EKG is observed for changes in the ST segment. The ST segment is normal if the needle is in the pericardial sac, and it is elevated if the needle touches the epicardium. The pericardial fluid then is aspirated and collected in labeled and numbered specimen tubes. The pericardial fluid is evaluated for color, turbidity, blood, white blood cell (WBC) and differential counts, hemoglobin, cultures, cytology, glucose, cholesterol, and protein.

When the needle is removed, pressure is applied immediately to the site with a sterile gauze pad for about 3 to 5 minutes. A bandage is then applied. Some patients with recurrent cardiac tamponade may need an indwelling pericardial catheter for continuous drainage.

A physician performs this procedure in approximately 10 to 20 minutes. Although the test is not considered painful, most patients will feel pressure as the needle is introduced into the pericardial sac.

Contraindications

Contraindications for pericardiocentesis are as follows:

- Patients who are uncooperative
  This is because of the risk of lacerations to the epicardium or coronary artery.
- Patients with a bleeding disorder
  Inadvertent puncture of the myocardium may cause uncontrollable bleeding into the pericardial sac, leading to tamponade.

Nursing implications with rationale

Before

☞ Explain the procedure to the patient. Pericardiocentesis is a frightening experience for most patients.

■ Ensure that written and informed consent is obtained before the procedure.

■ Administer pretest medications as ordered. Atropine is frequently given to prevent the vasovagal reflex, which may cause bradycardia and hypotension.

During

■ Assist the physician as necessary during the procedure. Observe the EKG for evidence of ST-segment elevation, which would indicate the needle has touched the epicardial wall. If this occurs, the needle should be retracted slightly.

■ Observe the aspirate for blood. Gross blood indicates inadvertent puncture of a cardiac chamber. The blood should not clot if it is from the pericardial space.

After

■ Carefully label and number the specimen tubes of pericardial fluid and send them to the laboratory immediately after the procedure. The specimen tubes usually contain an additive. If the proper additives are not used, the test results may be inaccurate.

■ If bacterial culture and sensitivity tests are scheduled, record on the laboratory requisition slip any antibiotic therapy that the patient is receiving.

■ Observe the puncture site for bleeding and hematoma formation.

■ Monitor the vital signs closely (normally every 15 minutes for four times, then every 30 minutes for four times, then every hour for four times, and then every 4 hours). A decreasing blood pressure and increasing heart rate may indicate bleeding. An increase in temperature may indicate infection.

■ If a catheter remains in place for continual drainage, it is usually sutured to the skin, and a sterile dressing is applied. The catheter is connected to a sterile drainage bag and secured safely below the level of the patient's midchest to prevent return of the drainage into the pericardial sac.

■ Because of the risk of infection, catheters are usually removed within 24 to 48 hours. After the sutures are cut, the catheter is withdrawn with a firm, continuous pull. A sterile dressing is applied to the puncture site.

Plethysmography, Venous (Cuff Pressure Test)

Test type Manometric

Normal values
Patent venous system without evidence of thrombosis or occlusion

Rationale
Plethysmography measures changes in the volume of an extremity and is usually performed on a leg to exclude deep vein thrombosis (DVT). During this test, blood pressure cuffs are placed on the proximal, middle, and distal portions of the extremity and attached to a pulse volume recorder. The leg volume then can be recorded as a baseline value. The venous system is occluded by inflating the proximal cuff (occlusion cuff); the distal cuff (recording cuff) should record a sudden increase in venous volume. When the occlusion cuff is released, the venous volume of the leg should return to preocclusion baseline levels. In patients with venous obstruction, however, no initial increase in leg volume is recorded. Also, because venous outflow is obstructed, the venous volume of the leg will not dissipate quickly after release of the proximal cuff.

Although the results of venous plethysmography are less accurate than those of venography (see p. 53), no complications are associated with this noninvasive study. Plethysmography can be performed easily and quickly on any patient with suspected venous disease. Furthermore, with the use of portable plethysmography, this test can be performed at the bedside for extremely ill patients.

Doppler flow studies (see p. 52) are now being performed to identify DVT but are less accurate than venous plethysmography in evaluating the venous system below the knee.

Interfering factors

Venous occlusion proximal to the site of the occlusion cuff interferes with plethysmography.

Procedure

No fasting is required. The patient is asked to lie supine on a bed. All clothing from the patient's extremity is removed. A large, inflatable occlusion cuff is placed on the proximal portion of the extremity (Figure 2-12). A second smaller plethysmographic monitor or recording cuff is placed distally on the leg. A third cuff may be placed in between the proximal and distal cuffs. The second cuff is inflated to 10 mm Hg to facilitate recognition of small changes in the leg's venous volume. The effects of respiration on the leg's venous volume are evaluated. If no significant changes occur with respiration, venous occlusion can be suspected.

The occlusion cuff is inflated to 50 mm Hg. The monitor cuff should demonstrate a rise in venous volume, displayed on the pulse volume recorder. After the highest volume is recorded in the monitor cuff, the occlusion cuff is deflated rapidly. The leg should return to its preocclusion volume within 1 second. If return to preocclusion baseline values is delayed, venous thrombosis is suspected.

This test is usually performed in the noninvasive vascular laboratory or at the patient's bedside by a noninvasive-vascular technologist in approximately 30 minutes. No discomfort is associated with this test.

Nursing implications with rationale

Before

☑ Explain the procedure to the patient. Assure the patient that no discomfort is associated with the procedure.

☑ Tell the patient that no fasting is required.

After

■ No special care is required after this test. However, if the results indicate DVT, immediate interventions, such as anticoagulation therapy, should be initiated.

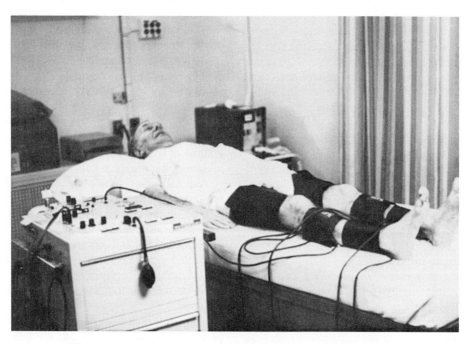

Figure 2-12 Placement of occlusion cuffs for plethysmography.

Case Study

Thrombophlebitis

Mrs. N. was a 32-year-old nursing assistant who was admitted to the hospital complaining of a painful, swollen right leg. She was otherwise in good health. On physical examination, her right leg was one and a half times the size of her left leg. The right calf was tender and 3+ pitting edema was present.

Studies	**Results**
Venous duplex, Doppler ultrasound, and plethysmography, pp. 52 and 47	Occlusion of the deep venous system in the right thigh and calf (normal: no occlusion)
Venography, p. 53	Same as above

Diagnostic Analysis

The diagnosis of acute vein thrombophlebitis was made. Normally all the studies noted above would not be ordered, but the tests are shown here to indicate their usage. Venous duplex and Doppler studies are the least invasive. However, venography is the most accurate, especially for suspected disease below the knee. Heparin therapy was prescribed. After anticoagulation, Mrs. N. was switched to warfarin (Coumadin) (see Heparin and Warfarin Monitoring, pp. 426 and 433). She was discharged and continued receiving warfarin therapy and PT monitoring. After 4 months, the warfarin was discontinued.

Critical Thinking Questions

1. If Mrs. N. were to develop an acute episode of shortness of breath, what would you do?
2. What would be included in the diagnostic evaluation of this problem?

Transesophageal Echocardiography (TEE)

Test type Endoscopy/ultrasound

Normal values

Normal position, size, and movement of the heart muscle, valves, and chambers

Rationale

Transesophageal echocardiography (TEE) provides ultrasonic imaging of the heart from a retrocardiac vantage point, which avoids interference of the ultrasound waves by the subcutaneous tissue, bony thorax, and lungs. It provides very accurate information about the heart structure and function and also about the thoracic aorta. In this procedure, a high-frequency ultrasound transducer placed in the esophagus by endoscopy provides better resolution than that of images obtained with routine transthoracic echocardiography (see p. 32). The transducer is positioned behind the heart (Figure 2-13). Controls on the handle of the endoscope permit the transducer to be rotated and flexed in both the anteroposterior and right-left lateral planes.

This test is performed for the following reasons:

1. To visualize the mitral valve
2. To differentiate between intracardiac and extracardiac masses and tumors

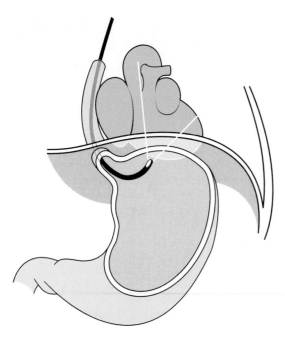

Figure 2-13 Transesophageal echocardiography (TEE). Diagram illustrates location of the transesophageal endoscope in the esophagus.

3. To visualize the atrial septum (for atrial septal defects)
4. To diagnose thoracic aortic dissection
5. To detect valvular vegetation indicative of endocarditis
6. To determine cardiac sources of arterial embolism
7. To detect coronary artery disease by identifying areas of muscle wall hypokinesia

Also, TEE can be used intraoperatively to monitor high-risk patients for ischemia. Ischemic muscle movement is much different from normal muscle movement; therefore, TEE is a very sensitive indicator of myocardial ischemia. TEE is more sensitive than EKG for detecting ischemia. TEE is also used intraoperatively to evaluate surgical results of valvular or congenital heart diseases. Furthermore, TEE is the most sensitive technique for detecting air emboli.

Potential complications

Potential complications of TEE are as follows:

■ Esophageal perforation or bleeding
These problems may occur from passage of the transducer.
■ Cardiac arrhythmias

Procedure

The patient must fast 4 to 6 hours before TEE is performed. Dentures are removed, and IV access is established. The short-acting benzodiazepine, midazolam, along with meperidine or butorphanol tartrate (Stadol), is commonly ordered to reduce patient anxiety, provide antegrade amnesia, and improve compliance. This is often referred to as *conscious sedation.* EKG leads are applied, and a rhythm strip is continually displayed on the EKG machine. Blood pressure is monitored periodically, and pulse oximetry is used to determine oxygen saturation.

The pharynx is anesthetized with benzocaine-tetracaine-butyl aminobenzoate (Cetacaine) or lidocaine to depress the gag reflex. For intubation, the patient is placed in the left lateral decubitus position. Intubation can also be performed with the patient in the supine or upright sitting position. A bite guard protects the patient's teeth from the endoscope. The transducer is slowly introduced into the throat. The patient is asked to swallow, and the transducer is advanced into position behind the heart. The room is darkened, and the ultrasound images are displayed on the monitor. After the desired images are visualized, the endoscope is removed.

This procedure is performed by a cardiologist in approximately 20 minutes in an endoscopy suite or at the bedside. Patients are observed closely for approximately 1 hour after the procedure until the effects of the sedatives have worn off. Very little discomfort is associated with this test.

Contraindications

Contraindications for TEE are as follows:

■ Patients with known upper esophageal pathology

This may prevent passage of the transducer down the esophagus.

- Patients with known esophageal varices
  They may experience bleeding from passage of the transducer.
- Patients with Zenker's diverticulum
  They may experience perforation from passage of the transducer into the diverticulum.
- Patients who cannot cooperate during the procedure

Nursing implications with rationale
Before
- Explain the procedure to the patient. Patients may be apprehensive about this study. Provide emotional support.
- Make sure the patient's written and informed consent is obtained.
- Keep the patient NPO (*nil per os,* nothing by mouth) for the designated time (usually 4 to 6 hours) before the test to prevent regurgitation when the scope is passed.
- Tell the patient that the test is not painful but may cause discomfort when the gag reflex is initiated. Inform the patient that the throat will be anesthetized to minimize discomfort.
- Remove the patient's dentures and eyeglasses before the test. Because the tube is passed through the mouth, oral hygiene procedures should be performed before and after the test.
- Explain to the patient that he or she will be unable to speak when the endoscope is passed.

After
- Do not allow the patient to eat or drink anything until the gag reflex returns (usually in about 2 hours) because the patient's throat has been anesthetized.
- Inform the patient that he or she may be hoarse or complain of a sore throat for several days. Drinking cool fluids and gargling may relieve some of the soreness.
- Observe safety precautions until the effects of the sedatives have worn off. Naloxone (Narcan) or flumazenil (Mazicon) may be ordered to reverse the sedative effects of the narcotics.
- Monitor the vital signs as ordered.

Triglycerides (TGs)

Test type Blood

Normal values
Adult/elderly
   Male: 40-160 mg/dl or 0.45-1.81 mmol/L (SI units)
   Female: 35-135 mg/dl or 0.40-1.52 mmol/L (SI units)

Children	Male	Female
0-5 years:	30-86 mg/dl	32-99 mg/dl
6-11 years:	31-108 mg/dl	35-114 mg/dl
12-15 years:	36-138 mg/dl	41-138 mg/dl
16-19 years:	40-163 mg/dl	40-128 mg/dl

Possible critical values: >400 mg/dl

Rationale
Triglycerides (TGs) are a form of fat within the bloodstream. They are transported by VLDLs and LDLs. TGs, composed of glycerol and other fatty acids, are produced in the liver. When blood levels of TGs are excessive, they are deposited into the fatty tissues, where they act as energy storage. TGs comprise most of the fat in the body and are part of a lipid profile that also evaluates cholesterol (see p. 27) and lipoproteins (see p. 43). A lipid profile is performed to assess the risk of coronary and vascular disease. This test also is performed on patients suspected to have fat metabolism disorders.

Interfering factors
Factors that interfere with determing triglyceride levels include the following:

- Ingestion of fatty meals
  This may cause *elevated* TG levels.
- Ingestion of alcohol
  This may cause *elevated* levels of TG by increasing the production of VLDL.
- Pregnancy may cause *increased* TG levels.
- Drugs that may cause *increased* TG levels
  These include cholestyramine, estrogens, and oral contraceptives.

Procedure

After eating a low-fat meal, the patient must fast 12 to 14 hours before testing. Only water is permitted. TGs are affected by meals eaten as early as 2 weeks before testing. Alcohol should not be taken 24 hours before the test. A peripheral venipuncture is performed, and 5 to 10 ml of blood are collected in a red-top tube.

Nursing implications with rationale

Before

☞ Instruct the patient to fast 12 to 14 hours before the test because blood levels are affected by meals. Tell the patient not to drink alcohol for 24 hours before testing because alcohol may cause TG elevations.

During

■ Indicate on the laboratory requisition slip any drugs that may affect test results.

After

■ After the venipuncture, apply pressure or a pressure dressing to the site to prevent further bleeding. Observe the site for bleeding.

☞ Instruct patients with elevated TG levels about diet, exercise, and appropriate body weight.

Vascular Doppler Studies (Venous Doppler Studies and Arterial Doppler Studies)

Test type Ultrasound

Normal values

Venous

Normal Doppler venous signal with spontaneous respiration

Normal venous system with no signs of occlusion

Arterial

Normal arterial Doppler signal with systolic and diastolic components

No reduction in blood pressure greater than 20 mm Hg compared with the normal extremity

Normal ankle-to-brachial arterial blood pressure index of 0.85 or greater

No evidence of arterial occlusion

Rationale

This ultrasound study provides information about arterial and venous patency without the use of invasive techniques. Arterial Doppler studies are used on patients with suspected arterial insufficiency (e.g., claudication; poorly healing skin ulcer; cold, pale leg; pulseless extremity; or rest pain). Venous ultrasound is used to evaluate the venous patency in patients with a swollen, painful leg; venous varicosities of the upper or lower extremity; or an edematous extremity. Venous Doppler studies are not accurate for venous occlusive disease of the lower calf.

With *single mode venous* Doppler studies, the blood flow can be augmented by an audio speaker as a swishing noise. If the vein is occluded, no swishing sounds are detected.

With *single mode arterial* Doppler studies, peripheral arteriosclerotic occlusive disease of the extremities can be identified and located by slowly deflating blood pressure cuffs placed on the calf and ankle. The systolic pressure in the various arteries of the extremities then can be accurately measured by detecting the first evidence of blood flow with the Doppler transducer. The extremely sensitive Doppler ultrasound detector can recognize the swishing sound of even the most minimal blood flow. Normally, there is a minimal drop in systolic blood pressure from the arteries of the arms compared with those of the legs. If the drop in blood pressure exceeds 20 mm Hg, occlusive disease is believed to exist immediately proximal to the area tested.

Duplex scanning provides an accurate representation of the appearance and patency of the arterial or venous vessel wall. In addition, this technique can measure the amplitude and waveform of the vascular pulse. Furthermore, a two-dimensional image of the vessel can be produced and allows direct visualization of possibly stenotic or occluded vessels with flow disruption. Additionally, lower extremity postsurgical arterial bypass graft patency can be assessed by using Doppler ultrasound technology.

Interfering factors

Factors that interfere with vascular Doppler studies include the following:

- Venous or arterial occlusive disease proximal to the site of testing
- Cigarette smoking
  Nicotine can cause spasms of the peripheral arteries and alter the results.

Procedure

No fasting or sedation is required. The tests can be performed equally well at the bedside or in the noninvasive vascular studies laboratory. The patient is placed in the supine position.

For *venous* Doppler studies, a conductive gel is applied in multiple areas to the skin overlying the venous system of the extremity. For the lower extremity, the deep venous system is identified in the ankle, calf, thigh, and groin. The characteristic swishing sound of the Doppler indicates a patent venous system. Failure to detect this signal indicates venous occlusion. Both the superficial and venous systems are evaluated. Duplex scanning can actually produce an image of the venous system and measure blood flow in the vessels.

For *arterial* Doppler studies, blood pressure cuffs are placed around the thigh, calf, and ankle. A conductive paste is applied to the skin overlying the artery distal to the cuffs. The proximal cuff is inflated to a level above systolic blood pressure in the normal extremity. The Doppler ultrasound transducer is placed immediately distal to the inflated cuff. The pressure in the cuff is slowly released. The highest pressure at which blood flow is detected by the characteristic swishing Doppler signal is recorded as the blood pressure of that artery. The test is repeated at each successive level. When the ankle pressure is divided by the arm (brachial artery) pressure, the result is known as the *AB index.* If the AB index is less than 0.85, significant arterial occlusive disease exists within the extremity. Duplex scanning can produce an image of the artery and its inner lining. Amplitude and blood flow can be accurately measured.

This study requires approximately 15 minutes to perform. It is usually performed by an ultra-sound technician and interpreted by a radiologist. No discomfort is associated with it.

Nursing implications with rationale

Before

- Explain the procedure to the patient. Reassure the patient that no discomfort is associated with this study.
- Tell the patient that he or she must lie still during the procedure. Movement can alter test results.
- Instruct the patient to avoid smoking for at least 30 minutes before this test. Nicotine causes constriction of the peripheral arteries and alters test results.
- Gently remove any occlusive dressings or stockings from the leg. The patient's leg may be tender to the touch.

After

- Gently remove the conduction lubricant from the patient's extremities. Massaging the legs is contraindicated because this action may dislodge thrombi.

Venography of the Lower Extremities (Phlebography, Venogram)

Test type X-ray with contrast dye

Normal values

No evidence of venous thrombosis or obstruction

Rationale

Venography is a radiographic study designed to identify and locate thrombi within the venous system of the lower extremities. During this study, dye is injected into the venous system of the affected extremity. Radiographic films are then taken at timed intervals to visualize the venous system. Obstruction to the flow of dye or a filling defect within the vein indicates thrombosis. A positive study accurately confirms the diagnosis of venous thrombosis; however, a normal study, although not as determinative, does make the diagnosis of venous thrombosis very unlikely. Often both extremities are studied, even though only

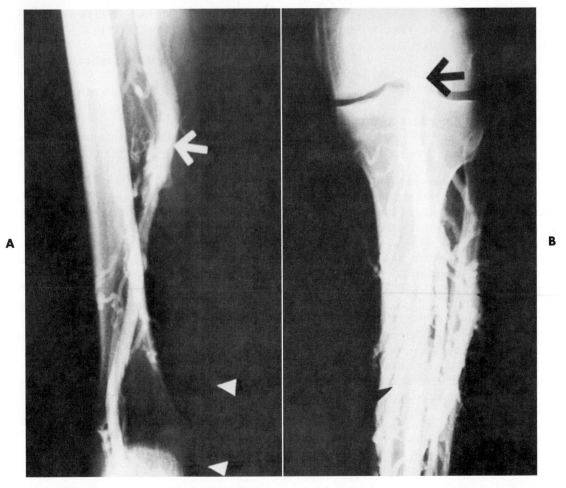

Figure 2-14 **A,** Normal venogram of the upper half of the leg. White arrow indicates normal deep femoral vein. Small white pointers indicate poorly visualized superficial saphenous vein. **B,** Normal venogram of the lower leg. Black arrow indicates normal popliteal vein. Small black pointer indicates one of many normal, unnamed deep veins in the calf.

one leg is suspected to contain a DVT. The normal extremity is used for comparison with the involved extremity (Figure 2-14). Unlike venous plethysmography or Doppler studies, (see pp. 47 and 52, respectively), venography is accurate even for thrombi in veins below the knee. Venography also is performed on the upper extremity to evaluate axillary, subclavian, and innominate veins.

Potential complications

Potential complications of venography of the lower extremities are as follows:

- Allergic reaction to iodinated dyes
  Allergic reactions vary from flushing, itching, and urticaria to life-threatening anaphylaxis (evidenced by respiratory distress, drop in blood pressure, shock). In the event of anaphylaxis,

the patient may be treated with diphenhydramine, steroids, and epinephrine. Oxygen and endotracheal equipment should be on hand for immediate use.

■ Renal failure, especially in elderly people who are chronically dehydrated or may have a mild degree of renal failure
■ Subcutaneous infiltration of the dye, causing cellulitis and pain

Procedure

No sedation or fasting is required. The patient is taken to the radiology department and placed in the supine position on the x-ray table. Catheterization of a superficial vein of the foot is performed, possibly requiring a surgical cutdown. The radiologist then injects an iodinated radiopaque dye into the vein and takes x-ray films to follow the dye's course. Frequently a tourniquet is placed on the leg to prevent filling of the superficial saphenous system. This study takes approximately 30 to 90 minutes. Often, both extremities are studied even though only one leg is suspected to contain a DVT. The normal extremity is used for comparison with the involved extremity. The venous catheterization is only as uncomfortable as a cutaneous needle stick.

The dye may cause the patient to feel a warm flush. (This is not as severe as that noted with arteriography.) Inform the patient that occasionally, mild degrees of nausea, vomiting, or skin itching may occur.

Contraindications

Contraindications for venography are as follows:

■ Severe edema of the legs, which makes venous access for dye injection impossible
■ Allergic reaction to iodinated dye or shellfish
■ Renal failure, because the iodinated dye is nephrotoxic

Nursing implications with rationale

Before
☞ Explain the procedure to the patient and allay the patient's fears regarding venography.

■ Assess the patient for allergies to dye or shellfish. Administer a steroid-antihistamine preparation, if ordered, for the patient allergic to the dye.
■ Ensure that the patient is adequately hydrated before testing. Iodinated dye can further impair renal function, especially if it is already compromised by dehydration or chronic renal disease.
■ Ensure that patients in a considerable amount of pain are medicated so that they can lie still during this procedure. Handle the affected extremity gently.

After
■ Assess the patient for cellulitis (redness, swelling, pain, tenderness), indicative of subcutaneous infiltration of dye.
■ Assess the patient for signs of bacteremia (elevated temperature, tachycardia, cutaneous flush, or chills).
■ Continue appropriate fluid administration to prevent dehydration caused by the diuretic action of the dye.

REVIEW QUESTIONS AND ANSWERS

1. **Question:** Your mother has just returned from an appointment with her doctor and asks you to help her understand her lipoprotein report. She does not understand why she needs to increase her HDLs and decrease her LDLs. What should you tell her?

   Answer: Explain to your mother that HDL is often called the *good cholesterol* because it removes cholesterol from the tissues and transports it to the liver for excretion. High levels are associated with a decreased risk of CHD. On the other hand, LDL is often called the *bad cholesterol* because it carries cholesterol and deposits it into the peripheral tissues. High levels are associated with an increased risk of CHD.

2. **Question:** Your patient is scheduled for a TEE.

Despite the fact that he was instructed to remain NPO for 4 to 6 hours before the test, you find him eating a sandwich 20 minutes before the test. He tells you he was allowed to eat before his last echocardiogram several years ago. What should you do?

Answer: Ask the patient to describe his previous echocardiogram. Most likely it was a TTE, which does not require fasting. Because the TEE requires inserting an endoscope through the mouth and into the esophagus, he should have remained NPO. Because he is at high risk for gagging and aspiration, the test should be cancelled.

3. **Question:** The physician has requested an EKG for a 6-week-old infant. What may be an appropriate method of quieting your patient during this procedure?

   Answer: Plan to record the EKG at a time when the infant usually receives a bottle feeding. If necessary, distract the infant's attention with toys or keys. If it is necessary to hold or touch the child, rubber gloves should be worn to avoid electrical interference.

4. **Question:** You are the nurse in the coronary care unit. While observing the cardiac monitors, you see a straight line for one of the patients. What should be your immediate reaction?

   Answer: Sometimes mechanical failure causes the equipment used for cardiac monitoring to display a straight or flat line on the cardiac monitor instead of the patient's normal heartbeat. Nevertheless, the possibility exists that the patient's heart has indeed stopped. Therefore, before notifying the appropriate personnel involved in cardiac resuscitation, you should go immediately to the patient's room and assess the patient for signs of cardiac arrest.

5. **Question:** Your patient has returned from undergoing femoral arteriography performed through the right groin. The patient begins to complain of right-leg pain, weakness, and tingling. You assess the patient and find a small hematoma in the groin. You note that the right leg is pale, pulseless, and cooler than the left. What are the appropriate nursing interventions?

   Answer: It appears that your patient has suffered an arteriocclusion of the right femoral vessels. The arterial puncture probably dislodged an intimal (inner arterial lining) atherosclerotic plaque, causing an embolus or dissection of the vessel. You should reassure the patient and do the following:
   a. Notify the physician of your present findings.
   b. Do not elevate the leg, because elevation will exacerbate the arterial ischemia.
   c. Prepare the patient for surgery, if this is directed by the physician.
      1. Shave and prepare both sides of the groin.
      2. Start an IV line.
      3. Keep the patient NPO.
      4. Obtain two red-top tubes for typing and cross-matching blood.
      5. Assist in obtaining written and informed consent for arterial embolectomy or arterial intimal repair.
      (This routine may vary from hospital to hospital.)
   d. Make the appropriate arrangements if a second femoral arteriogram is ordered before surgery.

6. **Question:** Your patient is admitted for an evaluation of increasingly frequent chest pains. In a review of other system complaints, you find that the patient has bilateral calf pain when walking two blocks (intermittent claudication). One of the studies ordered for this patient is an exercise stress test. Can you expect that this test will be completed reliably?

   Answer: No. The patient's peripheral vascular occlusive disease will cause the patient to have calf pain. This calf pain will probably precede exercise-induced chest pain or EKG changes and thus cause the stress test to be terminated prematurely. This patient may be a candidate for chemical stress testing.

7. **Question:** What is the purpose of determining

O_2 content in the blood obtained from the various heart chambers and arteries during cardiac catheterization?

Answer: Abnormal shunting of blood from one heart chamber to another can be diagnosed by the abnormal O_2 content of the blood withdrawn from a particular chamber. For example, in a patient with an atrial septal defect, the O_2 content of the blood in the right atrium is much higher than that of blood drawn from the superior vena cava. Normally, these areas have the same O_2 content. The elevated O_2 content in the right atrium is caused by the mixing of blood from the left atrium with the blood contained in the right atrium.

Bibliography

Antman EM: Magnesium in acute MI: timing is critical. *Circulation* 92:2367, 1995.

Antman EM, Braunwald E: Acute myocardial infarction. In Fauci AS et al, editors: Harrison's principles of internal medicine, ed 14, New York, 1998, McGraw-Hill.

Bain DS, Grossman W: Diagnostic cardiac catherization and angioplasty. In Fauci AS et al, editors: Harrison's principles of internal medicine, ed 14, New York, 1998, McGraw-Hill.

Braunwald E, editor: Heart disease: a textbook of cardiovascular medicine, ed 5, Philadelphia, 1997, WB Saunders.

Bubien RS et al: What you need to know about radiofrequency ablation. *Am J Nurs* 93(7):30-36, 1993.

Chaitman BR: Exercise stress testing. In Braunwald E, editor: Heart disease: a textbook of cardiovascular medicine, ed 5, Philadelphia, 1997, WB Saunders.

DiLucente L, Gorcsan J: Transesophageal echocardiography: application to the postoperative cardiac surgery patient. *Dimens Crit Care Nurs* 10(2):74-80, March-April, 1991.

Docker CS et al: Intraoperative echocardiography: an essential tool in cardiac surgery. *AORN* 55(1):167, 169-173, 1992.

Feigenbaum H: Echocardiography. In Braunwald E, editor: Heart disease: a textbook of cardiovascular medicine, ed 5, Philadelphia, 1997, WB Saunders.

Feldman T: Rheumatic heart disease, *Curr Opin Cardiol* 11:126, 1996.

Fisch C: Electrocardiography. In Braunwald E, editor: Heart disease: a textbook of cardiovascular medicine, ed 5, Philadelphia, 1997, WB Saunders.

Fisher EA et al: Transesophageal echocardiography: procedures and clinical applications, *J Am Coll Cardiol* 18(5):1338-1348, 1991.

Gibler WB et al: Chest pain: how many tests are enough? *Patient Care* 25(1):18-33, 1991.

Goldberger AL: Electrocardiography. In Fauci AS et al, editors: Harrison's principles of internal medicine, ed 14, New York, 1998, McGraw-Hill.

Goldman L: Cost and quality of life: thrombosis and primary angioplasty. *J Am Coll Cardiol* 25:38S, 1995.

Higgins CB: Newer cardiac imaging techniques. In Braunwald E, editor: Heart disease: a textbook of cardiovascular medicine, ed 5, Philadelphia, 1997, WB Saunders.

Kyle RA: Amyloidosis. *Circulation* 91:1269, 1995.

Lensing AW et al: A comparison of compression ultrasound with color Doppler ultrasound for diagnosis of symptomless postoperative deep vein thrombosis. *Arch Intern Med* 157(7):758-762, 1997.

Libby P: Atherosclerosis. In Fauci AS et al, editors: Harrison's principles of internal medicine, ed 14, New York, 1998, McGraw-Hill.

Massie BM, Shah NH: The heart failure epidemic: magnitude of the problem and potential mitigating approaches. *Curr Opin Cardiol* 11:221, 1996.

Merva J: A closer look at the heart SAECG, *RN* 56(5):50-53, 1993.

Myerburg RJ: Electrocardiography. In Wilson J et al, editors: Harrison's principles of internal medicine, ed 12, New York, 1991, McGraw-Hill.

Olaison L et al: Fever, C-reactive protein, and other acute-phase reactants during treatment of infective endocarditis. *Arch Intern Med* 157(8):885-892, 1997.

Pinner J: Patient teaching for x-ray and other diagnostics. *RN* 54(3):32-36, 1991.

Robie BH: Cardiovascular technology: noninvasive diagnosis of cardiovascular disease using ultrasound imaging. *J Cardiovasc Nurs* 6(2):36-42, 1992.

Selwyn AP, Braunwald E: Ischemic heart disease. In Fauci AS et al, editors: Harrison's principles of internal medicine, ed 14, New York, 1998, McGraw-Hill.

Smith MK: Transesophageal echocardiography in the diagnosis of rupture of the aorta. *N Engl J Med* 332:356, 1995.

Statton ML, Eichorn EJ: Beta-blocker therapy for heart failure. *Curr Opin Cardiol* 11:263, 1996.

Taylor DC: Duplex ultrasound in assessment of vascular disease in clinical hypertension. *Am J Hypertens* 4(6):550-556, 1991.

Thompson EJ: Transesophageal echocardiography: a new window on the heart and great vessels. *Crit Care Nurse* 13(10):55-56, 1993.

Wachers F et al: Nuclear cardiology. In Braunwald E, editor: Heart disease: a textbook of cardiovascular medicine, ed 5, Philadelphia, 1997, WB Saunders.

Watkins H, et al: Mutations in the genes for cardiac troponin T and alpha tropomyosin in hypertrophic cardiomyopathy. *N Engl J Med* 332:1058, 1995.

Chapter 3

Diagnostic Studies Used in the Assessment of the
Gastrointestinal System

ANATOMY AND PHYSIOLOGY

The primary function of the gastrointestinal (GI) tract (Figure 3-1) is to provide the body with water, electrolytes, and nutrients. To accomplish

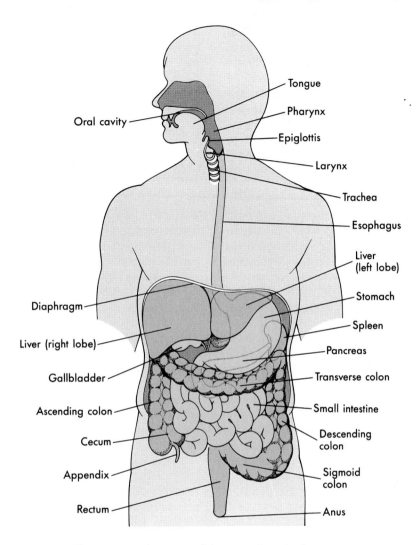

Figure 3-1   Anatomy of the gastrointestinal system.

this, food must be moved through the system while digestive enzymes are secreted to break down the food to a form that can easily be absorbed by the GI tract's lining cells.

The *esophagus* is a long muscular tube that, by successive and synchronized contractions, moves food from the pharynx (posterior mouth) through the lower esophageal sphincter and into the *stomach*. The stomach is a J-shaped structure that lies between the esophagus and the duodenum. In the stomach food is stored. Here the parietal and chief cells, located in the lining of the proximal stomach, secrete hydrochloric acid and pepsinogen, respectively. The acid and enzymes mix with the food, and the digestive process is begun. Intrinsic factor, essential to the absorption of vitamin B_{12}, is also secreted by the parietal cells.

Partially digested food (chyme) is expelled through the pyloric sphincter and into the *duodenum*. Here the pancreas and biliary tract enter the GI tract. The pancreas secretes proteolytic enzymes (trypsin and chymotrypsin), lipolytic enzymes (lipase), and amylatic enzymes (amylase). Because all digestive enzymes work best in an alkaline environment, water and bicarbonate also are secreted by the pancreas to provide an optimum basic pH. Water and bicarbonate are also secreted by the biliary system, along with bile salts, bilirubin, cholesterol, and phospholipids. The bile salts mix with the fatty acids and speed absorption of the fats. Bilirubin, cholesterol, and phospholipids have little or no digestive function and are merely excreta.

As the chyme moves through the *small bowel* (jejunum and ileum), further digestion and nutrient absorption occur. Finally, water and electrolytes (sodium, potassium, chloride, and bicarbonates) are absorbed in the *colon.* Undigested material (feces) is moved into the *rectum.* The rectum is a vault at the end of the GI tract where the feces are stored until evacuation.

The entire GI system is regulated by a neurohormonal feedback system. Gastrin (secreted in the mucosa of the distal stomach), along with the vagus nerve, stimulates hydrochloric acid secretion and propulsive muscular action of the stomach and intestines. The acid load in the duodenum stimulates the secretion of cholecystokinin and secretin from the duodenal mucosa. These in turn stimulate, respectively, secretions of biliary and pancreatic products of digestion. After digestion is completed, secretin and enterokinase (made by the intestinal mucosa) inhibit gastrin release and thereby slow the digestive process to its "between meal" activity.

Barium Enema (BE, Lower GI Series)

Test type X-ray with contrast dye

Normal values
Normal filling, contour, patency, and positioning of barium in the colon
Normal filling of the appendix and terminal ileum

Rationale
The barium enema (BE) study consists of a series of radiographic films visualizing the colon, distal small bowel, and, occasionally, the appendix. It is used to demonstrate the presence and location of polyps, tumors, and diverticula. Anatomic abnormalities (e.g., malrotation) also can be detected. BE is indicated for patients with:

Abdominal pain (It is contraindicated, however, in patients with acute abdominal pain.)
Obvious or occult blood in the stools
Inflammatory bowel diseases
Suspected cancer (bowel or other abdominal)
Abnormal obstruction series (see p. 80) indicating volvulus or colon obstruction

Therapeutically, the BE may be used to reduce nonstrangulated ileocolic intussusception in children. Bleeding from diverticula can cease after a barium enema.

The BE occasionally is used to assess filling of the appendix. When the clinical picture suggests possible appendicitis, failure of the appendix to fill with barium may support the diagnosis. Although the colon is the main organ evaluated by a BE, reflux of barium into the terminal ileum also will allow adequate visualization of the distal portion of the small intestine. Diseases that affect the terminal ileum, especially Crohn's disease (regional enteritis), can be identified. Inflammatory bowel disease and fistulas involving the colon can be detected with a BE.

In many instances, air is insufflated into the colon after the instillation of barium. This provides an air contrast to the barium. With air contrast, the colonic mucosa can be much more accurately visualized. This is called an *air-contrast barium enema (ACBE)* or *double-contrast barium enema.* It is used especially when small polyps are suspected. The accuracy of the regular BE in detecting small colonic tumors is approximately 60%. However, the accuracy of an ACBE in detecting small colonic tumors exceeds 85% (Figure 3-2).

Potential complications
Potential complications associated with BE are as follows:

- Colonic perforation, especially when the colon is weakened by inflammation, tumor, or infection
- Barium fecal impaction

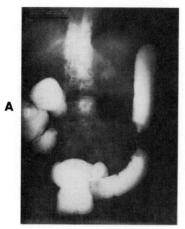
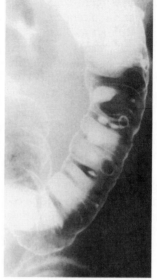

Figure 3-2 Barium enema. **A,** Single-contrast barium study illustrates obstructing circumferential carcinoma of the sigmoid colon. **B,** Double-contrast barium study shows multiple colonic diverticula. Diverticula on dependent surfaces are barium-filled; divertula on nondependent surfaces are seen as ring shadows.

Interfering factors

Factors that interfere with BE include the following:

- Barium within the abdomen from previous barium tests
  Barium in the abdomen may interfere with the visualization of portions of the colon.
- Significant residual stool within the colon
  This precludes adequate visualization of the entire bowel wall. Stool may be mistaken for polyps.
- Spasm of the colon
  Spasm can mimic the radiographic signs of a cancer. The use of intravenous (IV) glucagon minimizes spasm.

Procedure

The specific preparation of a BE study varies according to the protocol of the radiologist performing the test. A sample preparation follows:

One day before the examination
  Clear liquid diet

Evening before
  10 oz. of magnesium citrate or X-prep
Day of examination
  NPO (*nil per os,* nothing by mouth) after midnight
  Enema or suppository in the morning if the patient was unable to drink all of the colonic lavage

It is important to note that this procedure will vary depending on other medical conditions and age. For example, preparation for patients with a stoma would include stoma irrigation rather than an enema. In pediatric patients, preparation is diminished considerably. Dehydration must be avoided in the pediatric and geriatric patient.

The test begins with the rectal instillation of approximately 500 to 1500 ml of barium. Because the patient often has difficulty retaining the barium, a rectal tube with an inflatable balloon is used. The patient is placed in supine, prone, and lateral positions. The progress of the barium flow is followed on a fluoroscope. Small polyps and early changes in ulcerative colitis are more easily detected with an ACBE study. In this study, after the bowel mucosa is outlined with a thin coat of barium, air is insufflated to enhance the contrast and outline of small lesions. After the x-rays are taken, the patient is allowed to expel the barium. After the barium is expelled, another film is taken for retention of the barium. The colon is examined again for pathologic conditions in the post-evacuation film.

The method of administering a BE to a patient with a *colostomy* is to cover the stoma with a colostomy or bongart pouch to catch any backflow of barium. A cone from a colostomy irrigation kit is inserted into the stoma. This cone is then attached to irrigation tubing with a straight catheter. A clamp is turned on, and the contrast medium is instilled. A collection device, such as a bedpan, can be placed at the patient's side to collect any overflow of contrast medium from the stoma. The end of the pouch can be brought down to rest in the collecting device. When the radiographic studies are completed, a clamp is placed at the bottom of the pouch. This method is very effective because the barium does not get on the patient's skin and obscure the diagnostic radiographic films. Also, the patient is spared the embarrassment of having barium leak from the stoma.

This test is usually performed in the radiology department by a radiologist in approximately 45 minutes. Abdominal bloating and rectal pressure will occur during instillation of barium.

Contraindications

Contraindications for BE are as follows:

- Patients suspected of a perforation of the colon
  In these patients, diatrizoate meglumine (Gastrografin), a water-soluble iodine-containing contrast medium, is used. No bowel preparation is administered.
- Patients who are unable to cooperate
  This test requires the patient to hold the barium in the rectum and colon. This is especially difficult for elderly patients.

- Patients with megacolon
  Barium may worsen the disease.

Nursing implications with rationale
Before

- Explain the procedure to the patient. Tell the patient that it is not painful but that the preparation and procedure may be exhausting. Give written instructions.
- Tell the patient that his or her bowel must be free of fecal debris for the barium to outline the lumen of the bowel accurately.
- Assist the patient with the required preparation and chart the effects of the cathartics and suppository.
- Instruct the patient to remain NPO after midnight to provide optimum visualization of the bowel.
- Suggest that the patient take reading material to the radiology department so that he or she may read while expelling the barium.

After

- The patient may resume a regular diet. Instruct the patient to force oral fluids to avoid dehydration caused by cathartics.
- Assess the patient for complete evacuation of the barium. (Retained barium may cause a hardened impaction.) Stool will be light in color until all of the barium has been expelled. A cathartic, such as magnesium citrate, or an oil-retention enema, may be given.
- A local anesthetic ointment, such as dibucaine (Nupercainal), may be ordered to relieve anal discomfort.
- Allow the patient time to rest after the test. The cleansing regimen and the BE procedure may be exhausting.
- If a patient is not too tired, a warm bath may be soothing.

Barium Swallow (BS, Esophagogram)

Test type X-ray with contrast dye

Normal values

Normal size, contour, filling, patency, and positioning of the esophagus

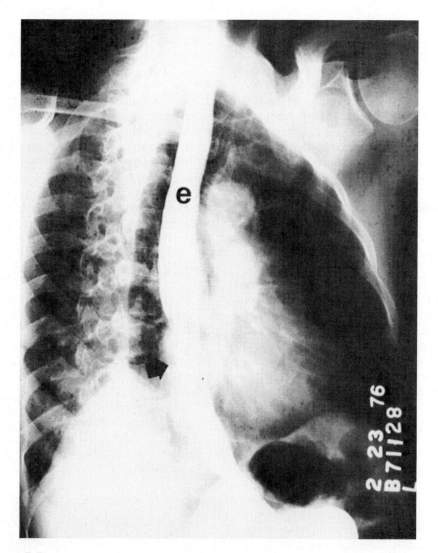

Figure 3-3 Barium swallow demonstrating an esophageal cancer *(black arrow)* within the esophagus *(e)*.

Rationale

This barium contrast study is a more thorough examination of the esophagus than that provided by most upper GI (UGI) series (see p. 92). It is indicated in patients with the following symptoms: dysphagia, noncardiac chest pain, painful swallowing, swallowing abnormalities (see videofluorosocopy swallowing examination, p. 91), and gastroesophageal reflux.

As in most barium contrast studies, defects in normal filling and narrowing of the barium column indicate tumor (Figure 3-3); strictures, or extrinsic compression from extraesophageal masses; or an abnormally enlarged heart and great vessels. Varices also can be seen as serpiginous, linear filling defects. Anatomic abnormalities, such as hiatal hernia, Schatzski's rings, and diverticula (Zenker's or epiphrenic) can be seen as well.

In patients with esophageal reflux, the radiologist may identify reflux of the barium from the stomach back into the esophagus. Muscular abnormalities, such as achalasia, as well as diffuse esophageal spasm, can be detected easily by a barium swallow. If perforations or rupture of the esophagus is suspected, it is best not to use barium. A water-soluble x-ray contrast should be used. Anatomic abnormalities, such as sliding or paraesophageal hiatal hernias, also can be detected.

Potential complication

A potential complication of barium swallow is barium-induced fecal impaction.

Procedure

The fasting patient swallows a flavored barium solution similar to that used in an upper gastrointestinal (UGI) study. The patient is secured to a tilt table and placed in various positions as x-ray films are taken. The radiologist follows the barium column through the entire esophagus. Both frontal and lateral views are taken. This procedure takes about 15 minutes to perform and is not uncomfortable. This procedure is usually performed in the radiology department by a radiologist. Refer to the swallowing examination (videofluoroscopy) for discussion on testing for swallowing function.

Contraindications

Contraindications for barium swallow are as follows:

- Patients with evidence of bowel obstruction or severe constipation
  Barium may create a stonelike impaction.
- Patients with a perforated viscus
  Barium can cause chronic abscess formation within the free peritoneum. Usually, when perforation is suspected, diatrizoate meglumine (Gastrografin) is used.
- Patients whose vital signs are unstable
- Patients who are unable to cooperate for the test

Nursing implications with rationale

Before

- Explain the procedure to the patient. Instruct the patient not to take anything by mouth for at least 8 hours before testing.
- Assess the patient's ability to swallow. If the patient tends to aspirate, inform the radiologist.

After

- Inform the patient of the need to evacuate all the barium. Cathartics are recommended. Initially, stools will be white but should return to normal color with complete evacuation.

Case Study

Esophageal Reflux

Ms. K. was a 45-year-old woman who complained of heartburn and frequent regurgitation of "sour" material into her mouth. Often, while sleeping, she would be awakened by a severe cough. The results of her physical examination were negative.

Studies	Results
Routine laboratory studies	Negative
Barium swallow (BS), p. 62	Hiatal hernia (see Figure 3-3)
Esophageal function studies	
(EFS), p. 69	
Lower esophageal sphincter (LES)	4 mm Hg
pressure	(normal: 10-20 mm Hg)

Acid reflux	Positive in all positions (normal: negative)
Acid clearing	Cleared to pH 5 after 20 swallows (normal: <10 swallows)
Swallowing waves	Normal amplitude and normal progression
Bernstein test	Positive for pain (normal: negative)
Esophagogastroduodenoscopy (EGD), p. 71	Reddened, hyperemic, esophageal mucosa
Gastric scan, p. 74	Reflux of gastric contents to the lungs
Swallowing function, p. 91	No aspiration during swallowing

Diagnostic Analysis

The barium swallow indicated a hiatal hernia. Although many patients with a hiatal hernia have no reflux, this patient's symptoms of reflux necessitated esophageal function studies. She was found to have a hypotensive LES pressure, along with severe acid reflux into her esophagus. The abnormal acid clearing and the positive Bernstein test result indicated esophagitis caused by severe reflux. The esophagitis was directly visualized during esophagoscopy. Her coughing and shortness of breath at night were due to aspiration of gastric contents at night, while sleeping. This was demonstrated by the gastric nuclear scan. When awake, she did not aspirate, as evident during the swallowing function study.

Ms. K. was given antacid (Maalox), omeprazole (Prilosec), and cisapride (Propulsid). She was told to avoid the use of tobacco and caffeine. Her diet was limited to small, frequent, bland feedings. She was instructed to sleep with the head of her bed elevated at night. Because Ms. K. had only minimal relief of her symptoms after 6 weeks of medical management, she underwent a laproscopic surgical antireflux procedure. She had no further symptoms.

Critical Thinking Questions

1. Why would Ms. K. be instructed to avoid tobacco and caffeine?
2. Why did the physician recommend 6 weeks of medical management?

Carcinoembryonic Antigen (CEA)

Test type Blood

Normal values

<5 ng/ml or 0.0-2.5 mg/L (SI units)

Rationale

Carcinoembryonic antigen (CEA) is a protein that normally occurs in fetal gut tissue. By birth, detectable serum levels disappear. CEA was originally thought to be a specific indicator of the presence of colorectal cancer. Subsequently, however, this tumor marker has been found in patients who have various carcinomas (e.g., breast, pancreatic, gastric, hepatobiliary), sarcomas, and even many benign diseases (e.g., ulcerative colitis, diverticulitis, cirrhosis). Chronic smokers also have elevated CEA levels.

Because the CEA level can be elevated in both benign and malignant diseases, it is not a specific test for colorectal cancer. Furthermore, not all colorectal cancers make CEA. Therefore, CEA is not a reliable screening test for the detection of colo-rectal cancer in the general population. Its use is limited to determining the prognosis and monitoring the response of tumor to antineoplastic therapy in a patient with cancer. This is especially helpful in patients with breast and GI cancers. The initial pretreatment CEA level is an indicator of tumor burden and therefore prognosis. Patients with smaller and early-staged tumors are likely to have low CEA levels, if not normal CEA levels. Patients with more advanced or metastatic tumors are likely to have high CEA levels. A drastic reduction of the preoperative CEA to normal levels indicates complete eradication of tumor. Therefore, this test is used to determine the efficacy of treatment.

This test also is used in the surveillance of patients with cancer. A steadily rising CEA level is occasionally the first sign of tumor recurrence. This makes CEA testing valuable in the follow-up of patients who already have had potentially curative therapy. It is important to reiterate that about 20% of patients with advanced breast or gastrointestinal tumors may not have elevated CEA levels.

CEA also can be detected in body fluid other than blood. Its presence in those body fluids indicates metastasis. This test is commonly performed on peritoneal fluid or chest effusions. Elevated CEA levels in these fluids indicate metastasis to the peritoneum or pleura, respectively. Likewise, elevated CEA levels in cerebrospinal fluid would indicate central nervous system metastasis.

Procedure

No fasting is required. A total of 6 to 10 ml of peripheral blood is collected. The collecting tube varies according to the commercial laboratory. Diagnostic kits are now available for CEA tests to be done at most hospitals.

Nursing implications with rationale

Before

☞ Explain the procedure to the patient and tell the patient that no fasting is required.

After

■ Apply pressure or a pressure dressing to the venipuncture site to prevent further bleeding. Observe the site for further bleeding.

Clostridial Toxin Assay (*Clostridium difficile*, Antibiotic-associated Colitis Assay, Pseudomembranous Colitis Toxic Assay, *C. diff.*)

Test type Stool

Normal values

Negative (no *Clostridium* toxin identified)

Rationale

Clostridium difficile bacterial infection of the intestine may occur in patients who are immuno-compromised or taking broad-spectrum antibiotics (e.g., clindamycin, ampicillin, and cephalosporins). The infection results from depression of the normal flora of the bowel through the administration of antibiotics. This increases the number of *C. difficile* bacteria within the intestines. The overgrowth of *C. difficile* causes diarrhea, which is usually watery and voluminous. Abdominal cramps, fever, and leukocytosis are noted in most patients. Symptoms usually begin 4 to 10 days after the initiation of antibiotic therapy.

The clostridial bacterium releases a toxin that causes necrosis of the colonic epithelium. The detection of this toxin in the stool is therefore diagnostic of clostridial enterocolitis (pseudomembranous colitis). This toxin is identified by stool immunoassay techniques. *C. difficile* also can be diagnosed by obtaining colonic-rectal tissue for this toxin. Finally, stool cultures (p. 89) for *C. difficile* can be performed. The latter take longer for results to be available.

Management of this antibiotic-associated colitis includes immediate cessation of the broad-spectrum antibiotics (if possible), IV replacement of fluid and electrolytes, and institution of metronidazole (Flagyl) or vancomycin (Vancocin) antibiotic therapy.

Procedure

Stool is collected in a clean, wide-mouth plastic or waxed container with a tight-fitting lid. A rectal swab cannot be used because an adequate amount of stool cannot be obtained by this method. A stool specimen also can be obtained during proctoscopy. The specimen should be transported immediately to the laboratory to prevent deterioration of the toxin. If the specimen cannot be processed immediately, it should then be refrigerated.

Nursing implications with rationale
Before
☞ Explain the method of stool collection to the patient. Be matter-of-fact to avoid any embarrassment to the patient.
☞ Instruct the patient not to mix urine or toilet paper with the specimen. Both can contaminate the specimen and alter test results.
During
■ Handle the specimen carefully, as though it were infectious. If the nurse is assisting with the specimen collection, he or she should wear gloves.
After
■ Indicate on the laboratory requisition slip if the patient is taking any medications, such as antibiotics, which can alter the intestinal flora.
■ Send the stool specimen to the laboratory as soon as possible after collection.

Colonoscopy

Test type Endoscopy

Normal values
Normal rectum, colon, and distal small bowel

Rationale
With fiberoptic colonoscopy, the entire colon from anus to cecum (and often a portion of terminal ileum) can be examined in most patients. Benign and malignant neoplasms, polyps, mucosal inflammation, ulceration, and sites of active hemorrhage can be visualized. Diseases, such as cancer, polyps, ulcers, and arteriovenous (AV) malformations, also can be visualized. Samples for biopsies of cancers, polyps, and inflammatory bowel diseases can be obtained through the colonoscope with cable-activated instruments.

Sites of active bleeding can be coagulated with the use of laser, electrocoagulation, and injection of sclerosing agents.

This test is recommended for patients who have Hemoccult-positive stools, lower GI bleeding, or a change in bowel habits. This test is also recommended for patients who are at high risk for colon cancer. This includes patients with a strong personal or family history of colon cancer, polyps, or ulcerative colitis.

Potential complications
Potential complications associated with colonoscopy are as follows:

■ Bowel perforation from forceful advancement of the scope
■ Persistent bleeding from a biopsy or polypectomy site
■ Oversedation resulting in respiratory depression

Interfering factors
Factors that interfere with colonoscopy include the following:

■ Poor bowel preparation
The stool immediately obstructs the lens and precludes adequate visualization of the colon.
■ Active bleeding
Blood obstructs the lens system and precludes adequate visualization of the colon.

Procedure
The patient's large intestine must be completely free of fecal material. Bowel preparations vary, yet a commonly used preparation is as follows:
Day before examination
Clear liquid diet is followed from morning until midnight.
Patient should drink 8 oz. of colonic lavage every 15 to 20 minutes over a 2- to 4-hour period beginning about 4 PM until 1 gallon of colonic lavage is consumed.
Day of examination
The patient is kept NPO after midnight.
If the patient was unable to drink all the colonic lavage, two saline enemas are given.

Elderly patients should be cautious because of the dehydration and exhaustion that may result from the test preparation. It may be helpful for someone to stay with the elderly patient if this is done on an outpatient basis. Patients need to drink lots of fluid to preclude dehydration from the test preparation. Patients with valvular heart disease should receive prophylactic antibiotics before the test.

The patient is usually premedicated with atropine 0.4 mg and meperidine (Demerol) 50 mg IM. The study is performed in a room specially equipped for this procedure. An IV infusion is begun, and the patient is given midazolam (Versed) 1 mg and meperidine 25 to 50 mg IV. With the patient in the left lateral decubitus (Sims') position, the scope is inserted into the anus (or colostomy) and slowly advanced to the cecum. For complete colonic examination all the way to the cecum, a significant amount of manipulation of the scope is required.

As in all endoscopy, air is insufflated to distend the bowel for better visualization. Endoscopic biopsy specimen or polyp removal is performed, and then the scope is removed.

This test is performed in approximately 30 to 60 minutes by a physician trained in endoscopy. It usually is performed in an endoscopy suite or the operating room. The patient is heavily sedated so very little discomfort is experienced.

Contraindications

Contraindications for colonoscopy are as follows:

- Patients who are uncooperative
  As in all studies that require technical finesse, patient cooperation is essential to successful completion of the test.
- Patients whose medical conditions are unstable
  This test requires sedation, which may induce hypotension in medically unstable patients.
- Patients who are bleeding profusely from the rectum
  The viewing lens will become covered with blood clots, preventing visualization of the lower intestinal tract.

- Patients with a suspected perforation of the colon
  The air insufflated during colonoscopy may worsen the fecal peritoneal soilage.
- Patients with toxic megacolon
  These patients may worsen with the test preparation.
- Patients with a recent colon anastomosis (within the past 14 to 21 days)
  The anastomosis may break down with significant insufflation of carbon dioxide (CO_2).

Nursing implications with rationale

Before

- Explain the procedure to the patient. Tell the patient that the examination is uncomfortable but that sedation will be given by injection and IV infusion. Provide emotional support.
- Obtain the patient's written consent for colonoscopy.
- Assist the patient with the preparation. Record the results from the cathartics and enemas.
- Tell the patient that he or she will be draped to avoid embarrassment.

After

- Inform the patient that because air is insufflated into the bowel during the procedure, he or she may have "gas pains."
- Monitor the patient's vital signs. Watch for a decrease in blood pressure and an increase in pulse rate as an indication of hemorrhage. Fever and chills may indicate a bowel perforation.
- Check for evidence of bowel perforation (abdominal pain, tenderness, and bleeding). Examine stool for gross blood.
- Unless further studies are needed or bowel perforation is suspected, the patient may resume a normal diet. Force fluids to avoid cathartic-induced dehydration.
- If the patient is not too tired, a warm bath may be soothing.
- Allow the patient time to rest after the test. The cleansing regimen and fasting may tire and weaken the patient.
- Ensure safety precautions until the effect of the medications has worn off.

Esophageal Function Studies
(Esophageal Manometry, Esophageal Motility Studies)

Test type Manometric

Normal values
Lower esophageal sphincter pressure:
  10-20 mm Hg
Swallowing pattern: normal peristaltic waves
Acid reflux: negative
Acid clearing: <10 swallows
Bernstein test: negative

Rationale
This test is used to identify and document the severity of diseases affecting the swallowing function of the esophagus. It is used also to document and quantify gastroesophageal reflux. Various motor disturbances can be identified. It is commonly used on patients with heartburn, chest pain, or difficulty in swallowing (dysphagia). Esophageal function studies include the following:

1. Determination of the lower esophageal sphincter (LES) pressure (manometry)
2. Graphic recording of esophageal swallowing waves, or swallowing pattern (manometry)
3. Detection of reflux of gastric acid back into the esophagus (acid reflux)
4. Detection of the ability of the esophagus to clear acid (acid clearing)
5. An attempt to reproduce symptoms of heartburn (Bernstein test)

Manometry studies
Two manometry studies are used in assessing esophageal function: (1) measurement of LES pressure and (2) graphic recording of swallowing waves (motility). The LES acts as a valve to prevent reflux of gastric acid into the esophagus. Free reflux of gastric acid occurs when the sphincter pressures are low. An example of such a disorder in adults is *gastroesophageal reflux;* in children, it is called *chalasia* (incompetent or relaxed LES).

With increased sphincter pressure, as found in patients with achalasia (failure of the LES to relax normally with swallowing), and with diffuse esophageal spasms, food cannot pass from the esophagus into the stomach. Increased LES pressures are noted on manometry. In achalasia, few, if any, swallowing waves are detected. In contrast, diffuse esophageal spasm is characterized by strong, frequent, asynchronous, and nonpropulsive waves.

Acid reflux with pH probe
Acid reflux is the primary component of gastroesophageal reflux. Patients with an incompetent LES will regurgitate gastric acid into the esophagus. This then will cause a drop in pH testing done by the pH probe. With the newer and smaller catheters, 24-hour pH monitoring can be performed. Episodes of acid reflux are evident. If they coincide with the patient's symptoms of chest pain, esophagitis can be incriminated.

Acid clearing
Patients with normal esophageal function can completely clear hydrochloric acid from the esophagus in fewer than 10 swallows. Patients with decreased esophageal motility (frequently caused by severe esophagitis) require more swallows to clear the acid.

Bernstein test (acid perfusion)
The Bernstein test is simply an attempt to reproduce the symptoms of gastroesophageal reflux. If the patient suffers pain with the instillation of hydrochloric acid into the esophagus, the test is positive and proves the patient's symptoms are caused by reflux esophagitis. If the patient has no discomfort, a cause other than esophageal reflux must be sought to explain the patient's discomfort.

Potential complication
A potential complication of esophageal function studies is aspiration of gastric contents, which is a result of gagging during the procedure.

Interfering factors

Factors that interfere with determining esophageal function studies include the following:

- Eating shortly before the test, which may affect results
- Drugs, such as sedatives, which can alter test results

Procedure

Esophageal studies usually are performed in a room specially equipped with appropriate instruments. The fasting, unsedated patient is asked to swallow three very thin tubes, the ends of which are 5 cm apart (Figure 3-4). The other ends of the tubes are attached to transducers for pressure recordings. The LES pressure is recorded as each of the three tubes reaches the esophagus.

With all tubes in the esophagus, the patient is asked to swallow. With normal motility the proximal tube registers a rapid rise and fall in pressure. This pattern is successively and graphically re-corded through the transducer of the middle and then of the distal tube (if three tubes are used). The tubes are then replaced into the stomach, and a fourth tube (pH indicator) is passed into the esophagus. The stomach is filled with approximately 100 ml of 0.1 N hydrochloric acid. If a drop in esophageal pH occurs, this indicates acid reflux from the stomach into the esophagus.

Next, the tubes are returned to the esophagus. Hydrochloric acid is instilled through them. Acid clearing is determined by counting the number of swallows required to clear the acid completely.

Finally 0.1 N hydrochloric acid and saline solution are alternately instilled into the esophagus for the Bernstein test. The patient is not told which solution is being infused. If the patient volunteers symptoms of discomfort while the acid is running, the test is positive. If no discomfort is recognized, the test is negative.

Surprisingly, the entire study is not uncomfortable despite some initial gagging. No significant complications have been reported. The duration of the study is approximately 30 minutes.

Contraindication

Esophageal function studies are contraindicated in patients who cannot cooperate by swallowing the tubes required for testing.

Nursing implications with rationale

Before

- ☞ Explain the procedure to the patient and describe the initial gagging associated with the study. Most patients are apprehensive about this test. Provide emotional support.
- ☞ Instruct the patient to remain NPO after midnight to prevent aspiration of gastric contents into the lungs during the study.
- Avoid sedating the patient, because sedation causes a false decrease in LES pressure. Also, the patient's participation is essential for swallowing the tubes, swallowing during acid clearance, and describing any discomfort during the instillation of hydrochloric acid.

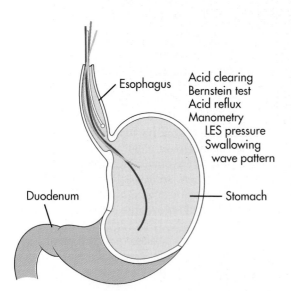

Figure 3-4 Esophageal function studies demonstrating placement of manometry tubes and a pH probe within the esophagus.

After

☞ Inform the patient that it is not unusual to have a mild sore throat after tube placement.

Esophagogastroduodenoscopy
(EGD, Upper Gastrointestinal [UGI] Endoscopy, Gastroscopy)

Test type Endoscopy

Normal values
Normal esophagus, stomach, and duodenum

Rationale
Endoscopy enables direct visualization of the UGI tract by means of a long, flexible, fiberoptic-lighted scope. The lumen of the esophagus, stomach, and duodenum are examined for tumors, varices, mucosal inflammations, hiatal hernias, polyps, ulcers, and obstructions. It is used to evaluate patients with the following: dysphagia, weight loss, early satiety, upper abdominal pain, "ulcer symptoms" or dyspepsia, alcoholism and suspected varices, and suspicious barium swallow or UGI x-rays.

The endoscope has one to three channels. The first channel is used for viewing, the second for insufflation of air and aspiration of fluid, and the third for passing cable-activated instruments to perform a biopsy of suspected pathologic tissue. Probes also can be passed through the third channel to allow for coagulation or injection of sclerosing agents to areas of active GI bleeding. A laser beam can pass through the endoscope to perform endoscopic surgery (e.g., obliteration of tumors or polyps, control of bleeding), and the fiberoptics of endoscopy are so refined that video images and photographs can be taken.

With endoscopy, one can not only evaluate the esophagus, stomach, and duodenum, but, with the use of an extra-long fiberoptic endoscope, can also visualize and perform a biopsy of tissue in the upper small intestinal tract. This procedure is referred to as *enteroscopy*. Abnormalities of the small intestine, such as AV malformations, tumors, enteropathies (e.g., celiac disease), and ulcerations, can be diagnosed with enteroscopy.

Besides being much more sensitive and specific than an UGI series (see p. 92) in diagnosing diseases of the esophagus, stomach, and duodenum, EGD also can be used therapeutically. An experienced endoscopist often can control active GI bleeding by electrocoagulation, laser coagulation, or the injection of sclerosing agents such as alcohol. Also, with the endoscope, benign and malignant strictures can be dilated to reestablish patency of the UGI tract. Biliary stents and a percutaneous gastrostomy can be placed with the use of EGD. The role of endoscopic surgery is expanding in light of its dramatic success and minimal morbidity.

Potential complications
Potential complications of EGD are as follows:

- Perforation of the esophagus, stomach, and duodenum by the scope
- Bleeding at a site from which a specimen was obtained for biopsy
- Pulmonary aspiration of gastric contents as a result of obtundation caused by administration of sedatives
- Hypotension induced by the sedative medication
  Sometimes patients with UGI bleeding or vomiting already have some significant element of hypovolemia or dehydration.

Interfering factors
Factors that interfere with EGD include the following:

- Food in the stomach
  This interferes with adequate visualization of all surfaces of the stomach wall.
- Excessive GI bleeding
  The blood obliterates the view through the lens.

Procedure

This examination is usually performed in an endoscopy room, with the patient in the Sims' position. The fasting patient is usually sedated with midazolam before the examination. Atropine is given to decrease secretions. The patient's posterior pharynx is anesthetized with lidocaine to inactivate the gag reflex and lessen the discomfort caused by passage of the scope. The scope then is passed slowly into the mouth, esophagus, stomach, and duodenum. Air is insufflated to maintain patency of the lumen. A gastroenterologist usually performs this procedure in 30 minutes. This procedure can be performed at the bedside under urgent conditions (e.g., UGI bleeding).

Contraindications

Contraindications for EGD are as follows:

- Patients who cannot cooperate fully
  As in all studies that require technical finesse, patient cooperation is essential for successful, safe, and accurate test completion.
- Patients with severe UGI bleeding
  The viewing lens will become covered with blood clots, preventing adequate visualization. If the stomach can be lavaged and aspirated to clear the blood clots, however, EGD can be performed.
- Patients with esophageal diverticula
  The scope can easily fall into the diverticulum and perforate the wall of the esophagus.
- Patients with suspected perforation
  The perforation can be worsened by the insufflation of pressurized air into the GI tract.
- Patients who have had recent UGI surgery
  The anastomosis may not be able to withstand the pressure of the required air insufflation. This may lead to anastomotic disruption.

Nursing implications with rationale

Before
- ☞ Explain the procedure to the patient and obtain written permission for this test. Tell the patient what drugs will be prescribed and what their effects will be.
- Keep the patient NPO after midnight to provide optimum visualization of the GI tract and prevent regurgitation when the gastroscope is passed.
- ☞ Tell the patient that the test is not painful but may cause discomfort and vomiting when the gag reflex is initiated. Encourage verbalization of the patient's fears. Provide emotional support.
- Remove the patient's dentures and eyeglasses before the test. Because the tube is passed through the mouth, oral hygiene procedures should be performed before and after the test.
- ☞ Explain to the patient that he or she will be unable to speak when the scope is positioned in the GI tract. Breathing will not be affected.

During
- Place tissue specimens into an appropriate specimen container and label the container correctly.
- Have an Ambu bag ready in case of respiratory arrest from midazolam overdose. Physostigmine (Antilirium) should be available to counteract serious respiratory depression.

After
- After the patient's throat has been anesthetized with lidocaine, do not allow him or her to eat or drink anything until the gag reflex returns (usually in about 2 to 4 hours).
- ☞ Inform the patient that after the anesthesia wears off, he or she may be hoarse and complain of a sore throat for several days. Drinking cool fluids and gargling will help relieve some of this soreness.
- Observe the patient for bleeding, fever, abdominal pain, dysphagia, and dyspnea. Monitor the vital signs as ordered.
- Observe safety precautions until the effects of the sedatives have worn off.
- ☞ Inform the patient that because of air insufflation it is normal to have some bloating, belching, and flatulence after the procedure.

Case Study

Peptic Ulcer Disease

A 35-year-old male executive had a 6-month history of epigastric discomfort that occurred at times of high stress and on an empty stomach. This pain frequently woke him at night and was relieved by antacids or food. The physical examination results were negative.

Studies	Results
Routine laboratory studies	Negative
UGI series, p 92	Large ulcer on lesser curvature of distal stomach
EGD, p 71	Large ulcer as described above
	Biopsies were negative for malignancy
Gastrin, p 73	90 pg/ml (normal: <100-200 pg/ml)
Helicobacter pylori antibodies, p 77	IgG antibodies present

Diagnostic Analysis

The results of the UGI and EGD clearly demonstrated that this man's symptoms were caused by an ulcer. No malignant cells were seen on the biopsy specimens taken through the gastroscope. Because the possibility of malignancy was excluded, a conservative medical regimen that included antacids (such as Maalox), a gastric acid pump inhibitor (omeprazole), and rest was prescribed. An aggressive anti-*H. pylori* antibiotic regimen was also instituted. Repeat UGI series that were performed 6 weeks later demonstrated near-total healing of the ulcer.

Critical Thinking Questions

1. Why would a patient with peptic ulcer disease be treated with an antibiotic?
2. What methods are used to detect *H. pylori* organisms in your hospital?

Gastrin

Test type Blood

Normal values

Adult: <100-200 pg/ml or <200 ng/L (SI units)
Levels are higher in elderly patients
Child: <10-125 pg/ml

Rationale

Gastrin is a hormone produced by the G cells located in the distal part of the stomach (antrum). Gastrin is a potent stimulator of gastric acid. In normal gastric physiology, an alkaline environment (created by food or antacids) stimulates the release of gastrin. Gastrin then stimulates the parietal cells of the stomach to secrete gastric acid. The pH environment in the stomach thereby is reduced. By negative feedback, this low-pH environment suppresses further gastrin secretion.

Zollinger-Ellison (ZE) syndrome (gastrin-producing pancreatic tumor) and *G-cell hyperplasia* (overfunctioning of G cells in the distal stomach) are associated with high serum gastrin levels. Patients with these tumors have aggressive peptic ulcer disease. Unlike the patient with routine peptic ulcers, the patient with ZE syndrome or G-cell hyperplasia has a high incidence of complicated and recurrent peptic ulcers. It is important to identify this latter group of patients to institute more appropriate, aggressive medical and surgical therapy. The serum gastrin level will be normal in the patient with routine peptic ulcer and greatly elevated in patients with ZE syndrome or G-cell hyperplasia.

It is important to note, however, that patients who are taking antacid peptic ulcer medicines, have had peptic ulcer surgery, or have atrophic gastritis will have a high serum gastrin level. Levels usually are not as high, however, as in patients with ZE syndrome or G-cell hyperplasia.

Not all patients with ZE syndrome exhibit increased levels of serum gastrin. Some patients may have "top" normal gastrin levels, making them difficult to differentiate from patients with routine peptic ulcer disease. ZE syndrome or G-cell hyperplasia can be diagnosed in these "top" normal patients by *gastrin stimulation tests* using calcium or secretin. Patients with these diseases will have greatly increased serum gastrin levels associated with the infusion of these drugs.

Interfering factors

Factors that interfere with gastrin testing include the following:

- Previous peptic ulcer surgery
  This creates a persistent alkaline environment, which is the strongest stimulant to gastrin.
- Calcium or insulin, because they *increase* gastrin levels by acting as a gastrin stimulant
- Drugs, such as catecholamines and caffeine, because they may *increase* gastrin levels

Procedure

Instruct the patient to fast for 12 hours. Water is permitted. A peripheral venipuncture is performed, and approximately 5 to 7 ml of venous blood is collected in a red-top tube.

For the *calcium infusion test,* calcium gluconate is administered intravenously for 3 hours. A preinfusion serum gastrin level is then compared with specimens taken every 30 minutes for 4 hours. For the *secretin test,* secretin is administered intravenously. Preinjection and postinjection serum gastrin levels are taken at 15-minute intervals for 1 hour after injection.

Nursing implications with rationale

Before
- Explain the procedure to the patient. Instruct the patient to fast for 12 hours. Only water is permitted.

After
- Apply pressure or a pressure dressing to the venipuncture site to prevent further bleeding. Observe the site for bleeding.

Gastroesophageal Reflux Scan (GE Reflux Scan, Aspiration Scan)

Test type Nuclear scan

Normal values

No evidence of gastroesophageal reflux

Rationale

Gastroesophageal (GE) reflux scans are used to evaluate patients with symptoms of heartburn, regurgitation, vomiting, and dysphagia. Also, these scans are used to evaluate the medical or surgical treatment of patients with GE reflux. Finally, aspiration scans may be used to detect aspiration of gastric contents into the lungs and evaluate swallowing function.

Procedure

For this procedure the patient eats a full meal just before the study. The patient assumes a supine position while images are taken over the chest. The patient then swallows a mouthful of a tracer cocktail, such as orange juice, dilute hydrochloric acid, or technetium 99m (Tc 99m)–labeled protein such as sulphur colloid, and images are taken. Then, after drinking the remainder of the cocktail and some water, the patient assumes an upright position, and images of the chest are taken.

A large binder (similar to a blood pressure cuff) is then placed around the abdomen to increase intraabdominal pressure, which stresses the sphincter at the GE junction. The patient is placed in the supine position while under the gamma ray detector camera. Examination for the presence of nuclear material in the esophagus is performed by taking images with no pressure applied to the abdomen and then with gradual increments in pressure up to 100 mm Hg.

Aspiration scans can also be performed by adding a radionuclide to the evening meal and then keeping the patient in a supine position until the next morning. Images then are made over the lungs to detect esophageal-tracheal aspiration of the tracer. Infants are evaluated for chalasia by adding the tracer into the formula and then taking films over the next hour, with delayed films as needed.

The entire procedure is completed in approximately 30 minutes in the nuclear medicine department. The only discomfort associated with the study is that of lying on a hard table and the application of some abdominal pressure from the binder.

Contraindications

Contraindications for the GE reflux scan are as follows:

- Patients who cannot tolerate the abdominal compression required for this test
- Patients who are pregnant or lactating, because the radionuclide could injure the fetus/newborn

Nursing implications with rationale

Before

☞ Explain the procedure to the patient. Assure the patient that no pain is associated with this study.
☞ Instruct the patient to eat a full meal just before the study.

After

☞ Ensure that the patient and/or family understand that only a small dose of nuclear material is used. No radiation precautions need to be taken against the patient or his or her bodily secretions.

Gastrointestinal Bleeding Scan
(Abdominal Scintigraphy, GI Scintigraphy)

Test types Nuclear scan

Normal values

No collection of radionuclide in GI tract

Rationale

The GI bleeding scan is used to localize the site of bleeding in patients who are having active GI hemorrhage. The scan also can be used in patients who have suspected intraabdominal (nongastrointestinal) hemorrhage from an unknown source. Localization of the source of GI or other bleeding can be difficult. When surgery is required under these circumstances, it is difficult, cumbersome, and prolonged. The surgeon may have extreme difficulty finding the source of bleeding. The bleeding scan helps localize the bleeding for the surgeon.

The GI bleeding scan has several advantages over arteriography. The GI bleeding scan can detect bleeding if the rate is in excess of 0.05ml/minute. Also, with the use of Tc 99m–labeled red blood cells (RBCs), delayed films (as long as 24 hours) can be obtained indicating the site of an intermittent or extremely slow intestinal bleed.

A GI scintigram is sensitive in locating the site of GI bleeding; however, it is not specific in pinpointing the site or the cause of bleeding. Usually, when positive, the exact source of bleeding cannot be localized any more accurately than by indicating the affected quadrant of the abdomen (e.g., right upper, left lower). This test usually is performed by injecting sulfur colloid labeled with Tc 99m or Tc 99m–labeled RBCs into the patient. If the patient is bleeding at a rate in excess of 0.05 ml/minute, pooling of the radionuclide will ultimately be detected in the abnormal segment of the intestine. Few false-positive results occur. Again, it is important to recognize that the test will only localize the bleeding; it will not indicate the exact pathologic condition causing the bleeding. With this test result, if surgery is required, the surgeon is directed to the abnormal area and hopefully can detect and resect the pathologic bleeding source.

It is important to realize that this test can take at least 1 to 4 hours to obtain useful information. Unstable patients should not leave the intensive care environment for that long a period. Furthermore, the unstable patient may need to go to surgery in minutes and may not have the luxury of taking several hours to determine the region of active bleeding.

Interfering factor
A factor that interferes with the GI bleeding scan is barium within the GI tract, which may mask a small source of bleeding.

Procedure
Ten mCi of freshly prepared Tc 99m–labeled sulfur colloid is administered intravenously to the patient. If RBCs are used, 3 ml of the patient's own whole blood is combined with technetium and reinjected into the patient. Immediately after the administration of the radionuclide, the patient is placed under a scintillation camera. Multiple images of the abdomen are obtained at short intervals. The scintigrams are recorded on film. Detection of the radionuclide in the abdomen indicates the site of bleeding.

Areas of the bowel hidden by the liver or spleen may not be adequately evaluated by this procedure. Also, the rectum cannot be easily evaluated because other pelvic structures (e.g., the bladder) obstruct the view. If the initial study is negative and subsequent films give clinical evidence of active bleeding, a repeat scan may be performed with the administration of another dose of Tc 99m.

The test takes about 10 to 20 minutes to perform and is usually done in the nuclear medicine department. No pretest preparation is required. The only discomfort associated with this study is that of injecting the radioisotope.

Contraindications
Contraindications for the GI bleeding scan are as follows:

- Patients who are pregnant or lactating, because the fetus or infant may experience significant radiation exposure
- Medically unstable patients, whose stay in the nuclear medicine department may be risky

Nursing implications with rationale
Before
- Explain the study to the patient. Encourage the patient to verbalize his or her fear of internal hemorrhage.
- Make sure the patient understands that only a small dose of nuclear material is administered.
- Instruct the patient to notify the technician if he or she has a bowel movement during the test. Blood in the GI tract can act as a cathartic. The technician may want to examine the stool for the presence of nuclear material. If nuclear material is present, this highly suggests that the source of the bleeding is in the distal colon or rectum.
- Assess the patient's vital signs to make sure the patient is stable for transfer to and from the nuclear medicine department.

During
- If the patient is having major GI bleeding, closely monitor his or her vital signs during the test.

After
- Reevaluate the patient's vital signs on return to the nursing unit.
- Inform the patient that only tracer doses of radioisotopes have been used and that no precautions against radiation exposure are necessary.

Helicobacter pylori Tests

(*Campylobacter pylori*, Anti-*Helicobacter pylori* Immunoglobulin G [IgG] Antibody, *Campylobacter*-like Organism [CLO] Test)

Test type Blood, microscopic examination, breath test

Normal values

Not present

Rationale

Helicobacter pylori tests are used to detect *H. pylori* infections. They are indicated in patients who have recurrent or chronic gastric or duodenal ulceration or inflammation. When *H. pylori* is successfully treated, the ulcer or inflammation will heal.

H. pylori, a bacteria that can be found in the mucus overlying the gastric mucosa and on the mucosal cells that line the stomach, has been recognized as a risk factor for gastric diseases such as duodenal ulcers or chronic gastritis. This gram-negative bacillus may also be a possible cause of gastric carcinoma. Gastric colonization by this organism has been reported in about 90% to 95% of patients with a duodenal ulcer, in 60% to 70% of patients with a gastric ulcer, and in about 20% to 25% of patients with gastric cancer.

Approximately 10% of healthy persons under age 30 have gastric colonization with *H. pylori*. Gastric colonization increases with age, with people older than 60 having rates similar to their ages. Most patients with gastric colonization by *H. pylori* remain asymptomatic and never develop ulceration.

Several methods are used to detect the presence of this organism. The organism can be cultured from a specimen of mucus obtained through a gastroscope. The organism also can be detected on a gastric mucosal biopsy. This method is slightly more accurate than culture techniques.

Newer methods now available to detect this organism are more easily performed and are more accurate. Immunoassays to antibodies to *H. pylori* have been developed and are very accurate in detecting the presence of the organism. The IgG anti-*H. pylori* antibody is most commonly used. It becomes elevated 2 months after infection and stays elevated for more than a year after treatment. The IgA anti-*H. pylori* antibody, like IgG, becomes elevated 2 months after infection but decreases 3 to 4 weeks after treatment. The IgM anti-*H. pylori* antibody is the first to become elevated (about 3 to 4 weeks) and is not detected after 2 to 3 months following treatment. These antibody titers are fast becoming the gold standard for *H. pylori* detection. A breath test also is available for the detection of *H. pylori*. It is based on *H. pylori*'s great ability to metabolize urea to CO_2.

Procedure

No fasting is required for the blood test. A venous blood sample is obtained according to the protocol of the laboratory performing the test. If a biopsy specimen or culture will be obtained by endoscopy, see the discussion of EGD (p. 71). The specimen must be kept moist by adding approximately 2 to 5 ml of sterile saline placed in a sterile container. It is then cultured on special media.

Nursing implications with rationale

Before

- Explain the method of collection to the patient. Tell the patient that no fasting is required for the blood test. If endoscopy will be used, see the preparation for EGD on p. 71.

After

- Apply pressure or a pressure dressing to the venipuncture site to prevent further bleeding.
- If endoscopy was performed, see the discussion of EGD on p. 71.

Lactose Tolerance Test

Test type Blood, microscopic examination, breath test

Normal values

Blood: Adult/elderly: Rise in plasma glucose levels >20 mg/dl. No abdominal cramps or diarrhea

Breath: Less than 50 ppm hydrogen increase over baseline

Rationale

The lactose tolerance test is performed to detect lactose intolerance. Lactose is a disaccharide typically found in dairy products. During digestion, lactose is broken down into glucose and galactose by the intestinal enzyme lactase. Because lactose-intolerant patients have an absence of lactase, lactose digestion will not occur. Thus the small bowel is flooded with a high lactose load. Bacterial metabolism of the lactose occurs within the intestine. This creates excess hydrogen ions and methane (flatus). It also creates a strong cathartic effect. Symptoms of lactose intolerance include abdominal cramping, flatus, abdominal bloating, and diarrhea.

Although all adults have some degree of lactase reduction, severe lactose intolerance can occur in patients with inflammatory bowel disease, short-gut syndrome, and other malabsorption syndromes. Lactase deficiency can be congenital and become apparent in the newborn. Affected infants present with vomiting, diarrhea, malabsorption, and failure to thrive.

In this test, the patient is given a lactose load. If lactase is not present in sufficient quantities, lactose is not metabolized to glucose and galactose. Plasma levels of glucose do not rise as expected. Therefore, lower-than-expected serum glucose levels suggest intestinal lactase deficiency. Patients who have malabsorption without lactase deficiency will also not have elevated blood glucose levels, not because the lactose was not broken down but because the glucose could not be absorbed. These patients can be excluded by following the lactose tolerance test with a glucose tolerance test. That is, after a positive lactose tolerance test, the patient returns and is given 25 g of a glucose/galactose preparation. A normal increase in glucose indicates that the patient can absorb glucose and that the problem is, indeed, lactase insufficiency.

This test also has a breath component, in which exhaled air is analyzed for hydrogen content. The hydrogen content is directly proportional to the amount of lactose not broken down and absorbed.

Interfering factors

Factors that interfere with the lactose tolerance test include the following:

- Enterogenous steatorrhea (i.e., malabsorption)
  This problem will diminish absorption of glucose from the gut even if the lactose is broken down by normal levels of lactase.
- Patients with diabetes
  These patients may have rising glucose levels that exceed 20 mg/dl despite lactase insufficiency.

Procedure

The patient is instructed to fast and to avoid strenuous exercise for 8 hours before the test. After a fasting blood sugar is obtained, the adult patient receives a specified dose (approximately 100 g) of lactose orally in 200 ml of water. Blood is then withdrawn from a peripheral vein and placed in a gray-top tube at 30, 60, and 120 minutes after the loading dose of lactose. Plasma glucose levels are then determined (see p. 305).

Nursing implications with rationale

Before

- Explain the procedure to the patient. Instruct the patient to drink the entire amount of lactose and not ingest anything else until the blood is drawn.
- Inform the patient that smoking is also prohibited, because it may increase the blood sugar level.

During

- Make sure the blood is drawn at the appropriate times.

After

- To prevent further bleeding, apply pressure or a pressure dressing to the venous puncture site after the blood is obtained. Observe the site for bleeding.

Case Study

Inflammatory Bowel Disease

Andrea is an 11-year-old girl who has been complaining of intermittent right lower quadrant pain and diarrhea for the past year. She is small for her age. Her physical examination indicates some mild right lower quadrant tenderness and fullness.

Studies	Results
Hemoglobin, p. 411	8.6 g/dl (normal: >12 g/dl)
Hematocrit, p. 411	28% (normal: 31%-43%)
Vitamin B_{12} level, p. 441	68 pg/ml (normal: 100-700 pg/ml)
Meckel's scan, p. 79	No evidence of Meckel's diverticulum
D-xylose absorption, p. 79	60 min: 8 mg/dl (normal: >15-20 mg/dl)
	120 min: 6 mg/dl (normal >20 mg/dl)
Lactose tolerance, p. 77	No change in glucose level
	(normal: >20 mg/dl rise in glucose)
Schilling test, p. 85	No excretion of radioactive B_{12}
	(normal: 8%-40%)
Small bowel series, p. 94	Constriction of multiple segments of the
	small intestine

Diagnostic Analysis

Andrea's small bowel series is compatible with Crohn's disease of the small intestine. Intestinal absorption is diminished as indicated by the abnormal D-xylose and lactose tolerance tests. Absorption is so bad that she cannot absorb vitamin B_{12}. As a result, she has vitamin B_{12} deficiency anemia. She was placed on an aggressive immunosuppressive regimen, and her condition improved significantly. Unfortunately, 2 years later she experienced unremitting obstructive symptoms and required surgery. One year after surgery, her GI function was normal and her anemia had resolved. Her growth status caught up to her peers. Her absorption tests were normal, as were her B_{12} levels. Her immunosuppressive drugs were discontinued, and she is doing well.

Critical Thinking Questions

1. Why was this patient placed on immunosuppressive therapy?
2. Why was the Meckel's scan ordered for this patient?

Meckel's Diverticulum Nuclear Scan

Test type Nuclear medicine

Normal values

No increased uptake of radionuclide in the right lower quadrant of the abdomen

Rationale

Meckel's diverticulum is the most common congenital abnormality of the intestinal tract. It is a persistent remnant of the omphalomesenteric tract. The diverticulum usually occurs in the ileum, approximately 2 feet proximal to the ileocecal valve. Approximately 20% to 25% of Meckel's diverticula are lined internally by ectopic gastric mucosa. This gastric mucosa can secrete acid and cause ulceration of the intestinal mucosa nearby. Bleeding, inflammation, and intussusception are other potential complications of this congenital abnormality. The majority of these complications occur by age 2. This test is indicated in young patients who have recurrent lower abdominal pain or in pediatric or young adult patients who have occult GI bleeding.

Both normal gastric mucosa within the stomach and ectopic gastric mucosa in Meckel's diverticulum concentrate Tc 99m pertechnetate. When this radionuclide is injected intravenously, it is concentrated in the ectopic gastric mucosa of Meckel's diverticulum. One can then expect to see a hot spot in the right lower quadrant of the abdomen at about the same time as the normal stomach mucosa is visualized. This test is sensitive and specific for this congenital abnormality.

Other conditions can simulate a hot spot compatible with Merkel's diverticulum containing ectopic gastric mucosa. These usually are associated with inflammatory processes within the abdomen (e.g., appendicitis, Crohn's inflammatory bowel disease, or ectopic pregnancy).

Procedure

The patient is advised to refrain from eating or drinking anything for 6 to 12 hours before the examination. A histamine H_2-receptor antagonist is usually given for 1 to 2 days before the scan. This blocks secretion of the radionuclide from the ectopic gastric mucosa and improves visualization of Meckel's diverticulum.

The patient lies in a supine position, and a large-view nuclear detector camera is placed over the patient's abdomen to identify concentration of nuclear material after intravenous injection. Images are taken at 5-minute intervals for 1 hour. Patients may be asked to lie on their left side to minimize the excretion of the radionuclide from the normal stomach and the flooding of the intestine with radionuclide, which precludes visualization of Meckel's diverticulum. Occasionally, glucagon is provided to prolong intestinal transit time and avoid downstream contamination with the radionuclide. Occasionally, gastrin is given to increase the uptake of the radionuclide by the ectopic gastric mucosa. At the conclusion of the test, the patient is asked to void, and a repeat image is obtained. This is to ensure that Meckel's diverticulum has not been hidden by a distended bladder.

This test is performed in the nuclear medicine department by a physician trained to interpret this study. It may take several hours to complete. There is no pain associated with this test.

Nursing implications with rationale

Before

☞ Explain the procedure to the patient. Tell the patient to fast for 6 to 12 hours before this test.

☞ Inform the patient of the importance of taking a histamine H_2 receptor antagonist for 1 to 2 days before the scan. This blocks secretion of the radionuclide from the ectopic gastric mucosa and improves visualization of Meckel's diverticulum.

After

☞ Because only tracer doses of radioisotopes are used, inform the patient that no precautions need to be taken against radiation exposure.

Obstruction Series (Flat Plate of the Abdomen, Plain Film of the Abdomen, Scout Film)

Test types X-ray

Normal values

No evidence of bowel obstruction
No abnormal calcifications
No free air

Rationale

The obstruction series is a group of x-ray films performed on the abdomen of patients with suspected bowel obstruction, paralytic ileus, perforated viscus, abdominal abscess, kidney stones, appendicitis, or foreign body ingestion. This series of films usually consists of at least two x-ray studies. The first is an *erect abdominal* film that should include visualization of both diaphragms. The film is examined for evidence of free air under either diaphragm, which is pathognomonic for a perforated viscus. This view is also used to detect air-fluid levels within the intestine; the presence of an air-fluid level is compatible with bowel obstruction or paralytic ileus. Occasionally, patients are too ill to stand erect. In this case, an x-ray film can be taken with the patient in the left lateral decubitus position. If free air is present, it will be seen between the liver and the right side of the abdominal wall. As with the erect-position film, air-fluid levels also can be detected.

The second view in the obstruction series is usually a *supine abdominal* x-ray study. This is similar to the kidney, ureter, and bladder (KUB) x-ray study (see p. 249). An abdominal abscess may be seen as a cluster of tiny bubbles within one localized area. A calcification within the course of the ureter could indicate a kidney ureteral stone. A small calcification in the right lower quadrant on the film of a patient complaining of pain in this quadrant may be an appendicolithiasis. A gas-filled, distended bowel is compatible with bowel obstruction or paralytic ileus.

The obstruction series can also be used to monitor the clinical course of patients with GI disease. For example, repeated obstruction series on patients who have a partial small-bowel obstruction or paralytic ileus can indicate worsening or improvement of the clinical situation.

Frequently, a *cross-table lateral* view of the abdomen is included in an obstruction series to detect abdominal aortic calcification, which often occurs in older patients. The calcification represents the anterior wall of the aorta. If an aortic aneurysm exists, this calcification will be seen to protrude from the spine.

Finally, the *supine abdominal* x-ray study can be used as a "scout film" before performing GI or abdominal x-ray studies that use contrast, such as a barium enema (see p. 60) or intravenous pyelogram (see p. 245), just to be sure there is nothing that is obstructing adequate visualization of what needs to be studied.

Interfering factor

A previous GI barium contrast study can interfere with an obstruction series. Although at times barium within the GI tract can preclude the identification of other important calcifications (e.g.,

kidney stones), barium can be helpful in outlining the GI anatomy.

Procedure

Although the procedure varies among hospitals, usually supine abdominal x-ray, erect abdominal x-ray, and, perhaps, low erect chest x-ray studies are taken. Often, a cross-table lateral x-ray study is also taken. An obstruction series is performed in the radiology department by an x-ray technician. A radiologist interprets the film. No discomfort is associated with this study. It takes only minutes to perform.

Contraindication

Pregnancy is a contraindication for an obstructive series because radiation may harm the fetus.

Nursing implications with rationale

Before

☞ Explain the procedure to the patient. Assure the patient that no contrast dye is used. For adequate visualization, ensure that this study is scheduled before any barium studies.

After

■ No special aftercare is needed. Based on test findings, other tests are often scheduled.

Paracentesis (Peritoneal Fluid Analysis, Abdominal Paracentesis, Ascitic Fluid Cytology, Peritoneal Tap)

Test type Fluid analysis

Normal values

Gross appearance: Clear, serous, light yellow, <50 ml
Red blood cells: None
White blood cells (WBCs): 300/ml
Protein: <4.1 g/dl
Glucose: 70-100 mg/dl
Amylase: 138-404 U/L
Ammonia: <50 mg/dl
Alkaline phosphatase
   Adult male: 90-240 U/L
   Female >45 years: 87-250 U/L
   Female <45 years: 76-196 U/L

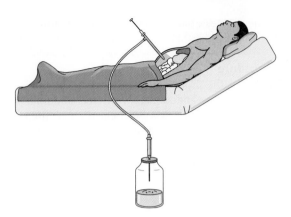

Figure 3-5 Paracentesis.

Lactate dehydrogenase (LDH): Similar to serum lactate dehydrogenase
Cytology: No malignant cells
Bacteria: None
Fungi: None
Carcinoembryonic antigen (CEA): <5.0 ng/ml

Rationale

Paracentesis is an invasive procedure in which a needle is inserted into the peritoneal cavity (Figure 3-5) to remove ascitic fluid. Peritoneal fluid is removed for diagnostic and therapeutic purposes. Diagnostically, paracentesis is performed to obtain and analyze fluid to determine the etiology of the peritoneal effusion. Peritoneal fluid is classified as transudate or exudate. See Table 3-1 for differentiation between transudate and exudate. This is an important differentiation and is helpful in determining the etiology of the effusion. Transudates are most frequently caused by congestive heart failure, cirrhosis, nephrotic syndrome, myxedema, peritoneal dialysis, hypoproteinemia, and acute glomerulonephritis. Exudates are most often found in infectious or neoplastic conditions. However, collagen vascular disease, pulmonary infarction, GI diseases, trauma, and drug hypersensitivity also may cause an exudative effusion.

Therapeutically, this procedure is done to remove large amounts of ascitic fluid from the abdominal cavity. Affected patients usually experience transient relief of symptoms (shortness of breath, distention, and early satiety) as a result of reduction of fluid within the abdominal cavity.

The peritoneal fluid usually is evaluated for gross appearance, RBCs, WBCs, protein, glucose, amylase, ammonia, alkaline phosphatase, LDH, cytology, bacteria, fungi, and other tests, such as CEA levels. Each is discussed separately. Urea and creatinine may be measured if there is a question that the fluid may represent urine from a perforated bladder.

Gross appearance

Transudative peritoneal fluid may be clear, serous, and light yellow, especially in patients with hepatic cirrhosis. Milk-colored peritoneal fluid may result from the escape of chyle from blocked abdominal or thoracic lymphatic ducts. Conditions that may cause lymphatic blockage include lymphoma, carcinoma, and tuberculosis involving the abdominal or thoracic lymph nodes. The triglyceride value in a chylous effusion exceeds 110 mg/dl.

Cloudy or turbid fluid may result from inflammatory or infectious conditions such as peritonitis, pancreatitis, and appendicitis. Bloody fluid may be the result of a traumatic tap (the aspirating needle penetrates a blood vessel), intraabdominal bleeding, tumor, or hemorrhagic pancreatitis. Bile-stained, green fluid may result from a ruptured gallbladder, acute pancreatitis, or perforated intestines.

Cell counts

Normally, no RBCs should be present. The presence of RBCs may indicate neoplasms, tuberculosis, or intraabdominal bleeding. Increased WBC counts may be seen with peritonitis, cirrhosis, and tuberculosis. These counts usually are performed manually, using a simple hemacytometer.

Protein count

Total protein levels greater than 3 g/dl are characteristic of exudates, whereas transudates usually have a protein content of less than 3 g/dl. It is now thought that the albumin gradient between

TABLE 3-1 Differentiation Between Transudate and Exudate

	Transudate	Exudate
Total protein fluid/serum ratio	<0.5	>0.5
Total protein level	<3 g/dl	>3 g/dl
LDH fluid/serum ratio	<0.6	>0.6
Serum − fluid = albumin gradient	>1.1	<1.1
Specific gravity	<1.015	>1.015
Clotting	None	Present
WBCs	<300/μl	>500/μl
Differential	Mononuclear	Neutrophils
Glucose	Equal to serum	<60 mg/dl
Serum − fluid = glucose difference	<30 mg/dl	>30 mg/dl
Appearance	Clear, thin fluid	Cloudy, viscous
Etiology	Cirrhosis, nephrosis, heart failure, low protein	Infection, inflammation, malignancy, collagen vascular diseases

serum and ascitic fluid can differentiate better between the transudate and exudate nature of ascites than can the total protein content. This gradient is obtained by subtracting the ascitic albumin value from the serum albumin value. Values of 1.1 g/dl or more suggest a transudate, which is usually caused by portal hypertension as a result of cirrhosis. Values less than 1.1 g/dl suggest an exudate but will not differentiate the potential cause of the exudate (malignancy, infection, or inflammation).

Glucose

Peritoneal glucose levels usually approximate serum glucose levels. Decreased levels may indicate tuberculous/bacterial peritonitis or peritoneal carcinomatosis.

Amylase

Increased amylase levels may be seen in patients with pancreatic trauma, pancreatic pseudocyst, acute pancreatitis, and intestinal necrosis, perforation, or strangulation. In these diseases, the amylase level is usually less than 1.5 times higher than serum levels.

Ammonia

High ammonia levels occur in ruptured or strangulated intestines and also with a ruptured appendix or ulcer.

Alkaline phosphatase

Levels of alkaline phosphatase are greatly increased in infarcted or strangulated intestines.

Lactate dehydrogenase

A peritoneal fluid/serum LDH ratio of greater than 0.6 is typical of an exudate. Exudates are identified with a higher degree of accuracy if the peritoneal fluid/serum protein ratio is greater than 0.5 and the peritoneal fluid/serum LDH ratio is greater than 0.6.

Cytology

A cytologic study is performed to detect tumors. The tumors most often seen are ovarian, pancreatic, colon, and gastric. The interpretation of cytologic changes requires that the pathologist have considerable experience in cytology. It can be difficult to differentiate malignancy from severely inflamed, mesothelial cells. Malignant cells generally tend to clump together and have a high nuclear/cytoplasm ratio, prominent and multiple nucleoli, and unevenly distributed chromatin.

Bacteria

The fluid usually is cultured, and the antibiotic sensitivities are determined. Gram stains (see p. 173) are often performed.

Gram stain and bacteriologic culture

The presence of bacteria may indicate a ruptured intestine, primary peritonitis, or infections such as appendicitis, pancreatitis, or tuberculosis. Culture and Gram stains identify the organisms involved in the infection and also provide information concerning antibiotic sensitivity. See p. 173 for a more thorough discussion of Gram stain, culture, and sensitivity. These tests are routinely performed to diagnose bacterial peritonitis. If possible, these tests should be done before initiation of antibiotic therapy.

Fungi

Fungi may indicate infections with histoplasmosis, candidiasis, or coccidioidomycosis.

Carcinoembryonic antigen

Peritoneal fluid levels for CEA are associated with abdominal malignancy, usually arising from the GI tract.

Potential complications

Potential complications associated with paracentesis are as follows:

- Hypovolemia, if a large volume of peritoneal fluid was removed
  The fluid may reaccumulate with the fluid from the intravascular volume.
- Peritonitis, caused by the needle penetrating the GI tract
- Seeding of the needle tract with tumor, when malignant ascites exists

Procedure

Obtain an informed consent for this procedure. No fasting or sedation is necessary. The patient should urinate before the test to avoid inadvertent puncture of the bladder with the aspirating needle.

The patient is placed in a high Fowler's position in bed or in a chair, with the back supported and the feet on a stool. Paracentesis is performed under strict sterile technique. A paracentesis tray usually contains all necessary supplies. The needle insertion site is aseptically cleansed and anesthetized locally. A scalpel may be used to make a small stab wound into the peritoneal cavity approximately 1 to 2 inches below the umbilicus. A trocar, cannula, or needle is threaded through the incision and into the peritoneal cavity. Tubing is attached to the cannula. The other end of the tubing is placed in the collection receptacle (usually a container with a pressurized vacuum), and fluid is aspirated. Usually the volume of peritoneal fluid removed is limited to 4 L to avoid hypovolemia if the ascitic fluid rapidly reaccumulates.

Paracentesis is performed by a physician at the patient's bedside, in a procedure room, or in the physician's office in fewer than 30 minutes. Although local anesthetics eliminate pain at the insertion site, the patient may feel a pressurelike pain as the needle is inserted.

Contraindications

Contraindications for paracentesis are as follows:

- Patients with coagulation abnormalities or bleeding tendencies
- Patients with only a small amount of fluid and extensive previous abdominal surgery
  The needle could easily penetrate the bowel and cause an acute infection.

Nursing implications with rationale

Before

- Explain the procedure to the patient. Tell the patient that no fasting or sedation is necessary.
- Obtain informed consent for this procedure.
- Instruct the patient to empty the bladder before this test to avoid inadvertent puncture by the aspirating needle during the procedure.
- Measure the abdominal girth and weight of the patient. Obtain baseline vital signs.

During
- If assisting with this procedure, review the procedural steps.

After
- All tests involving peritoneal fluid should be performed immediately to avoid false results caused by chemical or cellular deterioration.
- Place a small bandage over the needle site.
- Label the specimen with the patient's name, date, source of fluid, and diagnosis.
- Send the specimen promptly to the laboratory.
- Observe the puncture site for bleeding, continued drainage, or signs of inflammation.
- Measure the abdominal girth and weight of the patient; compare with baseline values.
- Monitor vital signs for evidence of hemodynamic changes. Watch for signs of hypotension if a large volume of fluid was removed.
- Write any recent antibiotic therapy on the laboratory requisition slip.
- Because of the high protein content of ascitic fluid, albumin infusions may be ordered after paracentesis to compensate for protein loss. Monitor serum protein and electrolyte (especially sodium) levels.
- Occasionally, ascitic fluid continues to leak out of the needle tract after removal of the needle. A suture can stop that. If a suture is unsuccessful, a collection bag should be applied to the skin to allow for measurement of the volume of fluid loss.

Schilling Test (Vitamin B_{12} Absorption Test)

Test type Urine

Normal values
Excretion of 8% to 40% of radioactive vitamin B_{12} within 24 hours

Rationale
The Schilling test is performed to detect vitamin B_{12} absorption. Normally, ingested vitamin B_{12} combines with intrinsic factor, which is produced by gastric mucosa, and is absorbed in the distal part of the ileum. Pernicious anemia results when absorption of vitamin B_{12} is inadequate. This may be caused by a primary malabsorption problem of the intestinal tract or from lack of intrinsic factor.

The Schilling test, which can be performed in one or two stages, can detect either defect in vitamin B_{12} absorption. With normal absorption, the ileum absorbs more vitamin B_{12} than the body needs and excretes the excess into the urine. With impaired absorption, however, little or no vitamin B_{12} is excreted into the urine.

In the Schilling test, urinary B_{12} levels are measured after the ingestion of radioactive vitamin B_{12}. The test can be performed in one stage (without intrinsic factor) or two stages (with intrinsic factor). Patients with pernicious anemia from lack of intrinsic factor will have an abnormal first-stage and a normal second-stage Schilling test. Patients with malabsorption from an intestinal source will have an abnormal first and second-stage Schilling test. A test that combines both stages now is commonly used.

Interfering factors
Factors that interfere with the Schilling test include the following:

- Radioactive nuclear material received 10 days before testing
- Renal insufficiency, which may cause reduced excretion of radioactive vitamin B_{12}
- Inadequate collection of urine, which can falsely reduce the vitamin B_{12} in the urine
- Stool contamination of the urine specimen

Procedure
Patients who excrete a normal amount of radioactive vitamin B_{12} in the first stage require no further testing. The second stage is performed if the first stage shows a decreased percentage of radioactive vitamin B_{12} in the urine. The second stage of the test is needed to confirm the diagnosis of pernicious anemia.

First stage (without intrinsic factor): After the patient is kept NPO for 8 to 12 hours before the test, a urine specimen is collected and discarded. The patient then receives an oral dose of radioactive vitamin B_{12} and begins a 24- to 48-hour urine collection. After 1 to 2 hours, the patient receives an intramuscular injection of nonradioactive vitamin B_{12} to saturate tissue-binding sites and permit some excretion of radioactive vitamin B_{12} in the urine. The patient may resume eating after the injection.

Second stage (with intrinsic factor): After being kept NPO for 8 to 12 hours before the test, the patient voids and discards the urine. The patient then receives an oral dose of radioactive vitamin B_{12} and human intrinsic factor. A 24-hour urine collection then is begun. After 2 hours, the patient receives an intramuscular dose of nonradioactive vitamin B_{12} to saturate tissue-binding sites and permit some excretion of radioactive vitamin B_{12} in the urine, if it is absorbed. The patient may resume eating after the injection. After administration of intrinsic factor and vitamin B_{12} in the second stage, patients who have B_{12} deficiency secondary to lack of intrinsic factor (e.g., chronic gastritis) excrete normal amounts of radioactive B_{12}. Patients who have B_{12} deficiency from primary bowel disease, however, do not have normal B_{12} urinary levels. The second stage is usually performed within 1 week after the first stage.

A combined assay also can be performed to incorporate stages one and two into one procedure. In this method the fasting patient receives a capsule of cobalt-57–labeled vitamin B_{12} plus intrinsic factor and a second capsule of cobalt-58. One hour later, an intramuscular injection of nonradioactive vitamin B_{12} is given. All urine is then collected for 24 hours, and the percentages of cobalt-57 and cobalt-58 are calculated. Cobalt-57–labeled vitamin B_{12} only will be present in patients with pernicious anemia secondary to lack of intrinsic factor. No vitamin B_{12} will be present in the urine of patients whose pernicious anemia is caused by primary bowel malabsorption.

Contraindication
The Schilling test is contraindicated for patients who are pregnant or lactating, because nuclear exposure could injure the fetus or infant.

Nursing implications with rationale
Before
- ☞ Explain the purpose and procedure of the Schilling test to the patient. Also provide written instructions.
- ■ Ensure that laxatives are not given to the patient the evening before the test, because they could decrease the rate of vitamin B_{12} absorption.
- ☞ Instruct the patient to remain NPO for 8 to 12 hours before the test. Food should not be given until after the patient receives the injection.
- ■ Be certain that the patient receives the injection of the nonradioactive vitamin B_{12} at the exact time specified. Otherwise, the radioactive vitamin B_{12} will be absorbed by the liver and not excreted in the urine.
- ☞ Explain the procedure for collection of the 24-hour urine specimen (see the creatinine clearance test, p. 237). Follow the laboratory guidelines with regard to refrigerating the specimen. Patients with elevated blood urea nitrogen (BUN) levels may be required to collect the urine specimens for longer periods, because impaired renal function may slow excretion of vitamin B_{12}.

After
- ☞ Inform the patient that the tracer dose of radioactive vitamin B_{12} is not harmful to them or others, because the radioactive dose is tiny.
- ☞ If the patient had a decreased excretion of vitamin B_{12} in the first stage of the test, explain that the second stage is usually performed within 1 week.
- ■ Make sure the urine specimen is transported promptly to the laboratory.

Sigmoidoscopy (Proctoscopy, Anoscopy)

Test type Endoscopy

Normal values
Normal anus, rectum, and sigmoid colon

Rationale

Endoscopy of the lower GI tract allows one to visualize and perform biopsies of tumors, polyps, hemorrhoids, or ulcers of the anus, rectum, and sigmoid colon. *Anoscopy* refers to examination of the anus; *proctoscopy* to examination of the anus and rectum; and *sigmoidoscopy* (the most frequent procedure) to examination of the anus, rectum, and sigmoid colon. This test can be performed with a rigid (to 25 cm from the anus) or flexible (to 60 cm from the anus) sigmoidoscope.

Sigmoidoscopy is recommended for patients who have had a change in bowel habits, who have obvious or occult blood in the stool, or who have abdominal pain. It is part of routine screening for colorectal cancer in people over age 50. The American Cancer Society recommends a sigmoidoscopy every 3 to 5 years after age 50.

Sigmoidoscopy, as with colonoscopy, can be therapeutic. Reduction of sigmoid volvulus, removal of polyps, and obliteration of hemorrhoids can be performed through the sigmoidoscope.

Potential complications

Potential complications associated with sigmoidoscopy are as follows:

- Perforation of the colon, caused by forceful advancement of the scope
- Bleeding from the rectum or colon, as a result of biopsy or polypectomy

Interfering factors

Factors that interfere with sigmoidoscopy include the following:

- Poor bowel preparation, which may obscure visualization of the bowel mucosa
- Rectal bleeding, which obstructs the lens system and precludes adequate visualization

Procedure

In most cases, two Fleet enemas are sufficient for examining the lower sigmoid colon and rectum. An oral cathartic is usually required to examine as far as 60 cm. Food should be limited to a light breakfast on the morning of the examination. The patient is placed on the endoscopy table or bed in the left lateral decubitus position. Some physicians often prefer the knee-chest position; many operating and examining tables are easily converted to make the knee-chest position more comfortable. This procedure also can be performed with the patient in the lithotomy position. Usually, no sedation is required. The anus is mildly dilated with a well-lubricated finger. The rigid or flexible sigmoidoscope is placed into the rectum and advanced to its point of maximal penetration. Air is insufflated during the procedure to distend more fully the lower intestinal tract. The sigmoid, rectum, and anus are visualized. Biopsy specimens can be obtained, and polypectomy can be performed at the time of sigmoidoscopy.

A physician trained in GI endoscopy usually performs this procedure in the GI laboratory, operating room, patient's bedside, or outpatient clinic setting in approximately 15 to 20 minutes. Very little discomfort is associated with the test. A sense of having to defecate during the procedure, caused by the scope within the rectum, is uncomfortable.

Contraindications

Contraindications for sigmoidoscopy are as follows:

- Patients who are uncooperative
- Patients with diverticulitis
  The insufflation of air needed to distend the rectum and colon for passage of the scope may cause a perforation of the inflamed diverticulum.
- Patients with painful anorectal conditions (e.g., fissures, fistulas, hemorrhoids)
  They will have anal pain associated with passage of the scope.
- Patients with severe bleeding
  Blood clots obstruct the view of the scope.
- Patients suspected of having perforated colon lesions
  The insufflation of air needed to distend the rectum and colon for passage of the scope may increase fecal soilage of the peritoneal cavity.

Nursing implications with rationale

Before

- Explain the procedure to the patient. Warn the patient that he or she will feel discomfort and the urge to defecate as the sigmoidoscope is passed. Encourage verbalization of the patient's fears. Provide emotional support.
- Obtain written consent for sigmoidoscopy and possible biopsy.
- Instruct the patient to have only a light breakfast on the morning of the examination.
- Assist the patient with enemas ordered on the morning of and on the evening before the test to ensure optimum visualization of the lower GI tract.
- Assure the patient that he or she will be properly draped to avoid exposure and embarrassment.

After

- Tell the patient that because air is insufflated into the bowel during the procedure, he or she may have "gas pains" and that ambulation will help.
- Observe the patient for fever, chills, abdominal distention, and unusual complaints of pain, which may indicate perforation. Slight rectal bleeding may occur if biopsy specimens are taken.

Case Study

Colon Cancer

An 85-year-old man with previously normal bowel function began to complain of constipation, rectal bleeding, and pencil-like stool. The results of a physical examination were negative.

Studies	Results
Routine laboratory studies	Normal, except hemoglobin (10 g/dl) and hematocrit (29%) (normal hemoglobin: 12-13 g/dl) (normal hematocrit: 36%-42%)
Examination of stool for occult blood, p. 90	Positive (normal: negative)
Carcinoembryonic antigen (CEA) test, p. 65	33 ng/ml (normal: <2 ng/ml)
Sigmoidoscopy, p. 86	No tumor seen
Barium enema (BE) study, p. 60	Stricture in left side of colon
Colonoscopy, p. 67	Tumor in left side of colon; no other synchronous lesion found
Colonoscopic biopsy	Adenocarcinoma

Diagnostic Analysis

The elevated CEA level and the occult (hidden) blood in the stool indicated serious colorectal disease. Because the sigmoidoscopy was normal, the disease was suspected to be beyond the reach of the 25-cm sigmoidoscope. The barium enema study demonstrated a narrowing in the left side of the colon, which could have been caused by infection, infestation, or neoplasm. Adenocarcinoma of the colon was diagnosed by means of a colonoscopic biopsy. The patient had surgery to resect the left side of his colon. Postoperatively, his CEA level was 1.8 ng/ml. On examination 3 years later, no evidence of disease was found. Five years after surgery, his CEA had risen to 38 ng/ml. He was found to have liver metastasis from his primary tumor in the colon. He died 18 months later.

Critical Thinking Question

1. How would you respond if one of the patient's children asked if he should be routinely screened for cancer by checking CEA levels?

Stool Culture (Stool for Culture and Sensitivity [C&S], Stool for Ova and Parasites [O&P])

Test type Stool

Normal values
Normal intestinal flora

Rationale
Stool normally contains bacteria and fungi. Bacteria are indigenous to the bowel; however, several bacteria act as pathogens within the bowel. These include *Salmonella, Shigella, Campylobacter, Yersinia,* pathogenic *Escherichia coli, Clostridium,* and *Staphylococcus.* Parasites also may affect the stool. Common parasites are *Ascaris* (hookworm), *Strongyloides* (tapeworm), *Giardia* (protozoans), and *Cryptosporidium* (especially in patients with acquired immunodeficiency syndrome [AIDS]). Identification of any of these pathogens in the stool incriminates that organism as the causative agent of the infectious enteritis. Sometimes the normal stool flora can become pathogenic if overgrowth of the bacteria occurs as a result of antibiotics, immunosuppression, or overaggressive catharsis (e.g., *Clostridium difficile,* [see p. 66]).

Stool cultures are indicated for patients who have unrelenting diarrhea, fever, and abdominal bloating. One is especially suspicious if the patient has been drinking well water, has been on prolonged antibiotics, or has traveled outside of the United States.

Interfering factors
Factors that interfere with stool culture include the following:

■ Contamination of the stool specimen by urine Because urine may inhibit the growth of bacteria, it should not be mixed with the feces during collection of a stool sample.
■ Recent barium studies, which may obscure the detection of parasites

Procedure
Stools for bacteria or parasites are collected in a clean, wide-mouth plastic or waxed container with a tight-fitting lid. The patient usually defecates into a clean bedpan and transfers either a walnut-size piece of the feces or the entire specimen (as directed by the laboratory) into the specimen container. Urine and toilet paper should not be mixed with the specimen. Because parasites or bacteria often are found in mucus or blood streaks, some of this material, if present, should be included with the sample.

The *tape test* can be done by placing cellophane tape over the perianal area to detect pinworms. Because the female worm lays her eggs at night around the perianal area, the tape is applied at bedtime and removed in the morning before the patient gets out of bed. The sticky surface is then applied directly to a glass slide and examined microscopically for pinworm ova.

If a rectal swab is to be used, the nurse (wearing gloves) inserts a sterile, cotton-tipped swab approximately 1 inch into the anal canal. The swab is gently moved from side to side and left in place for 30 seconds to absorb organisms. This sometimes is done to detect *Shigella* and gonorrhea (p. 387).

Nursing implications with rationale

Before

🖉 Explain the method of stool collection to the patient. Be matter-of-fact to avoid any embarrassment to the patient.

🖉 Instruct the patient not to mix urine or toilet paper with the specimen. Both can contaminate the specimen and alter test results.

■ Handle the specimen carefully, as though it were infectious. If the nurse is assisting with the specimen collection, he or she should wear gloves.

🖉 Inform the patient that barium, oil, or laxatives containing heavy metals usually are not given 7 days before the stool collection because they interfere with the detection of ova and parasites.

During

■ If the patient received a purgative medication, the complete stool specimen is usually collected.

■ If an enema must be administered to collect specimens, only normal saline or tap water should be administered. Soapsuds or any other substance could affect the viability of the organisms collected.

After

■ Indicate on the laboratory requisition slip whether the patient is taking any medications (such as antibiotics), which can alter the intestinal flora.

■ Send the stool specimen to the laboratory as soon as possible after collection.

Stool for Occult Blood (Stool for OB)

Test type Stool

Normal values
No occult blood within stool

Rationale

Normally, only minimal quantities of blood are passed into the GI tract. Usually, this bleeding is not significant enough to cause a positive result in stool for occult blood (OB) testing. Tumors of the intestine grow into the lumen and are subjected to repeated trauma by the fecal stream. Eventually, the friable tumor ulcerates and bleeding occurs. Most often, bleeding is so slight that gross blood is not seen in the stool. The blood can only be detected by chemical assay through the OB testing. This test can detect occult blood when as little as 5 ml of blood are lost per day.

Benign and malignant GI tumors, ulcers, inflammatory bowel disease, arteriovenous malformations, diverticulosis, and hematobilia (hemobilia) can all cause OB within the stool. Other more common abnormalities (e.g., hemorrhoids, swallowed blood from oral or nasal pharyngeal bleeding) may also cause OB within the stool.

It has been well documented that vigorous exercise can create OB within the stool. It is important to note that many drugs and the ingestion of red meats, such as beef and pork, may cause a false-positive OB stool test (red meats contain animal hemoglobin). The more sensitive the test, the more false positives will be obtained.

When OB testing is performed properly, a positive result obtained on multiple specimens performed on successive days warrants a thorough GI evaluation. No consensus exists, however, about how many specimens need to be positive before a thorough evaluation is indicated. Most would agree that four positives out of six specimens would constitute criteria for a more thorough evaluation. Patients with chronic and prolonged occult blood loss in the stool may present with iron-deficiency anemia.

This test is a part of every routine physical examination. It is an important part of the evaluation for abdominal pain. Its use in the screening of asymptomatic individuals over age 50 has significantly lowered the mortality rate from colorectal cancer by allowing neoplasms to be identified sooner in their clinical course.

Interfering factors

Factors that interfere with determining stool occult blood results include the following:

- Bleeding gums following a dental procedure
  This blood can cause false-positive results.
- Ingestion of red meat within 3 days before testing
  This can cause false-positive results.

Procedure

The preparation for collecting a stool for occult blood varies. Often the preparation involves prescribing a high-fiber diet and abstinence from red meats for 48 to 72 hours before the test. Medications, such as iron preparations, iodides, colchicine, salicylates, steroids, and ascorbic acid, may be withheld for 48 hours before testing. Eliminating meat decreases the incidence of weak false-positive test results. If patients on an unrestricted diet who are screened for occult blood manifest a weak positive result, they are usually studied again later on a restricted diet. Stool is obtained by digital retrieval by the nurse or physician. Alternatively, the patient can be asked to save his or her stool in a container or smear a specimen on a card or paper, which then can be sent to the laboratory or doctor's office. There are several methods of examining the stool for occult blood. The two most common ones are described below:

1. The first is a slide, card, or paper method. A stool sample is placed on one side of guaiac paper. Two drops of developer are placed on the other side. Bluish discoloration indicates the presence of occult blood in the stool.
2. The second type is the tablet method. A stool sample is placed on the developer paper. A tablet is placed on top of the stool specimen. Two to three drops of tap water are placed on the tablet and allowed to flow onto the paper. Again, a bluish discoloration indicates occult blood in the stool.

Nursing implications with rationale

Before

- Explain the procedure to the patient. If any special dietary restrictions are applicable, instruct the patient as indicated. Often the patient is instructed to avoid red meats for 3 days before testing.
- If the stool is to be obtained by digital examination, explain the procedure to the patient. It is important to be gentle during the rectal examination. The slightest mucosal trauma can cause a positive test result.
- Tell the patient how many stool specimens are required and supply specimen containers. Give the patient tongue blades to transfer the specimens from the bedpan to the specimen container.
- Instruct the patient not to mix urine or toilet paper with the specimen. Both can contaminate the specimen and alter test results.

During

- If checking the stool for occult blood on the nursing unit, follow the directions explicitly, or send the specimen to the laboratory for analysis.

After

- Indicate on the laboratory requisition slip any medications, such as anticoagulants, that can affect test results.
- If the results are positive, inquire whether the patient violated any of the preparation recommendations.

Swallowing Examination
(Videofluoroscopy Swallowing Examination)

Test type X-ray with contrast dye

Normal values

Normal swallowing function and complete clearing of radiographic material through the upper digestive tract

Rationale

Problems in swallowing may result from local structural diseases such as tumors, upper esophageal diverticula, inflammation, extrinsic compression of the UGI tract, or surgery to the oropharyngeal tract. Motility disorders of the UGI tract, such as Zenker's diverticulum, and neurologic disorders, such as stroke syndrome, Parkinson's disease, and neuropathies, also may cause difficulty in swallowing. Videofluoroscopy of the swallowing function allows the speech pathologist to delineate more clearly the exact pathology in the swallowing mechanism. This videofluoroscopy then can be used to determine the most appropriate treatment and teach the patient proper swallowing technique.

This test is performed by asking the patient to swallow barium or a barium-containing meal. With videofluoroscopy, the act of swallowing is visualized and documented. Morphologic abnormalities and functional impairment can be identified easily using the slow-framed progression and reversal that is available with videofluoroscopy. Although this test is similar to the barium swallow (see p. 62), finer details of swallowing can be evaluated with videofluoroscopy.

Procedure

No preparation is required. In the radiology department, the patient is asked to swallow a barium-containing meal. The consistency of the meal will be determined by the speech therapist and radiologist. The meal consistency simulates foods to which the patient will be reintroduced initially. The food may be in the form of a liquid, semisoft (e.g., applesauce), or solids (e.g., a tea biscuit). While the patient is swallowing, videofluoroscopy is recorded in both the lateral and anterior positions. The video then is repeatedly examined by the radiologist and speech pathologist.

Contraindication

Swallowing examinations are contraindicated for patients who obviously aspirate their saliva. They are not candidates for swallowing because they will require nonswallowing methods of alimentation.

Nursing implications with rationale

Before

☞ Explain the procedure to the patient. Tell the patient that no special preparation is required.

After

☞ Inform the patient that no catharsis is needed because of the small amount of barium used.

Upper Gastrointestinal X-ray Study (Upper GI Series, UGI)

Test type X-ray with contrast dye

Normal values

Normal size, contour, patency, filling, positioning, and transit of barium through the lower esophagus, stomach, and upper duodenum

Rationale

The UGI study consists of a series of x-ray films of the lower esophagus, stomach, and duodenum, usually using barium sulfate as the contrast medium. When leakage of x-ray contrast through a perforation of the GI tract is a concern, however, diatrizoate meglumine (Gastrografin), a water-soluble contrast, is used. This test can be performed in conjunction with a barium swallow or a small bowel series (see pp. 62 and 94), which can precede or succeed the upper GI study, respectively.

This examination is used to detect ulcerations (Figure 3-6), tumors, inflammations, or anatomic malpositions (e.g., hiatal hernia) within these organs. Obstruction of the UGI tract also is detected easily. In this test, the patient is asked to drink barium. As the contrast descends, the lower esophagus is examined for position, patency, and filling defects (e.g., tumors, scarring, varices). As the contrast enters the stomach, the gastric wall is examined for benign or malignant ulcerations, filling defects (most often in cancer), and anatomic abnormalities (e.g., hiatal hernia). The patient is placed in a flat or head-down position, and the gastroesophageal area is examined for evidence of gastroesophageal reflux of barium.

As the contrast leaves the stomach, patency of

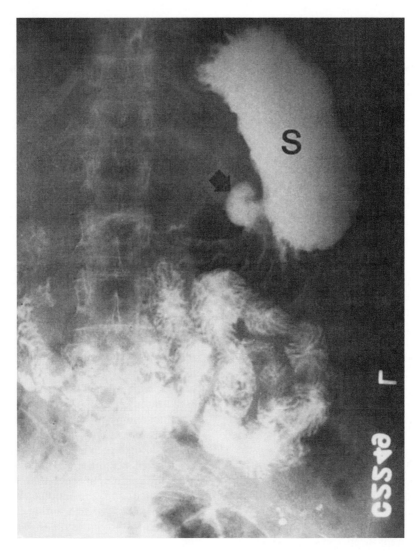

Figure 3-6 Upper gastrointestinal series demonstrating an ulcer *(black arrow)* on the lesser curvature of the stomach *(S)*.

the pyloric channel and the duodenum is evaluated. Benign peptic ulceration is the most common pathologic condition affecting these areas. Extrinsic compression caused by tumors, cysts, or enlarged pathologic organs (e.g., liver) near the stomach also can be identified by anatomic distortion of the outline of the UGI tract.

Potential complications

Potential complications associated with UGI are as follows:

■ Aspiration of barium, if the patient has swallowing problems
■ Constipation or partial bowel obstruction,

caused by inspissated barium in the small bowel or colon

Interfering factors

Factors that interfere with determining UGI results include the following:

- Previously administered barium
  This may block visualization of the UGI tract.
- Incapacitated patients, who cannot assume the multiple positions required for the study
- Food and fluid in the stomach
  This gives the false impression of filling defects within the stomach, precluding adequate evaluation of the gastric mucosa.

Procedure

To examine the UGI tract, the fasting patient is required to swallow approximately 8 ounces of barium, a white, chalky, radiopaque substance that is ingested in a suspension much like a milk shake. It usually is flavored to increase palatability. After drinking the barium, the patient is moved through several position changes, such as prone, supine, and lateral, to promote barium flow by gravity through the UGI tract. Small spot films are taken at the discretion of the radiologist. Large films are taken in standard, specified positions.

As this contrast medium descends, the lower esophagus (see barium swallow, p. 62) is examined for position, patency, and filling defects (which would indicate tumors, scarring, or varices). As the barium fills the stomach, the gastric wall is examined for ulcers (both benign and malignant), filling defects (tumors, most commonly malignant), and anatomic abnormalities such as hiatal hernia (Figure 3-7). As the barium leaves the stomach, the patency of the pyloric valve is evaluated. Benign ulcers are the most common pathologic condition seen in the duodenum. The duration of this study is about 30 minutes. The patient may be uncomfortable lying on the hard x-ray table.

If *air contrast* is requested, the patient is asked to swallow CO_2 powder. The CO_2 gas creates a contrast to the barium and provides more accurate visualization of the mucosa of the esophagus, stomach, and duodenum.

If desired, a *small-bowel follow-through* (small bowel series) *study* may be performed by instructing the patient to drink additional barium mixed with saline solution. Films then are taken at timed intervals to follow the progression of the barium through the small intestine. A significant delay in the transit time of barium may occur with benign or malignant obstruction. The flow of barium is faster in patients with hypermotility of the bowel (as in malabsorption). Sometimes transit time is so delayed (as in partial bowel obstruction) that x-ray films must be taken 24 hours later to see complete progression of the barium meal. Small-bowel follow-through studies are also helpful in identifying and defining the anatomy of small-bowel fistulas (i.e., abnormal connections between the small bowel and other abdominal organs or skin).

A more accurate radiographic evaluation of the small intestine is provided by the *small-bowel enema*. Unlike the small-bowel follow-through study, in which the barium is swallowed by the patient, with a small-bowel enema, a tube is placed through the mouth, esophagus, stomach, and duodenum, and into the small intestine. Barium is injected through this tube and allowed to flow through the small intestine. Visualization is improved with the small-bowel enema because the barium injected through the tube is concentrated and not diluted by gastric and duodenal juices as it is during UGI and small-bowel follow-through studies. The small intestine is therefore more accurately outlined by the dye and more easily evaluated radiographically. This test is especially useful in the evaluation of patients with partial small-bowel obstruction of unknown etiology. Tumors, inflammatory bowel disease, ulcers, and small-bowel fistula may be more easily identified and defined with this procedure.

The tube can be placed transorally with the use of a weighted tip. However, having the endoscopist deliver the tube to the upper small bowel via enteroscopy (see p. 71) is easier. After the barium has been injected through the tube, the small-

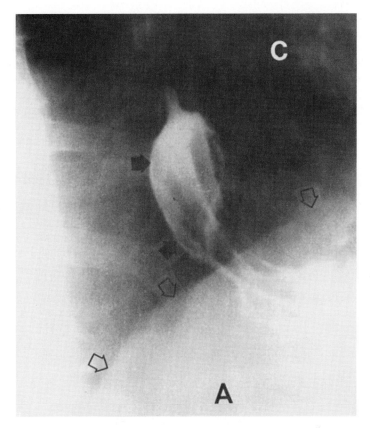

Figure 3-7 Upper gastrointestinal series demonstrating a hiatal hernia. Note that the proximal portion of the stomach *(solid black arrows)* is above the diaphragm *(arrow outlines)* and lying within the chest *(C)*. Abdominal cavity *(A)*.

bowel enema is carried out as described in the discussion concerning UGI and small-bowel follow-through studies.

Contraindications

Contraindications for UGI studies are as follows:

■ Patients with complete bowel obstructions, because the barium cannot be cleared
Retention of barium may worsen a bowel obstruction.

■ Patients suspected of UGI perforation
Barium in the peritoneal cavity can cause chronic abscess formation. Water-soluble diatrizoate meglumine (Gastrografin) should be used instead of barium.

■ Patients who are uncooperative, because of the necessity of frequent position changes

Nursing implications with rationale

Before

▱ Explain the procedure to the patient. Encourage verbalization of the patient's questions or fears. Assure the patient that the test will not cause discomfort other than that of lying on a hard table.

▱ Instruct the patient to remain NPO after midnight. Food and fluid in the stomach prevent the barium from accurately outlining the GI tract, and the radiographic results may be misleading.

Explain to the patient that the test may take several hours and that during that time he or she cannot eat or drink. The patient may eat as soon as the radiology department determines that the series is completed.

After

Explain to the patient the importance of rectally expelling all the barium. Stools will be light in color until all the barium is expelled.

Eventual absorption of fecal water may cause a hardened barium impaction. Increasing fluids is usually effective. Occasionally a mild laxative, such as magnesium citrate, or an enema may be needed to prevent this complication.

If diatrizoate meglumine was used, inform the patient that significant diarrhea may develop. This contrast agent is an osmotic diuretic.

Case Study

Anorexia Nervosa

Becky J., a 14-year-old white girl, was taken to her family nurse practitioner by her mother because of cessation of menses. Once an overweight child, Becky recently had a severe weight loss and was described by her mother as anxious, irritable, and depressed. Despite her weight of 85 pounds (and height of 64 inches), Becky was jogging long distances daily. The physical examination was compatible with signs of starvation (such as sparse, dry hair; dry, flaky skin; muscle wasting; and red, swollen lips).

Studies	Results
Triceps skinfold thickness (TSF) (Figure 3-8)	65% standard
Midarm circumference (MAC) (Figure 3-8)	65% standard
Midarm muscle circumference (MAMC) (Figure 3-8)	65% standard
Hemoglobin (p. 412)	10 g/dl (normal: 12 g/dl)
Hematocrit (p. 412)	31% (normal: 36%)
Total iron-binding capacity (TIBC) (p. 425)	210 µg/dl (normal: 250-420 µg/dl)
Serum albumin (p. 135)	2.8 g/dl (normal: 3.2-4.5 g/dl)
Total protein (p. 135)	4 g/dl (normal: 6-8 g/dl)
Total lymphocyte count (p. 413)	1200/mm³ (normal: 1500-3000/mm³)
Blood urea nitrogen (BUN) (p. 266)	30 mg/dl (normal: 5-20 mg/dl)
24-hour urine for creatinine (p. 237)	Decreased when compared with expected creatinine clearance based on height and sex
Serum triglycerides (p. 51)	200 mg/dl (normal: 40-150 mg/dl)
Skin testing with common antigens	Delayed sensitivity to mumps, purified protein derivative (PPD), and *Candida*

Diagnostic Analysis

The triceps skinfold thickness (TSF), which estimates the amount of subcutaneous fat, reflected the depleted caloric stores in the body. The midarm muscle circumference

(MAMC), which is calculated using the midarm circumference (MAC) and the TSF (Figure 3-8), reflected moderate to severe muscle protein depletion as a result of catabolism. The decreased hemoglobin and hematocrit levels reflected anemia because of iron and folic acid deficiency. The TIBC level reflected transferrin concentration (p. 423), which is a sensitive and early indicator of protein deficiency. The decreased plasma albumin and protein levels correlated with protein depletion, fatty liver, and edema. The elevated BUN level was the result of catabolism. The decreased lymphocyte count is further evidence of protein malnutrition. Because the 24-hour urinary excretion of creatinine is approximately proportional to lean body mass, its decrease reflected a severe degree of muscle protein depletion and decreased muscle mass. The antigen skin test showed decreased immunocompetence, which is seen in nutritional starvation. This also reflects the impaired ability of the white blood cells to fight infection.

Based on the results of these tests and a detailed family history, Becky was placed in the hospital in an adolescent unit for patients with anorexia. After several weeks of nutritional counseling and behavior modification, Becky was discharged to home. Individual and family counseling were continued over the next year.

Critical Thinking Question

1. What kind of questions were probably asked while obtaining the detailed family history?

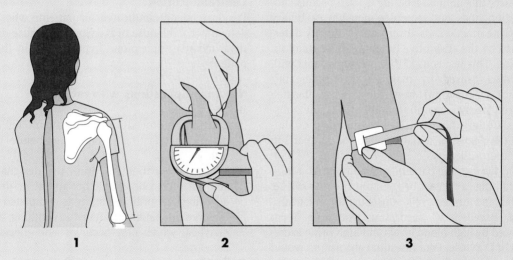

1   **2**   **3**

Figure 3-8 Techniques for obtaining anthropomorphic measurements. *Step 1,* Determine the midway point. With the patient sitting, determine the midway point of the upper arm by measuring the halfway point between the acromial process of the scapula and the olecranon process of the ulna. *Step 2,* Measure triceps skinfold. With the patient's arm extended, pull the skinfold gently away from the muscle and measure the thickness of the skinfold with calipers at the midway point determined in Step 1. *Step 3,* Measure midarm circumference. With the patient's arm extended, measure the circumference of the arm with a tape measure at the midway point determined in Step 1.

D-xylose Absorption Test (Xylose Tolerance Test)

Test type Blood

Normal values

Age	60 Min Plasma (mg/dl)	120 Min Plasma (mg/dl)	Urine (g/5 hr) [%]
Child	>15-20	>20	>4.0 (16-32)
Adult	20-57	30-58	>3.5-4.0 (>14)

Rationale

D-xylose is a monosaccharide that is absorbed easily by the normal intestine. In patients with malabsorption, intestinal D-xylose absorption is diminished, and, as a result, blood levels and urine excretion will be reduced. D-xylose is the monosaccharide chosen for the test because it is not metabolized by the body. Its serum levels directly reflect intestinal absorption.

Also, this monosaccharide is used because absorption does not require pancreatic or biliary exocrine function. Its absorption is directly determined by the absorptive function of the small intestine. This test is used to separate patients with diarrhea caused by maldigestion (pancreatic/biliary dysfunction) from those with diarrhea caused by malabsorption (sprue, Whipple's disease, Crohn's disease). It is also used to quantitate the degree of malabsorption for comparison to monitor therapy.

In this test, the patient is asked to drink a fluid containing a prescribed amount of D-xylose. Blood and urine levels subsequently are evaluated. Excellent GI absorption would be documented by high blood levels and high urine excretion of D-xylose. Poor intestinal absorption would be marked by low blood levels and low urine excretion.

Interfering factor

An interfering factor for D-xylose occurs with patients with abnormal kidney function. They may not be able to excrete the xylose. The urine measurement for xylose should not be performed, and the interpretation should be based on the blood results only.

Procedure

For the D-xylose absorption test, the patient is kept fasting at least 8 hours, usually from midnight on the day of the test. Before the monosaccharide D-xylose is administered, a peripheral venipuncture is performed, and approximately 7 ml of venous blood is placed in a red-top tube. A first-voided morning urine specimen also is collected.

The adult patient then receives 25 g D-xylose dissolved in 8 ounces of water, followed by another 8 ounces of water. For children, a calibrated dose of D-xylose is based on body weight. The patient should remain on bed rest during the test, because activity can affect the test results by altering digestive activity. The peripheral venipuncture then is repeated in 2 hours for an adult and in 1 hour for a child. All urine is collected for the designated period, usually 5 hours.

Contraindication

D-xylose is contraindicated for patients who are dehydrated. The dose of D-xylose can cause diarrhea and may precipitate hypovolemia in these patients.

Nursing implications with rationale

Before

- Explain the procedure to the patient. Tell the patient that fasting is necessary before this test.
- Instruct the patient to drink the designated amount of D-xylose and not to eat or drink anything else until the study is completed.
- Observe the patient for nausea, vomiting, and diarrhea, which may occur as side effects of D-xylose.
- Tell the patient to remain on bed rest during the testing period, because activity alters GI activity and may affect test results.

After

- Apply pressure or a pressure dressing to the venipuncture site to prevent further bleeding. Observe the site for further bleeding.

REVIEW QUESTIONS AND ANSWERS

1. **Question:** The UGI, barium swallow, and barium enema all use barium as a contrast agent. Why is barium used to visualize the GI tract radiographically?

   Answer: Diagnostic radiology is based entirely on contrasting densities. If no contrast medium were used, an x-ray film of the abdomen would show only general shadows, fluid levels, and gas. With barium, the inside of the gut can be evaluated for pathology.

2. **Question:** Mr. Smith was a patient with severe congestive heart failure and ascites. A paracentesis was performed to remove some of the fluid and relieve intraabdominal pressure. Why did the doctor order an albumin infusion after this procedure?

   Answer: Because of the high protein content of ascitic fluid, albumin is sometimes ordered to compensate for protein loss. The serum protein and electrolyte levels should be monitored.

3. **Question:** You are caring for an elderly patient taking antibiotics for pneumonia. After several days, she develops severe diarrhea. After a stool specimen for *Clostridium difficile* has been collected, her daughter asks how an antibiotic for pneumonia can cause diarrhea. What would be an appropriate response?

   Answer: Diarrhea may have resulted from a bowel infection caused by broad-spectrum antibiotic therapy. Antibiotics can depress the normal flora of the bowel and allow the overgrowth of other bacteria in the bowel, such as *C. difficile.* Infection results in watery and voluminous diarrhea.

4. **Question:** Your patient has just returned from getting a GI bleeding scan in the nuclear medicine department. Her pregnant daughter is afraid to visit because her mother received an injection of a radionuclide for this test. What would you advise?

   Answer: Tell the patient and her daughter that only tracer doses of radioisotopes are used for this procedure. No precautions against radiation exposure are necessary.

5. **Question:** Your patient has just completed a Schilling test, and the diagnosis of pernicious anemia was made. The results indicated that the patient has a lack of intrinsic factor. Can the patient be treated by taking large oral doses of vitamin B_{12}?

   Answer: No. The patient lacks intrinsic factor, which is needed to absorb vitamin B_{12} in the intestine. Therefore, vitamin B_{12} must be given by injection.

6. **Question:** Before his UGI study, your patient requests pain medication or a sedative. What effect would the administration of narcotics or sedatives have on the results of the UGI?

   Answer: Narcotics and sedatives often prolong gastric emptying time. If these drugs are administered before a UGI, the radiologist should be informed to prevent false attribution of the prolonged emptying time of the stomach to a pathologic cause.

7. **Question:** Often the patient admitted for evaluation of the GI tract needs various diagnostic procedures performed in the shortest amount of time possible. If your patient requires a UGI and a BE study, in what order should these procedures be performed and why?

   Answer: The BE study should precede the UGI because the ingested barium, descending through the intestine, would obstruct the visualization of the lower GI tract.

8. **Question:** Your patient is very anxious before having esophageal function studies. Since admission, the patient has had an order for diazepam (Valium), as needed, for anxiety. Should this drug be given the morning of the test?

   Answer: No. Sedation of any kind may reduce the LES pressure and cause greater acid reflux than what might have been present if the patient were not sedated.

9. **Question:** Is colonoscopy more accurate than barium enema studies in diagnosing pathologic colorectal conditions?

Answer: Yes. Several well-controlled studies have indicated the marked superiority of colonoscopy to barium enema studies. The accuracy of BE studies varies from 50% to 75%. Colonoscopy is accurate about 95% of the time.

10. **Question:** Your patient returns to the unit after having a colonoscopy and polypectomy. A regular diet is ordered. He tolerates his lunch well. Before eating supper, he begins to complain of severe abdominal pain and vomits. What nursing interventions are appropriate in this situation?

    Answer: Assessment of the symptomatology present and knowledge of the potential complications of colonoscopy should lead you to suspect perforated colon. The following interventions should be performed:
    a. Hold the supper meal and keep him NPO.
    b. Maintain the patency of the intravenous line, if one is running.
    c. Assess the patient's abdomen for distention.
    d. Record the vital signs.
    e. Contact the physician immediately.

Bibliography

Allen ML, DiMarino AJ: Manometric diagnosis of diffuse esophageal spasms, *Dig Dis Sci* 41:1346, 1996.

Alpers DH: Malabsorption. In Rakel RE, editor: Conn's current therapy, Philadelphia, 1998, WB Saunders.

Bentley DW: *Clostridium difficile*-associated disease in long-term care facilities, *Infect Control Hosp Epidemiol* 11(8):434-438, 1990.

Brooks MJ et al: The infectious etiology of peptic ulcer disease: diagnosis and implications for therapy, *Prim Care* 23(3), 443-454, 1996.

Christie JP et al: Flexible sigmoidoscopy screening. *Patient Care* 24(12):133-145, 1990.

Clouse RE: Irritable bowel syndrome. In Rakel RE, editor: Conn's current therapy, Philadelphia, 1998, WB Saunders.

Cohen S, Parkman H: Disease of the esophagus. In Bennet JC et al, editors: Cecil textbook of medicine, ed 20, Philadelphia, 1996, WB Saunders.

Fine KD: The prevalence of occult gastrointestinal bleeding in celiac sprue, *N Engl J Med* 334:1163, 1996.

Goyal RK: Diseases of the esophagus. In Fauci AS et al, editors: Harrison's principles of internal medicine, ed 14, New York, 1998, McGraw-Hill.

Greenberger NJ, Isselbacher KJ: Diseases of absorption. In Fauci AS et al, editors: Harrison's principles of internal medicine, ed 14, New York, 1998, McGraw-Hill.

Isenberg JI, Soll AH: Peptic ulcer: epidemiology, clinical manifestations, and diagnosis. In Bennet JC et al, editors: Cecil textbook of medicine, ed 20, Philadelphia, 1996, WB Saunders.

Isselbacher KJ, Podolsky DK: Approach to the patient with gastrointestinal disease. In Fauci JC et al, editors: Harrison's principles of internal medicine, ed 14, New York, 1998, McGraw-Hill.

Kikuchi S et al: Serum anti–*Helicobacter pylori* antibody and gastric carcinoma among young adults, *Cancer* 75(12):2789-2792, 1995.

Kuhlman JE: Oral and IV contrast-enhanced abdominal CT, *Appl Radiol* 21(10):20-21, 1992.

Lanza FL: Tumors of the stomach. In Rakel RE, editor: Conn's current therapy, Philadelphia, 1998, WB Saunders.

McGowan CC, et al: *Helicobacter pylori* and gastric acid: biological and therapeutic implications, *Gastroenterology* 110:926, 1996.

Mittal RF et al: Transient lower esophageal sphincter relaxation, *Gastroenterology* 109:601, 1995.

Rank JM, Vennes JA: Gastrointestinal endoscopy. In Bennet JC et al, editors: Cecil textbook of medicine, ed 20, Philadelphia, 1996, WB Saunders.

Sandowski DC, Rabeneck L: Gastric ulcers at endoscopy: brush, biopsy, or both? *Am J Gastroenterol* 92(4):608-613, 1997.

Silverstein FE: Gastrointestinal endoscopy. In Fauci AS et al, editors: Harrison's principles of internal medicine, ed 14, New York, 1998, McGraw-Hill.

Silverstein FE, Tytgat GNJ: Atlas of gastrointestinal endoscopy, ed 3, London, 1996, Mosby-Wolfe.

Taylor JL et al: Pharmacoeconomic comparison of treatments for the eradication of *Helicobacter pylori*, *Arch Intern Med* 157:87, 1997.

Trate D et al: Dysphagia: diagnosis and treatment, *Prim Care* 23(3):417-432, 1996.

Wall SD: Diagnostic imaging procedures in gastroenterology. In Bennet JC et al, editors: Cecil textbook of medicine, ed 20, Philadelphia, 1996, WB Saunders.

Webb WA: Management of foreign bodies of the upper GI tract: update. *Gastrointest Endosc* 41:39, 1995.

Winawer SJ: Tumors of the colon and rectum. In Rakel RE, editor: Conn's current therapy, Philadelphia, 1998, WB Saunders.

Yamada T et al: Textbook of gastroenterology, ed 2, Philadelphia, 1995, JB Lippincott.

Zeman PK et al: Gallbladder imaging: the state of the art, *Gastroenterol Clin North Am* 20(1):127-156, 1991.

Chapter 4

Diagnostic Studies Used in the Assessment of the

Hepatobiliary and Pancreatic Systems

Review Questions and Answers, p. 140

Bibliography, p. 142

ANATOMY AND PHYSIOLOGY

The liver, the biliary tract, and the pancreas (Figure 4-1) are being considered together because of their anatomic proximity, their closely related functions, and the similarity of the symptom complexes caused by their closely related functions. The liver is the largest gland in the body, occupying most of the right upper quadrant of the abdomen and lying directly beneath the diaphragm. In brief, the liver's main functions are the following:

1. Formation and secretion of bile. *Bile* is a collective term that includes bile salts, bilirubin, phospholipids, cholesterol, bicarbonate, and water. Bile salts mix with ingested lipids to provide fat absorption from the gastrointestinal (GI) tract. Bilirubin, cholesterol, and phospholipids are excretory products of metabolism. Bicarbonate and water are secreted into the alimentary tract and neutralize the stomach acid, because digestion and absorption require an alkaline environment.

2. Metabolism and storage of ingested carbohydrates, protein, and fats

3. Catabolism of many endogenous substances, including insulin, steroids, and gastrin

4. Detoxification of a variety of drugs

5. Formation of clotting factors II, VII, IX, and X

6. Filtration of portal venous blood

The biliary system consists of the gallbladder and the hepatic, cystic, and common bile ducts. The gallbladder is located directly beneath the right lobe of the liver. The principal function of the gallbladder is the storage and concentration of bile. Bile, formed within the liver, flows through an enlarging intrahepatic canalicular system that leads into the hepatic duct. The hepatic duct merges with the cystic duct of the gallbladder to form the common bile duct, which then enters the duodenum at the ampulla of Vater (Figure 4-1). The sphincter of Oddi surrounds the ampulla of Vater and is hormonally controlled to regulate bile

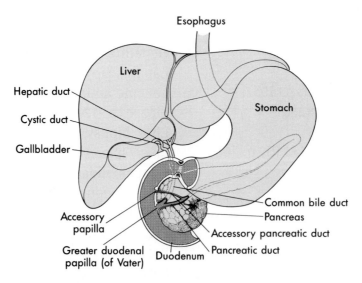

Figure 4-1   Liver, gallbladder, and pancreas.

flow into the gut. When the food in the alimentary canal flows into the duodenum, cholecystokinin is released from the duodenal mucosa and stimulates contraction of the gallbladder and common bile duct and stimulates relaxation of the sphincter of Oddi.

The pancreas lies directly adjacent to the stomach and duodenum and, like the liver, is a complex and multifunctional organ. The primary functions of the pancreas include:

1. Endocrine function: The islets of Langerhans produce and secrete into the bloodstream glucagon, insulin, and many unnamed, hormonally active peptides
2. Exocrine function: Pancreatic glandular cells (acini) produce and secrete digestive enzymes such as lipase, amylase, trypsin, and chymotrypsin into the GI tract via the pancreatic duct
3. Neutralizing function: Bicarbonate and water are secreted by the pancreatic glandular cells via the main pancreatic duct; they neutralize the stomach acid to provide an alkaline environment for digestion

The main pancreatic duct enters the ampulla of Vater beside the distal common bile duct (see Figure 4-1).

Bilirubin Metabolism and Excretion

To understand the diagnostic studies used in evaluating the patient with jaundice, one must first be familiar with normal bilirubin metabolism and the pathologic mechanisms of jaundice formation. In the spleen and other organs of the reticuloendothelial system, red blood cells (RBCs) are lysed. Hemoglobin then is released and broken down to heme and globin molecules. Heme is catabolized to form biliverdin and bilirubin. This form of bilirubin is called *unconjugated ("indirect") bilirubin.* In the liver this substance is conjugated with a glucuronide, resulting in *conjugated ("direct") bilirubin.* The conjugated bilirubin is then excreted from the liver cell and into intrahepatic canaliculi, which eventually lead to the major extrahepatic bile duct system and into the

gut. Once in the GI tract, the conjugated bilirubin is acted on by bacteria to form urobilinogen. Most of this urobilinogen is excreted in the stool. Some, however, is reabsorbed through the enterohepatic pathway and is either excreted in the urine or re-excreted in the bile (enterohepatic circulation of bile salts) (Figure 4-2).

Jaundice is the discoloration of body tissues caused by abnormally high blood levels of bilirubin. Jaundice usually can be recognized when the total serum bilirubin exceeds 2 to 2.5 mg/100 ml. Defects in bilirubin metabolism can occur during any stage of the catabolism of heme. Unconjugated hyperbilirubinemia results if the defect exists before glucuronide conjugation (Table 4-1). Unconjugated bilirubin is not water soluble and therefore cannot enter the urine and be excreted.

Physiologic jaundice of the newborn occurs because the immature liver does not have conjugating enzymes. This results in high circulating blood levels of unconjugated bilirubin, which

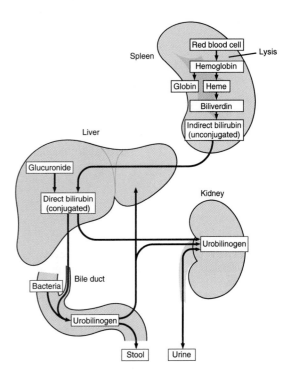

Figure 4-2 Bilirubin metabolism and excretion.

crosses the blood-brain barrier and is deposited in the brain cells, causing encephalopathy (kernicterus).

If the defect occurs after glucuronide addition, conjugated hyperbilirubinemia results (see Table 4-1). Conjugated bilirubin is water soluble and can be excreted in the urine by the kidney. It causes the urine to be very dark. Because bilirubin gives the stool its greenish-brown color, obstruction to bilirubin flow results in light yellow or clay-colored stools. In certain situations, as in hepatitis, bilirubin metabolism is interrupted in more than one site, causing a combined conjugated and unconjugated hyperbilirubinemia. When obstructive jaundice is of sufficient duration, hepatocellular dysfunction occurs and also may cause combined conjugated and unconjugated hyperbilirubinemia.

Once the jaundice is recognized, it is important in terms of therapy to differentiate whether it is predominately caused by unconjugated or conjugated hyperbilirubinemia. This determination helps to differentiate prehepatic and intrahepatic jaundice (requiring only medical treatment) from extrahepatic jaundice (usually requiring surgery or therapeutic endoscopy).

TABLE 4-1   Causes and Classification of Jaundice

Condition		Cause	Pathophysiology
Prehepatic cholestasis	Unconjugated (indirect) hyperbilirubinemia	Physiologic jaundice of newborn	Production of bilirubin exceeds liver function
		Hemolytic anemia	Overproduction of bilirubin
		Gilbert's disease	Inability to transport bilirubin into the cells
		Crigler-Najjar syndrome	Inability to conjugate bilirubin
Intrahepatic (medical) cholestasis	Combined conjugated and unconjugated hyperbilirubinemia	Hepatocellular disease (e.g., hepatitis)	Inability to transport bilirubin into the cells and to excrete it
		Dubin-Johnson syndrome	Inability to excrete bilirubin from hepatocytes
		Biliary cirrhosis	Obstruction of bilirubin at small intrahepatic bile canaliculi
		Drugs and viruses	
Extrahepatic (surgical) cholestasis	Conjugated (direct) hyperbilirubinemia	Gallstones in common duct	Obstruction of bilirubin at extrahepatic ducts
		Bile duct carcinoma	
		Choledochal cyst	
		Biliary atresia	
		Benign fibrous stricture	
		Periampullary (distal bile duct, pancreas, duodenum, ampulla) carcinoma	

Abdominal Ultrasound (Abdominal Sonogram; Echogram; Ultrasound of the Kidney, Liver, Pancreatobiliary System, Gallbladder, Pancreas, Biliary Tree)

Test type Ultrasound

Normal values

Normal abdominal aorta, liver, gallbladder, bile ducts, pancreas, kidneys, ureters, and bladder

Rationale

Ultrasonography uses reflected sound waves to provide accurate visualization of the abdominal aorta, liver, gallbladder, pancreas, bile ducts, spleen, kidneys, ureters, and bladder. A transducer emits high-frequency sound waves that penetrate the particular organ being studied. The sound waves are bounced back to the transducer and then are converted electronically into a pictorial image film. Real-time ultrasound provides an image of the organ being studied, whereas Doppler ultrasound provides information concerning the organ's blood flow.

The kidney is evaluated ultrasonographically to diagnose and locate renal cysts; to differentiate renal cysts from solid renal tumors; to demonstrate renal and pelvic calculi; to document hy-dronephrosis; and to guide a percutaneously inserted needle for cyst aspiration or to obtain a biopsy specimen. Ultrasonography of the urologic tract is also used to detect malformed or ectopic kidneys and perinephric abscesses. Surveillance of renal transplants is possible via ultrasound.

Sonography is used to assess the abdominal aorta for aneurysmal dilation. It also is an ideal way to assess aneurysms before and after surgery.

Ultrasonography is used to detect cystic structures of the liver (e.g., benign cysts, hepatic abscesses, dilated hepatic ducts) and solid, intrahepatic tumors (primary and metastatic). Hepatic ultrasonography can also be performed intraoperatively by using a sterile probe. This technique allows for accurate location of small, nonpalpable, hepatic tumors or abscesses. The gallbladder (Figure 4-3) and extrahepatic ducts can be examined for gallstones, polyps, or dilation secondary to obstructive strictures or tumors. The pancreas is examined for tumors, pseudocysts, acute inflammation, chronic inflammation, or pancreatic abscess. Ultrasound of the pancreas frequently is performed serially to document resolution of acute pancreatic inflammatory processes. The pancreas often is better visualized if the stomach and duodenum are filled with water.

Because this study requires no contrast material and has no associated radiation, it is espe-

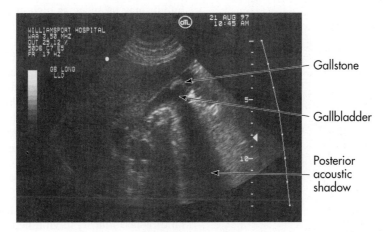

Figure 4-3 Ultrasonogram of the gallbladder. Long axis view of the gallbladder containing a gallstone. Note the posterior acoustic shadowing, typical of gallstones.

cially useful in patients who are allergic to contrast or who are pregnant. Although fasting may be preferred, it is not mandatory.

Interfering factors
Factors that interfere with abdominal ultrasound are barium or gas, which may distort the sound waves and alter test results. This test should be performed before any radiographic testing with barium.

Procedure
Fasting may or may not be required, depending on the organ to be examined. No fasting is required for ultrasonography of the abdominal aorta, kidney, liver, spleen, or pancreas. Fasting, however, is preferred for ultrasonography of the gallbladder and biliary tree. The patient is placed on the ultrasonography table in the prone or supine position, depending on the organ to be studied. A greasy conductive paste is applied to the patient's skin. This paste enhances sound wave transmission and reception. A transducer is placed over the skin (Figure 4-4), and the wave reflections from the organs being studied are photographed.

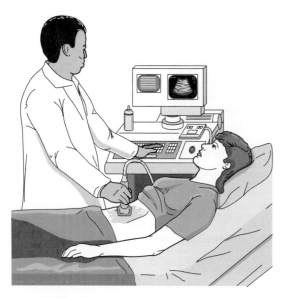

Figure 4-4   Abdominal ultrasonography.

To distend the stomach, the patient is asked to drink 8 to 10 oz of water while standing. The test is completed in approximately 20 minutes, usually by an ultrasound technologist, and interpreted by a radiologist. No discomfort is associated with the procedure.

Nursing implications with rationale
Before
- ☞ Explain the procedure to the patient. Assure the patient that no discomfort is associated with the procedure.
- ☞ Inform the patient that fasting may be required, depending on the organ to be studied.
After
- ■ Remove the coupling agent (grease) from the patient's skin.

Alanine Aminotransferase (ALT, Serum Glutamate Pyruvate Transaminase [SGPT])

Test type Blood

Normal values
Elderly: may be slightly higher than adult
Adult/child: 5-35 IU/L or 8-20 U/L (SI units) (values may be higher in men and in black Americans)
Infant: may be twice as high as adult

Rationale
Alanine aminotransferase (ALT) is found predominantly in the liver; lesser quantities are found in the kidneys, heart, and skeletal muscle. Injury or disease affecting the liver parenchyma will cause a release of this hepatocellular enzyme into the bloodstream, thus elevating serum ALT levels. Most ALT elevations are caused by impaired liver function. Therefore, this enzyme is not only a sensitive, but also a specific, indicator of liver disease. In liver diseases other than viral hepatitis, the ALT/AST (see p. 15) ratio (DeRitis ratio) is less than 1. In viral hepatitis, the ratio is greater than 1. This is helpful in the diagnosis of viral hepatitis.

This test also indicates improvement or worsening of liver diseases. In patients with jaundice, an abnormal ALT will incriminate the liver rather than RBC hemolysis as a source of the jaundice.

Interfering factors

Factors that interfere with determining ALT levels include intramuscular (IM) injections, which may cause *elevated* levels.

Procedure

No special preparation is necessary for these liver enzyme studies. Approximately 7 to 10 ml of blood is collected in a red-top tube and sent to the laboratory for analysis.

Nursing implications with rationale

Before

☞ Explain the procedure to the patient. Tell the patient that no fasting is required.

During

■ Because many of these liver enzyme tests are affected by medications, to aid in interpretation of test results, indicate on the laboratory requisition slip any medications that the patient is taking.

After

■ Apply pressure or a pressure dressing to the venipuncture site to prevent further bleeding. Assess the site for bleeding, because patients with liver dysfunction often have prolonged clotting times (see p. 432).

Case Study

Gallbladder and Common Duct Stones

Mrs. R., a 44-year-old mother of seven children, was an obese woman. Two weeks before she was admitted to the hospital, she began to complain of right upper quadrant abdominal pain associated with nausea and vomiting. Two days before admission she noticed that her urine was very dark, and her stools were lighter in color. The results of her physical examination revealed she was mildly icteric. Her abdominal examination results indicated mild upper abdominal tenderness and muscle guarding. No other abnormalities were noted during her physical examination.

Studies	Results
Complete blood count (CBC), electrolyte, glucose, and blood urea nitrogen (BUN) determinations	Normal
Total serum bilirubin determination, p. 111	3.8 mg/dl (normal: 0.1-1.0 mg/dl)
Indirect fraction	1.0 mg/dl (normal: 0.2-0.8 mg/dl)
Direct fraction	2.8 mg/dl (normal: 0.1-0.3 mg/dl)
Urine bilirubin test, p. 111	+3 (normal: negative)
Liver enzymes test	
Serum aspartate aminotransferase, p. 15	46 IU/L (normal: 5-40 IU/L)
Serum alanine aminotransferase, p. 106	40 IU/L (normal: 5-35 IU/L)
Lactic dehydrogenase (LDH), p. 42	228 ImU/ml (normal: 90-200 ImU/ml)
Alkaline phosphatase (ALP), p. 108	885 ImU/ml (normal: 30-85 ImU/ml)
5'-nucleotidase, p. 132	2.4 units (normal: 0-1.6 units)
Leucine aminopeptidase (LAP), p. 127	250 units/ml (normal: 75-185 units/ml)
Serum gamma glutamyl transpeptidase (GGTP), p. 123	250 U/l (normal: 5-27 U/l)
Total serum protein test, p. 135	7.2 g/dl (normal: 6-8 g/dl)

Continued

Gallbladder and Common Duct Stones—cont'd

Serum albumin test, p. 135

4.2 g/dl (normal: 3.2-4.5 g/dl)

Prothrombin time (PT) test, p. 432

14.2 seconds (patient);
12.0 seconds (control)

Ultrasound examination of the liver and gallbladder, p. 105

Dilated intrahepatic and extrahepatic bile ducts; presence of stones within the gallbladder

Endoscopic retrograde cholangiopancreatography (ERCP), p. 118

Dilated common bile duct containing a gallstone

Diagnostic Analysis

Obstructive jaundice was suspected as the cause of this patient's complaints because of the increased levels of direct bilirubin, alkaline phosphatase, 5'-nucleotidase, GGTP, and LAP, along with the minimally elevated levels of AST and LDH. The urine bilirubin level corroborated the clinical finding of a direct type of hyperbilirubinemia. The prolonged PT resulted from impaired intestinal absorption of vitamin K and impaired hepatic synthesis of prothrombin and factors VII, IX, and X.

Ultrasound examination of the gallbladder revealed the presence of gallstones. However, it had to be verified that gallstones alone were the cause of the common bile duct obstruction, because patients with gallstones may also have a tumor obstructing this duct. The ERCP results indicated that only a gallstone was causing the common bile duct obstruction.

The patient underwent a sphincterotomy (papillotomy) of the ampulla of Vater. Common bile duct stones were removed. Laparoscopic cholecystectomy then was performed. The patient's postoperative course was uneventful. Her serum bilirubin level returned to normal. She returned to her normal physical activity in 5 days.

Critical Thinking Questions

1. Why was the patient's urine dark-colored?
2. What is the difference between a direct and an indirect type of hyperbilirubinemia?

Alkaline Phosphatase (ALP)

Test type Blood

Normal values

Elderly: slightly higher than adults
Adult: 30-85 ImU/ml or 42-128 U/L (SI units)
Child/adolescent:
   <2 years: 85-235 ImU/ml
   2-8 years: 65-210 ImU/ml
   9-15 years: 60-300 ImU/ml
   16-21 years: 30-200 ImU/ml

Rationale

Although alkaline phosphatase (ALP) is found in many tissues, the highest concentrations are found in the liver, biliary tract epithelium, and bone. This phosphatase enzyme is called alkaline because its function is increased in an alkaline (pH of 9 to 10) environment. Detection of this enzyme is important for determining liver and bone disorders. Within the liver, ALP is present in Kupffer's cells, which line the biliary collecting system. ALP is excreted into the bile. Enzyme levels of ALP are greatly increased in both extrahepatic and intrahepatic obstructive biliary disease and cirrhosis. Other liver abnormalities (e.g., hepatic tumors, hepatitis) and hepatoxic drugs cause lesser elevations in ALP levels.

Bone is the most common source of ALP outside the liver; new bone growth is associated with elevated ALP levels. Pathologic new bone growth occurs with osteoblastic, metastatic (e.g., breast, prostate) tumors. Paget's disease, healing fractures, rheumatoid arthritis, hyperparathyroidism, and normal-growing bones are sources of elevated ALP levels as well.

Isoenzymes of ALP also are used to distinguish between liver and bone diseases. ALP_1 would be high when liver pathology is the source of the elevated total ALP. ALP_2 would be high when bone pathology is the source of the elevated total ALP. Another way to separate the source of elevated ALP is to test simultaneously for 5'-nucleotidase, an enzyme that is made predominantly in the liver. If total ALP and 5'-nucleotidase are concomitantly elevated, the disease is in the liver. If the 5'-nucleotidase is normal, the bone is the most probable source.

Interfering factor

A factor that interferes with determining ALP levels is age. Young children with rapid bone growth have *increased* ALP levels. This is most magnified during growth spurts.

Procedure

No special preparation is necessary for these liver enzyme studies. Fasting is preferred, but not required. Approximately 7 to 10 ml of blood is collected in a red-top tube and sent to the laboratory for analysis.

Nursing implications with rationale

Before

☞ Explain the procedure to the patient. Tell the patient that fasting is preferred, but not required. An overnight fast may be required for isoenzymes.

During

- Many of these liver enzyme tests are affected by medications. To aid in interpretation of test results, indicate on the laboratory requisition slip any medications that the patient may be taking.

After

- Apply pressure or a pressure dressing to the venipuncture site to prevent further bleeding. Assess the site for bleeding because patients with liver dysfunction often have prolonged clotting times (see p. 432).

Ammonia

Test type Blood

Normal values

Adult: 15-110 mg/dl or 47-65 mmol/L (SI units)
Child: 40-80 mg/dl
Newborn: 90-150 mg/dl

Rationale

Ammonia is a by-product of protein catabolism. Most of it is made by bacteria acting on proteins present in the gut. The portal vein transports ammonia to the liver, where it normally is converted into urea and then secreted by the kidneys. With severe hepatocellular dysfunction, ammonia cannot be catabolized. Furthermore, when portal blood flow to the liver is altered (e.g., in portal hypertension), ammonia cannot reach the liver to be catabolized. As a result ammonia in the peripheral bloodstream rises. Ammonia levels also are used in the diagnosis and follow-up of hepatic encephalopathy (obtundation secondary to liver disease). High levels of ammonia result in encephalopathy and coma.

Interfering factors

Factors that interfere with determining ammonia levels include the following:

- Hemolysis
  This *increases* ammonia levels because the RBCs have approximately 3 times the ammonia level content of plasma.
- Muscular exertion, which can *increase* ammonia
- Cigarette smoking
  This can significantly *increase* ammonia levels within 1 hour of inhalation.
- Tight tourniquet for venipuncture

Ammonia levels may be factitiously *increased* if the tourniquet is tied too tightly or left on the extremity too long.

Procedure

Fasting is not usually required. Venous blood (5 to 7 ml) is collected in a green-top tube and sent to the laboratory for analysis.

Nursing implications with rationale

Before

☞ Explain the procedure to the patient. Tell the patient that no fasting is required.

During

■ Because many of these liver enzyme tests are affected by medications, to aid in interpretation of test results, indicate on the laboratory requisition slip any medications that the patient is taking. Certain antibiotics can cause a decreased ammonia level.

After

■ Apply pressure or a pressure dressing to the venipuncture site to prevent further bleeding. Assess the site for bleeding because patients with liver dysfunction often have prolonged clotting times (see p. 434).

Amylase, Serum/Urine

Test type Blood, urine

Normal values

Serum:
Adult: 56-190 IU/L, 80-150 Somogyi units/dl, or 25-125 U/L (SI units)
Newborn: 6-65 U/L
Values may be slightly increased during normal pregnancy and in the elderly

Urine:
3-35 IU/hr or 6-30 Wohlgemuth units/ml, up to 5000 Somogyi units/24 hr or 6.5-48.1 U/hr (SI units)

Possible critical values: More than 3 times the upper limit of normal serum level (depending on the method)

Rationale

Serum amylase is an easily and rapidly performed test that is most sensitive for pancreatitis. It is used to detect and monitor the clinical course of this disease. It frequently is ordered when a patient presents with acute abdominal pain. Amylase is normally secreted from the pancreatic acinar cell into the pancreatic duct and then into the duodenum. Once in the intestine, it aids the digestion of carbohydrates (starch) to their component simple sugars. Damage to pancreatic acinar cells (as in pancreatitis) or obstruction of the pancreatic duct flow (as in pancreatic carcinoma or common bile duct gallstones) causes an outpouring of this enzyme into the intrapancreatic lymph system and the free peritoneum. Blood vessels draining the free peritoneum and absorbing the lymph pick up the excess amylase. An abnormal rise in the serum level of amylase occurs within 12 hours of the onset of disease. Because amylase is cleared within 2 hours by the kidney, serum levels return to normal 48 to 72 hours after the initial insult. Persistent pancreatitis, duct obstruction, or pancreatic duct leak (e.g., pseudocysts) will cause persistent elevated serum amylase levels.

Urine amylase also is used to assist in making the diagnosis of pancreatitis. The urine amylase levels rise later than the blood levels. Several days after the onset of the disease process, serum amylase levels may be normal, but urine levels are significantly elevated. Urine amylase is particularly useful in detecting pancreatitis late in the disease course. Levels of urine amylase remain elevated 5 to 7 days after the onset of disease.

Although amylase is a sensitive test for pancreatic disorders, it is not specific. Other nonpancreatic diseases can cause elevated serum amylase levels. For example, in a bowel perforation, intraluminal amylase leaks into the free peritoneum and is picked up by the peritoneal blood vessels, resulting in an elevated serum amylase level. Also, a peptic ulcer penetrating into the pancreas will cause elevated amylase levels. Duodenal obstruction can be associated with less significant elevations in amylase. Because salivary glands contain amylase, elevations can be expected in patients with parotiditis (mumps).

Amylase also is found, in low levels, in the ovaries and skeletal muscles. Ectopic pregnancy and severe diabetic ketoacidosis are also associated with hyperamylasemia.

A comparison of the renal clearance ratio of amylase to creatinine provides more specific diagnostic information than either the urine amylase level or the serum amylase level alone. When the amylase/creatinine clearance ratio is 5% or more, the diagnosis of pancreatitis can be made with certainty. With ratios less than 5% in a patient having elevated serum and urine amylase levels, nonpancreatic pathologic conditions should be suspected (e.g., perforated bowel, macroamylasemia).

Patients with chronic pancreatic disorders (e.g., chronic pancreatitis) that have previously resulted in pancreatic cell destruction or patients with massive hemorrhagic pancreatic necrosis often do not have high amylase levels because very few pancreatic cells may remain to produce amylase.

Interfering factors

Factors that interfere with determining amylase levels include the following:

- Serum lipemia, which factitiously *decreases* amylase with current laboratory methods
- Intravenous (IV) dextrose solutions, which can lower amylase levels and cause false-negative results
- Drugs that may cause *increased* serum amylase levels, such as glucocorticoids and loop diuretics (e.g., furosemide)

Procedure

Blood is withdrawn from a peripheral vein and placed in a red-top tube. No fasting is required.

For urine testing, a timed 2-hour or 24-hour urine collection is required. A standard specimen container is used, and the specimen is refrigerated or kept on ice during the collection period.

Nursing implications with rationale
Blood
Before

☞ Explain the procedure to the patient. Tell the patient that no fasting is required.

During
- To aid in interpretation of test results, indicate on the laboratory requisition slip any medications that the patient is taking.

After
- Apply pressure or a pressure dressing to the site to prevent further bleeding.
- Note on the laboratory requisition slip if the patient is receiving IV dextrose, because dextrose can cause a false-negative result.

Urine
Before

☞ Explain the procedure to the patient. Give the patient the appropriate urine containers.

During
- Record the exact times of the beginning and the end of the collection period. The collection begins after the patient empties his or her bladder and discards that specimen. All subsequent urine is collected, including the one at the end of the collection period.

☞ Instruct the patient to void before defecating so that the urine is not contaminated by stool.

☞ Instruct the patient not to put toilet paper in the urine container.

- Encourage the patient to drink fluids during the collection period unless fluids are restricted for medical reasons.
- Keep the specimen on ice or refrigerated during the collection period.

After
- Send the specimen to the laboratory promptly.

Bilirubin

Test type Blood, urine

Normal values
Blood:
Adult/elderly/child

Total bilirubin: 0.1-1.0 mg/dl or 5.1-17.0 mmol/L (SI units)

Indirect bilirubin: 0.2-0.8 mg/dl or 3.4-12.0 mmol/L (SI units)

Direct bilirubin: 0.1-0.3 mg/dl or 1.7-5.1 mmol/L (SI units)

Newborn total bilirubin: 1-12 mg/dl or 17.1-20.5 mmol/L (SI units)

Urine: 0-0.02 mg/dl

Possible critical values (blood): Adults: >12 mg/dl

Newborns: >15 mg/dl. In these newborns, immediate treatment is required to avoid kernicterus.

Rationale

The total serum bilirubin determination measures both direct (conjugated) and indirect (unconjugated) bilirubin. (See discussion of bilirubin metabolism and excretion, pp. 103.) The total serum bilirubin level is the sum of the direct and indirect bilirubin levels. Normally, the indirect (unconjugated) bilirubin makes up 70% to 85% of the total bilirubin. In patients with jaundice, when more than 50% of the bilirubin is direct (conjugated), it is considered a direct hyperbilirubinemia from gallstones, tumor, inflammation, scarring, or obstruction of the extrahepatic ducts. Indirect hyperbilirubinemia exists when less than 15% to 20% of the total bilirubin is direct bilirubin. Typical causes of this form of jaundice include diseases such as accelerated erythrocyte (RBC) hemolysis or hepatitis, and drugs such as antibiotics, diuretics, barbiturates, phenothiazines, or oral contraceptives.

When the defect in bilirubin metabolism occurs after conjugation, elevated levels of direct (conjugated) bilirubin result. Unlike the unconjugated form, direct bilirubin is water-soluble and can be excreted into the urine. Therefore, bilirubin in urine suggests disease affecting bilirubin metabolism after conjugation or defects in excretion (e.g., gallstones). There normally may be a small amount of bilirubin in the urine. Testing for bilirubin is a part of routine urine analysis.

Once the jaundice is recognized, it is important to differentiate for therapeutic purposes whether it is predominantly caused by indirect (unconjugated) or direct (conjugated) bilirubin. This, in turn, will help differentiate the etiology of the jaundice. In general, jaundice caused by hepato-cellular dysfunction (e.g., hepatitis) results in elevated levels of indirect bilirubin. This usually cannot be repaired surgically. On the other hand, jaundice resulting from extrahepatic dysfunction (e.g., gallstones or tumor blocking the bile ducts) results in elevated levels of direct bilirubin; this type of jaundice usually can be resolved surgically or endoscopically.

Procedure

For blood testing, a peripheral venipuncture is performed, and one red-top tube of blood is collected. A heel puncture is used for blood collection in infants, and two blood microtubes are filled. No fasting is required.

For urine testing, a spot urine test is performed. At least 10 ml of urine is collected for quick, simple testing. Reagent strips (e.g., Multistix) or tablets (e.g., Icotest) are used.

Nursing implications with rationale

Before

- Explain the purpose of the test to the patient and follow specific hospital guidelines regarding fasting. Some guidelines require fasting after midnight.
- Medications that affect the serum bilirubin level may be held as ordered for at least 24 hours before the test.

During

- The blood specimen should not be exposed to sunlight or artificial light because this may reduce the bilirubin content.
- List any medications that the patient is taking on the laboratory requisition slip to aid in test interpretation.
- If testing the urine with reagent strips, compare the strip to the color chart on the label of the bottle after 20 to 30 seconds, according to the directions.

After

- Apply pressure or a pressure dressing to the venipuncture site to prevent further bleeding. Assess the site for bleeding because patients with liver dysfunction often have prolonged clotting times (see p. 434).

■ Do not reuse reagent strips or Icotest tablets for urine testing.

Computed Tomography of the Abdomen (CAT Scan of the Abdomen, CT Scan of the Abdomen)

Test type X-ray with contrast dye

Normal values
No evidence of abnormality

Rationale
The computed tomography (CT) scan of the abdomen is a noninvasive, yet very accurate, radiographic procedure used to diagnose pathologic conditions (e.g., tumors, cysts, abscesses, inflammation, bowel perforation, intraabdominal bleeding, intestinal or ureteral obstruction, vascular aneurysms, and calculi) in the abdominal and retroperitoneal organs. The CT scan image results from passing x-rays through the abdominal organs at many angles. The variation in density of each tissue allows for a variable penetration of the x-rays. Each density is given a numeric value called a *density coefficient*, which is digitally computed into shades of gray. This then is displayed on a television screen as thousands of dots in various shades of gray. The final display appears as an actual photograph of the anatomic area sectioned by x-rays (Figure 4-5). The image can be enhanced by repeating the CT scan after IV administration of iodine-containing contrast dye. The image can be recorded on radiographic film.

Liver tumors, abscesses, trauma, cysts, and anatomic abnormalities can be seen. Pancreatic tumors, pseudocysts, inflammation, calcification, bleeding, and trauma can be detected. The kidneys and urinary outflow tract are well-visualized.

Renal tumors and cysts, ureteral obstruction, calculi, and congenital renal and ureteral abnormalities are seen easily with IV contrast injection. Extravasation of urine secondary to trauma or obstruction also can be easily demonstrated. Adrenal tumors and hyperplasia are best diagnosed with

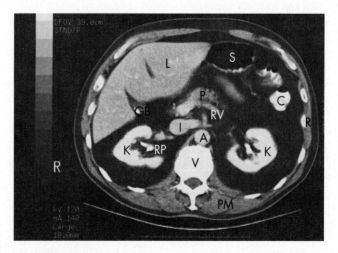

Figure 4-5 Computed tomography (CT) of the abdomen. Normally many abdominal structures can be seen on a CT scan. *L*, Liver; *GB*, gallbladder (containing a gallstone-radiolucent area); *K*, kidney; *RV*, left renal vein; *RP*, pelvis of the right renal collecting system; *V*, vertebra; *I*, inferior vena cava; *A*, aorta; *C*, the splenic flexure of the colon (contrast filled); *S*, air/contrast-filled stomach; *P*, pancreas; *R*, bony ribs of the lower chest; *PM* paraspinal muscles of the back.

CT. Some radiology literature indicates that the histology of the tumor can be suggested based on the density coefficients shown on the scan.

Although the bowel can be visualized better by an upper GI series, small-bowel follow-through, or barium enema, large tumors and bowel perforations can be identified with the CT scan, especially when oral contrast is ingested. The spleen can be well visualized for hematoma, laceration, fracture, tumor infiltration, and splenic vein thrombosis. The retroperitoneal lymph nodes can be evaluated. These nodes are present normally; however, all nodes with a diameter greater than 2 cm are considered abnormal. The abdominal aorta and its major branches can be evaluated for aneurysmal dilation and intramural thrombi, and the pelvic structures (including the uterus, ovaries, fallopian tubes, prostate, and rectum) and musculature can be evaluated for tumors, abscesses, infection, or hypertrophy. Ascites and hemoperitoneum can easily be demonstrated with the CT scan.

With the development of newer and faster scanners, dynamic scanning can be performed during arterial injection of dye to the organ being studied. Dynamic scanning can indicate the blood flow and degree of vascularity of an organ or part of an organ in the abdomen. This is called *dynamic CT scanning* (see CT portography, p. 117).

CT can be used to aspirate fluid from the abdomen, or one of the abdominal organs, for cultures and other studies; to guide needles into abdominal tumors to obtain tissue for biopsy; and to guide catheter placement for drainage of intraabdominal abscesses.

The CT scan is an important part of staging and monitoring many tumors before and after therapy. Treatment of tumors of the colon, rectum, liver, breast, lung, prostate, ovary, uterus, kidney, and lymph and adrenal glands commonly fails, and this can be detected early with the CT scan.

Potential complications

Potential complications associated with CT of the abdomen are as follows:

- Allergic reaction to iodinated dye
  Allergic reactions vary from flushing, itching,

and urticaria to life-threatening anaphylaxis (evidenced by respiratory distress, drop in blood pressure, and/or shock). In the unusual event of anaphylaxis, diphenhydramine (Benadryl), steroids, and epinephrine are added to routine resuscitative efforts. Oxygen and endotracheal equipment should be on hand for immediate use.
- Acute renal failure from dye infusion
  Adequate hydration before the test may reduce the likelihood of this complication occurring.

Interfering factors

Factors that interfere with CT of the abdomen include the following:

- Presence of metallic objects (e.g., hemostasis clips), which can obscure visualization
- Retained barium from previous studies, which can obscure visualization

Procedure

The patient is kept fasting for 4 hours before the test. Sedation is rarely required and is induced only with a patient who cannot remain still during the procedure. The patient is taken to the radiology department and asked to remain motionless, usually in the supine position, because any motion causes blurring and streaking of the final image. An encircling radiographic camera (body scanner) takes pictures at varying levels (usually 1 to 2 cm apart) of the abdomen from the pubis to the xiphoid process.

The patient may be given a radiographic water-soluble dye by mouth, by IV, or occasionally via the rectum, depending on the type of scan being performed. This contrast agent helps to delineate the margins of the abdominal structure.

The patient is asked to hold his or her breath for a few seconds while each x-ray is being taken. The images are immediately displayed on a monitor and are recorded on film. The procedure takes about 30 minutes and is painless.

Contraindications

Contraindications for CT of the abdomen are as follows:

- Allergies to iodinated dye or shellfish
- Pregnancy
- Unstable vital signs
- Obesity
  The CT table cannot hold patients who weigh more than 300 pounds.

Nursing implications with rationale

Before

☞ Explain the procedure to the patient. The patient's cooperation is necessary because he or she must lie still during the procedure.

☞ Show the patient a picture of the CT machine (Figure 4-6). Encourage the patient to verbalize his or her concerns because some patients may have claustrophobia. Most patients who are mildly claustrophobic can be scanned after premedication with antianxiety drugs.

☞ Instruct the patient to remain NPO (*nil per os*, nothing by mouth) for 4 hours before the test.

Food in the stomach or duodenum may confuse the final picture. Mild nausea may occur after injection of contrast dyes.

- Not all hospitals have CT equipment. You may have to make arrangements to transport the patient to another facility.
- Assess the patient for allergies to iodinated dye or shellfish. Inform the radiologist if an allergy to iodinated contrast is suspected. The radiologist may prescribe diphenhydramine and a steroid preparation to be administered before testing. Usually a hypoallergenic, nonionic contrast will be used during the test.

After

☞ Encourage the patient to drink fluids to avoid dye-induced renal failure and to promote dye excretion.

☞ Inform the patient that diarrhea may occur after ingestion of the oral contrast medium.

- Evaluate the patient for delayed reaction to dye (dyspnea, rashes, tachycardia, hives). This may occur 2 to 6 hours after the test.

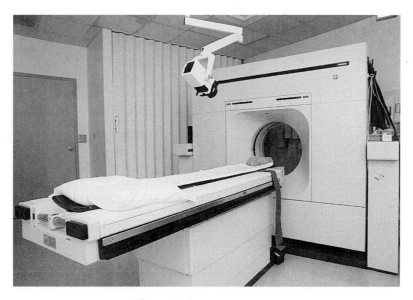

Figure 4-6 CT equipment.

Case Study

Pancreatitis

Mr. D., 52 years old, was admitted to the hospital complaining of severe epigastric pain with radiation to his back. The pain started on the day before admission and was associated with nausea and vomiting. On examination he was found to be dehydrated and to have only mild epigastric midline tenderness and guarding. He denied a recent alcohol debauch. Because of previous symptoms, Mr. D. had undergone an ultrasound of the gallbladder, the results of which were normal.

Studies	Results
Routine laboratory studies	Within normal limits (WNL) except for white blood cells (WBCs), which were 15,000/mm^3 (normal WBC: 5000-10,000/mm^3)
Serum amylase test, p. 110	640 IU/L (normal: 56-190 IU/L)
Urine amylase test, p. 110	1240 IU/hr (normal: 3-35 IU/hr)
Serum lipase test, p. 127	240 units/L (normal: 0-110 units/L)
Ultrasound examination of pancreas, p. 105	Edematous and enlarged head of the pancreas
CT scanning of abdomen, p. 113	Diffusely edematous and enlarged pancreas
ERCP, p. 118	Normal pancreatic duct

Diagnostic Analysis

The diagnosis of pancreatitis was certain in light of the elevation of both the serum and urine amylase levels and also of the serum lipase level. Alcohol and gallstones are the two most common causes of pancreatitis. However, the patient denied drinking alcohol, and previous ultrasound of the gallbladder excluded gallstones. Because cancer of the pancreas also can cause distal pancreatic inflammation, tumor had to be ruled out as a cause of this pancreatitic episode. Ultrasonography, which is occasionally inaccurate for pathologic pancreatic conditions, indicated an enlarged head of the pancreas that could be compatible with a tumor. However, CT scanning and ERCP results eliminated the possibility of cancer.

The patient was treated with nasogastric (NG) suction and IV infusions until his GI function returned to normal. His pancreatitis was subsequently found to be drug induced (by hydrochlorothiazide). The drug was stopped, and he had no further problems.

Critical Thinking Questions

1. Why was it important to question this patient about binge drinking?
2. What advantage is achieved by obtaining urine amylase levels in addition to serum amylase levels?

Computed Tomography Portogram (CT Portogram)

Test type X-ray wiht contrast dye

Normal values
No evidence of liver abnormalities

Rationale
A CT scan of the liver (see p. 113) is inaccurate in identifying hepatic tumors smaller than 2 cm. A CT portogram can accurately identify liver abnormalities as small as 5 mm. The difference between a CT scan of the liver and a CT portogram is the manner in which the contrast dye is injected. In a routine CT scan, dye is injected through a peripheral vein. In a CT portogram, dye is injected through a catheter that is placed in the splenic artery. The dye passes through the spleen and into the splenic vein and, subsequently, into the portal vein and its tributaries. Hepatic tumors and cysts, however, do not take up dye. On the portogram, these lesions appear as a filling defect (dark spots) in the liver.

Use of this test is limited to identification of suspected smaller neoplasms in the liver. It is used in cancer patients who are suspected to have liver metastasis.

Potential complications
Potential complications associated with CT portogram are as follows:

- Allergic reaction to iodinated dye
  Allergic reactions vary from flushing, itching, and urticaria to life-threatening anaphylaxis (evidenced by respiratory distress, drop in blood pressure, and/or shock). In the unusual event of anaphylaxis, diphenhydramine, steroids, and epinephrine are added to routine resuscitative efforts. Oxygen and endotracheal equipment should be on hand for immediate use.
- Hemorrhage from the arterial puncture site used for arterial access
- Arterial embolism from dislodgment of an arteriosclerotic plaque
- Soft tissue infection around the puncture site
- Renal failure, especially in elderly patients who are chronically dehydrated or have a mild degree of renal failure
- Pseudoaneurysm as a result of the puncture site's failure to seal

Procedure
The patient is kept NPO for at least 2 to 4 hours before testing. The patient may be sedated before being taken to the angiography room, usually located in the radiology department. The patient is placed on the x-ray table in the supine position. If the femoral artery is to be used, the groin is shaved, prepared, and draped in a sterile manner. The femoral artery is cannulated, and a wire is threaded up that artery and into or near the opening of the splenic artery. A catheter is placed over that wire and into the splenic artery. The patient is transferred to the CT scan unit, also usually located in the radiology department. Iodinated contrast material is injected through the catheter and into the splenic artery. CT scan images are taken immediately after the injection of dye.

Placement of the arterial catheter, which is done by a radiologist, takes about 30 minutes and is minimally uncomfortable. CT scan imaging takes about 15 minutes and is not uncomfortable.

Contraindications
Contraindications for CT portograms are patients with a bleeding propensity, which could lead to bleeding at the femoral arterial puncture site

Nursing implications with rationale
Before
- Explain the procedure to the patient. Instruct the patient to fast 2 to 4 hours before the test. Allay any fears and allow the patient to verbalize concerns.
- Ensure that written and informed consent for this procedure is in the patient's chart.
- Assess the patient for allergies to iodinated dye or shellfish. Inform the radiologist if an allergy to iodinated contrast is suspected. The

radiologist may prescribe diphenhydramine and a steroid preparation to be administered before the test. Usually, hypoallergenic, non-ionic contrast will be used during the test.

- Determine if the patient has been taking anti-coagulants. Abnormal coagulation studies may delay the study.
- Mark the site of the patient's peripheral pulses before arterial catheterization so that these pulses may be assessed easily after the procedure.

After

- Monitor the vital signs carefully for indications of hemorrhage (increased pulse and decreased blood pressure).
- Assess the peripheral pulses in the extremity used for vascular access and compare them with the preprocedural baseline values.
- Maintain pressure at the puncture site with a 1- to 2-pound sandbag or an IV bag for several hours.
- Instruct the patient to remain on bed rest for approximately 4 to 8 hours to allow for complete sealing of the arterial puncture site.
- Evaluate the patient for delayed allergic reaction to the dye (dyspnea, rash, tachycardia, hives). This usually occurs within 2 to 6 hours after the test. Treat the patient with antihistamines or steroids.

Endoscopic Retrograde Cholangiopancreatography (ERCP, ERCP of the Biliary and Pancreatic Ducts)

Test type Endoscopy

Normal values
Normal size of biliary and pancreatic ducts
No obstruction or filling defects within the biliary or pancreatic ducts

Rationale
With the use of a fiberoptic endoscope, endoscopic retrograde cholangiopancreatography (ERCP) provides radiographic visualization of the bile and pancreatic ducts. This is especially useful in patients with jaundice. If a partial or total obstruction of those ducts exists, characteristics of the obstructing lesion can be demonstrated. Stones, benign strictures, cysts, ampullary stenosis, anatomic variations, and malignant tumors can be identified. Only ERCP and percutaneous transhepatic cholangiography (PTHC) (see p. 133) can provide direct radiographic visualization of the biliary and pancreatic ducts. PTHC is an invasive procedure with significant morbidity; ERCP is associated with much less morbidity.

In contrast to oral cholecystogram or an IV cholangiogram, which are rarely performed anymore and do not visualize the biliary tree when high levels of bilirubin are present, the biliary ducts of patients with jaundice can be visualized by ERCP. As a result, this test is extremely important in the evaluation of such patients.

Incision of the sphincter muscle in the ampulla of Vater can be performed through the scope at the time of ERCP. This incision widens the distal common duct so that common bile duct gallstones can be removed. Stents can be placed through strictured bile ducts during ERCP and allow the bile of patients with jaundice to be drained into the duodenum. Pieces of tissue and brushings of the common bile duct can be obtained by ERCP for pathologic review.

Potential complications
Potential complications associated with ERCP are as follows:

- Perforation of the esophagus, stomach, or duodenum by forceful progression of the scope
- Gram-negative sepsis
  This results from introducing bacteria through the biliary system and into the blood. Usually, this occurs in patients who have obstructive jaundice.
- Pancreatitis
  This results from pressure of the dye injection.
- Aspiration of gastric contents into the lungs during the procedure

Interfering factor

A factor that interferes with ERCP is barium within the abdomen as a result of a previous upper GI series or barium enema studies. This precludes adequate visualization of the biliary and pancreatic ducts.

Procedure

The patient is kept NPO after midnight on the day of the test. The patient is placed in the supine or left lateral decubitus position. A flat plate of the abdomen (kidney, ureter, and bladder) may be done before this study to ensure that any barium from previous studies is not obscuring visualization. The patient is usually premedicated intravenously with diazepam (Valium) or midazolam (Versed) and meperidine (Demerol) or butorphanol (Stadol). A side-viewing fiberoptic duodenoscope is inserted through the oral pharynx and passed through the esophagus and stomach and into the duodenum (Figure 4-7). At this time, the patient is given 0.4 mg glucagon intravenously to paralyze the duodenum so that the ampulla of Vater can be located more easily. Through an accessory lumen within the scope, a small catheter

is passed through the ampulla of Vater and enters into either the common bile duct or pancreatic duct. Radiographic dye is injected, and films are taken. The patient does not feel any discomfort with the dye injection. The duration of this test is about 1 hour.

Contraindications

Contraindications for ERCP are as follows:

- Patients who are uncooperative
  Cannulation of the ampulla of Vater requires that the patient lie very still.
- Patients whose ampulla of Vater is not accessible endoscopically because of previous upper GI surgery
  An example is gastrectomy patients whose duodenum containing the ampulla is surgically separated from the stomach.
- Patients with esophageal diverticula
  The scope can fall into a diverticulum and perforate its wall.
- Patients with known acute pancreatitis
  ERCP can worsen this inflammation.

Nursing implications with rationale

Before

☞ Explain the procedure to the patient. Assure the patient that breathing will not be compromised by the insertion of the endoscope.

☞ Instruct the patient to remain NPO after midnight the day of the test.

■ Make sure the written and informed consent for this procedure is obtained before premedicating the patient.

☞ Tell the patient that the test takes approximately 1 hour, during which time he or she must lie completely motionless on a hard x-ray table. Remaining still for this period may be uncomfortable for the patient.

After

■ Do not give the patient anything to eat or drink until the gag reflex returns.

■ Maintain safety precautions until the effects of the sedatives have worn off.

■ If ordered, obtain a serum amylase determination the day following the procedure. Occa-

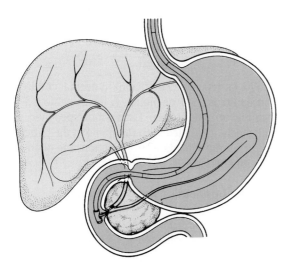

Figure 4-7 Endoscopic retrograde cholangiopancreatography. The fiberoptic scope is passed into the duodenum. Note the small catheter being advanced into the biliary duct.

sionally the pressure of the injection into the main pancreatic duct causes an acute bout of pancreatitis.

- Monitor the patient's temperature, heart rate, and blood pressure as ordered. Assess the patient for signs of bacteremia or septicemia. Notify the physician immediately if fever or shaking chills occur. These may indicate possible cholangitis.
- Notify the doctor immediately if increasing abdominal pain, nausea, or vomiting occurs. These may be the early signs of pancreatitis or gastroduodenal perforation.
- Inform the patient that a sore throat is expected. Drinking cool fluids and gargling with a soothing mouthwash may help.
- Encourage the patient to eat lightly for the next 12 to 24 hours.

Fecal Fat (Fat Absorption, Quantitative Stool Fat Determination)

Test type Stool

Normal values
Fat: 5 g/24 hr
Retention coefficient: ≥95%

Rationale
The fecal fat test is performed to confirm the diagnosis of steatorrhea. Steatorrhea is suspected when the patient has large, greasy, and foul-smelling stools. An abnormally high fecal fat content confirms the diagnosis. The total output of fecal fat per 24 hours in a 72-hour stool collection provides the most reliable measurement.

Children with cystic fibrosis have mucous plugs that obstruct the pancreatic ducts. The pancreatic enzymes (amylase, lipase, trypsin, and chymotrypsin) cannot be expelled into the duodenum and, therefore, are either completely absent or present only in diminished quantities within the GI tract. Lipase and bicarbonate are lipolytic, and without them fat is not digested for absorption. This results in impaired fat absorption (malabsorption) and steatorrhea.

Fecal fat analysis is not specific to cystic fibrosis. Any condition that may cause malabsorption (e.g., sprue, Crohn's disease, Whipple's disease) or maldigestion (e.g., bile duct obstruction, pancreatic duct obstruction secondary to tumor or gallstones) is also associated with increased fecal fat. Short-gut syndrome also increases fecal fat.

Interfering factors
Factors that interfere with fecal fat levels include laxatives, especially mineral oil, which may *increase* levels of fecal fat.

Procedure
For quantitative stool analysis, a timed stool collection and a standard amount of dietary fat are essential. Generally, a 3- to 5-day stool collection is obtained because of daily variations in the amount of fecal fat. The standard fat-content diet should begin 2 to 3 days before the stool collection and should continue throughout the collection period. Usually, 100 g of fat per day is recommended for adults. In children and infants who cannot eat 100 g of fat per day, a fat retention coefficient is determined by measuring the difference between ingested fat and fecal fat and then expressing that difference (the amount of fat retained) as a percentage of the ingested fat.

$$\frac{\text{Ingested fat} - \text{Fecal fat}}{\text{Ingested fat}} \times 100\%$$

The fat retention coefficient in normal children and adults is 95% or higher. A lower value is indicative of steatorrhea. Each stool specimen is collected and labeled with the name of the patient and the time and date of collection and then is sent immediately to the laboratory.

Nursing implications with rationale
Before
- Explain the purpose of this test and the procedure of stool collection to the patient (and to the parents).
- Instruct the patient to defecate into a dry, clean bedpan or container. Give the patient tongue blades to transfer the stool, if needed. For an infant, the diapers must be examined

for stools and the stools transferred to the container.

☞ Instruct the patient not to urinate into the stool container or bedpan.

☞ Inform the patient that diarrheal stools should also be collected.

☞ Explain to the patient that toilet paper should not be placed into the stool container because it interferes with stool analysis.

☞ Instruct the patient not to take any laxatives or enemas during this test, because they interfere with intestinal motility and alter test results.

After

■ Label all specimens appropriately and send them to the laboratory immediately after collection.

■ If the specimen is collected at home, give the patient a large stool container to keep in the freezer.

Gallbladder Nuclear Scanning
(Hepatobiliary Scintigraphy, Hepatobiliary Imaging, Biliary Tract Radionuclide Scan, Cholescintigraphy, DISIDA Scanning, HIDA Scanning, IDA Gallbladder Scanning)

Test type Nuclear scan

Normal values

Gallbladder, common bile duct, and duodenum visualize within 60 minutes after radionuclide injection

Rationale

Through the use of iminodiacetic acid analogues (IDAs) labeled with technetium 99m (Tc 99m), the biliary tract can be evaluated in a safe, accurate, and noninvasive manner. These radionuclide compounds are extracted by the liver and excreted into the bile. When gamma rays are emitted from the Tc 99m in the bile through the body, they are arranged in a spatial order and a realistic image of the biliary tree becomes apparent (Figure 4-8). Cholescintigraphy is valuable in evaluating patients for suspected gallbladder disease.

The primary use of this study is to diagnose acute cholecystitis in patients who have acute right upper quadrant abdominal pain. Failure to visualize the gallbladder 60 to 120 minutes after injection of the radionuclide dye is diagnostic of an obstruction of the cystic duct, which instigates acute cholecystitis. Delayed filling of the gallbladder is associated with chronic or acalculus cholecystitis. This procedure also is helpful in diagnosing biliary duct obstructions. The identification of the radionuclide in the biliary tree, but not in the bowel, is diagnostic of common bile duct obstruction.

This procedure is superior to oral cholecystography, IV cholangiography, ultrasonography, and CT of the gallbladder in the detection of cholecystitis. Also, with cholescintigraphy, gallbladder function can be determined numerically by calculating the capability of the gallbladder to eject its contents. It is believed that an ejection fraction below 35% indicates primary gallbladder disease.

Occasionally, morphine sulfate is given intravenously during nuclear scanning. The morphine causes increased ampullary contraction. Not only can this reproduce the patient's symptoms of biliary colic, but also it serves to force the bile containing the radionuclide into the gallbladder. If no radionuclide is seen in the gallbladder, with the use of morphine within 15 to 60 minutes, the diagnosis of acute cholecystitis is nearly certain.

Interfering factors

A factor that interferes with gallbladder nuclear scanning is prolonged fasting. If the patient has not eaten for more than 24 hours, the radionuclide may not fill the gallbladder. This would produce a false-positive result.

Procedure

After a 4-hour fast the patient reports to the radiology department and is placed in the supine position on an x-ray table. After an IV injection of Tc-99m–IDA derivative (e.g., DISIDA, PIPIDA, HIDA), the right upper quadrant of the abdomen is scanned. The HIDA or PIPIDA scans are

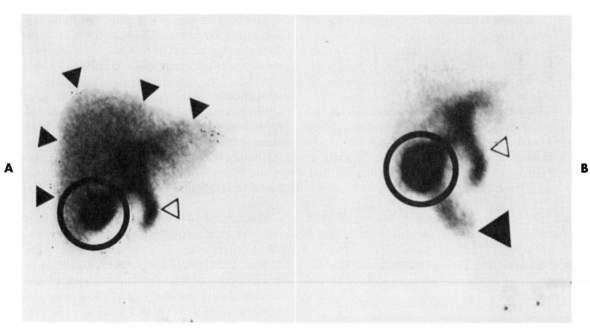

Figure 4-8   **A,** Normal gallbladder scan. Solid pointers indicate outline of the liver. Gallbladder is circled. Pointer outline indicates normal common bile duct. **B,** Normal gallbladder scan, later in time. Liver is now less well defined because most of the radionuclide is in the biliary tree. Duodenum *(solid black pointer)* now visibly contains radionuclide.

most useful in assessing the patency of the biliary tree since these radionuclides are secreted by the hepatocytes into the bile canaliculi. Serial images are obtained over an hour. Subsequent images can be obtained at 10- to 15-minute intervals. A right lateral view is taken to document the anterior position of the gallbladder. If the gallbladder, common bile duct, and duodenum are not seen within 60 minutes after the injection, delayed images up to 4 hours may be obtained. Some patients are given a fatty meal or cholecytokinin to evaluate the emptying of the gallbladder and the ejection fraction.

The only discomfort associated with this procedure is that of the IV injection of radionuclide. However, many patients complain about lying on the hard x-ray table. A radiologist or physician trained in nuclear medicine performs this study in approximately 1 to 4 hours.

Contraindications

A contraindication for gallbladder nuclear scanning is pregnancy, because of the risk of fetal injury.

Nursing implications with rationale

Before

☞ Explain the procedure to the patient. Instruct the patient to fast 4 hours before the procedure. Many patients without any cystic duct obstruction fail to demonstrate the gallbladder if they are not in the fasting state.

After

■ Obtain a meal for the patient.

☞ Assure the patient that he or she was not exposed to large amounts of radioactivity because only tracer doses of the radioisotopes are used.

Gamma-Glutamyl Transpeptidase
(GGTP, g-GTP, Gamma-Glutamyl Transferase [GGT])

Test type Blood

Normal values
Male and female over age 45: 8-38 U/L
Female under age 45: 5-27 U/L
Elderly: slightly higher than adult level
Child: similar to adult level
Newborn: 5 times higher than adult level

Rationale
The highest concentrations of gamma-glutamyl transpeptidase (GGTP) are found in the liver and biliary tract. Lesser concentrations are found in the kidney, spleen, heart, intestine, brain, and prostate. Tiny amounts have been detected in endothelial cells of capillaries. This test detects liver cell dysfunction, and it very accurately indicates even the slightest degree of cholestasis. GGTP is the most sensitive liver enzyme in detecting biliary obstruction, cholangitis, or cholecystitis. As with leucine aminopeptidase and 5′-nucleotidase, the elevation of GGTP generally parallels that of alkaline phosphatase; however, GGTP is more sensitive. Also, as with 5′-nucleotidase and leucine aminopeptidase, GGTP is not increased in bone diseases as is alkaline phosphatase. A normal GGTP level with an elevated alkaline phosphatase (ALP) level would imply skeletal disease. An elevated GGTP and elevated ALP level would imply hepatobiliary disease. GGTP also is not elevated in childhood or pregnancy as ALP usually is.

Another important clinical aspect of GGTP is that it can detect chronic alcohol ingestion. GGTP is elevated in approximately 75% of patients who chronically drink alcohol. Therefore, it is very useful in the screening and evaluation of alcoholic patients.

Why this enzyme is elevated after an acute myocardial infarction (MI) is not clear. It may represent the associated hepatic insult (if elevation occurs in the first 7 days) or the proliferation of capillary endothelial cells in the granulation tissue that replaces the infarcted myocardium. The elevation usually occurs 1 to 2 weeks after MI.

Procedure
No special preparation is necessary for these liver enzyme studies. Approximately 7 to 10 ml of blood is collected in a red-top tube and sent to the laboratory for analysis.

Nursing implications with rationale
Before
☞ Explain the procedure to the patient. Tell the patient that no fasting is required.
During
■ Because many of these liver enzyme tests are affected by medications, to aid in interpretation of test results, indicate on the laboratory requisition slip any medications that the patient is taking.
After
■ Apply pressure or a pressure dressing to the venipuncture site to prevent further bleeding. Assess the site for bleeding because patients with liver dysfunction often have prolonged clotting times (see p. 432).

Hepatitis Virus Studies
(Hepatitis-Associated Antigen [HAA], Australian Antigen)

Test type Blood

Normal values
Negative

Rationale
This group of tests is used to diagnose and identify serologically the type and current status of hepatitis. *Hepatitis* is an inflammation of the liver caused by viruses, alcohol ingestion, drugs, toxins, or overwhelming bacterial sepsis. The three most common viruses now recognized to cause disease are hepatitis A, hepatitis B, and hepatitis

non-A/non-B (also called hepatitis C) viruses. Hepatitis D and E viruses are much less common in the United States. The various types of hepatitis cannot be differentiated based on clinical presentation because they all may present as low-grade fever, malaise, anorexia, and tiredness. Usually, they are all associated with elevations of hepatocellular enzymes such as AST, ALT, and LDH (see p. 15, 106, 42, respectively).

Hepatitis A virus (HAV) originally was called *infectious hepatitis*. It has a short incubation period of 2 to 6 weeks and is highly contagious. During active infection, HAV is excreted in the stool and transmitted via the oral-fecal contamination of food and drink. Although immunologic tests are not yet available to detect HAV antigen, two types of antibodies to HAV can be detected.

The first type of antibody to HAV is immunoglobulin (Ig) M antibody (HAV-Ab/IgM), which appears approximately 3 to 4 weeks after exposure or just before hepatocellular enzyme elevations occur. These IgM levels usually return to normal in approximately 8 weeks.

The second type of antibody is IgG (HAV-Ab/IgG), which appears approximately 2 weeks after the beginning of the IgM increase and slowly returns to normal levels. The IgG enzyme can remain detectable for more than 10 years after the infection. If the IgM antibody is elevated in the absence of the IgG antibody, acute hepatitis is suspected. If, however, IgG is elevated in the absence of IgM elevation, this indicates the convalescent or chronic stage of HAV viral infection.

Hepatitis B virus (HBV) commonly is known as *serum hepatitis*. It has a long incubation period of 5 weeks to 6 months. HBV is most frequently transmitted by blood transfusion; however, it also can be contracted via exposure to other body fluids. HBV may cause a severe and unrelenting form of hepatitis ending in liver failure and death. Its incidence is increased among blood transfusion recipients, male homosexuals, patients receiving dialysis or transplants, IV drug abusers, and patients with leukemia or lymphoma. Hospital personnel are also at increased risk of infection, mostly as a result of needle stick contamination. Besides the acute phase of HBV, carrier

and chronic states of this disease have been recognized.

The HBV, also called the *Dane particle,* is composed of an inner core surrounded by an outer capsule. The outer capsule contains the hepatitis B surface antigen (HBsAg), formerly called *Australian antigen.* The inner core contains HBV core antigen (HBcAg). The hepatitis B e-antigen (HBeAg) is also found within the core. Antibodies to these antigens are called *hepatitis B surface antibody (HBsAb), hepatitis B core antibody (HBcAb),* and *hepatitis B e-antibody (HBeAb).* The tests used to detect these antigens and antibodies are as follows:

1. HBsAg. This is the most frequently and easily performed test for hepatitis B and is the first test to indicate abnormality. HBsAg rises before the onset of clinical symptoms, peaks during the first week of symptoms, and returns to normal by the time jaundice subsides. HBsAg generally indicates active infection by HBV. If the level of this antigen persists in the blood, the patient is considered to be a carrier.

2. HBsAb. This antibody appears approximately 4 weeks after the disappearance of the surface antigen and signifies the end of the acute infection phase. HBsAb also signifies immunity to subsequent infection. Concentrated forms of this agent constitute the hyperimmunoglobulin given to patients who have come in contact with HBV-infected patients (e.g., contact by an inadvertent needle prick from a needle used on a patient with HBV infection). HBsAb is the antibody that denotes immunity after administration of hepatitis B vaccine.

3. HBcAb. This antibody appears approximately 1 month after infection with HBsAg and declines (although it remains elevated) over several years. HBcAb is also present in patients with chronic hepatitis. The HBcAb level is elevated during the time lag between the disappearance of HBsAg and the appearance of HBsAb. This interval is called the *core window.* During the core window,

HBcAb is the only detectable marker of a recent hepatitis infection.

4. HBeAg. This antigen generally is not used for diagnostic purposes but rather as an index of infectivity. The presence of HBeAg correlates with early and active disease, as well as with high infectivity in acute HBV infection. The persistent presence of HBeAg in the blood predicts the development of chronic HBV infection.

5. HBeAb. This antibody indicates that an acute phase of HBV infection is over, or almost over, and that the chance of infectivity is greatly reduced.

No tests are currently available to detect HBcAg.

Non-A, non-B hepatitis (NANB), also called *hepatitis C (HCV),* is transmitted in a manner similar to HBV. Most hepatitis infections are caused by blood transfusions. The incubation period is 2 to 12 weeks after exposure. The clinical manifestations of the illness parallel HBV. An HCV titer to detect HCV IgG antibodies is now available to detect these infections; however, no vaccine protection exists against this form of hepatitis.

Hepatitis D virus (HDV) is known to cause "delta hepatitis." The HDV antigen can be detected by immunoassay within a few days after infection. The IgM and total antibodies to HDV are detected early in the disease also. A persistent elevation of these antibodies indicates a chronic or carrier state.

Procedure

No special preparation is necessary for these antigen-antibody studies. A peripheral venipuncture is performed, and generally one red-top tube of blood is obtained.

Nursing implications with rationale

Before

☞ Explain the procedure to the patient. Tell the patient that no fasting is required.

During

■ Handle the serum specimen as though it were capable of transmitting viral hepatitis. Wash your hands carefully after handling all equipment. Gloves should always be worn during venipuncture.

After

■ Apply pressure or a pressure dressing to the venipuncture site to prevent further bleeding. Observe the site for bleeding. Patients with liver dysfunction often have prolonged clotting times.

■ Advise patients suspected of having hepatitis that they should refrain from intimate contact with others. Until the serology indicates otherwise, they should be considered infective.

Laparoscopy (Pelvic Endoscopy, Gynecologic Video Laparoscopy, Peritoneoscopy)

Test type Endoscopy

Normal values

Normal-appearing female reproductive organs

Rationale

During laparoscopy, the abdominal organs can be visualized by inserting a scope through the abdominal wall and into the peritoneum (Figure 4-9). Usually, a television camera is attached to the scope, allowing the laparoscopist's view to be seen by others on color monitors. This is particularly helpful in diagnosing abdominal and pelvic

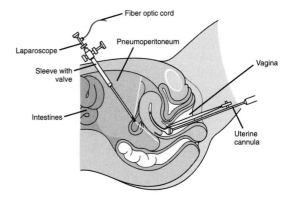

Figure 4-9 Gynecologic laparoscopy.

adhesions; tumors and cysts affecting any abdominal organ; and tubal and uterine causes of infertility. Endometriosis, ectopic pregnancy, ruptured ovarian cyst, and salpingitis also can be detected during an evaluation for pelvic pain. This procedure is also used to stage cancers and determine their resectability. Surgical procedures (e.g., cholecystectomy, appendectomy, hernia repair, tubal ligation, oophorectomy, hiatal hernia repair, and bowel resection) can be performed with the laparoscope. Laparoscopy has many advantages compared with an open laparotomy. With laparoscopy the incision is much smaller, and pain, immobility, and duration of hospitalization are reduced. Patients, therefore, can return to normal activities more rapidly.

Potential complications

Potential complications associated with laparoscopy are as follows:

- Perforation of the bowel, which spills intestinal contents into the peritoneum
- Hemorrhage, from the trocar site or surgical site

Procedure

The patient is kept NPO after midnight on the day of the test. After general anesthesia is induced, a urinary catheter and nasogastric tube are inserted to minimize the risk of penetrating a distended bladder or stomach with the initial needle placement. After the abdominal skin is cleansed, a blunt-tipped (Veress) needle is inserted through a small incision in the periumbilical area and into the peritoneal cavity. The peritoneal cavity is filled with approximately 3 to 4 L of carbon dioxide (CO_2) to separate the abdominal wall from the intraabdominal viscera, enhancing visualization of pelvic and abdominal structures. A laparoscope is inserted through a trocar to examine the abdomen (see Figure 4-9). Other trocars can be placed as conduits for other instrumentation. After the desired procedure is completed, the laparoscope is removed, and the CO_2 is allowed to escape. The incision(s) is closed with a few skin stitches and covered with an adhesive bandage.

Laparoscopy is performed by a surgeon. Because general anesthesia is used, no discomfort occurs during the procedure. Most patients will have mild to moderate incisional pain. However, patients may complain of shoulder or subcostal discomfort from diaphragmatic irritation caused by the pneumoperitoneum.

Contraindications

Contraindications for laparoscopy are as follows:

- Patients who have had multiple surgical procedures, because adhesions may have formed between the viscera and the abdominal wall, making safe access to the abdomen impossible. Limited laparoscopy may be done in these situations.
- Patients with suspected intraabdominal hemorrhage, because visualization through the scope will be obscured by the blood.

Nursing implications with rationale

Before
- Explain the procedure to the patient. Because of the possibility of intraabdominal injury, an open laparotomy may be required. Confirm that the patient is aware of this possibility.
- Ensure that a written and informed consent for this procedure is obtained.
- If enemas are ordered to clear the bowel, assist the patient as needed and record the results.
- Because the procedure usually is performed with the patient under general anesthesia, follow the routine general anesthesia precautions.
- Shave and prepare the patient's abdomen as ordered.
- Instruct the patient to void before going to the operating room, because a distended bladder can be penetrated easily.

After
- Assess the patient frequently for signs of bleeding (increased pulse rate, decreased blood pressure) and perforated viscus (abdominal tenderness, guarding, decreased bowel sounds). Report any significant findings to the physician.
- If patients have shoulder or subcostal discom-

fort from pneumoperitoneum, assure them that this usually lasts only 24 hours. Minor analgesics usually relieve this discomfort.

- If a surgical procedure has been performed laparoscopically, provide appropriate postsurgical care.

Leucine Aminopeptidase (LAP, Aminopeptidase Cytosol)

Test type Blood

Normal values
Blood:
   Male: 80-200 U/ml
   Female: 75-185 U/ml
Urine: 2-18 U/24 hr

Rationale
Leucine aminopeptidase (LAP) is an intracellular enzyme that exists in the hepatobiliary system and, to a much smaller degree, in the pancreas and small intestine. When disease or injury affects these organs, the cells lyse and LAP is spilled out into the bloodstream. Produced almost exclusively by the liver, LAP is used in diagnosing liver disorders and in the differential diagnosis of increased levels of ALP (see p. 108). LAP levels tend to parallel ALP levels in hepatic disease. LAP is a sensitive indicator of cholestasis; however, unlike ALP, LAP remains normal in bone disease. LAP can be detected in both blood and urine. Patients with elevated serum LAP levels always will show elevations in urine levels. When the urine LAP level is elevated, however, the blood level already may have returned to normal.

Interfering factors
A factor that interferes with LAP levels is pregnancy, which may cause *increased* values if tested by the enzyme method. Although there is no quantitative increase in this "LAP-like" enzyme, its activity is increased. This causes a false increase in the LAP if tested by the enzyme method.

Procedure
No special preparation is necessary for these liver enzyme studies. Approximately 7 to 10 ml of blood is collected in a red-top tube and sent to the laboratory for analysis.

Nursing implications with rationale
Before
- Explain the procedure to the patient. Tell the patient that no fasting is required.
During
- Because many of these liver enzyme tests are affected by medications, to aid in interpretation of test results, indicate on the laboratory requisition slip any medications that the patient is taking.
After
- Apply pressure or a pressure dressing to the venipuncture site to prevent further bleeding. Assess the site for bleeding because patients with liver dysfunction often have prolonged clotting times (see p. 434).

Lipase

Test type Blood

Normal values
0-110 units/L or 0-417 U/L (SI units)
   (values are method dependent)

Rationale
The most common cause of an elevated serum lipase level is acute pancreatitis. Lipase is an enzyme secreted by the pancreas into the duodenum to break down triglycerides into fatty acids. As with amylase (see p. 110), lipase appears in the bloodstream following damage to the pancreas or with disease affecting the pancreatic acinar cells.

Because lipase was thought to be produced only in the pancreas, elevated serum levels were considered to be specific to pathologic pancreatic conditions. It is now apparent that other conditions can be associated with elevated lipase levels. Lipase is excreted through the kidneys. Therefore, elevated lipase levels often are found in patients with renal failure. Intestinal infarction or obstruction also can be associated with lipase elevation. However, the lipase elevations in nonpancreatic diseases are less than 3 times the upper limit of normal, compared with pancreatitis, in which they are often 5 to 10 times normal values.

In acute pancreatitis, elevated lipase levels usually parallel serum amylase levels. The lipase levels usually rise a little later than amylase (24 to 48 hours after the onset of pancreatitis) and remain elevated for 5 to 7 days. Because they peak later and remain elevated longer than the serum amylase levels, serum lipase levels are more useful in the late diagnosis of acute pancreatitis. Lipase levels are less useful in more chronic pancreatic diseases (e.g., chronic pancreatitis, pancreatic carcinoma).

Procedure

Blood is withdrawn from a peripheral vein and collected in a red-top tube. The blood is drawn after an overnight fast. No water restrictions are necessary.

Nursing implications with rationale

Before

☞ Explain the procedure to the patient. Instruct the patient to remain NPO after midnight, except for water.

During

■ Many narcotics (e.g., morphine, codeine, meperidine) may interfere with test results if given within the 24 hours preceding the test. Note the time of their administration on the laboratory requisition slip if they were given during this period.

After

■ Apply pressure or a pressure dressing to the venipuncture site to prevent further bleeding.

Liver Biopsy

Test type Microscopic examination of tissue

Normal values

Normal liver histology

Rationale

Liver biopsy is a safe, simple, and valuable method of diagnosing pathologic liver conditions. For this study, a specially designed needle is inserted through the abdominal wall and into the liver. A piece of liver tissue is removed for microscopic examination. Percutaneous liver biopsy is used in the diagnosis of various liver disorders, such as cirrhosis, hepatitis, drug reaction, granuloma, and tumor. Biopsy is indicated for:

1. Patients with unexplained hepatomegaly
2. Patients with persistently elevated liver enzymes
3. Patients with suspected primary or metastatic tumor
4. Patients with unexplained jaundice
5. Patients with suspected hepatitis
6. Patients with suspected infiltrative diseases (e.g., sarcoidosis, amyloidosis)

The biopsy may be performed by a blind stick or may be directed with the use of a CT scan, magnetic resonance imaging (MRI) scan, or laparoscopy. Directed biopsy is used if there is a specific focal area of the liver that is suspicious and from which tissue must be obtained (e.g., a metastatic tumor). The blind stick is used if the liver is diffusely involved.

Potential complications

Potential complications associated with obtaining a liver specimen for biopsy are as follows:

■ Hemorrhage caused by inadvertent puncture of a blood vessel within the liver
■ Chemical peritonitis, caused by the inadvertent puncture of a bile duct with subsequent leakage of bile into the abdominal cavity
■ Pneumothorax (collapsed lung), caused by improper placement of the biopsy needle into the adjacent chest cavity

Procedure

Before the study a coagulation profile (PT, partial thromboplastin time [PTT], and platelet count) is performed to ensure adequate hemostasis if a small intrahepatic blood vessel is punctured. The patient's blood may be typed and crossmatched so that blood can be made available for transfusion if necessary.

The patient is kept NPO from midnight on the day of the examination. Meperidine and atropine often are administered 30 to 60 minutes before the study. The patient is placed in the supine or left lateral decubitus position. The skin overlying the area of the liver from which the biopsy specimen will be obtained is aseptically cleansed and anesthetized. The patient is asked to exhale and hold the exhalation, which causes the liver to descend and reduces the possibility of a pneumothorax. Frequently, the patient practices exhalation 2 or 3 times before the needle is inserted. During the patient's sustained exhalation, the physician rapidly introduces the biopsy needle into the liver and obtains liver tissue. The needle is then withdrawn from the liver.

This test is performed by a physician in approximately 15 minutes. Minor discomfort may be experienced during injection of the local anesthetic. Moderate discomfort is felt during needle insertion and biopsy.

Contraindications

Contraindications for obtaining a liver specimen for biopsy are as follows:

- Uncooperative patients who cannot remain still and hold their breath during sustained exhalation
- Patients with impaired hemostasis to avoid excessive bleeding from the liver puncture
- Patients with anemia
  These patients could not tolerate the major blood loss associated with inadvertent puncture of an intrahepatic blood vessel.
- Patients with infections in the right pleural space or right upper quadrant
  The infection may spread as an inadvertent consequence of obtaining a specimen for biopsy.
- Patients with obstructive jaundice
  In these patients, bile within the ducts is under pressure and may subsequently leak into the abdominal cavity after needle penetration.
- Patients with a hemangioma
  This is a highly vascular tumor, which may bleed profusely after a biopsy.

- Patients with ascites
  Persistent leakage of fluid may occur.

Nursing implications with rationale
Before
- ☞ Explain the procedure to the patient. Most patients are very apprehensive about this procedure. Encourage verbalization of the patient's fears.
- Confirm that the physician has obtained written and informed consent for this procedure.
- Check the results of the patient's hemostasis studies to make certain that the patient has no coagulation disorders. Many patients with liver disease have coagulation problems that make them prone to hemorrhage. Inform physician of any abnormal test results.
- ☞ Instruct the patient to remain NPO after midnight on the day of the procedure in case emergency surgery is needed to control hemorrhage or biliary leakage.
- ☞ Inform the patient that it is vital to lie very still during this procedure and to hold his or her breath during exhalation when instructed. Any movement of the chest may cause the needle to slip and lacerate the liver or diaphragm.
- Administer sedatives, if ordered.

During
- Support the patient during the procedure. Assist the physician as needed.
- Place the tissue into the appropriate specimen container and have it sent to the pathology department.
- Apply a small dressing over the needle insertion site.

After
- ☞ Instruct the patient to lie on the right side for 1 to 2 hours. In this position the liver capsule is compressed against the chest wall, thereby tamponading any hemorrhage or bile leak. The patient should remain on bed rest for 12 to 24 hours.
- Assess the patient's vital signs frequently for evidence of hemorrhage (increased pulse, decreased blood pressure) and peritonitis (increased temperature).
- Evaluate the patient for increasing abdominal pain. Be aware that some pain in the right up-

per quadrant of the abdomen and the top right shoulder area is common. This pain is caused by the inevitable leakage of blood or bile or both from the biopsy site in the liver. This fluid causes a localized and mild peritonitis. When the leak involves a large quantity of blood or bile, the peritoneal reaction is great, and the resulting pain is severe. Report this immediately.

Case Study

Cirrhosis

R.H. was a 48-year-old male, with a history of former drug abuse, who presented to the emergency room with abdominal swelling, lethargy, anorexia, and hemoptysis. On physical examination, he was noted to have mild ascites and was somewhat obtunded.

Studies	Results
ALT, p. 106	178 IU/L (normal: 5-35 IU/L)
ALP, p. 108	130 ImU/L (normal: 30-85 ImU/L)
AST, p. 15	176 U/L (normal: 5-40 U/L)
LDH, p. 42	240 U/L (normal: 45-90 U/L)
GGTP, p. 123	33 U/L (normal: 8-38 U/L)
Ammonia, p. 109	348 mg/dl (15-110 mg/dl)
CT scan of liver, p. 113	Shrunken fibrotic liver compatible with cirrhosis
Liver biopsy, p. 128	Posthepatitis cirrhosis
Hepatitis profile, p. 123	All negative, except HBVc-Ab
Esophagoscopy, p. 71	Esophageal varices

Diagnostic Analysis

R.H. presented with cirrhosis and ascites. His elevated liver enzymes were compatible with liver cellular disease. His elevated ammonia level indicated that he was susceptible to encephalopathy. The patient was somewhat obtunded. He was bleeding from his esophageal varices, and the blood in the gut increased the load on his liver's capability to metabolize protein. He became progressively encephalopathic. His coagulation studies were probably prolonged, thereby contributing to his esophageal bleeding. The etiology of his cirrhosis could have been prior hepatitis B infection. The acute phase sometimes goes unrecognized. He may have contracted the virus from a contaminated needle. He had no serologic evidence of acute infection. The HBVc-Ab indicated a previous infection.

Unfortunately, this man became progressively encephalopathic and expired during this hospitalization.

Critical Thinking Questions

1. Why do you think the coagulation studies would be elevated?
2. How are the ammonia results related to encephalopathy?

Liver/Spleen Scanning (Liver Scanning)

Test type Nuclear scan

Normal values
Normal size, shape, and position of the liver and spleen, containing no filling defects

Rationale
Liver scanning is used to detect and outline structural changes of the liver and spleen. A radionuclide, usually Tc sulfur-labeled albumin colloid, is administered intravenously. Later, a gamma ray scintillator is placed over the right and left upper quadrants of the patient's abdomen and records, on film, the distribution of the radioactive particles emitted from the liver and spleen.

This scan is indicated for patients with cancer to rule out metastatic liver tumors. It is a routine part of tumor staging. It also is indicated for patients with primary tumors (hepatomas) or in patients with cirrhosis who are at high risk for developing primary hepatomas. Liver scanning is used to visualize the liver of patients with abnormal liver enzymes. It is also used to monitor liver diseases and responses to therapy.

The liver scan can detect tumors, cysts, granulomas, abscesses, and diffuse infiltrative processes affecting the liver (e.g., amyloidosis, sarcoidosis). Because the scan can only demonstrate filling defects greater than 2 cm in diameter, false-negative results may occur in patients with space-occupying lesions smaller than 2 cm.

A Tc-labeled RBC liver scan is used to differentiate a benign hemangioma from a more serious tumor involving the liver. The patient's own RBCs are labeled with Tc and reinjected into the patient. Immediate uptake of the radionuclide by the filling defect suggests a benign hemangioma.

In general, CT and MRI scans have replaced the liver scan in diagnostics. Single photon emitting computed tomography (SPECT) has significantly improved the quality and accuracy of liver scanning. With SPECT scanning, the scintillator is positioned to receive images from multiple angles around the circumference of the liver. This greatly increases the sensitivity of nuclear liver scanning.

The liver scan also can identify portal hypertension. Normally, most of the radionuclide administered during a liver scan is taken up by the liver. If the liver-to-spleen ratio is reversed (i.e., the spleen takes up more of the radionuclide), the reversal of hepatic blood flow exists as a result of portal hypertension. Splenic hematomas, abscesses, cysts, tumors, infarctions, and infiltrate processes, such as granulomas, also can be detected.

Procedure
No special preparation is required. Thirty minutes after a peripheral IV injection of the radioisotope, a gamma ray detecting device is passed slowly over the patient while he or she is moved in multiple positions to visualize all surfaces of the liver (Figure 4-10).

This procedure is performed in the nuclear medicine department by a trained technician in approximately 1 hour. A physician trained in nuclear medicine interprets the reports. The only discomfort is associated with the IV injection of the radioisotope. Because only tracer doses of radioisotopes are used, no precautions need to be taken against radioactive exposure.

Contraindication
A contraindication for liver scanning is pregnancy or lactation, because of risk of damage to the fetus or infant.

Nursing implications with rationale
Before
☞ Explain the procedure to the patient. Encourage verbalization of the patient's fears. Because of the possibility of intraabdominal injury, an open laparotomy may be required. Be sure the patient is aware of that. Tell the patient that no fasting or premedication is required.
☞ Assure the patient that he or she will not be exposed to large amounts of radioactivity because only tracer doses of isotopes are used.

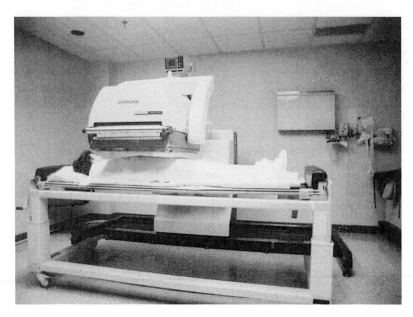

Figure 4-10   Patient prepared for a liver scan.

After

☞ Instruct the patient that no precautions against radiation exposure need to be taken.

5′-Nucleotidase

Test type Blood

Normal values

0.0-1.6 U or 27-233 nmol/sec/L (SI units)

Rationale

5′-nucleotidase is an enzyme specific to the liver. The 5′-nucleotidase level is elevated in patients with liver diseases, especially those associated with cholestasis (obstruction to the formation and flow of bile). It provides information similar to ALP; however, ALP is not specific to the liver. Diseases of the bone, other diseases, sepsis, and pregnancy can cause ALP to be elevated. When the cause of an elevated ALP is unclear, 5′-nucleotidase is recommended. If this enzyme is elevated along with ALP, the source of the pathology is certainly in the liver. If the 5′-nucleotidase

is normal in the face of an elevated ALP, the source of pathology is outside the liver (bone, kidney, or spleen). GGTP (see p. 123) is used similarly because it is also specific to the liver.

Procedure

No special preparation is necessary for these liver enzyme studies. Approximately 7 to 10 ml of blood is collected in a red-top tube and sent to the laboratory for analysis.

Nursing implications with rationale

Before

☞ Explain the procedure to the patient. Tell the patient that no fasting is required.

During

■ Because many of these liver enzyme tests are affected by medications, to aid in interpretation of test results, indicate on the laboratory requisition slip any medications that the patient is taking.

After

■ Apply pressure or a pressure dressing to the venipuncture site to prevent further bleeding. Assess the site for bleeding because patients with liver dysfunction often have prolonged clotting times (see p. 432).

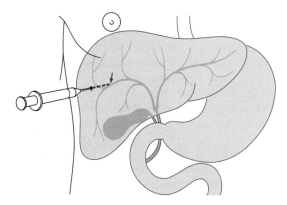

Percutaneous Transhepatic Cholangiography (PTC, PTHC)

Test type X-ray with contrast dye

Normal values
Normal gallbladder and biliary ducts

Rationale
By passing a needle through the liver and into a bile duct, the biliary system can be directly injected with iodinated radiographic contrast dye. The bile ducts within and outside the liver, and occasionally the gallbladder, can be visualized and studied for partial or total obstruction caused by gallstones, benign strictures, malignant tumors, congenital cysts, and anatomic variations. This is especially helpful in patients with jaundice. If the jaundice is found to result from extrahepatic obstruction, a catheter can be left in the bile duct and used for external drainage of bile. Furthermore, a stent can be placed across a stricture to internally decompress the biliary system.

Both percutaneous transhepatic cholangiography (PTC) and ERCP, (see p. 118) are the only methods available to visualize the biliary tree in patients with jaundice. ERCP is used more frequently because of its lower complication rate. PTC, however, is the only way to visualize the biliary tree after most gastric surgeries.

Potential complications
Potential complications associated with PTC are as follows:

- Allergic reaction to iodinated dye
  This is rare because the dye is not administered intravenously but rather into the bile duct.
- Peritonitis, caused by bile extravasation from the liver after the needle has been removed
- Bleeding, caused by inadvertent puncture of a large hepatic blood vessel
- Sepsis and cholangitis, resulting from injection

Figure 4-11 Percutaneous transhepatic cholangiography.

of the dye into an already infected and obstructed bile duct, which pushes the bacteria into the bloodstream, causing bacteremia

Interfering factors
A factor that interferes with PTC is the presence of barium from a previous radiographic study, which may preclude visualization of the biliary tree.

Procedure
A bile duct ultrasound usually is performed. If the bile ducts are found to be dilated, the patient proceeds to PTC. However, if the bile ducts are not dilated, the chance of gaining bile duct access is small, and the PTC is not attempted.

If the PTC is to be done, the patient is kept NPO after midnight on the day of the study. Before the patient reports to the radiology department, an IV infusion is started for venous access and the injection of sedatives. In the radiology department the patient is placed in a supine position on an x-ray table. The abdominal wall over the liver is anesthetized with lidocaine (Xylocaine). With the use of televised fluoroscopic monitoring, the needle is advanced through the skin and into the liver (Figure 4-11), and the physician aspirates bile. When bile flows freely into the syringe, a wire is advanced through the needle and well into the biliary system. A catheter is placed over the wire. An antibiotic-containing dye is injected, and radiographic films are taken immediately. If complete obstruction is found, the catheter may be temporarily left in place to establish drainage and decompression of the biliary tract.

PTC takes about 1 hour, during which time the patient must lie completely still. If repeated needle sticks must be made to obtain biliary access, the patient may become uncomfortable. If hemorrhage or bile extravasation occurs, the patient may have severe right upper quadrant abdominal pain. Shoulder pain, referred from the right upper quadrant, may be present. After returning to the nursing floor, the patient is kept on bed rest and NPO in the event that surgery becomes necessary to control hemorrhage or significant bile extravasation.

Contraindications

Contraindications for PTC are as follows:

- Patients with evidence of mild cholangitis
  Dye injections increase biliary pressure and cause bacteremia, which may lead to septicemia and shock.
- Patients who cannot cooperate and remain still
  This procedure requires that the patient lie still for more than 1 hour.
- Patients with prolonged clotting times
  Bleeding can occur from the liver puncture.

Nursing implications with rationale

Before

- Explain the procedure to the patient. Tell the patient that he or she will feel slight discomfort when the abdomen is anesthetized locally. Pressure may be felt when the needle is placed into the liver.
- Assess the patient for an allergy to iodine or shellfish.
- Ensure that written and informed consent for PTHC is obtained before premedicating the patient.
- If GI contrast studies recently were performed, obtain a physician's order for a cathartic to remove any residual barium.
- Prepare the patient as if for surgery because emergency surgical intervention may become necessary to control hemorrhage or bile leak-

age. Type and crossmatch the patient's blood before this test. The patient's platelet count and the PT should be normal.

After

- Instruct the patient to remain NPO and on bed rest.
- Place a sandbag over the site of needle insertion, if ordered. Observe the site for bile leakage or hemorrhage. A small amount of bleeding is usually present.
- Assess the patient's vital signs frequently (every 15 minutes for four times, then every 30 minutes for four times, then every hour for four times, and then every 4 hours). Assess for signs of hemorrhage (a decrease in blood pressure or an increase in pulse). A hemoglobin and hematocrit determination may be ordered 6 hours after PTC.
- Assess the patient's temperature for signs of bacteremia or sepsis.
- If the catheter is left in the biliary tract, establish a sterile closed system of drainage.
- Withhold pain medications to avoid blunting the abdominal signs associated with hemorrhage or bile extravasation. Observe the patient for increasing abdominal pain.

Prealbumin (PAB, Thyroxine-binding Prealbumin [TBPA], Thyretin, Transthyretin)

Test type Blood

Normal values
Blood:
Adult/elderly: 15-36 mg/dl or 150-360 mg/L (SI units)
Child:
    Umbilical cord: 13 mg/dl or 130 mg/L (SI units)
    1 year: 10 mg/dl or 100 mg/L (SI units)
    2-36 months: 16-28 mg/dl or 160-280 mg/L (SI units)
Urine (24-hour):
0.017-0.047 mg/day
Cerebrospinal fluid (CSF):
Approximately 2% of total CSF protein

Possible critical values: Serum prealbumin levels <10.7 mg/dl indicate severe nutritional deficiency

Rationale

Prealbumin is one of the major plasma proteins. Because prealbumin can bind with thyroxine, it is also called *thyroxine-binding prealbumin* (TBPA). This test is used to indicate the level of a person's nutritional status. It also is used to indicate the status of liver function.

Because serum prealbumin levels fluctuate more rapidly in response to alterations in the synthetic rate than do those of other serum proteins, clinical interest has centered on prealbumin's use as a marker of nutritional status. Its half-life of 1.9 days is much less than the 21-day half-life of albumin (see p. 135). Because of prealbumin's short half-life, it is a sensitive indicator of any change affecting protein synthesis and catabolism. As a result, prealbumin is frequently ordered to monitor the effectiveness of total parenteral nutrition (TPN).

Prealbumin is reduced significantly in diseases of the liver because of impaired synthesis. Serum levels of prealbumin serve as a better indicator of liver function than do albumin levels. Prealbumin also is a negative acute-phase reactant protein; that is, serum levels decrease in inflammation, malignancy, and protein-wasting diseases of the intestines or kidneys. Because zinc is required for synthesis of prealbumin, low levels occur with a zinc deficiency. Increased levels of prealbumin occur in Hodgkin's disease and chronic kidney disease.

Because of the low level of prealbumin in the serum, this protein often is not detected on serum protein electrophoresis. However, because prealbumin crosses the blood-brain barrier, it is found in the CSF and can be seen on CSF electrophoresis (see discussion of lumbar puncture, p. 208).

Procedure

No food or fluid restrictions are needed. Collect a venous blood sample in a red-top tube. If a urine sample is requested, a 24-hour urine specimen is obtained.

Nursing implications with rationale

Before

☞ Explain the procedure to the patient. Tell the patient that no food or fluid restrictions are necessary.

■ If a 24-hour urine collection is needed, provide a collection bottle. Review this procedure with the patient.

After

■ Apply pressure or a pressure dressing to the venipuncture site to prevent further bleeding.

■ Transport the 24-hour urine to the laboratory promptly.

Protein Electrophoresis (Serum Protein Electrophoresis, SPEP, Urine Electrophoresis)

Test type Blood, urine

Normal values

Total protein: 6.4-8.3 g/dl or 64-83 g/L (SI units)
Albumin: 3.5-5.0 g/dl or 35-50 g/L (SI units)
Alpha$_1$ globulin: 0.1-0.3 g/dl or 1-3 g/L (SI units)
Alpha$_2$ globulin: 0.6-1.0 g/dl or 6-10 g/L (SI units)
Beta globulin: 0.7-1.1 g/dl or 7-11 g/L (SI units)

Rationale

Evaluation and fractionation of serum proteins are used to diagnose, evaluate, and monitor the disease course in patients with cancer (lymphoma, myeloma), intestinal/renal–protein losing states, immune disorders, impaired liver function, impaired nutrition, and chronic edematous states.

Proteins are constituents of muscle, enzymes, hormones, transport proteins, hemoglobin, and several other key functional and structural entities within the body. Total serum protein is a combination of prealbumin (see p. 134), albumin, and globulins.

Albumin is a small protein molecule that is most important in maintaining the oncotic pressure (the pressure that acts to keep water within the vascular space) of plasma. Albumin also acts as a carrier protein for drugs and hormones. The second type of protein in the blood, *globulins,* are larger molecules and are subclassified into three main groups: alpha, beta, and gamma. The globulins have very little effect on oncotic pressure. Alpha$_1$ globulins are mostly alpha 1 antitrypsin. Some transporting proteins, such as thyroid and cortisol-binding globulin, also contribute to this zone. Alpha$_2$ globulins include serum haptoglobins (glycoproteins that bind hemoglobin during hemolysis), ceruloplasmin (a carrier for copper), prothrombin, and cholinesterase (an enzyme used in the catabolism of acetylcholine). Beta$_1$ globulins include lipoproteins, transferrin, plasminogen, and complement proteins; beta$_2$ globulins include fibrinogen. Gamma globulins are the immune globulins (antibodies) (see p. 479).

Albumin is synthesized within the liver and therefore, is a measure of hepatic function. Prealbumin (see p. 134) may be a somewhat better test of liver function. When disease affects the liver cell, the hepatocyte loses its ability to synthesize albumin, and the serum albumin level is diminished. Because the half-life of albumin is approximately 21 days, however, severe impairment of hepatic albumin synthesis may not be recognized for several weeks or even months.

Serum albumin and globulin also are measures of nutrition. Malnourished patients, especially after surgery, have a greatly decreased level of serum proteins. Patients with burns and patients who have protein-losing enteropathies and uropathies have low levels of protein, despite normal synthesis. Pregnancy, especially the third trimester, usually is associated with reduced total proteins.

In some diseases, albumin is selectively diminished, and globulins are normal or increased to maintain a normal total protein level. For example, in collagen vascular diseases (e.g., systemic lupus erythematosus [SLE]), capillary permeability is increased. Albumin, a molecule much smaller than globulin, is selectively lost into the extravascular space. Therefore, albumin levels will be low, but globulin levels will be normal or even high. Another group of diseases similarly associated with low albumin, high globulin, and normal total protein levels is chronic liver diseases. In these diseases the liver cannot produce albumin, but globulin is made mostly in the reticuloendothelial system. In both of these types of diseases, the albumin level is low, but the total protein level is normal because of increased globulin levels. These changes can be detected if one measures the albumin/globulin ratio or protein electrophoresis. Normally, this ratio exceeds 1. In SLE or severe chronic hepatocellular dysfunction, the ratios diminish.

The albumin fraction of the total protein can be factitiously elevated in dehydrated patients. Increased total protein levels, particularly the globulin fraction, occur with multiple myeloma and other gammopathies.

Interfering factors

A factor that interferes with protein electrophoresis is sampling of peripheral venous blood proximal to an IV administration site. This can result in an inaccurately low protein level because of a local dilution caused by the IV fluid. Likewise, massive IV infusion of crystalloid fluid can result in acute hypoproteinemia from dilution.

Procedure

No fasting is required. Approximately 7 to 10 ml of venous blood is collected in a red-top tube. For a urine specimen, collect a first-morning voided specimen or a 24-hour specimen (preferred). No preservative is required if the specimen is kept refrigerated.

Nursing implications with rationale

Before

🖎 Explain the procedure to the patient. Inform the patient that no fasting is required.

After

■ Apply pressure or a pressure dressing to the venipuncture site to prevent further bleeding. Observe the site for bleeding because patients with liver dysfunction often have prolonged clotting times.

Secretin-Pancreozymin (Pancreatic Enzymes)

Test type Fluid analysis

Normal values
Volume: 2-4 ml/kg body weight
HCO_3 (bicarbonate): 90-130 mEq/L
Amylase: 6.6-35.2 U/kg

Rationale
Secretin-pancreozymin is a corroborative test used in the evaluation of cystic fibrosis. This test is indicated in children with recurrent respiratory tract infections, malabsorption syndromes, or failure to thrive.

Cystic fibrosis is an inherited disease characterized by abnormal secretions by exocrine glands within the bronchi, small intestines, pancreatic ducts, bile ducts, and skin (sweat glands). Because of this abnormal exocrine secretion, children with cystic fibrosis develop mucous plugs that obstruct their pancreatic ducts. The pancreatic enzymes (e.g., amylase, lipase, trypsin, chymotrypsin) cannot be expelled into the duodenum and, therefore, are either completely absent or present only in diminished quantities within the duodenal aspirate. For the same reason, bicarbonate and other neutralizing fluids cannot be secreted from the pancreas. In this test, secretin and pancreozymin are used to stimulate pancreatic secretion of these enzymes and bicarbonate into the duodenum. The duodenal contents then are aspirated and examined for pH, bicarbonate, and enzyme levels; amylase is the most frequently measured enzyme. Diminished values are suggestive of cystic fibrosis.

Procedure
After a 12-hour fast, the patient goes to the radiology department. With the use of fluoroscopy (a radiographic image displayed immediately on a television screen), a Dreiling tube is passed through the nose. The distal lumen is placed within the duodenum; the proximal lumen lies within the stomach. Both lumens are aspirated separately to avoid mixing of gastric contents with duodenal contents, which can alter the test results. The duodenum is aspirated until the contents are clear and the pH is basic. This ensures that no gastric (acid) contents are within the duodenum. A baseline specimen is collected for 20 minutes. The patient then is tested intradermally for sensitivity to secretin and pancreozymin. If no sensitivity is present, these hormones are administered intravenously. Secretin stimulates pancreatic water and bicarbonate secretions. Pancreozymin stimulates pancreatic enzyme secretion. Four duodenal aspirates are collected at 20-minute intervals and placed in specimen containers. These are placed on ice and sent to the laboratory for analysis of volume, bicarbonate content, pH level, and enzyme determination. A pH reading of less than 7 indicates contamination by gastric contents and thus invalidates the test results.

This test takes approximately 2 hours. It can be performed in the laboratory or on the ward. The patient may have discomfort and gagging during placement of the nasogastric (NG) tube.

Nursing implications with rationale
Before
- Explain the procedure to the patient (and to parents, if appropriate).
- Instruct the adult patient to remain NPO for 12 hours before the study to avoid the presence in the duodenum of food, which may block the aspirating lumen. The NPO time for children varies according to age.
- Tell the patient (and the parents) that he or she will receive an intradermal injection to identify sensitivities to the drugs before they are administered intravenously.

After
- Clamp and withdraw the NG tube. Give mouth and nose care.
- Allow the patient to resume a normal diet.

Cystic Fibrosis

R.T., 9 months old, was brought to his pediatrician by his mother for evaluation of recurrent respiratory tract infections. During the examination the doctor noted the infant's thin extremities and distended abdomen. No weight gain was evident since the child's checkup at the age of 6 months. When questioned about the baby's stools, his mother said they were large and foul smelling since she had started him on solid foods.

Studies	Results
Chest x-ray, p. 155	Patchy atelectasis, segmental hyperaeration, and air trapping
Sweat electrolytes test (by iontophoresis), p. 139	
Sodium	95 mEq/L (normal: <70 mEq/L)
Chloride	65 mEq/L (normal: <50 mEq/L)
Secretin-pancreozymin test (duodenal aspirate), p. 137	Absence of trypsin
Fecal fat (fat absorption) test	
72-hour collection, p. 120	Fat retention coefficient: 80% (normal: ≥95%)

Diagnostic Analysis

The chest x-ray findings indicated a significant degree of bronchiolar obstruction, causing atelectasis distally. Compensatory hyperaeration also was seen. With the history compatible with fat malabsorption and the bronchiolar obstruction (most probably caused by thickened mucus), the diagnosis of cystic fibrosis was considered. The sweat electrolytes test confirmed the diagnosis, as did the secretin-pancreozymin and fat absorption tests.

The parents were instructed in appropriate pulmonary therapy. A high-protein, low-fat diet (with medium-chain triglycerides) and pancreatic enzyme replacement were prescribed. Water-soluble vitamins were started. The patient gradually gained weight and returned to a near-normal growth pattern.

Critical Thinking Questions

1. Why were R.T.'s stools large and foul smelling?
2. Why did therapy for R.T. include pancreatic enzyme replacement?

Sweat Electrolytes Test
(Iontophoretic Sweat Test)

Test type Fluid analysis

Normal values
Sodium values in children
    Normal: <70 mEq/L
    Abnormal: >90 mEq/L
    Equivocal: 70-90 mEq/L
Chloride values in children
    Normal: <50 mEq/L
    Abnormal: >60 mEq/L
    Equivocal: 50-60 mEq/L

Rationale
Cystic fibrosis is an inherited disease (autosomal recessive) characterized by abnormal secretion by exocrine glands within the bronchi, small intestines, pancreatic ducts, bile ducts, and skin (sweat glands). Patients with cystic fibrosis have increased sodium and chloride contents in their sweat; that increase forms the basis of this test, which is both sensitive and specific for cystic fibrosis. This test is indicated in children with recurrent respiratory tract infections, chronic cough, early-onset asthma, malabsorption syndromes, late passage of meconium stool, or failure to thrive. This test also is used to screen children or siblings of cystic fibrosis patients for the disease.

  Sweat, induced by electrical current (pilocarpine iontophoresis), is collected, and its sodium and chloride contents are measured. The degree of abnormality is no indication of the severity of cystic fibrosis; it merely indicates that the patient has the disease. Almost all patients with cystic fibrosis have sweat sodium and chloride contents 2 to 5 times greater than normal values. In patients with suspicious clinical manifestations, these levels are diagnostic of cystic fibrosis. Abnormal sweat tests can also occur in patients with glycogen storage diseases, adrenal hypofunction, or glucose-6-phosphate dehydrogenase (G6PD) deficiency. The sweat test is not reliable during the first few weeks of life.

Interfering factors
Factors that interfere with sweat electrolytes tests include the following:

- A cold examination or testing room, because sweating is inhibited
  The room should be warmed or the child covered to maintain body heat.
- Dehydration
  Test results will not be accurate because dehydration is associated with a *decreased* volume of sweat and an *increased* concentration of sodium and chlorides.
- Values in pubertal adolescents, which may vary significantly and are not accurate

Procedure
No fluid or food restrictions are necessary. The test usually is performed in a laboratory by an experienced technician. For iontophoresis, a low level of electrical current is applied to the test area (the thigh in infants, the forearm in older children) (Figure 4-12). The iontophoresis unit contains two electrodes. The positive electrode is covered by gauze saturated with pilocarpine hydrochloride, a stimulating drug that induces sweating. The negative electrode is covered by gauze saturated with a bicarbonate solution. The electrodes are strapped onto the test area, and the iontophoresis unit is turned on for 5 to 12 minutes. The electrodes are then removed, the arm is washed with distilled water, and paper disks are placed over the test site with dry, clean forceps. The disks then are covered with paraffin to obtain an airtight seal to prevent evaporation. After 1 hour, the paraffin is removed, and the paper disks are transferred immediately by forceps to a weighing jar and sent for sodium and chloride analysis.

  The sweat test takes about 1 to 1½ hours to perform. The electrical current is small, and no discomfort or pain generally is associated with the test. However, some patients report a slight stinging sensation. Inadvertent contact of the elec-

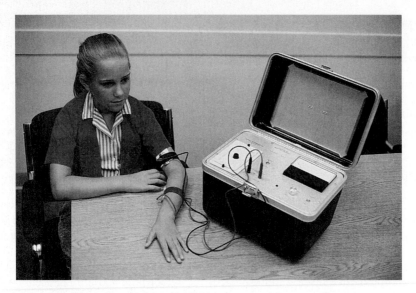

Figure 4-12 Child undergoing sweat test for cystic fibrosis.

trodes with the skin may cause a low-voltage shock or burn.

A screening test now can be done to detect sweat chloride levels. For this procedure a test paper containing silver nitrate is pressed against the child's hand for several seconds. The test is positive when the excess chloride combines with the silver nitrate to form white silver chloride on the paper. The child with cystic fibrosis will leave a heavy handprint on the paper. A positive screening test usually is validated by iontophoresis.

Nursing implications with rationale

Before

- ☞ Explain the procedure to the parent and child (depending on the child's age). Role-playing with a doll may be helpful.
- ☞ Tell the patient and/or parents that no fastingis required.
- ☞ Assure the parents and child that the child willnot be shocked by the electrical current.

After

- ■ Initiate extensive education, emotional support, and counseling for the patient and/or parents if the results indicate cystic fibrosis.

REVIEW QUESTIONS AND ANSWERS

1. **Question:** Your patient was scheduled for a liver biopsy, but the physician cancelled the test because no coagulation studies were done. Why was this done?

   Answer: Many patients with liver disorders have coagulation problems that make them prone to hemorrhage. If hemostasis is impaired, liver biopsy is contraindicated to avoid excessive bleeding from the liver puncture. Therefore, coagulation studies should be done before this test.

2. **Question:** Your patient has just returned from having a laparoscopy to detect abdominal adhesions. She asks you why she is having shoulder discomfort. What would you say?

   Answer: During the procedure carbon dioxide is inserted into the peritoneal cavity to separate the abdominal wall from the intraabdominal viscera. This enhances visualization of pelvic and abdominal structures. After the procedure, the residual carbon dioxide irritates the diaphragm and causes the shoulder pain.

3. **Question:** A patient in the emergency room is suspected of having hepatic encephalopathy. To confirm this problem, you have drawn blood for ammonia levels. Later, you receive a call from the laboratory requesting another blood sample because of hemolysis. Why is it necessary to obtain another blood test?

   Answer: Hemolysis increases ammonia levels because RBCs have about three times the amount of ammonia content than plasma does.

4. **Question:** Your patient is scheduled to have an upper GI series and ultrasound examination of the gallbladder. Which should be done first and why?

   Answer: Because ultrasound cannot penetrate the radiopaque contrast medium used in an upper GI series, the ultrasonography should be done first. The upper GI series is done next.

5. **Question:** Your patient is 2 months pregnant and is being evaluated for pancreatitis. An ultrasound examination of her gallbladder and pancreas has been ordered. The patient is concerned that the test may harm her unborn child. What is the appropriate intervention?

   Answer: Reassure the patient that ultrasound has been proven to be harmless to pregnant women and unborn children. Explain that ultrasonography is based on sound-wave transmission and that no radiographic films are taken.

6. **Question:** Your patient was admitted in severe pain with a diagnosis of acute pancreatitis. Do you think he will be scheduled for an ERCP?

   Answer: No. On the contrary, ERCP is rarely performed on patients with acute pancreatitis because the cause of the inflammation is usually obvious (gallstones, alcohol, or penetrating peptic ulcer). However, when the cause of pancreatitis is not obvious, tumor must be ruled out. ERCP is the most reliable method to rule out pancreatic tumor.

7. **Question:** A patient with jaundice is scheduled for ERCP. He has been complaining of vague right upper quadrant abdominal pain. He tells you that he needs a shot for pain before he goes for ERCP. (Morphine has been ordered for him every 4 hours as needed.) What is the appropriate intervention?

   Answer: Explain that morphine sulfate cannot be given because it causes severe spasm of the sphincter of Oddi and the endoscopist could not catheterize the sphincter and perform the ERCP. Inform the patient that he will receive meperidine before the test and that this will alleviate his pain.

8. **Question:** Before sending your jaundiced patient for PTHC, you receive his PT test results. The PT is 50% of the normal value. What should you do?

   Answer: Notify the physician. He or she probably will want to cancel the study because inadvertent puncture of a large blood vessel in a patient with a coagulation disorder could be disastrous. The physician probably will recommend that vitamin K be given for 2 to 3 days. Then the PT test should be repeated. If the PT test results are normal, the PTHC can be performed.

9. **Question:** On returning from having PTHC, your patient becomes hypotensive. What are the appropriate nursing interventions?

   Answer:
   a. Notify the physician.
   b. Increase the IV rate and place the patient in the Trendelenburg position.
   c. Assess the patient for signs of gram-negative septic shock (fever, chills, warm and flushed skin, disorientation).
   d. Assess the patient for signs of hemorrhagic shock secondary to inadvertent puncture of a large blood vessel (coldness, clamminess, pallor, air hunger, tachycardia).
   e. Draw blood for a CBC and a hemoglobin/hematocrit count. If the WBC is elevated, consider sepsis. If the hemoglobin/hematocrit count is decreased, consider hemorrhage.

f. If septic shock exists, the physician will order appropriate antibiotics.

g. If hemorrhagic shock exists, blood and volume replacement should be given. Surgery may be necessary for repair of the ruptured blood vessel.

10. **Question:** Your patient has an increase in urine amylase level and a normal serum amylase level. Could this patient have pancreatitis?

    Answer: Yes. The early transient rise in the serum level amylase may have been missed. The urine level stays elevated for a longer period.

Bibliography

Alter HJ: To C or not to C: these are the questions, *Blood* 85:1681, 1995.

Barrera JM et al: Persistent hepatitis C viremia after acute self-limiting posttransfusion hepatitis C, *Hepatology* 21:639, 1995.

Boat TF: Cystic fibrosis. In Behrman RE, editor: Nelson textbook of pediatrics, ed 15, Philadelphia, 1996, WB Saunders.

Bone R: Cystic fibrosis. In Bennet JC et al, editors: Cecil textbook of medicine, ed 20, Philadelphia, 1996, WB Saunders.

Burch JM: Acute pancreatitis. In Rakel RF, editor: Conn's current therapy, Philadelphia, 1998, WB Saunders.

Dienstag JL, Isselbacher KJ: Acute viral hepatitis. In Fauci AS et al, editors: Harrison's principles of internal medicine, ed 14, New York, 1998, McGraw-Hill.

Innis BL et al: Protection against hepatitis A by an inactivated vaccine, *JAMA* 271:1328, 1994.

Kaplan MM: Medical prognosis: primary biliary cirrhosis, *N Engl J Med* 335:1570, 1996.

Krawczynski K: Hepatitis E, *Hepatology* 17:932, 1993.

Lemon SM, Thomas DL: Vaccines to prevent viral hepatitis, *N Engl J Med* 336:196, 1997.

Metcalf JV et al: Natural history of early primary biliary cirrhosis, *Lancet* 348:1399, 1996.

Nahrwold DL: Cholelithiasis and cholecystitis. In Rakel RF, editor: Conn's current therapy, Philadelphia, 1998, WB Saunders.

Podolsky DK, Isselbacher KJ: Evaluation of liver function. In Fauci AS et al, editors: Harrison's principles of internal medicine, ed 14, New York, 1998, McGraw-Hill.

Reynolds TB: Cirrhosis. In Rakel RF, editor: Conn's current therapy, Philadelphia, 1998, WB Saunders.

Rossi RL et al: Chronic pancreatitis. In Rakel RE, editor: Conn's current therapy, Philadelphia, 1998, WB Saunders.

Scharschmidt BF: Hepatic tumors. In Bennet JC et al, editors: Cecil textbook of medicine, ed 20, Philadelphia, 1996, WB Saunders.

Sheth SG et al: Nonalcoholic steatohepatitis, *Ann Intern Med* 126:137, 1997.

Simmonds P: Variability of hepatitis C virus, *Hepatology* 21:570, 1995.

Tahahashi M et al: Natural history of chronic hepatitis C, *Am J Gastroenterol* 88:240, 1993.

Thoeni RF: Imaging of the liver, *Curr Opin Radiol* 3(3):427-439, 1991.

Toskes PP, Greenberger NJ: Approach to the patient with pancreatic disease. In Fauci AS et al, editors: Harrison's principles of internal medicine, ed 14, New York, 1998, McGraw-Hill.

Vlahcevic ZR, Heuman DM: Diseases of the gallbladder and bile duct. In Bennet JC et al, editors: Cecil textbook of medicine, ed 20, Philadelphia, 1996, WB Saunders.

Weisinger RA: Laboratory tests in liver disease. In Bennet JC et al, editors: Cecil textbook of medicine, ed 20, Philadelphia, 1996, WB Saunders.

Chapter 5

Diagnostic Studies Used in the Assessment of the
Pulmonary System

ANATOMY AND PHYSIOLOGY

The lungs are elastic, spongelike structures located within the thoracic cavity, one on either side of the chest. Their outer surface is enveloped by a two-layered membrane (pleura) that covers each lung and lines the thoracic cavity. The pleura is termed *visceral* when it covers the lungs and *parietal* when it lines the thorax. Between the two layers is a potential space called the *pleural space*. A small amount of fluid lubricates the pleural surfaces and prevents any friction between the lungs and the thorax during respiration.

Each lung is divided into subsections called *lobes.* The right lung has three lobes (upper, middle, lower); the left lung has two lobes (upper and lower). Each lobe is further divided into segments. Each pulmonary segment is ventilated by its own bronchiole, perfused by its own pulmonary arteriole, and drained by its own pulmonary venule. These structures are branches of the bronchus, pulmonary artery, and pulmonary vein, respectively. These structures enter the lung at its root (hilus) (Figure 5-1).

Air travels through the nose, trachea, bronchus, and bronchiole to end up in the alveoli (tiny air sacs). Each alveolus is in close association with a pulmonary arteriole and venule. Together the alveoli and their blood supply form the basic unit of the pulmonary system, where the exchange of oxygen (O_2) and carbon dioxide (CO_2) ultimately takes place. The human lung contains approximately 300 million of these microscopic units (alveoli). Cells contained within the alveolar walls secrete a lipoprotein called *surfactant.* This substance prevents complete alveolar collapse at the end of expiration. If this collapse were to occur, high inflating pressures would be required for reexpansion. This would increase the work of respiration.

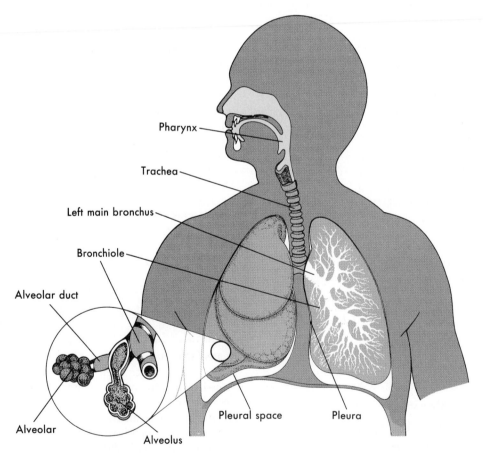

Figure 5-1 Normal anatomy of the pulmonary system.

Ventilation

The process of ventilation includes two phases: inspiration and expiration. During inspiration, contraction of the diaphragm and intercostal muscles causes the thoracic cavity to enlarge and thus to decrease intrathoracic pressure below atmospheric pressure. Air then is drawn into the lungs.

During expiration the muscles of respiration relax, causing the thoracic cavity to decrease in size. The intrathoracic pressure then becomes greater than atmospheric pressure, causing air to flow from the lungs into the atmosphere.

The stimulus for respiration is controlled by the respiratory center in the medulla of the brain. Chemoreceptors located in the aortic arch and the carotid bifurcation assess the level of CO_2 and O_2 in the blood. CO_2 is most important in respiratory control. When the CO_2 level of the blood increases (hypercapnia), the chemoreceptors relay that message to the medulla. The medulla then stimulates the person to breathe. Central (brain) chemoreceptors sensitive to CO_2 and O_2 are also in the cerebrospinal fluid (CSF). O_2 normally is a much less forceful chemoreceptor stimulant. Yet in patients with chronic obstructive pulmonary disease (COPD), these chemoreceptors get used to chronically high blood-CO_2 levels and become insensitive to CO_2. O_2 then assumes the role of respiratory stimulant. This is important because when the O_2 level in a patient with COPD is artificially raised (e.g., by use of an O_2 mask) to high levels, the stimulus for breathing (i.e., a low O_2 level, or hypoxemia) is lost, and the patient may stop breathing.

In addition to the effect of pressure gradients existing between the thoracic cavity and the atmosphere, inspiration and expiration are also affected by lung and thoracic cavity compliance. The term *compliance* refers to the ease with which lung tissue may be stretched. Compliance is expressed as the volume inhaled per unit of pressure required to expand the lung during that inhalation (volume in cubic centimeters and pressure in centimeters of water). A compliant lung (high compliance) expands easily when pressure is applied. A noncompliant, or stiff, lung (low compliance) requires greater than normal amounts of pressure for reexpansion; therefore, the patient must expend greater energy to achieve normal ventilation.

Pulmonary Circulation

Almost the entire cardiac output of the right ventricle passes through the capillaries of the lung and comes into close contact with the alveoli. Here the O_2 moves from the alveoli to the blood, and CO_2 moves in reverse. A small percentage of the right ventricle's output does not participate in gas exchange and bypasses the alveoli. This unoxygenated blood returns to the left atrium, where it mixes with the oxygenated blood. The movement of this blood, which bypasses the pulmonary circulation, is referred to as a *right-to-left shunt*. The end result of this shunt, although it is physiologically normal, is to lower the O_2 in the arterial blood. If the amount of shunted blood were to increase, severe hypoxia could result. Examples of this include pneumonia, in which some of the alveoli are filled with pus, and adult respiratory distress syndrome (ARDS [as in shock lung and pulmonary edema]), in which alveoli are filled with fluid. When the alveoli are filled, no air can ventilate them; therefore, the blood supplying those alveoli must return to the left atrium without the opportunity for gas exchange and oxygenation. This causes an increase in the amount of blood shunted from the right to the left side of the heart, and profound hypoxemia results.

Arterial Blood Gases (Blood Gases, ABGs)

Test type Blood

Normal values
pH (arterial)
Adult/child: 7.35-7.45
2 months-2 years: 7.34-7.46
Newborn: 7.32-7.49
pH (venous) 7.31-7.41

Pco$_2$ (arterial)
Adult/child: 35-45 mm Hg (torr)
Child <2 years: 26-41 mm Hg (torr)
Pco$_2$ (venous) 40-50 mm Hg (torr)
HCO$_3$
Adult/child: 21-28 mEq/L
Newborn/infant: 16-24 mEq/L
Po$_2$ (arterial)
Adult/child: 80-100 mm Hg (torr)
Newborn: 60-70 mm Hg (torr)
Po$_2$ (venous) 40-50 mm Hg (torr)
O$_2$ saturation
Elderly: 95%
Adult/child: 95% to 100%
Newborn: 40% to 90%
O$_2$ content (arterial) 15-22 vol %
O$_2$ content (venous) 11-16 vol %

Possible critical arterial values

pH: <7.25, >7.55
Pco$_2$: <20, >60
HCO$_3$: <15, >40
Po$_2$: <40
O$_2$ saturation: 75% or lower
Base Excess ± 3 mEq/L

Rationale

Measurement of arterial blood gases (ABGs) provides valuable information in assessing and managing a patient's respiratory (ventilation) and metabolic (renal) acid-base and electrolyte homeostasis. It also is used to assess oxygenation.

ABGs are used to monitor patients on ventilators; monitor critically ill, nonventilated patients; establish preoperative baseline parameters; and regulate electrolyte therapy. Although O$_2$ saturation monitors can accurately indicate O$_2$ saturation, ABGs still are used to monitor O$_2$ flow rates in the hospital and at home. ABGs often are performed in conjunction with pulmonary function studies.

pH

The pH is the negative logarithm of the hydrogen ion concentration in the blood. It is inversely proportional to the actual hydrogen ion concentration. Therefore, as the hydrogen ion concentration decreases, the pH increases, and vice versa. The

acids normally in the blood include carbonic acid (H$_2$CO$_3$), dietary acids, lactic acid, and ketoacids. The pH is a measure of alkalinity (pH >7.4) and acidity (pH <7.35). In respiratory or metabolic alkalosis, the pH is elevated; in respiratory or metabolic acidosis, the pH is decreased. The pH usually is calculated by a machine that directly measures pH.

Pco$_2$

The Pco$_2$ is a measure of the partial pressure of CO$_2$ in the blood. Pco$_2$ is a measurement of ventilation. The faster and more deeply the patient breathes, the more CO$_2$ is blown off and Pco$_2$ levels drop. Pco$_2$ therefore is referred to as the *respiratory* component in acid-base determination because this value is controlled primarily by the lungs. As the CO$_2$ level increases, the pH decreases. The CO$_2$ level and the pH are inversely proportional. The Pco$_2$ in the blood and in the CSF is a major stimulant to the breathing center in the brain. As Pco$_2$ levels rise, breathing is stimulated. If Pco$_2$ levels rise too high, the lungs cannot keep up with the demand to blow off or ventilate. As Pco$_2$ levels rise further, the brain is depressed and ventilation decreases further, causing coma.

The Pco$_2$ level is elevated in primary respiratory acidosis and decreased in primary respiratory alkalosis. Because the lungs compensate for primary metabolic acid-base derangements, Pco$_2$ levels are affected by metabolic disturbances as well. In metabolic acidosis, the lungs attempt to compensate by blowing off CO$_2$ to raise pH. In metabolic alkalosis, the lungs attempt to compensate by retaining CO$_2$ to lower pH.

HCO$_3$ or CO$_2$ content

Most of the CO$_2$ content in the blood is in the form of bicarbonate (HCO$_3$). HCO$_3$ is a measure of the metabolic (renal) component of the acid-base equilibrium and is regulated by the kidneys. This ion can be measured directly by the HCO$_3$ value or indirectly by the CO$_2$ content (see p. 518). It is important not to confuse CO$_2$ content with Pco$_2$. CO$_2$ content is an indirect measurement of HCO$_3$. Pco$_2$ is a direct measurement of the tension (pressure) of CO$_2$ in the blood and is regulated by the lungs.

As the HCO_3 level increases, the pH also increases; therefore, the relationship of HCO_3 to pH is directly proportional. HCO_3 is elevated in metabolic alkalosis and decreased in metabolic acidosis. The kidneys also are used to compensate for primary respiratory acid-base derangements. For example, in respiratory acidosis the kidneys attempt to compensate by reabsorbing increased amounts of HCO_3. In respiratory alkalosis, the kidneys excrete HCO_3 in increased amounts in a compensatory attempt to lower pH. In diabetic ketoacidosis, HCO_3 decreases because it is directly used to neutralize the plasma diabetic acids.

Po_2

The partial oxygen pressure (Po_2) is an indirect measure of the O_2 content of the arterial blood. Po_2 is a measure of the tension (pressure) of O_2 dissolved in the plasma. This pressure determines the force of O_2 to diffuse across the pulmonary alveoli membrane. The Po_2 level is decreased in:

1. Patients who are unable to oxygenate the arterial blood because of O_2 diffusion difficulties (e.g., pneumonia, shock lung, congestive failure)
2. Patients who have premature mixing of venous blood with arterial blood (e.g., in right-sided to left-sided shunting of blood associated with congenital heart defects)
3. Patients who have underventilated and overperfused pulmonary alveoli (in pickwickian syndrome [i.e., obese patients who cannot breathe properly in the supine position] or patients with significant atelectasis). The unoxygenated blood passes through that lung area and does not get oxygenated. The unoxygenated blood gets dumped back into the left side of the heart and dilutes the oxygenated blood.

Po_2 is one of the measures used to determine the effectiveness of O_2 therapy.

O_2 saturation

O_2 saturation indicates the percentage of hemoglobin (Hgb) saturated with O_2. When 92% to 100% of the Hgb carries O_2, the tissues are adequately provided with O_2 (assuming normal O_2

dissociation). As the Po_2 level decreases, the percentage of Hgb saturation also decreases. This decrease (on an oxyhemoglobin [O_2Hb] dissociation curve) is linear to a certain value. However, when the Po_2 level drops below 60 mm Hg, small decreases in the Po_2 level will cause large decreases in O_2 saturation. At O_2 saturation levels of 70% or lower, the tissues are unable to extract enough O_2 to carry out their vital functions.

O_2 saturation is calculated by a blood gas machine utilizing the following formula:

$$O_2 \text{ sat } \% = 100 \times \frac{\text{vol of } O_2 \text{ content Hgb}}{\text{vol of } O_2 \text{ capacity Hgb}}$$

O_2 content

O_2 content represents the amount of O_2 in the blood. The numeric formula is:

$$O_2 \text{ content} = O_2 \text{ sat} \times \text{Hgb} \times 1.34 + Po_2 \times 0.003$$

Nearly all O_2 in the blood is bound to Hgb. O_2 content decreases with the same diseases that diminish Po_2.

Base excess/deficit

The base excess/deficit is calculated by a blood gas machine using the pH, Pco_2, and hematocrit. This number represents the amount of buffering anions in the blood, with HCO_3 having the largest representation. Other buffering anions include Hgb, proteins, and phosphates. Base excess reflects all these anions and assists in determining acid-base treatment based on the metabolic component. Negative base excess (deficit) indicates a metabolic acidosis (e.g., lactic acidosis). A positive base excess indicates metabolic alkalosis or compensation to prolonged respiratory acidosis.

Alveolar to arterial O_2 difference (A-a gradient)

The A-a gradient indicates the difference between alveolar O_2 and arterial O_2. The normal value is less than 10 torr (mm of Hg). If the A-a gradient is abnormally high, there is either a problem diffus-

Acid-Base Disturbances	pH	Pco$_2$ (mm Hg)	HCO$_3^-$ (mEq/L)	Common Cause
None (normal values)	7.35-7.45	35-45	22-26	
Respiratory acidosis	↓	↑	Normal	Respiratory depression (drugs, central nervous system trauma)
				Pulmonary disease (pneumonia, chronic obstructive pulmonary disease, respiratory underventilation)
Respiratory alkalosis	↑	↓	Normal	Hyperventilation (emotions, pain, respirator overventilation)
Metabolic acidosis	↓	Normal	↓	Diabetes, shock, renal failure, intestinal fistula
Metabolic alkalosis	↑	Normal	↑	Sodium bicarbonate overdose, prolonged vomiting, nasogastric drainage

TABLE 5-1 Normal Values for Arterial Blood Gases and Abnormal Values in Uncompensated Acid-Base Disturbances

ing O$_2$ across the alveolar membrane (thickened edematous alveoli) or unoxygenated blood is mixing with the oxygenated blood, as previously described. Thickened alveolar membranes can occur in patients with pulmonary edema, pulmonary fibrosis, and ARDS. Mixing of unoxygenated blood occurs with congenital cardiac septal defects, arterial-venous shunts, or underventilated alveoli that are still being perfused (atelectasis, mucous plug).

Interpretation of ABGs may seem difficult but really is easy when one follows a system of evaluation (Tables 5-1 and 5-2). One such system is as follows:

1. Evaluate the pH.
   If the pH is less than 7.4, acidosis is present.
   If the pH is more than 7.4, alkalosis is present.
2. Next, look at the Pco$_2$.
   A. If the Pco$_2$ is high in a patient said to have acidosis (by step 1), the patient has a respiratory acidosis.
   B. If the Pco$_2$ is low in a patient said to have acidosis (by step 1), the patient has a metabolic acidosis and is compensating for that situation by blowing off CO$_2$.
   C. If the Pco$_2$ is low in a patient said to have

TABLE 5-2 Acid-Base Disturbances and Compensatory Mechanisms

Acid-base Disturbance	Mode of Compensation
Respiratory acidosis	Kidneys will retain increased amounts of HCO$_3^-$ to increase pH
Respiratory alkalosis	Kidneys will excrete increased amounts of HCO$_3^-$ to lower pH
Metabolic acidosis	Lungs blow off CO$_2$ to raise pH
Metabolic alkalosis	Lungs retain CO$_2$ to lower pH

alkalosis (by step 1), the patient has a respiratory alkalosis.
   D. If the Pco$_2$ is high in a patient said to have alkalosis (by step 1), the patient has a metabolic alkalosis and is compensating for that situation by retaining CO$_2$.

3. Next, look at the bicarbonate ion (HCO_3).
   In patient A, HCO_3 can be expected to be high in an attempt to compensate for the respiratory acidosis.
   In patient B, HCO_3 can be expected to be low as a reflection of the metabolic acidosis.
   In patient C, HCO_3 can be expected to be low to compensate for the respiratory alkalosis.
   In patient D, HCO_3 can be expected to be high as a reflection of the metabolic alkalosis.

Potential complications

Potential complications associated with ABGs are as follows:

- Occlusion of the artery used for access
  It is preferable to avoid use of end arteries such as the brachial or femoral artery.
- Penetration of other important structures anatomically juxtaposed to the artery (e.g., nerve)

Interfering factor

A factor that interferes with determining ABG levels is inhalation of carbon monoxide (CO). This *increases* the carboxyhemoglobin (COHb) level and can falsely *increase* the O_2 saturation.

Procedure

The arterial blood can be obtained from any area of the body in which pulses are palpable (usually the radial, brachial, or femoral artery). The arterial site is cleaned with povidone-iodine (Betadine) or alcohol. A 20-gauge needle is attached to a syringe containing approximately 0.2 ml of heparin (to ensure adequate heparinization of the syringe) and inserted into the artery. After 3 to 5 ml of blood are drawn, the needle is removed and pressure is applied to the arterial site for 3 to 5 minutes. The syringe is capped and gently rotated to mix the blood and heparin. The arterial blood sample is placed in an iced container and immediately taken to the chemistry laboratory for analysis.

This arterial puncture is performed by laboratory technicians, respiratory therapists, nurses, or physicians. The patient is placed in a sitting or supine position. The arterial puncture takes 5 to 10 minutes, depending on the skill of the person drawing the blood. An ABG test is more painful than a venous puncture. For ongoing respiratory monitoring an arterial line can be inserted to avoid multiple punctures.

Contraindications

Contraindications for ABGs are as follows:

- There is no palpable pulse.
- Cellulitis or open infection is present in the area considered for access.
- The Allen test is negative, indicating that there is no ulnar circulation. If the radial artery is used for the access, thrombosis may occur and jeopardize the viability of the hand.
- There is an arteriovenous (AV) fistula proximal to the site of proposed access.
- The patient has a severe coagulopathy.

Nursing implications with rationale

Before

- Explain the procedure to the patient and indicate that it will cause more discomfort than a venous puncture.
- If you are drawing the blood, know the anatomy of the arterial sites to avoid nerve damage.
- If you plan to use the radial artery, perform an Allen test to evaluate the presence of the ulnar circulation (Figure 5-2). The Allen test is performed by obliterating both the radial and ulnar pulses, which causes the hand to blanch. The pressure then is released only over the ulnar artery. If circulation through the ulnar artery is good, flushing will be seen immediately. The Allen test is then positive, and the radial artery can be used for puncture. If the Allen test is negative (no flushing), repeat the test on the other arm. If both arms give a negative result, choose another artery for puncture. The Allen test ensures collateral circulation to the hand if thrombosis of the radial artery should follow the puncture.
- Notify the laboratory before drawing the ABGs so that the necessary equipment can be calibrated before the blood sample arrives.

During

- Expel any air bubbles present in the blood sample immediately. Air bubbles affect the O_2 level of the ABGs measurement.

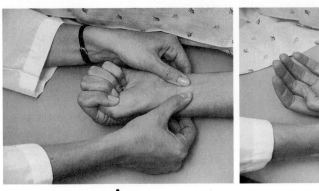
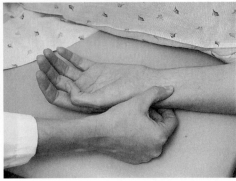

A   B

Figure 5-2 The Allen test for evaluating collateral circulation of the radial artery. **A,** *Step 1,* While the patient's fist is closed tightly, simultaneously obliterate both the radial and ulnar arteries. Instruct the patient to relax the hand, and watch for blanching of the palm and fingers. **B,** *Step 2,* Release the obstructing pressure from only the ulnar artery. Wait 15 seconds, observing the hand for flushing caused by capillary refilling. This indicates a positive Allen test, verifying that the ulnar artery alone is capable of supplying the entire hand. If flushing does not occur within 15 seconds, the Allen test is negative and the radial artery cannot be used.

■ Place the blood sample in an iced container. The lower temperature reduces blood cell metabolism, which may alter the pH, Pco_2, and HCO_3 values.

After
■ Maintain pressure to the arterial site for 3 to 5 minutes to avoid hematoma formation. If the patient has an abnormal clotting time or is taking anticoagulants, apply pressure longer (approximately 15 minutes). Remember that an artery, rather than a vein, has been accessed. Ensure that no active subcutaneous bleeding exists before leaving the patient.

Bronchoscopy

Test type Endoscopy

Normal values
Normal larynx, trachea, bronchi, and alveoli

Rationale
Bronchoscopy permits endoscopic visualization of the larynx, trachea, and bronchi by either a flexible fiberoptic bronchoscope or a rigid bronchoscope.

Bronchoscopy is used for many diagnostic and therapeutic purposes. Diagnostic uses of bronchoscopy include:

1. Direct visualization of the tracheobronchial tree for abnormalities (e.g., tumors, inflammation, strictures)
2. Biopsy of tissue from observed lesions
3. Aspiration of deep sputum for culture and sensitivity and for cytology determinations
4. Direct visualization of the larynx for suspected vocal cord paralysis. With pronunciation of "eeee" the cords normally move toward the midline.

Therapeutic uses of bronchoscopy include:

1. Aspiration of retained secretions in patients with airway obstruction or postoperative atelectasis
2. Control of bleeding within the bronchus
3. Removal of aspirated foreign bodies
4. Brachytherapy, which is endobronchial ra-

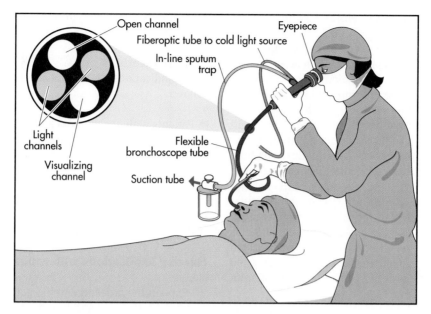

Figure 5-3 Flexible fiberoptic bronchoscope. The four channels consist of two that provide a light source, one vision channel, and one open channel that accommodates instruments or allows administration of an anesthetic or oxygen.

diation therapy using an iridium wire placed via the bronchoscope
5. Palliative laser obliteration of bronchial neoplastic obstruction

The bronchoscope has accessory lumens through which cable-activated instruments can remove biopsy specimens of pathologic lesions (Figure 5-3). The collection of bronchial washings (obtained by flushing the airways with saline solution), pulmonary toilet (removal of mucus), and the instillation of anesthetic agents also can be carried out through these extra lumens. Double-sheathed, plugged-protected brushes also can be passed through this accessory lumen. Specimens for cytology and bacteriology can be obtained with these brushes. Needles can be placed through the scope to obtain biopsy specimens by aspiration from tissue immediately adjacent to the bronchi. Laser therapy now can be performed through the bronchoscope to burn out endotracheal lesions.

Potential complications

Potential complications associated with bronchoscopy are as follows:

- Laryngospasm, induced by the scope passing over the vocal cords
- Bronchospasm, induced by the scope in the bronchi
- Pneumothorax, caused by needle aspiration of lung tissue
- Hemorrhage, caused by biopsy

Procedure

The patient is kept NPO (*nil per os,* nothing by mouth) after midnight on the day of the bronchoscopy. Fiberoptic bronchoscopy is performed by a surgeon or pulmonary specialist at the bedside or, preferably, in an endoscopy room. Preoperative medications, such as atropine, 0.6 to 1.0 mg, and meperidine (Demerol), 50 mg, may be administered intramuscularly (IM) approximately 1 hour before the study.

The patient's nasopharynx and oropharynx are anesthetized topically with lidocaine (Xylocaine) spray before insertion of the bronchoscope. This topical spray often is preceded by an aerosol treatment with lidocaine. The patient then is placed in the sitting or supine position, and the tube is inserted through the nose or mouth and into the pharynx. After the tube passes into the larynx and through the glottis, more lidocaine is sprayed into the trachea to prevent the cough reflex. The tube is passed farther, well into the trachea, the bronchi (Figure 5-4), and the first- and second-generation bronchioles for systematic examination of the bronchial tree. Biopsy specimens and washings are taken if a pathologic condition is seen or suspected. If bronchoscopy is performed for pulmonary toilet, each bronchus is aspirated until clear. This procedure takes less than 30 minutes and is somewhat uncomfortable for most patients.

Contraindications

Contraindications for bronchoscopy are as follows:

- Patients with hypercapnia and severe shortness of breath, who cannot tolerate interruption of high-flow O_2
  Bronchoscopy, however, can be performed through a special O_2 mask or an endotracheal tube so that the patient can receive O_2 if required.
- Severe tracheal stenosis, which may make it difficult to pass the scope

Nursing implications with rationale

Before

☞ Explain the procedure to the patient to reduce anxiety and enhance patient cooperation. Reassure the patient that he or she will be able to breathe during this procedure.
■ Ensure that written and informed consent for this procedure is obtained before the patient is premedicated.
☞ Instruct the patient to remain NPO after midnight on the day of the study to prevent possible aspiration of gastric contents induced by gagging.
■ Administer the preoperative medications as ordered. Atropine is used to prevent vagally induced bradycardia and to minimize secretions. (The patient may complain of having a dry mouth.) Meperidine or morphine is used to sedate the patient and relieve anxiety.
■ Remove and store the patient's dentures, glasses, or contact lenses before administering the preprocedure medication.
☞ Instruct the patient not to swallow the local anesthetic sprayed into the throat. An emesis basin should be provided for expectoration of the lidocaine.

After

☞ Instruct the patient not to eat or drink anything until the tracheobronchial anesthesia has worn off and the gag reflex has returned, usually in about 2 hours. A patient who eats or

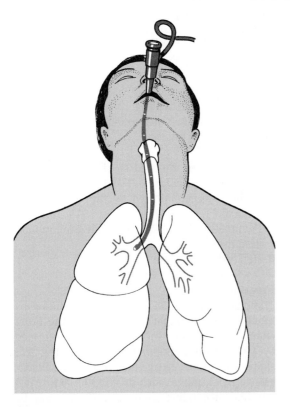

Figure 5-4 Bronchoscopy. A bronchoscope is inserted through the trachea and into the bronchus.

drinks anything before that time could un-knowingly aspirate the food or fluid and develop pneumonia.

- Observe the patient's sputum for blood if biopsy specimens were removed. A small amount of blood streaking is to be expected for several hours after bronchoscopy. Large amounts of bleeding (several ounces within 30 minutes) are disconcerting because this blood may be drawn into the pulmonary alveoli and create a chemical pneumonitis.
- Monitor vital signs frequently, as ordered. Fever may be seen for 2 to 6 hours after the procedure because of chemical pneumonitis.
- Observe the patient closely for evidence of impaired respiration or laryngospasm. Transient

hoarseness is a complication. The vocal cords may become spastic after intubation. Emergency resuscitation equipment (including tracheal tube, laryngoscope, and medications such as steroids and epinephrine) should be readily available.

- Enforce postanesthesia precautions until the effect of the sedative medications ceases.
- Instruct the patient that warm saline gargles and lozenges may soothe a sore throat.
- If a tumor is suspected, collect a postbronchoscopy sputum sample for cytologic determination.
- Note that a chest x-ray may be ordered to identify a pneumothorax if a deep biopsy specimen was obtained.

Case Study

Lung Cancer

Mr. N., 63 years old, had a long history of cigarette smoking. He had a chronic cough but more recently had noticed blood-streaked sputum. The results of his physical examination were normal.

Studies	Results
Routine laboratory work	Normal
Chest radiographic film, p. 155	Soft tissue mass in left lower lobe
Computed tomography (CT) scan of the chest, p. 157	3-cm soft tissue mass in the left lower lobe, no calcification, no mediastinal lymph node enlargement, no other pulmonary lesions
Bronchoscopy, p. 150	Partially obstructing tumor in basal segment of left lower lobe
Lung biopsy, p. 159	Squamous cell carcinoma
Mediastinoscopy, p. 164	No lymph nodes affected by tumor
Pulmonary function studies, p. 168	
Forced vital capacity	3400 cc (predicted: 3800 cc)
Forced expiratory volume	2600 cc (predicted: 3000 cc)
Maximal midexpiratory flow	340 L/min (predicted: 360 L/min)
Maximal volume ventilation	120 L/min (predicted: 130 L/min)
ABGs study p. 145	
pH	7.41 (normal: 7.35-7.45)
Po_2	70 mm Hg (normal: 80-100 mm Hg)
Pco_2	33 mm Hg (normal: 35-45 mm Hg)
HCO_3	24 mEq/L (normal: 22-26 mEq/L)

Continued

Case Study

Lung Cancer—cont'd

Diagnostic Analysis

The mass seen in the lung on radiographic examination and CT scan was considered to be malignant based on the bronchoscopy and the lung biopsy results, which indicated squamous cell carcinoma. Mediastinoscopy showed no involved mediastinal lymph nodes. If positive for metastasis, the tumor would have been considered inoperable. Preoperative pulmonary functions indicated that the patient could tolerate an aggressive surgical approach to this tumor, and a left lower-lobe lung resection, by means of a thoracotomy, was performed. Postoperatively Mr. N. had no problems. He died of unrelated problems 6 years later.

Critical Thinking Questions

1. Why was mediastinoscopy a key study in considering whether this patient was a candidate for surgery?
2. Based on the size of the tumor and the absence of nodal involvement and metastasis, how would you stage this lung cancer?

Carboxyhemoglobin (COHb, Carbon Monoxide)

Test type Blood

Normal values
Nonsmoker: <3% of total Hgb
Light smoker: 2%-5%
Heavy smoker: 5%-10%
Newborn: ≥12%

Possible critical values >20%

Rationale

Carboxyhemoglobin (COHgb) measures the amount of serum COHb, which is formed by the combination of carbon monoxide (CO) and Hgb. CO combines with Hgb 200 times more readily than O_2 can combine with Hgb (oxyhemoglobin), resulting in fewer Hgb bonds available to combine with O_2. Furthermore, when CO occupies the O_2 binding sites, the Hgb molecule is altered to bind the remaining O_2 more tightly. This greater affinity of CO for Hgb and the change in O_2-binding strength does not allow the O_2 to pass readily from the RBCs to the tissue. Less O_2, therefore, is available for tissue cell respiration, which results in hypoxemia.

CO poisoning is documented by Hgb analysis for COHb. A specimen should be drawn as soon as possible after CO exposure, because CO is cleared rapidly from the Hgb by breathing normal air. O_2 saturation studies (see p. 147) and oximetry (see p. 164) are inaccurate in CO-exposed patients because they measure all forms of oxygen-saturated hemoglobin, including COHb. In these circumstances, the patient's oximetry is normal, yet the patient is hypoxemic because the Hgb is saturated with CO rather than O_2.

This test also can be used to evaluate patients with complaints of headache, irritability, nausea, vomiting, and vertigo, who unknowingly may have been exposed to CO. Its greatest use, however, is in patients exposed to smoke inhalation, exhaust fumes, and fires. Other sources of CO include tobacco smoke; petroleum and natural gas fumes; automobile exhaust; unvented, natural-gas heaters; and defective gas stoves. Symptoms

TABLE 5-3	Symptoms of CO Poisoning by Level of Hgb Saturation

CO-Saturated Hgb (%)	Symptoms
10	Slight dyspnea
20	Headache
30	Irritability, disturbed judgment, memory loss
40	Confusion, weakness, dimness of vision
50	Fainting, ataxia, collapse
60	Coma
>60	Death

of CO poisoning correlated with blood levels are shown in Table 5-3. CO toxicity is treated by administering high concentrations of O_2 to displace the COHb.

Procedure
Approximately 5 to 10 ml of venous blood is collected in a lavender- or green-top tube.

Nursing implications with rationale
Before
☞ Explain the procedure to the patient or family.
■ Obtain the patient history related to any possible source of CO inhalation.
■ Assess the patient for signs and symptoms of mild CO toxicity (e.g., headache, weakness, dizziness, malaise, dyspnea) and moderate to severe CO toxicity (e.g., severe headache, bright-red mucous membranes, cherry-red blood). Maintain safety precautions if confusion is present.
After
■ Apply pressure or a pressure dressing to the venipuncture site to prevent further bleeding.
■ Treat the patient as indicated by the physician. Usually, the patient receives high concentrations of O_2.

☞ Instruct the patient to take deep breaths to clear the CO from the Hgb.

Chest X-ray (CXR, Chest Radiography)

Test type X-ray

Normal values
Normal lungs and surrounding structures

Rationale
The chest radiographic film is important in the complete evaluation of the pulmonary and cardiac systems. This procedure often is part of the general admission screening workup in adult patients. Chest x-rays can provide much information (Figure 5-5). With repeated chest x-rays, the following can be identified or monitored:

1. Tumors of the lung (primary and metastatic), heart (myxoma), chest wall (soft-tissue sarcomas), and bony thorax (osteogenic sarcoma)
2. Inflammation of the lung (pneumonia), pleura (pleuritis), and pericardium (pericarditis)
3. Fluid accumulation in the pleura (pleural effusion), pericardium (pericardial effusion), and lung (pulmonary edema)
4. Air accumulation in the lung (chronic obstructive pulmonary disease [COPD]) and pleura (pneumothorax)
5. Thoracic or vertebral bone fractures
6. Diaphragmatic hernia
7. Heart size, which may vary depending on cardiac function
8. Calcification, which may indicate large-vessel deterioration or old lung granulomas
9. Location of centrally placed intravenous (IV) access devices

Most chest radiographic films are taken with the patient standing (Figure 5-6). The sitting or supine position also can be used, but radiographic films taken with the patient in the supine position will not demonstrate fluid levels (resulting from

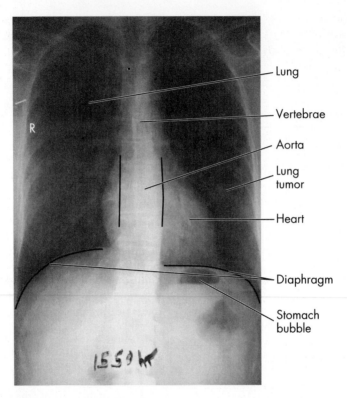

Lung

Vertebrae

Aorta

Lung tumor

Heart

Diaphragm

Stomach bubble

R

Figure 5-5 Chest x-ray. The diaphragm separates the abdominal contents (including the stomach) from the chest. The heart is situated in the middle of the chest. A tumor is noted in the left lung. The air-filled lungs are represented as dark spaces on either side of the chest. The tubular, opaque structure running vertically along the vertebrae represents the aorta. The ribs, clavicle, and other bony structures can also be seen as part of the thoracic cage.

pleural effusion) or pneumothorax (collapsed lung).

Interfering factors
Factors that interfere with chest x-ray include the following:

- Conditions (e.g., severe pain), that prevent the patient from taking and holding a deep breath
- Obesity, which requires more x-rays to penetrate the body to provide a readable radiographic picture

Procedure
Chest radiographic studies are best performed in the radiology department. Studies using a por-table camera may be done at the bedside and commonly are performed on critically ill patients who cannot leave the nursing unit. The patient's clothing is removed down to the waist, and a gown or drape is put on the patient. Metal objects (e.g., necklaces, watches, and pins) must be removed; otherwise, they will show up on the radiographic film and obscure visualization of part of the chest.

Most chest radiographic films are taken at a distance of 6 feet, with the patient standing. A *posteroanterior (PA)* view, with the x-rays passing through the back of the body (posterior) to the front of the body (anterior), is taken first. Then a *lateral* view, with the x-rays passing through the patient's side, is taken.

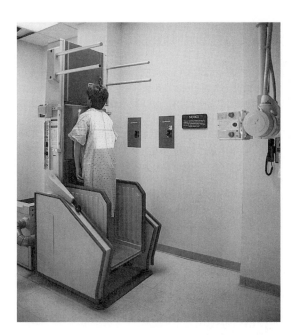

Figure 5-6 Patient positioned for chest x-ray study.

Oblique views may be taken with the x-rays slanted at specific angles as they pass through the body. *Lordotic* views provide visualization of the apices (rounded upper portions) of the lungs and are commonly used for tuberculosis detection. *Decubitus* films are taken with the patient in the recumbent lateral position to localize fluid in the pleural space (pleural effusion). After the patient is correctly positioned, he or she is told to take a deep breath and hold it until the radiographic film is taken. Films are taken by a radiologic technician in several minutes. The patient feels no discomfort.

Contraindication
Pregnancy is a contraindication for chest x-ray because of radiation exposure to the fetus.

Nursing implications with rationale
Before
☞ Explain the procedure to the patient. Tell the patient that no fasting is required.
☞ Inform the patient that clothing above the waist needs to be removed and that a gown will be supplied. If the patient will be going from a nursing unit to the radiology department, it is recommended that the patient put on a gown before leaving the nursing unit. This eliminates the need for dressing and undressing in the radiology department.
☞ Inform the patient that any metal objects, such as necklaces, need to be removed. Metal objects block the body structures that they cover and appear on the film.
☞ Inform the patient that he or she will be asked to take a deep breath and hold it while the radiographic film is being taken. This ensures that a maximum amount of air fills the lungs and allows a clear view of the pulmonary system. Any movement will blur the film.
☞ Instruct premenopausal women who are not presently in their menstrual cycle to wear a metal apron over their abdominal organs. This prevents radiation exposure to a fetus, should the woman be pregnant.
☞ Instruct men to cover their testes and women to cover their ovaries with a lead shield to prevent radiation-induced abnormalities that may result in congenital abnormalities in future children.

Computed Tomography of the Chest (Chest CT Scan)

Test type X-ray with contrast dye

Normal values
No evidence of pathologic conditions

Rationale
Computed tomography (CT) of the chest is a non-invasive, yet very accurate, radiographic procedure for diagnosing and evaluating pathologic conditions (e.g., tumors, lung nodules, hematomas, parenchymal coin lesions, cysts, abscesses, pleural effusion, and enlarged lymph nodes affecting the lungs and mediastinum). Tumors and cysts of the pleura and fractures of the ribs also can be seen. When an IV contrast material is

given, vascular structures can be identified, and a diagnosis of aortic aneurysm or other vascular abnormality can be made. With oral contrast, the esophagus and upper gastrointestinal (GI) structures can be evaluated for tumors and other conditions.

The radiographic image results from using a body scanner (radiographic tube held in a circular gantry) to deliver x-rays through the patient's chest at many different angles. The variation in density of each tissue allows for a variable penetration of the x-rays. Each density is given a numeric value called a *coefficient,* which is digitally computed into shades of gray. This is then displayed on a television screen as thousands of dots in various shades of gray. The final display appears as an actual photograph of the anatomic area sectioned by the x-rays.

Potential complications

Potential complications associated with CT of the chest are as follows:

- Allergic reaction to iodinated dye
  Allergic reactions may vary from mild flushing, itching, and urticaria to life-threatening anaphylaxis (evidenced by respiratory distress, drop in blood pressure, shock). In the unusual event of anaphylaxis, diphenhydramine (Benadryl), steroids, and epinephrine are added to routine resuscitation. O_2 and endotracheal equipment should be on hand for immediate use.
- Acute renal failure from dye infusion
  Adequate hydration beforehand may reduce this likelihood.

Procedure

The patient usually fasts for 4 hours before the CT of the lung in case contrast dye is administered. Sedation rarely is required and is given only to the patient who cannot remain still during the procedure. The patient is taken to the radiology department and is asked to remain motionless in the supine position because any motion causes blurring and streaking of the final picture. An encircling radiographic camera (body scanner) takes images at varying positions (usually 1

to 4 cm apart). Television equipment allows for immediate display, and the image is recorded on film.

The procedure takes 30 to 45 minutes to perform and is painless. However, many patients are uncomfortable lying on a hard table for this amount of time.

Often, intravenous dye is administered to the patient, and the radiographic studies are repeated. This adds an additional 30 to 45 minutes to the procedural time. During the dye injection the patient may feel a warm flush of the face or body. Many patients have momentary nausea with the dye injection.

Contraindications

Contraindications for CT of the chest are as follows:

- Pregnancy, because of radiation exposure to the fetus
- Patients who are allergic to iodinated dye or shellfish
- Patients who are claustrophobic
- Patients who are very obese (more than 300 pounds), because the CT table cannot hold large patients
- Patients whose vital signs are unstable

Nursing implications with rationale

Before

- Explain the procedure to the patient. Assure the patient that CT scanning of the lungs is a safe and painless radiographic method that incurs no more radiation than a series of regular radiographic studies.
- If possible, show the patient a photograph of the doughnut-like scanner. Tell the patient that he or she will be alone in the x-ray room but will be observed from a control room by a specialized technician. The patient and technician can communicate through an intercom system. Inform the patient that clicking noises from the scanner will be heard. People often describe the clicking noise as sounding similar to that of a washing machine. The patient will not be able to feel the scanning machine rotate.

☞ Instruct the patient to remain NPO for 4 hours before the test, because the iodine dye may cause nausea. It usually is not known before the test if enhanced visualization by the dye injection is needed.

■ Assess the patient for allergies to iodinated dye or shellfish to prevent dye-induced anaphylaxis. Sometimes the patient is pretested for dye allergies. Observe the patient for signs of anaphylaxis (such as respiratory distress, palpitations, blood pressure drop, itching, urticaria, or diaphoresis). Emergency drugs should always be available to counteract any severe allergic reaction. If iodine allergy is suspected and is not severe, diphenhydramine and steroids can be administered before scanning.

☞ Inform the patient that lying motionless is required during the study. Even talking or sighing may cause artifacts on the computer image.

After

☞ Encourage patients who received the dye injection to increase their fluid intake because the dye is excreted by the kidneys and causes diuresis.

Lung Biopsy

Test type Microscopic examination of tissue

Normal values
No evidence of pathology

Rationale
Lung biopsy is indicated to determine the pathology of pulmonary parenchymal disease, which has been identified on plain chest x-ray or chest CT scan. Carcinomas, granulomas, infections, and sarcoidosis can be diagnosed with this procedure. This procedure also is useful in detecting environmental exposures, infections, or familial disease, which may lead to better prevention and treatment.

The open method involves a limited thoracotomy or video-assisted thoracoscopy (VAT). The closed technique includes methods such as transbronchial lung biopsy, transbronchial needle aspiration biopsy, transcatheter bronchial brushing, and percutaneous needle aspiration biopsy.

Potential complications
Potential complications associated with lung biopsy are as follows:

■ Pneumothorax from the biopsy needle
■ Pulmonary hemorrhage from the biopsy needle

Procedure
The patient generally is kept NPO after midnight on the day of the biopsy. The patient usually is sedated 30 minutes to 1 hour before the procedure. The position of the patient depends on the method used. The histologic specimen may be obtained by several different methods.

A *transbronchial lung biopsy* is performed via a flexible fiberoptic bronchoscope, using cutting forceps. Fluoroscopy may be used to ensure the proper opening and positioning of the forceps on the lesion. Fluoroscopy also permits visualization of the tug of the lung as the specimen is removed.

Another technique of obtaining a lung specimen is by *transbronchial needle aspiration biopsy*, in which the specimen is obtained via a fiberoptic bronchoscope using a needle. After the target site has been identified by fluoroscopy, the needle is inserted through the bronchoscope and into the tumor, and aspiration is performed with the attached syringe and catheter. The needle then is retracted within its sheath, and the entire catheter is withdrawn from the fiberoptic bronchoscope. The bronchoscope then is removed.

A *transcatheter bronchial brushing* is performed also via a fiberoptic bronchoscope. During bronchoscopy a small brush is moved back and forth over the suspicious area. The cells adhere to the brush, which is removed and wiped on microscopic slides. The bronchoscope then is removed.

Another method of obtaining a lung specimen is by *percutaneous needle biopsy*. First, an x-ray of the desired site is obtained. Then, a specimen is obtained by using a cutting needle or by aspiration with a spinal-type needle. The main problem with this procedure is potential damage to major blood vessels and pneumothorax.

Open-lung biopsy is another method of obtaining lung tissue. For this procedure the patient is taken to the operating room, and general anesthesia is used. The patient is placed in the supine position, and a small thoracic incision is made in the chest wall. After a piece of lung tissue is removed, the lung is closed. Chest tube drainage is used for about 24 hours after an open-lung biopsy. More recently, lung tissue can be obtained without open thoracotomy (see video-assisted thoracoscopy [VAT], p. 179).

These procedures are performed by a surgeon or pulmonologist in 30 to 60 minutes. Most patients describe the percutaneous biopsy procedure as painful. Postoperative incisional pain can be expected if open or VAT techniques are used.

Contraindications

Contraindications for lung biopsy are as follows:

- Patients with bullae or cysts of the lung, because they have a greater risk of pneumothorax
- Patients with suspected vascular anomalies of the lung, because bleeding may occur
- Patients with bleeding abnormalities, because bleeding may occur
- Patients with pulmonary hypertension, because bleeding is more likely to occur
- Patients with respiratory insufficiency, because they are not likely to survive a pneumothorax if it were to occur

Nursing implications with rationale

Before
- ☞ Explain the procedure to the patient and describe the method of obtaining a specimen.
- Ensure that written and informed consent is obtained.
- ☞ Instruct the patient to fast as ordered. Usually the patient is kept NPO after midnight on the day of the test to prevent aspiration during the procedure.
- Administer the preprocedure medications as ordered 30 to 60 minutes before the test. Atropine usually is given before bronchoscopic examinations to decrease the bronchial secretions. Meperidine may be given to sedate anxious patients.

During
- ☞ Instruct the patient to remain still. Any movement or coughing could cause perforation of the lung by the biopsy needle.
- Observe the patient carefully for signs of respiratory distress (e.g., shortness of breath, rapid pulse, or cyanosis). If these symptoms are observed, immediately report them to the physician.

After
- After the specimens are obtained, place them in the appropriate jars for histologic and microbiologic examinations to ensure appropriate test results.
- Assess the vital signs frequently (usually every 15 minutes for four times, then every 30 minutes for four times, and then every hour for four times, and then every 4 hours). The patient should be evaluated for signs of bleeding (increased pulse and decreased blood pressure) and for shortness of breath. The patient's breath sounds should be evaluated, and any decrease noted on the biopsy site should be reported immediately.
- After the lung biopsy a chest x-ray usually is ordered to check for complications such as pneumothorax. Observe the patient for signs of pneumothorax (e.g., dyspnea, tachypnea, decrease in breath sounds, anxiety, and restlessness).

Lung Scan (Ventilation/Perfusion Scanning [VPS], Pulmonary Scintiphotography, V/Q Scan)

Test type Nuclear scan

Normal values

Diffuse and homogeneous uptake of nuclear material by the lungs

Rationale

This nuclear medicine procedure is used to identify defects in blood perfusion of the lung in patients with suspected pulmonary embolism. It is easily and rapidly performed on patients who have sudden onset of noncardiac chest pain or short-

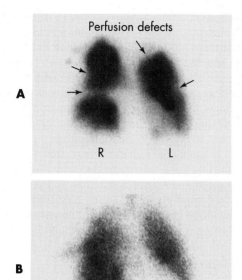

Perfusion defects

A

R   L

B

R   L

Figure 5-7 Lung scan. **A,** Perfusion. **B,** Ventilation. Multiple perfusion defects are noted on the perfusion lung scan. However, the uptake of radionuclide on the ventilation scan is normal. This combination of findings is due to pulmonary emboli.

fluid, emphysematous bullae) can distort the lung tissue to cause a similar picture. Therefore, although the scan may be sensitive, it is not specific, because many different pathologic conditions can cause the same abnormal results.

The chest radiographic film aids in the interpretation of the perfusion scan, because a defect on the perfusion scan seen in the same area as a pulmonary parenchymal abnormality on the chest x-ray does not indicate pulmonary embolism (PE). Rather, the defect may represent pneumonia, atelectasis, or effusion, for instance. When a perfusion defect occurs in an area of the lung that is normal on a chest radiographic study, however, PE is likely.

Specificity of a perfusion scan also can be enhanced by the concomitant performance of a ventilation lung scan, which detects parenchymal abnormalities in ventilation (e.g., pneumonia, pleural fluid, emphysematous bullae). The ventilation scan reflects the patency of the pulmonary airways using a radioactive aerosol. When vascular obstruction (embolism) is present by perfusion scan, ventilation scans will demonstrate a normal wash-in and wash-out of radioactivity from the embolized lung area. If parenchymal disease (e.g., pneumonia) is responsible for the abnormality on perfusion scan, the wash-in or wash-out will be abnormal. Therefore, the mismatch of perfusion and ventilation is characteristic of embolic disorders, whereas the match is indicative of parenchymal disease. When ventilation and perfusion scans are performed synchronously, this is called a *ventilation/perfusion (V/Q) scan.*

It is important to obtain a chest x-ray film around the same time as a perfusion lung scan to identify any parenchymal abnormalities that may affect perfusion. If the lung scan results are suspicious or equivocal, a pulmonary angiogram should be performed. Likewise, if anticoagulation is risky to the patient, an angiogram is required to diagnose pulmonary embolus with certainty. Most physicians trained in nuclear medicine report the lung scan results as follows: negative for PE, low probability for PE, high probability of PE, or positive for PE.

ness of breath. Blood flow to the lungs is evaluated using a macroaggregated albumin (MAA) tagged with technetium (Tc), which is injected into the patient's peripheral vein. Because the diameter of the radionuclide aggregates is larger than that of the pulmonary capillaries, the aggregates temporarily become lodged in the pulmonary vasculature. A scintillator detects the gamma-rays from within the lung microvasculature and converts it into a realistic image of the lung.

A homogeneous uptake of particles that fills the entire pulmonary vasculature conclusively rules out pulmonary embolism. If a defect in an otherwise smooth and diffusely homogeneous pattern is seen, a perfusion embolus exists (Figure 5-7). Unfortunately, many other pulmonary parenchymal lesions (e.g., pneumonia, pleural

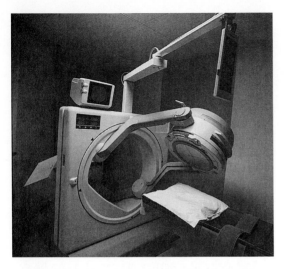

Figure 5-8 Clinical setting for lung scanning.

Procedure

The unsedated, nonfasting patient suspected of having a PE is taken to the nuclear medicine department (Figure 5-8). A peripheral IV injection of radionucleotide-tagged albumin aggregate is given for the perfusion portion of the scan. During scanning the patient lies in the supine, prone, and various lateral positions, to obtain anterior, posterior, and lateral views, respectively. A gamma camera is passed over the patient and records nucleotide uptake on film. The results are interpreted by a physician trained in diagnostic nuclear medicine. The procedure is painless except for the initial injection.

For the ventilation scan, the patient breathes the radionuclide tracer through a face mask with a mouthpiece. Less patient cooperation is needed with a krypton tracer. Ventilation scans using krypton can even be performed on comatose patients. Krypton images can be obtained before, during, or after perfusion images. In contrast, Tc 99m DTPA images are usually done before perfusion images and require patient cooperation, with deep breathing and appropriate use of breathing equipment to prevent contamination.

The amount of radiation that the patient receives is minimal. The test takes about 30 minutes. If an iodine-tagged agent (^{131}I) is used, the patient's thyroid gland should be blocked by administration of Lugol's solution (10 drops) several hours before the administration of the iodine.

Contraindication

Pregnancy is a contraindication for a lung scan because of radiation exposure to the fetus.

Nursing implications with rationale

Before

- ☞ Explain the procedure to the patient. Tell the patient that no fasting is required.
- ■ Obtain written and informed consent for this procedure if required by the institution.
- ☞ Instruct the patient to remove jewelry from the chest area.
- ■ If ^{131}I will be used, obtain the physician's order and administer 10 drops of Lugol's solution several hours before the test. This will block thyroid uptake of the iodine.

After

- ☞ Inform the patient that no radiation precautions are necessary.

Case Study

Pulmonary Embolism

Mrs. K., 68 years old, fell on the ice while shopping. She was taken to the local hospital, where a fracture of her hip was diagnosed and repaired. She had been doing well until the sixth postoperative day, when she complained of an acute onset of right-sided chest pain, shortness of breath, and palpitations. Physical examination revealed her to be tachypneic and anxious. Her pulse rate was 140 beats per minute. Her chest was clear, with minimal wheezing noted on the right side. Her heart was normal except for the tachycardia and an accentuated pulmonic sound.

Studies	Results
Routine laboratory work	Normal
Chest x-ray study, p. 155	Positive lucent area on the right side of her chest
Lactose dehydrogenase (LDH) determination, p. 42	600 ImU/ml (normal: 90-200 ImU/ml)
Total bilirubin determination, p. 111	1.9 mg/dl (normal: 0.1-1.0 mg/dl)
Aspartate aminotransferase (AST) determination, p. 15	33 IU/L (normal: 5-40 IU/L)
Electrocardiogram (EKG), p. 34	Severe right-sided heart strain
ABGs, p. 145	
pH	7.44 (normal: 7.35-7.45)
Pco_2	22 mm Hg (normal: 35-45 mm Hg)
Po_2	48 mm Hg (normal: 80-100 mm Hg)
HCO_3^-	23 mEq/L (normal: 22-26 mEq/L)
Lung scanning, p. 160	Multiple filling defects: right side worse than left side
Pulmonary angiography, p. 167	Complete obstruction of right pulmonary artery and upper branch of left pulmonary artery

Diagnostic Analysis

In light of the clinical findings, pulmonary embolism was highly suspected. Lucency on the chest radiographic film was compatible with pulmonary embolism, as were the features shown on the lung scan and the pulmonary angiogram. The trend of elevated LDH and bilirubin levels in the presence of a normal AST level is considered classic for pulmonary embolism. The ABG levels indicate severe hypoxemia compatible with a significant pulmonary embolism. Heparin was prescribed. One day later the patient's partial thromboplastin time (PTT) was 72 seconds (control value: 32 seconds; normal value: 30-40 seconds). Warfarin (Coumadin) was started 5 days after the heparin was begun. Four days after starting warfarin therapy, the patient's prothrombin time (PT) was 15 seconds (control value: 12 seconds; normal value: 11.0-12.5 seconds). The heparin was stopped, and the patient was discharged with continuing warfarin therapy. She had no further problems, and warfarin was discontinued after 6 months.

Critical Thinking Questions

1. What was Mrs. K's major risk factor for the development of a pulmonary embolism?
2. Why was the heparin started before coumadin for anticoagulation?

Mediastinoscopy

Test type Endoscopy

Normal values
No mediastinal tumors or abnormal lymph nodes

Rationale
Mediastinoscopy is a surgical procedure in which a mediastinoscope (a lighted instrument scope) is inserted through a small incision made at the suprasternal notch. The scope is passed into the superior mediastinum to inspect the mediastinal lymph nodes and to remove biopsy specimens. Because these lymph nodes receive lymphatic drainage from the lungs, their assessment can provide information on intrathoracic diseases such as carcinoma, granulomatous infections, and sarcoidosis; therefore, mediastinoscopy is used in diagnosing various intrathoracic diseases. This procedure also is used to stage lung cancers and to assess whether the patients are surgical candidates. Evidence of metastasis to the mediastinal lymph nodes usually is a contraindication to surgery because the tumor is considered inoperable. Tumors occurring in the mediastinum (e.g., thymoma or lymphoma) can also be sampled for biopsy through the mediastinoscope.

Potential complications
Potential complications associated with mediastinoscopy are as follows:

- Puncture of the esophagus, trachea, or great blood vessels by the scope
- Pneumothorax caused by the biopsy instrument

Procedure
Mediastinoscopy is a surgical procedure that is performed in the operating room. The patient is kept NPO after midnight on the day of the study. With the patient under general anesthesia, an incision is made in the suprasternal notch, and the mediastinoscope is passed through this neck incision into the superior mediastinum. After the lymph nodes are examined and biopsy specimens are removed, the scope is withdrawn and the incision is sutured closed. This procedure is performed by a surgeon in approximately 1 hour. A chest x-ray usually is performed after the procedure to ensure that a pneumothorax or hemorrhage has not occurred.

Contraindications
Contraindications for mediastinoscopy are patients who have superior vena cava obstruction. These patients have tremendous venous collaterization in the mediastinum. Mediastinoscopy in this group of patients is dangerous because of the risk of hemorrhage.

Nursing implications with rationale
Before
- Explain the procedure to the patient. Encourage verbalization of the patient's feelings, fears, and anxieties regarding mediastinoscopy.
- Ensure that the physician has obtained written and informed consent for the procedure before premedicating the patient.
- Provide the same preoperative and postoperative care as for any other surgical procedure.
- Instruct the patient to remain NPO after midnight on the day of the test.
- Ensure that the patient's blood has been typed and crossmatched, that several units of blood are available, and that the patient is ready for thoracotomy if necessary.

After
- Note that a chest x-ray examination usually is performed after the procedure to ensure that pneumothorax or hemorrhage has not occurred.

Oximetry (Pulse Oximetry, Ear Oximetry, Oxygen Saturation)

Test type Photodiagnostic

Normal values
95% or higher

Possible critical values ≤75%

Rationale

Oximetry is a noninvasive method of monitoring O_2 saturation levels (SaO_2) for patients at risk for developing hypoxemia. This includes patients who are undergoing surgery, cardiac stress testing, mechanical ventilation, heavy sedation, multiple trauma, or lung function testing. It also is used as an indicator of Po_2 in patients who may experience hypoventilation, sleep apnea, or dyspnea. This test is commonly used to titrate O_2 administration.

The SaO_2 is the ratio of oxygenated Hgb to the total amount of Hgb. The SaO_2 is expressed as a percentage; for example, a saturation of 95% indicates that 95% of the total Hgb attachments for O_2 have O_2 attached to them. The SaO_2 is an accurate approximation of O_2 saturation obtained from ABG studies (see p. 145). Through correlation of the SaO_2 and the patient's physiologic status, a close estimate of the Po_2 can be obtained.

Interfering factors

Factors that interfere with oximetry are as follows:

- Extreme vasoconstriction, which diminishes the blood flow to the periphery
  This *decreases* the accuracy of oximetry.
- Extreme alterations in temperature, which may *diminish* the accuracy of the procedure
- CoHb saturation (Hgb saturated with CO)
  Oximetry cannot differentiate COHb saturation from O_2 Hb saturation. Therefore, in cases of suspected smoke or CO inhalation, oximetry should not be used to monitor oxygenation because the levels will be falsely *elevated*.
- Digital motion, which can alter accurate reading
- Severe anemia, which affects the accurate comparison of oximetry and Po_2 levels
- Fingernail polish, which will interrupt the digital readings
  The earlobe is used as an alternative to the finger.

Procedure

The earlobe, pinna (upper portion of the ear), or the fingertip is rubbed to increase blood flow. The

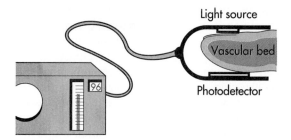

Figure 5-9 Oximetry. The pulse oximeter passes a beam of light through the tissue. The amount of light absorbed by the oxygen-saturated hemoglobin is measured by the sensor.

monitoring probe or sensor is then clipped to the ear or finger. The sensor warms and increases blood flow to the tissue. A beam of light passes through the tissue, and the sensor measures the amount of light the tissue absorbs (Figure 5-9). SaO_2 values are recorded. The study usually is performed by a respiratory therapist or nurse at the bedside and takes only a few minutes to carry out.

Nursing implications with rationale

Before

- Explain the procedure to the patient, assuring him or her that this is a noninvasive test that entails no discomfort.
- Inform the patient that no fasting is required.

Pleural Biopsy

Test type Microscopic examination of tissue

Normal values

No evidence of pathology

Rationale

Pleural biopsy is the removal of pleural tissue for histologic examination. This test is indicated when the pleural fluid obtained by thoracentesis (see p. 174) is exudative fluid, which suggests infection, neoplasm, or tuberculosis. The pleural biopsy is indicated to distinguish among these disease processes. It also is performed when a chest x-ray film indicates a pleural-based tumor, reaction, or thickening. Pleural biopsy usually is performed by a percutaneous needle biopsy. It also can be performed via thoracoscopy, which is done by inserting a scope into the pleural space for inspection and biopsy of the pleura. Pleural tissue also may be obtained by an open pleural biopsy, which involves a limited thoracotomy and requires general anesthesia. For this procedure, a small intercostal incision is made, and the biopsy of the pleura is done under direct observation. The advantage of these open procedures is that a larger piece of pleura can be obtained.

Potential complications

Potential complications associated with pleural biopsy are as follows:

- Bleeding or injury to the lung, caused by the aspirating needle
- Pneumothorax, caused by puncture of the lung by the aspirating needle

Procedure

No fasting or sedation is required before pleural biopsy unless an open biopsy is to be performed surgically. This procedure usually is performed with the patient in a sitting position, with the shoulders and arms elevated and supported by a padded overhead table. The patient should be instructed to remain still during the procedure.

Several special needles are available for performing biopsy of the parietal pleura. All have a cutting edge and a device for obtaining the biopsy specimen. After a thoracentesis confirms the presence of exudative fluid, the skin overlying the biopsy site is anesthetized. The Copelike needle then is inserted within the cannula until fluid is removed (some fluid is left in the pleural space after the thoracentesis to make the procedure easier). The inner needle is then removed, and the blunt-tipped, hooked biopsy trocar, attached to a three-way stopcock, is substituted in the cannula. The patient is instructed to expire all air and then to perform the Valsalva maneuver to prevent air

from entering the pleural space. The cannula and the biopsy trocar then are withdrawn, while the hook catches the parietal wall and removes a specimen with its cutting edge. Usually three specimens are taken from different sites during the same session. The specimens are placed in a fixative solution and sent to the laboratory immediately. After the specimens are taken, additional parietal fluid can be removed. However, postbiopsy bleeding may obscure the true character of the fluid. An adhesive bandage is applied to the site. A chest x-ray usually is performed after the study to detect the potential complication of pneumothorax.

This procedure is done by a physician at the bedside, in a special procedures room, or at the physician's office in approximately 30 minutes. Because of the local anesthetic, little discomfort is associated with this procedure.

Contraindications

Pleural biopsy is contraindicated for patients with prolonged bleeding or clotting times.

Nursing implications with rationale

Before

- Explain the procedure to the patient. Instruct him or her to remain still during the procedure. Any movement can cause inadvertent needle damage.
- Ensure that signed and informed consent is obtained before the procedure.
- Inform the patient that no fasting or sedation is necessary.

After

- Apply an adhesive bandage to the biopsy site.
- Check the vital signs frequently (usually every 15 minutes for four times, then every 30 minutes for four times, then every hour for four times, and then every 4 hours).
- Observe the patient for signs of respiratory distress (e.g., shortness of breath and diminished breath sounds on the side of the biopsy site). Make sure the chest x-ray examination is repeated if ordered to check for pneumothorax.
- Ensure that the biopsy specimen is placed in the proper fixative solution and immediately

sent to the laboratory. Failure to do so may interfere with accurate test result interpretation.

- Note that a chest x-ray usually is taken to detect a possible pneumothorax.

Pulmonary Angiography (Pulmonary Arteriography, Bronchial Angiography)

Test type X-ray with contrast dye

Normal values
Normal pulmonary vasculature

Rationale
A pulmonary angiogram is indicated most commonly when patients are suspected to have had a pulmonary embolism; the lung scan is inconclusive; and anticoagulation represents a moderate risk. Pulmonary angiography permits visualization of the pulmonary vasculature by means of injection of a radiographic contrast material into the pulmonary arteries. Angiography is used to detect pulmonary embolism and various congenital and acquired lesions of the pulmonary vessels.

When PE is suspected, lung scanning (see p. 160) should be performed first. If the lung scan is normal, PE is ruled out. If the scan is equivocal, however, the diagnosis of PE is questionable because pathologic parenchymal processes (e.g., emphysema, pneumonia) also may cause abnormalities on the lung scan. Definitive diagnosis for PE may require pulmonary angiography. This may be especially important in patients with peptic ulcers or bleeding disorders for whom anticoagulant treatment for PE may be associated with significant risks. Also, in rare instances, pulmonary embolectomy, rather than anticoagulation, is considered critical for patient survival. In these cases, the angiographic location of the clot is important.

Potential complication
Allergic reaction to iodinated dye is a potential complication associated with pulmonary angiography. Allergic reactions may vary from mild flushing, itching, and urticaria to life-threatening anaphylaxis (evidenced by respiratory distress, drop in blood pressure, or shock). In the unusual event of anaphylaxis, the patient may be treated with diphenhydramine, steroids, and epinephrine. O_2 and endotracheal equipment should be immediately available.

Procedure
Preferably, the patient is kept NPO after midnight on the day of the examination. He or she is sedated. In the angiography room, usually located in the radiology department, the patient is placed on an x-ray table. The groin is prepared and draped in a sterile manner. A catheter is placed into the femoral vein and passed into the inferior vena cava. With fluoroscopic visualization (motion picture radiographic images displayed on a television monitor), the catheter is advanced to the right atrium and right ventricle. With expertise, the angiographer (a physician) can manipulate the catheter into the main pulmonary artery, where the dye is injected through the catheter. Radiographic films of the chest are immediately taken in a timed sequence, allowing all vessels visualized by the injection to be photographed. If filling defects are seen in the contrast-filled vessels, a PE is present.

During the actual injection of dye material, the patient may feel a burning and flush throughout the body. This is transient, usually passing within seconds. The test takes about 1 hour. Lying on the hard table for that time is uncomfortable for the patient.

Contraindications
Contraindications for pulmonary angiography are as follows:

- Allergies to iodinated dye and shellfish
- Pregnancy, because of radiation exposure of the fetus
- Bleeding disorders

Nursing implications with rationale
Before
- Explain the procedure to the patient. Tell the patient where the catheter will be inserted (usually the femoral vein). Inform the patient

that a warm flush may be felt when the dye is injected.

- Ensure that written and informed consent for this procedure is obtained before premedicating the patient.
- Assess the patient for allergies to the iodine dye.
- ☞ Instruct the patient to remain NPO after midnight on the day of the study.
- Administer the preprocedure medications as ordered. Atropine may be ordered to decrease secretions, and meperidine is often used to sedate the patient and relieve anxiety.

After

- Observe the catheter insertion site for inflammation, hemorrhage, hematoma, or absence of a peripheral pulse.
- Assess the vital signs for evidence of bleeding (decreased blood pressure and increased pulse). Vital signs are usually taken every 15 minutes for 4 times, then every 30 minutes for 4 times, and then every 4 hours.
- ☞ Educate the patient regarding the need for bed rest for 12 to 24 hours after the test.
- Evaluate the patient for a delayed reaction to the dye (rash, dyspnea, tachycardia, hives). This usually occurs 2 to 6 hours after the test. Treat with antihistamines.

Pulmonary Function Tests (PFTs)

Test type Airflow assessment

Normal values

Vary with the patient's age, sex, height, and weight

Rationale

The main reasons for performing pulmonary function tests (PFTs) include the following:

1. Preoperative evaluation of the lungs and pulmonary reserve. When planned thoracic surgery will result in loss of functional pulmonary tissue, as in lobectomy (removal of part of a lung) or pneumonectomy (removal of an entire lung), a significant risk of pulmonary failure exists if the preoperative pulmonary function already is severely compromised by other diseases, such as COPD.
2. Evaluation of response to bronchodilator therapy. Some patients with COPD have a spastic component to their obstructive disease that may respond to long-term use of bronchodilators. Pulmonary function studies performed before and after the use of bronchodilators will identify that group of patients.
3. Differentiation between restrictive and obstructive forms of chronic pulmonary disease. *Restrictive defects* (e.g., pulmonary fibrosis, tumors, chest-wall trauma) occur when ventilation is disturbed by a limitation in chest expansion. Inspiration is primarily affected. *Obstructive defects* (e.g., emphysema, bronchitis, asthma) occur when ventilation is disturbed by an increase in airway resistance. Expiration is primarily affected.
4. Determination of the diffusing capacity of the lungs (DL). Rates are based on the difference in concentration of gases in inspired and expired air.
5. Performance of inhalation tests in patients with inhalation allergies.

PFTs routinely include spirometry, measurement of air flow rates, and calculation of lung volumes and capacities. Gas diffusion and inhalation (bronchial provocation) tests are also done when requested, but not routinely. Exercise pulmonary stress testing also can be performed to provide data concerning the patient's pulmonary reserve. During this staged test, the patient performs an aerobic function, such as stationary bicycling or walking on a treadmill.

Spirometry is performed first. A spirometer is a machine that can measure air volumes. When a time element is added to the tracing, airflow rates can be determined. Based on age, height, weight, race, and sex, normal values for the volumes and flow rates can be predicted. Values greater than 80% of predicted values are considered normal.

Measurement of airflow rates provides information about airway obstruction. This portion of the study adds a time element to spirometry. If airflow rates are significantly diminished ($<60\%$ of normal) or if requested by the physician, the test can be repeated after bronchodilators are administered with a nebulizer. If the airflow rates are improved by 20%, the prolonged use of bronchodilators may be recommended to the patient. Patients with an asthmatic component to their COPD will benefit from bronchodilators.

Measurement of lung capacities (combination of two or more lung volumes) can be performed by nitrogen or helium washout techniques. This provides further information about air trapping within the lung.

Gas exchange studies measure the DL, that is, the amount of gas exchanged across the alveolar-capillary membrane per minute. Gas exchange is abnormal in patients with diseases that fill the alveoli with fluid or exudate (congestive heart failure [CHF], pneumonia). Also, any disease that causes material to be deposited in the interstitium of the lung (ARDS, collagen vascular disease, Goodpasture's syndrome, or pulmonary fibrosis) will decrease gas exchange.

ABGs (see p. 145) also are a part of pulmonary function studies because the information obtained is used in calculations of lung function data.

PFTs routinely include determination of the following:

1. Forced vital capacity (FVC)
2. Forced expiratory volume in 1 second (FEV_1)
3. Maximal midexpiratory flow (MMEF)
4. Maximal volume ventilation (MVV)

Forced vital capacity (FVC)

FVC is the amount of air that can be forcefully expelled from a maximally inflated lung position. Lower than expected values occur in obstructive and restrictive pulmonary diseases.

Forced expiratory volume in 1 second (FEV_1)

FEV_1 is the volume of air expelled during the first second of the FVC. In patients with obstructive disease, airways are narrowed and resistance to flow is high. Therefore, not as much air can be expelled in 1 second, and FEV_1 will be reduced below the predicted value. In restrictive lung disease, FEV_1 is decreased not because of airway resistance but because the amount of air originally inhaled is less. One should therefore measure the FEV_1/FVC ratio. A normal value of 80% is found in patients with restrictive lung disease. In obstructive lung disease, this ratio is considerably less than 80%.

Maximal midexpiratory flow (MMEF)

MMEF is the maximal rate of airflow through the pulmonary tree during forced expiration. This is also called *forced midexpiratory flow.* This test is independent of the patient's effort or cooperation. MMEF is reduced below expected values in obstructive diseases and is normal in restrictive diseases.

Maximal volume ventilation (MVV)

MVV, formerly called *maximal breathing capacity,* is the maximal volume of air that the patient can breathe in and out during 1 minute. MVV is decreased below the expected value in both restrictive and obstructive pulmonary disease.

A comprehensive pulmonary function study also may include evaluation of the following lung volumes and capacities, many of which are illustrated in Figure 5-10:

Tidal volume (TV or V_T)

   TV or V_T is the volume of air inspired and expired with each normal respiration.

Inspiratory reserve volume (IRV)

   IRV is the maximal volume of air that can be inspired from the end of a normal inspiration. It represents forced inspiration over and beyond the tidal volume.

Expiratory reserve volume (ERV)

   ERV is the maximal volume of air that can be exhaled after a normal expiration.

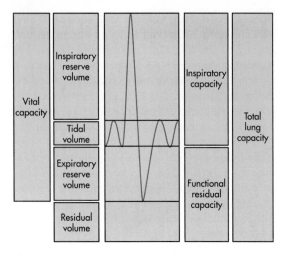

Figure 5-10 Relationship of lung volumes and capacities.

Residual volume (RV)
RV is the volume of air remaining in the lungs following forced expiration.

Inspiratory capacity (IC)
IC is the maximal amount of air that can be inspired after a normal expiration (IC = TV + IRV).

Functional residual volume (FRV)
FRV is the amount of air left in the lungs after a normal expiration (FRV = ERV + RV).

Vital capacity (VC)
VC is the maximal amount of air that can be expired after a maximal inspiration (VC = TV + IRV + ERV).

Total lung capacity (TLC)
TLC is the volume to which the lungs can be expanded with the greatest inspiratory effort (TLC = TV + IRV + ERV + RV).

Minute volume (MV)
MV, sometimes called *minute ventilation,* is the volume of air inhaled and exhaled per minute.

Dead space
Dead space is the part of the V_T that does not participate in alveolar gas exchange. This would include the air within the trachea.

Forced expiratory flow (FEF)
FEF is the portion of the airflow curve that is most affected by airway obstruction.
$FEF_{200-1200}$: Rate of expired air between 200 and 1200 ml during the FVC.
FEF_{25-75}: Rate of expired air between 25% and 75% of flow during the FVC.

Peak inspiratory flow rate (PIFR)
PIFR is the flow rate of inspired air during maximum inspiration. This is used to indicate large-airway (trachea and bronchi) disease.

Potential complications

Potential complications associated with PFTs are as follows:

- Light-headedness during the test, caused by the relative hyperventilation
- Fainting during the FVC maneuver, caused by the Valsalva effect that sometimes occurs
- Asthmatic attack, which can be precipitated during inhalation studies
Bronchodilators may be necessary to begin immediate treatment.

Procedure

The unsedated patient is taken to the pulmonary function laboratory. The patient breathes into a sterile cylinder, which is connected to a computerized machine able to measure and record the desired values. The patient is asked to inhale as deeply as possible and then to exhale as much air as possible. The machine then computes FVC, FEV_1, FEV_1/FVC, PIFR, and MMEF. Next, the patient is asked to breathe in and out as deeply and frequently as possible for 15 seconds. The total volume breathed is recorded and multiplied by 4 to obtain the MVV.

This test takes approximately 10 minutes and is painless. It usually is performed by an inhalation therapist or technician.

The DL for any gas can be measured as part of a pulmonary function study. The DL measures the diffusion of gases per minute across the alveolar-capillary membrane.

Inhalation tests also may be performed during

pulmonary function studies to establish a cause-and-effect relationship in some patients with inhalant allergies. The methacholine, or histamine challenge, test commonly is used to detect the presence of hyperactive airway diseases. This test would not be indicated for a patient known to have asthma. A positive methacholine challenge is a greater than 20% reduction in the patient's FEV_1 after the administration of that drug. Care is taken during this challenge test to reverse any severe bronchospasm with prompt administration of an inhalant bronchodilator (e.g., isoproterenol).

Contraindications

Contraindications for PFTs are as follows:

- Patients who are in pain, because of inability to cooperate with deep inspiration and expiration
- Patients who are unable to cooperate, because of age or mental incapability

Nursing implications with rationale

Before

☞ Explain the test to the patient. The patient's cooperation is necessary to obtain accurate results.

☞ Assure the patient that his or her air supply will be adequate during this procedure. Many people with respiratory disorders are anxious about undergoing breathing tests.

☞ Instruct the patient not to use bronchodilators and not to smoke for 6 hours before this study.

- Withhold the use of small-dose meter inhalers and aerosol therapy before this study.
- Measure and record the patient's height and weight before this study to determine the predicted values.

After

- To aid in test interpretation, list any medications on the laboratory requisition slip.
- Plan needed periods of rest because occasionally patients with severe respiratory problems are exhausted after the testing.

Sleep Studies (Polysomnography, PSG)

Test type Sleep evaluation

Normal values

Respiratory disturbance index (RDI): fewer than 5-10 episodes per study

Rationale

Sleep studies are indicated for any person who snores excessively; experiences narcolepsy, excessive daytime sleeping, or insomnia; or has motor spasms while sleeping. They also are indicated for patients who have cardiac rhythm disturbances limited to sleeping times as determined by a Holter monitor (see p. 40).

Sleep apnea is a disease that now is becoming increasingly recognized through sleep time signs and the daytime sequelae. Its economic impact in the workplace has demanded improved methods of diagnosis and treatment. Obstructive sleep apnea (OSA) occurs as a result of complete upper airway obstruction associated with no ventilation for at least 10 seconds. These apneic spells may be associated with significant O_2 desaturation, cardiac rhythm disturbances, muscle spasms or seizures (restless leg syndrome), sleep interruption, and insomnia. As a result of these symptoms, sleep is frequently interrupted. The preceding partial or nearly complete upper airway obstruction causes excessive snoring, that is so pronounced that the home life of these patients may be severely affected. The daytime sequelae of sleep apnea is excessive daytime sleeping or narcolepsy.

Other nonairway obstructive forms of sleep apnea exist. Central sleep apnea is highlighted by simple cessation of breathing not caused by obstructed airway. Primary cardiac events that lead to significant and transient reduction in cardiac output also can cause apnea.

Testing for OSA is performed in a specially constructed sleep laboratory. This is a well-insulated room in which external sounds are eliminated and room temperature is easily controlled. During the observation period (usually during normal sleep hours), the patient is monitored by EKG, pulse oximetry, electroencephalogram (EEG), electromyography, (see pp. 34, 164, 199, 201, respectively). Airflow in the mouth and nose is monitored. Chest and abdominal wall impedance as a measure of respiratory effort also is monitored.

Interfering factors

Factors that interfere with sleep studies include the following:

- Psychologically induced insomnia associated with the laboratory environment compared with home
- Environmental noises, temperature changes, or other sensations

Procedure

The patient is asked to abstain from caffeine for several days before testing. Electrodes for EKG, EEG, and electromyography are applied to the patient. Excess body hair may need to be shaved on male patients. Airflow, oximetry, and impedance monitors also are applied. Once the patient is comfortable, he or she is allowed to sleep normally. The lights are turned off, and monitoring begins before sleep ensues. The test takes about 8 to 12 hours to complete. Although some anxiety may be noted during the study, it is not painful.

Nursing implications with rationale

Before

- ☞ Explain the procedure to the patient. Allow the patient to express concerns about videotaping and other forms of monitoring.
- ☞ Reassure the patient that monitoring equipment should not interrupt the patient's sleeping pattern.

After

- Remove the monitors and electrodes on completion of the sleep cycle.

Case Study

Sleep Apnea

Mr. E.K., 47 years old, constantly fell asleep whenever he sat in his living room and read. He slept very soundly and snored all night. He was concerned that his family napped often during the day. Because the home was heated by a kerosene heater, he wondered if they had CO poisoning.

Studies	Results
COHb, p. 154	2% (normal: Nonsmoker: <3% of total hemoglobin)
Sleep apnea studies, p. 171	Respiratory disturbance index 22 (normal <5-10 episodes per study), associated with bouts of hypoxemia

Diagnostic Analysis

Mr. E.K. did not have any evidence of CO poisoning. Rather, he had classic sleep apnea. His wife and family learned to live with his snoring but were sleep-deprived because of his snoring. Mr. E.K. was becoming apneic 22 times per night. This created frequent sleep interruptions. Despite the use of gadgets designed to stop snoring, his sleep apnea continued. Finally, nasopharyngeal surgery was performed, and his snoring abated. His apneic spells stopped. He and his family slept soundly and woke well rested. The narcolepsy ceased.

Critical Thinking Questions

1. Where and how are sleep apnea studies performed?
2. Describe some of the signs and symptoms of CO poisoning. Were any noted in Mr. E.K. and his family?

Sputum Culture and Sensitivity
(C&S, Culture and Gram Stain)

Test type Sputum

Normal values
Normal upper respiratory tract

Rationale
Sputum culture is indicated in any patient with a persistent productive cough, fever, hemoptysis, or a chest x-ray compatible with a pulmonary infection. This test is used to diagnose pneumonia, bronchiectasis, bronchitis, or pulmonary abscess. Bacterium, fungus, or virus can be cultured.

Sputum cultures are obtained to determine the presence of pathogenic bacteria in patients with respiratory infections, such as pneumonia. A Gram stain is the first step in the microbiologic analysis of sputum. By Gram staining, bacteria are classified as gram positive or gram negative. This may be used to guide drug therapy until the C&S report is complete. The sputum sample is applied to a series of bacterial culture plates. The bacteria that grow on those plates 1 to 3 days later then are identified. Determinations of bacterial sensitivity to various antibiotics (also called *drug sensitivity testing*) are done to identify the most appropriate antimicrobial drug therapy. This is done by observing a ring of growth inhibition around an antibiotic plug in the culture medium. Sputum for C&S should be collected before antimicrobial therapy is initiated. Preliminary reports usually are available in 24 hours. Cultures require at least 48 hours for completion. Sputum cultures for fungus and *Mycobacterium tuberculosis* may take 6 to 8 weeks (see tuberculosis [TB] culture/ smear, p. 181).

Interfering factors
Factors that interfere with sputum culture and sensitivity are antiseptic mouthwashes, which may affect test results.

Procedure
Sputum specimens are best collected when the patient wakes and before he or she eats or drinks. Only sputum that has come from deep within the lungs should be collected. At least one teaspoon of sputum must be collected in a sterile, wide-mouth sputum container. Sputum usually is obtained by having the patient cough after taking several deep breaths. If the patient is unable to produce a sputum specimen, coughing can be stimulated by lowering the head of the patient's bed or by giving the patient an aerosol administration of a warm hypertonic solution. Other methods used to collect sputum include endotracheal aspiration, fiberoptic bronchoscopy (direct visualization and aspiration of bronchial secretion), and transtracheal aspiration (needle puncture into the trachea and aspiration through a catheter). These methods exclude oropharyngeal contamination of the specimen.

Nursing implications with rationale
Before

☞ Explain the procedure for sputum collection to the patient. Remind the patient that the sputum must be coughed up from the lungs and that saliva is not sputum. The laboratory technician will evaluate the specimen according to specific criteria, such as the number of epithelial cells, to determine whether the specimen is sputum or saliva before studying it. Sputum contains columnar (bronchial) cells; saliva is identified by squamous (mouth) cells.

■ Hold antibiotics until after the sputum has been collected. If the patient has been taking these drugs, they should be listed on the laboratory requisition slip.

- Give the patient a sterile sputum container on the night before the sputum is to be collected, so that the morning specimen may be obtained on the patient's arising. Obtaining an early-morning specimen is best because secretions pool and collect in the lungs during sleep. The early-morning specimen is likely to be the most productive.
- Instruct the patient to rinse out his or her mouth with water before the sputum collection to decrease contamination of the sputum specimen by particles in the oropharynx. The patient should not use toothpaste or mouthwash because they can affect the viability of microorganisms in the sputum specimen.
- If an aerosol treatment is necessary, explain the procedure to the patient and point out that it will stimulate coughing and sputum expectoration.

After

- Inform the patient to notify the nurse as soon as the specimen is collected so it can be labeled appropriately and sent to the laboratory as soon as possible. For aesthetic reasons the sputum container should be wrapped in paper towels so that the contents cannot be seen.
- Provide the patient with an ample supply of tissues with which to wipe his or her mouth after expectorating.

Thoracentesis and Pleural Fluid Analysis (Pleural Tap)

Test type Fluid analysis

Normal values

Gross appearance: Clear, serous, light yellow, 50 ml
Red blood cells (RBCs): None
White blood cells (WBCs): 300/ml
Protein: <4.1 g/dl
Glucose: 70-100 mg/dl
Amylase: 138-404 U/L

Alkaline phosphatase (ALP)
  Adult male: 90-240 U/L
  Female >45 years: 87-250 U/L
  Female <45 years: 76-196 U/L
Lactate dehydrogenase (LDH): Similar to serum lactate dehydrogenase, see p. 42
Cytology: No malignant cells
Bacteria: None
Fungi: None
Carcinoembryonic antigen (CEA): <5.0 ng/mL

Rationale

Thoracentesis is an invasive procedure that entails insertion of a needle into the pleural space for removal of fluid (Figure 5-11). The *pleural space* is defined as the space between the visceral pleura (thin membrane covering the lungs) and the parietal pleura (thin membrane covering the inside of the thoracic cavity).

Pleural fluid is removed for diagnostic and therapeutic purposes. Therapeutically, it is done to relieve pain, dyspnea, and other symptoms of pleural pressure. Removal of this fluid also permits better radiographic visualization of the lung.

Diagnostically, thoracentesis is performed to obtain and analyze fluid to determine the etiology of the pleural effusion. Pleural fluid is classified as *transudate* or *exudate*. This is an important differentiation and is very helpful in determining the

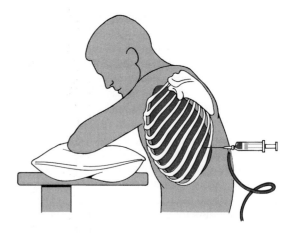

Figure 5-11 Thoracentesis.

etiology of the effusion. Transudates are most frequently caused by CHF, cirrhosis, nephrotic syndrome (a protein-losing renal disease), and hypoproteinemia. Exudates are most often found in inflammatory, infectious, or neoplastic conditions. However, collagen vascular disease, pulmonary infarction, trauma, and drug hypersensitivity also may cause an exudative effusion.

Pleural fluid is usually evaluated for gross appearance; cell counts; protein, LDH, glucose, triglyceride, and amylase levels; Gram stain and bacteriologic cultures; *M. tuberculosis* and fungus; cytology; CEA levels; and sometimes for other specific tests. Each is discussed separately.

Gross appearance

The color, optical density, and viscosity are noted as the pleural fluid appears in the aspirating syringe. Transudative pleural fluid may be clear, serous, and light yellow, especially in patients with hepatic cirrhosis. Milk-colored pleural fluid may result from the escape of chyle from blocked thoracic lymphatic ducts. An opalescent, pearly fluid is characteristic of chylothorax (chyle in the pleural cavity). Conditions that may cause lymphatic blockage include lymphoma, carcinoma, and TB involving the thoracic lymph nodes.

Cloudy or turbid fluid may result from inflammatory or infectious conditions such as empyema. Empyema is characterized by the presence of a foul odor and thick, puslike fluid. Bloody fluid may be the result of a traumatic tap (the aspirating needle penetrates a blood vessel), intrathoracic bleeding, or tumor.

Cell counts

The WBC and differential counts are determined. A WBC count exceeding 1000/ml is suggestive of an exudate. The predominance of polymorphonuclear leukocytes (see p. 416) usually is an indication of an acute inflammatory condition (e.g., pneumonia, pulmonary infarction, early TB effusion). When more than 50% of the WBCs are small lymphocytes, the effusion is usually caused by TB or tumor. Normally, no RBCs should be present. The presence of RBCs may indicate neo-

plasms, TB, or intrathoracic bleeding. Usually these counts are performed manually using a simple hemacytometer.

Protein content

Total protein levels greater than 3 g/dl are characteristic of exudates, whereas transudates usually have a protein content of less than 3 g/dl. It is now thought that the albumin gradient between serum and pleural fluid can differentiate between the transudate and exudate nature of pleural fluid better than can the total protein content. This gradient is obtained by subtracting the pleural albumin value from the serum albumin value. Values of 1.1 g/dl or more suggest a transudate. Values less than 1.1 g/dl suggest an exudate but will not differentiate the potential cause of the exudate (malignancy from infection or inflammation).

Because there is a significant overlap in protein values differentiating transudate from exudate, the total protein ratio (fluid/serum) is considered to be a more accurate criterion. A total protein ratio of fluid to serum greater than 0.5 is considered to be an exudate.

Lactic dehydrogenase

A pleural fluid/serum LDH ratio greater than 0.6 is typical of an exudate. An exudate is identified with a high degree of accuracy if the pleural fluid/serum protein ratio is greater than 0.5, and the pleural fluid/serum LDH ratio is greater than 0.6.

Glucose

Pleural glucose levels usually approximate serum levels. Low values appear to be a combination of glycolysis by the extra cells within an exudate and impairment of glucose diffusion because of damage to the pleural membrane. Values less than 60 mg/dl also indicate exudate.

Amylase

In a malignant effusion, the amylase concentration is slightly elevated. Amylase levels above the normal range for serum or two times the serum level are seen when the effusion is caused by pancreatitis or rupture of the esophagus associated with leakage of salivary amylase into the chest cavity.

Triglyceride

Measurement of triglyceride levels is an important part of identifying chylous effusions. These effusions usually are produced by obstruction or transection of the lymphatic system caused by lymphoma, neoplasm, trauma, or recent surgery. The triglyceride value in a chylous effusion exceeds 110 mg/dL.

Gram stain and bacteriologic culture

Culture and Gram stains identify the organisms involved in the infection and also provide information concerning antibiotic sensitivity. (See p. 173 for a more thorough discussion of Gram stain, cultures, and sensitivity.) These tests are routinely performed when bacterial pneumonia or empyema is a possible cause of the effusion. If possible, these tests should be done before initiation of antibiotic therapy.

Cultures for *Mycobacterium tuberculosis* and fungus

TB is less often a cause for pleural effusion in the United States today than it was in the past (although its incidence is back on the rise, especially among immunosuppressed patients). Fungus may be a cause of pulmonary effusion in patients with compromised immunologic defenses. (See p. 184 for more information about TB culture techniques.)

Cytology

A cytologic study is performed to detect tumors. It is positive in approximately 50% to 60% of patients with malignant effusions. Breast and lung are the two most frequent tumors; lymphoma is the third.

CEA

Pleural fluid CEA levels are elevated in various malignant (gastrointestinal [GI], breast) conditions.

Special tests

The pH of pleural fluid is usually 7.4 or greater. The pH is typically less than 7.2 when empyema is present. The pH may be 7.2 to 7.4 in TB or malignancy. In some instances, the rheumatoid factor (see p. 485) and the complement levels (see p. 472) are also measured in pleural fluid. Pleural fluid antinuclear antibody (ANA) and pleural fluid/serum ANA ratios are often used to evaluate pleural effusion secondary to systemic lupus erythematosus.

Potential complications

Potential complications associated with thoracentesis are as follows:

- Pneumothorax
  This results from puncture of the lung or entry of air into the pleural space through the aspirating needle.
- Intrapleural bleeding, because of puncture of a blood vessel
- Seeding of the needle tract with tumor, when malignant pleural effusion exists
- Empyema, caused by infection delivered by the aspirating needle

Procedure

No fasting or sedation is necessary for thoracentesis. If the patient has a troublesome cough, a suppressant, such as codeine, may be given before the procedure. The patient usually is placed in an upright position with the arms and shoulders raised and supported on a padded overbed table. This position spreads the ribs and enlarges the intercostal space for insertion of the needle. Patients who cannot sit upright are placed in a side-lying position on the unaffected side, with the side to be tapped uppermost.

The thoracentesis is performed under strict sterile technique. The needle insertion site, which is determined by percussion, auscultation, and examination of a chest radiographic film, ultrasound scanning, or fluoroscopy, is aseptically cleansed and anesthetized with a local anesthetic such as lidocaine. The site is dull on percussion because of the fluid accumulation. The presence of this fluid indicates that the needle should enter the pleural space and not the lung. After the needle is positioned in the pleural space, the fluid is withdrawn with a syringe and a three-way stopcock. A spring or Kelly clamp may be placed on the needle at the chest wall to stabilize the needle depth during fluid collection. A short polyethylene catheter may be inserted into the pleural space for fluid aspiration. The advantage of inserting this catheter is that it decreases the risk of puncturing the visceral pleura and inducing a pneumothorax. Also, large volumes of fluid may be collected by connecting the catheter to a gravity-drainage system.

After the fluid is obtained, the needle is removed and a small bandage is placed over the site. The patient is then usually turned on the unaffected side for 1 hour to allow the pleural puncture site to heal.

This procedure can be performed by a physician at the patient's bedside, in a procedure room, or in the physician's office. Although the local anesthetic eliminates pain at the insertion site, some patients complain of feeling pressure when the pleura is entered and the fluid is removed.

Contraindication

Thoracentesis is contraindicated for patients with significant thrombocytopenia because the aspirating needle may initiate bleeding.

Nursing implications with rationale

Before

☞ Explain the purpose of the test and the procedure to the patient. Be certain that the patient knows that movement or coughing during the procedure is prohibited to avoid inadvertent needle damage to the lung or pleura.

■ Administer a cough suppressant before the procedure if the patient has a troublesome cough. If the patient must cough during the procedure, the physician may withdraw the needle slightly to avoid puncture.

■ Ensure that written and informed consent for this procedure is obtained.

■ Assess the patient's lung sounds as a baseline for comparison after the study.

■ A decubitus chest radiographic film (see p. 155) is often obtained before thoracentesis to ensure that the pleural fluid is mobile and accessible to a needle placed within the pleural space. Fluoroscopy also may be used.

■ Help position the patient appropriately (usually in a sitting position) to enhance the patient's comfort and allow the fluid to pool in the base of the pleural space.

During

■ Monitor the pulse for reflex bradycardia and evaluate the patient for diaphoresis and a feeling of faintness. If these occur, the procedure should be terminated and the patient placed in the recumbent position. A second attempt at thoracentesis may be tried several hours later.

■ Label the specimen with the patient's name, date, source of fluid, and diagnosis. Record the exact location of the thoracentesis, the quantity of the fluid obtained, and the gross appearance of the fluid.

After

■ Obtain a chest radiographic study as ordered to check for the complication of pneumothorax, which could be induced by the pleural tap.

■ Monitor the vital signs as ordered. Observe the patient for coughing or for the expectoration of blood (hemoptysis), which might indicate trauma to the lung. Evaluate the patient for signs and symptoms of pneumothorax, tension pneumothorax, subcutaneous emphysema, and pyogenic infection (e.g., tachypnea, dyspnea, decrease in breath sounds, anxiety, restlessness, or fever). Pulmonary edema or cardiac distress may also be produced because of a sudden shift of mediastinal contents if a large amount of fluid was aspirated.

■ Assess the patient's lungs for diminished breath sounds, which could be a sign of pneumothorax. Compare these sounds to the baseline breath sounds auscultated before thoracentesis.

■ If the patient has no complaints of dyspnea, normal activity usually can be resumed 1 hour after the procedure.

Case Study

Pleural Effusion

Mr. D.L., 54 years old, developed shortness of breath. He was otherwise in good health. He had no chest pain. His physical examination indicated that he had decreased breath sounds in the left lung and also dullness to percussion in this area.

Studies	Results
Routine laboratory work	Within normal limits (WNL)
Chest radiographic study, p. 155	Possible pleural effusion (noted on decubitus views)
CT scan of the chest, p. 157	No intraparenchymal lung tumor; there is, however, free fluid in the pleural cavity and a thickened parietal pleura, especially in the lower chest cavity

Thoracentesis and pleural fluid analysis, p. 174

Gross appearance	Bloody
Cell count	WBC >1000 mm^3; 70% of WBCs are small lymphocytes
	RBCs $>100,000$/mm^3 (all suggestive of exudate)
Specific gravity	1.016 (suggestive of exudate)
Protein content	3.9 g/dl (characteristic of exudate)
LDH	Pleural fluid to serum LDH ratio 0.7 (typical of exudate)
Glucose	80 mg/dl (serum: 90 mg/dl)
C&S	No growth
Mycobacterium and fungus	Negative
Cytology	Malignant-appearing mesothelial cells
Pleural biopsy, p. 165	Undifferentiated mesothelium

Diagnostic Analysis

The pleural effusion suspected on the chest x-ray film and documented on the CT scan could have been caused by infection, tumor, or other forms of inflammation. The thickening of the parietal pleura on the CT scan did, however, strongly point to a tumor affecting the parietal mesothelial pleural surface. The thoracentesis analysis indicated that it was an exudative type of fluid consistent with either an infection or tumor. Because the pleural fluid glucose was not markedly diminished, infection was an unlikely possibility. The negative cultures for bacteria, TB, and fungus ruled out the possibility for these infections. Cytology strongly pointed toward a mesothelial type of tumor. Thoracoscopic pleural biopsy, however, made the definitive diagnosis of mesothelioma.

The patient was treated with chemotherapy, which unfortunately did not help. He attempted, ineffectually, several unconventional forms of anticancerous therapy outside the country. He died 3 months after the diagnosis of his neoplastic disease.

Critical Thinking Questions
1. What is the difference between an exudate and a transudate?
2. Thoracentesis can be performed for both diagnostic and therapeutic purposes. What was the reason for the thoracentesis in this patient?

Thoracoscopy

Test type Endoscopy

Normal values
Normal pleura and lung

Rationale
This procedure is used to directly visualize the pleura, lung, and mediastinum. Tissue can be obtained for testing. It also is helpful in assisting in the staging and dissection of lung cancers. Any tissue abnormality can be removed for biopsy. Fluid can be drained and aspirated for testing. Dissection for lung resection can be carried out with the thoracoscope (video-assisted thoracotomy [VAT]), thereby minimizing the extent of a thoracotomy incision VAT is especially helpful for lung biopsy in patients with pulmonary nodules of uncertain etiology or for suspected pneumocystis infections in immunocompromised patients.

The patient must be aware of the possibility of undergoing an open thoracotomy if the procedure cannot be performed thoracoscopically or if bleeding occurs that cannot be controlled any other way. Any patient who can have an open thoracotomy can have a thoracoscopy.

Potential complications
Potential complications associated with thoracoscopy are as follows:

- Bleeding from surgical dissection
- Infection or empyema

Procedure
Thoracoscopy is performed in the operating room. The patient initially is placed in the lateral decubitus position. After the thorax is cleansed, a blunt-tipped (Veress) needle is inserted through a small incision, and the lung is collapsed. A thoracoscope is inserted through a trocar to examine the chest cavity. Additional trocars can be placed as conduits for other instrumentation. After the desired procedure is completed, the scope and trocars are removed. Usually a small chest tube is placed to ensure full reexpansion of the lung. The incision(s) is closed with a few skin stitches and covered with an adhesive bandage. The procedure is performed by a surgeon in about 1 to 2 hours. Postoperative pain is much less than with an open thoracotomy.

Contraindications
Thoracoscopy is contraindicated for patients who underwent previous lung surgery, because it is difficult to obtain access to the free pleural space.

Nursing implications with rationale

Before

☞ Explain the procedure to the patient. Because the procedure usually is performed with general anesthesia, follow the routine precautions for general anesthesia.

▪ Ensure that written and informed consent for this procedure is obtained. Because of the possibility of intrathoracic injury, an open thoracotomy may be required. Verify that the patient is aware of that.

▪ Shave and prepare the patient's chest as ordered.

☞ Instruct the patient to remain NPO after midnight on the day of the test. IV fluids may be given.

After

▪ Assess the patient frequently for signs of bleeding (increased pulse rate, decreased blood pressure). Report any significant findings to the physician.

▪ Provide analgesics to relieve the minor to moderate pain that may be experienced.

▪ If a surgical procedure has been performed thoracoscopically, provide appropriate postsurgical care.

▪ A chest x-ray examination is performed after the procedure to ensure complete reexpansion of the lung.

Throat Culture and Sensitivity
(C&S, Strept screen)

Test type Microscopic evaluation

Normal values
Negative

Rationale

A throat culture is obtained to diagnose bacterial, viral, gonococcal, or candidal pharyngitis. It is indicated for patients who have a sore throat or a fever of unknown etiology, or who may be chronic carriers of recurrent infection.

Because the throat normally is colonized by many organisms, culture of this area serves only to isolate and identify a few particular pathogens (e.g., streptococci, meningococci, gonococci, *Bordetella pertussis*, *Corynebacterium diphtheriae*). Recognition of these organisms requires treatment. Streptococci are most often sought because a beta-hemolytic streptococcal pharyngitis may be followed by rheumatic fever or glomerulonephritis. This type of streptococcal infection most frequently affects children between ages 3 and 15. Therefore, all children with a sore throat and fever should have a throat culture done to identify any streptococcal infections. In adults, however, fewer than 5% of patients with pharyngitis have a streptococcal infection. Therefore, throat cultures in adults only are indicated when the patient has severe or recurrent sore throat, often associated with fever and palpable lymphadenopathy. These adults often have a history of previous streptococcal infections.

Rapid immunologic tests (strept screen) with antiserum against group A streptococcal antigen are now available and are very accurate for the identification of the organism without culture. With these newer kits, the streptococcal organism can be identified directly from the swab specimen. If the strept screen is negative, the specimen still may be cultured for *Streptococcus*. If that culture is negative, no streptococcal infection exists. The rapid serologic tests can be performed in approximately 15 minutes. The final culture report requires at least 2 days.

All cultures should be performed before antibiotic therapy is initiated; otherwise, the antibiotic may interrupt the growth of the organism in the laboratory. Most organisms take approximately 24 hours to grow in the laboratory, and a preliminary report can be given at that time. Occasionally, a period of 48 to 72 hours is required for growth and identification of the organism. Cultures may be repeated on completion of appropriate antibiotic therapy to identify resolution of the infection.

Interfering factor

Factors that interfere with throat culture and sensitivity are antiseptic mouthwashes, which may affect test results.

Procedure

A throat culture specimen can best be obtained by depressing the tongue with a wooden tongue blade and touching the posterior wall of the throat and areas of inflammation, exudation, or ulceration with a sterile cotton swab (Figure 5-12). One should avoid touching any other part of the mouth. Two swabs are preferred. Growth of *Streptococcus* from both swabs is more accurate, and the second swab also can be used in the strept screen. The swab is placed in a sterile container and sent to the microbiology laboratory. When a specimen is obtained from young children, an adult should hold the child on his or her lap. The person obtaining the specimen places one hand on the child's forehead to stabilize the head. The culture then is taken as previously described.

Nursing implications with rationale

Before

☞ Explain the procedure to the patient.

During

■ Wear gloves and handle the specimen as if it were infectious.

After

■ Indicate on the laboratory requisition slip any medications that the patient may be taking that could affect test results.

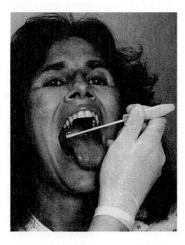

Figure 5-12 Throat culture. Collection of specimen from posterior pharynx.

■ Notify the physician of any positive results so that appropriate antibiotic therapy can be initiated.

Tuberculin Test (PPD Skin Test, Mantoux Test)

Test type Skin

Normal values
Negative; reaction <5 mm

Rationale
Purified protein derivative (PPD) testing is performed on patients who are suspected to have had recent TB exposure or active TB infection. This includes patients with suspicious chest radiographic findings, productive coughs with negative routine cultures, hemoptysis, or undetermined weight loss. PPD testing is also performed on high-risk populations such as immunocompromised or malnourished patients; people who have had close, recent contact with TB patients; people who abuse IV drugs; or foreigners from continents with high TB rates (Africa, South America, and Asia).

A PPD of the tubercle bacillus (0.1 ml, or 5 tuberculin units) is injected intradermally. If the patient is infected with or has been exposed to TB (whether active or dormant), lymphocytes will recognize the PPD antigen and cause a local inflammatory reaction at the site of injection. If the patient has had no exposure, no reaction will occur. Although this test is used to detect TB infection, it is unable to indicate whether the infection is active or dormant. If the test is negative and the physician strongly suspects TB, a second-strength PPD can be used. If this test is then negative, the patient has not been exposed to TB. The PPD skin test usually becomes positive 6 weeks after infection. Once positive, the reaction usually persists for life.

The PPD test also can be used as part of a series of skin tests done to assess the immune system. If the immune system is nonfunctioning because of poor nutrition or chronic illness (e.g., neoplasia, infection, or acquired immunodeficiency syndrome [AIDS]), the PPD test will be negative despite the patient having been previously exposed to TB. Other skin tests used to test immune function include *Candida,* mumps virus, and *Trichophyton,* organisms to which most people in the United States have been exposed. The PPD test will not cause active TB, because no live organisms exist in the test solution.

Potential complication

Skin slough is a potential complication associated with tuberculin testing. When a patient known to have active TB or a patient who has received a TB vaccination receives a PPD test, the local reaction may be so severe as to cause a complete skin slough requiring surgical care. When these patients are eliminated from PPD testing, the test has no complications.

Interfering factors

Factors that interfere with tuberculin testing include the following:

- Subcutaneous injection of PPD, which may cause a negative reaction
  The injection must be intradermal for induration to occur.
- Immunocompromised patients, who will not react to PPD despite exposure to TB
- Improper storage of PPD material, which can cause false-negative results
- Improper dosage of PPD, which can cause false-negative results

Procedure

A nurse prepares the volar (inner) aspect of the forearm with alcohol and intradermally injects 0.1 ml of PPD with a tuberculin syringe (Figure 5-13). A skin wheal should result. The test site should be marked with indelible ink. A nurse or physician reads the test 48 to 72 hours later. The test site is examined for induration (hardening), and the hardened area (*not* the reddened area) is marked and measured. If the thickened, swollen area

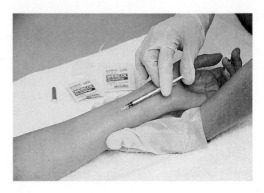

Figure 5-13   Tuberculin testing. Intradermal injection in forearm for skin testing.

measures more than 10 mm, the test is considered positive. Induration measurements between 5 and 10 mm are considered doubtful, and results less than 5 mm are labeled negative.

Contraindications

Contraindications for tuberculin testing are as follows:

- Patients with known active TB
- Patients who have received bacille Calmette-Guérin (BCG) immunization against PPD
  These patients will demonstrate a positive reaction to the PPD vaccination even though they have never had TB infection.

Nursing implications with rationale

Before

- Explain the procedure to the patient. Assure the patient that he or she will not contract TB from this test.
- Assess the patient for a previous history of TB. Report significant findings to the physician.
- Evaluate the patient's history of previous PPD results and BCG immunization.

During

- Prepare the forearm with alcohol and allow it to dry. Intradermally inject the PPD and then circle the area with indelible ink. Record the time at which the PPD was injected.

- If the patient is an outpatient, do not give the PPD test when the reading time (48 to 72 hours later) falls on a weekend. Frequently, no one is available then to read the results.

After

- Read the results in 48 to 72 hours and record the results. Some hospitals require readings at both 48- and 72-hour intervals.
- If the test is positive, confirm that the physician is notified and that the patient is treated appropriately.
- If the test is positive, check the arm 4 to 5 days after the test in case a severe skin reaction has occurred and requires surgical debridement.

Case Study

Tuberculosis

Ms. N., a 32-year-old nurse, worked in an inner-city hospital. She had a 3-month history of weight loss, cough, hemoptysis, low-grade fever, and drenching night sweats over the upper half of her body several times a week.

Studies

Routine laboratory work
  Hemoglobin
  Hematocrit
Erythrocyte sedimentation rate (sed rate), p. 476
Chest x-ray, p. 155

Sputum culture, p. 173

Acid-fast bacilli (AFB) smear

Tuberculin skin test, p. 181

Results

WNL except for:
  10.5 g/dl (normal: 12-16 g/dl)
32% (normal: 37-47%)
30 mm/hour (normal: up to 20 mm/ hour)
Multinodular infiltration in the apical posterior segments of the upper lobes and superior segments of the lower lobes (normal: no pathology)
Mycobacterium tuberculosis (normal: none)
Positive for acid-fast bacilli (normal: none)
17-mm tranverse diameter of induration (normal: <5 mm)

Diagnostic Analysis

The diagnosis of TB was confirmed in light of the sputum culture, tuberculin test, and chest x-ray examination. An elevated sedimentation rate and modest anemia are common components of the clinical picture. The mainstay for the treatment of TB is pharmacologic. The patient was placed on a 9- to 12-month regimen of isoniazid and rifampin therapy.

Critical Thinking Questions

1. What kind of infectious disease precautions should be initiated with this patient?
2. Why is TB usually treated with combination drug therapy?
3. What laboratory tests are used in the follow-up care of patients being treated for TB?

Tuberculosis Culture (TB Culture, BACTEC Method, Polymerase Chain Reaction, Acid-fast Bacilli Smear [AFB])

Test type Microbiology culture

Normal values
Negative for TB
No acid-fast bacilli seen

Rationale
TB culture is indicated in any patient with a persistent productive cough, night sweats, anorexia, weight loss, fever, and hemoptysis. This diagnosis should be considered especially in high-risk patients, such as those who are immunocompromised, alcoholic, or have recently been exposed to TB.

The diagnosis of TB (see p. 181 for other TB testing) can be made only by identification and culture of *Mycobacterium tuberculosis* in the specimen. Conventional culture techniques for growth, identification, and susceptibility testing of acid-fast mycobacteria take 4 to 6 weeks. Because the patient suspected of having TB cannot be isolated from society for that duration, the disease may spread to many other people while awaiting results. With the resurgence and increasing incidence of TB in the United States population (especially among immunocompromised patients with AIDS), newer, more rapid culture techniques, such as the BACTEC and polymerase chain reaction culture methods, have been developed to permit quick identification of mycobacterial growth. With these newer techniques, *M. tuberculosis* can be identified in as little as 36 to 48 hours.

Sputum and other fluids can be specially stained to allow microscopic identification of TB. The acid-fast smear (usually of sputum) is used to support the diagnosis of TB. The diagnosis of TB cannot be made with only a positive AFB; TB cultures are also required. After taking up a dye such as fuchsin, *M. tuberculosis* is not decolorized by acid alcohol (i.e., it is acid-fast). It is seen under the microscope as a red, rod-shaped organism. If this bacillus is seen, the patient may have active TB. However, other species of mycobacteria, *Nocardia,* and some fungi are acid-fast. Smears may be negative as often as 50% of the time even with positive cultures. AFB smears also are used to monitor treatment of TB. If after adequate therapy (2 months), the sputum still contains AFB (even though the culture may be negative as a result of antituberculosis drugs), treatment failure should be considered.

Interfering factors
Factors that interfere with TB culture are antituberculosis drugs that were started before culture, which could interfere with the growth of TB.

Procedure
See sputum C&S, p. 173. Obtain three to five early-morning specimens. All specimens must contain mycobacteria to make the diagnosis of TB. For urine collection, obtain three to five single, clean-voided specimens early in the morning.

Nursing implications with rationale
See Sputum C&S, p. 173.
Before
- Explain the procedure to the patient.
- Instruct the patient about appropriate isolation of sputum and other body fluids to avoid potential spread of suspected TB.

After
- Transport the swabs, intestinal washings, and biopsy specimens to the laboratory immediately for preparation.
- Follow the institution's policy for universal specimen handling.

REVIEW QUESTIONS AND ANSWERS

1. **Question:** One hour after having a thoracentesis, your patient's breath sounds are markedly diminished. You also note dyspnea, tachypnea, anxiety, and restlessness. Why does the physician order a chest x-ray?

Answer: The patient may have developed a pneumothorax as a complication of this test. This would be noted on a chest x-ray.

2. **Question:** Your patient has just returned from the x-ray department where he had a pulmonary angiogram to detect a PE. His left femoral vein was used for the catheter insertion site. He had begun to complain of severe left calf pain. What assessments should receive priority?

   Answer: His catheter insertion site should be evaluated for inflammation, hemorrhage, hematoma, and the presence of the femoral pulse. Peripheral pulses should be evaluated, along with the color and temperature of the extremity. Most likely, he has lost his pulses as a result of a blood clot. An embolectomy is probably needed.

3. **Question:** Your clinic is screening factory workers for TB by the tuberculin test. Why should patients with a past history of TB be excluded from this screening?

   Answer: These patients could have a local reaction that may be so severe as to cause a complete skin slough. Because of this potential complication, these patients should not be screened with this test.

4. **Question:** Your patient with pneumonia is scheduled for a portable chest x-ray examination to be done on the nursing unit. What precautions should the staff observe to prevent radiation exposure?

   Answer: The nursing staff should, if necessary, assist the radiologic technician in the placement of the radiographic film cassette behind the patient. Then, the nursing staff, visitors, and other patients should leave the room before the radiographic films are taken. If constant bedside care is needed, a lead apron should be worn for protection from exposure.

5. **Question:** A 42-year-old patient develops a clinical picture compatible with a PE. Lung scanning is done and is positive. Does this patient need pulmonary angiography?

   Answer: Not necessarily. A positive lung scan is not definitive evidence of PE, because other pathologic pulmonary conditions (pneumonia or pleural effusion) can create the same results. However, angiography is not always necessary. If the chest x-ray study results are normal (i.e., no pneumonia or pleural effusion), then one can be confident that the patient has a PE. If the chest x-ray study results are abnormal, pulmonary angiography is needed to establish the diagnosis of PE.

6. **Question:** The physician orders O_2 for your patient, who is short of breath. How long after the start of O_2 would ABGs be drawn to evaluate the patient's Po_2 level?

   Answer: Twenty to 30 minutes. It takes this long for any change in inspired O_2 concentration to be reflected in the Po_2 level. Whenever O_2 therapy is initiated or changed, an ABG study should be done 10 to 40 minutes later, depending on the patient's underlying lung disease, to evaluate the effect of the new O_2 therapy. Likewise, when a patient is started on a respirator or a respiratory setting is changed, an ABG study should be performed 30 to 40 minutes later.

7. **Question:** Interpret the following ABG results on a patient admitted to your unit with uncontrolled diabetes mellitus: pH, 7.25; Pco_2, 36 mm Hg; HCO_3^-, 19 mEq/L; Po_2, 84 mm Hg.

   Answer: The patient's ABGs show metabolic acidosis. This is because the pH is acidotic, the Pco_2 level is within the normal range, and the HCO_3^- is altered in a way (decreased) compatible with acidosis.

8. **Question:** One hour later, before therapy is initiated, the ABGs of the patient described in Question 7 show the following: pH, 7.32; Pco_2, 28; HCO_3^-, 19. Interpret these results.

   Answer: The results indicate persistent metabolic acidosis with partial respiratory compensation. The Pco_2 level is decreased because the lungs are blowing off CO_2 in an attempt to compensate for the acid-base derangement.

9. **Question:** Interpret the ABG results on this patient seen in the emergency room with pneumonia: pH, 7.28; Pco_2, 60 mm Hg; HCO_3^-, 32 mEq/L.

Answer: The results indicate respiratory acidosis with partial metabolic compensation. Respiratory acidosis is present because the increased CO_2 level is compatible with the acidotic pH. The kidneys are retaining bicarbonate to attempt to compensate for the acidotic pH.

10. **Question:** Your patient, who is being evaluated for lung surgery, is scheduled for PFTs. Shortly before leaving for these tests, the patient complains of severe back pain. The patient has an order for meperidine, 50 mg IM for pain. Should the drug be given?

    Answer: Yes. Remember that sedation should not be given to a patient before PFTs, because many of these tests are effort-related and the sedated patient cannot cooperate completely. However, a patient in severe pain cannot cooperate either. Therefore, the drug should be given to alleviate the pain, and the studies should be canceled and rescheduled for another time.

Bibliography

Ball EM et al: Diagnosis and treatment of sleep apnea within the community: the Walla Walla project, *Arch Intern Med* 157(4):419-424, 1997.

Bitran JB: Primary lung cancer. In Rakel RF, editor: Conn's current therapy, Philadelphia, 1998, WB Saunders.

Blue PN et al: The need for oblique or lateral ventilation images in the diagnosis of pulmonary embolism, *Clin Nucl Med* 15(12):917-919, 1990.

Bordow RA, Moser KM: Manual of clinical problems in pulmonary medicine, ed 3, Boston, 1991, Little, Brown.

Breiman RF et al: Emergence of drug-resistant pneumococcal infections in the United States, *JAMA* 271:1831, 1994.

Cheney AM, Maquindang ML: Patient teaching for x-ray and other diagnostics, *RN* 56(4):54-56, 1993.

Drazen JM, Weinberger SE: Approach to the patient with disease of the respiratory system. In Fauci AS et al, editors: Harrison's principles of internal medicine, ed 14, New York, 1998, McGraw-Hill.

Geerts WH: Pulmonary embolism. In Rakel RE, editor: Conn's current therapy, Philadelphia, 1998, WB Saunders.

Greenberg SB: Bacterial pneumonia. In Rakel RE, editor: Conn's current therapy, Philadelphia, 1998, WB Saunders.

Harris A, Argent BE: The cystic fibrosis gene and its product CFTR, *Semin Cell Biol* 4:37, 1993.

Harris RJ et al: The diagnostic and therapeutic utility of thoracoscopy: a review, *Chest* 108:828, 1995.

Hiratzka LF: Atelectasis. In Rakel RE, editor: Conn's current therapy, Philadelphia, 1998, WB Saunders.

Konstan MW et al: Effect of high-dose ibuprofen in patients with cystic fibrosis, *N Engl J Med* 332:848, 1995.

McFadden ER et al: Asthma, *Lancet* 345:1215, 1995.

McFadden ER, Gilbert IA: Exercise-induced asthma, *N Engl J Med* 330:1362, 1994.

Miller YE: Pulmonary neoplasms. In Bennet JC et al, editors: Cecil textbook of medicine, ed 20, Philadelphia, 1996, WB Saunders.

Senior RM: Pulmonary embolism. In Bennet JC et al, editors: Cecil textbook of medicine, ed 20, Philadelphia, 1996, WB Saunders.

Sferra TJ, Collins FS: The molecular biology of cystic fibrosis, *Annu Rev Med* 44:133, 1995.

Stark JR: Tuberculosis in children, *Primary Care* 23(4), 861-881, 1996.

Stein PD et al: Diagnostic utility of ventilation/perfusion lung scan in acute pulmonary embolism is not diminished by pre-existing cardiac or pulmonary disease, *Chest* 100(3):604-606, 1991.

Weinberger SE: Bronchiectasis. In Fauci AS et al, editors: Harrison's principles of internal medicine, ed 14, New York, 1998, McGraw-Hill.

Weinberger SE, Drazen JM: Diagnostic procedures in respiratory diseases. In Fauci AS et al, editors: Harrison's principles of internal medicine, ed 14, New York, 1998, McGraw-Hill.

Weinberger SE, Drazen JM: Disturbances of respiratory function. In Fauci AS et al, editors: Harrison's principles of internal medicine, ed 14, New York, 1998, McGraw-Hill.

Zoloth SR: Anergy compromise screening for tuberculosis in high-risk populations, *Am J Public Health* 83(5):749-751, 1993.

Chapter 6

Diagnostic Studies Used in the Assessment of the
Nervous System

ANATOMY AND PHYSIOLOGY

The nervous system may be divided conveniently into three areas:

1. The central nervous system (CNS), consisting of the brain and spinal cord
2. The peripheral nervous system, which includes the cranial and spinal nerves
3. The autonomic nervous system, made up of the sympathetic and parasympathetic nerves

Because the diagnostic procedures discussed in this chapter relate primarily to the brain and spinal cord, this brief discussion of anatomy and physiology is limited to these areas.

The brain is encased and protected by the bony skull, which is a composite of the frontal, parietal,

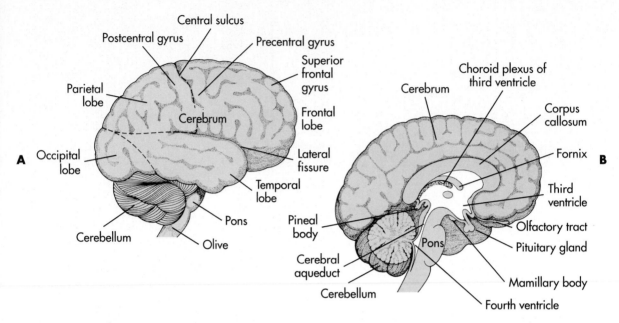

Figure 6-1 Right hemisphere of cerebrum. **A,** Lateral surface. **B,** Medial surface.

occipital, and temporal bones. At the base of the skull is the foramen magnum, through which the spinal cord passes. Numerous small openings in the skull permit the passage of cranial nerves and blood vessels.

The brain is divided into the cerebrum, cerebellum, and brainstem (Figure 6-1). The cerebrum is the largest part of the brain. It is divided into two hemispheres, each consisting of five lobes. The frontal lobe, located anteriorly, contains nerves that primarily affect emotional responses, attitudes (personality), and thought processes (e.g., judgment, volition, ethical values, and abstract and creative thinking). The parietal lobe, located in the midcentral area, contains nerves associated with somatic sensations such as pain and temperature. The temporal lobe is located laterally and inferiorly to the frontal and parietal lobes. It contains the hearing center. The posterior part of each cerebral hemisphere is the occipital lobe, which is primarily concerned with visual perception. A fifth lobe, the insula (island of Reil), lies hidden from view in the lateral fissure.

Within the cerebrum are fluid-filled spaces called *ventricles.* The large lateral ventricles empty into a smaller central, or third, ventricle. This, in turn, drains into a fourth ventricle located within the brainstem. The fluid within the four ventricles normally flows into the subarachnoid space.

The cerebellum is located just below the cerebral occipital lobe (see Figure 6-1). It is separated from the cerebrum by the tentorium cerebelli and is responsible for the control and coordination of skeletal function and spatial equilibrium.

The brainstem extends from the cerebral hemispheres through the foramen magnum, where it then is called the *spinal cord.* The brainstem includes the midbrain, pons, and medulla oblongata (see Figure 6-1) and neurologically controls breathing, heart rate, blood pressure, and consciousness.

The vertebral column (Figure 6-2) supports the head and protects the spinal cord contained within the column. The vertebral column consists of cervical, thoracic, lumbar, sacral, and coccygeal vertebrae. Between two vertebrae is an open-

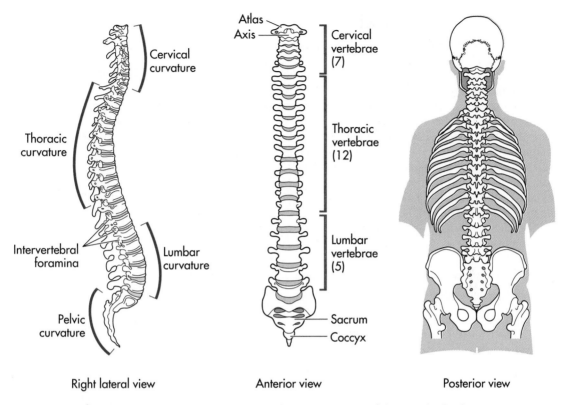

Right lateral view   Anterior view   Posterior view

Figure 6-2 Right lateral, anterior, and posterior views of the vertebral column.

ing called a *vertebral foramen,* through which spinal nerves leave the spinal cord. The vertebrae are held together by strong ligaments. True joint spaces separate the vertebrae. Within these joints are vertebral disks. Each disk is composed of a central core called the *nucleus pulposus* and an outer rim called the *anulus fibrosus.*

The spinal cord, which is contained within the spinal canal, is approximately 45 cm (18 inches) in length and approximately the width of a finger. The spinal cord is a direct continuation of the medulla oblongata. It contains the motor and sensory relay fibers to and from the higher centers within the cord and brain.

Because the brain and spinal cord are vital yet delicate organs, they are well protected by three membranes called *meninges* (dura mater, arachnoid, and pia mater). The dura mater is the dense fibrous outer layer. The arachnoid lies next to the dura mater. The pia mater is that layer most closely adherent to the brain and spinal cord. The space between the arachnoid mater and the pia mater is called the *subarachnoid* space. Within this space cerebrospinal fluid (CSF) circulates.

The choroid plexuses, found in the lateral and third and fourth ventricles of the brain, are the sites of CSF formation. CSF is secreted from the blood as the blood circulates through the capillaries of the choroid plexuses. The CSF passes through the channels from the lateral ventricles to the third and fourth ventricles and then into the subarachnoid space surrounding the brain and spinal cord. Subsequently, the CSF is reabsorbed by the venous circulation of the skull.

The function of the CSF is to cushion and support the brain and spinal cord within the skull and vertebral column. This fluid acts as a shock absorber and therefore reduces the impact of trauma to the CNS. CSF also carries nutrients to various areas of the brain and spinal cord. The average person has approximately 150 ml of CSF in the ventricular and subarchnoid systems.

The brain has a dual blood supply (i.e., carotid and vertebral). There are left and right carotid and vertebral arteries. This double blood supply serves to protect the brain from tissue necrosis in the event of occlusion of one of the four vessels. Unique to the brain is the blood-brain barrier, which prevents the movement of large molecules from the blood into the extracellular fluid surrounding the brain cell. This barrier eliminates the need for the brain to compensate rapidly for sudden and transient changes in blood volume and composition.

Brain Scan (Cerebral Blood Flow)

Test type Nuclear scan

Normal values
No areas of increased radionuclide uptake within the brain

Rationale
In the past, the brain scan was the only test available to study the brain. Since the advent of the computed tomography (CT) scan of the brain (see p. 196), magnetic resonance imaging (MRI) (see p. 213), and positron emission tomography (PET) (see p. 525) scan, the brain scan has diminished in usefulness. This test is utilized to identify pathology (e.g., tumor, infarction, infection) involving the cortex.

Brain scanning is accomplished by means of a camera that scans the brain after intravenous (IV) injection of a radionuclide material, usually technetium (Tc) 99m. A realistic image of the blood vessels, gray matter, meninges, and any pathologic deposits becomes apparent. Patients with suspected stroke (cerebrovascular accident [CVA] syndrome) or other neurologic complaints are candidates for this type of study.

Normally, the blood-brain barrier does not allow blood (containing the radionuclide) to come in direct contact with brain tissue. However, in lo-

calized pathologic conditions, this normal barrier is disrupted. The isotopes are then preferentially localized or concentrated in abnormal regions of the brain.

The precise cause of the disruption of the blood-brain barrier can be any of various pathologic processes. Study of the location, size, and shape of the abnormality, along with the timing of the scan, may help specify the pathologic process.

The timing of brain scanning in relation to the onset of CVA-like symptoms is usually significant. For example, in cerebral infarction, scanning performed soon after the onset of symptoms may be normal and then become abnormal 2 weeks later; this combination is virtually pathognomonic of infarction. Tumors (Figure 6-3) and abscesses will show abnormalities on the initial scan.

The injection of isotopes followed by immediate scanning can be used to detect changes in the dynamics of cerebral blood flow by comparing one side of the brain with the other. For example, cerebrovascular occlusive disease is characterized by a decreased flow, in contrast to an arteriovenous (AV) malformation, which is associated with an increased flow rate. A cerebral blood flow scan often is used to support the findings of "brain death" by demonstrating lack of blood flow to the brain while still demonstrating blood flow to the scalp.

The technique of single photon emission computed tomography (SPECT) has significantly improved the quality of brain scanning. With SPECT scanning, the radionuclide is injected, and the scintillator is placed to receive images from multiple angles (around the circumference of the head). This technique greatly increases the usefulness of nuclear brain scanning. In general, CT, MRI, and carotid duplex scans have replaced the brain scan in diagnostic neurology.

Procedure
The nonfasting, unsedated patient is given a potassium chloride capsule 2 hours before the IV injection of technetium-99m pertechnetate (Tc 99m pertechnetate). The potassium chloride prevents an inordinate amount of Tc 99m pertechnetate uptake by the choroid plexus, which would simulate a pathologic cerebral condition. Shortly after

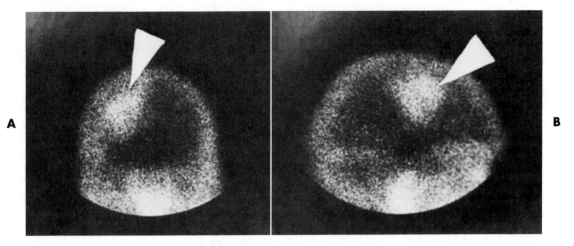

Figure 6-3   Brain scans. **A,** Anteroposterior view. **B,** Lateral view. White pointers indicate a tumor seen in both views.

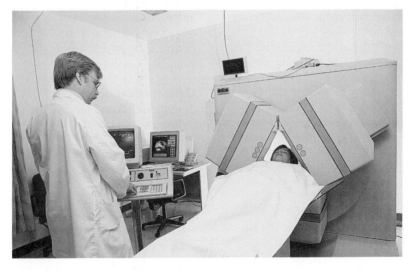

Figure 6-4   Patient positioned for a radionuclide scan of the brain. In this diagnostic study, a small amount of radioactive material crosses the blood-brain barrier to produce an image. This study is known as *single-photon emission computed tomography (SPECT).*

the injection, the patient is placed in the supine, lateral, and prone positions while a gamma camera is passed over the patient's head, and an image is obtained (Figure 6-4).

When cerebral flow studies are performed, the patient is placed in the supine position and injected with isotopes. A counter is placed immediately over the head. The counts are anatomically recorded in a timed sequence to follow the isotope during its flow through the brain.

Brain scanning is performed by a technician in the nuclear medicine department. The duration of this study is approximately 35 to 45 minutes. No discomfort is associated with this study other than that of the peripheral IV puncture required for the injection of the radioisotopes.

Contraindications

A contraindication for brain scanning is pregnancy because radionuclear material can be harmful to the development of the fetus.

Nursing implications with rationale

Before

☞ Explain the procedure to the patient. Tell the patient that no fasting or sedation is necessary.

■ Administer blocking agents (e.g., potassium chloride) as ordered before the scanning.

■ Assess for iodine allergy in case an iodinated solution will be used.

During

■ Monitor confused or unstable patients throughout the procedure.

After

☞ Because only tracer doses of radioisotopes are used, inform the patient that no precautions need to be taken to prevent radioactive exposure to others.

☞ Assure the patient that the radioactive material will be excreted from the body within 24 hours. Encourage fluids to aid the excretion of the isotope.

Caloric Study (Oculovestibular Reflex Study)

Test type Electrodiagnostic

Normal values

Nystagmus with irrigation

Rationale

Caloric studies are used to evaluate the vestibular (inner ear) portion of the eighth cranial nerve (CN VIII) by irrigating the external auditory canal with hot or cold water. Normally, stimulation with cold water causes rotary nystagmus (involuntary rapid eye movement) away from the ear being irrigated; hot water induces nystagmus toward the side of the ear being irrigated. If the labyrinth (inner ear) is diseased or CN VIII is not functioning (e.g., from tumor compression), no nystagmus is induced. This study aids in the differential diagnosis of abnormalities

that may occur in the vestibular system, brainstem, or cerebellum. When results are inconclusive, electronystagmography (see p. 205) may be performed.

Procedure

Solid food usually is held for several hours before this study to reduce the possibility of vomiting. This procedure usually takes place in a treatment room. The exact procedure for caloric studies varies. The ear canal should be examined and cleaned by a physician before testing to ensure that the water will freely flow to the middle ear area.

The ear on the affected side is irrigated first, because the client's response may be minimal. After an emesis basin is placed under the ear, the irrigation solution is directed into the external auditory canal until the client complains of nausea and dizziness or until nystagmus is seen. Usually this occurs within 20 to 30 seconds. If, after 3 minutes, no symptoms occur, the irrigation is stopped.

Contraindications

Contraindications for caloric studies are as follows:

■ Patients with a perforated eardrum
Cold air, however, may be substituted for the fluid.

■ Patients with an acute disease of the labyrinth (e.g., Meniere's syndrome)
The test can be performed when the acute attack subsides.

Nursing implications with rationale

Before

☞ Explain the procedure to the patient. Instruct the patient to avoid solid foods before the test to reduce the incidence of vomiting.

After

☞ Inform the patient that bed rest is prescribed until the nausea and vomiting subsides, usually in 30 to 60 minutes. After that time, fluid, food, and normal activities may be resumed.

■ Ensure safety precautions related to dizziness.

Cerebral Arteriography
(Cerebral Angiography)

Test type X-ray with contrast dye

Normal values
Normal arterial vasculature

Rationale
Cerebral angiography provides radiographic visualization of the cerebral vascular system after the intraarterial injection of radiopaque dye into the carotid or vertebral arteries. This procedure is used to detect abnormalities of the cerebral circulation (e.g., aneurysms, occlusion, or AV malformations) (Figure 6-5). Vascular tumors are seen

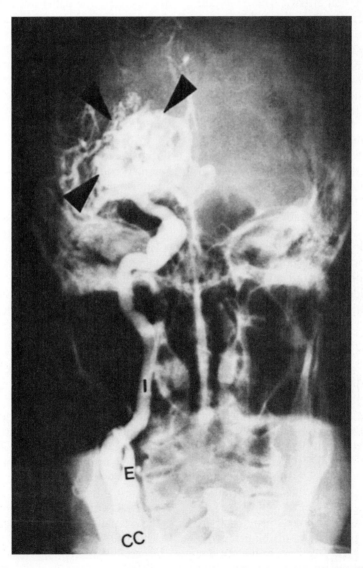

Figure 6-5   Cerebral angiogram. Black pointers indicate large arteriovenous malformation. *CC,* common carotid artery; *E,* external carotid artery; *I,* internal carotid artery.

as masses containing multiple, small AV fistulas. Nonvascular tumors, abscesses, and hematomas present as an avascular mass, distorting the normal vascular location.

A relatively new procedure called *digital subtraction angiography* (DSA), or *digital venous subtraction angiography* (DVSA), is a type of computerized fluoroscopy that uses venous or arterial catheterization to visualize the arteries, especially the carotid and cerebral arteries. This procedure enables small differences in radiographic absorption between an artery and the surrounding tissues to be converted to digital information and stored. DSA is especially useful when bone blocks visualization of the blood vessels under study. This study is valuable in the preoperative and postoperative evaluation of patients having vascular and tumor surgery. For DSA, an image "mask" is made of the area of clinical interest and then stored in the computer. After the IV injection of the contrast material, subsequent images are made. The computer then subtracts the preinjection mask image from the postinjection image. This removes all undesired tissue images, such as bone, and leaves an arterial image of high contrast and quality. If venous injection of the dye is used rather than arterial injection, the complications and risk associated with conventional arteriography are avoided. However, DSA is more often performed with an arterial injection of contrast material.

Procedure

The patient usually is kept NPO (*nil per os,* nothing by mouth) for solid foods after midnight on the day of cerebral angiography. The patient usually is sedated 30 minutes before the study and taken to the angiography room, located in the radiology department. This procedure usually is performed with the patient under local anesthesia. If DSA is to be performed, a mask film of the region is performed before contrast injection.

The puncture site usually is the femoral artery in the groin. A cannula may be placed percutaneously into the vessel. Selective catheterization also may be performed to cannulate any of the major cervical vessels. The catheter is followed under fluoroscopy as it passes into the desired artery. Radiopaque contrast material then is injected, and the flow of blood through the cranial cavity is seen. Serial radiographic films are taken in a timed sequence to show the arterial and venous phases of the cerebral circulation.

The patient is required to lie quietly in the supine and lateral positions (Figure 6-6). During the dye injection, the patient will feel a severe, transient burning sensation and flush. The only other discomfort associated with this study is from the arterial puncture needed for dye injection. After the radiographic films are completed, the catheter is removed, and a pressure dressing is applied to the puncture site. Conventional angiography and DSA are usually performed by an angiographer (radiologist) in approximately 1 hour.

Potential complications

Potential complications associated with cerebral arteriography are as follows:

- Anaphylaxis, caused by an allergic reaction to the iodinated contrast material
- Hemorrhage or hematoma formation at the puncture site used for arterial access
- Neurologic deficits, caused by the angiocatheter dislodging an atherosclerotic plaque, which can travel to the brain and cause infarction

Contraindications

Contraindications for cerebral arteriography are as follows:

- Patients with allergies to iodinated dye
- Patients who are uncooperative or agitated
- Patients who are pregnant, because radiation can be harmful to a developing fetus
- Patients with renal disorders, because iodinated contrast is nephrotoxic
- Patients with a bleeding propensity, because the arterial puncture site may not stop bleeding
- Patients who are dehydrated, because they are especially susceptible to dye-induced renal failure

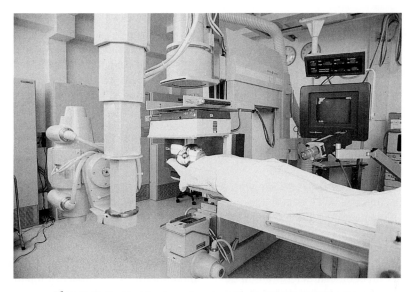

Figure 6-6 Positioning of patient for cerebral angiography.

Nursing implications with rationale

Before

☞ Explain the procedure to the patient. Most patients are very frightened about this procedure. Encourage verbalization of the patient's fears and provide emotional support.

☞ Instruct the patient to fast from solid foods after midnight on the day of the test.

■ Ensure that the written, informed consent for this procedure is in the patient's chart.

☞ Tell the patient where the catheter will be inserted (usually into the femoral artery). Inform the patient that an uncomfortably warm flush during dye insertion will be felt.

■ Assess the patient for allergies to iodine dye. A sensitivity test may be performed on the day before the study.

■ Assess the patient for anticoagulant therapy because of the potential complication of bleeding. If the procedure is not postponed, it is done with the awareness that severe bleeding can occur.

■ Perform a baseline neurologic assessment for comparison with subsequent assessment. Baseline data should include vital signs, level of consciousness, pupil reaction, facial symmetry, strength and motion of the extremities, and distal pulses (if the femoral artery approach is to be used).

■ If a sedative has been ordered, administer it on the evening before the study to ensure that the patient sleeps well.

■ Administer the preprocedure drugs, as ordered, before angiography.

After

■ Monitor vital signs and perform a neurologic evaluation frequently (every 15 minutes for 4 times, then every 30 minutes for 4 times, then every hour for 4 times, and then every 4 hours) and compare these findings with the preprocedure database. An increase in pulse rate and a decrease in blood pressure may indicate bleeding. Notify the physician immediately of any signs of hemorrhage or embolism.

■ Assess the catheter insertion site for hemorrhage, hematoma, and inflammation each time the vital signs are taken. If the neck arteries were used for arterial access, assess the neck region for swelling or hematoma that could compromise respiration. If the brachial or femoral arteries were cannulated, assess the involved extremity for peripheral pulses, numbness, tingling, pain, color, temperature, and loss of function. Any abnormalities should be reported immediately to the physician.

☞ Instruct the patient to remain on bed rest for 12 hours after the procedure to allow for complete sealing of the arterial puncture. During this time, the involved extremity should be extended and immobilized to prevent kinking of the vessel and clot formation.

■ Apply an ice bag to the puncture site to reduce swelling and pain.

■ Maintain pressure at the puncture site with a 1- to 2-pound sand bag or IV bag.

■ Check if the patient can resume a regular diet after the procedure.

☞ Unless prohibited for medical purposes, encourage fluids to promote dye excretion by the kidneys. Renal function can deteriorate in dehydrated patients who receive iodine dye injection.

■ Assess the patient for a delayed reaction to the dye.

Computed Tomography of the Brain (CT Scan of the Brain, Computerized Axial Transverse Tomography [CATT])

Test type X-ray with contrast dye

Normal values

No evidence of pathologic conditions

Rationale

Computed tomography (CT) scan of the brain is indicated when CNS pathology is suspected. Specifically, CT scanning is useful in the diagnosis of brain tumors, infarction, bleeding, and hematomas. Information about the ventricular system also can be obtained by CT scanning. Multiple sclerosis (MS) and other degenerative abnormalities can be identified also.

CT of the brain consists of a computerized analysis of multiple tomographic, radiographic films taken of the brain tissue at successive layers, providing a three-dimensional view of the cranial

contents. The CT image provides a view of the head as though one were looking down through its top. The computer also allows images to be presented on sagittal and fascial views. The variation in density of each tissue allows for variable penetration of the x-ray beam. The computer calculates the amount of x-ray penetration of each tissue and displays this as shades of gray. An image is obtained.

The CT scan is used in the differential diagnosis of intracranial neoplasms, cerebral infarctions, ventricular displacement or enlargement, cortical atrophy, cerebral aneurysms, intracranial hemorrhage and hematoma, and arteriovenous (AV) malformation.

Visualization of a neoplasm, previous infarction, or any pathologic process that destroys the blood-brain barrier may be enhanced by IV injection of an iodinated contrast dye. CT scans may be repeated serially to monitor the progress of disease or the healing process. In many cases, CT scanning has eliminated the need for more invasive procedures, such as cerebral arteriography and pneumoencephalography. In many localities, MRI scanning of the brain has replaced the use of computed axial tomography (CAT) scan of the brain.

Potential complications

Potential complications associated with CT scanning are as follows:

■ Allergic reaction to iodinated dye
Allergic reactions vary from mild flushing, itching, and urticaria to life-threatening anaphylaxis (evidenced by respiratory distress, drop in blood pressure, shock). In the unusual event of anaphylaxis, diphenhydramine (Benadryl), steroids, and epinephrine are added to routine resuscitation. Oxygen and endotracheal equipment should be on hand for immediate use.

■ Acute renal failure from dye infusion
Adequate hydration beforehand may reduce this likelihood.

Procedure

Sedation is required only for young children and other patients who cannot remain still during the procedure. Wigs and hairpins are removed from the patient's head. The patient lies in the supine position on an examining table with his or her head resting in a snug-fitting rubber cap within a water-filled box. The patient's head is enclosed only to the hair line (as in a hair dryer). Sponges are placed along the side of the head to ensure that it is cushioned but does not move during this study. Any movement causes computer-generated artifacts on the image produced. The scanner passes a small x-ray beam through the brain from one side to the other. The machine then rotates 1 degree; the procedure is repeated at each degree through a 180-degree arc. The machine is then moved down approximately 0.5 to 2 cm, and the entire procedure is repeated for a total of about 3 to 7 "slices," or planes. Usually an iodinated dye is then used. A peripheral IV line is started, and the iodine dye is administered through it. The entire scanning process is repeated. The patient may feel facial flushing with the dye injection. The image is available in a few minutes.

CT scanning is performed by a technician in approximately 45 to 60 minutes. This is a painless procedure. The only discomforts associated with this study are those of lying still on a table and of the peripheral venipuncture.

Contraindications

Contraindications for CT scanning are as follows:

- Patients who are allergic to iodinated dye
- Patients who are claustrophobic
- Patients who are pregnant
- Patients whose vital signs are unstable
- Patients who are very obese, usually weighing more than 300 pounds, because the CT table cannot hold that weight

Nursing implications with rationale

Before

☞ Explain the procedure to the patient. Assure the patient that CT scanning is a safe and painless x-ray method of studying the structures of the brain. If possible, show the patient a picture of the scanning machine and encourage verbalization of anxieties.

☞ Instruct the patient to remain NPO for 4 hours before the study, because the iodine dye may cause nausea. It is not usually known before the test if enhanced visualization by dye injection will be indicated.

☞ Instruct the parents if their child should be sleep deprived before this study. This is done by keeping the child awake until midnight the night before the study. The child then is awakened every hour beginning at 4 AM for a 5-minute to 10-minute period. The child should not be allowed to fall asleep in the car on the way to the hospital.

☞ Instruct the patient that wigs, hairpins, or clips cannot be worn during this procedure because they hamper visualization of the brain.

■ Assess the patient for allergies to iodinated dye to prevent dye-induced anaphylaxis. Sometimes the patient is pretested for dye allergies. Observe the patient for signs of anaphylaxis (such as respiratory distress, palpitations, or diaphoresis).

■ Sedate the patient, if ordered. Sedation is used for children and other patients who cannot lie still during the procedure.

☞ Inform the patient that he or she must lie motionless during the study. Even talking or sighing may cause artifacts on the computer image.

☞ Tell the patient that during the procedure he or she will hear a clicking noise as the scanner moves around the head. Some describe the sound as being like that of a washing machine. The patient will not be able to feel the scanner rotate.

After

■ The patient can resume all activities. If the patient was sedated, however, observe safety precautions until the effects of the sedative have worn off.

☞ Encourage patients who received a dye injection to increase their fluid intake, because iodine contrast can cause renal function deterioration, especially in the dehydrated patient.

Case Study

Seizure Disorder

J.C., a 12-year-old boy, began to complain of frequent headaches 4 months before his hospital admission. On the day of his admission, he had a major motor seizure, which his parents observed. During the seizure he lost bladder and bowel control. On physical examination he appeared to be in deep postictal sleep. He had no focal neurologic signs. On examination of the optic fundi, no evidence of papilledema was found.

Studies	Results
Routine laboratory work	Within normal limits (WNL)
Skull x-ray study, p. 220	No evidence of skull fracture
Lumbar puncture, p. 208	
Opening pressure	250 cm H_2O (normal: <200 cm H_2O)
Closing pressure	220 cm H_2O (normal: <200 cm H_2O)
Cerebrospinal fluid (CSF) examination, p. 208	
Blood	Negative
Color	Clear
Cells	
Lymphocytes	0-2/mm^3 (normal: <5/mm^3)
Polymorphonuclear leukocytes	None (normal: none)
Protein	120 mg/dl (normal: 15-45 mg/dl)
Glucose	50 mg/dl (normal: 50-75 mg/dl)
Cytology	Questionably malignant cells
Serologic test for venereal disease	Negative (normal: negative)
Electroencephalography (EEG), p. 205	Focal slowing of wave pattern in posterior aspect of the cerebrum (normal: regular, rhythmic, electrical waves)
Brain scanning, p. 190	Increase in radioactivity in the posterior aspect of the brain (normal: homogenous and minimal uptake of radioactive material)
Cerebral angiography, p. 193	Neovascularity (tumor vessels) in the posterior aspect of the brain, involving the cerebellum and the occipital lobe of the cerebrum (normal: normal carotid vessels and terminal branches)
CT (computed tomography) scanning, p. 196	A soft-tissue mass arising out of the cerebellum and invading the occipital lobe of the cerebrum

Diagnostic Analysis

The skull x-ray study ruled out the possibility of a skull fracture as the cause of the boy's problem. Lumbar puncture excluded the possibility of meningitis or subarachnoid hemorrhage. However, the high protein count and questionably positive cytology indicated a possible neoplasm. An electroencephalogram (EEG) located an area of nonspecific abnormality in the posterior aspect of the brain. Brain scanning, cerebral angiography, and CT scanning all indicated a posterior fossa tumor.

Because of these findings, the patient underwent a craniotomy. A very invasive medulloblastoma was found to be arising from the patient's cerebellum and involving the occipital lobe of the cerebrum. The tumor was unresectable. Postoperatively, the patient was given phenytoin (Dilantin) and radiation therapy to the involved area. A chemotherapy regimen was administered. The patient's tumor did not respond to the therapy, and he died 4 months after the onset of disease.

Critical Thinking Questions

1. What are the major assessments that the nurse should make during seizure activity?
2. Why is the EEG a priority study for patients with seizure disorders?

Electroencephalography
(Electroencephalogram [EEG])

Test type Electrodiagnostic

Normal values

Normal frequency, amplitude, and characteristics of brain waves

Rationale

The electroencephalogram (EEG) is a graphic recording of the electrical activity of the brain. EEG electrodes are placed on the scalp overlying multiple areas of the brain to detect and record electrical impulses within the brain. This study is invaluable in the investigation of epileptic (seizure) states, in which the focus of seizure activity is characterized by rapid, spiking waves seen on the graph. Patients with cerebral lesions (e.g., tumors, infarctions) will have abnormally slow EEG waves depending on the size and location of the lesion. Because this study determines the overall electrical activity of the brain, it can be used to evaluate trauma and drug intoxication and also to determine cerebral death in comatose patients.

The EEG also can be used to monitor cerebral blood flow during surgical procedures. For ex-

ample, during carotid endarterectomy, the carotid vessel must be occluded temporarily. When this surgery is performed with the patient under general anesthesia, the EEG can be used for the early detection of cerebral tissue ischemia, which would indicate that continued carotid occlusion will result in a CVA (stroke) syndrome. Temporary shunting of the blood during the surgery then is required. Finally, the EEG is a confirmatory test for determination of brain death.

Interfering factors

Factors that interfere with the EEG include the following:

- Fasting, which may cause hypoglycemia and modify the EEG pattern
- Drinks containing caffeine (e.g., coffee, tea, cocoa, cola), which interfere with the test results
- Body and eye movements during the test, which can cause changes in the brain wave patterns
- Lights, especially bright or flashing, which can alter test results
  Photostimulation may be a part of EEG testing to see if seizure activity can be induced by a flashing strobe light.
- Sedative medications, which may affect test results

Procedure

The patient is instructed to shampoo his or her hair the night before the study. No oils, sprays, or lotions may be used. The patient should not fast before this study. Coffee, tea, and cola are not permitted on the morning of the procedure. Usually only a limited amount of sleep is allowed the night before the study.

EEG is often performed in a specially constructed room that is shielded from outside disturbances (electrical, auditory, and visual). EEG can be done at the bedside if the patient is too ill to be moved.

The patient is placed in a supine position on a bed or reclining in a chair. Sixteen or more electrodes are applied to the scalp with electrode paste in a uniform pattern over both sides of the head, covering the prefrontal, frontal, temporal, parietal, and occipital areas. One electrode may be applied to each earlobe for grounding (Figure 6-7).

The patient is instructed to lie still with his or her eyes closed. The technician continuously observes the patient during the EEG recording for any movements that could alter the results. Approximately every 5 minutes the recording is interrupted to permit the client to move, if desired.

In addition to the resting EEG, a number of activating procedures can be performed:

1. The patient is hyperventilated (asked to breathe deeply 20 times a minute for 3 minutes) to induce alkalosis and cerebral vasoconstriction, which may activate abnormalities.

2. Photostimulation is performed by flashing a light (stroboscope) over the patient's face with the patient's eyes opened or closed. Photostimulated seizure activity may be seen on the EEG.

3. A sleep EEG may be performed to detect abnormal brain waves that are seen only if the patient is sleeping (such as frontal lobe epilepsy). The sleep EEG is performed after orally administering methyprylon (Noludar) and secobarbital (Seconal). (Secobarbital should not be administered to children.) A recording is performed while the patient is falling asleep, while the patient is asleep, and while the patient is waking.

After the study, the electrode paste and the electrodes are removed. This study is performed by an EEG technician in approximately 45 min-

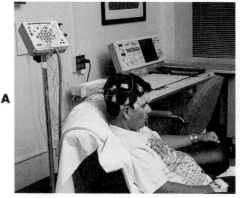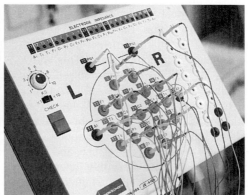

Figure 6-7 Electroencephalography. **A,** Patient with electrodes attached to the head, with wires leading to corresponding areas on the equipment. **B,** Equipment used to record brain wave activity.

utes to 2 hours. Other than the fatigue caused by missing sleep before and the discomfort of remaining still during the study, no pain is associated with this study.

Nursing implications with rationale

Before

☞ Explain the procedure to the patient. Many patients fear that the EEG can read the mind or detect senility. Some patients fear that the EEG is a form of electric shock therapy. Reassure the patient that these ideas are false. Encourage verbalization of the patient's fears.

☞ Assure the patient that the flow of electrical current is *from* the patient. He or she will feel no electrical impulses during this study.

☞ Instruct the patient to wash his or her hair the night before the study. No hair oils, sprays, or lotions should be used because these can cause movement of the scalp electrodes.

■ Confirm with the physician whether any medications should be discontinued before the study.

☞ Instruct the patient if sleep time should be shortened on the night before the test. Adults should sleep no more than 4 to 5 hours and children no more than 5 to 7 hours. This allows the patient to relax and possibly fall asleep during the study.

■ Administer the sedatives or hypnotics before the study, as indicated, for the sleep EEG. (These are usually given in the EEG room.) Otherwise, sedatives or hypnotics should not be given, because they cause abnormally low-voltage, fast waves to appear on the EEG.

☞ Instruct the patient to fast before the study. Fasting may cause hypoglycemia, which could modify the EEG pattern. Coffee, tea, and cola are not permitted on the morning of the study because of their stimulating effect.

☞ Tell the patient that during the recording of the EEG, his or her activity should be minimal, if any. Movement, including opening of the eyes, creates interference and alters the EEG recording.

After

■ Help the patient remove the electrode paste. The paste may be removed with acetone or witch hazel, and the hair should be shampooed.

■ Follow safety precautions (side rails up) until the effects of any sedatives have worn off. If the patient is having the study done as an outpatient, an adult should accompany the patient and provide transportation home after the study.

Electromyography (EMG)

Test type Electrodiagnostic

Normal values
No evidence of neuromuscular abnormalities

Rationale
By placing a recording electrode into a skeletal muscle, one can monitor the electrical activity of a skeletal muscle in a manner similar to electrocardiography. The electrical activity is displayed as an electrical waveform. An audio electrical amplifier can be added to the system so that both the appearance and sound of the electrical potentials can be analyzed and compared simultaneously. Electromyography (EMG) is used to detect primary muscular disorders, along with muscular abnormalities caused by other system diseases (e.g., nerve dysfunction, sarcoidosis, paraneoplastic syndrome).

Spontaneous muscle movement, such as fibrillation and fasciculation, can be detected during EMG. When evident, these rapid waveforms indicate injury or disease of the nerve innervating that muscle. Spastic myotonic muscle (jerky muscle contraction) is also evidence of nerve injury or disease. Reduced amplitude (size) of the electrical waveform is indicative of a primary muscle disorder (e.g., polymyositis, muscular dystrophies, various myopathies). A progressive decrease in amplitude of the electrical waveform during contraction is a classic sign of myasthenia gravis. A decrease in the number of muscle fibers able to contract is seen with peripheral nerve damage. This study is usually done in conjunction with nerve conduction studies (see p. 202) and also may be called *electromyoneurography*.

Potential complication

Hematoma at the needle insertion site is a rare complication associated with EMG.

Interfering factors

Factors that interfere with EMG include the following:

- Edema, hemorrhage, or thick subcutaneous fat
  These conditions can interfere with the transmission of electrical waves to the electrodes and alter test results.
- Excessive pain, which can cause false results

Procedure

No fasting or preparation is required. Although this study can be done at the bedside, the patient usually is taken to the EMG laboratory. The position in which the patient is placed depends on the muscle being studied. A needle that acts as a recording electrode is inserted into the muscle being examined. A reference electrode is placed nearby on the skin surface. The patient is asked to keep the muscle at rest. The oscilloscopic display is viewed for any evidence of spontaneous electrical activity, such as fasciculation or fibrillation. Next, the patient is asked to contract the muscle slowly and progressively. The electrical waves produced are examined for their number and form. Maximum muscle contraction against an opposing resistance allows the opportunity to detect a complete interference pattern.

EMG is performed by a physical therapist, physiatrist, or neurologist in about 20 minutes. Results are interpreted by the physician. The test is moderately uncomfortable; pain may occur with the insertion of the needle electrode. The patient may have some muscle soreness after the procedure.

Contraindications

Contraindications for EMG are as follows:

- Patients receiving anticoagulant therapy
  The electrodes may induce intramuscular bleeding.
- Patients with extensive skin infection
  The electrodes may penetrate the infected skin and spread the infection to the muscle.

Nursing implications with rationale

Before

- ☞ Thoroughly explain the procedure to the patient. Assure the patient that the needle will not cause electrocution. Encourage verbalization of the patient's fears.
- Obtain written, informed consent if required by the institution.

After

- Observe the needle site for hematoma or inflammation.

Electroneurography (ENeG, Nerve Conduction Studies)

Test type Electrodiagnostic

Normal values

No evidence of peripheral nerve injury or disease (Conduction velocity is usually decreased in the elderly.)

Rationale

Electroneurography (ENeG) is performed to identify peripheral nerve injury in patients with localized or diffuse weakness. It also is used to differentiate primary peripheral nerve pathology from muscular injury. This test is helpful in documenting the severity of injury in legal cases. Finally, it is used to monitor response of the nerve injury to treatment.

ENeG, or nerve conduction studies, can identify the localization of peripheral nerve injury or disease. By initiating an electrical impulse at one site (proximal) of a nerve and recording the time required for that impulse to travel to a second site (distal) of the same nerve, the conduction velocity of any impulse in that nerve can be determined. This study usually is done in conjunction with EMG (see p. 201) and also may be called *electromyoneurography.*

The normal value for conduction velocity varies from one nerve to another. Individual variation also exists. It is always best to compare the conduction velocity of the suspected side with the nerve conduction velocity of the opposite (normal) side. In general, a range of normal conduction velocity will be approximately 50 to 60 m/second.

Traumatic nerve transection, contusion, or neuropathy usually will cause maximal slowing of conduction velocity in the affected side compared with that in the normal side. A velocity greater than normal does not indicate a pathologic condition.

Because conduction velocity may require contraction of a muscle as an indication of an impulse arriving at the recording electrode, primary muscular disorders may cause a falsely slow nerve conduction velocity. This variable is eliminated if one evaluates the involved muscle group before performing nerve conduction studies. This muscular factor can be evaluated by measuring *distal latency* (i.e., the time required for stimulation of the distal end of the nerve to cause muscular contraction). Once the distal latency is calculated, the nerve conduction study is performed, usually by stimulating the proximal portion of the nerve bundle. Conduction velocity then can be determined by the following equation:

$$\text{Conduction velocity (in meters per second)}$$
$$= \frac{\text{Distance (in meters)}}{\text{Total latency} - \text{Distal latency}}$$

Procedure

No fasting or sedation is required. The patient is taken to the nerve conduction laboratory (in the physiatrist's or neurologist's office, or in the physical rehabilitation department). Because the machine is portable, the study also can be performed at the bedside.

The patient is placed in whatever position is best for studying the area of suspected peripheral nerve injury or disease. A recording electrode is placed on the skin overlying a muscle innervated solely by the relevant nerve. A reference electrode is placed nearby (Figures 6-8 and 6-9). Electrical paste is used to connect the electrodes to the skin. The nerve then is stimulated by a shock-emitter device at an adjacent location. The time between nerve impulse and muscular contraction (distal latency) is measured in milliseconds on an oscilloscope (electromyograph). Next, the nerve is similarly stimulated at a location proximal (i.e., more central) to the area of suspected injury or disease. The time required for the impulse to travel from the site of initiation to muscle contraction (total latency) is recorded in milliseconds. The distance between the site of stimulation and recording electrode is measured in centimeters. Conduction velocity is converted to meters per second and is computed as in the equation provided earlier.

This test is uncomfortable because a mild electrical shock (comparable to that obtained in most household electrical outlet accidents) is required for nerve impulse stimulation. The test is performed by a neurologist, physiatrist, physical therapist, or technician in approximately 15 minutes. No complications are associated with it.

Nursing implications with rationale

Before

☞ Explain the procedure to the patient. Tell the patient that no fasting or sedation is required.

■ Allow the patient to verbalize his or her fears regarding the electrical stimulation (shock) necessary for this study. Provide emotional support.

After

■ Remove the electrode gel from the patient's skin.

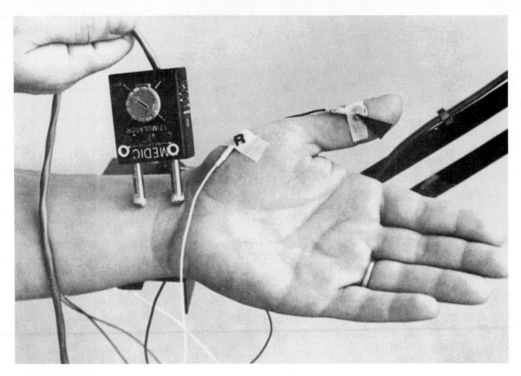

Figure 6-8 Electroneurography: measurement of distal latency. Pointer indicates reference electrode. *R*, Recording electrode.

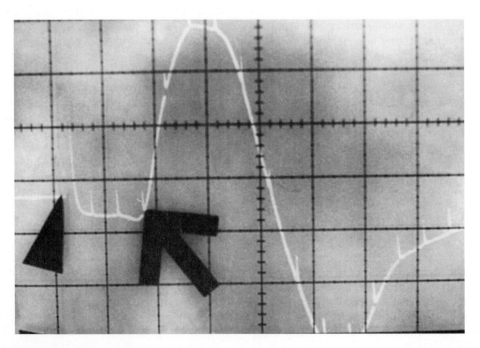

Figure 6-9 Electroneurography: electromyogram. Pointer indicates shock stimulation. Arrow indicates initiation of muscular contraction (the wave that follows the arrow). Distal latency is measured from pointer to arrow (1.2 m/second).

Electronystagmography (ENG)

Test type Electrodiagnostic

Normal values
Normal nystagmus response
Normal oculovestibular reflex

Rationale
This electrodiagnostic test is used to evaluate patients with vertigo (dizziness) and to differentiate organic from psychogenic vertigo. With ENG, central (cerebellum/brainstem, and eighth cranial nerve) pathology can be differentiated from peripheral (vestibular-cochlear/inner ear) pathology. If a known lesion exists, ENG can identify the side of the pathology. This test also is used to evaluate unilateral deafness.

ENG detects nystagmus (involuntary, rapid eye movement) and evaluates the muscles controlling eye movement. By measuring changes in the electrical field around the eye, ENG can make a permanent recording of eye movement at rest, with a change in head position, and in response to various stimuli. The test delineates the presence or absence of nystagmus, which is caused by the initiation of the oculovestibular reflex. Nystagmus should occur when initiated by positional, visual, or caloric stimuli (see p. 192). Unlike caloric studies, in which nystagmus usually is determined visually, with ENG, the direction, velocity, and degree of nystagmus can be recorded. If nystagmus does not occur with stimulation, the vestibular-cochlear apparatus, cerebral cortex (temporal lobe), auditory nerve, or brainstem is abnormal. Tumors, infection, ischemia, and degeneration can cause such abnormalities. The pattern of nystagmus, in addition to the entire clinical picture, helps differentiate between central and peripheral vertigo. This test also is used in the differential diagnosis of lesions in the vestibular system, brainstem, and cerebellum.

ENG also may help evaluate unilateral hearing loss and vertigo. Unilateral hearing loss may be due to middle ear problems or nerve injury. If the patient experiences nystagmus with stimulation, the auditory nerve is working, and hearing loss can be blamed on the middle ear.

Interfering factors
A factor that interferes with ENG is blinking of the eyes, which can alter test results.

Procedure
Solid foods are held before the test to reduce the likelihood of vomiting. Instruct the patient not to drink caffeine or alcoholic beverages for approximately 24 to 48 hours (as ordered) before the test. This procedure usually is performed in a darkened room, with the patient seated or lying down on an examination table. Any wax in the ear is removed. Electrodes are taped to the skin around the eyes. Various procedures, such as changing head position, changing gaze position, and caloric tests (see p. 192), are used to stimulate nystagmus. Several recordings are made with the patient at rest and when stimulated. Nystagmus response is compared with the expected ranges; and the results are recorded as normal, borderline, or abnormal. This procedure is performed by a physician or audiologist in approximately 1 hour.

Contraindications
Contraindications for ENG are as follows:

- Patients with perforated eardrums, who should not have water irrigation
- Patients with pacemakers

Nursing implications with rationale
Before
- Explain the procedure to the patient. Instruct the patient to avoid solid foods before the test to reduce the likelihood of nausea and vomiting during the test.
- Instruct the patient not to apply facial makeup before the test, because electrodes will be taped to the skin around the eyes.
- Withhold any medications (e.g., sedatives, stimulants, and antivertigo agents) as ordered before the test.

After
■ Recommend bed rest until nausea, vertigo, or weakness subsides.

Evoked Potential Studies (EP Studies, Evoked Brain Potentials, Evoked Responses, Visual-Evoked Potentials [VEP], Auditory Brainstem-Evoked Potentials [ABEP], Somatosensory-Evoked Responses [SER])

Test type Electrodiagnostic

Normal values
No neural conduction delay

Rationale
Evoked potential (EP) studies are indicated for patients who are suspected of having a sensory deficit but who are unable to indicate or are unreliable in indicating recognition of a stimulus (i.e., infants, comatose patients, or patients who are unable to communicate). These tests are used to evaluate specific areas of the cortex that receive incoming stimulus from the sensory nerves of the eyes, ears, and lower or upper extremities. EP studies are used to monitor the natural progression or the treatment of deteriorating neurologic diseases (e.g., MS). Finally, they also are used to identify histrionic or malingering patients who have sensory deficit complaints.

EP studies focus on the changes and responses in brain waves that are evoked from stimulation of a sensory pathway. Whereas the EEG measures spontaneous brain electrical activity, the sensory EP study measures minute voltage changes produced in response to a specific stimulus, such as a light pattern, click, or shock. A computer averages out (or cancels) unwanted random waves to sum up the evoked response that occurs at a specific time after a given stimulus. EP studies allow one to measure and assess the entire sensory pathway from the peripheral sensory organ (e.g., the eye) to the brain cortex (recognition of the stimulus).

Clinical abnormalities usually are detected by an increase in *latency*, which refers to a delay between the stimulus and the wave response. Normal latency times are calculated depending on body size, body position where the stimulus is applied, conduction velocity of axons in the neural pathways, number of synapses in the system, location of nerve generators of EP components (brainstem or cortex), and presence of CNS pathology. Conduction delays indicate damage or disease anywhere along the neural pathway from the sensory organ to the cortex. Sensory stimuli used for the EP study can be visual, auditory, or somatosensory.

The sensory stimulus chosen depends on what sensory system is suspected to be pathologic (e.g., questionable blindness, deafness, or numbness). Also, the sensory stimulus chosen may depend on the area of the brain where pathology is suspected. (Auditory stimuli check the brainstem and temporal lobes of the brain; visual stimuli test the optic nerve, central neural visual pathway, and occipital portions of the brain; somatosensory stimuli check the peripheral nerves, spinal cord, and parietal lobe of the brain.)

Visual-evoked potentials (VEPs) are usually stimulated by a strobe light flash, reversible checkerboard pattern, or retinal stimuli. A visual stimulus to the eye causes an electrical response in the occipital area that can be recorded with EEG-like electrodes placed on the scalp overlying the vertex and on the occipital lobes. Ninety percent of patients with MS show abnormal latencies in VEPs, a phenomenon attributed to demyelination of nerve fibers. In addition, patients with other neurologic disorders (e.g., Parkinson's disease) show an abnormal latency with VEPs. The degree of latency seems to correlate with the disease severity. Abnormal results also may be seen in patients with lesions of the optic nerve, optic tract, visual center, and the eye itself. Eyesight problems or blindness can be detected in infants through VEPs or electroretinography. VEPs also can be used during eye surgery to provide a warning of possible damage to the optic nerve. An infant's gross visual acuity can be checked with VEPs.

Auditory brainstem-evoked potentials (ABEPs)

are usually stimulated by clicking sounds to evaluate the central auditory pathways of the brainstem. Either ear can be evoked, without affecting hearing, to detect lesions in the brainstem that involve the auditory pathway. One of the most successful applications of ABEPs has been screening low-birth–weight newborns and other infants for hearing disorders. Recognition of deafness enables infants to be fitted with corrective devices as soon as possible before learning to speak (to prevent speech pathology). ABEPs also have great therapeutic implications in the early detection of posterior fossa brain tumors.

Somatosensory-evoked responses (SERs) are usually produced by sensory stimulus to an area of the body. The time for the current of the stimulus to travel along the nerve to the cortex of the brain is then measured. SERs are used to evaluate patients with spinal cord injuries and to monitor spinal cord functioning during spinal surgery. They also are used to monitor treatment of diseases (e.g., MS), evaluate the location and extent of areas of brain dysfunction after head injury, and pinpoint tumors at an early stage. These tests also can be used to identify malingering or hysterical numbness. The latency is normal in these patients despite the fact that they indicated numbness.

One of the main benefits of EP studies is their objectivity because voluntary patient response is not needed. This makes EP studies useful with nonverbal and uncooperative patients. This objectivity distinguishes between organic and psychogenic problems and is invaluable in settling lawsuits concerning workmen's compensation insurance.

Procedure

No fasting or sedation is required before administration of EP studies. The position of the electrode depends on the type of EP study to be done.

For VEPs, electrodes are placed on the scalp along the vertex and the occipital areas. Stimulation occurs by using a strobe light, checkerboard patterns, or retinal stimuli.

ABEPs are stimulated with clicking noises or tone bursts delivered with earphones. The responses are detected by scalp electrodes placed on the vertex and on each earlobe.

SERs are performed using electrical stimuli applied to nerves at the wrist (medial nerve) or the knee (peroneal). The response is detected by electrodes placed over the sensory cortex of the opposite hemisphere on the scalp.

Nursing implications with rationale

Before

- Explain the procedure to the patient. Tell the patient that no fasting or sedation is necessary. Allow verbalization of the patient's fears and questions. Many patients fear the diagnosis that may be substantiated by EP studies.
- Instruct the patient to shampoo his or her hair before the test and avoid oils and sprays.

After

- Remove the gel used for adherence of the electrodes.

Case Study

Multiple Sclerosis

Mrs. W., 35 years old, was active in jogging and horseback riding until 1 year ago. During the past year she began to notice severe weakness and paresthesias in her legs. Her gait became unsteady, and she developed loss of vision in one eye. A neurologist suspected MS and ordered the following studies:

Studies	Results
Routine laboratory work	WNL

Continued

Case Study

Multiple Sclerosis—cont'd

Lumbar puncture with CSF examination
(see p. 208)

Immunoglobulin G (IgG) index	0.8 (normal: 0.3-0.7)
IgG determination	20% (normal: 0%-11% of total protein)
Oligoclonal bands	Present (normal: none)

Evoked potentials, p. 206

Visual-evoked potentials	Abnormal latency
Auditory brainstem-evoked potentials	Normal
Somatosensory-evoked responses	Abnormal latency
Magnetic resonance imaging, p. 213	Plaques indicative of multiple sclerosis

Diagnostic Analysis

The wide variety of symptom manifestation often makes MS difficult to diagnose. However, the above studies clearly identified MS as Mrs. W.'s problem. The CSF study results were classic for the diagnosis of MS. The abnormal latency demonstrated on the EP studies was the result of the demyelination process of MS. MRI revealed plaques indicative of MS.

  Mrs. W. was given prednisone to decrease the inflammation and associated edema of the myelin sheath. When remission occurred, she was instructed about factors that exacerbate, prevent, or ameliorate symptoms.

Critical Thinking Questions

1. Why were the results of the CSF study classic for the diagnosis of MS?
2. What is *latency* and why is it increased in MS?

Lumbar Puncture and Cerebrospinal Fluid Examination
 (LP and CSF Examination, Spinal Tap, Spinal Puncture, Cerebrospinal Fluid Analysis, Cisternal Puncture)

Test type Fluid analysis

Normal values
Pressure: <200 cm H_2O
Color: clear and colorless
Blood: none
Blood cells:
  Red blood cell (RBC): 0

White blood cell (WBC):
  Total
  Adult 0-5 cells/ul
  6-18 years 0-10 cells/ul
  1-5 years 0-20 cells/ul
  Neonate 0-30 cells/ul
  Differential
  Neutrophils 0%-6%
  Lymphocytes 40%-80%
  Monocytes 15%-45%
Culture and sensitivity: no organisms present
Protein: 15-45 mg/dl CSF (up to 70 mg/dl in elderly adults and children)
Protein electrophoresis:
  Prealbumin: 2%-7%

Albumin: 56%-76%

Alpha$_1$ globulin: 2%-7%

Alpha$_2$ globulin: 4%-12%

Beta globulin: 8%-18%

Gamma globulin: 3%-12%

Oligoclonal bands: none

IgG: 0.0-4.5 mg/dl

Glucose: 50-75 mg/dl CSF or 60%-70% of blood glucose level

Chloride: 700-750 mg/dl

Lactic dehydrogenase (LDH): <2.0-7.2 U/ml

Lactic acid: 10-25 mg/dl

Cytology: no malignant cells

Serology for syphilis: negative

Glutamine: 6-15 mg/dl

Rationale

Lumbar puncture (LP) and cerebrospinal (CSF) fluid examination may assist in the diagnosis of primary or metastatic brain or spinal cord neoplasm, cerebral hemorrhage, meningitis, encephalitis, degenerative brain disease, autoimmune diseases involving the CNS, neurosyphilis, and demyelinating disorders (e.g., MS, acute demyelinating polyneuropathy).

By placing a needle in the subarachnoid space of the spinal column (Figure 6-10), one can measure the pressure of that space and obtain CSF for

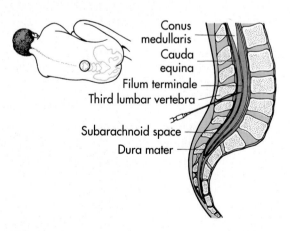

Figure 6-10 Patient position for a lumbar puncture.

Conus medullaris

Cauda equina

Filum terminale

Third lumbar vertebra

Subarachnoid space

Dura mater

examination and diagnosis. Lumbar puncture also may be used to inject therapeutic or diagnostic agents and to administer spinal anesthetics.

Examination of the CSF includes evaluation for the presence of blood, bacteria, and malignant cells, along with quantification of the amount of glucose and protein present. Color is noted, and various other tests, such as a serologic test for syphilis (see p. 392), are performed. Because the CSF is made from plasma, its constituents are approximately the same as plasma. Chloride levels are higher, however. Blood constituents of larger molecular size cannot be secreted by the choroid plexus (blood-brain barrier).

Pressure

By attaching a sterile manometer to the needle used for LP, the pressure within the subarachnoid space can be measured. A pressure greater than 200 cm H$_2$O is considered abnormal and indicative of increased spinal pressure. Because the subarachnoid space surrounding the brain is freely connected to the subarachnoid space of the spinal cord, any increase in intracranial pressure will be directly reflected as an increase at the lumbar site. Tumors, infection, hydrocephalus, and intracranial bleeding can cause increased intracranial and spinal pressure. If this normal connection is suspected to be obstructed by tumor or postinfection scarring, a Queckenstedt-Stookey test is performed (see Procedure, p. 212).

Decreased pressure is noted in hypovolemia (dehydration or shock). A chronic leakage of CSF through a previous LP or through a nasal sinus fracture with a dura tear also is associated with reduced pressures.

Pressures routinely are measured at the beginning and the end of an LP. If there is a significant difference in these values, one must suspect a spinal cord obstruction (i.e., tumor). If high opening pressures are noted, normal volumes of CSF should not be removed in order to prevent the risk of cerebellar herniation. One must be aware that a child who is crying and holding his or her breath may have transient elevations of pressure that reduce as the child relaxes.

Color

Normal CSF is clear and colorless. The term *xanthochromia* is commonly used to describe an abnormal yellowish discoloration of CSF. Color differences can occur with hyperbilirubinemia, hypercarotenemia, melanoma, or elevated proteins.

A cloudy appearance may indicate an increase in the WBC count or protein. Normally, CSF contains no blood cells. A red tinge to the CSF indicates the presence of blood. Blood may be present because of bleeding into the subarachnoid space or because the needle used in the LP has inadvertently penetrated a blood vessel on the way into the subarachnoid space. Bloody CSF caused by a traumatic tap is evident if the opening CSF pressures are low, the redness diminishes as more CSF is withdrawn, and the color clears with centrifugation.

Blood

Blood within the CSF indicates cerebral hemorrhage into the subarachnoid space or a traumatic tap, as just described.

Cells

The number of RBCs is merely an indication of the amount of blood present within the CSF. Except for a few lymphocytes, the presence of WBCs in the CSF is abnormal. The presence of polymorphonuclear leukocytes (neutrophils) is indicative of bacterial meningitis or cerebral abscess. When mononuclear leukocytes are present, viral or tubercular meningitis or encephalitis is suspected. Eosinophils may indicate parasitic infection. Leukemia or primary or metastatic malignant tumors also may cause elevated WBCs in the CSF. *Pleocytosis* is a term used to indicate turbidity of CSF resulting from an increased number of blood cells within the fluid.

Culture and sensitivity

The organisms that cause meningitis or brain abscess can be cultured from the CSF. Cultured organisms may include atypical bacteria, fungi, or *Mycobacterium tuberculosis*. The most common causes of meningitis include *Haemophilus influenzae* (in children) and *Neisseria* or *Streptococcus* in adults.

Protein

Normally, very little protein is found in CSF because it is a large molecule that does not cross the blood-brain barrier. The proportion of albumin to globulin normally is higher in CSF than in blood plasma (see p. 135) because albumin is smaller in size than globulin and therefore can pass more easily through the blood-brain barrier. Disease processes, however, can alter the permeability of the blood-brain barrier, allowing protein to leak into the CSF. Diseases associated with a more permeable blood-brain barrier include infectious or inflammatory processes such as meningitis, encephalitis, or myelitis. Furthermore, CNS tumors may produce and secrete protein into the CSF. Obstruction of CSF flow in the spinal canal caused by tumors or a vertebra disk also is associated with high protein counts because normal CSF circulation and resorption is impaired by the obstruction.

CSF protein electrophoresis is very important in the diagnosis of CNS diseases. Patients with MS, neurosyphilis, or other immunogenic, degenerative, central neurologic diseases have elevated immunoglobulins in their CSF. Myelin basic protein, a component of myelin (the substance that surrounds normal nerve tissue) is elevated when demyelinating diseases, such as MS or amyotrophic lateral sclerosis, occur. This protein can be used to monitor the course of these deteriorating diseases.

Glucose

The glucose level is decreased when the bacteria or cells within the CSF increase in number and catabolize the glucose. The cells may be inflammatory cells in response to infection or inflammation or cells that are shed by tumors. A blood sample for glucose (see p. 305) usually is drawn before the spinal tap is performed. A CSF glucose level less than 60% of the blood glucose may indicate meningitis or neoplasm.

Chloride

The chloride concentration in CSF may be decreased in patients with meningeal infections, tubercular meningitis, and conditions of low blood chloride levels.

Lactic dehydrogenase

Quantification of LDH (specifically, fractions 4 and 5; see p. 42) is helpful in diagnosing bacterial meningitis. The source of LDH is the neutrophils that fight the invading bacteria. When the LDH level is elevated, infection or inflammation is suspected.

Lactic acid

Elevated levels of lactic acid indicate anaerobic metabolism associated with decreased oxygenation of the brain. CSF lactic acid is increased in both bacterial and fungal meningitis but not in viral meningitis. Chronic cerebral hypoxemia or cerebral ischemia (hypoxic encephalopathy) also is associated with elevated CSF lactic acid levels.

Cytology

Examination of cells found in the CSF can determine if they are malignant. Tumors (mostly metastatic) in the CNS may shed cells from their surface. These cells can float freely in CSF. Their presence suggests neoplasm as the cause of any neurologic symptoms.

Tumor markers

Increased levels of tumor markers such as carcinoembryonic antigen (CEA), alpha-fetoprotein, or human chorionic gonadotropin (HCG) may indicate metastatic tumor.

Serology for syphilis

Latent syphilis is diagnosed by performing one of many currently available serologic tests on CSF. These include (1) the Wasserman test, (2) the Venereal Disease Research Laboratory test (see p. 392), and (3) the fluorescent treponemal antibody (FTA) test (see p. 392). The FTA test is currently considered to be the most sensitive and specific test for syphilis.

Glutamine

Elevated glutamine levels are helpful in the detection and evaluation of hepatic encephalopathy and hepatic coma. The glutamine results from increased ammonia levels, which commonly are associated with liver failure (see serum ammonia, p. 109). Glutamine levels are also often elevated in patients with Reye's syndrome.

Potential complications

Potential complications associated with LP and CSF examination are as follows:

- Persistent CSF leak, causing severe headache
- Introduction of bacteria into CSF, causing suppurative meningitis
- Herniation of the brain through the tentorium cerebelli or herniation of the cerebellum through the foramen magnum
  In patients with increased intracranial pressure, the quick reduction of pressure in the spinal column by release through the LP may induce herniation of the brain. This can cause compression of the brainstem, which may result in deterioration of the patient's neurologic status and death.
- Inadvertent puncture of the spinal cord, caused by inappropriately high puncture of the spinal cord
- Puncture of the aorta or vena cava, causing serious retroperitoneal hemorrhage

Procedure

No fasting or sedation is required for lumbar puncture. This study is a sterile procedure that can easily be performed at the bedside by a qualified physician. The patient usually is placed in the lateral decubitus (fetal) position (see Figure 6-10). The patient should clasp the hands on the knees to maintain this position. It is important that the lumbar area be flexed as much as possible to assure maximum bowing of the spine and to allow as much space as possible between the vertebrae. A vertebral interspace between L2 and S1 is chosen for the puncture, because the spinal cord ends near L2.

A local anesthetic (usually 1% lidocaine) is injected into the skin and subcutaneous tissues after the site has been aseptically cleansed. Next, a spinal needle containing an inner obturator is placed through the skin and into the spinal canal. The subarachnoid space is entered. The inner obturator is removed, and CSF can be seen slowly dripping from the needle. The needle is then attached to a sterile manometer, and the pressure (called the *opening pressure*) is recorded. Before the pressure reading is taken, the patient is asked to relax and straighten the legs to reduce the intraabdominal pressure, which causes an increase in CSF pressure. Next, three sterile test tubes are filled with 5 to 10 ml of CSF and sent for appropriate testing. Finally, the pressure (called the *closing pressure*) is measured.

If blockage in CSF circulation in the spinal (subarachnoid) space is suspected, a Queckenstedt-Stookey test is performed. For this test the jugular veins are occluded, either manually by digital pressure or by a medium-sized blood pressure cuff inflated to approximately 20 mm Hg. Within 10 seconds after jugular vein occlusion, CSF pressure should increase from 15 to 40 cm H_2O and then promptly return to normal within 10 seconds after release of the pressure. A sluggish rise or fall of CSF pressure with venous compression suggests partial blockage of CSF circulation. No rise after 10 seconds suggests complete obstruction within the spinal canal.

After the procedure, the spinal needle is removed, and digital pressure is placed over the area of needle insertion. An adhesive bandage can be placed over the puncture site. The patient is then placed in the prone position, with a pillow under the abdomen to increase the intraabdominal pressure, which indirectly increases the pressure on the tissues surrounding the spinal canal. This acts to retard continued CSF flow from the spinal canal. The patient is encouraged to drink increased amounts of fluid to replace the CSF removed during the lumbar puncture. The patient is asked to maintain the reclining position, usually for 4 to 12 hours, to avoid the discomfort of potential postpuncture spinal headache.

This procedure usually is described as painful by the patient, who usually complains of a feeling of pressure from the needle. The procedure lasts approximately 20 minutes.

Contraindications

Contraindications for LP and CSF examination are as follows:

- Patients with increased intracranial pressure
  The LP may induce cerebral or cerebellar herniation through the foramen magnum.
- Patients who have severe degenerative vertebral joint disease
  It is very difficult to pass the needle through the degenerated, arthritic, intervertebral space.
- Patients with infection near the LP site
  Meningitis can result from contamination of CSF with infected material.

Nursing implications with rationale

Before

- ☝ Explain the procedure and the postprocedure routine to the patient to minimize anxiety and ensure his or her cooperation. Many patients have misconceptions regarding this procedure. Assure the patient that insertion of the needle will not cause paralysis because the needle is inserted into the area below the spinal cord.
- Ensure that the physician has obtained written and informed consent for this procedure.
- Order the necessary lumbar puncture tray from the hospital's central supply department.
- ☝ Tell the patient that no fasting or sedation is necessary.
- Perform a baseline neurologic assessment of the legs by evaluating the patient's strength, sensation, and movement.
- ☝ Instruct the patient to empty the bladder before the procedure. A misdirected needle may puncture a bladder distended with urine.
- ☝ Explain to the patient that he or she must lie very still throughout this procedure. Movement may cause traumatic injury.

During

- Assist the patient in assuming the appropriate position. The patient's head and neck are flexed into the chest, and the knees are pulled up into the chest. You may place a pillow between the patient's legs to prevent the upper part of the legs from rolling forward. Stand facing the patient, with one hand on the patient's shoulder and the other hand on the patient's knees.

- You may be required to assist the physician by holding the manometer straight. If you are not wearing sterile gloves, hold the very top of the manometer with your fingertips.

After

- Label and number the specimen jars appropriately and have them delivered immediately to the appropriate laboratory. A delay between collection time and testing can invalidate results, especially cell counts.
- Place the patient in the prone position, with a pillow under the abdomen to increase the intraabdominal pressure, which will indirectly increase the pressure in the tissues surrounding the spinal cord.
- ☞ Instruct the patient to remain on bed rest with his or her head flat because of the high risk of spinal headache. This headache is probably caused by the loss of CSF at the puncture site. The patient may turn from side to side.
- ☞ Encourage the patient to drink fluids through a straw. Drinking with a straw will enable the patient to keep his or her head flat.
- Assess the patient for numbness, tingling, and decreased movement of the extremities; pain at the injection site; drainage of blood or CSF at the injection site; and the ability to void. Notify the physician of any unusual occurrences.

Magnetic Resonance Imaging
(MRI, Nuclear Magnetic Resonance [NMRI])

Test type Magnetic field study

Normal values
No evidence of pathology

Rationale
Magnetic resonance imaging (MRI) is a noninvasive, diagnostic scanning technique that utilizes a magnetic field to provide valuable information about the body's anatomy. Significant indications for MRI include evaluation of patients with headaches or other neurologic signs for CNS lesions. Patients with neck and back pain are evaluated for disk herniation. Bones and joints, especially the knees, are evaluated after traumatic injury or for chronic pain. As this relatively new technique evolves, more indications for its usage will become apparent.

MRI technology is based on how hydrogen atoms react when they are placed in a magnetic field and then are disturbed by radiofrequency signals. The unique feature of MRI is that it does not require exposure to ionizing radiation. MRI has several advantages over CT scanning, including the following:

1. MRI provides better contrast between normal and pathologic tissue.
2. The obscuring bone artifacts that occur in CT scanning do not occur in MRI scanning.
3. MRI provides a natural contrast to the blood vessels because the rapid motion of blood flow appears as a dark image, thereby delineating many blood vessels.
4. Because magnetic fields can be varied in space, it is possible to directly image the transverse, sagittal, and coronal planes with MRI.
5. Because serial studies can be performed on the patient without risk of radiation exposure, MRI is useful in assessing the response of cancer to radiotherapy and chemotherapy.

Although the most common uses of MRI are visualization of the CNS (Figure 6-11) and bony spine, joints and extremities, and liver, this scanning technique also shows promise in the evaluation of the following areas:

1. Head and surrounding structures
2. Spinal cord and surrounding structures
3. Face and surrounding structures
4. Neck
5. Mediastinum

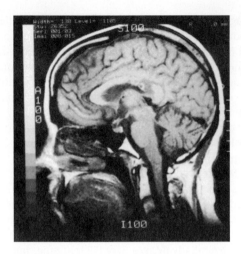

Figure 6-11 Midline sagittal view of the brain using MRI.

6. Heart and great vessels
7. Liver
8. Kidney
9. Prostate
10. Bone and joints
11. Breast
12. Extremities and soft tissues

MRI is not useful, however, for visualization of the abdomen because a contrast agent is needed before the abdomen can be evaluated well.

A major disadvantage of MRI is that patient eligibility is reduced compared with CT scanning. For example, MRI scanning is contraindicated in patients who require cardiac monitoring or have metal implants, pacemakers, or cerebral aneurysm clips. The presence of these objects can result in MRI image degradation and may endanger the patient.

Interfering factors
A factor that interferes with MRI is movement during the scan which causes significant image distortion.

Procedure
The patient lies on a platform that slides into a tube containing the doughnut-shaped magnet. The patient is instructed to lie still during the procedure. During the scan, the patient can communicate with the staff, using a microphone placed in the scanner. A new contrast medium called gadolinium (Magnevist) has been approved by the United States Food and Drug Administration. It is a paramagnetic enhancement agent that crosses the blood-brain barrier and is especially useful for distinguishing edema from tumors. When it is used in MRI scanning, approximately 10 to 15 ml of gadolinium is injected intravenously. Imaging can begin shortly thereafter.

This procedure is performed by a qualified radiologic technologist in approximately 30 to 90 minutes. The only discomfort associated with this procedure may be that of lying still on a hard surface. A tingling sensation may be felt in teeth containing metal fillings. Some patients may become claustrophobic in the tubelike MRI unit. This problem is decreased if the newer open scanners are used.

Contraindications
Contraindications for MRI are as follows:

- Patients who are extremely obese
  The table will not hold weight greater than 300 pounds.
- Patients who are pregnant
  The long-term effects of MRI are not known at this time. A risk of heating the amniotic fluid and injuring the fetus exists.
- Patients who are confused or agitated, because they cannot remain still
- Patients who are claustrophobic, because they are enclosed in a tube
- Patients who are unstable and require continuous life-support equipment
  Monitoring equipment cannot be used inside the scanner room because it will be affected by the magnet.
- Patients with implantable metal objects such as pacemakers, infusion pumps, aneurysm clips, inner-ear implants, and metal fragments in one or both eyes
  The magnet may move the object within the body and injure the patient

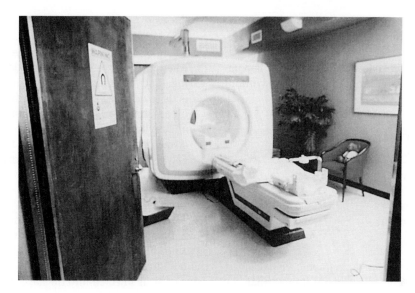

Figure 6-12 MRI equipment.

Nursing implications with rationale

Before

☞ Explain the procedure to the patient. Inform the patient that there is no exposure to radiation. Inform the adult patient that no fluid or food restrictions are necessary before MRI. Inform the parents whether the child should fast for 4 hours before the test. This is done because children are often sedated.

■ Obtain written and informed consent, if required by the institution.

☞ Tell parents that they may read or talk to a child in the scanning room during the procedure, because no risk of radiation exists.

■ Assess the patient for any contraindications for testing (e.g., aneurysm clips).

■ If possible, show the patient a picture of the scanning machine and encourage verbalization of anxieties (Figure 6-12). Some patients may experience claustrophobia. Antianxiety medications may be helpful for patients with mild claustrophobia.

☞ Instruct the patient to remove all metal objects (e.g., dental bridges, jewelry, hair clips, belts, credit cards), because they will create artifacts on the scan. The magnetic field can damage watches and credit cards. Also, movement of metal objects within the magnetic field can be detrimental to anyone within the field.

☞ Inform the patient that he or she will be required to remain motionless during this study. Any movement can distort the scan. Young children often are sedated during this procedure. For head and neck MRI scans, the patient's head may be placed in a cradle, which prohibits significant motion.

☞ Inform the patient that during the procedure, he or she may hear a thumping sound. Earplugs are available if the patient wishes to use them.

☞ Remind the patient that a microphone inside the MRI tube enables him or her to communicate with personnel.

☞ For comfort, instruct the patient to empty his or her bladder before the test.

☞ Inform the parents if the child should be sleep deprived for this study. This is done by keeping the child awake until midnight the night before the study. The child then is awakened for 5 to 10 minutes every hour beginning at 4

AM. The child should not be allowed to sleep in the car on the way to the hospital.

After

No special postprocedure care is needed. The patient can drive to and from the procedure without assistance.

Myelography (Myelogram)

Test type X-ray with contrast dye

Normal values

Normal spinal canal

Rationale

Myelography provides radiographic visualization of the subarachnoid space of the spinal canal, the spinal cord, nerve roots, and surrounding meninges. This test is indicated in patients with severe back pain or localized neurologic signs that suggest disease in the canal (e.g., herniated lumbar disk). This test is less commonly performed than MRI (see p. 213), which provides better visualization and is less invasive.

By placing radiopaque dye or air into the subarachnoid space, the contents of the spinal canal can be radiographically outlined. Cord tumors, meningeal tumors, metastatic spinal tumors, herniated intervertebral disks, and arthritic bone spurs can be detected by this study. These lesions appear as spinal canal narrowing or as varying degrees of obstruction to the flow of the dye column within the canal (Figure 6-13). The entire canal (from lumbar to cervical areas) can be examined. Because this test is usually performed by LP (see p. 208), all the potential complications of that procedure exist.

Potential complications

Potential complications associated with myelography are as follows:

- Headache, as a result of the lumbar puncture required for the test
- Meningitis, as a result of microbes introduced with the lumbar puncture
- Herniation of the brain

- Seizures, precipitated by the contrast medium injected into the spinal space
- Allergic reaction to iodinated dye
  Allergic reactions vary from mild flushing, itching, and urticaria to life-threatening anaphylaxis (evidenced by respiratory distress, drop in blood pressure, shock). In the unusual event of anaphylaxis, the patient may be treated with diphenhydramine, steroids, and epinephrine. Oxygen and endotracheal equipment should be on hand for immediate use.

Procedure

The patient usually fasts for 4 hours before the myelography. A lumbar puncture is performed on the nonsedated patient. Fifteen milliliters of CSF is withdrawn, and 15 ml or more of radiographic dye or air is injected into the subarachnoid space. Because the specific gravity of the dye is greater than that of the CSF, the direction of dye flow depends on the tilt of the table and patient position. With the needle in place, the patient is placed on a tilt table in the prone position, with the head downward. A foot support and shoulder brace or harness keep the patient from sliding. The column of dye is followed under fluoroscopy. Radiographic films are taken. Obstructions to the flow of dye are evident, and the level of the lesion is easily determined.

Metrizamide (Amipaque), a water-soluble contrast material, is now commonly used for myelography. This dye is absorbed by the blood and excreted by the kidneys. It has two advantages over the oil-based dyes that formerly were used. First, it does not need to be removed at the end of the procedure because it is water-soluble and completely reabsorbed. This feature reduces the length of the procedure and minimizes the discomfort associated with oil-based dye removal. Second, metrizamide is less viscous than the iodinated oil-based dyes and therefore permits better visualization of small areas (e.g., nerves, nerve roots, and sheaths), affording better differentiation of complete and incomplete spinal blockages. The disadvantage associated with metrizamide is that it may precipitate postprocedure seizure activity. Iohexol (omnipaque), another water-soluble contrast agent, has a significantly lower

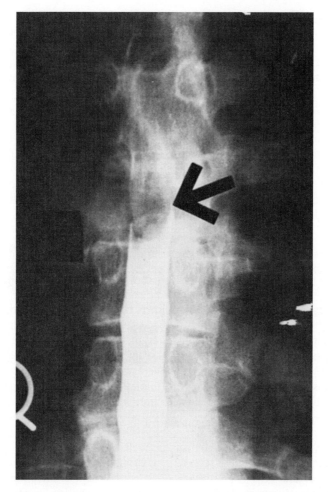

Figure 6-13   Abnormal myelogram. Obstruction of radiographic dye column at high lumbar level (*arrow*) is caused by metastatic tumor compressing the canal.

risk of CNS toxicity than does metrizamide. After the procedure, the patient's head and thorax should be elevated 30 to 50 degrees for approximately 6 to 8 hours to prevent contact of the water-soluble agent with the cerebral meninges, which could precipitate a seizure. Headache, nausea, and vomiting often occur 4 to 8 hours after the procedure and may persist for 24 to 36 hours.

After myelography is performed, the needle is removed and a dressing is applied. The procedure lasts approximately 45 minutes. Patient response to myelography varies from mild dis-comfort to severe pain. Many patients having this procedure already are experiencing back pain, which is then exacerbated by the LP and dye injection.

Contraindications
Contraindications for myelography are as follows:

- Patients with MS, because symptom exacerbation may be precipitated by myelography
- Patients with increased intracranial pressure, because LP may cause herniation of the brain
- Patients who are allergic to iodinated dye

Nursing implications with rationale

See LP, p. 212.

Before

☞ Instruct the patient to fast approximately 4 hours before the study to avoid vomiting during the study.

☞ Inform the patient that he or she will be tilted up and down on a table so that the dye can properly fill the spinal canal and provide adequate visualization of the desired area.

After

■ Proper positioning of the patient depends on the type of dye used. Specific positioning (see pp. 216-217) should be prescribed by the physician after consultation with the radiologist.

■ Observe the patient for signs and symptoms of meningeal irritation (e.g., fever, stiff neck, occipital headache, or photophobia).

■ Monitor the patient's vital signs and his or her ability to void.

■ If metrizamide was used, observe the patient for seizure activity. Do not administer medications that may precipitate seizure activity (e.g., phenothiazines).

☞ Instruct the patient to drink fluids to enhance excretion of the dye and hasten replacement of CSF.

Case Study

Herniated Disk

Mr. S., 38 years old, had a 3-year history of lower back pain. Although the pain was intermittent and transient, he missed many work days during the preceding year. In the 2 months before his admission to the hospital, increasing paresthesia (numbness and tingling) had developed in his toes and was associated with mild weakness of his right foot. All results of his physical examination were normal except for right-sided, lumbar paraspinal muscle spasm. His neurologic examination also indicated hypoesthesia (decreased sensation to pinprick) and anterior tibial muscle weakness.

Studies	Results
Routine laboratory work	WNL
Lumbosacral spinal x-ray study (LS spine), p. 208	Normal (no evidence of lumbosacral arthritic degenerative joint disease)
Nerve conduction studies, p. 202	No abnormalities in the distal sacral nerve or its branches
EMG, p. 201	Decrease in number of muscle fibers contracting in the anterior tibial muscle
Myelography, p. 216	Narrowing of the radiographic dye column at the area of lumbar vertebrae 4-5 (L4-L5), indicating herniated disk
MRI of lumbar spine, p. 213	Herniated disk at L4. Nerve root compression of L4 and L5

Diagnostic Analysis

The normal results of the lumbosacral spinal x-ray study ruled out degenerative joint disease as a cause for this patient's back pain. Nerve conduction studies and EMG indicated nerve-root compression at L5. Both myelography and MRI showed that this patient's symptoms were caused by a herniated lumbar intervertebral disk.

The patient underwent a posterior decompressive laminectomy of the L4 and L5 region. Postoperatively he had only minimal back pain, which did not interrupt his normal physical activities.

Critical Thinking Questions

1. What are the advantages of performing both an MRI and a myelogram on this patient?
2. What postoperative assessments will be done after Mr. S's surgery?

Oculoplethysmography (OPG, Ocular Pressures)

Test type Manometric

Normal values
Normal and equal blood flow in both carotid arteries

Rationale
Oculoplethysmography (OPG) is a noninvasive study used to indirectly measure blood flow in the ophthalmic artery. Because the ophthalmic artery is the first major branch of the internal carotid artery, its blood flow reflects the carotid blood flow and the alternative blood flow to the brain. OPG is indicated in patients who have symptoms of carotid atherosclerotic occlusive disease (e.g., transient ischemic attacks, carotid bruits, neurologic symptoms [e.g., dizziness, fainting]). This test also is often performed to monitor the success of carotid endarterectomy.

For OPG, eye pressures are measured with suction cups placed on the eyes. If the pressures are lower than normal or as compared with the other eye, carotid atherosclerotic occlusive disease is suspected. If indicated, this procedure may be followed by cerebral angiography. Carotid Doppler flow studies (see p. 26), however, are easier to perform, less invasive, and therefore are being used more frequently.

Procedure
No fasting or sedation is necessary before OPG. This study usually is performed in a special room designed for neurologic studies. The patient lies on his or her back on a table or bed. The blood pressure in both arms is taken before the test. Electrocardiogram (EKG) electrodes are applied to the patient's extremities to demonstrate any abnormal cardiac rhythms during the study.

Anesthetic eyedrops then are instilled in both eyes to minimize discomfort during OPG. Small pulse sensors are attached to the earlobes to detect blood flow to the ear through the external carotid artery. Tracings for both ears are recorded and compared. Suction cups resembling contact lenses are applied directly to the eyeballs (Figure 6-14). Tracings of the pulsations within each eye are recorded. A vacuum source then is applied to the suction cup. This increased pressure causes the pulse in both eyes to disappear temporarily because all the blood flow to the eye is interrupted. When the suction source is stopped, the blood flow returns to the eyes; both pulses should return simultaneously. Time difference in the pulse return from one eye to the other, from one ear to the other, and from the ear to the eye on each side is measured in milliseconds. If internal carotid stenosis is present, blood flow to the eye would be delayed. A trained technician is able to perform this test in approximately 20 to 30 minutes. The patient's eyes usually burn slightly when the ophthalmic drops are applied. When suction is applied to the suction cup, the patient may feel a pulling sensation. During the suction application, vision may be lost temporarily; however, it will immediately return after the suction is discontinued. After the study, vision should be unaffected.

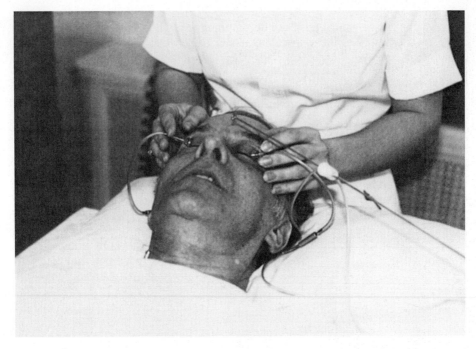

Figure 6-14   Suction cups ready to be placed on the eyeballs for OPG.

Contraindications

OPG is contraindicated in patients who have had eye surgery within the last 2 to 6 months or other eye problems.

Nursing implications with rationale

Before

☞ Explain the procedure to the patient. Tell the patient that no fasting or sedation is required.

☞ If the patient is wearing contact lenses, instruct him or her to remove them before the study.

After

☞ Inform the patient that the eye anesthesia usually wears off in approximately 30 minutes. Instruct the patient not to rub the eyes for at least 2 hours. If tears appear, the eye should only be blotted dry.

☞ If the patient wears contact lenses, inform him or her that lenses should not be reinserted for at least 2 hours after OPG.

☞ Explain to the patient that it is normal for the patient's eyes to appear bloodshot for several hours after the test. Artificial tears may be instilled to soothe any eye irritation.

☞ Instruct the patient to wear sunglasses, if photophobia is present.

Skull X-ray

Test type X-ray

Normal values

Normal skull and surrounding structures

Rationale

An x-ray study of the skull provides visualization of the bones making up the skull, the nasal sinuses, and any cerebral calcification. The study is indicated when a pathologic condition is suspected in any of these structures. When head trauma occurs, a CT scan of the head (see p. 196) usually is ordered instead of a skull x-ray. How-

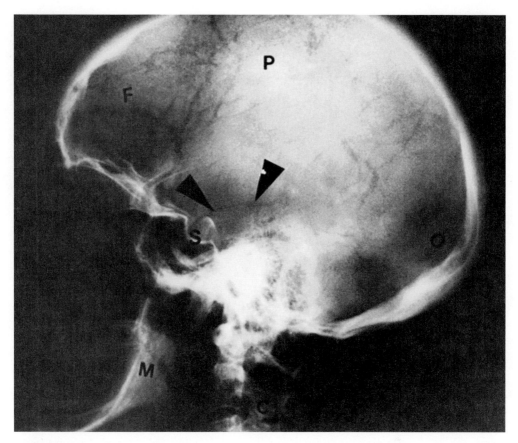

Figure 6-15 Skull x-ray, lateral view. Pointers indicate fracture line in temporal bone. *F,* Frontal bone; *P,* parietal bone; *O,* occipital bone; *S,* sella turcica; *M,* mandible; *C,* cervical vertebrae.

ever, fractures of the skull are easily seen as abnormal radiolucent lines in an otherwise radiopaque skull bone (Figure 6-15). Metastatic tumors of the skull can easily be seen as radiolucent spots in an otherwise normal skull (Figure 6-16). Opacification of the nasal sinuses may indicate sinusitis, hemorrhage, or tumor.

The pineal gland, located in the midline of the brain, is thought to regulate the biorhythms of mammals. This gland may become calcified at any time after puberty. When calcified, it is a very useful marker and allows the midline of the brain to be easily identified on a skull x-ray film. Conditions such as unilateral hematoma or tumor cause

a shift of the calcified pineal gland to the side opposite the site of the pathologic condition.

The sella turcica is the bony structure surrounding and protecting the pituitary gland. Tumors of the pituitary gland may cause an increase in size or erosion of the sella turcica. These changes can be detected by skull x-ray studies.

Procedure

The unsedated patient is taken to the radiology department and placed on an x-ray table. Axial (submentovertical [i.e., chin to top of head]), half-axial (Towne's projection), posteroante-

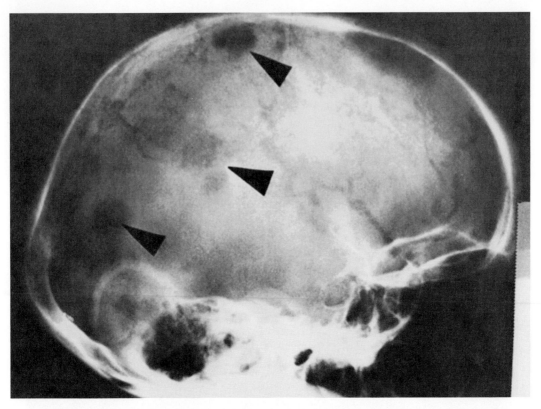

Figure 6-16   Skull x-ray, lateral view. Pointers indicate osteolytic metastasis to the skull.

rior, and lateral views of the skull usually are taken.

Nursing implications with rationale
Before
- ☞ Explain the procedure to the patient. Tell the patient that no fasting or sedation is necessary.
- ☞ Inform the patient that all objects above the neck must be removed. Metal objects and dentures prevent radiographic visualization of the structures they cover.
- ■ Avoid hyperextension and manipulation of the head until cervical injuries are ruled out.
- ■ If the scalp has been lacerated, dress the wound in a sterile manner before the radiographic film is taken.

Spinal X-rays (Cervical, Thoracic, Lumbar, Sacral, or Coccygeal X-ray Studies)

Test type X-ray

Normal values
Normal spinal vertebrae

Rationale
Spinal x-ray studies may be performed to evaluate any area of the spine and usually include anteroposterior, lateral, and oblique views. These radiographic films often are done to assess back or neck pain, degenerative arthritic changes, traumatic fractures, tumor metastasis, spondylosis

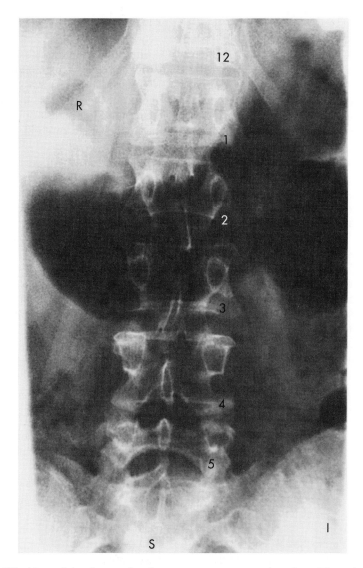

Figure 6-17 Normal lumbosacral spine x-ray, anteroposterior view. Thoracic vertebrae number 12. Lumbar vertebral bodies number *1* through *5*. *R*, Rib; *S*, fused sacrum; *I*, iliac bone.

(stress fracture of the vertebrae), and spondylolisthesis (slipping of one vertebral disk over the other). Cervical spine x-ray studies are routinely performed in cases of multiple trauma to ensure that no fracture exists before the patient is moved or the neck is manipulated. Spinal x-rays are very helpful in evaluating children and adults for spinal alignment abnormalities (e.g., kyphosis, scoliosis).

Procedure

The patient is taken to the radiology department and dressed in a long x-ray gown. Metal objects must be removed, or they will obscure visualization of the LS spinal area. The patient is then placed on an x-ray table. Anterior, posterior, lateral, and oblique radiographic films are taken of the lumbar and sacral areas (Figure 6-17). Radiographic films are taken by a radiologic technician in only a few minutes. The patient feels no discomfort. Cervical and thoracic areas can also be studied. To visualize the upper levels of the cervical spine adequately, both the patient's arms may need to be pulled down as the film is being taken.

Contraindications

Spinal x-ray studies are contraindicated in patients who are pregnant.

Nursing implications with rationale

Before

☞ Explain the procedure to the patient. Tell the patient that no discomfort is associated with this study.

☞ Instruct the patient to remove all clothing above and below the waist for adequate radiographic visualization.

■ If the patient has a confirmed or suspected spinal fracture, assist the physician in safely moving the patient. Unnecessary movement is avoided until the extent of the damage is determined. Ensure that the patient is appropriately positioned during transportation to and from the radiology department and during the study.

■ If the patient is having severe back pain and cannot cooperate, administer sedation as ordered.

■ Assess the patient's menstrual status to prevent radiation exposure to a possible fetus.

After

■ Patient positioning and activity depend on test results.

REVIEW QUESTIONS AND ANSWERS

1. **Question:** Your patient is scheduled for a carotid endarterectomy. After speaking to her doctor, she asks you why she will have an EEG during the operation. What is the reason for this?

   Answer: One of the reasons for an EEG is to monitor cerebral blood flow during major surgical procedures. During a carotid endarterectomy, the carotid vessel must be occluded temporarily. Because of this, the EEG is used to detect early cerebral tissue ischemia and prevent a CVA.

2. **Question:** Your patient appears to be brain dead. What role does EEG play in establishing brain death before organs can be obtained for transplantation?

   Answer: A patient is considered brain dead if all of the following conditions apply:

   a. The patient is unaware and unresponsive.

   b. The patient has no natural spontaneous respiration.

   c. The patient has no brainstem reflexes (e.g., doll's eye, papillary, and oculovestibular).

   d. The patient has not had recent anesthesia, drug overdose, or hypothermia.

   e. The patient registers a flat line on each of two EEG (isoelectric) recordings taken 24 hours apart.

3. **Question:** Your patient is scheduled to have CT scanning and is complaining of severe backache. What is the appropriate nursing intervention?

   Answer: The patient must be comfortable in order to lie still for long periods during CT scanning. Therefore, you should obtain a physician's order to administer an analgesic to the patient. However, it is important that analgesics or sedatives never be administered to a patient who has an altered level of consciousness. If the analgesic is given and no relief is obtained, the study should be canceled.

4. **Question:** Your patient is admitted for evaluation of a brain tumor. CT scanning is ordered. On the morning of the examination you are informed that the CT scanner is broken indefinitely. What study probably will be ordered at this time?

   Answer: Although less sensitive and specific,

brain scanning may be adequate in detecting a brain tumor and therefore will probably be ordered.

5. **Question:** Your patient is scheduled for CT scanning, and you find that he has an allergy to iodine dye. Should you cancel the study?
   Answer: No. Although the IV injection of iodine enhances the quality and sensitivity of the CT scan, it is not necessary. An adequate study usually can be obtained without the dye. Be certain that the test request form indicates the patient is allergic to this dye.

6. **Question:** Your patient returns to the floor after having cerebral angiography. He suddenly has right-sided upper and lower extremity weakness and expressive dysphasia. What might be the cause of this patient's problem?
   Answer: Thrombotic or atherosclerotic plaques along the cerebral arterial wall may have been dislodged when the angiocatheter was passed, thus creating the stroke syndrome. Cerebral arterial vasospasm also could cause these symptoms, but in such a case the symptoms are usually transient and milder in degree. Assess the patient and report your findings to the physician immediately.

7. **Question:** Your 29-year-old patient is admitted with the complaint of sudden onset of paralysis of the right hand. While talking with the patient, you discover that she has severe guilt feelings relating to abuse of her infant son. You strongly suspect a conversion reaction. Would either nerve conduction studies or EMG be indicated?
   Answer: An accurately performed nerve conduction study of the median, ulnar, and radial nerves can virtually eliminate any possibility of neurologic deficit to the hand. EMG would be less helpful because patient cooperation is required. Therefore, nerve conduction studies should be recommended, along with psychiatric evaluation.

8. **Question:** A 50-year-old patient is admitted to the emergency room and found to be febrile and comatose. The physician prepares for an LP. What should be evaluated before the LP is performed?

Answer: Before an LP is performed on any patient, the presence of increased intracranial pressure must be ruled out. This can be done by visualizing the optic fundi and assessing for the presence of papilledema.

9. **Question:** A 22-year-old Army private is being evaluated for meningitis. Several hours after an LP is performed, he begins to complain of severe headache when standing erect. What is the probable cause of this headache, and what are the appropriate nursing interventions?
   Answer: The most probable cause of this type of headache is a continued leak of the CSF through the puncture site in the dura mater. Appropriate nursing interventions include keeping the patient on bed rest, forcing fluids, and administering analgesics as ordered. This patient should not have been out of bed for at least 12 hours after this procedure. Explain the reasons for bed rest to the patient.

10. **Question:** A 48-year-old patient is admitted to your unit with the diagnosis of a possible herniated lumbar disk. Myelography is ordered. During routine physical examination, occult blood was found in the patient's stools, and the physician has ordered a barium enema study. In what sequence should these tests be performed?
    Answer: Myelography should precede the barium enema study. If the barium enema study were done first, visualization of the radiographic dye used in myelography would be obscured by the barium used in the lower gastrointestinal series.

Bibliography

Adams RD, Victor M: Principles of neurology, ed 6, New York, 1997, McGraw-Hill.

Aminoff MJ: Electrophysiologic studies of the central and peripheral nervous systems. In Fauci AS et al, editors: Harrison's principles of internal medicine, ed 14, New York, 1998, McGraw-Hill.

Bird TD, Bennet RL: Why do DNA testing? Practical and ethical implications of new neurogenetic tests, *Ann Neurol* 38:141, 1995.

Bird TD: Apolipoprotein E genotyping in the diagnosis of Alzheimer's disease: a cautionary view, *Ann Neurol* 38:2, 1995.

Dillon WP: Neuroimaging in neurologic disorders. In Fauci AS et al, editors: Harrison's principles of internal medicine, ed 14, New York, 1998, McGraw-Hill.

Dumitru D: Electrodiagnostic medicine, Philadelphia, 1995, Hanley and Belfus, 1995.

Dyck PJ: Peripheral neuropathy. In Rakel RE, editor: Conn's current therapy, Philadelphia, 1998, WB Saunders.

Easin JD et al: Cerebrovascular disorders. In Fauci AS et al, editors: Harrison's principles of internal medicine, ed 14, New York, 1998, McGraw-Hill.

Engel J, Jr: Surgery for seizures, *N Engl J Med* 334:647, 1996.

Fahn S: Parkinsonism. In Rakel RE, editor: Conn's current therapy, Philadelphia, 1998, WB Saunders.

Hauser SL, Goodkin DE: Multiple sclerosis and other demyelinating diseases. In Fauci AS et al, editors: Harrison's principles of internal medicine, ed 14, New York, 1998, McGraw-Hill.

Litofsky NS, Recht LD: Brain tumors. In Rakel RE, editor: Conn's current therapy, Philadelphia, 1998, WB Saunders.

Martin JB, Hauser SL: Approach to the patient with neurologic disease. In Fauci AS et al, editors: Harrison's principles of internal medicine, ed 14, New York, 1998, McGraw-Hill.

Mattay VS et al: Whole-brain functional mapping with isotropic MR imaging, *Radiology* 201(2):399, 1996.

Riederer SJ et al: New technical developments in magnetic resonance imaging of epilepsy, *Magn Reson Imaging* 13(8):1095, 1995.

Roses AD: Apolipoprotein E genotyping in the differential diagnosis, not prediction, of Alzheimer's disease, *Ann Neurol* 38:6, 1995.

Silberberg DH: Multiple sclerosis. In Rakel RE, editor: Conn's current therapy, Philadelphia, 1998, WB Saunders.

Tharp BR: Epilepsy in infants and children. In Rakel RE, editor: Conn's current therapy, Philadelphia, 1998, WB Saunders.

Chapter 7

Diagnostic Studies Used in the Assessment of the
Urinary System

ANATOMY AND PHYSIOLOGY

The urinary system consists of the kidneys, ureters, bladder, and urethra (Figure 7-1). The kidneys are paired organs located on either side of the vertebral column just above the waistline. The blood supply to each kidney comes from the renal arteries, which branch off from the abdominal aorta. The renal veins drain the kidneys and empty blood into the inferior vena cava.

The primary function of the kidneys is to regulate the internal environment of the body. Nitrogenous wastes, along with excess fluid and electrolytes, are filtered out by the kidneys. The filtrate (urine) is formed within the kidney's functional units, called *nephrons*. Each kidney is composed of approximately one million of these nephrons. The nephron (Figure 7-2) includes Bowman's capsule, with its invaginated glomeruli, and the renal tubules (proximal and distal convoluted tubules, loop of Henle, and collecting tubules). A glomerulus is a tuft of capillaries fed by an afferent arteriole. As blood flows through the glomerular capillaries, it is filtered. The filtered material (consisting of nitrogenous wastes, water, and electrolytes) is forced into Bowman's capsule because of the pressure gradient existing between these two areas. The filtrate then successively passes through the proximal convoluted tubules, the loop of Henle, the distal convoluted tubule, and finally the collecting tubule. As the filtrate passes through these renal tubules, materials needed by the body can be reabsorbed. With reabsorption, substances move out of the tubular fluid and back into the blood by both active and passive transport. A major portion of water, electrolytes (sodium chloride and bicarbonate), and nutrients (glucose and amino acids) is reabsorbed in the proximal tubule. Within the loops of Henle, sodium chloride is reabsorbed. Sodium and water are also reabsorbed in the distal and collecting tubules. Nitrogenous wastes generally are not reabsorbed. Not only can the tubular cells absorb substances, but they can also secrete substances. With tubular secretion, substances such as ammonia, potassium, hydrogen, and certain drugs

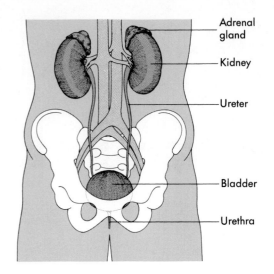

Figure 7-1 Location of the urinary system organs.

(e.g., penicillin) move out of the blood and into the tubular fluid by both active and passive transport. Although secretion occurs primarily in the distal and collecting tubules, 90% of hydrogen ion and penicillin secretion occurs in the proximal tubules.

The relatively dilute urine received into the distal convoluted and collecting tubules is either excreted unchanged into the renal calyces or further concentrated, depending on the individual's state of hydration. These calyces then empty the urine into the pelvis of the kidney (Figure 7-3). The urine passes from the pelvis into the ureters and finally into the urinary bladder. The bladder is a collapsible vesicle located directly behind the symphysis pubis. It serves as a temporary reservoir for urine. The bladder walls consist primarily of smooth muscle called *detrusor* muscle. Contraction of this muscle is mainly responsible for emptying the bladder during urination (micturition). During micturition the urine is emptied through the urethra. In the male, the urethra is also the terminal point of the reproductive tract and serves as the conduit for expelling semen.

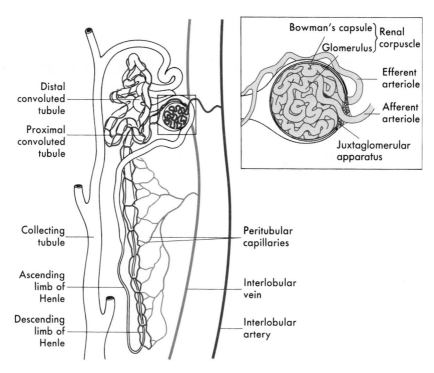

Figure 7-2 The nephron unit with its blood vessels. Blood flows through nephron vessels as follows: interlobular artery → afferent arteriole → glomerulus → efferent arteriole → peritubular capillaries (around the tubules) → venules → interlobular vein.

Electrolyte and Water Regulation

The amount of electrolytes and water excreted by the kidney and other sites of insensible loss (e.g., skin and lung) must equal the daily intake to maintain balance (homeostasis). Sodium and potassium excretion is regulated by aldosterone through the renin-angiotensin system. When the sodium level falls or when the potassium level rises, specialized cells within the kidney, collectively called the *macula densa,* stimulate the juxtaglomerular cells (found in the walls of the renal afferent arterioles) to secrete renin into the blood. Within the liver, renin converts angiotensinogen to angiotensin I. In the pulmonary tissue, angiotensin I is converted to angiotensin II. Angiotensin II stimulates the adrenal cortex to secrete aldosterone. This final hormone stimulates the renal tubule to reab-

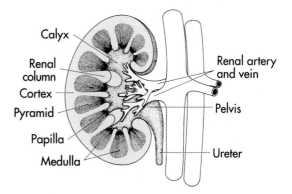

Figure 7-3 Cross section of the kidney.

sorb increased amounts of the sodium and secrete potassium. When electrolyte levels approach normal, the renin-angiotensin system is deactivated.

Regulation of water excretion takes place in the kidney, primarily by way of two regulatory mechanisms: renin-angiotensin and antidiuretic hormone (ADH).

Renin-angiotensin

When the patient is dehydrated, the renal blood flow drops. Specialized, pressure-sensitive cells within the juxtaglomerular apparatus recognize this drop in renal blood pressure. These cells surround the glomerular afferent arteriole in the kidney and secrete renin when renal blood flow decreases. The renin-angiotensin mechanism (as previously described) is activated (Figure 7-4). The end result of sodium reabsorption causes the obligatory reabsorption of water. The patient becomes euhydrated, and the renin system is deactivated.

Antidiuretic hormone

When a patient becomes dehydrated, the serum osmolality increases (i.e., the amount of solute per unit of water increases). This increase in osmolality stimulates the posterior pituitary gland to release ADH. This hormone stimulates water reabsorption in the renal collecting–tubule cells. The patient becomes euhydrated, osmolality returns to normal, and the feedback system is deactivated.

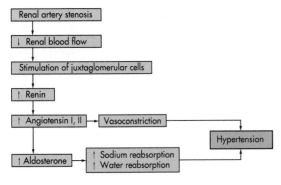

Figure 7-4 Physiology of renovascular hypertension.

Acid Phosphatase (Prostatic Acid Phosphatase [PAP], Tartrate-Resistant Acid Phosphatase [TRAP])

Test type Blood

Normal values

Adult/elderly: 0.11-0.60 U/L (Roy, Brower, Hayden; 37° C) or 0.11-0.60 U/L (SI units)
Child: 8.6-12.6 U/ml (30° C)
Newborn: 10.4-16.4 U/ml (30° C)

Rationale

Total acid phosphatase (specifically, the prostatic acid phosphatase [PAP] isoenzyme) primarily is used to diagnose and stage prostatic carcinoma and monitor treatment efficacy.

Elevated levels usually (but not always) are seen in patients with prostatic cancer that has metastasized to other parts of the body, especially bone. The degree of elevation indicates the extent of disease. Because PAP is not elevated in the early stage of prostate disease, this test is not recommended for screening. With successful treatment, PAP levels fall. Rising levels of PAP may indicate a recurrent tumor.

Because acid phosphatase also is found in high concentrations in seminal fluid, this test can be performed on vaginal secretions to investigate alleged rape. High levels of acid phosphatase also exist in white blood cells (WBCs), primarily in monocytes and lymphocytes. Acid phosphatase levels, especially tartrate-resistant acid phosphatase (TRAP), are helpful in determining the clinical course of patients with lymphoproliferative diseases and hairy-cell leukemia.

Interfering factors

A factor that interferes with determining acid phosphatase levels is prostatic stimulation, which may occur in males after a digital rectal examination or after instrumentation of the prostate (e.g., cystoscopy). This stimulation may cause falsely high levels of acid phosphatase, specifically PAP.

Procedure

No food or fluid restrictions are associated with this test. Peripheral venipuncture is performed, and 5 to 10 ml of blood is collected in a red-top tube. Hemolysis should be avoided. The enzyme can be fractionated to specify the amount secreted by the prostate gland in contrast to the total enzyme activity, which is also present in the bone, liver, kidney, red blood cells (RBCs), platelets, and spleen.

Nursing implications with rationale

Before

☞ Explain the purpose of the test to the patient. Tell the patient that no fasting is necessary.

■ Note on the laboratory requisition slip if the patient has had a prostatic examination or instrumentation of the prostate gland (e.g., cystoscopy) within 24 hours. Prostatic manipulation may elevate the serum acid phosphatase level.

■ Some laboratories request that they be notified before the blood sample is drawn so that immediate attention (within 1 hour) can be given to the sample. The specimen can be kept at room temperature for up to 1 hour because the enzyme is heat and pH sensitive.

After

■ Apply pressure or a pressure dressing to the venipuncture site to prevent further bleeding. Observe the site for bleeding.

Aldosterone

Test type Blood, urine

Normal values

Blood:
  Supine: 3-10 ng/dl or
    0.08-0.30 nmol/L (SI units)
  Upright (sitting for at least 2 hours):
    Female: 5-30 ng/dl or
      0.14-0.80 nmol/L (SI units)
    Male: 6-22 ng/dl or
      0.17-0.61 nmol/L (SI units)

Children:
  11-15 years: 5-50 ng/dl
  7-11 years: 5-70 ng/dl
  5-7 years: 5-50 ng/dl
  3-5 years: 5-80 ng/dl
  1-3 years: 5-60 ng/dl
  1 week-1 year: 1-160 ng/dl
  Newborn: 5-60 ng/dl
Urine:
  2-80 mg/24 hr or
  5.5-72.0 nmol/24 hr (SI units)

Rationale

Aldosterone, a hormone produced by the adrenal cortex, is a potent mineralocorticoid (i.e., this hormone affects the blood minerals, sodium and potassium). Production of aldosterone is regulated primarily by the renin-angiotensin system. This system works as follows: a decreased renal blood flow triggers pressure-sensitive renal glomeruli elements to release renin. The renin then stimulates the liver to secrete angiotensin I, which is converted to angiotensin II in the lung and kidney. Angiotensin II is a potent stimulator of aldosterone. Secondarily, aldosterone is stimulated by adrenocorticotropic hormone (ACTH), low serum sodium levels, and high serum potassium levels.

Aldosterone stimulates the renal tubules to absorb sodium (and, in turn, water) and secrete potassium into the urine. In this way, aldosterone regulates serum sodium and potassium levels. Because water follows sodium transport, aldosterone also partially regulates water absorption and plasma volume.

Increased aldosterone levels are associated with primary aldosteronism, in which a tumor (usually an adenoma) of the adrenal cortex (Conn's syndrome) or bilateral adrenal nodular hyperplasia causes increased production of aldosterone. The typical pattern for primary aldosteronism is an increased aldosterone level and a decreased renin level. The renin level is low because the increased aldosterone level deactivates the renin-angiotensin system. Patients with primary aldosteronism characteristically have hypertension, weakness, polyuria, and hypokalemia.

Increased aldosterone levels also occur with secondary aldosteronism caused by nonadrenal conditions, which include the following:

Renal vascular stenosis or occlusion
Hyponatremia (from diuretic or laxative abuse, or low salt intake)
Hypovolemia
Generalized fluid overload (edema) (e.g., congestive heart failure, cirrhosis, or nephrotic syndrome)

In secondary aldosteronism, aldosterone and renin levels are high.

The aldosterone assay can be done on a 24-hour urine specimen or a plasma blood sample. The advantage of the 24-hour urine sample is that short-term fluctuations are eliminated. Factors that cause fluctuations include:

Diurnal variation: peak aldosterone levels occur in early morning. In the later afternoon, aldosterone levels are cut in half.
Body position: upright position greatly increases plasma aldosterone.
Diet: levels of both urine and plasma aldosterone are increased by low-sodium diets and decreased by high-sodium diets. Diets high and low in potassium have the opposite effects.

Patients with primary aldosteronism demonstrate very little or no rise in renin or aldosterone with aldosterone stimulation (using salt restriction as the stimulant) and very little decrease in aldosterone with aldosterone suppression (1.5-2.0 L of normal saline solution (NSS) infused between 8 and 10 AM).

Interfering factors
Factors that interfere with determining aldosterone levels include the following:

- Excessive licorice ingestion
  This can cause *decreased* levels, because it produces an aldosterone-like effect
- Posture, diet, and diurnal variations (as previously described)

- Drugs that may cause *increased* levels include: hydralazine (Apresoline), diuretics, potassium, and spironolactone
- Drugs that may cause *decreased* levels include: propranolol, angiotensin-converting inhibitors (e.g., captopril)

Procedure

Blood collection
The patient should maintain a normal sodium diet (approximately 3 g/day) for at least 2 weeks before the blood collection. Excess salt should not be consumed before the test. Drugs that alter sodium, potassium, and fluid balance should be withheld at least 2 weeks before the test. Licorice should be avoided at least 2 weeks before the test because of its aldosterone-like effect. A fasting blood sample is withdrawn with the patient in a supine position. The blood is collected in a red-top tube and sent to the laboratory. Occasionally, a second sample is drawn 4 hours later with the patient in the standing position and after he or she has been moving.

Urine collection
A normal sodium diet (approximately 3 g/day) should be followed 2 weeks before the test. During the 24-hour collection period the patient should avoid strenuous exercise and stressful situations. Any medication restrictions that applied to the blood test also apply to the urine test. Keep the urine specimen refrigerated. The normal values for urine depend on total urinary sodium.

Nursing implications with rationale

Blood
Before
- Explain the procedure to the patient. Usually the patient is asked to be in the upright position for at least 2 hours before blood is drawn.
- Instruct the patient that no fasting is necessary.
- Instruct the patient regarding medication restrictions.

Instruct the patient to avoid licorice for at least 2 weeks before the test because of its aldosterone-like effect.

During

- Indicate on the laboratory requisition slip if the patient was supine or standing during the venipuncture.
- Handle the blood sample gently. Rough handling may cause hemolysis and alter the test results.

After

- Apply pressure or a pressure dressing to the venipuncture site to prevent further bleeding. Observe the site for bleeding.

Urine

Before

- Explain to the patient the procedure for collecting a 24-hour urine sample.
- Instruct the patient that no fasting is necessary.
- Instruct the patient regarding medication restrictions.
- Instruct the patient to avoid licorice for at least 2 weeks before the test because of its aldosterone-like effect.
- Instruct the patient to avoid strenuous exercise and stress because both can stimulate adrenocortical secretions and increase aldosterone levels.

During

- Instruct the patient to begin the 24-hour urine collection after discarding the first morning specimen. This is the start time of the 24-hour collection.
- Collect all urine passed over the next 24 hours into a container in which a boric acid preservative has been added.
- Instruct the patient to void before defecating so that the urine is not contaminated by feces.
- Remind the patient not to put toilet paper in the collection container.
- Keep the urine specimen on ice or refrigerated during the 24 hours.
- Collect the last specimen as close as possible to the end of the 24 hours.

After

- Transport the urine specimen promptly to the laboratory.

Antegrade Pyelography

Test type X-ray with contrast dye

Normal values

Normal outline, size, and position of the ureters and bladder

Rationale

Occasionally a kidney with very poor dye excretion following intravenous pyelography (IVP) cannot be adequately examined by retrograde pyelography, either because the ureter is impassable from below (e.g., from obstruction) or because a cystoscopic procedure is clinically contraindicated. For this patient, the upper collecting system may be opacified by antegrade pyelography with an injection of contrast material by percutaneous needle puncture of the renal pelvis or calyx. This test usually is performed when attempts at retrograde catheterization (retrograde pyelography, see p. 262) have been unsuccessful. Antegrade pyelography is specifically indicated in the following conditions:

1. Localization of ureteral obstruction caused by a stricture, nonopaque ureteral stone, or tumor
2. Evaluation of ureteral obstruction after a urinary diversion procedure
3. Hydronephrosis in a child with poor IVP dye excretion, to identify ureteropelvic and ureterovesical obstruction

This test is performed by a radiologist or urologist in less than 1 hour. The only uncomfortable aspect of this test is the local anesthesia used to numb the skin overlying the pelvis.

Potential complication

Hemorrhage from the needle is a potential complication associated with antegrade pyelography.

Procedure

The patient is placed in a prone position. The renal pelvis is localized by ultrasound or fluoroscopy. Skin overlying the desired site is marked and prepared. After a local anesthetic is injected, the skin is incised, and a needle with a stylet is inserted toward the renal pelvis. While the patient holds his or her breath, a wire is advanced through the needle and into the lumen of the renal pelvis. A catheter is advanced over the wire. Flexible tubing connects the syringe to the catheter, which is used to aspirate urine. Contrast medium is injected to outline the upper collecting system to the point of obstruction below. Posteroanterior, oblique, and anteroposterior radiographic images are taken. Antibiotics usually are recommended for several days after the procedure because of the risk of infection introduced by instrumentation above the ureteral obstructed area. Occasionally the catheter is left in place as is done with nephrostomy. Sometimes the catheter can be passed through the area of ureteral obstruction, and the nephrostomy catheter can be capped, while allowing urine to proceed through the holes of the ureteral catheter.

The only uncomfortable aspect of this test is the use of a local anesthetic to numb the skin overlying the pelvis. This test is performed by a radiologist or urologist in less than an hour.

Nursing implications with rationale

Before

☞ Explain the purpose and procedure of this test to the patient. Allow time for verbalization of questions regarding this procedure.
- Obtain written and informed consent.

After
- Apply a small pressure dressing to the incisional site. Assess the site for bleeding.
- Because the kidney is a highly vascular area, check the vital signs as ordered to detect any evidence of bleeding (increased pulse, decreased blood pressure).
- Note that antibiotics are often ordered for several days to prevent infection, which may be caused by instrumentation at a level above the ureteral obstruction.

ANTISTREPTOCOCCAL ANTIBODIES
Antistreptolysin O Titer (ASO)
Antideoxyribonuclease-B Titer
(Anti-DNase-B [ADB], ADNase-B)

Test type Blood

Normal values

ASO titer
Adult/elderly: ≤160 Todd units/ml
Children:
  5-12 years: 170-330 Todd units/ml
  2-4 years: ≤160 Todd units/ml
  2 years-6 months: ≤50 Todd units/ml
  Newborn: similar to mother's value

ADB
Adult: ≤85 U
Children:
  School age: ≤170 U
  Preschool: ≤60 U

Rationale

Antistreptococcal antibodies are used primarily to determine that a previous *Streptococcus* infection has caused a poststreptococcal disease, such as glomerulonephritis, rheumatic fever, bacterial endocarditis, and scarlet fever. Levels are highest in glomerulonephritis and rheumatic fever.

The *Streptococcus* organism produces an enzyme called *streptolysin O,* which is able to destroy (lyse) red blood corpuscles. Because streptolysin O is antigenic, the body reacts by producing antistreptolysin O (ASO), a neutralizing antibody. When the ASO elevation is seen in a patient with glomerulonephritis or endocarditis, one can safely assume that the disease was caused by streptococcal infection. ASO is of no value for diagnosing acute streptococcal infection. Serial ASO testing, however, may be done to detect the difference between the acute and convalescent phase of disease.

Serial testing that exhibits rising ASO titers over a period of several weeks, followed by a slow fall in titers, is much more significant in the diagnosis of a previous streptococcal infection than is a single titer. The highest incidence of positive results occurs during the third week after the onset of acute symptoms of the post-streptococcal disease. By 6 months, only approximately 30% of patients have abnormal titers.

Antideoxyribonuclease B (ADB), another immunologic test, also detects antigens produced by group A streptococci. The ADB level is elevated in most patients with acute rheumatic fever and poststreptococcal glomerulonephritis. When ASO and ADB are performed concurrently, 95% of previous streptococcal infections are detected.

Procedure

Peripheral venipuncture is performed, and one red-top tube of blood is collected. No fasting is required.

Nursing implications with rationale

Before

☞ Explain the test to the patient. Tell the patient that no fasting is necessary.

After

■ Apply pressure or a pressure dressing to the venipuncture site to prevent further bleeding. Observe the site for bleeding.

Case Study

Glomerulonephritis

A 7-year-old boy was brought to his pediatrician because he had developed hematuria, which required hospitalization. Approximately 6 weeks before his admission he had a severe sore throat but received no treatment for it. Subsequently, he did well except for complaints of mild lethargy and decreased appetite. Approximately 3 weeks before admission he had a temperature of 101° F daily for 7 days. He complained of minimal bilateral back pain. Physical examination revealed a well-developed young boy with moderate bilateral costovertebral angle (CVA) tenderness. The remainder of the physical examination results were negative. His blood pressure was 140/100 mm Hg in both arms and legs.

Studies	Results
Urinalysis, p. 268	Blood, +4; protein, +1; RBC casts, positive; specific gravity, 1.025; color, red-tinged urine (normal: negative for blood, protein, and RBC casts; specific gravity, 1.010-1.025; color, amber-yellow urine)
Urine culture and sensitivity (C&S), p. 273	No growth after 48 hours
Blood urea nitrogen (BUN), p. 266	42 mg/dl (normal: 7-20 mg/dl)
Creatinine, p. 237	1.8 mg/dl (normal: 0.7-1.5 mg/dl)
Creatinine clearance test, p. 237	64 ml/min (normal: approximately 120 ml/min)
Renal ultrasound, p. 105	No tumor. Kidneys diffusely enlarged and edematous

Continued

Case Study

Glomerulonephritis—cont'd

IVP, p. 245	Delayed visualization bilaterally; enlarged kidneys, no tumor; no obstruction seen
Renal biopsy, p. 256	Swelling of glomerular tuft, along with polymorphonuclear leukocyte infiltrates in Bowman's capsule (findings compatible with glomerulonephritis); immunofluorescent staining, positive for IgG
ASO titer, p. 234	210 Todd units/ml (normal: ≤200 Todd units/ml)
ADB titer, p. 234	200 units (normal: ≤170 units)

Diagnostic Analysis

The blood, protein, and RBC casts in this child's urine indicated a primary renal disorder. The elevated creatinine and BUN levels indicated that the problem was severe and that it was markedly affecting his renal function. Both kidneys were probably equally impaired. IVP was helpful only in ruling out Wilms' tumor or congenital abnormality. One normally would not do an IVP in light of this boy's impaired renal function. It is presented here for demonstration of the information it can provide. Renal ultrasound is a much safer test to visualize the kidney to exclude neoplasm. The ultrasound findings were compatible with an inflammatory process involving both kidneys. Renal biopsy was most helpful in suggesting glomerulonephritis. The history of recent pharyngitis, fever, the positive ASO titer, the positive ADB titer, and the finding of IgG antibodies on the immunofluorescent stain all suggested poststreptococcal glomerulonephritis.

The patient was placed on a 10-day course of penicillin. He was given antihypertensive medication, and his fluid and electrolyte balance was closely monitored. At no time did his creatinine or BUN level rise to a point requiring dialysis. After 6 weeks, the child's renal function returned to normal (creatinine, 0.7 mg/dl; BUN, 7 mg/dl). His antihypertensive medications were discontinued. He remained normotensive and returned to normal activity.

Critical Thinking Questions

1. At what point would the BUN and creatinine have signified the need for dialysis?
2. What was the cause of this child's hypertension?
3. What would you do if this child had developed a swollen mouth and neck after the IVP?

Creatinine, Blood (Serum Creatinine)

Test type Blood

Normal values
Elderly: decrease in muscle mass may cause decreased values
Adult:
  Female: 0.5-1.1 mg/dl or 44-97 mmol/L (SI units)
  Male: 0.6-1.2 mg/dl
Adolescent: 0.5-1.0 mg/dl
Child: 0.3-0.7 mg/dl
Infant: 0.2-0.4 mg/dl
Newborn: 0.3-1.2 mg/dl

Possible critical values >4 mg/dl (indicates serious impairment in renal function)

Rationale
Serum creatinine measures the amount of creatinine in the blood. Creatinine is a catabolic product of creatine phosphate and is used in skeletal muscle contraction. The daily production of creatine, and subsequently creatinine, depends on muscle mass, which fluctuates very little. Creatinine, as with BUN (see p. 266), is excreted entirely by the kidneys and therefore is directly proportional to renal excretory function. Thus, with normal renal excretory function, the serum creatinine level should remain constant and normal. Only renal disorders (e.g., glomerulonephritis, pyelonephritis, acute tubular necrosis, and urinary obstruction) will cause an abnormal elevation in creatinine.

Unlike the BUN, however, the creatinine level is affected very little by hepatic function. The serum creatinine level has much the same significance as the BUN level but tends to rise later. Therefore, elevations in creatinine suggest chronicity of the disease process. In general, a doubling of creatinine suggests a 50% reduction in the glomerular filtration rate. The creatinine level is interpreted in conjunction with the BUN. These tests are referred to as *renal function studies*.

Interfering factor
A factor that interferes with creatinine levels is a diet high in meat content, which can cause *elevated* creatinine levels.

Procedure
One red-top tube of blood is drawn from a peripheral vein and sent to the chemistry laboratory.

Nursing implications with rationale
Before
☞ Explain the procedure to the patient. Tell the patient that no fasting is needed.
After
■ Apply pressure or a pressure dressing to the venipuncture site to prevent further bleeding. Observe the site for bleeding.

Creatinine Clearance (CC)

Test type Urine

Normal values
Adult (<20 years)*
  Male: 90-139 ml/min or 0.87-1.34 ml/sec/m^2
  Female: 80-125 ml/min or 0.77-1.20 ml/sec/m^2
Newborn: 40-65 ml/min

Rationale
Creatinine is a catabolic product of creatine phosphate, which is used in skeletal muscle contraction. The daily production of creatine, and subsequently creatinine, depends on muscle mass, which fluctuates very little. Creatinine is excreted entirely by the kidneys and therefore is directly proportional to the GFR (i.e., the number of milliliters of filtrate made by the kidneys per minute). The creatinine clearance (CC) is a measure of the GFR. Urine and serum creatinine levels are assessed, and the clearance rate is calculated.

The amount of filtrate made in the kidney depends on the amount of blood present to be fil-

---

*Values decrease 6.5 ml/min/decade of life after age 20 because of a decline in glomerular filtration rate (GFR).

tered and on the ability of the glomeruli to act as a filter. The amount of blood present for filtration is decreased in renal artery atherosclerosis, dehydration, or shock. The ability of the glomeruli to act as a filter is decreased by certain diseases (e.g., glomerulonephritis, acute tubular necrosis, and most other primary renal disease). Significant bilateral obstruction to urinary outflow affects GFR and CC only after the obstruction is long-standing.

When one kidney alone becomes diseased, the opposite kidney, if normal, is able to compensate by increasing its filtration rate. Therefore, with unilateral kidney disease or nephrectomy, a decrease in CC is not expected if the other kidney is normal.

The CC test requires a 24-hour urine collection and a serum creatinine level. A 24-hour urine collection for creatinine is often measured along with other urine collections to assess the completeness of the other 24-hour collection. In patients with normal creatinine, the CC should indicate whether all the urine has been collected for the full 24 hours.

Interfering factors

Factors that interfere with determining CC include the following:

- Age
  With each decade of age, the CC *decreases* 6.5 ml/minute because of a decrease in the GFR
- Muscle mass
  Decreased muscle mass will cause *decreased* CC values
- Exercise, which may cause *increased* CC values
- Incomplete urine collection, which may give a falsely *decreased* value
- Pregnancy, which *increases* CC
  In part, this is due to the increased load placed by the growing fetus on the kidney

Procedure

The patient's urine is collected in an appropriate specimen container over a 24-hour period. It is then sent to the chemistry laboratory for measurement of volume and quantity of creatinine. No special diet is necessary. During the 24-hour col-

lection period, a blood specimen is obtained for a serum creatinine level. CC is then computed from the above measurements using the following formula:

$$UV/P = \text{creatinine clearance}$$

U = Number of mg/dl of creatinine excreted in the urine over 24 hours
V = Volume of urine in ml/min (total volume [in ml] of urine in 24 hours is divided by 1440 minutes to get the ml/min
P = Serum creatinine in mg/dl
  For example, when U = 96 mg/dl, V = 1800 ml/24 hours, and P = 1.0 mg/dl, the equation would be:

$$\frac{(96\text{mg/dl})(1800\text{ml/24hours})/}{(1.0\text{mg/dl})(1440\text{min})} = 120\text{ml/min}$$

Nursing implications with rationale

Before
- Explain the procedure to the patient. Show the patient where to store the urine specimen. The 24-hour urine specimen for creatinine is usually kept on ice or refrigerated.
- Inform the patient that the 24-hour collection period begins after he or she urinates. Indicate the starting time on the urine container or laboratory requisition slip. Discard the first sample. Make sure that all urine passed by the patient during the next 24 hours is collected. Test results are calculated based on a 24-hour output, and results will be inaccurate if any specimens are missed. If one voided specimen is accidentally discarded, the 24-hour collection usually must begin again. However, some hospitals allow the specimen to be sent if the amount of discarded urine is indicated on the laboratory requisition slip and is less than 250 ml.
- Post the hours for the urine collection on the patient's door, on the bedpan hopper, and in the utility room to prevent accidental discarding of a specimen.
- It is not necessary to measure each urine specimen (24-hour collection of some other specimens may require this measurement).

☞ Instruct the patient to void before defecating so that the urine is not contaminated by feces. Toilet paper should not be placed in the collection container.

■ Encourage the patient to drink fluids during the 24-hour period unless this is contraindicated for medical purposes.

■ Draw a venous blood sample in a red-top tube for a serum creatinine test during the 24-hour collection period.

■ Collect the last specimen as close as possible to the end of the 24-hour period. Remind the patient when the last sample is needed. Indicate the time of the last specimen on the laboratory requisition slip or urine container.

After

■ Send the specimen to the laboratory when the test is completed.

Cystography (Cystourethrography, Voiding Cystography, Voiding Cystourethrography)

Test type X-ray with contrast dye

Normal values
Normal bladder structure and function

Rationale
Filling the bladder with radiopaque contrast material provides visualization of the bladder for radiographic study. Either fluoroscopic or radiographic films demonstrate bladder filling and collapse after emptying. Filling defects or shadows within the bladder indicate primary bladder tumors (Figure 7-5). Extrinsic compression or distortion of the bladder is seen with pelvic tumor (e.g., rectal, cervical) or hematoma (secondary to pelvic bone fractures). Extravasation of the dye outside the bladder is seen with traumatic rupture, perforation, and fistula of the bladder. Vesicoureteral reflux (abnormal backflow of urine from bladder to ureters), which can cause persistent or recurrent pyelonephritis, also may be demonstrated during cystography. Although the bladder is visualized during an IVP (see p. 245),

primary pathologic bladder conditions are best studied by cystography.

Potential complications
Potential complications associated with cystography are as follows:

■ Urinary tract infection
This may result from catheter placement or the instillation of contaminated contrast material.

■ Allergic reaction to iodinated dye
This rarely occurs, because the dye is not administered intravenously.

Procedure
The patient is given only clear liquids for breakfast on the day of the examination. No cathartics are necessary. The patient is taken to the radiology department and placed in the supine or lithotomy position. If a urinary catheter is not already present, one is placed through the urethra and into the bladder. Approximately 300 cc (much less for children) of air or radiopaque dye is injected through the catheter and into the bladder, and the catheter is clamped. Radiographic films are then taken. If the patient is able to void, the catheter is removed, and the patient is asked to micturate. Further radiographic films are taken.

This test is moderately uncomfortable if bladder catheterization is required. A radiologist performs this study in approximately 15 to 30 minutes.

Contraindications
Cystography is contraindicated in patients with urethral or bladder infection or injury. Gram-negative sepsis can occur because of the catheterization. Any known bladder injury may be exacerbated by dye instillation.

Nursing implications with rationale
Before
☞ Explain the procedure to the patient. Embarrassment may inhibit the patient's ability to void on command. Assure the patient that he or she will be draped to prevent unnecessary exposure.

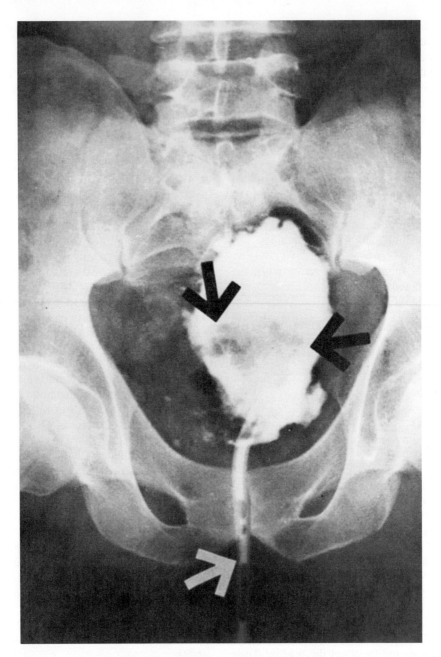

Figure 7-5   Cystography. Black arrows indicate large bladder tumor distorting normal bladder. White arrow indicates Foley catheter in urethra.

- Males should wear a lead shield over the testes to prevent irradiation of the gonads. Female patients cannot shield the ovaries without blocking bladder visualization.

After

- Instruct the patient to drink fluids to eliminate the dye and prevent accumulation of bacteria.
- Assess the patient for signs of urinary tract infection.

Cystometry (Cystometrogram [CMG])

Test type Manometric

Normal values

Normal sensations of fullness and temperature
Normal pressures and volumes
Maximal cystometric capacity
  Male: 350-750 ml
  Female: 250-550 ml
Intravesical pressure when bladder is empty: usually 40 cm H_2O
Detrusor pressure: <10 cm H_2O
Residual urine: <30 ml

Rationale

The purpose of cystometry is to evaluate the motor and sensory function of the bladder when incontinence is present or neurologic bladder dysfunction is suspected. It also is used to evaluate treatment efficacy for these abnormalities. A graphic recording of the pressure exerted at varying phases of the filling of the urinary bladder is produced. A pressure/volume relationship of the bladder is made. This study assesses the neuromuscular function of the bladder by measuring the efficiency of the bladder (detrusor) muscle, pressure and capacity within the bladder, and the bladder's response to thermal stimulation.

Cystometry can determine whether bladder function pathology is caused by neurologic, infectious, or obstructive diseases. Cystometry is indicated, especially before surgery on the urologic outflow tract, to elucidate the causes for urinary frequency and urgency. Cystometry also is part of the evaluation for the following: incontinence,

persistent residual urine; vesicoureteral reflux (i.e., abnormal backward urine flow from the bladder to the ureters), motor and sensory disorders affecting the bladder, and the effect of certain drugs on bladder function. Cystometry often is performed at the same time as cystoscopy.

Procedure

No food or fluid restrictions are necessary for cystometry. The test is usually performed in a urologist's office or in a special procedure room. The test begins with the patient being asked to void. The amount of time required to initiate voiding and the size, force, and continuity of the urinary stream are recorded. The amount of urine, the time of voiding, and the presence of any straining, hesitancy, and terminal urine dribbling also are recorded. The patient then is placed in a lithotomy or supine position. A retention catheter is inserted through the urethra and into the bladder. (The catheter also can be inserted suprapubically.) Residual urine volume is measured and recorded.

Thermal sensation is evaluated by the installation of approximately 30 ml of room temperature sterile saline solution or water into the bladder, followed by an equal amount of warm water. The patient reports any sensations. This fluid then is withdrawn from the bladder.

The urethral catheter then is connected to a cystometer (a tube used to monitor bladder pressure). With the patient usually in a seated position, sterile water, NSS, or carbon dioxide gas is slowly introduced into the bladder at a controlled rate. Patients then are asked to indicate (1) the first urge to void (usually after 100 to 200 ml has been instilled) and (2) the sensation that they must void (approximately 350 to 450 ml). The bladder is full at this point. The pressures and volumes are plotted on a graph. The patient is asked to void, and the maximal intravesical voiding pressure is recorded. The bladder is drained for any residual urine. If no additional studies are to be done, the urethral catheter is removed. Throughout the study the patient should report sensations such as pain, flushing, sweating, nausea, bladder filling, and an urgency to void.

Certain drugs may be administered during the cystometric examination to distinguish between underactivity of the bladder because of muscle failure and underactivity associated with denervation. Cholinergic drugs (e.g., terazosin [Hytrin], bethanechol [Urecholine]) may be given to enhance the tone of a flaccid bladder. Anticholinergic drugs (e.g., atropine) may be given to promote relaxation of a hyperactive bladder. If these drugs are to be given, the catheter is left in place. After the medications are administered, the examination is repeated in 20 to 30 minutes, using the first test as a control value.

This test is performed by a urologist in about 45 minutes. The only discomfort is that associated with the urethral catheterization.

Contraindications

Cystometry is contraindicated for patients with urinary tract infections because of the possibility of false results and the potential for the spread of infection.

Nursing implications with rationale

Before

☞ Explain the purpose of the test and the procedure to the patient. Many patients are embarrassed by this procedure. Assure them that they will be draped to ensure privacy.

■ Assess the patient for signs and symptoms of urinary tract infection, which is a contraindication for cystometry because of the possibility of false results and the potential for the spread of infection.

☞ Instruct the patient not to strain while voiding because doing so can skew the results.

■ If the patient has a spinal cord injury, ensure that he or she is transported to the testing area on a gurney. The test then will be performed with the patient on the gurney.

After

☞ Recommend a warm sitz bath or tub bath, which may be comforting to the patient.

■ Observe the patient for manifestations of infection (e.g., elevated temperature or chills), which may indicate sepsis.

■ Examine the urine for hematuria. Notify the

physician if the hematuria persists after several voidings.

Cystoscopy (Endourology)

Test type Endoscopy

Normal values

Normal structure and function of the urethra, bladder, ureters, and prostate

Rationale

Cystoscopy is used to evaluate patients with suspected pathology involving the urethra, bladder, and lower ureters. It also is used to obtain biopsy specimens and treat pathology related to those structures. This procedure is commonly performed for patients with the following problems:

1. Hematuria
2. Recurrent or resistant urinary tract infections
3. Urinary symptoms of dysuria, frequency, urinary retention, inadequate urinary stream, urgency, and incontinence

Cystoscopy provides direct visualization of the urethra and bladder through the transurethral insertion of a cystoscope into the bladder (Figure 7-6). Cystoscopy is used *diagnostically* to allow:

1. Direct inspection and obtainment of a biopsy specimen of the prostate, bladder, and urethra
2. Collection of separate urine specimens taken directly from each ureter by the placement of ureteral catheters
3. Measurement of bladder capacity and determination of ureteral reflux
4. Identification of bladder and ureteral calculi
5. Placement of ureteral catheters (Figure 7-7) for retrograde pyelography (see p. 262)
6. Identification of the source of hematuria

Cystoscopy is used *therapeutically* to provide:

1. Resection of small, superficial bladder tumors (transurethral resection of bladder [TURB])

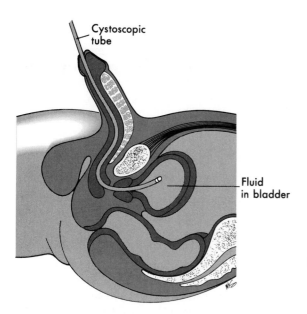

Figure 7-6 Cystoscopic examination of the male bladder.

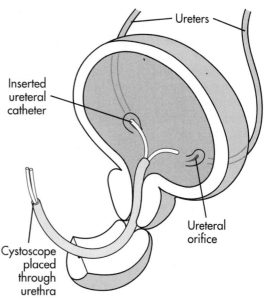

Figure 7-7 Ureteral catheterization through the cystoscope. Note the ureteral catheter inserted into the right orifice. The left ureteral catheter is ready to be inserted.

2. Removal of foreign bodies and kidney stones
3. Dilation of the urethra and ureters
4. Placement of catheters to drain urine from the renal pelvis
5. Coagulation of bleeding areas
6. Implantation of radium seeds into a tumor
7. Resection of hypertrophied or malignant prostate gland overgrowth (transurethral resection of prostate [TURP])
8. Placement of ureteral stents for identification of ureters during pelvic surgery

The cystoscope consists primarily of an obturator and telescope. The obturator is used to insert the cystoscope atraumatically. After the cystoscope is within the bladder, the obturator is removed, and the telescope is passed through the cystoscope. The lens and lighting system of the telescope permit adequate visualization of the lower genitourinary tract. Transendoscopic instruments, such as forceps, scissors, needles, and electrodes, are used when needed. *Endourology* is a term used to indicate procedures designed to visualize the bladder (cystoscopy) and urethra. Included in this term are endoscopic surgical procedures.

Potential complications
Potential complications associated with cystoscopy are as follows:

- Perforation of the bladder, from forceful advancement of the scope
- Sepsis, caused by seeding the bloodstream with bacteria from infected urine
- Hematuria from sites of tissue removal for biopsy
- Urinary retention related to overdistention of the bladder during the procedure

Procedure
Cystoscopy usually is performed in a surgical cystoscopy room or in a urologist's office, using local or general anesthesia. Fluids are forced several hours before the procedure to maintain a continu-

ous flow of urine for collection and prevent multiplication of bacteria that may be introduced during this technique. General anesthetics can be used for children and for the uncooperative or overly anxious adult. If general anesthetics are used, the patient is kept NPO (*nil per os,* nothing by mouth) after midnight (or a shorter time period for children). Fluids are given intravenously during the procedure.

Patients are sedated before the study. The patient is placed in the lithotomy position with his or her feet in stirrups. The external genitalia are cleansed with an antiseptic solution (e.g., providone-iodine [Betadine]). A local anesthetic is instilled into the urethra. The patient is instructed to lie very still during the entire procedure to prevent trauma to the urinary tract. The patient will have the desire to void as the cystoscope passes through the bladder neck. When the procedure is completed, the patient remains on bed rest for a short time.

When performed using local anesthesia, this test is uncomfortable (much more so than with urethral catheterization). This procedure is performed by a urologist in approximately 25 minutes.

Nursing implications with rationale

Before

☞ Explain the procedure to the patient. Tell the patient that the cystoscope is inserted into the bladder in the same manner as a Foley catheter. Encourage verbalization of the patient's fears.

■ Ensure that written and informed consent for this procedure is obtained by the physician.

■ If enemas are ordered to clear the bowel, assist the patient as needed and record the results.

☞ If the procedure will be done using local anesthesia, instruct the patient to have a liquid breakfast. Encourage fluids to provide urine samples as needed and prevent stasis of urine in the event that bacteria are introduced during cystoscopy.

☞ If the procedure is performed using general anesthesia, follow routine anesthesia precautions. Instruct the patient to remain NPO after midnight. You may give fluids intravenously.

■ Administer the preprocedure medications as ordered before the study. In addition to reducing anxiety, the sedatives decrease the spasm of the bladder sphincter, thereby decreasing the patient's discomfort. Deep-breathing exercises also can minimize spasms.

After

☞ Instruct the patient not to stand or walk unattended immediately after his or her legs have been removed from the stirrups. The sudden change in circulatory blood volume may cause dizziness and fainting.

■ Assess the patient's ability to void for at least 24 hours after the procedure. Urinary retention may be secondary to edema caused by instrumentation. If urinary retention does occur, an indwelling catheter may need to be inserted. Record the urine color, and test the urine for blood. Pink-tinged urine is common. The presence of bright red blood or clots should be reported to the physician.

■ The patient may complain of back pain, bladder spasms, urinary frequency, and burning upon urination. Warm sitz baths and mild analgesics may be ordered. Sometimes belladonna and opium (B&O) suppositories are given to relieve bladder spasms. Warm, moist heat to the lower abdomen may help relieve pain and promote muscle relaxation.

☞ Instruct the patient to increase his or her fluid intake. A dilute urine causes less burning upon urination. Fluids also maintain a constant flow of urine to prevent stasis and the accumulation of bacteria in the bladder.

■ Assess and record the patient's vital signs as ordered. Watch for a decrease in blood pressure and an increase in pulse, which would indication hemorrhage. Observe for signs and symptoms of sepsis (e.g., elevated temperature, flush, chills, decreased blood pressure, and increased pulse).

■ Antibiotics occasionally are ordered 1 day before and 3 days after the procedure to reduce the incidence of bacteremia, which may occur with instrumentation of the urethra and bladder.

☞ Encourage the patient to use cathartics, especially after cystoscopic surgery. Increases in intraabdominal pressure caused by constipation may initiate severe lower urologic bleeding.

☞ If a catheter is left in place after the procedure, provide catheter care instructions.

Intravenous Pyelography (IVP, Excretory Urography [EUG], Intravenous Urography [IUG, IVU])

Test type X-ray with contrast dye

Normal values
Normal size, shape, and position of the kidneys, renal pelvis, ureters, and bladder
Normal kidney excretory function as evidenced by the length of time for passage of contrast material through the kidneys

Rationale
Intravenous pyelography (IVP) is the most common radiographic test used to evaluate the urinary system. Much information concerning the kidneys, ureters, bladder, and prostate can be obtained with an IVP. This test is indicated for patients with:

Pain compatible with urinary stones
Blood in the urine
Proposed pelvic surgery, to locate the ureters
Trauma to the urinary system
Urinary outlet obstruction
Suspected kidney tumor

IVP is a radiographic study that uses radiopaque contrast material to visualize the kidneys, renal pelvis, ureters, and bladder. The dye is injected intravenously, filtered by the glomeruli, and then passed through the renal tubules. Radiographic films taken at specific intervals over the next 30 minutes will show passage of the dye through the kidneys and ureters and into the bladder (Figure 7-8).

If the artery leading to one of the kidneys is blocked, the dye cannot enter that part of the renal system, and that section of the kidney will not be visualized. If the artery is partially blocked, the length of time required for the appearance of the contrast material will be prolonged.

With primary glomerular disease (e.g., glomerulonephritis), the glomerular filtrate is reduced, which causes a reduction in the quantity of dye filtered. More time, therefore, is required for enough dye to enter the kidney filtrate and provide renal opacification. As a result, kidney visualization is delayed. This indicates an estimate of renal function.

Defects in dye-filling of the kidney can indicate renal tumors or cysts. Intrinsic tumors, stones, extrinsic tumors, and scarring often can partially or completely obstruct the flow of dye through the collecting system (pelvis, ureters, bladder). If the obstruction has been of sufficient duration, the collecting system proximal to the obstruction will be dilated (hydronephrosis). Retroperitoneal and pelvic tumors, aneurysms, and enlarged lymph nodes also can produce extrinsic compression and distortions of the opacified collecting system.

IVP also is used to assess the effect of trauma on the urinary system. Renal hematomas distort the renal contour. Renal artery laceration is suggested by nonopacification of one kidney. Laceration of the kidneys, pelvis, ureters, or bladder often causes urine leaks, which are identified by dye extravasation from the urinary system.

IVP also is used to assess a patient for congenital absence or malposition of the kidneys. Horseshoe kidneys (connection of the two kidneys), double ureters, and pelvic kidneys are typical congenital abnormalities.

Nephrotomography is a radiographic technique by which a sequence of films, each representing a visual "slice" through the organ, is taken.

Potential complications
Potential complications associated with IVP are as follows:

■ Allergic reaction to iodinated dye
Allergic reactions vary from mild flushing, itching, and urticaria to life-threatening anaphy-

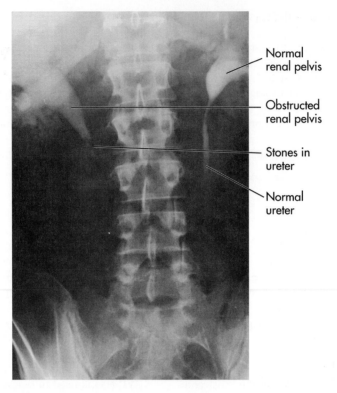

Normal renal pelvis

Obstructed renal pelvis

Stones in ureter

Normal ureter

Figure 7-8   IVP. Note distention of the urinary collecting system resulting from obstruction by a stone in the right ureter *(left side of figure)*. The left collecting system is normal in size and unobstructed.

laxis (evidenced by respiratory distress, drop in blood pressure, or shock). In the unusual event of anaphylaxis, the patient may be treated with diphenhydramine (Benadryl), steroids, and epinephrine. Oxygen and endotracheal equipment should be on hand for immediate use.

■ Renal failure
This occurs most often in elderly patients who are chronically dehydrated before the dye injection.

Interfering factors

Factors that interfere with IVP include the following:

■ Fecal material, gas, or barium in the bowel
Visualization of the renal system may be obscured. Studies using barium (e.g., barium enema) should be scheduled after an IVP.

■ Abnormal renal function studies
These may prevent adequate visualization of the urinary tract.

Procedure

In the afternoon or evening before the examination, the patient is given a strong laxative (e.g., castor oil) or a cathartic. No laxatives are usually required in the young child or infant. The patient is kept NPO after midnight. In the radiology department, the patient is placed in the supine position. A plain film of the patient's abdomen (see KUB, p. 249) is taken to confirm that no residual stool obscures visualization of the renal system. This also screens for calculi in the renal collecting system. Skin testing for iodine allergy is often done. In some institutions, a small dose of contrast is administered, and the patient is observed for allergic reactions. These precautions, however, do not ensure that a reaction will not occur during the IVP.

As much as 1 ml of contrast dye (diatrizoates [e.g., Hypaque or Renografin]) per pound of body weight is given by intravenous (IV) push. Larger doses of dye can be given by an IV infusion drip (infusion drip pyelography or drip-infusion IVP) to produce opacification of the renal parenchyma and complete filling of the urinary tract. Radiographic films are taken at specified times, usually at 1, 5, 10, 15, 20, and 30 minutes, and sometimes longer, to follow the dye's course from the cortex of the kidney to the bladder. Tomograms may be taken to identify a mass. The patient is then transported to the bathroom and asked to void. A postvoid film is taken to assess bladder emptying.

Occasionally, it is necessary to partially occlude the ureters temporarily to get a better filling of the collective system and the upper part of the ureters. This is done by compressing the abdomen with an inflatable rubber tube wrapped tightly around the abdomen slightly below the umbilicus.

Initial IV needle placement and lying on a hard x-ray table are the only discomforts associated with IVP. Patients occasionally become dizzy or have some other idiosyncratic reaction with injection of the dye. This test takes approximately 45 minutes and is performed by a radiologist.

Contraindications

Contraindications for IVP are as follows:

- Patients who are allergic to shellfish or iodinated dyes
  However, this test can be done if the patient has received premedication with prednisone and diphenhydramine.
- Patients who are severely dehydrated
  This can cause renal shutdown and failure. Geriatric patients are particularly vulnerable.

- Patients with renal insufficiency
  If the BUN value is greater than 40 mg/dl, the iodinated, nephrotoxic dye can worsen kidney function.
- Patients with multiple myeloma
  The iodinated, nephrotoxic dye can worsen renal function.
- Patients who are pregnant, because of radiation exposure to the fetus

Nursing implications with rationale

Before

- Explain the purpose of the test and the procedure to the patient. Written instructions should be given as a reminder.
- Give the patient cathartics or laxatives, as ordered, on the evening before the test. Stool or gas in the bowel may obscure visualization of the renal system. Children and infants usually are not given cathartics.
- Instruct the patient to remain NPO after midnight. Moderate dehydration is necessary for the concentration of the contrast dye within the urinary system. The oral fasting time in infants and children varies and will be ordered specifically for each child. The oral fasting time for elderly and debilitated patients also varies according to the patient. If the patient is receiving IV fluids, the infusion rate may be decreased for several hours before the study.
- Assess serum BUN and creatinine levels before the test. Abnormal renal function could make the IVP hazardous because the dye is excreted via the kidney.
- Instruct the patient to void before the test to prevent dilution of the contrast medium in the bladder.
- Assess the patient for allergy to iodine dye or shellfish. If the patient has a history of allergy to iodine dye or shellfish, administer prednisone and diphenhydramine, as ordered, for 1 to 3 days before and as many days after the procedure.
- Instruct the patient that the dye injection often causes a flushing of the face, a feeling of

warmth, and a salty taste in the mouth. These effects are transitory.

During

- Assess the IV site for infiltration by the contrast agent. Extravasation of iodine can cause sloughing of the tissue. If extravasation occurs, a local injection of hyaluronidase may be used to hasten absorption of iodine and resolution of the reaction.
- After the dye injection, look for signs and symptoms of anaphylaxis (e.g., respiratory distress, shock, and a drop in blood pressure). Emergency drugs (diphenhydramine, steroids, epinephrine) and equipment (oxygen and endotracheal equipment) should be on hand for immediate use in the event of anaphylaxis.

After

- ☞ Instruct the patient to drink fluids to counteract the fluid depletion caused by the preparation for this test.
- Maintain adequate oral or IV hydration for several hours.
- Assess the elderly and debilitated patient for weakness because of the combination of fasting and catharsis necessary for test preparation. Encourage bed rest and ambulation only with assistance.
- Evaluate the patient for delayed reaction to the dye (e.g. dyspnea, rash, tachycardia, hives). Reactions usually occur within the first 2 to 6 hours after the test. Treat with antihistamines or steroids.

Case Study

Hematuria

Mr. N., 55 years old, developed painless hematuria. He was otherwise completely asymptomatic. The results of his physical examination were within normal limits (WNL).

Studies	Results
Routine laboratory studies	WNL
Urinalysis, p. 268	Positive for blood (normal: no blood)
	RBCs: too numerous to count (TNTC) (normal: up to 2)
IVP, p. 245	1. Distortion of renal outline, compatible with a right renal mass
	2. Questionable bladder tumor
	3. Mild right ureteral dilation
CT scanning of the mass, p. 113	Normal kidneys, probable renal cyst present
Renal ultrasound, p. 105	Mass in the right kidney is a fluid-filled cyst
Cystography, p. 239	Bladder tumor
Cystoscopy, p. 242	Bladder tumor seen lying near the right ureteral orifice
Renal biopsy, p. 256	Transitional cell carcinoma
Retrograde pyelography, p. 262	Bladder tumor involving right distal ureter

Diagnostic Analysis

The urinalysis results documented this patient's hematuria. Three distinct abnormalities on IVP could have been responsible for the hematuria. The renal mass could have been a solid tumor or a benign cyst. CT scanning and ultrasonography indicated that the mass was the result of a benign renal cyst and was not the cause of the hematuria. No treatment was required for the cyst.

The questionable bladder tumor seen on IVP was more clearly demonstrated by cystography, and a specimen for biopsy was taken during cystoscopy. The diagnosis was transitional cell carcinoma of the bladder. Right ureteral dilation (seen on IVP) implied possible ureteral involvement by the bladder tumor. A retrograde pyelography study indicated that this was indeed the situation.

After 2 months of preoperative radiation, the patient had a total cystectomy and ileal urinary diversion. Six years later this man was found to have right-sided CVA tenderness and diminished renal function.

Studies	Results
BUN, p. 266	58 mg/dl (normal: 7-20 mg/dl)
Creatinine, p. 237	3.2 mg/dl (normal: 0.7-1.5 mg/dl)
Renal ultrasound, p. 105	Dilated ureters bilaterally
Antegrade pyelography	Obstruction of both ureters where the ureters join into the ileal conduit (new bladder made at the time of the previous surgery) caused by recurrent tumor

Bilateral nephrostomies (tubes placed in the ureter to relieve obstruction) were placed at the time of antegrade pyelography. Mr. N. died of his recurrent bladder cancer 8 months later.

Critical Thinking Questions

1. Why did this patient require a retrograde pyelography and an antegrade pyelography?
2. If, after cystoscopy, this patient had complained of lower abdominal pain and had developed a temperature, what would you suspect?

Kidney, Ureter, and Bladder X-ray Study (KUB)

Test type X-ray

Normal values

No evidence of calculi
Normal gastrointestinal (GI) gas pattern

Rationale

The kidney, ureter, and bladder x-ray study (KUB) is a screening x-ray used to rapidly evaluate the abdomen in patients with abdominal pain or abdominal trauma. It can demonstrate pathology of the urinary or GI system.

The KUB is a *"flat plate,"* or simple, radiographic film of the abdomen. It is often referred to as a *plain film,* or *scout film,* of the abdomen. The

KUB is similar to the supine view on an obstruction series (see p. 80) and can be performed to demonstrate the size, shape, location, and malformations of the kidneys and bladder. The KUB also can be used to identify calculi in these organs and in the ureters. This is often one of the first studies done to diagnose other intraabdominal diseases (e.g., intestinal obstruction, soft tissue masses, and a ruptured viscus) (Figure 7-9). The KUB also is useful in detecting abnormal accumulations of gas within the GI tract and identifying ascites. This study involves no contrast medium and poses no radiation risk to the patient.

Interfering factor

A factor that interferes with KUB is retained barium from previous studies, which can obscure visualization.

Procedure

No fasting or sedation is necessary. In the radiology department the patient is placed in the supine position, with the arms extended overhead. Radiographic films are taken of the patient's lower

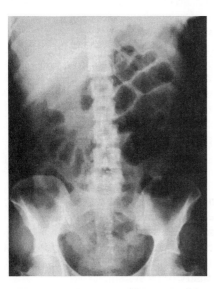

Figure 7-9 KUB depicting multiple, somewhat dilated loops of small bowel consistent with postoperative ileus.

abdomen. Other films can be taken with the patient standing up and turned to the side. No discomfort is associated with this study. KUB is performed by a radiologic technician in a few minutes. A KUB should be taken before IVP or GI studies.

Contraindications

KUB is contraindicated for patients who are pregnant, because of radiation exposure of the fetus.

Nursing implications with rationale
Before
- Explain the procedure to the patient. Tell the patient that no fasting or sedation is necessary.
- For adequate visualization, ensure that this test is scheduled before any barium studies.
- Ensure that the male patient has a lead shield over his gonads to prevent irradiation of the testes. In the female patient, the ovaries cannot be shielded because of their proximity to the kidneys, ureters, and bladder.

After
- If indicated, schedule IVPs or GI studies after completion of the KUB.

Pelvic Floor Sphincter Electromyography (EMG) (Pelvic Floor Sphincter EMG, Rectal EMG Procedure)

Test type Electrodiagnostic

Normal values
Increased EMG signal during bladder filling
Silent EMG signal on voluntary micturition
Increased EMG signal at the end of voiding
Increased EMG signal with voluntary contraction of the anal sphincter

Rationale

This urodynamic test uses the placement of electrodes on or in the pelvic floor musculature to evaluate the neuromuscular function of the urinary or anal sphincter. The main benefit of this study is to evaluate the external sphincter (skeletal muscle) activity during voiding or defecation. This test also is used to evaluate the bulbocavernous reflex and voluntary control of external sphincter or pelvic floor muscles. The pelvic floor sphincter EMG also aids in the investigation of functional or psychologic disturbances of voiding. Fecal incontinence caused by muscular dysfunction also can be identified by rectal sphincter EMG.

Procedure

Three electrodes, most commonly surface electrodes, are used for this procedure. Two electrodes, which may be pediatric surface electrocardiographic electrodes, are placed at the 2 o'clock and 10 o'clock positions on the perianal skin and monitor the pelvic floor muscular activity during voiding. The third electrode usually is placed on the thigh and serves as a grounding plate. These electrodes allow for observation of any change in the muscle activity before and during voiding.

This test begins by recording the electrical activity with the bladder empty and the patient's muscles relaxed. Reflex activity then is evaluated by asking the patient to cough and by stimulating the urethra and trigone by gently tugging on a Foley catheter (bulbocavernous reflex). Voluntary activity then is evaluated by asking the patient to contract and relax the sphincter muscle. The bladder is filled at 100 ml/minute with sterile water at room temperature. The EMG responses to filling and detrusor hyperreflexia (if present) are recorded. Finally, when the bladder is full and the patient is in the voiding position, the filling catheter is removed, and the patient is asked to urinate. In the normal patient, the EMG signals increase during bladder filling and cease promptly on voluntary micturition, remaining silent until the pelvic floor contracts at the end of voiding. The electrical waves are examined for their number and form.

This study is slightly more uncomfortable than urethral catheterization. A urologist performs this study in less than 30 minutes.

Nursing implications with rationale

Before

✏ Explain the purpose and procedure of pelvic floor sphincter EMG to the patient. Patient cooperation is essential to facilitate interpretation of the test results.

■ If the perianal area is soiled, ensure that it is washed before the placement of the electrodes.

After

■ If needle electrodes were used, observe the needle site for hematoma or inflammation.

Prostate/Rectal Sonogram
(Ultrasound Prostate)

Test type Ultrasound

Normal values

Normal size, contour, and consistency of the prostate gland

Rationale

Rectal ultrasound of the prostate is a valuable tool in the early diagnosis of prostate cancer. When combined with rectal digital examination and prostate-specific antigen (PSA) (see p. 252), very small prostate cancers can be identified. Rectal prostate sonography also is helpful in evaluating the seminal vessels and other perirectal tissue. Ultrasonography is very helpful in guiding the direction of a prostate biopsy procedure and can be very helpful in quantifying the volume of prostate cancer. When radiation therapy implantation is required for treatment, ultrasonography is used to map the exact location of the prostate cancer. Rectal ultrasound also is very helpful in staging rectal cancers. The depth of transmural involvement and presence of extrarectal extension can be accurately assessed.

Procedure

No food or fluid restrictions are necessary. However, 1 hour before the test an enema is administered to eliminate feces from the rectum. The patient is then placed on the ultrasonography table on the left side with the knees bent toward the chest. The ultrasonographer applies a greasy conductive paste to the probe. A digital rectal examination usually precedes insertion of the rectal transducer. After insertion of the lubricated rectal probe, water may be introduced into the sheaths surrounding the transducer. Scans are performed in various planes by a slight rotation of the transducer.

This procedure is mildly uncomfortable because of the rectal examination and the rectal insertion of the transducer. Patients also may complain of slight pressure when water is inserted during the procedure. This procedure is performed by an ultrasonographer or urologist in approximately 30 minutes.

Contraindications

Prostate/rectal sonogram is contraindicated for patients with latex allergies. Rectal ultrasound requires placement of the probe in a latex, condom-like sac. Patients with latex allergies may react significantly to that contact.

Nursing implications with rationale
Before
- Explain the procedure to the patient. No fasting is required.
- Administer an enema 1 hour before the study to eliminate feces from the bowel.

After
- Remove the lubricant from the rectal area.

Prostate-Specific Antigen (PSA)

Test type Blood

Normal values
<4 ng/ml

Rationale
Prostate-specific antigen (PSA) can be normally detected in all males; however, its level is greatly increased in patients with prostatic cancer. The higher the levels, the greater the tumor bur-

den. Furthermore, the PSA assay is a sensitive test for monitoring response to therapy. Successful surgery, radiation, or hormone therapy is associated with a marked reduction in the PSA blood level. Response of prostatic disease to treatment is indicated by PSA reductions. Significant elevation in PSA subsequently indicates the recurrence of prostatic cancer. PSA also is used to monitor therapy for benign prostatic hypertrophy (BPH).

PSA is more sensitive and specific than PAP (see p. 230). PSA levels may be minimally elevated in patients with BPH and prostatitis; however, PSA levels greater than 10 ng/ml indicate a high probability for prostate cancer. Lower values may be compatible with BPH or early prostate cancer. Several formulas have been created to partially correct for BPH, which normally occurs in elderly men. The following equation is one example of such a formula:

$$\text{Predicted PSA} = 0.12 \times \text{Gland volume [in cubic centimeters] as determined by ultrasound}$$

A PSA level greater than that predicted would indicate cancer. PSA has been recommended for routine use in screening men over age 50. When combined with digital rectal examination, it can detect approximately 90% of prostate cancers.

Interfering factors
A factor that interferes with determining PSA levels is prostatic manipulation. Obtaining specimens for biopsy or TURP will significantly elevate the PSA levels. The blood test should be done before the surgery just mentioned or 6 weeks after manipulation.

Procedure
No food or drug restrictions are associated with this test. Peripheral venipuncture is performed, and 5 ml of blood is collected in a red-top tube.

Nursing implications with rationale
Before
- Explain the procedure to the patient. Tell the patient that no fasting is needed.

After
- Apply pressure or a pressure dressing to the venipuncture site to prevent further bleeding. Observe the site for bleeding.

Renal Angiography
(Renal Arteriography)

Test type X-ray with contrast dye

Normal value
Normal renal vasculature

Rationale
Through the injection of radiopaque contrast material into the renal arteries, renal angiography permits visualization of the large and small renal vasculature. This permits evaluation of blood flow dynamics, demonstration of abnormal blood vessels, and differentiation of primary renal cysts (avascular) from tumors (very vascular). Atherosclerotic narrowing (stenosis) of the renal artery is best demonstrated with this study. The angiographic location of the stenotic area is helpful to the vascular surgeon considering repair. Complete transection of the renal artery by blunt or penetrating trauma will be seen as a total vascular obstruction. Highly vascular renal tumors produce a "blush" of contrast material during angiography.

Potential complications
Potential complications associated with renal angiography are as follows:

- Allergic reaction to iodinated dye
  These reactions may vary from mild flushing, itching, and urticaria to life-threatening anaphylaxis (evidenced by respiratory distress, drop in blood pressure, and shock). In the unusual event of anaphylaxis, diphenhydramine, steroids, and epinephrine are added to routine resuscitative efforts. Oxygen and endotracheal equipment should be on hand for immediate use.
- Renal failure
  This is common in elderly patients who are chronically dehydrated or have a mild degree of renal failure.
- Hemorrhage from the arterial puncture site used for arterial access
- Arterial embolism from dislodgment of an arteriosclerotic plaque
- Pseudoaneurysm development as a result of failure of the puncture site to seal

Procedure
The patient is kept NPO after midnight on the day of the examination. Because the contrast medium is an osmotic diuretic, the patient should void immediately before the test to avoid developing an overdistended bladder. The patient usually is sedated. In the angiography room, located in the radiology department, the patient is placed on an x-ray table in the supine position. Because access to the renal arteries usually is obtained through the femoral artery, the groin is prepared and draped in a sterile manner. The catheter is passed into the femoral artery and advanced into the aorta. With fluoroscopic visualization (motion picture radiographic images displayed on a television monitor) the catheter is manipulated into the renal artery (Figure 7-10). Dye is injected, and radiographic films are taken in a timed sequence over several seconds. This allows all portions of the injection to be photographed. Delayed films may be taken to visualize subsequent filling of the renal vein. After the radiographic films are taken, the catheter is removed, and a pressure dressing is applied to the puncture site.

The procedure usually is performed by an angiographer (radiologist) in approximately 1 hour. During the dye injection, the patient may feel an intense burning flush throughout the body, but this is gone in seconds. The only other discomfort is the groin puncture necessary for arterial access.

Contraindications
Contraindications for renal angiography are as follows:

- Patients with dye allergies
- Patients who are pregnant, because of radiation exposure to the fetus

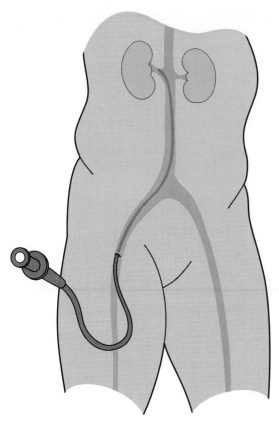

Figure 7-10 Catheter insertion for a renal angiogram.

- Patients with bleeding disorders
  They may bleed excessively from the arterial puncture site

Nursing implications with rationale

Before

- Explain the procedure to the patient. Tell the patient where the catheter will be inserted (usually the femoral artery). Inform the patient that a warm flush will be felt when the dye is injected. Encourage verbalization of the patient's feelings regarding angiography. This test is frightening for most patients.
- Ensure that written and informed consent for this procedure is in the chart.

- Assess the patient for allergies to iodine dye.
- Determine if the patient has been taking anticoagulants.
- Instruct the patient to remain NPO after midnight on the day of the study.
- Administer cathartics as ordered. The presence of feces or gas in the GI tract may impair clarity of the radiographic films and hinder interpretation of test results.
- Mark the patient's peripheral pulses with a pen before catheterization. This permits quicker assessment of the pulses after the procedure. Note and record the quality of the pulses as baseline data.
- Administer the preprocedure medications as ordered. Have the patient void before this study, because the dye acts as an osmotic diuretic. Bladder distention may cause patient discomfort during this study.

After

- Observe the arterial puncture site frequently for hematoma, hemorrhage, or absence of pulse. Assess the extremity for signs of ischemia (numbness, tingling, pain, absence of peripheral pulses, and loss of function). Compare these assessments with the preprocedure baseline values. The color and temperature of the extremity are compared with those of the uninvolved extremity.
- Assess the pulses and vital signs frequently (every 15 minutes for four times, then every 30 minutes for four times, and then every hour for four times, and then every 4 hours) because embolism or bleeding requires immediate intervention. Notify the physician of any abnormalities.
- Keep the patient on bed rest for 12 to 24 hours after the procedure to allow complete sealing of the arterial puncture.
- Apply cold compresses to the puncture site if these are needed to reduce discomfort and swelling.
- Encourage fluids after the study to prevent diuretic-induced dehydration caused by the dye.

Renovascular Hypertension

Mr. V., 65 years old, had a 2-year history of hypertension. He had been treated with antihypertensive medications. Recently, he came to the emergency room with complaints of headache and mild chest pain. The results of his physical examination were essentially normal, except for a blood pressure reading of 210/120 mm Hg and an S_4 heart sound heard on auscultation. He was admitted to the hospital for evaluation; the following studies were conducted.

Studies	Results
Routine laboratory work	WNL
Chest x-ray study, p. 155	Normal
Electrocardiogram (EKG), p. 34	Mild left ventricular hypertrophy
IVP, p. 245	Delayed visualization of the right kidney
Urine test (24-hour) for vanillylmandelic acid (VMA) and catecholamines, p. 276	VMA: 6 mg/24 hours (normal: 2-7 mg/24 hours) Catecholamines Epinephrine: 1.6 mg/24 hours (normal: 0.5-20 mg/24 hours) Norepinephrine: 16 mg/24 hours (normal: 15-18 mg/24 hours) Metanephrine: 53 mg/24 hours (normal: 24-96 mg/24 hours) Normetanephrine: 128 mg/24 hours (normal 75-375 μg/24 hours)
17-hydroxycorticosteroids test	8.3 mg/24 hours (normal 5.5-14.5 mg/24 hours)
Renal scanning, p. 258	Delayed visualization of the right kidney
Renal angiography, p. 253	Stenosis of right renal artery
Plasma renin assay (PRA), p. 259	22 ng/ml/hr (normal: 0.1-3.0 ng/ml/hr)
Renal vein renin assay, p. 261	Right: 78 ng/ml/hr Left: 18 ng/ml/hr
Renal vein renin ratio, p. 261	4.3 (normal: <1.4)

Diagnostic Analysis

The normal values for VMA, catecholamines, and 17-hydroxycorticosteroids ruled out the possibility of pheochromocytoma and Cushing's syndrome as causes of the hypertension. The increased aldosterone and renin indicated secondary hyperaldosteronism resulting from abnormal stimulation of the renin-angiotensin system as a cause of the hypertension. The IVP, renal scanning, renal angiography, and renin assay indicated that right renal artery stenosis was the cause of the patient's increased blood pressure. The patient underwent an aorta-to-renal artery bypass of the stenotic area. Postoperatively, his blood pressure returned to normal, and he required no antihypertensive medication.

Continued

Renal Biopsy (Kidney Biopsy)

Test type Microscopic examination

Normal values
No pathologic conditions

Rationale
Renal biopsy is performed for the following purposes:

1. To diagnose the cause of renal disease (e.g., poststreptococcal glomerulonephritis, Goodpasture's syndrome, lupus nephritis)
2. To detect primary and metastatic malignancy of the kidney in patients who may not be candidates for surgery
3. To evaluate kidney transplantation rejection, which enables the physician to determine the appropriate dose of immunosuppressive drugs

Through renal biopsy, tissue may be examined microscopically. Tissue for renal biopsy is most often obtained percutaneously (Figure 7-11) by inserting a biopsy needle through the skin and into the kidney. The needle, when guided by ultrasonography or fluoroscopy, is more accurately placed for precise localization of the desired tissue.

Occasionally, open renal biopsy is performed. This involves an incision through the flank and dissection to expose the kidney surgically.

Potential complications
Potential complications associated with renal biopsy are as follows:

■ Hemorrhage from the highly vascular renal tissue

■ Inadvertent puncture of the liver, lung, bowel, aorta, and inferior vena cava

Procedure
The patient is kept NPO after midnight on the day of the procedure. No sedative is required. The needle stick may be done at the bedside. If fluoroscopic or ultrasound guidance is to be used, the needle stick is performed in the radiology or ultrasonography department. The patient is placed in a prone position with a sandbag or pillow under the abdomen to straighten the spine. Under sterile conditions, the skin overlying the kidney is anesthetized. While the patient holds his or her breath to prevent kidney movement, the physician inserts the biopsy needle into the kidney and takes a specimen. After this procedure is completed, the

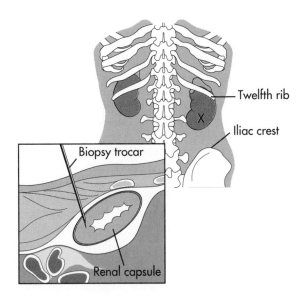

Figure 7-11   Renal biopsy.

needle is removed, and pressure is applied to the site for approximately 20 minutes. A pressure dressing is then applied, and the patient is turned on his or her back and remains on bed rest for approximately 4 to 6 hours. The vital signs, puncture site, and hematocrit values are assessed frequently during this period. The biopsy specimen is placed in a container filled with a fixative solution and sent to the pathology department for appropriate staining and microscopic review.

This procedure is only minimally uncomfortable, if enough lidocaine is used. The procedure is performed by a physician in approximately 10 minutes.

Contraindications

Contraindications for renal biopsy are as follows:

- Patients with coagulation disorders, because of the risk of excessive bleeding
- Patients with operable kidney tumors
  Tumor cells may be disseminated during the procedure
- Patients with hydronephrosis
  The enlarged renal pelvis can be entered easily and cause a persistent urine leak requiring surgical repair
- Patients with urinary tract infections
  The needle insertion may disseminate the active infection throughout the retroperitoneum

Nursing implications with rationale
Before

☞ Explain the procedure to the patient. Keep the patient NPO in the event that bleeding necessitates surgical intervention. Describe the postprocedure routine.
- Ensure that written and informed consent for this procedure is obtained by the physician.
- Check the results of the patient's coagulation studies (prothrombin time and partial thromboplastin time). The patient's hemoglobin and hematocrit values also should be checked.
- Be aware that the patient also may be typed and cross-matched for blood in the event of severe hemorrhage requiring transfusions.

After

- After the removal of the biopsy specimen, apply pressure to the site of the needle stick. The patient is kept on bed rest for 24 hours. Any activity that increases abdominal venous pressure (e.g., coughing) should be avoided.
- Check the vital signs and puncture site every 15 minutes for the first hour after the needle stick and then with decreasing frequency, as ordered. Assess the patient for signs and symptoms of hemorrhage (e.g., a decrease in blood pressure, increase in pulse, pallor, backache, shoulder pain, and lightheadedness). Evaluate the abdomen for signs of bowel or liver penetration (e.g., abdominal pain and tenderness, abdominal muscle guarding and rigidity, and decreased bowel sounds).
- Inspect all urine specimens for gross hematuria. The patient's urine may contain blood initially, but this does not usually continue after the first 24 hours. Urine samples may be placed in chronologic order to compare for hematuria. This is referred to as *rack,* or *serial,* urines.
☞ Instruct the patient to drink large amounts of fluid to prevent clot formation and urine retention. (However, an oliguric patient in renal failure could develop pulmonary edema with increased fluid intake.)
- Draw blood for a hemoglobin and hematocrit determination 8 hours after removal of the biopsy specimen to assess for active bleeding. One purple-top tube of blood is needed.
☞ Instruct the patient to avoid strenuous activities (e.g., heavy lifting, contact sports, horseback riding, or any other activity that causes jolting of the kidney) for at least 2 weeks. Teach the patient the signs and symptoms of renal bleeding and instruct him or her to call the physician if any of these symptoms occur.
☞ Instruct the patient to report burning on urination or any body temperature elevations. These could indicate a urinary tract infection.

Renal Scanning (Kidney Scan, Radiorenography, Renography, Radionuclide Renal Imaging, Nuclear Imaging of the Kidney, Dimercaptosuccinic Acid [DMSA] Renal Scan, Diethylenetriaminepentaacetic Acid [DTPA] Renal Scan, Captopril Renal Scan)

Test type Nuclear scan

Normal values
Normal size, shape, and function of the kidney

Rationale
Renal scans are used to indicate the perfusion, function, and structure of the kidneys. They also are used to indicate the presence of ureteral obstruction or renovascular hypertension. Renal scans are used to monitor renal function in patients with known renal disease. This scan also aids in the diagnosis of renal transplant rejection. Because this study uses no iodinated dyes (except when iodohippurate sodium is used), it is safe to use on patients who have iodine allergies or compromised renal function.

This nuclear medicine procedure provides visualization of the urinary tract after IV administration of a radioisotope. The radioactive material is detected by a gamma ray camera and creates a realistic image of the renal structure. The resultant image (scan) indicates distribution of the radionuclide within the kidney and ureters. This information also can be collated by a computer, and the amount of gamma ray emission per unit of time can be calculated to determine renal function, vascular insufficiency, or renal ureteral obstruction. Scans do not interfere with the normal physiologic process of the kidney.

A variety of renal scans can be used, depending on what information is needed. Different isotopes may be more suitable for different scans based on how the kidney handles the radioisotope.

Renal blood flow (perfusion) scan
This type of renal scan is used to evaluate the blood flow to each kidney. It is used to identify renal artery stenosis and renovascular hypertension and to assess rejection of a transplanted kidney. Hypervascular tumors (renal cell carcinoma) in the kidney also can be visualized.

The basic test is performed by rapidly injecting the radionuclide intravenously while the patient is under the scintography camera. Computers collate the data obtained by the camera and create a gamma activity-per-unit time curve. The kidneys are compared with each other and with the aorta. Decreased gamma activity is noted in the kidney with arterial stenosis or in rejection of a transplanted kidney. Increased gamma activity is noted in the kidney that contains a hypervascular tumor (cancer).

Renal structural scan
This type of renal scan outlines the structure of the kidney in order to identify pathology that may alter normal anatomic structure (e.g., tumor, cyst, abscess). Congenital disorders (e.g., hypoplasia or aplasia of the kidney, malposition of the kidney) also can be detected. Anatomic alterations in the parenchymal distribution of tracer may indicate transplant rejection.

Renal function scan (renogram)
Renal function can be determined by documenting the capability of the kidney to take up a particular radioisotope and excrete it. A well-functioning kidney can be expected to rapidly assimilate, and then excrete, the isotope. A poorly functioning kidney will not be able to take up the isotope rapidly nor excrete it in a timely manner. Each particular radioactive tracer is handled by the kidney in a different manner.

After the injection of the radionuclide, the activity detected by the gamma camera per unit of time equals the function of the kidney, which is plotted on graph paper. This is called a *renogram curve (isotope renography)*. Renal function can be monitored by serially repeating this test and comparing results.

Renal hypertension scan
This scan is used to determine the presence and location of renal artery stenosis, which leads to hypertension. This scan usually uses an

angiotensin-converting enzyme (ACE) inhibitor (e.g., captopril). The captopril scan (captopril renography/scintigraphy) determines the functional significance of a renal artery or arteriole stenosis. These scans may predict the response of the blood pressure to medical treatment, angioplasty, or surgery.

Renal obstruction scan

This scan is performed to identify obstruction of the outflow tract of the kidney caused by obstruction of the renal pelvis, ureter, or bladder outlet. Approximately 10 minutes after the injection of a radionuclide, a diuretic (e.g., furosemide [Lasix]) is administered. The radionuclide in the unobstructed kidney can be seen to rapidly "wash out" (be excreted) from the kidney. A slow excretion without a wash out is seen in an obstructed, but still functioning, kidney. Furthermore, when the collecting system does become visible, it is observed to be dilated.

Procedure

The unsedated, nonfasting patient is taken to the nuclear medicine department. A peripheral IV injection of a radionuclide is given. It takes only minutes for the radioisotope to be concentrated in the kidneys. While the patient assumes a supine, prone, or sitting position, a gamma-ray detecting device is passed over the kidney area and records the radioactive uptake on film.

The patient feels no discomfort during this procedure. The patient must lie still during the study. The duration of this test varies from 1 to 4 hours, depending on the specific information required. Perfusion scans are done in approximately 20 minutes, and functional scans in less than 1 hour. Static structure scans require 20 minutes to 4 hours for completion. This study is performed by a nuclear medicine technologist. Because only tracer doses of radioisotopes are used, no precautions need to be taken against radioactive exposure.

Contraindications

Renal scanning is contraindicated in patients who are pregnant, because of the risk of fetal injury.

Nursing implications with rationale

Before

☞ Explain the procedure to the patient. Tell the patient that no sedation or fasting is required but that good hydration is essential.

☞ Instruct the patient to drink two to three glasses of water before the scan.

■ Assure the patient that he or she will not be exposed to large amounts of radioactivity because only tracer doses of isotopes are used. The radioactive substance usually is excreted from the body within 6 to 24 hours.

■ Do not schedule a renal scan within 24 hours after an IVP. The iodinated dye may temporarily diminish renal function.

After

☞ Encourage the patient to drink fluids to aid in excretion of the radioisotopes.

Renin Assay, Plasma (Plasma Renin Activity [PRA], Plasma Renin Concentration [PRC])

Test type Blood

Normal values

Adult/elderly:

Upright position, sodium depleted (sodium-restricted diet):

>40 years: 2.9-10.8 ng/ml/hr

20-39 years: 2.9-24.0 ng/ml/hr

Upright position, sodium replaced (normal sodium diet):

>40 years: 0.1-3.0 ng/ml/hr

20-39 years: 0.1-4.3 ng/ml/hr

Children:

15-18 years: <4.3 ng/ml/hr

12-15 years: <4.2 ng/ml/hr

9-12 years: <5.9 ng/ml/hr

6-9 years: <4.4 ng/ml/hr

3-6 years: <6.7 ng/ml/hr

0-3 years: <16.6 ng/ml/hr

Rationale

Renin is an enzyme released by the juxtaglomerular apparatus of the kidney into the renal veins in response to hyperkalemia, sodium depletion, decreased renal blood perfusion, or hypovolemia. Renin activates the renin-angiotensin system, which results in the production of angiotensin II, a powerful vasoconstrictor that also stimulates aldosterone production from the adrenal cortex. Angiotensin and aldosterone increase the blood volume, blood pressure, and serum sodium (see Figure 7-4).

The plasma renin activity (PRA) is a screening procedure for the detection of essential, renal, or renovascular hypertension (RVH). The information obtained by PRA is supported by other tests, such as aldosterone and renal vein renin assay (see p. 261). A determination of the PRA and a measurement of the plasma aldosterone level (see p. 231) are used in the differential diagnosis of primary versus secondary hyperaldosteronism. Patients with primary hyperaldosteronism (adrenal adenoma overproducing aldosterone or Conn's syndrome) will have increased aldosterone production associated with decreased renin activity. Patients with secondary hyperaldosteronism (caused by renovascular occlusive disease or primary renal disease) will have increased levels of aldosterone and increased PRA.

The renin stimulation test can be performed to more clearly diagnose and separate primary from secondary hyperaldosteronism. In the stimulation test, PRA is compared with the patient in the recumbent position and while the patient is standing erect. In primary hyperaldosteronism, the blood volume is extensively expanded. A change in position will not result in decreased renal perfusion or sodium level. Therefore, renin levels do not increase. In secondary hyperaldosteronism (or in normal persons with essential hypertension), the renal perfusion decreases while in the upright position, and sodium levels decrease with decreased intake. Therefore, renin levels increase.

The captopril test is a screening test for RVH. Patients with RVH have greater decreases in blood pressure and increases in PRA after administration of ACE inhibitors than do those with essential hypertension. For the captopril test, the patient receives an oral dose of captopril (ACE inhibitor) after baseline PRA and blood pressure measure-

ments are taken. Subsequent blood pressure measurements and a repeat PRA at 60 minutes are used for test interpretation. This is an excellent screening procedure to determine the need for a more invasive radiographic evaluation (bilateral renal arteriography, see p. 253).

It should be noted that the PRA test does not actually measure renin but rather the rate of angiotensin I generation per unit of time.

Interfering factors
Factors that interfere with determining PRA include the following:

- Pregnancy
  Renin is *increased* during pregnancy by virtue of increased substrate proteins concomitantly present in the serum during testing
- Reduced salt intake
  Renin is *increased* with reduced salt intake. Reduced sodium acts as a direct stimulant to renin production.
- High licorice intake
  Renin is *increased* by high licorice ingestion. Licorice has an aldosterone-like effect. This increases sodium reabsorption in the kidney and raises blood pressure, which, in turn, inhibits renin production.
- Time of day
  Renin production varies diurnally, with *increased* values occurring early in the day.
- Positioning
  Renin levels are *increased* when the patient is in an upright position. Normally, the upright position decreases renal perfusion because the blood pools in the veins of the lower extremities. This decreased renal perfusion is a strong stimulant to renin production. Renin levels are decreased in the recumbent position for the same reason (i.e., renal perfusion is increased in the recumbent position and renin levels diminish).
- Drugs that *increase* levels of renin include antihypertensives, ACE inhibitors, diuretics, estrogens, oral contraceptives, and vasodilators.
- Drugs that *decrease* renin levels include beta blockers, clonidine, and reserpine.

Procedure

Random samples of PRA are useless because of marked fluctuations in renin activity caused by salt intake, time of the day, and positioning. For this reason, the patient must maintain a normal diet with a restricted amount of sodium (approximately 3 g/day) for 3 days before the test. Medications (such as diuretics, antihypertensives, and vasodilators) and licorice are usually discontinued 2 to 4 weeks before the test. The patient must stand or sit upright for 2 hours before the blood is drawn. If a recumbent sample is ordered, the patient should remain in bed in the morning until the blood sample has been obtained.

Because the renin values are higher in the morning, a fasting blood sample usually is drawn. Approximately 7 to 12 ml of peripheral venous blood is obtained and placed in a chilled, lavender-top tube to which ethylenediamine tetraacetic acid (EDTA) has been added as an anticoagulant. The tube should be gently inverted to allow adequate mixing of the blood sample and the anticoagulant. The tube of blood then is placed on ice and immediately sent to the laboratory. After the test, a normal diet usually may be resumed, and medications that were withheld may be reordered.

Nursing implications with rationale

Before

☞ Explain the test to the patient. Renin levels are affected by failure to observe diet restrictions before the test. A high sodium diet causes a decrease in renin activity.

☞ Explain the importance of positioning. Improper patient positioning before the test affects the results. The renin levels are decreased in supine patients; therefore, patients usually should be in the upright position.

■ Confirm that the patient has discontinued diuretics, oral contraceptives, antihypertensives, vasodilators, and licorice, as ordered. These can affect the plasma renin levels.

During

■ Chill the collection tube (containing EDTA) before withdrawing the blood sample. After the blood is drawn, the tube is inverted gently and

placed on ice. If these measures are not taken, renin breakdown occurs because the enzyme is very unstable.

■ Record the position of the patient, the time of the day, and any medications that the patient may be taking on the laboratory requisition slip.

After

■ Apply pressure or a pressure dressing to the venipuncture site to prevent further bleeding. Observe the site for bleeding.

Renin Assay, Renal Vein

Test type Blood

Normal values

Renin activity ratio of involved kidney to uninvolved kidney <1.4

Rationale

Renin is an enzyme released by the juxtaglomerular apparatus of the kidney into the renal veins in response to hyperkalemia, sodium depletion, decreased renal blood perfusion, or hypovolemia. Renin activates the renin-angiotensin system, which results in the production of angiotensin II, a powerful vasoconstrictor that also stimulates aldosterone production from the adrenal cortex. Angiotensin and aldosterone increase the blood volume, blood pressure, and serum sodium (see Figure 7-4).

Renal vein assays for renin are used to diagnose RVH. This form of hypertension is due to inappropriately high renin levels, which are made in a diseased or hypoperfused kidney. By injection of a radiopaque dye into the inferior vena cava, the renal veins can be identified and catheterized. Blood is withdrawn from each vein. If hypertension is caused by renal artery stenosis or primary renal pathology, the renal vein renin level of the affected kidney should be 1.4 or more times greater than that of the unaffected kidney. If the levels are the same, the hypertension is not caused by a renovascular source. This is very helpful in determining whether a stenosis seen on a renal angiogram is significant enough to contribute to hypertension. Any stenosis identified on an arteriogram would not be considered severe enough to cause renin-related hypertension if renin levels from that renal vein were not at least 1.4 times greater than those of the opposite kidney. Therefore, another cause for the patient's elevated blood pressure should be considered.

Potential complications

Potential complications associated with renal vein assays are allergic reactions to iodinated dye. Allergic reactions may vary from mild flushing, itching, and urticaria to life-threatening anaphylaxis (evidenced by respiratory distress, drop in blood pressure, shock). In the unusual event of anaphylaxis, the patient may be treated with diphenhydramine, steroids, and epinephrine. Oxygen and endotracheal equipment should be on hand for immediate use.

Procedure

The fasting patient usually is premedicated with meperidine and atropine and taken to the radiology department. The patient is placed on the fluoroscopy table in the supine position. The patient's groin is prepared and draped in a sterile manner and then anesthetized. The femoral vein is punctured, and a catheter is placed into the vein and advanced into the inferior vena cava. Fluoroscopy is used to monitor catheter placement. Dye is injected, and the renal veins are identified. The catheter is placed into one renal vein at a time, and separate blood specimens are withdrawn.

The catheter is removed, and a pressure dressing is applied to the puncture site. The blood usually is sent to a commercial laboratory for analysis. This procedure usually is performed by a radiologist in less than 1 hour. The groin puncture needed for arterial access is uncomfortable.

Contraindications

Renal vein assays are contraindicated for patients who are allergic to iodinated dye. These patients can have an allergic reaction to the radiopaque dye required to visualize the renal vein.

Nursing implications

Before

☞ Explain the procedure to the patient. Instruct the patient to remain NPO after midnight on the day of the test.

■ Ensure that written and informed consent for this procedure is obtained by the physician.

■ Assess the patient for allergies to iodine.

☞ Instruct the patient to remain in the upright position for 2 hours before the test because the renin level is at its maximum in this position.

■ Give the preprocedure medications as ordered, usually 1 hour before the procedure.

After

■ Maintain the patient on bed rest for several hours.

■ Monitor the vital signs. Assess the patient for bleeding.

■ Observe the venous puncture frequently for hematoma and hemorrhage.

■ Apply cold compresses to the puncture site, if needed, to reduce discomfort and swelling.

■ Assess the patient for renal vein thrombosis, which may occur 1 to 7 days after the procedure and is manifested by CVA tenderness, hematuria, and elevated creatinine levels.

Retrograde Pyelography

Test type X-ray with contrast dye

Normal values

Normal outline and size of the ureters and bladder
No evidence of ureteral obstruction

Rationale

Retrograde pyelography refers to radiographic visualization of the urinary tract through ureteral catheterization and the injection of contrast material. The ureters are catheterized during cystoscopy. A radiopaque material is injected into the ureters, and radiographic films are taken (Figure 7-12). This test can be performed even if the patient has an allergy to IV contrast dye, because

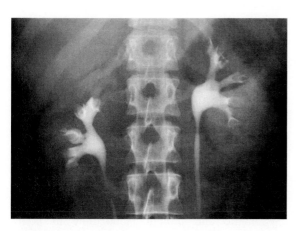

Figure 7-12 Retrograde pyelography with patient in lithotomy position.

none of the dye injected into the ureters is absorbed.

Retrograde pyelography is helpful in radiographically examining the ureters in patients when visualization with IVP (see p. 245) is inadequate or contraindicated. When a ureter is obstructed, IVP will visualize only the ureter proximal to the obstruction. To visualize the distal portion of the ureter, retrograde pyelography is necessary. Also, in patients with unilateral renal disease, the involved kidney and collecting system are not visualized on the IVP because renal function is so poor. As a result, no dye will be filtered into the collecting system by the nonfunctioning kidney. To rule out ureteral obstruction as a cause of the unilateral kidney disease, retrograde pyelography must be done. Tumors, benign strictures, tortuous ureters, stones, scarring, and extrinsic compression may cause ureteral obstruction. Retrograde pyelography provides complete visualization of the ureters so that these disorders can be diagnosed.

Potential complications

Potential complications associated with retrograde pyelography are as follows:

- Urinary tract infection, caused by the invasive nature of this procedure

- Sepsis, caused by bacteria from infected urine seeding the bloodstream
- Perforation of the bladder or ureter, from forceful advancement of the scope
- Hematuria, as a result of urologic instrumentation
- Temporary obstruction to ureteral urine flow Manipulation of the ureters may cause edema, which can result in temporary, partial obstruction to urine flow.

Interfering factor

A factor that interferes with retrograde pyelography is retained barium from previous x-ray studies, which can obscure visualization.

Procedure

The ureteral catheters (see Figure 7-6) are passed into the ureters by means of cystoscopy (see p. 242). Radiopaque contrast material (Hypaque or Renografin) is injected, and radiographic films are taken. The entire ureter and the renal pelvis are demonstrated. As the catheters are withdrawn, more dye is injected, and more radiographic films are taken to visualize the complete outline of the ureter. The procedure is uncomfortable. It is performed by a urologist, usually in the operating room, in approximately 15 minutes.

Nursing implications with rationale
Before

☞ Explain the procedure to the patient. Tell the patient that the cystoscope is inserted into the bladder in the same manner as a Foley catheter. Encourage verbalization of the patient's fears.
- Ensure that written and informed consent for this procedure is obtained by the physician.
- If enemas are ordered to clear the bowel, assist the patient as needed and record the results.
☞ If the procedure will be done with the patient under local anesthesia, instruct the patient to have a liquid breakfast. Encourage fluids to provide urine samples as needed and to prevent urinary stasis in the event that bacteria are introduced during cystoscopy.
☞ If the procedure is performed with the patient

under general anesthesia, follow routine anesthesia precautions. Instruct the patient to remain NPO after midnight. You may give fluids intravenously.

■ Administer the preprocedure medications, as ordered, before the study. In addition to reducing anxiety, the sedatives decrease the spasm of the bladder sphincter, thereby decreasing the patient's discomfort. Deep-breathing exercises also can minimize spasms.

After

☞ Instruct the patient not to stand or walk alone immediately after his or her legs have been removed from the stirrups. The sudden change in circulatory blood volume may cause dizziness and fainting.

■ Assess the patient's ability to void for at least 24 hours after the procedure. Urinary retention may be secondary to edema caused by instrumentation. If urinary retention does occur, an indwelling catheter may need to be inserted.

■ Note the color of the urine. Pink-tinged urine is common. The presence of bright red blood or clots should be reported to the physician.

■ The patient may complain of back pain, bladder spasms, urinary frequency, and burning upon urination. Warm sitz baths and mild analgesics may be ordered and given. Sometimes belladonna and opium suppositories are given to relieve bladder spasms. Warm, moist heat to the lower abdomen may help relieve pain and promote muscle relaxation.

☞ Instruct the patient to increase his or her fluid intake. A dilute urine decreases burning upon urination. Fluids also maintain a constant flow of urine to prevent stasis and the accumulation of bacteria in the bladder.

■ Check and record the patient's vital signs as ordered. Watch for a decrease in blood pressure and an increase in pulse as an indication of hemorrhage. Observe for signs and symptoms of sepsis (e.g., elevated temperature, flush, chills, decreased blood pressure, and increased pulse).

■ Note that antibiotics occasionally are ordered 1 day before and 3 days after the procedure to reduce the incidence of bacteremia that may occur with instrumentation of the urethra and bladder.

Scrotal Nuclear Imaging (Scrotal Scan, Testicular Imaging)

Test type Nuclear scan

Normal values
Symmetric and prompt blood flow to both testicles

Rationale
Scrotal imaging is helpful in the diagnosis of patients with a sudden onset of unilateral testicular swelling and pain. Scrotal imaging can differentiate unilateral testicular torsion from other causes of testicular pain (e.g., acute epididymitis, torsion of the testicular appendage, orchitis, strangulated hernia, testicular hemorrhage).

Testicular torsion is a surgical emergency requiring prompt surgical exploration to salvage the involved testicle. It must be differentiated from other causes of testicular pain in order to provide immediate surgical care. The other causes of painful testicular swelling, however, do not require surgery. Use of radionuclide scrotal imaging enables the surgeon to diagnose testicular torsion. This study usually is performed on an emergency basis and in the nuclear medicine department.

The patient is positioned under the gamma ray detector camera, with the scrotum supported between the abducted thighs. Technetium-99m pertechnetate (Tc-99m pertechnetate) is administered, and a dynamic radionuclide nuclear angiogram is obtained. Static images are obtained immediately. An area of decreased perfusion corresponding to the involved testes indicates a high probability of testicular torsion. If the clinically involved testis is normally perfused or hypervascular, a disease other than testicular torsion (as previously described) exists. In 95% of all cases of testicular torsion, the scrotal image will confirm the diagnosis.

Procedure

The patient is placed on a padded table in the supine position. The patient's legs are abducted, and the testicles are supported with tape or a lead shield. The penis is taped to the lower abdomen. A small IV injection of Tc-99m pertechnetate is administered. Radionuclide imaging is then immediately performed over both testicles. Both dynamic and static images are obtained. This information can be obtained in 30 to 45 minutes after injection of the nuclear material.

Nursing implications with rationale

Before

☞ Explain the procedure to the patient. Tell the patient that no fasting or premedication is required.

■ Assure the patient that he will not be exposed to large amounts of radiation, because only tracer doses of isotope are used.

■ If the patient is a child, encourage the parent(s) to be present.

After

☞ Because only tracer doses of radioisotopes are used, inform the patient that no precautions need to be taken by others against radiation exposure.

■ If the patient is identified as having testicular torsion, prepare the patient for surgery.

Case Study

Torsion of the Testicle

T.P., 22 years old, developed severe, left-sided testicular pain 2 hours before his emergency room visit. He denies any other symptoms. He has no back pain. His physical examination reveals a slightly enlarged and very tender left testicle.

Studies	Results
Routine laboratory studies	Normal
Urinalysis, p. 268	Normal
Testicle ultrasound, p. 266	Diffusely edematous left testicle
Scrotal scan, p. 264	No blood flow to the left testicle

Diagnostic Analysis

The urinalysis failed to indicate blood suggesting a ureteral stone, which can sometimes present as testicular pain. The ultrasound failed to show any localized testicular pathology (e.g., tumor, hematoma [from acute bleeding] or hydrocele). The scrotal scan, however, made the diagnosis of testicular torsion. The blood supply to the testicle was impaired because of the torsion. Emergency scrotal surgery was carried out. The testicle was repositioned, and the blood flow returned. The patient was discharged the following day and remained asymptomatic.

Critical Thinking Questions

1. Scrotal imaging was able to differentiate unilateral testicular torsion from other causes of testicular pain. What are some other possible causes of testicular pain that were ruled out by this procedure?
2. Why was emergency surgery performed based on the scrotal scan results?

Scrotal Ultrasound (Ultrasound of Testes)

Test type Ultrasound

Normal values
Normal size, shape, and configuration of the testicles

Rationale
Ultrasound of the scrotum allows for thorough evaluation of the testicle and other scrotal structures for evidence of suspected pathology. Uses for scrotal ultrasound include:

1. Evaluation of scrotal masses
2. Measurement of testicular size
3. Evaluation of scrotal trauma
4. Evaluation of scrotal pain
5. Evaluation of occult testicular neoplasm
6. Surveillance of patients with prior primary or metastatic contralateral testicular neoplasms
7. Follow-up for testicular infections
8. Location of undescended testicles
9. Ultrasound-guided needle biopsy of a suspected testicle tumor

The scrotum is examined with the real-time ultrasound transducer. The testicle and extratesticular, intrascrotal tissues are examined. The accuracy of scrotal ultrasound is 90% to 95%. Both benign and malignant tumors (primary and metastatic) can be identified with ultrasound. Benign abnormalities (e.g., testicular abscess, orchitis, testicular infarction, and testicular torsion) also can be identified. Extratesticular lesions (e.g., hydrocele, hematocele [blood in the scrotum], and pyocele [pus in the scrotum]) can be identified as well. Scrotal and groin ultrasound also can locate cryptorchid (undescended) testicles.

Procedure
The scrotum is supported by a towel or cradled by the examiner's gloved hand. A greasy, conductive paste is applied to the scrotum before scanning. This paste enhances sound wave transmission and reception. Thorough scanning in the sagittal, transverse, and oblique projections is performed. Very little discomfort is associated with testicular ultrasound, which takes approximately 20 to 30 minutes to complete. The test usually is performed by an ultrasound technologist and interpreted by a physician trained in ultrasonography.

Nursing implications with rationale
Before
☞ Explain the procedure to the patient. Tell the patient that no fasting is required.
After
■ Remove the coupling agent (grease) from the patient's scrotum.

Urea Nitrogen Blood (Blood Urea Nitrogen [BUN], Serum Urea Nitrogen)

Test type Blood

Normal values
Elderly: may be slightly higher than those of adults
Adult: 10-20 mg/dl or 3.6-7.1 mmol/L (SI units)
Child: 5-18 mg/dl
Infant: 5-18 mg/dl
Newborn: 3-12 mg/dl
Umbilical cord: 21-40 mg/dl

Possible critical values >100 mg/dl (indicates serious impairment of renal function)

Rationale
Blood urea nitrogen (BUN) is an indirect and rough measurement of renal function and GFR (if normal liver function exists). It also is a measurement of liver function. It is routinely performed on patients who are undergoing routine laboratory testing. It usually is performed as part of a multiphasic automated testing process.

The BUN measures the amount of urea nitrogen in the blood. Urea is formed in the liver as the end product of protein metabolism and digestion. During ingestion, protein is broken down into amino acids. In the liver, these amino acids are catabolized, and free ammonia is formed. The ammonia molecules are combined to form urea, which then is deposited into the blood and transported to the kidneys for excretion. Therefore, the BUN is directly related to the metabolic function of the liver and the excretory function of the kidney, and it serves as a functional index of these organs. Patients who have elevated BUN levels are said to have *azotemia* or to be *azotemic.*

Nearly all bilateral renal diseases cause an inadequate excretion of urea, which causes the blood concentration to rise above normal. If the disease is unilateral, however, the unaffected kidney can compensate for the diseased kidney, and the BUN may not become elevated. The BUN also increases in conditions other than primary renal disease. *Prerenal azotemia* refers to elevation of the BUN as a result of pathology affecting urea nitrogen before it gets to the kidney. Examples of prerenal azotemia include shock, dehydration, congestive heart failure (CHF), or excessive protein catabolism. *Postrenal azotemia* refers to pathology that affects urea nitrogen after it gets to the kidney. Examples of this include ureteral or urethral obstruction.

Finally, one must be aware that the synthesis of urea depends on the liver. Patients with severe primary liver disease will have a decreased BUN. With combined liver and renal disease (as in hepatorenal syndrome), the BUN can be normal not because renal excretory function is good, but because poor hepatic functioning resulted in decreased formation of urea.

The BUN is interpreted in conjunction with the creatinine test (see p. 237). These tests are referred to as *renal function studies.* The BUN is less accurate than creatinine as an indicator of renal disease.

Interfering factors

Factors that interfere with determining BUN levels include the following:

■ Changes in protein intake, which may affect BUN levels
Low protein diets will *decrease* BUN if caloric intake is maintained with carbohydrates. High

protein diets or alimentary tube feedings are associated with *elevated* BUN levels.
■ Muscle mass
Women and children tend to have *lower* BUN levels than men.
■ Hydration status
Overhydrated patients tend to dilute the BUN and have *decreased* levels. Dehydrated patients tend to concentrate BUN and have *increased* levels.

Procedure
One red-top tube of blood is drawn from a peripheral vein and sent to the chemistry laboratory.

Nursing implications with rationale
Before
☞ Explain the procedure to the patient. Tell the patient that no fasting is needed.
After
■ Apply pressure or a pressure dressing to the venipuncture site to prevent further bleeding. Observe the site for bleeding.

Urethral Pressure Profile (UPP, Urethral Pressure Measurements)

Test type Manometric

Normal values

Maximal Urethral Pressures in Normal Patients (cm H₂O):		
Age	*Male*	*Female*
>64 years	35-105	35-75
45-64 years	40-123	40-100
25-44 years	35-113	31-115
<25 years	37-126	55-103

Rationale
Urethral pressure profile (UPP) often is a part of cystometry (see p. 241). It is used to document reduced urethral pressures in incontinent patients (females with stress incontinence or males after prostatectomy). It also is used to indicate the degree of compression applied to the urethra from

an abnormally enlarged prostate (which will increase UPP).

The UPP indicates the intraluminal pressure along the length of the urethra with the bladder at rest. Indications for this test include the following:

1. Assessment of prostatic obstruction
2. Assessment of stress incontinence in females
3. Assessment of postprostatectomy sequelae of incontinence
4. Assessment of the adequacy of external sphincterotomy
5. Analysis of the effects of drugs on the urethra
6. Analysis of the effects of stimulation on urethral flow
7. Assessment of the adequacy of implanted artificial urethral sphincter devices

Procedure

No fasting or sedation is required. A catheter is passed into the bladder and withdrawn slowly through the urethra. Fluids (or gas) are instilled through the catheter, which is withdrawn while the pressures along the urethral wall are obtained. A constant infusion of the fluids or gas is maintained by a motorized syringe pump. The catheter is removed, and the test is completed in less than 15 minutes.

This test is slightly more uncomfortable than urethral catheterization. It usually is performed by a urologist during an office visit.

Contraindications

UPP is contraindicated for patients with urinary tract infections because catheterization may induce bacteremia.

Nursing implications with rationale

Before
- ☞ Explain the procedure to the patient. Many patients are embarrassed by this procedure. Assure them that they will be draped to ensure privacy.
- ☞ Inform the patient that no fasting or sedation is necessary.

After
- ▪ Suggest a warm tub bath or a sitz bath, which may be comforting to the patient.

Urinalysis (UA)

Test type Urine

Normal values

Appearance: clear
Color: amber yellow
Odor: aromatic
pH: 4.6-8.0 (average 6.0)
Protein:
   0 to 8 mg/dl
   50-80 mg/day (at rest)
   <250 mg/day (exercise)
Specific gravity:
   Elderly: values decrease with age
   Adult: 1.005-1.030 (usually 1.010-1.025)
   Newborn: 1.001-1.020
Leukocyte esterase: negative
Nitrites: negative
Ketones: negative
Crystals: negative
Casts: none present
Glucose (see urine glucose discussion, p. 313)
   Fresh specimen: negative
   24-hour specimen: <0.5 g/day or <2.78 mmol/day (SI units)
WBCs: 0-4 per low-power field
WBC casts: none
RBCs: up to 2
RBC casts: none

Rationale

A total urinalysis (UA) involves multiple routine tests on a urine specimen. This specimen is not necessarily a clean-catch specimen. However, if urinary tract infection is suspected, a midstream, clean-catch specimen often is obtained. This urine then is split into two portions. One is sent for UA, and the other is held in the laboratory refrigerator and cultured if the UA indicates infection. A UA routinely includes remarks about the color, appearance, and odor of the urine. The pH is determined. The urine is tested for the presence of proteins, glucose, ketones, blood, and leukocyte esterase. The urine is examined microscopically for RBCs, WBCs, casts, crystals, and bacteria.

Examination of the urine sediment provides a significant amount of information about the urinary system. The test is done on centrifuged urinary sediment. Because of the many different methods of preparing the sediment for microscopic review, normal values may vary significantly among laboratories. Reference ranges have been provided in order to recognize marked abnormalities.

Appearance and color

Urine appearance and color are noted as part of routine UA. The appearance of a normal urine specimen should be clear. Cloudy urine may be caused by the presence of pus, RBCs, or bacteria; however, normal urine also may be cloudy because of ingestion of certain foods (e.g., large amounts of fat, ureates, or phosphates). The color of urine ranges from pale yellow to amber because of the pigment, *urochrome*. The color indicates the concentration of the urine and varies with specific gravity. Dilute urine is straw-colored, and concentrated urine is deep amber.

Abnormally colored urine may result from a pathologic condition or the ingestion of certain foods or medicines. For example, bleeding from the kidney produces dark-red urine, whereas bleeding from the lower urinary tract produces bright-red urine. Dark-yellow urine may indicate the presence of urobilinogen or bilirubin. *Pseudomonas* organisms may produce green urine. Ingesting beets may cause red urine, and ingesting rhubarb may cause brown urine. Many frequently used drugs also may affect urine color (Table 7-1).

Odor

Determination of urine odor is a part of routine UA. The aromatic odor of fresh, normal urine is

---

TABLE 7-1 Commonly Used Drugs that Can Affect Urine Color

Generic and Brand Names	Drug Classification	Urine Color
Cascara sagrada	Stimulant laxative	Red in alkaline urine; yellow-brown in acid urine
Chloroquine (Aralen)	Antimalarial	Rusty yellow or brown
Docusate calcium (Doxidan, Surfak)	Laxative	Pink to red to red-brown
Iron preparations (Ferotran, Imferon)	Hematinic	Dark brown or black on standing
Levodopa	Antiparkinsonian	Dark brown on standing
Methylene blue (Urolene Blue)	Antimethemoglobinemic	Blue-green
Nitrofurantoin (Macrodantin, Nitrodan)	Antibacterial	Brown
Phenazopyridine (Pyridium)	Urinary tract analgesic	Orange to red
Phenolphthalein (Ex-Lax)	Contact laxative	Red or purplish pink in alkaline urine
Phenothiazines (e.g., prochlorperazine [Compazine])	Antipsychotic, neuroleptic, antiemetic	Red-brown
Phenytoin (Dilantin)	Anticonvulsant	Pink, red, red-brown
Riboflavin (vitamin B_2)	Vitamin	Intense yellow
Rifampin	Antibiotic	Red-orange
Sulfasalazine (Azulfidine)	Antibacterial	Orange-yellow in alkaline urine
Triamterene (Dyrenium)	Diuretic	Pale blue fluorescence

caused by the presence of volatile acids. Urine of patients with diabetic ketoacidosis has the strong, sweet smell of acetone. In patients with a urinary tract infection, the urine may have a very foul odor. Patients with a fecal odor to their urine may have an enterovesical fistula.

pH

The pH analysis of a freshly voided urine specimen indicates the acid-base balance of the patient. An alkaline pH is obtained in a patient with alkalemia. Also, bacteria, urinary tract infection, or a diet high in citrus fruits or vegetables may cause an increased urine pH. Certain medications (e.g., streptomycin, neomycin, kanamycin) are effective in treating urinary tract infections when the urine is alkaline. Acidic urine generally is obtained in patients with acidemia, which can result from metabolic or respiratory acidosis, starvation, dehydration, or a diet high in meat products or cranberries.

The urine pH is useful in identifying crystals in the urine and determining the predisposition to form a given type of stone. Acidic urine is associated with xanthine, cystine, uric acid, and calcium oxalate stones. To treat or prevent these injurious calculi, urine should be kept alkaline. Alkaline urine is associated with calcium carbonate, calcium phosphate, and magnesium phosphate stones. To prevent or treat these stones, urine should be kept acidic.

Protein

Evaluation of protein is a sensitive indicator of kidney function. Protein normally is not present in the urine because the spaces in the normal glomerular membrane are too small to allow its passage. If the glomerular membrane is injured or diseased, as in glomerulonephritis, the spaces become much larger, and protein seeps into the filtrate and then into the urine. If this persists at a significant rate, the patient can become hypoproteinemic because of the severe protein loss through the kidneys. This decreases the normal capillary oncotic pressure that holds fluid within the vasculature and causes severe interstitial edema. The combination of proteinuria and edema is known as the *nephrotic syndrome*.

Proteinuria is probably the most important indicator of renal disease. The urine of all pregnant women is routinely checked for proteinuria, which can be an indicator of preeclampsia. In addition to screening for nephrotic syndrome, urinary protein also screens for complications of the following diseases: diabetes mellitus, glomerulonephritis, amyloidosis, and multiple melanoma.

Glucose

See discussion on p. 313.

Specific gravity

The specific gravity is a measure of the concentration of particles (including wastes and electrolytes) in the urine. A high specific gravity indicates a concentrated urine; a low specific gravity indicates dilute urine. *Specific gravity* refers to the weight of the urine compared with distilled water (which has a specific gravity of 1.000). It is the particles in the urine that give the urine its weight or specific gravity.

The specific gravity is used to evaluate the concentrating and excretory power of the kidney. Renal disease tends to diminish the concentrating capability of the kidney. As a result, chronic renal diseases are associated with a low specific gravity. The specific gravity must be interpreted in light of the presence or absence of glycosuria and proteinuria. The specific gravity also is a measurement of the hydration status of the patient. An overhydrated patient will have a more dilute urine with a lower specific gravity. The specific gravity of the urine in a dehydrated patient can be expected to be abnormally high. The measurement of urine specific gravity is easier and more convenient than the measurement of osmolality (see p. 323). The specific gravity correlates roughly with osmolality. Knowledge of the specific gravity is needed for interpreting the results of most parts of the urinalysis. Specific gravity usually is evaluated with a refractometer or dipstick.

Leukocyte esterase (WBC esterase)

Leukocyte (WBC) esterase is a screening test used to detect leukocytes in the urine. When positive, this test indicates a urinary tract infection. This examination employs chemical testing with a leukocyte esterase dipstick; a shade of purple is considered positive. Some laboratories have established screening protocols in which a microscopic examination (see p. 273) is performed only if a leukocyte esterase test is positive.

Nitrites

Like the leukocyte esterase, the nitrite test is a screening test for the identification of urinary tract infections. This test is based on the principle that many bacteria produce an enzyme called *reductase,* which can reduce urinary nitrates to nitrites. Chemical testing is done with a dipstick containing a reagent that reacts with nitrites to produce a pink color, thereby indirectly suggesting the presence of bacteria. A positive test result would indicate the need for a urine culture. Nitrite screening enhances the sensitivity of the leukocyte esterase test to detect urinary tract infections.

Ketones

Ketones normally are not present in the urine; however, a patient with poorly controlled diabetes who is hyperglycemic may have massive fatty acid catabolism. The purpose of this catabolism is to provide an energy source when glucose cannot be transferred into the cell because of an insufficiency of insulin. Ketones (beta-hydroxybutyric acid, acetoacetic acid, and acetone) are the end products of this fatty acid breakdown. As with glucose, ketones spill over into the urine when the blood levels of patients with diabetes are elevated. The excess production of ketones in the urine usually is associated with poorly controlled diabetes. This test for ketonuria also is important in evaluating ketoacidosis associated with alcoholism, fasting, starvation, high-protein diets, and isopropanol ingestion. Ketonuria may occur with acute febrile illnesses, especially in infants and children.

Crystals

Crystals found in urinary sediment on microscopic examination indicate that renal stone formulation is imminent, if not already present. Urea crystals occur in patients with high serum uric acid levels (gout). Phosphate and calcium oxalate crystals occur in the urine of patients with parathyroid abnormalities or malabsorption states. The type of crystal found varies with the disease and the pH of the urine (see previous discussion on urinary pH, p. 270).

Casts

Casts are clumps of materials or cells. They are formed in the renal distal and collecting tubules where the material is maximally concentrated. These amorphous clumps of material and cells have the shape of the tubule, thus the term *cast.* Casts are most usually associated with some degree of proteinuria and stasis within the renal tubules. There are two kinds of casts: hyaline and cellular. *Hyaline casts* are conglomerations of protein and indicate proteinuria. A few hyaline casts are normally found, especially after strenuous exercise. *Cellular casts* are conglomerations of degenerated cells. The following are types of cellular casts:

Granular casts. These result from the disintegration of cellular material into granular particles within a WBC or epithelial cell cast. Granular casts are found after exercise and in patients with various renal diseases. The basic etiology is the same as that of their cellular component.

Fatty casts. In some diseases, the epithelial cells are shed into the renal tubule. As the cell degenerates, fatty deposits within the cell coalesce and become incorporated with protein into fatty casts. These casts are all associated with the nephrotic syndrome or nephrosis.

Waxy casts. These probably represent further degeneration of granular casts. They occur when urine flow through the renal tubule is diminished, giving the time for granular casts to degenerate. Waxy casts are found especially in patients with chronic renal diseases and are associated with chronic renal failure. They also occur in patients with diabetic nephropathy, malignant hypertension, and glomerulonephritis.

Epithelial cells and casts. Epithelial cells can enter the urine at any point during urinary excretion. The presence of occasional epithelial cells is not remarkable. Large numbers, however, are abnormal and can conglomerate into *tubular (epi-*

thelial) casts. These are most suggestive of glomerulonephritis.

WBCs and casts. Normally, few WBCs are found in the urine sediment on microscopic examination. The presence of five or more WBCs in the urine indicates a urinary tract infection (UTI) involving the bladder, kidney, or both. A clean-catch urine culture should be done for further evaluation. WBC casts are most frequently found in patients with infections within the kidney (e.g., acute pyelonephritis).

RBCs and casts. Any disruption in the blood-urine barrier, whether at the glomerular, tubular, or bladder level, will cause RBCs to enter the urine. The bleeding can be microscopic or gross. RBC casts suggest glomerulonephritis. RBC casts also are seen in patients with acute necrosis, pyelonephritis, renal trauma, or renal tumor.

Interfering factors

Factors that interfere with UA include the following:

- Certain foods affect urine color.
  Carrots may cause a dark-yellow color. Beets may cause a red-colored urine. Rhubarb may cause a red or brown discoloration.
- Some foods (e.g., asparagus) produce characteristic urine odors.
- The urine pH becomes alkaline on standing because of urea-splitting bacteria, whose actions produce ammonia.
- Dietary factors affect urine pH.
  An alkaline urine is observed in people who eat large quantities of citrus fruits, dairy products, and vegetables. Acidic urine is observed with a diet high in meat and certain foods (e.g., cranberries).
- Radiopaque contrast media received within the last 3 days may cause false-positive results for proteinuria.
- Urine contaminated with vaginal secretions may cause proteinuria.
- False-positive leukocyte esterase results may occur in specimens contaminated with vaginal secretions (e.g., heavy menstrual discharge, *Trichomonas* infection, and parasites).

- Special diets (e.g., carbohydrate-free, high-protein, high-fat) may cause ketonuria.
- Vaginal discharge may contaminate the urine specimen and factitiously cause WBCs in the urine.
- Traumatic urethral catheterization may cause RBCs in the urine.

Procedure

A reliable UA depends on properly collecting the urine specimen and immediately performing the analysis. The first-voided morning specimen is the ideal specimen for analysis because of its concentration and characteristic acidity. However, a fresh urine specimen collected at any other time usually is reliable. For a routine urinalysis, no special preparation of the patient is needed. The patient voids into a clean bedpan, urinal, or preferably, a urine container. This specimen cannot be used for a culture and sensitivity. If a culture and sensitivity test (see p. 273) also is required, a "clean-catch," or midstream, specimen is collected.

Specimens from infants and young children can be collected in a disposable bag called a U-*bag*. This bag has an adhesive backing around the opening to attach to the child. Composite urine specimens are collected over a period of 2 to 24 hours. Composite specimens are examined for specific components (e.g., electrolytes, catecholamines, and creatinine). To collect a composite specimen, the patient is instructed to void and discard the urine. The test period then begins. All subsequent urine is saved in a container for the designated time. At the end of this period, the patient urinates and adds this urine to the collection container.

The pH and the presence of protein, glucose, ketones, or blood (hemoglobin) can be detected easily by using reagent dipsticks or other multiple test strips for UA. The reagent strip is completely immersed in the well-mixed urine and removed immediately to avoid dissolving the reagents. The strip is held in a horizontal position to prevent possible mixing of the chemical reagents and then is compared with the test chart at the time specified.

For microscopic examination, an aliquot (approximately 10 ml) of the urine specimen is placed in a test tube and centrifuged. The sediment is resuspended in the last few drops of urine by vigorous agitation of the tube. A drop of the sediment then is examined microscopically.

Nursing implications with rationale

Before
- Explain the purpose and specific method of urine collection to the patient. Give the patient the proper specimen jars and cleansing agents, if necessary. The perianal area should be washed if it is soiled with feces.
- If possible, obtain the first-voided specimen of the day, because it is usually more concentrated than other specimens.

During
- If the specimen cannot be tested immediately, cover and refrigerate it. Refrigeration may reduce the bacterial cell proliferation and retard deterioration of casts and cells. The pH of uncovered specimens becomes alkaline, because CO_2 diffuses into the air.
- If the patient is menstruating, indicate that on the laboratory requisition slip. Hematuria is then discounted.
- When using dipsticks or tablets, read the directions on the bottle or package insert and follow the directions precisely. The color reaction must be compared with the manufacturer's color chart at the *exact* time specified. After removing the dipstick from the bottle, close the bottle tightly to prevent the remaining dipstick from absorbing moisture and altering results.
- Check the expiration date on the bottle before use.
- Inform the patient that, because of contamination, toilet paper or feces should not be placed in the container.

After
- Transport the urine specimen to the laboratory promptly.
- Casts will break up as urine is allowed to sit. Urine examinations for casts should be performed with fresh specimens.

Urine Culture and Sensitivity (C&S)

Test type Urine

Normal values
Negative: fewer than 10,000 bacteria/ml of urine
Positive: greater than 100,000 bacteria/ml of urine

Rationale
Urine cultures and sensitivities are obtained to determine the presence of pathogenic bacteria in patients with suspected UTIs. This test is used to diagnose UTIs in patients who complain of dysuria, frequency, or urgency. It also is indicated when patients have a fever of unknown origin or when their UA indicates infection. All cultures should be performed before antibiotic therapy is initiated; otherwise, the antibiotic may interrupt the growth of the organism in the laboratory. Most organisms require approximately 24 hours to grow in the laboratory, and a preliminary report can be given at that time. Occasionally, 48 to 72 hours are required for growth and identification of the organism. Cultures may be repeated after appropriate antibiotic therapy to assess for complete resolution of the infection (especially in UTIs).

To reduce costs, some institutions require urine cultures only if the UA suggests a possible infection (e.g., increased number of WBCs, bacteria, high pH, positive leukocyte esterase). In these institutions, urine is collected and divided. Half the sample is sent for UA, and half is held in the laboratory refrigerator and evaluated only if the UA indicates a possible infection.

Assessment of the sensitivity of any bacteria growing within the urine to various antibiotics is an important part of any routine culture. This assessment aids the physician in prescribing the correct antibiotic therapy. Antibiotics that are the safest, least expensive, and most effective treatment for the specific bacteria present are prescribed.

Interfering factor
A factor that interferes with urine C&S is contamination of the urine with stool, vaginal secretions,

or infected hands or clothing. Such contamination will cause false-positive results.

Procedure

A clean-catch or midstream urine collection is required for C&S testing. This procedure requires meticulous cleansing of the perineal area or penis with an iodine preparation to reduce contamination of the specimen by external organisms. The cleansing agent then must be completely removed, or it will contaminate the urine specimen. The midstream collection is obtained by having the patient begin to urinate into a bedpan, urinal, or toilet, and then stop. (This washes the urine out of the distal urethra.) A sterile urine container then is correctly positioned, and the patient voids 3 to 4 ounces of urine into the container. The container is capped. The patient finishes voiding. For patients unable to void, urinary catheterization may be needed; however, this procedure is not commonly performed because of the risk of introducing infectious organisms and because of patient discomfort.

In patients with an *indwelling urinary catheter,* a specimen can be obtained by attaching a small-gauge needle to a syringe and aseptically inserting the needle into the catheter at a point distal to the sleeve leading to the balloon. Urine is aspirated and placed into the container. The catheter tubing distal to the puncture site usually needs to be clamped for 15 to 30 minutes before the aspiration of urine to allow urine to fill the tubing. After the specimen is withdrawn, the clamp is removed.

Suprapubic aspiration is a safe method of collecting urine in neonates and infants. For this technique, the abdomen is prepared with an antiseptic, and a 25-gauge needle (attached to a 5-ml syringe) is inserted into the suprapubic area, 1 inch above the symphysis pubis. Urine is aspirated into the syringe and transferred to a sterile urine container.

For patients with a *urinary diversion* (e.g., an ileal conduit), catheterization should be done through the stoma. Urine should not be collected from the ostomy pouch. The urine from a urinary diversion rarely is sterile. Bacteria is expected. Overgrowth of just one type of bacteria may indicate upper UTI.

Nursing implications with rationale

Before

- ☞ Explain to the patient the procedure for collecting a clean-catch (midstream) urine specimen.
- ■ Hold antibiotics until after the urine specimen has been collected.
- ■ Provide the patient with the necessary supplies for the collection.
- ☞ Remind the patient that, to avoid contamination, urine should not be taken from a bedpan or a jar from home for C&S testing.

After

- ■ Transport the specimen to the laboratory within 30 minutes. If this is not possible, the specimen may be refrigerated up to 2 hours. Cultures for cytomegalovirus, however, will be destroyed by refrigeration.
- ■ Notify the physician of any positive results so that appropriate antibiotic therapy can be initiated.

Urine Flow Studies (Uroflowmetry, Urodynamic Studies)

Test type Urodynamic

Normal values

Depends on the patient's age, gender, and volume voided

Age (years)	Minimum Volume (ml)	Male (ml/sec)	Female (ml/sec)
66-80	200	>9	>10
46-65	200	>12	>15
14-45	200	>21	>18
4-13	100	>10-12	>10-15

Rationale

Uroflowmetry is the simplest of the urodynamic techniques, because it is noninvasive and requires uncomplicated and relatively inexpensive equipment. This study measures the volume of urine expelled from the bladder per second, and it is indicated to investigate dysfunctional voiding or suspicious outflow tract obstruction. It also is done before and after any procedure designed to modify the function of the urologic outflow tract.

It is used to monitor micturition for decisions concerning timing and adequacy of treatment. Together with clinical observation, this test provides valuable information on the severity of outflow obstruction, the likelihood of urinary retention, and the state of compensation or decompensation of the detrusor muscle.

The urine flow depends greatly on the volume of urine voided. The flow rates are highest and most predictable when the urine volume ranges from 200 to 400 ml. When the bladder contains more than 400 ml of urine, the efficiency of the bladder muscle is greatly decreased. Nomograms of maximal flow versus voided volume may be used for accurate test result interpretation, taking into account the patient's gender and age. If the flow rates are abnormally low, the test should be repeated to check for accuracy. This test often is performed in conjunction with cystometry (see p. 241).

Procedure

This test should be performed when the patient has a normal desire to void and in conditions suitable for privacy. The bladder should be adequately full. If urine samples are needed for another test, there should be a separate voiding. All the patient essentially has to do is urinate into the flowmeter. Several different types of flowmeters are available.

Nursing implications with rationale

Before

- Explain the procedure to the patient. Ensure that the patient knows how to void into the urine flowmeter. Ensure privacy during voiding.
- Determine the number of flow rates that are needed.
- Inform the patient that no discomfort is associated with this test.
- If a series of flow rates are needed, explain this procedure to the patient.

After

- Record the position of the patient, the method of filling the bladder, and whether this study was part of another evaluation. Uroflowmetry is usually the first of the urodynamic investigations performed. In many instances, urine flow studies alone allow for a confident urodynamic diagnosis.

Case Study

Urinary Obstruction

Mr. M.P., 57 years old, noted urinary hesitancy and a decrease in the force of his urinary stream for several months. Both had progressively become worse. His physical examination was essentially negative except for an enlarged prostate, which was bulky and soft.

Studies	Results
Routine laboratory studies	WNL
IVP, p. 245	Mild indentation of the interior aspect of the bladder, indicating an enlarged prostate
Uroflowmetry with total voided flow of 225 ml, p. 274	8 ml/sec (normal: >12 ml/sec)
Cystometry, p. 241	Resting bladder pressure: 35 cm H_2O (normal: <40 cm H_2O)
	Peak bladder pressure: 50 cm H_2O (normal: 40-90 cm H_2O)
Electromyography of the pelvic sphincter muscle, p. 250	Normal resting bladder with a positive tonus limb

Continued

Urinary Obstruction—cont'd

Cystoscopy, p. 242
PAP, p. 230
PSA, p. 252
Prostate ultrasound, p. 251

BPH
1.0 U/L (normal: 0.11-0.60 U/L)
6 ng/ml (normal: <4 ng/ml)
Diffusely enlarged prostate. No localized
tumor

Diagnostic Analysis

Because of the patient's symptoms, bladder outlet obstruction was highly suspected. Physical examination indicated an enlarged prostate. IVP studies corroborated that finding. The reduced urine flow rate indicated an obstruction distal to the urinary bladder. Because the patient was found to have a normal total voided volume, one could not say that the reduced flow rate was the result of an inadequately distended bladder. Rather, the bladder was appropriately distended, yet the flow rate was decreased. This indicated outlet obstruction. The cystogram indicated that the bladder was capable of mounting an effective pressure and was not an atonic bladder compatible with neurologic disease. The tonus limb again indicated the bladder was able to contract. The peak bladder pressure of 50 cm H_2O was normal, again indicating appropriate muscular function of the bladder. Based on these studies, the patient was diagnosed with a urinary outlet obstruction. The PAP and PSA indicated BPH. The ultrasound supported that diagnosis. Cystoscopy documented that finding, and the patient was appropriately treated by transurethral prostatectomy (TURP). This patient did well postoperatively and had no major problems.

Critical Thinking Questions

1. Does BPH predispose this patient to cancer?
2. Why are patients with BPH at increased risk for UTIs?
3. What would you expect the patient's PSA level to be after surgery?

Vanillylmandelic Acid and Catecholamines (VMA and Epinephrine, Norepinephrine, Metanephrine, Normetanephrine, Dopamine)

Test type Urine

Normal values
VMA
Adult/elderly: 2-7 mg/24 hr or 10-35 mmol/24 hr
(SI units)

Adolescent: 1-5 mg/24 hr
Child: 1-3 mg/24 hr
Infant: <2.0 mg/24 hr
Newborn: <1.0 mg/24 hr
Catecholamines
Epinephrine
Adult/elderly: 0.5-20.0 µg/24 hr or
<275 nmol/24 hr (SI units)
Children:
7-10 years: 0.5-14.0 µg/24 hr
4-7 years: 0.2-10.0 µg/24 hr
2-4 years: 0.0-6.0 µg/24 hr
1-2 years: 0-3.5 µg/24 hr
0-1 year: 0-2.5 µg/24 hr

Norepinephrine
Adult/elderly: 15-80 μg/24 hr
Children:
    7-10 years: 13-65 μg/24 hr
    4-7 years: 8-45 μg/24 hr
    2-4 years: 4-29 μg/24 hr
    1-2 years: 0-17 μg/24 hr
    0-1 year: 0-10 μg/24 hr
Dopamine
Adult/elderly: 65-400 μg/24 hr
Children:
    >4 years: 65-400 μg/24 hr
    2-4 years: 40-260 μg/24 hr
    1-2 years: 10-140 μg/24 hr
    0-1 year: 0-85 μg/24 hr
Metanephrine
    24-96 μg/24 hr
Normetanephrine
    75-375 μg/24 hr

Rationale

This 24-hour urine test for vanillylmandelic acid (VMA) and catecholamines is performed primarily to diagnose hypertension secondary to pheochromocytoma. This test also is used to detect the presence of neuroblastomas and other rare adrenal tumors.

A pheochromocytoma is a tumor of the chromaffin cells within the adrenal medulla. It frequently secretes abnormally high levels of epinephrine and norepinephrine. These hormones cause episodic or persistent severe hypertension by causing peripheral arterial vasoconstriction. Dopamine is the precursor of epinephrine and norepinephrine. Metanephrine and normetanephrine are catabolic products of epinephrine and norepinephrine, respectively. VMA (or 3-methoxy-4-hydroxymandelic acid) is the product of catabolism of both metanephrine and normetanephrine. In patients with pheochromocytoma, one or all of these substances will be present in excessive quantities in a 24-hour urine collection. These hormones may be measured singularly in the urine, but the collective metabolic end product, VMA, is more easily detected because VMA concentration is much higher than any one catecholamine component.

A 24-hour urine test is preferable to a blood test because catecholamine secretion from the tumor may be episodic and could be potentially missed at any one time during the day. The 24-hour urine specimen reflects catecholamine production over an entire day. It is best to perform testing when the symptoms (e.g., hypertension) of the potential adrenal tumor are significant because catecholamine production is greatest at that time and, therefore, is more easily identified.

Interfering factors

Factors that interfere with determining VMA and catecholamine levels include the following:

- Certain foods
  Tea, coffee, cocoa, vanilla, chocolate, cider vinegar, soda, and licorice are examples of foods that may cause *increased* levels of VMA.
- Vigorous exercise, stress, and starvation, which may cause *increased* VMA levels
- Caffeine and levodopa, which may cause *increased* VMA or catecholamine levels

Procedure

For 2 or 3 days before the 24-hour urine collection and throughout the collection period, the patient is placed on a VMA-restricted diet. The food restrictions generally include coffee, tea, bananas, chocolate, cocoa, licorice, citrus fruit, all foods and fluids containing vanilla, and aspirin. Dietary restrictions may vary among different laboratories. No special diet is needed for catecholamine testing. Antihypertensive medications, and sometimes all medications, are also prohibited during this period and possibly even longer (depending on the laboratory). A 24-hour urine specimen is collected in a container into which a preservative has been added.

Nursing implications with rationale

Before
- Explain the procedure for collecting a 24-hour urine sample. Show the patient where to store the urine specimen. The 24-hour urine specimen for VMA requires a preservative.
- Inform the patient that no fasting is necessary.

☞ Instruct the patient regarding medication restrictions.

☞ Instruct the patient to follow a VMA-restricted diet for 2 or 3 days before and throughout the 24-hour collection period. Instruct the patient to avoid coffee, tea, bananas, chocolate, cocoa, licorice, citrus fruits, all foods and fluids containing vanilla, and aspirin. Check with the laboratory for specific restrictions.

☞ Inform the patient that excessive physical exercise and emotion can alter catecholamine test results by causing an increased secretion of epinephrine and norepinephrine. Therefore, identify and minimize factors contributing to patient stress and anxiety.

During

☞ Instruct the patient to begin the 24-hour urine collection after discarding the first morning specimen. This is the start time of the 24-hour collection.

☞ Collect all urine voided over the next 24 hours into a container into which a boric acid preservative has been added.

☞ Instruct the patient to void before defecating so that the urine is not contaminated by feces.

☞ Remind the patient not to put toilet paper in the collection container.

☞ Keep the urine specimen on ice or refrigerated during the 24 hours.

☞ Collect the last specimen as close as possible to the end of the 24 hours.

After

■ Transport the urine specimen promptly to the laboratory.

☞ After the 24-hour collection for VMA is completed, instruct the patient that the food and drug restrictions can be discontinued.

REVIEW QUESTIONS AND ANSWERS

1. **Question:** Your patient returns from her doctor's appointment and discusses her scheduled workup for hypertension with you. She asks why she needs to avoid ingesting licorice before several tests. What would you tell her?

Answer: Licorice has an aldosterone-like effect, which increases sodium reabsorption in the kidney and raises blood pressure. Licorice ingestion would affect renin and aldosterone studies.

2. **Question:** Today, your father had his annual physical examination, which included a digital rectal examination. He was annoyed that his doctor wanted a blood test for PAP, but told him he had to wait and get it drawn on another day. Do you have any explanation for this inconvenience?

Answer: Yes. The rectal examination causes prostate manipulation, which would elevate PAP levels. At least 24 hours must pass before this blood test can be drawn.

3. **Question:** Your patient had a cystoscopy for evaluation of hematuria. Upon return to the unit, you encourage him to drink fluids. He reports burning with urination, however, and does not want to drink fluids. How will you handle this problem?

Answer: Patient education is essential in this situation. Instruct the patient to increase fluids because a dilute urine will decrease burning with urination. Also instruct him that fluids are needed to maintain a constant flow of urine to prevent stasis and the accumulation of bacteria in the bladder.

4. **Question:** A healthy, 28-year-old construction worker was just admitted to the emergency room for evaluation following a fall. Part of his laboratory results indicate an increased BUN. Is renal failure a possibility?

Answer: Probably not. Given his age and type of work, dehydration must be considered. Levels of BUN are increased with dehydration and decreased with overhydration.

5. **Question:** IVP is ordered for a trauma patient whose vital signs are stable. After the injection of the iodinated dye, the patient becomes flushed, hypotensive, and develops severe bronchospasms. What should be done?

Answer: This patient is having an anaphylactic reaction to the dye. You should reassure the patient and do the following:

a. Place the patient in the Trendelenburg position.

b. Increase the IV rate to treat the hypotension.

c. Administer oxygen by mask or nasal cannula.

d. Notify the physician. The physician will most probably order epinephrine, 0.3 ml subcutaneously (SQ), methylprednisolone sodium succinate (Solu-Medrol), 2 g IV, and diphenhydramine, 25 mg IV or intramuscularly (IM).

e. Draw blood to determine hemoglobin and hematocrit values to ascertain whether the hypotension is related to unrecognized, trauma-induced intraabdominal bleeding.

f. The patient may require endotracheal intubation for respiratory support. Dopamine may be required for circulatory support.

6. **Question:** Your patient is scheduled for IVP. His creatinine level is 2.4 mg/dl, and his BUN level is 49 mg/dl. Will the kidneys be visualized by IVP?

   Answer: Yes. Even with the decreased renal function, the kidneys will be visualized. More time, however, will be required for visualization. (e.g., instead of visualizing the kidney on a 5-minute film, you may not see anything for 15 minutes.)

7. **Question:** Your patient has had a renal biopsy. Shortly afterward, he develops severe back and leg pain on the side from which the biopsy specimen was obtained. He begins to have nausea and vomiting. His blood pressure drops from 140/100 mm Hg to 100/68 mm Hg. What should be done for this patient?

   Answer: An expanding retroperitoneal hematoma secondary to inadvertent puncture of a blood vessel is probably causing the back and leg pain and also the hypotension. The nausea and vomiting is a result of the paralytic ileus that usually occurs with retroperitoneal hematoma. You should reassure the patient and do the following:

   a. Monitor the vital signs every 15 minutes and notify the physician. Ask the physician to examine the patient.

b. Obtain IV access, because the patient will require fluid volume replacement.

c. Draw blood for a hemoglobin and hematocrit determination to document the bleeding.

d. Type and cross-match the patient for several units of blood, as ordered. Transfusion may become necessary.

e. Draw blood for prothrombin and partial thromboplastin times to determine whether the patient has the clotting ability to plug the puncture hole in the vessel.

f. Keep the patient NPO; surgical repair may be required if the hypotension persists. The physician will probably order a radiographic film of the abdomen because these clinical symptoms also could occur with inadvertent puncture of the bowel. In that case, free air may be seen on the radiographic film.

8. **Question:** What precautions are necessary before performing CT scanning of the kidneys in a patient who is allergic to iodinated dyes?

   Answer: For CT scanning of the kidney, the patient frequently is injected with an iodinated contrast material to aid in renal visualization. The physician should be notified of the patient's allergy. If the patient requires CT scanning with iodinated contrast material, he or she will need a diphenhydramine-prednisone preparation. CT scanning without contrast material can be done without any precautions.

9. **Question:** Your patient returns to the unit after having had transcystoscopic biopsy specimen removal. A Foley catheter is in place. On his return, you note gross hematuria and blood clots. Two hours later you notice that the patient has not produced any urine. He begins to complain of lower abdominal midline pain and is mildly hypotensive. What are the appropriate interventions for this patient?

   Answer: The hematuria and blood clots indicate postprocedure bleeding. The clots should have concerned you because urine is a mild anticoagulant and clotting occurs only with brisk urinary bleeding. A clot probably has occluded the catheter and caused acute urinary retention, resulting in the lower abdominal pain. You should reassure the patient and do the following:

a. Flush the Foley catheter with a premeasured amount of sterile saline solution, using sterile technique.

b. After patency is established, monitor the urine output.

c. Notify the physician.

d. Increase the rate of the IV infusion, as ordered. This is done to increase urine output, which will flush out the bladder. Maintain accurate intake and output.

e. Begin Foley irrigation, as ordered, to attempt to clear the bladder of clots.

f. Draw blood for a hemoglobin and hematocrit determination to measure the severity of the blood loss.

g. Draw, type, and cross-match blood, as ordered, in the event that a transfusion is required. Surgery or recystoscopy may be necessary to terminate the bleeding.

10. **Question:** Your patient is scheduled to receive a nephrotoxic drug. She has no suspected renal disease or injury, yet her creatinine clearance is only 52 ml/minute. What should be done?

Answer: Do not administer the drug. In a young adult who has no suspected renal disease or injury, the most likely cause of the abnormal creatinine clearance is error in the collection (e.g., not all of the urine samples were collected). The creatinine clearance test should be repeated. If the results are within the normal range, administer the drug. If the results still indicate 52 ml/minute, the renal function is truly impaired, and the drug should not be given. A complete workup will be required to elucidate the patient's renal problem.

11. **Question:** A 28-year-old woman who is menstruating comes to the emergency room complaining of a sudden onset of colicky, left-sided back pain with radiation to the groin. A ureteral calculus (stone) is suspected. The physician orders a UA. What should be done?

Answer: You should remind the physician that the patient is menstruating and suggest that the patient be catheterized for a urine specimen. RBCs are diagnostic of a ureteral stone. However, one has to expect RBCs in a quantity too numerous to count in a voided specimen from a menstruating patient. The only way to obtain an adequate specimen is by urethral catheterization.

12. **Question:** Your patient develops bleeding from a peptic ulcer. His routine laboratory studies indicate a BUN level of 68 mg/dl and a creatinine level of 1 mg/dl. Does this patient have renal disease?

Answer: No. The creatinine level is normal. The BUN level is elevated because there is an increased GI absorption of protein (blood), which is metabolized to urea. Patients with normal renal function who develop GI bleeding will have elevated BUN levels. The BUN level returns to normal as soon as the GI hemorrhage ceases.

Bibliography

Bolton WK: Primary glomerular disease. In Rakel RE, editor: Conn's current therapy, Philadelphia, 1998, WB Saunders.

Brady HR, O'Meara YM, Brenner BM: The major glomerulopathies. In Fauci AS et al, editors: Harrison's principles of internal medicine, ed 14, New York, 1998, McGraw-Hill.

Brenner BM, editor: Brenner and Rector's the kidney, ed 5, Philadelphia, 1996, Ardmore Medical Books.

Brunzel NA: Fundamentals of urine and body fluid analysis, Philadelphia, 1994, WB Saunders.

Carpenter CB: Long-term failure of renal transplants: adding insult to injury, Kidney Int 48(suppl 50):40, 1995.

Coe FL, Brenner BM: Approach to the patient with diseases of the kidneys and urinary tract. In Fauci AS et al, editors: Harrison's principles of internal medicine, ed 14, New York, 1998, McGraw-Hill.

Couser WG: Glomerular disease. In Wyngaarden JB et al, editors: Cecil textbook of medicine, ed 19, Philadelphia, 1992, WB Saunders.

Freeman NJ et al: Elevated prostate markers in metastatic small cell carcinoma of unknown primary, Cancer 68(5):1118-1120, 1991.

Guasch A et al: Early detection of the course of glomerular injury in patients with sickle cell anemia, Kidney Int 49:786, 1996.

Hricak H, White SS: Radiologic assessment of the kidney. In Brenner BM, editor: Brenner and Rector's the kidney, ed 5, Philadelphia, 1996, Ardmore Medical Books.

Humphreys MH: Human immunodeficiency virus-associated glomerlosclerosis, *Kidney Int* 48:311, 1995.

Johnson CP et al: Evaluation of renal transplant dysfunction using color Doppler sonography, *Surg Gynecol Obstet* 173(4):279-284, 1991.

Johnson R et al: Renal manifestations of hepatitis C infection, *Kidney Int* 46:1265, 1994.

Kasiske BK, Keane WF: Laboratory assessment of renal disease. In Brenner BM, editor: Brenner and Rector's the kidney, ed 5, Philadelphia, 1996, Ardmore Medical Books.

Lakkis FG et al: Microvascular diseases of the kidney. In Brenner BM, editor: Brenner and Rector's the kidney, ed 5, Philadelphia, 1996, Ardmore Medical Books.

Mata JA: Bacterial infections of the urinary tract in females. In Rakel RE, editor: Conn's current therapy, Philadelphia, 1998, WB Saunders.

McGuire EJ: Urinary incontinence. In Rakel RE, editor: Conn's current therapy, Philadelphia, 1998, WB Saunders.

Pak CY: Renal calculi. In Wyngaarden JB et al, editors: Cecil textbook of medicine, ed 19, Philadelphia, 1992, WB Saunders.

Schaeffer AJ: Prostatitis. In Rakel RE, editor: Conn's current therapy, Philadelphia, 1998, WB Saunders.

Seifter JL, Brenner BM: Urinary tract obstruction. In Fauci AS et al, editors: Harrison's principles of internal medicine, ed 14, New York, 1998, McGraw-Hill.

Silverblatt FS: Bacterial infections of the urinary tract in males. In Rakel RE, editor: Conn's current therapy, Philadelphia, 1998, WB Saunders.

Tanagho EA, McAninch JW, editors: Smith's general urology, ed 13, Norwalk, Conn, 1992, Appleton & Lange.

Williams RD: Tumors of the kidney, ureter, and bladder. In Wyngaarden JB et al, editors: Cecil textbook of medicine, ed 19, Philadelphia, 1992, WB Saunders.

Wozniak-Petrofsky J: Basics of urodynamics, *J Urol Nurs* 12(2):434-463, 1993.

Diagnostic Studies Used in the Assessment of the
Endocrine System

Review Questions and Answers, p. 339

Bibliography, p. 341

ANATOMY AND PHYSIOLOGY

The endocrine system functions to maintain homeostasis of the body's internal environment. Endocrine glands secrete their products directly into the bloodstream. The endocrine system secretes chemical substances called *hormones.* Figure 8-1 shows the anatomy and location of the endocrine glands. The concentration of most hormones is maintained at an appropriate level in the bloodstream by a feedback-control mechanism. If the

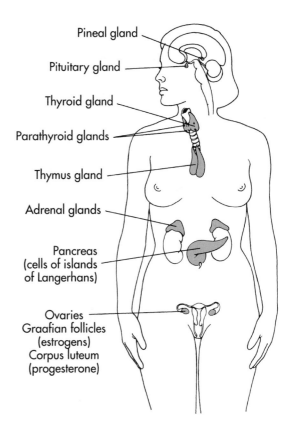

Figure 8-1 Location of endocrine glands.

hormone concentration increases, further production of the hormone is inhibited. When the hormone concentration decreases, production of that hormone then is stimulated.

Hormones are the main regulators of metabolism, growth and development, reproduction, and stress response. An excess or deficiency of hormones causes various types of abnormalities. This chapter focuses on the diagnostic studies related to the pituitary, thyroid, parathyroid, adrenal glands, and the endocrine pancreas. The anatomy and physiology of each gland are discussed briefly.

Pituitary Gland

The pituitary gland is a small gland located at the base of the brain within the bony cavity called the *sella turcica.* Because of its position under the hypothalamus, it is also called the *hypophysis.* The pituitary gland is divided into regions that function as distinct and separate endocrine glands. The pituitary gland consists of an anterior lobe (adenohypophysis), a smaller posterior lobe (neurohypophysis), and a poorly developed intermediate lobe (pars intermedia) lying between the anterior and posterior lobes.

The anterior pituitary gland (Figure 8-2) has multiple functions, and because it regulates the functions of many other glands, it is also known as the *master gland.* Seven anterior pituitary hormones have been identified (Table 8-1). The posterior gland stores two hormones: antidiuretic hormone and oxytocin. See Table 8-1 for a brief overview of pituitary hormones, target organs, and principal functions.

Disorders of the pituitary gland

Growth hormone is the only hormone secreted by the anterior pituitary that has no specific target organ. All body cells are affected by growth hormone. Growth hormone is regulated by hormones released from the hypothalamus and by somatomedins, which are synthesized in the liver. The action of growth hormone is influenced by many other hormones (e.g., thyroid hormone, insulin, steroids, and androgens). Nutritional status, exercise, stress, sleep, and diurnal rhythm also affect growth hormone secretion.

Overproduction of growth hormone, which is usually from a benign pituitary adenoma, causes gigantism or acromegaly.

Hyposecretion of growth hormone during childhood results in growth retardation, or dwarfism.

Thyroid Gland

The thyroid gland (Figure 8-3) is located in the neck anterior to the thyroid-laryngeal cartilage. It is bilobal, with a narrow strip (isthmus) of glandular tissue connecting the lateral lobes and giv-

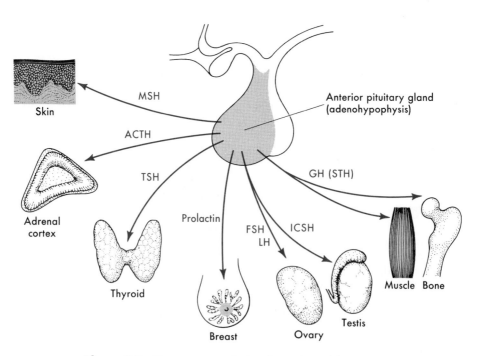

Figure 8-2 Target organs of adenohypophyseal hormones.

TABLE 8-1   Pituitary Gland Hormones

Hormones	Target Organ or Tissue	Principal Function
Anterior Pituitary		
Growth hormone (somatotropin)	General	Accelerates rate of body growth, regulates organic metabolism
Thyroid-stimulating hormone (TSH, thyrotropin)	Thyroid gland	Synthesizes and releases thyroid hormone, promotes bone growth
Adrenocorticotropic hormone (ACTH)	Adrenal cortex	Promotes growth of adrenal cortex, secretion of cortisol
Follicle-stimulating hormone (FSH)	Ovaries, testes	Stimulates growth of ovarian follicle in women; spermatogenesis in men
Luteinizing hormone (LH)	Ovaries, testes	Promotes maturation of ovaries, ovulation, and secretion of progesterone in women; stimulates development of the testes and secretion of androgens in men
Prolactin (luteotropic hormone, mammotropin)	Mammary glands	Causes proliferation of breast tissue, initiation of milk secretion
Interstitial cell–stimulating hormone (ICSH)	Testes	Promotes secretion of testosterone
Posterior Pituitary		
Antidiuretic hormone (ADH, vasopressin)	Renal tubules, arterioles	Facilitates water resorption, produces vasoconstriction
Oxytocin	Uterus	Contracts pregnant uterus

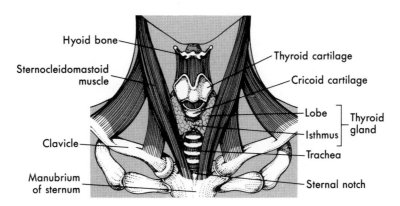

Figure 8-3   Landmarks of the thyroid.

ing the gland an H-shaped appearance. The thyroid originates embryologically near the foramen cecum of the tongue and descends caudally to its place in the neck. Ectopic thyroid tissue frequently is found along that tract of descent or more distally in the chest.

The thyroid is microscopically composed of follicles lined by cuboidal-shaped epithelial cells. In the center of these follicles is a colloidal material (thyroglobulin) in which thyroid hormones are stored. These follicular cells produce triiodothyronine (T_3) and thyroxine (T_4) hormones. Next to these follicular cells are parafollicular cells, or C cells. These C cells probably produce calcitonin, a calcium-lowering hormone.

Production, storage, and secretion of thyroid hormone

Dietary ingestion of iodine provides the iodide necessary for thyroid hormone synthesis. The plasma iodide is actively transformed to its organic form, I_2, which immediately becomes bound to thyroglobulin. The tyrosine radical of the thyroglobulin molecule combines with the organic iodine and becomes monoiodotyrosine or diiodotyrosine. A complicated coupling of a monoiodotyrosine and a diiodotyrosine results in T_3. A similar coupling of two diiodotyrosines produces T_4. T_4 contains four iodine atoms in each molecule, whereas T_3 contains only three. The hormones, still bound to thyroglobulin, are stored in their inactive states. When secretion is required, the thyroglobulin is broken off by proteinases secreted by the thyroid cells, and the free hormone is secreted into the plasma (Figure 8-4).

Regulation of thyroid hormone production

When the blood levels of T_4 and T_3 fall, thyrotropin-releasing hormone (TRH) is secreted by the hypothalamus. TRH stimulates the anterior pituitary gland to secrete thyroid-stimulating hormone (TSH). TSH enhances many of the chemical reactions that occur during thyroid hormone synthesis (see Figure 8-4). When the blood levels of T_3 and T_4 return to normal, the secretion of TRH

is inhibited by a negative feedback mechanism. This feedback system promotes hormone regulation in a normal (or euthyroid) person.

In a normally functioning thyroid regulation system, one would expect the following:

1. When T_3 and T_4 levels are decreased, TRH and TSH levels should be increased, unless the pituitary is not functional (e.g., panhypopituitarism or cretinism).
2. When T_3 and T_4 levels are increased, TRH and TSH levels should be decreased.

When adenomas or carcinomas of the thyroid are present, this regulatory function may be lost.

Thyroid disorders

Hyperthyroidism, or thyrotoxicosis, is the hypermetabolic state that occurs with excessive production of thyroid hormone. The most common cause of hyperthyroidism is Graves' disease. Other causes of hyperthyroidism include nodular toxic goiter (Plummer's disease), overtreatment with thyroid drugs, thyroid adenoma or carcinoma, and excessive secretion of TSH by a pituitary adenoma.

Hypothyroidism results when the thyroid gland produces too little of either or both of its hormones (T_3 and T_4). Major causes of hypothyroidism include:

1. Cretinism (a disorder of infancy and childhood caused by insufficient thyroid hormone during fetal or neonatal life); newborn screening programs for the diagnosis of hypothyroidism include assays of T_4 and TSH
2. Myxedema (the deficient synthesis of thyroid hormone in the adult)
3. Surgical removal of all thyroid tissue
4. Radioactive iodine ablation of the thyroid
5. Autoimmune destruction of the thyroid

Parathyroid Glands

Most people have four parathyroid glands, with a pair located behind each lobe of the thyroid

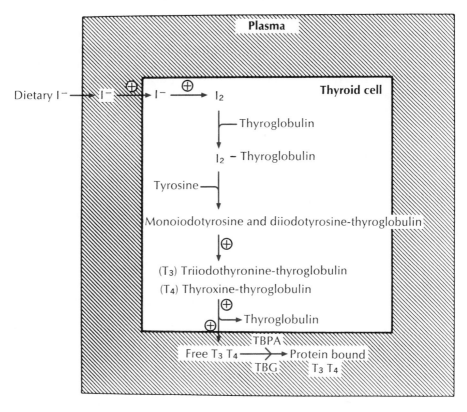

Figure 8-4   Thyroid hormone synthesis. Plus signs (+) indicate steps that are enhanced or stimulated by thyroid-stimulating hormone. *TBPA,* thyroid-binding prealbumin; *TBG,* thyroid-binding globulin.

gland. The location of the parathyroid glands is not constant, although in most people all four glands are found in the neck. The parathyroid glands can, however, occur anywhere from the base of the tongue to the mediastinum. This sometimes presents a problem when a surgeon attempts to locate these glands, which measure 7 mm.

The glands are microscopically composed of oxyphil cells, chief cells, and water-clear cells. Oxyphil cells are considered by some to be inactive, whereas the other cells actively secrete parathormone (parathyroid hormone [PTH]). PTH is one of the major factors in the control of calcium metabolism (see the following sec-

tion). PTH increases serum calcium levels by causing:

1. Increased bone resorption
2. Increased calcium absorption from the intestines
3. Increased calcium resorption in the kidney tubules
4. Increased phosphate excretion, which indirectly raises the serum calcium level

The most potent stimulus to PTH secretion is low serum calcium levels. As the serum calcium level decreases, the parathyroids are stimulated to secrete PTH. This, in turn, raises the serum calcium level. The increased calcium level then acts as a negative feedback inhibitor and deactivates PTH secretion, thus maintaining normal calcium levels.

So-called primary hyperparathyroidism can be the result of parathyroid hyperplasia or tumor (adenoma or carcinoma). In these diseases, both the serum calcium and serum PTH levels are high (Figure 8-5).

Secondary hyperparathyroidism occurs in patients with a buildup of serum phosphates (e.g., because of renal failure). The phosphate levels vary inversely with calcium levels; the chronic increase in phosphate levels causes a chronically low serum calcium level. The resulting hypocalcemia acts as a powerful stimulus for PTH secre-

tion and causes the parathyroid glands to become maximally stimulated to produce PTH, resulting in compensatory parathyroid hyperplasia. Thus, in patients with renal failure, the serum calcium level is usually low despite the high serum PTH level. The patient experiences severe bone weakening.

Phosphate and calcium levels return to normal when the patient is no longer in renal failure (because of transplant, dialysis, or healing of the primary renal injury or disease). However, the parathyroid glands are occasionally unable to decrease their overstimulation despite the new (normal) calcium levels. Therefore, they continue to secrete high levels of PTH. This is called *tertiary*

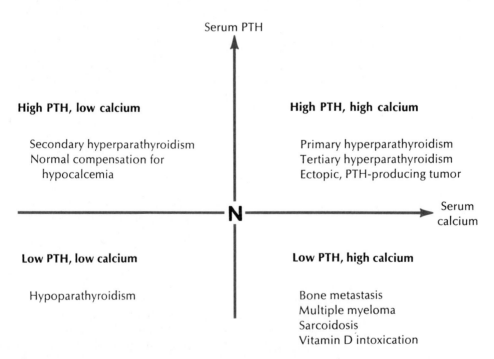

DIFFERENTIAL DIAGNOSIS USING CONCOMITANT SERUM PTH AND SERUM CALCIUM ASSAYS

Serum PTH

High PTH, low calcium

Secondary hyperparathyroidism
Normal compensation for
  hypocalcemia

High PTH, high calcium

Primary hyperparathyroidism
Tertiary hyperparathyroidism
Ectopic, PTH-producing tumor

N — Serum calcium

Low PTH, low calcium

Hypoparathyroidism

Low PTH, high calcium

Bone metastasis
Multiple myeloma
Sarcoidosis
Vitamin D intoxication

Figure 8-5 Graph showing various disease entities associated with concomitantly abnormal PTH and calcium levels. *N*, Normality, which is marked by eucalcemia and a normal PTH level.

hyperparathyroidism. It results in hypercalcemia and high PTH levels, much the same as in primary hyperparathyroidism.

Tumor of the lung, thymus, kidney, or pancreas can secrete a PTH-like substance that can cause severe hypercalcemia (paraneoplastic syndrome). Patients with this disorder also will have increased levels of calcium and PTH.

The most common cause of hypoparathyroidism is infarction or removal of the parathyroid during thyroid or parathyroid surgery. Autoimmune destruction has rarely been reported and is seen only in young patients when it does occur.

Calcium metabolism

Ingested calcium is actively absorbed by the intestinal mucosa. This absorption is facilitated by the action of activated vitamin D and PTH. Calcium exists in the blood in a free-ionized form and in a bound (to albumin) form. The ionized calcium is the physiologically active form. There are large stores of calcium in the bone. PTH can mobilize these stores by stimulating bone resorption, thus raising serum calcium levels. Calcitonin (secreted by the parafollicular cells of the thyroid glands) lowers the serum calcium and phosphate levels by inhibiting bone resorption, thus acting as an antagonist to PTH. Calcium is excreted in the urine and stool. Again, PTH acts to increase serum calcium levels.

Vitamin D is another principal factor in calcium homeostasis. Vitamin D is produced by sunlight irradiation of the skin. This inactive form of the vitamin is then hydroxylated, first in the liver and then in the kidney. The hydroxylated form is the active form that increases intestinal absorption of calcium. Patients with renal failure are unable to hydroxylate vitamin D, which contributes to their hypocalcemia.

Hypercalcemia can be caused by many disorders other than hyperparathyroidism. These include metastatic and primary tumors of the bone; nonparathyroid, ectopic, PTH-producing tumors; vitamin D intoxication; sarcoidosis; and milk-alkali syndrome. These disorders can be differentiated by determinations of concomitant serum calcium and PTH levels.

With the widespread use of multichannel, serum-testing machines, more asymptomatic patients are being recognized. Hypocalcemia is most frequently caused by renal disease, hypoparathyroidism, or low serum albumin levels.

Adrenal Glands

The adrenal glands (see Figure 8-1) lie in the retroperitoneum, immediately superior to the kidneys. Because of this anatomic relationship with the kidneys, any significant enlargement in the adrenal glands displaces the kidneys (as can be seen during intravenous pyelogram [IVP]). The arterial supply to the glands is variable and multiple. The venous drainage is more constant. The right adrenal vein enters the inferior vena cava directly, whereas the left adrenal vein enters the left renal vein directly. The adrenal glands are microscopically composed of an inner medulla and an outer cortex, which has three layers (zona glomerulosa, zona fasciculata, and zona reticularis).

The adrenal glands are able to secrete many hormones. Glucocorticoids (e.g., cortisol), mineralocorticoids (e.g., aldosterone), androgens (e.g., testosterone), and estrogens are secreted by the adrenal cortex. (See Table 8-2 for the action of each hormone.) The adrenal medulla is responsible for production of epinephrine and norepinephrine.

Glucocorticoid secretion

Cortisol is the primary, and physiologically the most important, glucocorticoid. The hypothalamus normally secretes corticotropin-releasing factor (CRF), which travels down to the anterior pituitary gland by way of the pituitary portal blood system. Adrenocorticotropic hormone (ACTH) secretion from the anterior pituitary is then stimulated by CRF. ACTH directly stimulates the adrenal glands to produce and secrete cortisol and, to a lesser degree, aldosterone. Cortisol then acts as described in Table 8-2. As the levels of cortisol increase, CRF secretion is inhibited by a negative feedback mechanism to maintain appropriate levels of cortisol.

With any physical or emotional stress (e.g.,

TABLE 8-2 Action of Adrenal Hormones and Symptoms of Excess and Deficiency

Hormone	Function	Excess	Deficiency
Cortisol	Glycogenesis:	Diabetes, polyuria	Hypoglycemia, asthenia, weakness
	Mobilization of protein	Destruction of protein material in bone, connective tissue, and muscle Muscle weakness, osteoporosis, back pain, pathologic fractures, cutaneous striae, increased bruising	
	Mobilization and redeposition of adipose tissue	Buffalo hump, moon facies, truncal obesity	
	Increased resorption of sodium	Hypertension, edema, plethora	Orthostatic hypotension
	Increased potassium excretion	Hypokalemic alkalosis	Hyperkalemic acidosis
	Reduction of inflammation	Increased susceptibility to infection	
	Maintenance of integrity of personality	Emotional lability	Irritability
	Suppression of ACTH		Excess ACTH (melanocyte-stimulating hormone (MSH)-like hyperpigmentation)

Androgen	Secondary male sex characteristics	Hirsutism
		Acne
		Precocious puberty
		Baldness
		In women:
		  Amenorrhea
		  Deepening of voice
		  Atrophy of uterus
		  Atrophy of breast
		  Enlargement of clitoris
		  Increased sex drive
			In men:
			  Lack of body hair
			  Decreased sex drive

Estrogen	Secondary female sex characteristics	In men:
		  Gynecomastia
		  Reduction of body hair
		  Increased subcutaneous fat
		In women:
		  Uterine bleeding
		  Uterine cancer
		  Precocious puberty
		  Cystic breast
			In women:
			  Hot flashes
			  Amenorrhea

Aldosterone	Increased water resorption Increased sodium resorption Increased potassium excretion	Hypertension, edema Hypernatremia Hypokalemia	Hyponatremia Hyperkalemia

trauma, infection, chronic illness, or high levels of anxiety), this negative-feedback, cortisol-control system can be overcome by other central nervous system (CNS) mechanisms. Therefore, CRF and ACTH can be secreted, at times of stress, despite high levels of cortisol. These elevated cortisol levels are apparently protective, supplying the body with extra sources of glucose and other substances.

Normally, there is diurnal variation in the secretion of CRF and ACTH and, therefore, in cortisol secretion. This is a biologic circadian rhythm. As a result, cortisol is maximally secreted at approximately 6 to 8 AM, and the level falls to its nadir at approximately 12 AM. An important feature of Cushing's syndrome (adrenal hyperfunction) is failure of this circadian rhythm and resultant variation in cortisol levels.

Mineralocorticoid secretion

Aldosterone is the mineralocorticoid of primary physiologic importance. Of this hormone secretion, 25% to 30% is influenced by ACTH, whereas the majority of its secretion depends on the renin-angiotensin system, as described in Chapter 7, p. 230.

Androgen and estrogen secretion

The quantity of androgen and estrogen produced by the adrenal glands (in contrast to the gonads) is a subject of ongoing debate. However, it is sufficient to say that adrenal production of these hormones is secondary to gonadal production. In men the adrenal gland is the primary source of estrogen, and in women the adrenal gland is the primary source of androgen. After menopause, the adrenal glands become the only source of estrogen production in women.

Epinephrine secretion

Epinephrine is secreted by the adrenal medulla. This hormone affects smooth and cardiac muscle, as well as many other tissues. Epinephrine is sympathomimetic. Increased secretion of epinephrine is one of the body's first responses to physical and emotional stress.

Diseases affecting the adrenal glands

Many diseases affect the adrenal glands. Cushing's syndrome is the result of adrenal gland hypersecretion of cortisol. Bilateral adrenal hyperplasia (Cushing's disease), adrenal adenomas and carcinomas, and nonadrenal, ACTH-producing tumors (e.g., of the lung or thymus) can all produce Cushing's syndrome. One must be aware that exogenously administered pharmacologic doses of steroids can also cause the signs and symptoms of cortisol excess (see Table 8-2).

Addison's disease (reduced cortisol secretion) is the result of adrenal gland hypofunction and can be caused by destruction of the adrenal gland by hemorrhage, infarction, metastatic tumor invasion, or autoimmunity. Congenital enzyme deficiency and enzyme blockers, such as metyrapone, also cause adrenal hypofunction. Pituitary hypofunction may result not only in adrenal hypofunction but also in a decrease in thyroid growth and sexual function. Addison's disease is most commonly found in patients who have had their adrenal glands surgically removed and are taking inadequate cortisol replacement.

Endocrine Pancreas

The pancreas, located in the abdomen (see Figure 8-1), has both exocrine (digestive enzymes) and endocrine functions. The islets of Langerhans are clusters of endocrine-secreting cells embedded in the pancreatic tissue. Many different and distinct cells make up the islets of Langerhans: alpha cells secrete glucagon; beta cells secrete insulin; gamma cells (or C cells) secrete gastrin; and delta cells secrete vasoactive intestinal polypeptide (VIP).

The major action of insulin is to lower the blood glucose level by facilitating the movement of glucose out of the bloodstream and into the cells of the liver, muscle, or other tissue, where glucose is either used for immediate energy or stored as glycogen for later energy requirements. Insulin also promotes the storage of fat in adipose tissue and aids in the synthesis of body proteins.

In the absence of insulin, serum glucose levels

rise because glucose cannot enter the cells. When the levels of glucose reach approximately 180 mg/dl (renal threshold), glucose spills over into the urine. Diabetes mellitus is both a chronic metabolic disorder, involving glucose metabolism, and a disturbance of fat and protein metabolism because these substances are catabolized and used as a source of immediate energy instead of glucose. Patients with diabetes have more than just a deficiency of insulin quantitatively; they also have a disturbance in the production, action, or metabolic use of insulin.

Glucagon, on the other hand, tends to raise the blood glucose level, primarily by promoting the conversion of glycogen to glucose in the liver. Glucagon is secreted by the pancreas in response to a fall in the serum glucose level. Gastrin is a hormone that affects the gastrointestinal (GI) tract. It stimulates gastric acid secretion, intestinal motility, and sphincter contraction. VIP, also an active GI hormone, is thought to be responsible for a watery diarrhea syndrome.

Adrenal Venography

Test type X-ray with contrast dye

Normal values
Normal adrenal veins and normal adrenal vein hormone assay

Rationale
Adrenal venography is a radiologic test performed to obtain blood samples from the adrenal veins and detect adrenal pathology. Once the veins are identified, a catheter can be placed in the veins and blood selectively obtained from each adrenal vein.

In patients with Cushing's syndrome, the blood is analyzed for plasma cortisol. If the plasma cortisol level in the blood obtained from one side is much higher than that of the other, a unilateral adrenal tumor is causing Cushing's syndrome. If, on the other hand, plasma cortisol levels are bilaterally elevated, one can safely conclude that Cushing's syndrome is caused by bilateral adrenal hyperplasia.

In patients with a pheochromocytoma, the adrenal venous blood is analyzed for catecholamines. If the catecholamine level on one side is much higher than that of the other, a unilateral pheochromocytoma exists on the side with the elevated levels. If blood obtained from both sides is equally elevated, the patient probably has bilateral adrenal pheochromocytoma. If the adrenal venous blood samples are not elevated on either side in a patient who has elevated peripheral blood catecholamine levels, the pheochromocytoma exists outside the adrenal gland (i.e., extra-adrenal pheochromocytoma). The venous blood also can be evaluated for aldosterone, androgens, and other substances.

Potential complications
Potential complications associated with adrenal venography are as follows:

- Allergic reaction to iodinated dye
  Allergic reactions may vary from flushing, itching, and urticaria to life-threatening anaphylaxis (evidenced by respiratory distress, drop in blood pressure, or shock). In the unusual event of anaphylaxis, the patient is treated with diphenhydramine (Benadryl), steroids, and epinephrine. Oxygen and endotracheal equipment should be on hand for immediate use.
- Adrenal hemorrhage or necrosis
  This is caused by the pressure of the dye injection and may cause Addison's disease (adrenal insufficiency).

Procedure
The fasting patient is brought to the special studies angiography laboratory (usually in the radiology department). The patient is placed in the supine position on the x-ray table. The patient's groin is prepared in a sterile manner. After the venipuncture site is locally anesthetized, the femoral vein is catheterized. The catheter is passed into the adrenal vein. Dye is injected to visualize the adrenal veins and to ensure that the catheter

is in the adrenal vein. Blood is obtained and sent to the chemistry laboratory for assays.

In a patient suspected of having a pheochromocytoma, appropriate pharmacologic beta- and alpha-adrenergic blocking agents are administered, propranolol (Inderal) and phenoxybenzamine (Dibenzyline), respectively. This prevents the occurrence of a catecholamine-initiated malignant hypertensive episode.

The duration of the study is approximately 1 hour. Venous catheterization is as uncomfortable as any cutaneous needle stick. A burning sensation is associated with the dye injection.

Contraindications

Complications associated with adrenal venography are as follows:

- Patients with allergies to iodinated dye
- Patients with bleeding disorders
  They may not be able to stop bleeding at the venous puncture site (usually in the groin).

Nursing implications with rationale

Before

☞ Explain the procedure to the patient and allay the patient's fears regarding venography. Provide emotional support.

- Ensure that written and informed consent for this procedure is obtained before the study.
- Assess the patient for allergies to dye. Administer a steroid and antihistamine preparation, as ordered, to the patient allergic to dye (see Contraindications).
- Administer propranolol and phenoxybenzamine, as ordered.

After

- Assess the patient's vital signs frequently (normally every 15 minutes for four times, then every 30 minutes for four times, then every hour for four times, and then every 4 hours). Assess the patient suspected of having a pheochromocytoma for signs and symptoms of a hypertensive episode. If such an episode occurs, notify

the physician immediately to obtain an order for appropriate alpha- and beta-adrenergic blocking agents.

- Assess the groin site for redness, pain, swelling, and bleeding with each vital sign check.
- Apply cold compresses to the puncture site as needed to reduce discomfort or swelling.

Adrenocorticotropic Hormone
(ACTH, Corticotropin)

Test type Blood

Normal values

AM: 15-100 pg/ml or 10-80 ng/L (SI units)
PM: <50 pg/ml or <50 ng/L (SI units)

Rationale

The serum ACTH study is a test of anterior pituitary gland function, which affords the greatest insight into the causes of either Cushing's syndrome (overproduction of cortisol) or Addison's disease (underproduction of cortisol).

An elaborate feedback mechanism for cortisol exists to coordinate the function of the hypothalamus, pituitary gland, and the adrenal glands. ACTH is an important part of this mechanism. In the patient with Cushing's syndrome, an elevated ACTH level can be caused by a pituitary ACTH-producing tumor, or a nonpituitary (ectopic) ACTH-producing tumor, usually in the lung, pancreas, thymus, or ovary. ACTH levels greater than 200 pg/ml usually indicate ectopic ACTH production. If the ACTH level is below normal in a patient with Cushing's syndrome, an adrenal adenoma or carcinoma is probably the cause of the hyperfunction (Table 8-3).

In patients with Addison's disease, an elevated ACTH level indicates primary adrenal gland failure, as in adrenal gland destruction caused by infarction, hemorrhage, or autoimmunity; surgical removal of the adrenal gland; congenital enzyme deficiency; or adrenal suppression after prolonged ingestion of exogenous steroids. If the ACTH level is below normal in a patient with adrenal insuffi-

TABLE 8-3   Cortisol/ACTH Levels in Diagnosis of Adrenal Dysfunction

Disease	Cortisol Level	ACTH Level

Cushing's syndrome
  Adrenal micronodular
    hyperplasia
  Adrenal tumor
    (adenoma, cancer)
	High	Low

Cushing's syndrome
  Cushing's disease
    (ACTH-producing
    pituitary tumor)
  Ectopic ACTH-
    producing tumor
    (e.g., lung cancer)
	High	High

Addison's disease
  Adrenal gland failure
    (e.g., infarction,
    hemorrhage, or
    congenital adrenal
    hyperplasia)
	Low	High

Hypopituitarism	Low	Low

ciency, hypopituitarism is most probably the cause of the hypofunction.

ACTH can be directly measured by immunoassay in many large reference laboratories. Because it is not done in most average laboratories, it requires several days to obtain results. One must be aware that there is a diurnal variation of ACTH levels that correspond to cortisol levels. Levels in evening (8 to 10 PM) samples are usually half to two-thirds less than those of morning (4 to 8 AM) specimens. This diurnal variation is lost when disease (especially neoplasm) affects the pituitary or adrenal glands. Likewise, stress can blunt or eliminate this normal diurnal variation.

ACTH is measured in amniotic fluid when anencephaly is suspected. Decreased levels are noted with anencephalic fetuses.

Interfering factors
Factors that interfere with determining ACTH levels include the following:

- Stress (trauma, pyrogen, or hypoglycemia), menses, and pregnancy, which cause *increased* levels of cortisol
  ACTH levels are artificially elevated in these situations.
- Recently administered radioisotope scans, which can affect levels determined by either radioimmunoassay or immunoradiometry
- Exogenously administered corticosteroids *decrease* ACTH levels.

Procedure
A chilled, plastic, heparinized syringe is used to collect a 20-ml fasting sample of peripheral venous blood, usually between 8 and 10 AM. The blood is placed on ice and sent immediately to the chemistry laboratory for radioimmunoassay. As with cortisol, stress of any kind can artificially increase the ACTH level. Therefore one must try to minimize the psychologic trauma of venipuncture.

Nursing implications with rationale
Before
- Explain the procedure to the patient. Allow plenty of time to answer questions so that stress is diminished.
- Instruct the patient to remain NPO (*nil per os,* nothing by mouth) after midnight the day of the test.
- Evaluate the patient for stress factors that would invalidate the test results.
- Evaluate the patient for sleep pattern abnormalities. With a normal sleep pattern, the ACTH level is highest between 4 and 8 AM and lowest at approximately 9 PM.
After
- Apply pressure or a pressure dressing to the venipuncture site to prevent further bleeding. Observe the site for bleeding.

Case Study

Cushing's Syndrome

Ms. D., a 22-year-old nurse, complained of weakness, tiredness, easy bruising, leg edema, recent acne, and hirsutism. Her menses became irregular. Her family commented that she was emotionally labile. They also believed that her face had become fuller. On physical examination she was found to be mildly hypertensive with a moon facies, buffalo hump, truncal obesity, diffuse cutaneous striae, and +2 pitting pretibial edema. The results of a recent chest x-ray study performed at work were reported as normal.

Studies	Results
Routine laboratory work	Within normal limits (WNL) except glucose: 240 mg/dl (normal: 60-120 mg/dl)
Urine test for 17-hydroxycorticosteroids (OHCS), p. 338	28 mg/24 hours (normal: 4.5-10.0 mg/24 hr)
Urine test for 17-ketosteroids, p. 338	14 mg/24 hours (normal: 4-15 mg/24 hr)
Plasma cortisol test, p. 301	
8 AM	88 mg/dl (normal: 6-28 mg/dl)
4 PM	78 mg/dl (normal: 2-12 mg/dl)
Dexamethasone suppression test, p. 303	
Plasma cortisol level after 2 mg/day	60 mg/dl (normal: <10 mg/dl)
Plasma cortisol level after 8 mg/day	8 mg/dl (normal: <10 mg/dl)
Plasma ACTH test, p. 293	140 pg/ml (normal: 15-100 pg/ml)
Plasma cortisol level after ACTH stimulation test, p. 296	140 mg/dl (normal: >40 mg/dl, <60 mg/dl)
Urine 17-OHCS level after metyrapone stimulation test, p. 338	Stimulated excretion of 17-OHCS tripled (normal: doubled) baseline values
Computed tomography (CT) scan of head, p. 196	No pituitary tumor
Adrenal CT scan, p. 113	Bilaterally enlarged adrenal gland; no tumor

Diagnostic Analysis

The patient had the classic signs and symptoms of Cushing's syndrome (adrenal gland hyperactivity). Her elevated urinary 17-OHCS level and the elevation and loss of normal diurnal variation in her plasma cortisol levels substantiated the diagnosis. The underlying pathologic condition causing the adrenal gland hyperfunctioning had to be determined to permit appropriate therapy. The causes could have been bilateral adrenal hyperplasia, adrenal adenoma or carcinoma, a pituitary tumor, or an ACTH-secreting tumor. Lack of adrenal gland suppression with 2 mg of dexamethasone, combined with complete suppression with 8 mg of dexamethasone, strongly indicated that adrenal hyperplasia (abnormally high secretion of ACTH), rather than an adrenal tu-

Continued

Case Study

Cushing's Syndrome—cont'd

mor, was causing the Cushing's syndrome. The patient's elevated levels on the plasma ACTH, metyrapone suppression, and ACTH stimulation tests were all consistent with bilateral adrenal hyperplasia. The CT studies of the head and the adrenal glands eliminated the possibility of pituitary and adrenal tumors. The CT scan of the adrenal glands was compatible with adrenal hyperplasia. The patient underwent bilateral adrenalectomy and became asymptomatic. She was given physiologic steroid-replacement medications and had no further difficulties.

Critical Thinking Questions

1. If Ms. D. did not have adrenal hyperfunction, metyrapone could instigate an adrenal crisis. How might that present clinically?
2. What nonpathologic factors might influence ACTH levels?

Adrenocorticotropic Hormone Stimulation Test (ACTH Stimulation Test, Cortisol Stimulation Test, Cosyntropin Test)

Test type Blood

Normal values

Rapid test: cortisol levels >7 μg/dl above baseline
24-hour test: cortisol levels >40 μg/dl
3-day test: cortisol levels >40 μg/dl

Rationale

The ACTH stimulation test is performed on patients found to have an adrenal insufficiency. An increase in plasma cortisol levels after the infusion of an ACTH-like drug indicates that the adrenal gland is normal and capable of functioning if stimulated. In that case, the cause of the adrenal insufficiency would lie within the pituitary gland (hypopituitarism, which is called *secondary adrenal insufficiency*). If little or no rise in cortisol levels occurs after the administration of the ACTH-like drug, the adrenal gland is the source of the problem and cannot secrete cortisol. This is called *primary adrenal insufficiency* (Addison's disease), which may be caused by adrenal hemorrhage, infarction, autoimmunity, metastatic tu-

mor, surgical removal of the adrenal glands, or congenital adrenal enzyme deficiency.

This test also can be used to evaluate patients with Cushing's syndrome. Patients with Cushing's syndrome caused by bilateral adrenal hyperplasia have an exaggerated cortisol elevation in response to the administration of the ACTH-like drug. Those experiencing Cushing's syndrome as a result of hyperfunctioning adrenal tumors (which are usually autonomous and relatively insensitive to ACTH) have little or no increase in cortisol levels over baseline values.

Cosyntropin (Cortrosyn) is a synthetic subunit of ACTH that has the same corticosteroid-stimulating effect as does endogenous ACTH in healthy persons. During this test, cosyntropin is administered to the patient, and the ability of the adrenal gland to respond is measured by plasma cortisol levels.

The rapid stimulation test is only a screening test. A normal response excludes adrenal insufficiency. An abnormal response, however, requires a 1- to 3-day prolonged ACTH stimulation test to differentiate primary insufficiency from secondary insufficiency. It should be noted that the adrenal gland also can be stimulated by insulin-induced hypoglycemia as a stressing agent. When insulin is the stimulant, cortisol and glucose levels are measured.

Interfering factors

Factors that interfere with determining ACTH stimulation test levels include drugs that may cause artificially *increased* cortisol levels (e.g., prolonged corticosteroid administration and spironolactone).

Procedure

After a baseline plasma cortisol level (see p. 301) is obtained, an intravenous (IV) infusion of synthetic alpha-ACTH (cosyntropin) in 1 L of normal saline solution is administered at the rate of 2 U/hour for 24 hours. Peripheral venous blood for plasma cortisol level determination is again obtained 24 hours later and sent to the chemistry laboratory. This test also can be performed by comparing the baseline urine hydroxysteroid excretion with stimulated hydroxycorticosteroid excretion. In normal patients, stimulated hydroxysteroid excretion should exceed 25 mg/day.

The ACTH stimulation test also can be performed by IV administration of 25 U of cosyntropin over an 8-hour period on 2 to 3 consecutive days. The response seen at the end of the second and third 8-hour period should approximate that seen after the continuous 24-hour infusion.

For the sake of convenience, the most widely used test is the rapid ACTH stimulation test, which is done by giving an intramuscular (IM) injection of 25 U (0.25 mg) of cosyntropin and measuring plasma cortisol levels before and at 30- and 60-minute intervals after drug administration. Normal patients have an increase of cortisol of more than 7 mg/dl above baseline values.

Nursing implications with rationale

Before
- ☞ Explain the method of testing to the patient.
- ☞ Instruct the patient to remain NPO after midnight the day of the test.

During
- ■ Accurately administer the cosyntropin, as ordered. Perform the venipuncture for cortisol level determination or obtain a urine specimen at the exact time indicated.

After
- ■ Apply pressure or a pressure dressing to the venipuncture site to prevent further bleeding. Observe the site for bleeding.

Antidiuretic Hormone (ADH, Vasopressin, Arginine Vasopressin [AVP])

Test type Blood

Normal values

1-5 pg/ml or 1.5 ng/L (SI units)

Rationale

Antidiuretic hormone (ADH) is performed to assist in the diagnosis of patients suspected to have diabetes insipidus (DI) or the syndrome of inappropriate ADH (SIADH). It is often performed on patients who complain of polyuria or polydipsia and are found to have marked variation in blood and osmolarity or sodium levels.

ADH, also known as *vasopressin,* is formed by the hypothalamus and stored in the posterior pituitary gland. It controls the amount of water reabsorbed by the kidney. ADH release is stimulated by an increase in serum osmolality or a decrease in intravascular blood volume. Physical stress, surgery, and even high levels of anxiety also may stimulate ADH release. With a release of ADH, more water is reabsorbed from the kidneys. This increases the amount of free water within the bloodstream (decreased sodium and serum osmolality) and causes a very concentrated urine (increased urine osmolality). With low ADH levels, water is allowed to be excreted, thereby producing hemoconcentration and a more dilute urine.

DI occurs when ADH secretion is inadequate or when the kidney is unresponsive to ADH stimulation. Inadequate ADH secretion is usually associated with central neurologic abnormalities (neurogenic DI) such as trauma, tumor, or inflammation of the hypothalamus. Surgical ablation of the pituitary gland also will result in the neurogenic form of DI; such patients excrete large volumes of free water within a dilute urine. Their blood is hemoconcentrated, causing them to have a strong thirst. Primary renal diseases may make the kidneys less sensitive to ADH stimulation (nephrogenic DI). Again, in this instance, a dilute urine created by excretion of high volumes of free water may occur.

High serum ADH levels are also associated with SIADH. In response to this inappropriately high level of ADH secretion, water is reabsorbed by the kidneys greatly in excess of normal amounts. Thus the patient becomes very hemodiluted, and the urine is concentrated. Blood levels of important serum ions diminish, causing severe neurologic, cardiac, and metabolic alterations. The most frequent cause of SIADH is the paraneoplastic syndrome of ectopic ADH production. The most common tumors associated with SIADH include carcinomas of the lung, thymus, pancreas, urologic tract, and intestine; lymphomas; and leukemia. SIADH also is associated with pulmonary diseases (e.g., tuberculosis, bacterial pneumonia), severe stress (e.g., surgery, trauma), CNS tumor, infection, or trauma.

Interfering factors
Factors that interfere with determining ADH levels include the following:

- Dehydration, hypovolemia, or stress, which may cause *increased* ADH levels
- Overhydration, decreased serum osmolality, and hypervolemia, which may cause *decreased* ADH levels
- Use of a glass syringe or collection tube, which causes degradation of ADH

Procedure
The patient should be adequately hydrated. Instruct the patient to fast (except for water) for 12 hours before testing. Approximately 7 ml of venous blood is collected in a plastic, prechilled anticoagulant tube while the patient is in the sitting or recumbent position.

Nursing implications with rationale
Before
- ☞ Explain the procedure to the patient.
- ☞ Instruct the patient to fast for 12 hours.
- ■ Ensure that the patient is adequately hydrated.

- ■ Evaluate the patient for high levels of physical or emotional stress.

After
- ■ Apply pressure or a pressure dressing to the venipuncture site to prevent further bleeding. Observe the site for bleeding.

Calcitonin (Human Calcitonin [HCT], Thyrocalcitonin)

Test type Blood

Normal values
Basal:
    Males: ≤19 pg/ml or ≤19 ng/L (SI units)
    Females: ≤14 pg/ml or ≤14 ng/L (SI units)
Calcium infusion (2.4 mg/kg):
    Males: ≤190 pg/ml or ≤190 ng/L
    Females: ≤130 pg/ml or ≤130 ng/L
Pentagastrin injection (0.5 mg/kg):
    Males: ≤110 pg/ml or ≤110 ng/L
    Females: ≤30 pg/ml or ≤30 ng/L

Rationale
Calcitonin is a hormone secreted by the parafollicular, or C cells, of the thyroid. Its secretion is stimulated by elevated serum calcium levels. The purpose of calcitonin is to contribute to calcium homeostasis. It decreases serum calcium levels by inhibiting bone resorption and increasing calcium excretion by the kidneys.

This test usually is used to evaluate patients with, or suspected to have, medullary carcinoma of the thyroid. This cancer has a familial tendency and, if found late, a poor prognosis. Seventy-five percent of patients with medullary thyroid cancer have hypersecretion of calcitonin despite normal serum calcium levels. Calcitonin is a useful tumor marker in monitoring response to therapy and predicting recurrences of medullary thyroid cancer. It also is useful as a screening test for those with a family history of medullary cancer and, therefore, are at high risk (20%). Routine screening for elevated calcitonin levels can detect medullary cancer early and improve chances for cure. C-cell hyperplasia, a benign calcitonin-producing disease that also has a familial tendency, also is associated with elevated calcitonin levels.

Equivocal elevations in calcitonin levels should be followed with additional provocative testing, using pentagastrin or calcium to stimulate calcitonin secretion.

Procedure

An overnight fast is required. Water is permitted. Approximately 7 ml of venous blood is collected in a heparinized green-top or a chilled red-top tube, according to the laboratory's protocol. The specimen should be placed on ice immediately. The blood is frozen and sent to a reference laboratory.

Nursing implications with rationale

Before

☞ Explain the procedure to the patient. Tell the patient that an overnight fast is required.

After

■ Apply pressure or a pressure dressing to the venipuncture site to prevent further bleeding. Observe the site for bleeding.

☞ Tell the patient that results may not be available for several days, because this test is often sent to a reference lab for analysis.

Calcium, Blood (Total/Ionized Calcium, Ca⁺⁺)
Calcium, Urine (Urine Calcium, Quantitative Calcium)

Test type Blood, urine

Normal values
Blood:
Total calcium:
Elderly: values tend to decrease
Adult: 9.0-10.5 mg/dl or 2.25-2.75 mmol/L (SI units)
Child: 8.8-10.8 mg/dl or 2.2-2.7 mmol/L (SI units)
10 days-2 years: 9.0-10.6 mg/dl or 2.30-2.65 mmol/L (SI units)
<10 days: 7.6-10.4 mg/dl or 1.9-2.6 mmol/L (SI units)

Umbilical: 9.0-11.5 mg/dl or 2.25-2.88 mmol/L (SI units)
Ionized calcium:
Adult: 4.5-5.6 mg/dl or 1.05-1.30 mmol/L
2 months-18 years: 4.80-5.52 mg/dl or 1.20-1.38 mmol/L (SI units)
Newborn: 4.20-5.58 mg/dl or 1.05-1.37 mmol/L (SI units)
Urine:
Values vary with diet.
Normal diet: 100-400 mg/day or 2.5-7.5 mmol/day (SI units)
Low-calcium diet: 50-150 mg/day or 1.25-3.75 mmol/day (SI units)

Possible critical values
Blood:
Total Calcium: <6 or >13 mg/dl or <1.50 or >3.25 mmol/L (SI units)
Ionized Calcium: <2.2 or >7.0 mg/dl or <0.78 or >1.58 mmol/L (SI units)

Rationale

The serum calcium test is used to evaluate parathyroid function and calcium metabolism by directly measuring the total amount of calcium in the blood. Serum calcium is necessary in many metabolic enzymatic pathways. It is vital for muscle contractility, cardiac function, neural transmission, and blood clotting. Approximately half of the total calcium exists in the blood in its free (ionized) form, and approximately half exists in its protein-bound form (mostly with albumin). The serum calcium level is a measure of both forms. As a result, when the serum albumin level is low (as in malnourished patients), the serum calcium level also will be low, and vice versa. As a rule of thumb, the total serum calcium level decreases by approximately 0.8 mg for every 1-g decrease in the serum albumin level. Serum albumin should be measured with serum calcium.

The ionized form of calcium also can be measured by ion-selective electrode techniques or can be calculated from several available formulas. An advantage of measuring the ionized form is that it is unaffected by changes in serum albumin levels.

When the serum calcium level is elevated on at least three separate determinations, the patient is said to have *hypercalcemia*. Symptoms of hypercalcemia may include anorexia, nausea, vomiting, somnolence, and coma. The most common cause of hypercalcemia is hyperparathyroidism. Parathormone (see p. 287) causes elevated calcium levels by increasing GI absorption, decreasing urinary excretion, and increasing bone resorption. Malignancy, the second most common cause of hypercalcemia, can cause elevated calcium levels in two ways. First, tumor metastasis (myeloma, lung, breast, renal cell) to the bone can cause resorption and push calcium into the blood. Second, the cancer (lung, breast, renal cell) can produce a parathyroid hormonelike substance that drives the serum calcium up (ectopic PTH). Excess vitamin D ingestion can increase serum calcium by increasing renal and GI absorption. Granulomatous infections, such as sarcoidosis or tuberculosis, are associated with hypercalcemia.

Large blood transfusions are associated with low serum calcium levels because the citrate additives used in banked blood for anticoagulation bind the free calcium in the recipient's bloodstream. Intestinal malabsorption, rhabdomyolysis, alkalosis, and acute pancreatitis (caused by saponification of fat) also are known to be associated with low serum calcium levels. Symptoms of hypocalcemia include nervousness, excitability, and tetany.

Excretion of calcium in the urine is increased in all patients with hypercalcemia. The test is still helpful in determining the cause of recurrent nephrolithiasis. When calcium is excreted in the urine at high levels, nephrolithiasis and nephrocalcinosis is possible.

Interfering factors

Factors that interfere with determining calcium levels include the following:

- Vitamin D intoxication, which may cause *increased* serum calcium levels
- Excessive ingestion of milk, which may cause *increased* levels
- Serum pH
  A decrease in pH causes *increased* calcium levels.

- Prolonged tourniquet time
  This will lower pH and factitiously *increase* calcium levels.
- Diurnal variation
  A small diurnal variation in calcium normally occurs, with peak levels occurring at approximately 9 PM.
- Hypoalbuminemia, which is associated with *decreased* levels of total calcium
- An alkaline urine, which *decreases* urine calcium
- Prolonged immobilization
  This can be associated with mobilization of calcium from the bones and, therefore, with *increased* urine calcium levels.

Procedure
Blood:

Approximately 7 ml of peripheral venous blood is obtained from a nonfasting patient and placed in a red-top tube. The serum calcium determinations usually are part of a multiple-chemical analysis done automatically by a machine. The patient may be kept fasting for multichannel examinations. The only discomfort associated with this test is that of the venipuncture.

Urine:

Begin the 24-hour urine collection after the patient urinates. The first sample is discarded. This is the start time of the collection. All urine passed by the patient during the next 24 hours is saved.

Nursing implications with rationale
Blood:
Before

- ☞ Explain the test to the patient. If fasting is required (for multichannel determinations), inform the patient.
- Assess the patient for concurrent use of thiazide diuretics, which can cause hypercalcemia.

During

- Note that this test usually is done on a multichannel laboratory machine that is only in operation during working hours from Monday through Friday. If a calcium determination is needed on a weekend, be certain that the laboratory is aware of this and prepared to perform the serum calcium test separately.

After

- Apply pressure or a pressure dressing to the venipuncture site to prevent further bleeding. Observe the site for bleeding.

Urine:

Before

- ☞ Explain the procedure to the patient. Determine the diet regimen recommended by the specific laboratory.
- ☞ Give the patient written and oral instructions regarding dietary restrictions.

During

- ☞ Instruct the patient not to place toilet paper in the collection container.
- ☞ Remind the patient to void before defecating so that the urine is not contaminated by feces.
- Encourage the patient to drink fluids during the 24 hours, unless contraindicated for medical purposes.
- Keep the urine on ice or refrigerated during the collection period.
- Check with the laboratory regarding the need for a preservative.

After

- Send the 24-hour specimen to the laboratory as soon as it is complete.

Cortisol, Blood (Hydrocortisone, Serum Cortisol)

Test type Blood

Normal values

Adult/elderly:
    8 AM: 6-28 mg/dl or 170-625 nmol/L (SI units)
    4 PM: 2-12 mg/dl or 80-413 nmol/L (SI units)
Child (1-16 years):
    8 AM: 3-21 mg/dl
    4 PM: 3-10 mg/dl
Newborn: 1-24 mg/dl

Rationale

Cortisol is a potent glucocorticoid released from the adrenal cortex. The best method of evaluating adrenal activity is by directly measuring plasma cortisol levels. Cortisol levels normally rise and fall during the day; this is called the *diurnal variation*. Cortisol levels are highest at approximately 6 to 8 AM and gradually fall during the day to their lowest point at approximately 12 AM. Occasionally, the earliest sign of adrenal hyperfunction is only the loss of this diurnal variation, even though the cortisol levels are not yet elevated. For example, individuals with Cushing's syndrome often have top-normal plasma cortisol levels in the morning and do not exhibit a decline as the day proceeds. High levels of cortisol indicate Cushing's syndrome, and low levels of plasma cortisol are suggestive of Addison's disease.

For this test, blood usually is collected at 8 AM and again at approximately 4 PM. One would expect the 4 PM value to be one third to two thirds of the 8 AM value. Normal values may be transposed in individuals who have worked during the night and slept during the day for long periods. Cortisol can be measured in the urine. With the use of a 24-hour urine specimen, the problem of diurnal variation is eliminated.

Interfering factors

Factors that interfere with determining cortisol levels include the following:

- Pregnancy, which is associated with *increased* levels
- Physical and emotional stress, which can cause *increased* cortisol levels
  Stress is stimulatory to the pituitary-cortical mechanism, which thereby stimulates cortisol production.
- Drugs that *increase* cortisol include cortisone and spironolactone (Aldactone).
- Drugs that *decrease* cortisol include aminoglutethimide, betamethasone and other exogenous steroid medications, and metyrapone.

Procedure

At 8 AM, after the patient has had a restful sleep, 7 to 10 ml of peripheral blood is obtained in a red-top tube. It is then sent to the chemistry laboratory for analysis. A second specimen usually is taken later in the day to identify the normal diurnal variation of the plasma cortisol levels. It is important that very little anxiety be associated with the venipuncture because physical and emotional stress can artificially elevate the cortisol level.

Nursing implications with rationale

Before

☞ Explain the procedure to the patient to minimize anxiety. Stress causes elevated cortisol levels and complicates the test interpretation.

■ Assess the patient for signs of physical stress (e.g., infection or acute illness) or emotional stress, and report these to the physician.

During

■ Obtain a specimen with minimal trauma to the patient. Indicate the time of the venipuncture on the laboratory requisition slip.

After

■ Apply pressure or a pressure dressing to the venipuncture site to prevent further bleeding. Observe the site for bleeding.

C-peptide (Connecting Peptide Insulin, Insulin C-peptide, Proinsulin C-peptide)

Test type Blood

Normal values

Fasting: 0.78-1.89 ng/ml or 0.26-0.62 nmol/L (SI units)
1 hour after glucose load: 5-12 ng/ml

Rationale

C-peptide (connecting peptide) is a protein that connects the beta and alpha chains of proinsulin together. In the beta cells of the pancreatic islets of Langerhans, the chains of proinsulin are separated during the conversion of proinsulin to insulin and C-peptide. C-peptide is released into the portal vein in nearly equal amounts. Because it has a longer half-life than insulin, more C-peptide exists in the peripheral circulation. In general, C-peptide levels correlate with insulin levels in the blood. The capacity of the pancreatic beta cells to secrete insulin can be evaluated by directly measuring either insulin or C-peptide. C-peptide levels more accurately reflect islet cell function in the following situations:

1. Patients with diabetes who are treated with insulin and who have antiinsulin antibodies. This most often occurs in patients treated with bovine or pork insulin. These antibodies falsely increase insulin levels.

2. Patients who secretly administer insulin to themselves (factitious hypoglycemia). Insulin levels will be elevated. Direct insulin measurement in these patients tends to be high because the insulin measured is the self-administered exogenous insulin. C-peptide levels in that same specimen, however, will be low because exogenously administered insulin suppresses endogenous insulin (and C-peptide) production.

3. Patients with diabetes who are taking insulin. The exogenously administered insulin suppresses endogenous insulin production. Insulin levels would only measure the exogenously administered insulin, but they would not accurately reflect true islet cell function. C-peptide would be a more accurate test of islet cell function. This test is done to see if the patient with diabetes is in remission and may not need exogenous insulin.

C-peptide testing also is used to evaluate patients who are suspected of having an insulinoma (a tumor of the pancreatic islet cells that secretes insulin). It can differentiate patients with insulinoma from those with factitious hypoglycemia. In the latter group of patients, C-peptide levels are suppressed by exogenous insulin challenge. In patients with an autonomous secreting insulinoma, C-peptide levels are significantly elevated. C-peptide also can be used to monitor treatment of patients with insulinoma. A rise in C-peptide levels indicates a recurrence or progression of the insulinoma. Likewise, some clinicians use C-peptide testing as an indicator of the adequacy of therapeutic surgical pancreatectomy in patients with pancreatic tumors.

Interfering factor

A factor that interferes with determining C-peptide levels is renal failure because the majority of C-peptide is degraded in the kidney and renal failure can cause *increased* levels of C-peptide.

Procedure

After an 8- to 10-hour fast from food and medications, venipuncture is performed, and 1 red-top tube of blood is collected.

Nursing implications with rationale

Before

☞ Explain the procedure to the patient. Instruct the patient to fast for 8 to 10 hours before the test. Only water is permitted.

After

■ Apply pressure or a pressure dressing to the venipuncture site to prevent further bleeding. Observe the site for bleeding.

Dexamethasone Suppression Test
(DST, Prolonged/Rapid DST, Cortisol Suppression Test, ACTH Suppression Test)

Test type Blood

Normal values
Prolonged method:
  Low dose: >50% reduction of plasma cortisol and 17-OHCS levels
  High dose: >50% reduction of plasma cortisol and 17-OHCS levels
Rapid method:
  Nearly 0 cortisol levels

Rationale

The dexamethasone suppression test (DST) is important for diagnosing adrenal hyperfunction (Cushing's syndrome) and distinguishing its cause. The DST is based on the fact that pituitary ACTH secretion is dependent on the plasma cortisol feedback mechanism. As plasma cortisol levels increase, ACTH secretion is suppressed; as cortisol levels decrease, ACTH secretion is stimulated. Dexamethasone is a synthetic steroid (similar to cortisol) that will suppress ACTH secretion. Under normal circumstances, dexamethasone administration results in reduced stimulation to the adrenal glands and, ultimately, a drop of 50% or more in plasma cortisol and urinary 17-OHCS levels. This important feedback system does not function properly in patients with Cushing's syndrome.

In Cushing's syndrome caused by bilateral adrenal hyperplasia (Cushing's disease), the pituitary gland responds only to high plasma levels of cortisol and other steroids. In Cushing's syndrome caused by adrenal adenoma or cancer (which acts autonomously), cortisol secretion will continue despite a decrease in ACTH. When Cushing's syndrome is caused by an ectopic, ACTH-producing tumor (as in lung cancer), that tumor also is considered autonomous and will continue to secrete ACTH despite high cortisol levels. Again, no decrease occurs in plasma cortisol. The following list outlines the causes for Cushing's syndrome and their respective DST levels:

1. Cushing's syndrome caused by bilateral adrenal hyperplasia
   Low dose: no change
   High dose: 50% reduction of plasma cortisol and 17-OHCS levels
2. Cushing's syndrome caused by adrenal adenoma or carcinoma
   Low dose: no change
   High dose: no change
3. Cushing's syndrome caused by ectopic, ACTH-producing tumor
   Low dose: no change
   High dose: no change

The DST also may identify patients with depression who are likely to respond to electroconvulsive therapy or antidepressants rather than to psychologic or social interventions. ACTH production will not be suppressed after administration of low-dose dexamethasone in these patients.

The prolonged DST can be performed over a 6-day period on an outpatient basis. The rapid DST is easily and quickly performed and is used primarily as a screening test to diagnose Cushing's syndrome. It is less accurate and less informative than the prolonged DST, but when its results are normal, the diagnosis of Cushing's syndrome can safely be excluded. The ease with which the rapid DST can be performed makes it useful in clinical medicine.

Interfering factor

A factor that interferes with determining DST levels is stress. Physical and emotional stress can elevate ACTH release and obscure interpretation of test results. Stress is stimulatory to the pituitary, which secretes ACTH.

Procedure

In the prolonged test, urinary 17-OHCS levels usually are measured. However, with the increased ease in obtaining plasma cortisol levels, this measurement is gradually replacing the urine determination. Specific protocols vary among laboratories performing this test. The following description, however, is a classic example of a dexamethasone suppression test:

Day 1: A baseline 24-hour urine test for corticosteroids (urinary 17-OHCS or urinary cortisol) is done.
Day 2: Same as Day 1.
Day 3: A low dose (0.5 mg) of dexamethasone is given by mouth every 6 hours, for a total of 2 mg/day. A 24-hour urine test for corticosteroids is done (as on Days 1 and 2).
Day 4: Same as Day 3.
Day 5: A high dose (2 mg) of dexamethasone is given by mouth every 6 hours, for a total of 8 mg/day. A 24-hour urine test for corticosteroids is done.
Day 6: Same as Day 5.

The creatinine clearance (see p. 237) should be measured in all 24-hour urine collections to demonstrate the accuracy and adequacy of the collection period. Creatinine excretion varies very little from day to day. The urine sample for cortisol and 17-OHCS should not contain a preservative. The specimen is kept refrigerated or on ice during the collection period and is sent to the chemistry laboratory at the end of each 24-hour period.

For the rapid dexamethasone suppression test, 1 mg of dexamethasone is given to the patient by mouth at 11 PM. The patient also is sedated with a barbiturate to ensure a restful sleep. At 8 AM the next morning, the patient's plasma cortisol level is determined before he or she rises, as described on p. 301. If there is no cortisol suppression after 1 mg of dexamethasone, 8 mg may be given to suppress ACTH production. This is often referred to as the *overnight 8 mg dexamethasone suppression test.*

Nursing implications with rationale

Before

☞ Explain the procedure to the patient. Allow plenty of time to answer questions so that anxiety (stress) is diminished as much as possible. Stress can cause ACTH release and obscure the interpretation of test results.

■ Obtain the patient's weight as a baseline for evaluating side effects of steroids.

■ Administer the dexamethasone orally at the exact time it is ordered, with milk or an antacid (if ordered) to prevent gastric irritation. Administer a hypnotic, if ordered, to ensure that the patient sleeps restfully.

During

☞ Instruct the patient to begin the 24-hour urine collection after discarding the first morning specimen. This is the start time of the 24-hour collection.

■ Instruct the patient to void before defecating so that the urine is not contaminated by feces.

■ Remind the patient not to put toilet paper in the collection container.

■ Keep the urine specimen on ice or refrigerated during the 24 hours.

■ Collect the last specimen as close as possible to the end of the 24 hours.

■ In studies such as the DST, when six continuous 24-hour urine collections are needed, no urine specimens are discarded except for the first one, after which the collection begins.

After

■ Send specimens to the laboratory promptly.

■ Assess the patient for steroid-induced side effects by monitoring the patient's weight daily, checking the urine for glucose and acetone, as-

sessing serum potassium levels, and evaluating the patient for evidence of gastric irritation.
- Apply pressure or a pressure dressing to the venipuncture site to prevent further bleeding. Observe the site for bleeding.

Glucagon

Test type Blood

Normal values
30-210 pg/ml or 30-210 ng/L (SI units)

Rationale
Glucagon is a hormone secreted by the alpha cells of the pancreatic islets of Langerhans. Glucagon is secreted in response to hypoglycemia and increases the blood glucose. As serum glucose levels rise in the blood, glucagon is inhibited by a negative feedback mechanism.

Elevated glucagon levels may indicate the diagnosis of a glucagonoma (i.e., an alpha islet cell neoplasm). Glucagon deficiency occurs with extensive pancreatic resection or with burned out pancreatitis. Arginine is a potent stimulator of glucagon. If the glucagon levels fail to rise even with arginine infusion, the diagnosis of glucagon deficiency as a result of pancreatic insufficiency is confirmed.

Glucagon normally decreases after ingestion of a carbohydrate-loaded meal through an elaborate negative feedback mechanism. In patients with diabetes, this does not occur. Furthermore, in the patient with insulin-dependent diabetes, glucagon stimulation caused by hypoglycemia does not occur. To differentiate between pancreatic insufficiency and diabetes, arginine stimulation is performed. The patient with diabetes will have an exaggerated elevation of glucagon with arginine. In pancreatic insufficiency, glucagon is not stimulated with arginine.

Because glucagon is thought to be metabolized by the kidneys, renal failure is associated with high glucagon levels and, as a result, high glucose levels. When rejection of a transplanted kidney occurs, one of the first signs of rejection may be increased serum glucagon levels.

Interfering factors
Factors that interfere with determining glucagon levels include the following:

- Recent radioactive scan
  Test results may be invalidated if a patient has undergone a radioactive scan within the previous 48 hours. Glucagon is measured by radioimmunoassay (RIA). Administration of radionuclides can affect results.
- Prolonged fasting, stress, or moderate to severe exercise, because they cause *increased* levels

Procedure
Fasting is necessary for 10 to 12 hours before the test. Only water is permitted. Approximately 7 ml of venous blood is collected in a lavender-top tube.

Nursing implications with rationale
Before
- Explain the procedure to the patient. Tell the patient that fasting, except for water, is necessary for 10 to 12 hours before the test.

After
- Apply pressure or a pressure dressing to the venipuncture site to prevent further bleeding. Observe the site for bleeding.
- Place the specimen on ice and send it immediately to the laboratory.

Glucose, Blood (Blood Sugar, Fasting Blood Sugar, FBS)

Test type Blood

Normal values
Elderly: increase in normal range after age 50
Child >2 years to adult: 70-105 mg/dl or 3.9-5.8 mmol/L
Child <2 years: 60-100 mg/dl or 3.3-5.5 mmol/L
Infant: 40-90 mg/dl or 2.2-5.0 mmol/L
Neonate: 30-60 mg/dl or 1.7-3.3 mmol/L
Premature infant: 20-60 mg/dl or 1.1-3.3 mmol/L
Cord: 45-96 mg/dl or 2.5-5.3 mmol/L (SI units)

Possible critical values
Adult male: <50 and >400 mg/dl

Adult female: <40 and >400 mg/dl

Infant: <40 mg/dl

Newborn: <30 and >300 mg/dl

Rationale

The serum glucose test is helpful in diagnosing many metabolic diseases. Serum glucose levels must be evaluated according to the time of the day they are performed. For example, a glucose level of 135 mg/dl may be abnormal if the patient is in the fasting state. However, it would be within normal limits if the patient had eaten a meal within the last hour. In general, true glucose elevations indicate diabetes mellitus (DM). However, one must be aware of other possible causes of hyperglycemia. These include:

1. Acute stress response (e.g., to surgery), mediated through epinephrine and glucocorticosteroid secretion
2. Cushing's disease, which causes elevated glucocorticoid levels (see Table 8-2, p. 290)
3. Pheochromocytoma, a tumor that causes increased levels of epinephrine
4. Hyperthyroidism, which is associated with increased levels of catecholamine
5. Adenoma (glucagonoma) of the pancreas, which causes pancreatic secretion of glucagon (a hyperglycemic agent)
6. Pancreatitis, in which there is destruction of islet cells (where insulin is produced)
7. Diuretics (e.g., furosemide and thiazides), which suppress insulin release by inducing hypokalemia
8. Corticosteroid therapy, which causes a chemically induced diabetes
9. IV administration of dextrose
10. Drugs associated with elevated glucose levels, including steroids, isoniazid, tricyclic antidepressants, beta-blockers, and phenothiazines

Similarly, hypoglycemia (i.e., low serum glucose levels) has many causes. The most common cause, however, is insulin overdose. Glucose determinations must be performed frequently in patients with newly diagnosed diabetes to monitor constantly the dosage of insulin being administered. Other causes of hypoglycemia include:

1. Insulinoma, an insulin-producing tumor of the pancreatic islet cells
2. Hypothyroidism, as a result of decreased levels of thyroid hormones
3. Hypopituitarism, as a result of decreased levels of glucose-elevating hormones (growth hormone, thyroid hormone, and ACTH)
4. Addison's disease, as a result of cortisol deficiency (see Table 8-2, p. 290)
5. Extensive liver disease, as a result of the inability of the liver to produce glycogen (a storage form of glucose)
6. An overdose of insulin or oral hypoglycemic agents

Procedure

For a fasting blood sugar (FBS) test, the patient fasts for at least 8 hours, usually from midnight on the day of the test. Water is permitted. The patient should not fast longer than 16 hours before the study is performed to prevent starvation effects, which may artificially raise the glucose level. A peripheral venipuncture is performed, and approximately 7 ml of venous blood is placed in a red- or gray-top tube and sent to the chemistry laboratory. The blood should be obtained before insulin or hypoglycemic agents are administered.

Serum glucose levels should be obtained on any diabetic patient suspected of having an insulin reaction. The blood should be obtained before oral or IV glucose administration. Glucose determinations now are a part of most multichannel specimen analyses. Blood glucose self-monitoring (as described in the following section) is widely done, with some diabetic patients evaluating their glucose levels as often as before every meal and at bedtime.

Blood glucose self-monitoring

Today blood glucose self-monitoring is replacing urine testing for many diabetic patients. Blood monitoring is important because it directly reflects the current serum glucose level. This is in contrast to urine glucose testing (see p. 313), which indirectly assesses the serum glucose level of several hours earlier and which is affected by renal threshold. Self-monitoring of glucose is especially important for the detection of hypoglycemia, which is not detected in urine specimens. A diabetic patient can test his or her blood independently whenever hypoglycemia is suspected.

To benefit from blood glucose self-monitoring, the diabetic patient must learn how to correctly perform the blood test, keep accurate records, and interpret the test results. Having written guidelines describing any alteration in his or her diabetic regimen also is essential. The correct method for accurately self-monitoring blood glucose levels is as follows:

1. Wash both hands with soap and water.
2. Let one arm hang below the level of the heart, and "milk" the finger to be used for the blood sample.
3. Prick the side of the finger, rather than the middle of the finger, to minimize pain and increase blood flow. A lancet or a needle may be used, but a device such as an Autolet, Autoclix, Hemalet, Monojet, or Penlet that has a spring-loaded lancet and a platform to control the depth of penetration is easier to use.
4. "Milk" the finger until a ¼-inch wide drop of blood hangs from the finger.
5. Hold the finger over the reagent strip and touch the reagent area of the strip to the drop of blood. The drop must cover the entire reagent area.

There are two types of self-glucose monitoring tests: the visually read tests and the reflectance meters. Examples of the visually read test, which allows the diabetic patient to make the glucose determination by sight, include Chemstrip bG, Dextrostix, and Visidex. The advantage of the visually read test is that it does not require expensive machinery, machinery calibration, or controlled testing. The disadvantage is that the patient must visually interpret the test results. The color of the reagent strip must be compared with the color chart on the bottle from which it came, *not* from another bottle even of the same brand. If the color falls between two reference blocks, the patient must estimate the results.

The second type of self-glucose monitoring is the reflectance meters. Product examples include the Dextrometer, Glucometer, AccuChek bG, Glucoscan-II, and the Stat Tek. Although these meters may improve the accuracy of the blood glucose determination, the process is far more complex. The machine must first be calibrated, then a control test must be done to check the accuracy of the calibration, and, finally, the test is performed using the patient's blood.

Nursing implications with rationale
Before
- Explain the procedure to the patient. Verify that the patient understands the timing of the test in relation to meals. If fasting is required, instruct the patient not to eat breakfast until the blood is obtained.
- Explain to the patient that insulin or oral hypoglycemic agents will be withheld until after the blood is obtained because these drugs lower the blood glucose level.
- If the patient will have repeated blood glucose determinations (e.g., daily fasting and 3 PM blood glucose tests), explain the reasoning for this. Allow the patient time to verbalize his or her feelings regarding repeated venous punctures.

After
- Apply pressure or a pressure dressing to the venipuncture site to prevent further bleeding. Observe the site for bleeding.

Case Study
Adolescent with Diabetes Mellitus

M.F., a 16-year-old high-school football player, was brought to the emergency room in a coma. His mother said that during the past month he had lost 12 pounds. She reported that he also had had excessive thirst associated with voluminous urination that

Continued

Case Study

Adolescent with Diabetes Mellitus—cont'd

often required voiding several times during the night. There was a strong family history of DM. The results of physical examination were essentially negative except for sinus tachycardia and Kussmaul respirations.

Studies	Results
Serum glucose test (on admission), p. 305	1100 mg/dl (normal: 60-120 mg/dl)
Arterial blood gases (ABGs) test (on admission), p. 145	
pH	7.23 (normal: 7.35-7.45)
Pco_2	30 mm Hg (normal: 35-45 mm Hg)
HCO_2	12 mEq/L (normal: 22-26 mEq/L)
Serum osmolality test, p. 323	440 mOsm/kg (normal: 275-300 mOsm/kg)
Serum glucose test, p. 305	250 mg/dl (normal: 70-115 mg/dl)
2-hour postprandial glucose test (2-hour PPG), p. 309	500 mg/dl (normal: <140 mg/dl)
Glucose tolerance test (GTT), p. 310	
Fasting blood glucose	150 mg/dl (normal: 70-115 mg/dl)
30 minutes	300 mg/dl (normal: <200 mg/dl)
1 hour	325 mg/dl (normal: <200 mg/dl)
2 hours	390 mg/dl (normal: <140 mg/dl)
3 hours	300 mg/dl (normal: 70-115 mg/dl)
4 hours	260 mg/dl (normal: 70-115 mg/dl)
Glycosylated hemoglobin, p. 315	9% (normal: <7%)

Diagnostic Analysis

M.F.'s symptoms and diagnostic studies were classic for hyperglycemic ketoacidosis associated with DM. The glycosylated hemoglobin showed that he had been hyperglycemic over the last several months. The results of his ABGs test on admission indicated metabolic acidosis with some respiratory compensation. He was treated in the emergency room with IV regular insulin and IV fluids.

During the first 72 hours of hospitalization, M.F. was monitored with frequent serum glucose determinations. Insulin was administered according to the results of these studies. M.F.'s condition was eventually stabilized on 40 U of Humulin N insulin daily. Comprehensive patient instruction regarding self-blood glucose monitoring (see p. 307), insulin administration, diet, exercise, foot care, and recognition of the signs and symptoms of hyperglycemia and hypoglycemia was given.

Critical Thinking Questions

1. Why was this patient in metabolic acidosis?
2. Do you think M.F. will be switched eventually to an oral hypoglycemic agent?

Glucose, Postprandial (2-Hour Postprandial Glucose [2-Hour PPG], 2-Hour Postprandial Blood Sugar, 1-Hour Glucose Screen for Gestational Diabetes Mellitus [GDM])

Test type Blood

Normal values

2-hour PPG:
>60 years: <160 mg/dl
50-60 years: <150 mg/dl
0-50 years: <140 mg/dl or
<7.8 mmol/L (SI units)
1-hour glucose screen for gestational diabetes:
<140 mg/dl

Rationale

The 2-hour postprandial glucose (PPG) test is a measurement of the amount of glucose in the patient's blood 2 hours after a meal (postprandial) is ingested. It is used to diagnose DM. For this study, a meal acts as a glucose challenge to the body's metabolism. Insulin normally is secreted immediately after a meal in response to the elevated blood glucose level and causes the level to return to the preprandial range within 2 hours. In patients with diabetes, the glucose level usually is still elevated 2 hours after the meal. The PPG is an easily performed screening test for DM. If the results are greater than 140 mg/dl and less than 200 mg/dl, a glucose tolerance test (see p. 310) may be performed to confirm the diagnosis. If the 2-hour PPG is greater than 200 mg/dl, the diagnosis of DM is confirmed. A GTT or glycosylated hemoglobin also can be performed to corroborate and better evaluate the disease.

The 1-hour glucose screen is used to detect gestational diabetes mellitus (GDM), which is the most common medical complication of pregnancy. GDM is a carbohydrate intolerance first recognized during pregnancy. GDM affects 3% to 8% of pregnant women, with up to half of these women developing overt diabetes later in life. The detection and treatment of GDM may reduce the risk for several adverse perinatal outcomes (e.g., excessive fetal growth and birth trauma, fetal death, or neonatal morbidity). Screening for GDM is performed with a 50-g oral glucose load followed by a glucose level determination 1 hour later. Screening is done between weeks 24 and 28 of gestation.

Interfering factors

Factors that interfere with determining postprandial glucose levels include the following:

- Smoking during the testing period, which may *increase* the blood glucose level
- Stress
  This can *increase* glucose levels through the catecholamine affect of increasing serum glucose.
- Eating
  If the patient eats a small snack or eats candy during the 2-hour interval, glucose levels will be falsely *increased.*
- Incomplete test meal
  If the patient is not able to eat the entire test meal or vomits some or all of the meal, levels will be falsely *decreased.*

Procedure

The patient is given a routine meal, consisting of at least 50 to 75 g of carbohydrates. Two hours after the meal, 7 ml of peripheral venous blood is obtained in a gray- or red-top tube and taken to the chemistry laboratory for glucose determination.

Nursing implications with rationale

Before
- Explain the procedure to the patient. Instruct the patient to eat the entire meal and then not to eat anything else until the blood is drawn.
- Inform the patient that smoking is prohibited, because it may increase the blood sugar level.

During
- Make sure the blood is drawn at the appropriate time.

After
- Apply pressure or a pressure dressing to the venipuncture site to prevent further bleeding. Observe the site for bleeding.

Glucose Tolerance Test (GTT, Oral Glucose Tolerance Test [OGTT])

Test type Blood, urine

Normal values

Serum test:
Fasting: 70-115 mg/dl or <6.4 mmol/L (SI units)
30 minutes: <200 mg/dl or <11.1 mmol/L (SI units)
1 hour: <200 mg/dl or <11.1 mmol/L (SI units)
2 hours: <140 mg/dl or <7.8 mmol/L (SI units)
3 hours: 70-115 mg/dl or <6.4 mmol/L (SI units)
4 hours: 70-115 mg/dl or <6.4 mmol/L (SI units)

Urine test: Negative

Rationale

The National Diabetes Data Group (NDDG) has defined criteria for the diagnosis of DM (Table 8-4). These include the following:

1. Sufficient clinical symptoms (polydipsia, polyuria, ketonuria, and weight loss), plus unequivocal elevation in FBS or a non-FBS of greater than 200 mg/100 ml
2. Elevated FBS of greater than 140 mg/100 ml on more than one occasion
3. A normal FBS, but a GTT peak and 2-hour value of greater than 200 mg/100 ml on more than one occasion

The GTT, then, is used when diabetes is suspected (retinopathy, neuropathy, diabetic-type renal diseases), but the criteria for the diagnosis cannot be met without the data obtained by the GTT.

The GTT also is suggested for the following:

1. Patients with a family history of diabetes
2. Patients who are massively obese
3. Patients with a history of recurrent infections
4. Patients with delayed healing of wounds, especially on the lower legs or feet
5. Women who have a history of delivering large babies, still births, or premature births
6. Patients who have transient glycosuria or hyperglycemia during pregnancy or following myocardial infarction, surgery, or stress

TABLE 8-4 **National Diabetes Data Group's Reclassification of Diabetic Patients**

NDDG Classification	Diagnosis*	Old Classification
Diabetes mellitus (insulin- and noninsulin-dependent)	Unequivocal signs/symptoms	Overt diabetes
	FBS >140 more than once; glucose tolerance peak or 2 hour >200 more than once	
Impaired glucose tolerance test	FBS normal and *either* glucose tolerance peak or 2 hour >200	Latent (chemical) diabetes
Previous abnormality of glucose tolerance	Normal glucose tolerance test but previous abnormal glucose tolerance test	Subclinical diabetes
Potential abnormality of glucose tolerance test	Genetic predisposition to diabetes (family history)	Prediabetes
Gestational diabetes mellitus	Onset of unequivocal diabetes or glucose tolerance test results exceeding pregnancy criteria†	Diabetes of pregnancy

*Glucose levels are recorded in mg/100 ml.
†Onset or recognition of criteria during pregnancy but not before.

In the GTT, the patient's ability to tolerate a standard oral glucose load is evaluated by obtaining serum and urine specimens for glucose level determinations before glucose administration and then at 30 minutes, 1 hour, 2 hours, 3 hours, and sometimes 4 hours after the administration. A rapid insulin response normally occurs after the ingestion of a large oral glucose load. This response peaks in 30 to 60 minutes and returns to normal in approximately 3 hours. Patients with an appropriate insulin response are able to tolerate the glucose dose easily, with only a minimal and transient rise in serum glucose levels within 1 to 2 hours after ingestion. In normal patients, glucose will not spill over into the urine.

Patients with diabetes, however, will not be able to tolerate this load. As a result, their serum glucose levels will be greatly elevated from 1 to 5 hours (Figure 8-6). Glucose also can be detected in their urine.

Gestational diabetes also can be diagnosed by the GTT. Generally, the diagnosis of diabetes can be made if two or more of the results exceed the following values:

Fasting: 105 mg/dl
1 hour: 190 mg/dl
2 hours: 165 mg/dl
3 hours: 145 mg/dl

GI absorption can vary among individuals. For that reason, some health care centers prefer the administration of an IV glucose load rather than an oral glucose load, which depends on GI absorption. In addition, patients occasionally are unable to tolerate the oral glucose load (e.g., patients with prior gastrectomy, short-bowel syndrome, or malabsorption). In these instances, an intravenous glucose tolerance test (IV-GTT) can be performed by intravenously administering the glucose load. The values for the IV-GTT differ slightly from those of the oral GTT because the IV glucose is absorbed faster.

The GTT also is used to evaluate patients with hypoglycemia. This hypoglycemia may occur as late as 5 hours after the initial glucose load.

Potential complications
Potential complications associated with GTT are as follows:

■ Dizziness, tremors, anxiety, sweating, euphoria, or fainting
  If these symptoms occur, a blood specimen is obtained. If the glucose level is too high, the test may need to be stopped, and insulin may need to be administered.

Interfering factors
Factors that interfere with GTT include the following:

■ Stress (e.g., from surgery, infection), because it can *increase* glucose levels
■ Exercise during the testing, which can affect glucose levels
■ Fasting or reduced caloric intake before GTT, which can cause glucose intolerance

Procedure
After at least 3 days of consuming a high-carbohydrate diet (at least 200 to 300 g), the patient is kept NPO except for water after midnight on the day of the test. A specimen for an FBS test is obtained, and the patient's urine is tested for glucose and acetone (see p. 313). The patient is then given a 100-g carbohydrate load, usually in the form of a carbonated sugar beverage (Glucola) or a cherry-flavored gelatin (Gel-a-dex). If

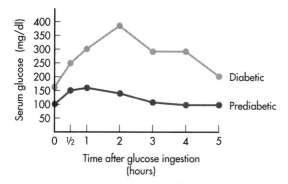

Figure 8-6 Glucose tolerance test curve for a diabetic patient and a prediabetic patient.

these commercial preparations are unavailable, 100 g of glucose is dissolved in water and flavored with lemon juice to increase its palatability. The entire glucose load must be ingested by the patient, because the GTT normal values are based on consumption of the standard 100 g of glucose. For children weighing less than 100 pounds, 1 g of glucose/pound of body weight is given. Serum and urine specimens for glucose level determination are obtained at 30 minutes, 1 hour, 2 hours, 3 hours, 4 hours, and sometimes 5 hours after ingestion of the carbohydrate load. During the testing period (approximately 5 hours) the patient is not permitted to eat or smoke. The patient is encouraged to drink water, however, so that urine specimens can be obtained more easily.

During the testing period, especially between the second and third hours, the patient should be assessed for reactions such as dizziness, sweating, weakness, and giddiness. These reactions are usually transient. This study can be performed in the outpatient department or in the patient's hospital room. The duration of this study is approximately 5 hours.

To perform an IV-GTT, a specimen for fasting blood glucose level determination is obtained. A 50% glucose solution (or glucose, 0.33 g/kg of ideal body weight in adults, or 0.5 g/kg body weight in children) is administered intravenously over a 3- to 4-minute period. Blood samples are obtained as indicated by the laboratory. These usually are obtained at 30-minute and 1-, 2-, and 3-hour intervals. The values for the IV-GTT differ slightly from those for the oral-GTT, because the IV glucose is absorbed faster. Both the oral- and IV-GTTs are uncomfortable because of the number of venipunctures required for blood glucose determinations.

Nursing implications with rationale
Before
- Explain the procedure to the patient. Allow the patient ample time to express his or her fears concerning this study and the potential diagnosis of DM. Many patients are anxious regarding the procedure for this study, because approximately six venipunctures are required in a 4- to 5-hour period. Outpatients who feel faint during blood withdrawal should be placed on a bed or gurney in the supine position during venipuncture.
- Give the patient written instructions explaining the pretest dietary requirements. An inadequate diet before the GTT may diminish carbohydrate tolerance and cause high glucose levels, simulating those found in DM.
- Instruct the patient to fast for 12 hours before the test.
- Obtain the patient's weight to determine the appropriate glucose loading dose.
- Encourage the patient to bring reading material or craft work to alleviate some of the boredom associated with this study.
- Give the patient the necessary urine containers, and write down the times at which specimens are needed. Encourage the patient to drink water to help obtain the urine specimens.
- Instruct the patient not to have anything by mouth during the study except for water. Tobacco, coffee, and tea are not allowed because they cause physiologic stimulation, which can alter the test results.
- Instruct the patient not to take any drugs (e.g., steroids) during the test period that may alter GTT results.

During
- Collect the blood samples at the designated times.
- If the patient has tremors, dizziness, euphoria, or other reactions during the study, obtain a blood specimen immediately. If the glucose level is too high, the test may need to be stopped, and insulin may need to be administered.

After
- Apply pressure or a pressure dressing to the venipuncture site to prevent further bleeding. Observe the site for bleeding.
- Instruct the patient to eat and drink normally. Insulin or oral hypoglycemics may be administered, if ordered.

Glucose, Urine (Urine Sugar, Urine Glucose)

Ketones, Urine (Beta-Hydroxybutyric Acid, Acetoacetic Acid, and Acetone)

Test type Urine

Normal values

Random specimen for glucose and ketones: negative

24-hour specimen for glucose: <0.5 g/day or <2.78 mmol/day (SI units)

Rationale

Glucose

A qualitative glucose test usually is part of a routine urinalysis (see p. 268). This screening test for the presence of glucose in the urine may indicate the likelihood of DM or other causes of glucose intolerance (see p. 306). This diagnosis must be confirmed by other tests (e.g., fasting glucose, GTT, glycosylated hemoglobin test). Urine glucose tests also can be used to monitor the effectiveness of diabetes therapy.

Glucose normally is filtered from the blood by the glomeruli of the kidney. The glucose concentration in the glomerular filtrate is the same as in the blood. Normally, all of the glucose is reabsorbed in the proximal renal tubules. When the blood glucose level exceeds the capability of the renal threshold to reabsorb the glucose (approximately 180 mg/dl), it begins to spill over into the urine (glycosuria). As the blood glucose level increases further, the amount of glucose spilling into the urine also increases.

Glucosuria is not always abnormal. It may occur immediately after eating a high-carbohydrate meal. It can also occur in normal or prediabetic patients who are receiving dextrose-containing IV fluids. Furthermore, glucosuria does not always indicate diabetes, but can occur normally or in diseases that affect the renal tubule or in genetic defects in metabolism and excretion of glucose. In these diseases, the renal threshold for glucose is abnormally low. Despite a normal blood glucose, the kidney cannot reabsorb the normal glucose load. As a result, the surplus of glucose is spilled into the urine. These patients have normal GTT results.

Ketones

When a patient with poorly controlled diabetes becomes hyperglycemic, massive fatty acid catabolism occurs. This catabolism occurs in order to provide an energy source when glucose cannot be transferred into the cell because of an insufficiency of insulin. Ketones (beta-hydroxybutyric acid, acetoacetic acid, and acetone) are the end products of this fatty acid breakdown. Like glucose, ketones spill over into the urine when their levels are elevated in the blood. (Nondiabetic causes of ketonuria are described in Chapter 7, under ketones, p. 271).

Because urine glucose and acetone determinations are easy to perform and painless to obtain and accurately reflect serum glucose levels, they are used to monitor insulin therapy in diabetic patients. These determinations, however, are being supplanted by self-monitoring of blood glucose (see p. 307). Negative results for glucose and acetone are not necessarily indicative of a stable condition. Although these results would rule out hyperglycemia, the patient could be hypoglycemic. As a result, many physicians prefer that juvenile diabetic patients show a trace of glucose in their urine because glucose levels in young diabetic patients are very difficult to regulate and often swing rapidly from hyperglycemic to hypoglycemic.

Interfering factors

Factors that interfere with determining urine glucose and acetone levels include the following:

- Drugs that may cause false-positive tests with Clinitest, but not with Clinistix or Tes-Tape, include acetylsalicylic acid, aminosalicylic acid, ascorbic acid, cephalothin, chloral hydrate, nitrofurantoin, streptomycin, and sulfonamides.

■ Any substance that can reduce the copper in Clinitest can produce positive results. This may include other sugars such as galactose, fructose, or lactose.

Procedure

Fractional urine tests for glucose and acetone are performed at specified times during the day, generally before meals and at bedtime. Test results are used to determine the patient's insulin requirements.

Because accuracy is necessary, the urine specimen for testing should contain fresh urine only. Stagnant urine that has been in the patient's bladder for several hours does not accurately reveal the amount of urine glucose and acetone at the time of the testing because such a specimen may contain a mixture of glucose-free and glucose-containing urine. For this reason, a double-voided specimen is preferred. This is obtained by collecting a urine specimen 30 to 40 minutes before the time the test specimen is actually needed. This first specimen is discarded, and the patient is given a glass of water (approximately 8 ounces) to drink. A second specimen is then obtained at the required time and tested for glucose and acetone. The result obtained from this double-voided, or second, specimen accurately reflects the amount of glucose in urine recently filtered by the kidney.

Urine glucose and acetone are easily detected by using a Keto-diastix or Multistix reagent strip. The reagent strip is completely immersed in a well-mixed urine specimen and removed immediately to avoid diluting the reagents. The strip is held in a horizontal position to prevent possible mixing of the chemical reagents and, at the time indicated, is compared with the test chart located on the jar of reagent strips. The ketone reading is made at exactly 15 seconds, and the glucose reading is made at exactly 30 seconds. The ketone results vary from negative to 3+ (large). The glucose results range from negative to 4+, or 2%.

Urine glucose testing also can be performed quickly and easily by the Clinitest method (a copper-reducing method). For this study, a test tube, medicine dropper, Clinitest tablet, and color chart are required. Five drops of well-mixed urine are placed in a test tube containing 10 drops of water. After the Clinitest tablet is placed into the test tube, boiling ensues for a few seconds. The resultant color change (pea green to yellow-green to yellow or brown) permits estimation of the approximate content of sugar up to 2%. This test can be modified to allow estimation of sugar concentrations up to 5% by using 2 (instead of 5) drops of urine and 10 drops of water. A special color chart is used, with a scale ranging from 0% to 5%. This modification is particularly useful in children, in whom marked glycosuria may escape recognition by the standard (5-drop) procedure.

Acetone in the urine can be detected by Acetest tablets. For this test, a drop of urine is placed on an Acetest tablet. If acetone is present, varying shades of lavender appear; these can be compared with a color chart after the time period indicated in the instructions.

Nursing implications with rationale

Before

🖋 Explain the purpose of urine glucose and acetone testing. Teach the diabetic patient how to perform this test accurately.

🖋 Inform the patient that urine tests for glucose and ketones may be performed at specified times during the day, generally before meals and at bedtime, and that test results may be used to determine insulin requirements.

■ Read the directions on the container of the reagent strips or tablets. Compare the color reaction with the manufacturer's color chart at the exact time specified. Check the expiration date on the bottle before use. Tightly close the bottle after removing the reagent strips or tablets to prevent them from absorbing moisture and altering future results.

■ If the patient is receiving cephalothin (Keflin) intravenously or cephalexin (Keflex) orally, do not use Clinitest tablets, because false-positive results can be obtained. Therefore, use reagent strips for these patients.

After

■ Record the urine glucose and/or ketones results. Treat as indicated.

Glycosylated Hemoglobin (GHb, GHB, Glycohemoglobin, Hemoglobin [Hb] A_{1c}, Diabetic Control Index)

Test type Blood

Normal values
Adult/elderly: 4% to 8%
Child: <7%
Good diabetic control: 7% to 10%
Fair diabetic control: 11% to 13%
Poor diabetic control: >13%
Values vary with the laboratory method employed.

Rationale
The glycosylated hemoglobin (GHb) test is used to monitor diabetes treatment because it provides an accurate, long-term index of the patient's average blood glucose level. GHb measures the amount of hemoglobin A_{1c} (Hb A_{1c}) in the blood. In adults, about 98% of the Hb in the red blood cell (RBC) is Hb A. About 7% of Hb A consists of a type of Hb (Hb A_1) that can bind strongly with glucose in a process called *glycosylation.* Once glycosylation occurs, it is not easily reversible. Hb A_1 is actually made up of three components: Hb A_{1a}, A_{1b}, and A_{1c}. Hb A_{1c} is the component that most strongly binds with glucose. Hb A_{1c} makes up the majority of the Hb A_1. About 70% of Hb A_{1c} is glycosylated. Only 20% of A_{1a} and A_{1b} are glycosylated. Hb A_{1c} is the most accurate measurement because it represents the majority of GHb. If total Hb A_1 is measured, its value is always 2% to 4% higher than that of the Hb A_{1c} component. Most often, total Hb A_1 is measured and reported as a percentage of total Hb A. Hb A_{1c} is fast becoming the more common measurement.

As the RBC circulates, it combines its Hb A_1 with some of the glucose in the bloodstream to form GHb. The amount of GHb depends on the amount of glucose available in the bloodstream over the 120-day life span of the RBC. Therefore, determination of the GHb value reflects the average blood sugar level for the 100- to 120-day period before the test. The more glucose the RBC was exposed to, the greater the GHb percentage. One important advantage of this test is that the sample can be drawn at any time because it is not affected by short-term variations (e.g., food intake, exercise, stress, hypoglycemic agents, patient cooperation). It is possible, however, for very high, short-term blood glucose levels to cause an elevation of GHb; the degree of glucose elevation usually results not from a transient high level, but from a persistent, moderate elevation over the entire life of the RBC.

The elevation in GHb occurs approximately 3 weeks after the sustained elevation in blood glucose. It takes at least 4 weeks for the GHb to decrease after a sustained reduction in blood glucose.

The GHb test is particularly beneficial for:

1. Evaluating the success of and patient compliance with diabetic treatment
2. Comparing and contrasting the success of past and new forms of diabetic therapy
3. Determining the duration of hyperglycemia in patients with newly diagnosed diabetes
4. Providing a sensitive estimate of glucose imbalance in patients with mild diabetes
5. Individualizing diabetic control regimens
6. Encouraging patients when the test shows achievement of good diabetic control
7. Evaluating the diabetic whose glucose levels change significantly day to day (brittle diabetic)
8. Differentiating short-term hyperglycemia in nondiabetic patients (e.g., recent stress or MI) from diabetes (in which the glucose has been persistently elevated).

Interfering factors
Factors that interfere with determining GHb levels include the following:

■ Hemoglobinopathies
The quantity of Hb A (and, as a result, Hb A_1) varies considerably in these diseases.
■ Increased RBC life span
Falsely *elevated* values occur when the RBC life span is lengthened because the Hb A_1 has a longer period available for glycosylation.

Procedure

No fasting is required. Peripheral venipuncture is performed, and approximately 3 to 5 ml of blood is obtained.

Nursing implications with rationale

Before

☞ Explain to the patient what the GHb test is and how it helps monitor his or her therapy. This test motivates most patients to follow their control regimen and to take a more active part in their self-care.

☞ Explain to the patient why fasting is not indicated. Most diabetic patients are accustomed to fasting for blood tests.

After

■ Apply pressure or a pressure dressing to the venipuncture site to prevent further bleeding. Observe the site for bleeding.

Growth Hormone (GH, Human Growth Hormone [HGH], Somatotropin Hormone [SH])

Somatomedin C (Insulin-like Growth Factor I, IGF-I)

Growth Hormone Stimulation Test (GH Provocation Test, Insulin Tolerance Test [ITT], Arginine Test)

Test type Blood

Normal values

GH:
Men: <5 ng/ml or <5 μg/L (SI units)
Women: <10 ng/ml or <10 μg/L
Children: 0-10 ng/ml or 0-10 μg/L
Newborn: 10-40 ng/ml or 10-40 μg/L
Somatomedin C:
Adults: 42-110 ng/ml

Somatomedin C (cont'd) Children: Ages (Years)	Girls (ng/ml)	Boys (ng/ml)
14-16	96-256	48-255
11-13	66-215	44-207
9-10	39-186	26-98
0-8	7-110	4-87

GH Stimulation:
Growth hormone levels >10 ng/ml or 10 μg/L (SI units)

Rationale

These three tests are used to identify growth hormone (GH) deficiency in adolescents who have short stature, delayed sexual maturity, or other growth deficiencies. They also are used to document the diagnosis of GH excess in patients with gigantism or acromegaly. Finally, they are often used as screening tests for pituitary hypofunction.

GH, or somatotropin, is secreted by the acidophil cells in the anterior pituitary gland and plays a central role in modulating growth from birth until the end of puberty. An elaborate feedback mechanism is associated with the secretion of GH. The hypothalamus secretes growth hormone–releasing hormone (GHRH), which stimulates GH release from the pituitary. GH affects many tissues through a group of peptides called *somatomedins*. High levels of somatomedins stimulate the production of somatostatin from the hypothalamus. Somatostatin inhibits further secretion of GH from the pituitary. GH is maximally secreted during sleep, exercise and ingestion of protein and in response to hypoglycemia.

In the total absence of GH, linear growth occurs at half to one third of the normal rate. GH also plays a role in the control of body cell anabolism throughout life by increasing protein synthesis, increasing the breakdown of fatty acids in adipose tissue, and increasing the blood glucose level.

If GH secretion is insufficient during childhood, limited growth and dwarfism may result. Also, a delay in sexual maturity in adolescents may be the result of reduced GH levels. Conversely, overproduction of GH during childhood results in gigantism, and affected individuals can reach nearly 7 to 8 feet in height. An excess of GH during adulthood (after closure of long-bone end plates) results in acromegaly, which is characterized by an increase in bone thickness and width, but no increase in height.

GH tests also are used to confirm hypopituitarism or hyperpituitarism. GH assay is the most widely used test for GH deficiency or excess. Because GH secretion is episodic, random assays for GH are not adequate determinants of GH deficiency. Normal GH levels overlap significantly with deficient levels. Low GH levels may indicate deficiency or may be normal for some individuals at certain times of the day. To negate time variables in GH testing, GH can be drawn 1 to 1½ hours after deep sleep has occurred, because levels increase during sleep. Also, strenuous exercise can be performed for 30 minutes in an effort to stimulate GH production.

To negate the common variations in GH secretion, screening for insulin-like growth factor I (IGF-I), or somatomedin C, provides a more accurate reflection of the mean plasma concentration of GH. Unlike GH, these proteins are not affected by the time of day or food intake because they circulate bound to proteins that are durable or long-lasting. IGF-I, or somatomedin C, levels increase significantly during the pubertal growth spurt.

Levels of somatomedin C depend on levels of GH. As a result, somatomedin C levels are low when GH levels are deficient. Nonpituitary causes of reduced somatomedin C levels include malnutrition, severe chronic illnesses, severe liver disease, and Laron's dwarfism. Abnormally low somatomedin C results still require an abnormally reduced or absent GH during a GH stimulation test to make the diagnosis of GH deficiency.

One of the most reliable GH stimulators is insulin-induced hypoglycemia, in which the blood glucose declines to less than 40 mg/dl. A GH concentration more than 10 mg/L after stimulation effectively excludes GH deficiencies. At present, the best method of identifying patients deficient in GH is a positive stimulation test followed by a positive response to a therapeutic GH trial. GH deficiency also is suspected when bone age, as determined by x-rays of the long bones (see p. 457), indicates retarded growth when compared with chronologic age.

Potential complications

Potential complications associated with GH stimulation testing are as follows:

■ Ketosis, acidosis, and shock
  These conditions may result from severe hypoglycemia during the GH stimulation test. With close observation, these complications are unlikely.

Interfering factors

Factors that interfere with GH testing include the following:

■ Random testing
  Because GH secretion is episodic, random measurements of GH are not adequate determinants of GH deficiency.
■ Recent radioactive scan
  A radioactive scan performed within the week before the test may affect GH and somatomedin C test results because levels are determined by radioimmunoassay.

Procedure

Peripheral venipuncture is performed, and one red-top tube of blood is collected for GH and somatomedin C. It is preferred that the patient be fasting and well rested. The patient should not be under physical or mental stress because this can increase GH levels.

GH stimulation test

Various agents, such as insulin, arginine, glucagon, levodopa, and clonidine, can be used to stimulate GH production. For a GH stimulation test, the patient remains NPO except for water after midnight on the morning of the test. A heparin or saline lock IV line is inserted for administration of medications and withdrawal of frequent blood samples. Baseline blood levels are obtained for GH, glucose, and cortisol. Venous samples for GH are obtained at 0, 60, and 90 minutes after injection of insulin or arginine. Blood glucose levels are monitored at 15- to 30-minute intervals with a glucometer. The blood glucose should drop to less than 40 mg/dl for effective measurement of GH reserve. The patient is monitored for signs of hypoglycemia, postural hypotension, and somnolence. At the end of the test, the patient receives cookies and punch or an IV glucose infusion.

GH also can be stimulated by vigorous exercise. This entails running or walking up stairs for 20 minutes. Blood samples of GH are obtained at 0, 20, and 40 minutes.

Contraindications

GH stimulation tests are contraindicated for patients with epilepsy, cerebrovascular disease, MI, and low basal plasma cortisol levels.

Nursing implications with rationale

Before

☞ Explain the procedure very carefully to the patient and parents, if appropriate. Most patients and their families are anxious regarding the possible diagnosis of GH deficiency.

☞ Instruct the patient to remain NPO, except for water, after midnight on the morning of the test.

During

■ During the stimulation test, monitor the patient for diaphoresis, nervousness, somnolence, and hypotension. Ice chips are often given during the test for patient comfort.

After

■ Indicate the patient's fasting status and the time blood is collected on the laboratory requisition slip. Remember, random levels do not permit a firm diagnosis to be established.

■ Apply pressure or a pressure dressing to the venipuncture site to prevent further bleeding. Observe the site for bleeding.

■ Inform the patient and family that the results are generally not available for approximately 10 to 14 days. Most laboratories only run GH tests once a week.

Case Study

Partial Growth Hormone Deficiency

E.L., a 14-year-old girl, was 4 feet 9 inches tall and had no signs of pubertal development. Her parents were both tall. Because of her drop on the growth chart for both height and weight, her pediatrician ordered a complete diagnostic workup to investigate her short stature.

Studies	Results
Routine laboratory studies	WNL
GH, p. 316	5.1 ng/ml (normal: 0-10 ng/ml)
GH stimulation test, p. 316	8 ng/ml (normal: >10 ng/ml)
Somatomedin C, p. 316	98 ng/ml (normal: 96-256 ng/ml)
Wrist and hand radiographic film, p. 457	Bone age of $11^1/_2$ years (normal: similar to chronologic age)
Serum T$_4$, p. 329	6.3 µg/dl (normal: 5-12 µg/dl)
Magnetic resonance imaging (MRI), p. 299	No evidence of craniopharyngioma or other CNS lesion
Serum calcium, p. 299	9.2 mg/dl (normal: 8.8-10.8 mg/dl)
Blood urea nitrogen (BUN), p. 266	12.2 mg/dl (normal: 5-18 mg/dl)

Erythrocyte sedimentation rate (ESR), p. 476   8 mm/hr (normal: ≤10 mm/hr)

Diagnostic Analysis

The T_4 level ruled out the possibility of hypothyroidism. An adequate T_4 level is a prerequisite for normal growth. The MRI ruled out a craniopharyngioma, which destroys the pituitary gland and impairs secretion of GH. The calcium level excluded the possibility of pseudohypoparathyroidism. The possibility of renal failure was excluded based on the normal BUN. The normal sedimentation rate eliminated the possibility of inflammatory bowel disease. The low-normal levels of GH and somatomedin C suggested the possibility of a partial deficiency of GH. The GH stimulation test confirmed the diagnosis. The child was placed on daily subcutaneous (SC) injection of GH for 2 years. She eventually reached the height of 5 feet 4 inches and began her menses at age 16.

Critical Thinking Questions

1. While undergoing a GH stimulation test, your pediatric patient becomes progressively lethargic and loses consciousness. The parents are very anxious for their child's welfare. How might you prioritize your nursing interventions?
2. Your small, thin pediatric patient, who is exposed to inner-city poverty, has been dropping progressively on the growth charts. How might the diagnosis of malnutrition be differentiated from a diagnosis of GH deficiency? Consider what tests the nurse should prepare the patient for if malnutrition were to be identified as the source of the patient's failure to grow.
3. How would you prepare a 9-year-old patient for an MRI scan of the brain?

Insulin Antibody (Antiinsulin Antibody)

Test type Blood

Normal values

No antibody detected for bovine or porcine insulin

Rationale

The insulin antibody test is used to evaluate insulin resistance. It also is used to identify type I diabetes. It is used when allergy to insulin is suspected. Insulin antibodies appear in nearly all patients with diabetes treated with exogenous (human, bovine, or porcine) insulin. These antibodies develop from impurities in animal insulin or from antigenic stimulation of the insulin molecule. With the increased use of human insulin, the frequency of development of antiinsulin antibodies has significantly decreased. Insulin antibodies also may be produced in patients who have never received exogenous insulin. These autoantibodies are present in nearly 50% of children at the time of diagnosis of juvenile diabetes.

The most common type of antiinsulin antibody is Immunoglobulin (Ig) G, but IgA, IgM, IgD, and IgE also have been reported. Most of these insulin antibodies do not cause clinical problems, but they may complicate most insulin assays (see p. 320). Antiinsulin antibodies act as insulin-transporting proteins and bind the free insulin. This can reduce the amount of insulin available for glucose metabolism. Furthermore, they may contribute to insulin resistance (daily insulin requirements exceeding 200 U per day for 2 days). IgM, especially, may cause insulin resistance. Insulin allergy (most common with animal insulin) may result from IgE antibodies to insulin.

Procedure

Seven ml of venous blood is collected in a red-top tube.

Nursing implications and rationale

Before

☞ Explain the procedure to the patient.

■ Inform the patient that no fasting is necessary.

After

■ Apply pressure or a pressure dressing to the venipuncture site to prevent further bleeding. Observe the site for bleeding.

■ In most hospitals or laboratories, the specimen is refrigerated and sent to a reference laboratory.

Insulin Assay

Test type Blood

Normal values

Adult: 5-24 mU/ml or 36-179 pmol/L (SI units)
Newborn: 3-20 mU/ml

Possible critical values >30 mU/ml

Rationale

The insulin assay is used to diagnose insulinoma (tumor of the islets of Langerhans) and evaluate abnormal lipid and carbohydrate metabolism. It also is used to evaluate patients with fasting hypoglycemia. Insulin regulates blood glucose levels by facilitating the movement of glucose out of the bloodstream and into the cells. Insulin secretion is primarily reactive to the blood glucose level. Normally, as the blood glucose level increases, the insulin level also increases; as the glucose level decreases, insulin release stops.

Some investigators believe that measuring the ratio of the blood glucose and insulin levels on the same specimen obtained during the OGTT (see p. 310) is more reliable than measuring insulin levels alone. Combined with the OGTT, the insulin assay can show characteristic curves. For example, patients with juvenile diabetes have low fasting insulin levels and display flat GTT insulin curves because of little or no increase in insulin levels. Patients who are mildly diabetic have normal fasting insulin levels and display GTT glucose curves with a delayed rise.

When combined with an FBG test, insulin assay is very accurate in detecting insulinoma. After the patient fasts 12 to 14 hours, the insulin/glucose ratio should be less than 0.3. Patients with insulinoma have ratios greater than this value. To increase the sensitivity and specificity of these combined tests for insulinoma, Turner et al. have proposed the amended insulin/glucose ratios using variable mathematic "fudge" factors:

$$\frac{\text{Serum insulin level} \times 100}{\text{Serum glucose} - 30 \text{ mg/100 ml}}$$

A Turner amended ratio of greater than 50 suggests insulinoma.

Interfering factors

Factors that interfere with insulin assay include the following:

■ Insulin therapy
Most patients being treated with insulin for diabetes develop antiinsulin antibodies (see p. 319) within a few months. These antibodies can interfere with insulin radioimmunoassay results by competing with the insulin antibodies used in the insulin assay.

■ Food intake and obesity, which may cause *increased* insulin levels

■ Recent administration of radioisotopes
This may affect test results by interfering with the radioimmunoassay method to detect insulin.

Procedure

After the patient is kept NPO, except for water, for 8 hours, a fasting blood sample is obtained by peripheral venipuncture. If the serum insulin level is to be measured during the GTT, the blood samples should be drawn before the oral ingestion of the glucose load.

Nursing implications with rationale
Before

☞ Explain the procedure to the patient. This test is usually done concurrently with the OGTT (see p. 310).

☞ Instruct the patient to remain NPO except for water for 8 hours.

After

■ Apply pressure or a pressure dressing to the venipuncture site to prevent further bleeding. Observe the site for bleeding.

Long-Acting Thyroid Stimulator
(LATS, Thyroid-Stimulating Immunoglobulin [TSIG or TSI])

Test type Blood

Normal values
Negative

Rationale
The long-acting thyroid stimulator (LATS) antibody is a part of a group of IgG antibodies directed against the thyroid cell membrane. LATS initially was thought to mimic the action of TSH. All of these immunoglobulins are associated with Graves' disease and some cases of Hashimoto's thyroiditis. They are helpful in the evaluation of patients in whom the diagnosis of Graves' disease is complicated by borderline data or conflicting data needed to support the diagnosis. Other components of this system include thyroid-stimulating immunoglobulin (TSI) and TSH binding inhibiting immunoglobulin (TBII).

Like TSI and TBII, LATS can be found in 75% of the patients with Graves' disease. It also can be found in some patients with Hashimoto's thyroiditis and hyperparathyroidism. LATS is found most frequently in patients with Graves'

disease associated with exophthalmos and/or pretibial edema. Its effect on the thyroid is long-lasting, and titers do not decrease until nearly 1 year after successful treatment of the thyroid disease. Because LATS crosses the placenta, it may be found in neonates whose mothers have Graves' disease.

Procedure
No fasting or special preparation is required. A peripheral venipuncture is done, and approximately 5 ml of blood is collected in a red-top tube and sent to the laboratory for analysis. The laboratory should be notified if ^{131}I has been administered to the patient within the preceding 2 days.

Interfering factor
A factor that interferes with LATS values is the recent administration of radioactive iodine.

Nursing implications with rationale
Before

☞ Explain the procedure to the patient. Inform the patient that no fasting is necessary.

■ Assess whether radioactive iodine has been administered to the patient within the past 2 days because this may affect the test results.

After

■ Apply pressure or a pressure dressing to the venipuncture site to prevent further bleeding. Observe the site for bleeding.

■ Handle the blood sample gently. Hemolysis may interfere with test result interpretation.

Metyrapone

Test type Blood, urine

Normal values
24-hour urine: baseline excretion of urinary 17-OHCS more than doubled
Blood: 11-deoxycortisol increased to >7 mg/dl and cortisol <10 mg/dl

Rationale

Metyrapone (Metopirone) is a potent blocker of an enzyme involved in cortisol production. Cortisol production therefore falls when this drug is given; the resulting fall should stimulate pituitary secretion of ACTH by way of a negative feedback mechanism. Cortisol itself cannot be synthesized because of the metyrapone inhibition at the 11-beta-hydroxylation step, but an abundance of cortisol precursors (11-deoxycortisol and OHCS) will be formed. These cortisol precursors can be detected in the urine or blood. This test is similar to the ACTH stimulation test (see p. 296).

The cortisol precursors are significantly increased with metyrapone stimulation in patients with adrenal hyperplasia caused by pituitary overproduction of ACTH. This increase occurs because the normal adrenal/pituitary feedback response mechanism is still intact. No response to metyrapone occurs in patients with Cushing's syndrome resulting from adrenal adenoma or carcinoma because the tumors are autonomous and, therefore, insensitive to changes in ACTH secretion.

Interfering factors

Factors that interfere with determining metyrapone levels include the following:

- Recent radioactive scan
  Recent administration of radioisotopes will interfere with test results performed by radioimmunoassay.
- Chlorpromazine (Thorazine) interferes with the response to metyrapone and should not be administered during the testing.

Procedure

Before this study is performed, a baseline 24-hour urine specimen for 17-OHCS (see p. 338) should be collected. A 24-hour urine collection for 17-OHCS also is obtained during and 1 day after the oral administration of 500 to 750 mg of metyrapone, which is given every 4 hours for 24 hours. The 24-hour excretion of 17-OHCS on the last day of collection should at least double the baseline excretion.

Contraindications

Contraindications associated with metyrapone are as follows:

- Patients with possible primary adrenal insufficiency, because metyrapone could further reduce the production of what little cortisol already is produced and precipitate an adrenal crisis
- Addison's disease and Addisonian crisis, because metyrapone inhibits cortisol production

Nursing implications with rationale

Before
- Explain the test to the patient. Verify that the patient knows how to collect the three 24-hour urine specimens required for this study.
- Obtain a baseline 24-hour urine specimen for the 17-OHCS level for the urine test.
- Obtain a baseline cortisol level for the blood test.

During
- Administer 2 to 3 g of metyrapone the night before the blood specimen is to be collected. Collect a blood specimen in the morning.
- Instruct the patient to begin the 24-hour urine collection after discarding the first morning specimen. This is the start time of the 24-hour collection.
- Collect all urine passed over the next 24 hours.
- Instruct the patient to void before defecating so that the urine is not contaminated by feces.
- Remind the patient not to put toilet paper in the collection container.
- Keep the urine specimen on ice or refrigerated during the 24 hours.
- Collect the last specimen as close as possible to the end of the 24 hours.

After
- Transport the urine specimen promptly to the laboratory.
- Because metyrapone inhibits cortisol production, assess the patient for impending signs of Addisonian crisis (muscle weakness, mental and emotional changes, anorexia, nausea, vomiting, hypotension, hyperkalemia, and vascular collapse). Addisonian crisis is a medical

emergency that must be treated vigorously. The immediate treatment basically includes replenishing steroids, reversing shock, and restoring blood circulation.

- Apply pressure or a pressure dressing to the venipuncture site to prevent further bleeding. Observe the site for bleeding.

Osmolality, Blood (Serum Osmolality)
Osmolality, Urine (Urine Osmolality)

Test type Blood, urine

Normal values
Serum osmolality:
Adult/elderly: 285-295 mOsm/kg H_2O
Child: 275-290 mOsm/kg H_2O
Urine osmolality:
12- to 14-hour fluid restriction: >850 mOsm/ kg H_2O (SI units)
Random specimen: 50-1400 mOsm/kg H_2O, depending on fluid intake (SI units)

Possible critical values
Serum osmolality:
<265 mOsm/kg H_2O
>320 mOsm/kg H_2O

Rationale
Osmolality measures the concentration of dissolved particles in blood. As the amount of free water in the blood increases or the amount of particles decreases, osmolality decreases. As the amount of water in the blood decreases or the amount of particles increases, osmolality increases. Osmolality increases with dehydration and decreases with overhydration.

The simultaneous use of urine and serum osmolality helps in the interpretation and evaluation of problems with osmolality. The serum osmolality test is useful in evaluating fluid and electrolyte imbalance and is very helpful in evaluating patients with seizures, ascites, hydration status, acid-base balance, and suspected ADH abnormalities.

Serum osmolality also is helpful in identifying the presence of organic acids, sugars, or ethanol. In these cases, there is an osmolal gap. This gap represents the difference between what the osmolality should be, based on calculations of serum sodium, glucose, and BUN (the three most important solutes in the blood), and what the osmolality is, as truly measured. If the gap is large, solutes (e.g., organic acids [ketones]), unusually high levels of glucose, or ethanol by-products are suspected to be present.

Urine osmolality is the measurement of the number of dissolved particles in the urine. Urine osmolality is used in the precise evaluation of the concentrating ability of the kidney. This test also is used to monitor fluid and electrolyte balance. Osmolality is valuable in the workup of patients with renal disease, SIADH, and DI. Osmolality may be used as part of the urinalysis when the patient has glycosuria or proteinuria, or has had tests that use radiopaque substances.

Procedure
Blood:
Approximately 7 ml of peripheral venous blood is obtained in a red-top tube from a nonfasting patient and sent to the chemistry laboratory for serum osmolality measurement. The only discomfort associated with this test is the venipuncture.
Urine:
The patient is instructed to eat a dry supper the evening before the test and to drink no fluids until the test is completed the next morning. The first-voided urine specimen is collected.

Nursing implications with rationale
Before
- ☞ Explain the method of testing to the patient. No fasting is required for the blood test. Fasting from fluids is necessary for the urine test.
After
- Apply pressure or a pressure dressing to the venipuncture site to prevent further bleeding. Observe the site for bleeding.
- Send the urine specimen to the laboratory promptly.

Parathyroid Hormone (PTH, Parathormone)

Test type Blood

Normal values
10-65 pg/mL

Rationale
Parathyroid hormone (PTH) is the only hormone secreted by the parathyroid gland in response to hypocalcemia. When serum calcium levels return to normal, PTH levels diminish. PTH, therefore, is one of the major factors affecting calcium metabolism. This test is useful in establishing a diagnosis of hyperparathyroidism and distinguishing non-parathyroid from parathyroid causes of hypercalcemia. Increased PTH levels are seen in patients with hyperparathyroidism (primary, secondary, or tertiary); in patients with nonparathyroid, ectopic, PTH-producing tumors (pseudohyperparathyroidism); or in patients with malabsorption or vitamin D deficiency as a normal compensatory response to hypocalcemia.

Primary hyperparathyroidism most often is caused by a parathyroid adenoma or hyperplasia, and, only rarely, parathyroid cancer. Patients with primary hyperparathyroidism have high PTH and calcium levels. Secondary hyperparathyroidism is the exaggerated response of the parathyroid gland to kidney insensitivity to PTH in patients with chronic renal failure (CRF). CRF patients have a chronically low serum calcium in reaction to persistently high phosphates, which the kidney fails to excrete. In response to this persistently low calcium, the parathyroid is constantly stimulated to produce PTH in an effort to maintain a normal calcium level. This is called *secondary hyperparathyroidism*. These patients have high PTH and normal to slightly low calcium levels. Occasionally the patient with CRF overshoots the compensatory process and autonomously develops unnecessarily high PTH production, which leads to hypercalcemia. This is called *tertiary hyperparathyroidism*. These patients have high PTH and high calcium levels.

It is important to measure serum calcium simultaneously with the measurement of PTH. Most laboratories have a PTH/calcium nomogram that indicates what PTH level is considered normal for each calcium level.

Decreased PTH levels are seen in patients with hypoparathyroidism or as a compensatory response to hypercalcemia in patients with metastatic bone tumors, sarcoidosis, vitamin D intoxication, or milk-alkali syndrome. Of course, surgical ablation of the parathyroid glands is another cause of hypoparathyroidism.

Interfering factor
A factor that interferes with determining PTH levels is the recent injection of radioisotopes.

Procedure
The procedure for acquiring blood for this study varies according to the laboratory performing the study. Peripheral venous blood is obtained from the fasting patient (usually in the morning). Some laboratories require 15 ml of blood in an iced, plastic syringe; others require only 7 ml in a red-top tube placed on ice. The blood then is taken to the chemistry laboratory, where it is often sent out to a commercial laboratory. Because of this procedure, test results typically are not available for several days. Testing is done by radioimmunoassay. The serum calcium level determination (see p. 299) should be obtained at the same time that the PTH specimen is drawn.

The only discomfort associated with this study is the venipuncture.

Nursing implications with rationale
Before
- Explain the procedure to the patient. Instruct the patient to remain NPO, except for water, after midnight on the day of the test.
- Obtain a serum calcium level determination at the same time, if ordered. The serum PTH and serum calcium levels are important in differential diagnosis.

After
- Apply pressure or a pressure dressing to the venipuncture site to prevent further bleeding. Observe the site for bleeding.

Case Study

Hyperparathyroidism

Mr. O., 42 years old, complaining of weakness, loss of appetite, and nausea, was found to have hypercalcemia after a blood test taken during a routine physical examination at work. He was completely asymptomatic, and the results of a physical examination were negative.

Studies	Results
Routine laboratory work	*Normal except for:*
Serum calcium, p. 299	12.8 mg/dl (normal: 9.0-10.5 mg/dl)
Phosphorus, p. 326	1.4 mg/dl (normal: 3.0-4.5 mg/dl)
PTH test, p. 324	232 pg/ml (normal: 10-65 pg/mL)
X-ray study of skull and hands, p. 457	Moderate bone resorption

Diagnostic Analysis

Although Mr. O. was completely asymptomatic, he had significant hypercalcemia. Concomitantly elevated PTH levels indicated that his hypercalcemia was the result of primary hyperparathyroidism. The serum phosphorus reinforced this diagnosis. Radiographic films of the skull and hands (the most common locations of bone resorption caused by hyperparathyroidism) showed moderate changes, indicating that the hyperparathyroidism was not an acute process. Mr. O. underwent extensive surgical exploration of the neck, and only three small parathyroid glands were found. No further surgery was performed.

Neck and chest venous PTH assays were performed postoperatively. PTH levels in all neck veins were below 10 pg/ml. However, the PTH in the superior vena cava was 308 pg/ml. This indicated that a fourth parathyroid gland was still encased in the chest. The patient underwent surgical exploration of the mediastinum. A large parathyroid benign adenoma was found and excised. Postoperatively, Mr. O. had no difficulties, and his calcium level returned to normal.

Critical Thinking Questions

1. What caused the bone resorption in this patient?
2. Mr. O. developed hypocalcemia 2 days after the operation. What symptoms of hypocalcemia should the nurse look for? What are the most likely causes of the hypocalcemia?
3. Elevated PTH levels can be considered a normal physiologic response in a patient with renal failure. Explain the pathophysiology for this process.

Phosphorus (Inorganic Phosphorus [PO$_4$], Phosphate [P])

Test type Blood

Normal values
Elderly: values slightly lower than adult
Adult: 3.0-4.5 mg/dl or 0.97-1.45 mmol/L
  (SI units)
Child: 4.5-6.5 mg/dl or 1.45-2.10 mmol/L
  (SI units)
Newborn: 4.3-9.3 mg/dl or 1.4-3.0 mmol/L
  (SI units)

Possible critical values <1 mg/dl

Rationale
Phosphorus found in the body is in the form of a phosphate. Phosphorus and phosphate will be used interchangeably throughout this and other discussions. Most body phosphate is a part of organic compounds. Only a small part of total body phosphate is inorganic phosphate (i.e., not part of another organic compound). It is the inorganic phosphate that is measured when one requests a phosphate, phosphorus, inorganic phosphorus, or inorganic phosphate test. Most of the body's inorganic phosphorus is combined with calcium within the skeleton; however, approximately 15% of the phosphorus exists in the blood as a phosphate salt. The inorganic phosphate (measured in this test) contributes to electrical and acid-base homeostasis. This test is performed to assist in the interpretation of studies investigating parathyroid and calcium abnormalities.

Dietary phosphorus is absorbed in the small bowel. The absorption is very efficient, and only rarely is hypophosphatemia caused by GI malabsorption. Renal excretion of phosphorus should equal dietary intake to maintain a normal serum phosphate level. Phosphate levels vary significantly during the day, with the lowest values occurring at approximately 10 AM and the highest occurring 12 hours later.

Phosphorus levels are determined by calcium metabolism, parathormone (PTH), renal excretion, and, to a lesser degree, by intestinal absorption. Because an inverse relationship exists between calcium and phosphorus, a decrease of one mineral results in an increase in the other. Serum phosphorus levels, therefore, depend on calcium metabolism, and vice versa. The regulation of phosphate by PTH is such that PTH tends to decrease phosphate reabsorption in the kidney. PTH and vitamin D, however, tend to weakly stimulate phosphate absorption within the gut.

Procedure
Testing for phosphorus usually is included in a multiphasic, automated system analysis of serum. Some hospitals require the patient to be fasting. For these multiphasic analyses, usually two red-top tubes are filled with peripheral venous blood. Hemolysis must be avoided because, if it occurs, intracellular phosphate can be released, which would artificially raise the phosphate level. The test is done in the chemistry laboratory.

Nursing implications with rationale
Before
☞ Explain the procedure to the patient. Instruct the patient to fast, if recommended by the laboratory.
After
■ Apply pressure or a pressure dressing to the venipuncture site to prevent further bleeding. Observe the site for bleeding.
■ Prevent hemolysis of the blood specimen.

Prolactin Levels (PRLs)

Test type Blood

Normal values
Adult male: 0-20 ng/ml
Adult female: 0-20 ng/ml
Pregnant female: 20-400 ng/ml

Rationale

Prolactin is a hormone secreted by the anterior pituitary gland (adenohypophysis). In females, prolactin promotes lactation. Its role in males is not demonstrated. This hormone is elevated in patients with prolactin-secreting pituitary acidophilic or chromophobic adenomas. To a lesser extent, moderately high prolactin levels have been observed in women with secondary amenorrhea (i.e., postpubertal), galactorrhea, and anorexia. In general, very high prolactin levels are more likely to be due to pituitary adenoma than to other causes.

The prolactin level is helpful in the diagnosis and monitoring of pituitary adenomas. Successful treatment is associated with a reduction in serum prolactin levels.

Interfering factor

A factor that interferes with determining prolactin levels is stress. Any source of stress from illness, trauma, surgery, or even the fear of a blood test can elevate prolactin levels. If the patient is fearful of venipuncture, it is recommended that a heparin lock be inserted and the blood specimen withdrawn 2 hours later.

Procedure

No fasting or special preparation is required. The blood sample should be drawn in the morning. Approximately 5 to 7 ml of venous blood is obtained in a red-top tube and sent to the laboratory as soon as possible. If a delay occurs, the specimen should be placed on ice.

Nursing implications with rationale

Before

☞ Explain the procedure to the patient. Inform the patient that no fasting is necessary.

After

■ Apply pressure or a pressure dressing to the venipuncture site to prevent further bleeding. Observe the site for bleeding.

Testosterone (Total Testosterone Serum Level)

Test type Blood

Normal values

Age	ng/dl	
	Male	*Female*
adult	280-1100	15-70
puberty	5-800	2-40
6-9 yrs	3-30	2-20
1-5 yrs	2-25	2-10
6-12 mos	2-7	2-5
1-5 mos	1-177	1-5
newborn	75-400	20-64

Rationale

Testosterone levels are used to evaluate ambiguous sex characteristics, precocious puberty, virilizing syndromes in the female, and infertility in the male. This test also can be used as a tumor marker for rare tumors of the ovary and testicle.

In the male, most of the testosterone is made by Leydig's cells in the testicle; this accounts for 95% of the circulating testosterone in men. In the female, approximately half of the testosterone is made by the conversion of dehydroepiandrosterone (DHEA) to testosterone in the peripheral fat tissue. Another 30% is made by the same conversion of DHEA in the adrenal gland, and 20% is directly made by the ovaries.

In males, a biofeedback mechanism for testosterone production exists. It starts in the hypothalamus, where gonadotropin-releasing hormone (GnRH) induces the pituitary to produce LH (called *interstitial cell-stimulating hormone* in the male) and FSH. LH stimulates Leydig's cells to produce testosterone. FSH stimulates the Sertoli cells to produce sperm. Testosterone then acts to inhibit further secretion of GnRH.

Physiologically, testosterone stimulates spermatogenesis and influences the development of male secondary sexual characteristics. Overproduction of this hormone in the young male may cause precocious puberty. This hormone overproduction can be caused by testicular, adrenal, or pituitary tumors. Overproduction of this hormone in females causes masculinization, which is demonstrated by amenorrhea and excessive growth of body hair (hirsutism). Ovarian and adrenal tumors/hyperplasia are all potential causes of masculinization in the female. Reduced levels of testosterone in the male suggest hypogonadism or Klinefelter's syndrome. Androstenedione also can be measured and provides similar information as does the testosterone assay.

Several testosterone stimulation tests can be performed to more accurately evaluate hypogonadism. Human chorionic gonadotropin (HCG), clomiphene citrate, and GnRH can be used to stimulate testosterone secretion.

Procedure
No fasting is required. Because testosterone levels are highest in early morning, blood should be drawn in the morning. Approximately 7 ml of peripheral venous blood is collected in a red-top tube.

Nursing implications with rationale
Before
☞ Explain the procedure to the patient. Inform the patient that no fasting is necessary.
After
■ Apply pressure or a pressure dressing to the venipuncture site to prevent further bleeding. Observe the site for bleeding.

THYROID ANTIBODIES
Antithyroglobulin Antibody
(Thyroid Autoantibody, Thyroid Antithyroglobulin Antibody, Thyroglobulin Antibody)

Antithyroid Microsomal Antibody
(Antimicrosomal Antibody, Microsomal Antibody, Thyroid Autoantibody, Thyroid Antimicrosomal Antibody)

Test type Blood

Normal values
Antithyroglobulin antibody:
Titer <1:100
Antithyroid microsomal antibody:
Titer <1:100

Rationale
The thyroid antibodies tests are primarily used in the differential diagnosis of thyroid diseases such as Hashimoto's thyroiditis and chronic lymphocytic thyroiditis (in children). Several antibodies correlate to various thyroid gland components. The two most common include antithyroglobulin antibody and antithyroid microsomal antibody.

Antithyroglobulin antibody occurs when thyroglobulin (thyroxine-binding globulin), which normally exists in the blood (as a thyroid hormone carrier) and in the thyroid, acts as an immune-stimulating antigen. Autoantibodies are developed and react against the thyroglobulin in the thyroid cells, leading to thyroid inflammation and destruction. Antithyroglobulin antibody is present in only approximately 50% of patients with Hashimoto's thyroiditis.

Thyroid microsomal antibodies also are commonly found in patients with various thyroid diseases. They are found in 70% to 90% of patients with Hashimoto's thyroiditis. Microsomal antibodies are produced in response to microsomes escaping from the thyroid epithelial cells surrounding the thyroid follicle. These escaped microsomes then act as antigens and stimulate the production of antibodies. These immune complexes initiate inflammatory and cytotoxic (cell-killing) effects on the thyroid follicle.

Although many different thyroid diseases are associated with elevated levels of these antibodies, the most frequently associated disease is chronic thyroiditis (Hashimoto's thyroiditis in the adult and lymphocytic thyroiditis in children and young adults). The antithyroglobulin test usually is performed in conjunction with the antithyroid microsomal antibody test. When performed in this manner, the specificity and sensitivity is greatly increased.

Procedure

Peripheral venipuncture is performed, and approximately 3 to 5 ml of blood is obtained in a red-top tube.

Nursing implications with rationale

Before

☞ Explain the procedure to the patient. Inform the patient that no fasting is necessary.

After

■ Apply pressure or a pressure dressing to the venipuncture site to prevent further bleeding. Observe the site for bleeding.

THYROID HORMONES

Thyroxine (T_4, Thyroxine Screen)

Thyroxine, Free (FT_4)

Thyroxine Index, Free (FTI, T7, FT_4 Index, FT_4I)

Triiodothyronine (Total T_3 Radioimmunoassay [T_3 by RIA], Free T_3)

Test type Blood

Normal values

Total T_4:
>60 years: 5-11 μg/dl
Adult male: 4-12 μg/dl
Adult female: 5-12 μg/dl
10-15 years: 5-12 μg/dl
5-10 years: 6-13 μg/dl
1-5 years: 7-15 μg/dl
1-4 months: 8-16 μg/dl
1-2 weeks: 10-16 μg/dl
1-3 days: 11-22 μg/dl

Free T_4:
Adult 0.8-2.7 ng/dL
2 weeks-20 years 0.8-2 ng/dL
0-4 days 2-6 ng/dL

Free T_4 Index:
0.8-2.4 ng/dl or 10-31 pmol/L (SI units)
Adult index = 1.5 to 4.5 if units are eliminated

T_3:
>50 years: 40-180 ng/dl
20-50 years: 70-205 ng/dl
16-19 years: 80-210 ng/dl
11-15 years: 80-215 ng/dl
6-10 years: 95-240 ng/dl
1-5 years: 105-270 ng/dl
1-11 months: 105-245 ng/dl
1-3 days: 100-740 ng/dl

Possible critical values

Total T_4:
Adult: <2 μg/dl if myxedema coma possible; >20 μg/dl if thyroid storm possible
Newborn: <7 μg/dl

Rationale

Thyroid hormones are produced when tyrosine incorporates organic iodine to form a monoiodotyrosine. This complex incorporates another iodine and becomes diiodotyrosine. Two diiodotyrosines combine to form tetraiodothyronine (also called *T_4 thyroid hormone*). If a diiodotyrosine combines with a monoiodotyrosine, triiodothyronine (also called *T_3 thyroid hormone*) is formed. T_4 makes up nearly all of what is known as *thyroid hormone*. Nearly all of T_4 and T_3 is bound to protein. Thyroid-binding globulin (TBG) binds most of T_3 and T_4. Albumin and prealbumin bind the rest. It is the unbound, or free, hormone that is metabolically active.

The serum *thyroxine test* is a measure of total T_4, (i.e., bound and free T_4). Greater-than-normal levels indicate hyperthyroid states, and subnormal values are seen in hypothyroid states. Newborns are screened with T_4 tests to detect hypothyroidism. Mental retardation can be prevented by early diagnosis. This test also is used to monitor replacement and suppressive therapy.

Because T_4 is bound by serum proteins, such as TBG, any increase in these proteins (as in pregnant women and patients taking oral contraceptives) will cause factitiously elevated levels of T_4 and T_3. The *free thyroxine* (FT_4) is used to evaluate thyroid function in patients who may have protein abnormalities that could affect total T_4 levels. Free T_4 measurement in these patients is a more accurate indicator of thyroid function than is total T_4.

The *FT_4 index* is another measure, although indirect, of free thyroxine. This measurement is calculated from the total T_4 and T_3 resin uptake (see pp. 329 and 337):

$$FT_4I = \frac{T_4 \text{ (total)} \times T_3 \text{ uptake (THBR*) (\%)}}{100}$$

Its use is similar to FT_4 in patients who may have protein abnormalities.

T_3 makes up less than 10% of thyroid hormone. A large proportion of T_3 is formed in the liver by conversion of T_4 to T_3. As with the thyroxine test, the serum T_3 test is an accurate indicator of thyroid function. The serum T_3 test measures the total bound and unbound (free) T_3. T_3 is less stable than T_4 because it is much less tightly bound to serum proteins. A total of 70% of T_3 is bound to the proteins TBG and albumin. Only minute quantities are unbound, or free. It is the free T_3 that is metabolically active. As with FT_4, measurement of *free T_3* is unaffected by the alterations that serum proteins have on the total T_3 measurement.

Generally, when the T_3 level is below normal, the patient is in a hypothyroid state. Because of the considerable overlap between hypothyroid states and normal thyroid function, T_3 levels are primarily used to diagnose hyperthyroid states. An elevated T_3 level indicates hyperthyroidism, especially when the T_4 also is elevated. A rare form of hyperthyroidism called *T_3 toxicosis* exhibits normal T_4 levels and elevated T_3 levels. Measurement of T_3 should not be confused with the T_3 uptake test (see p. 337).

---

*Thyroid hormone-binding ratio

Interfering factors

Factors that interfere with determining thyroid hormone levels include the following:

- Age
  Neonates have higher levels than do older children and adults.
- Prior use of radioisotopes
  This can alter test results because the method used to determine free T_4 levels is radioimmunoassay.
- Exogenously administered thyroxine, which will cause *increased* FT_4 results.
- Pregnancy, because it will cause *increased* levels.

Procedure

No special preparation is required. A peripheral venous blood specimen is obtained in a red-top tube and sent to the chemistry laboratory. A heel stick is done on newborns. For the newborn procedure, thoroughly saturate the circles on the filter paper with blood. Prompt specimen collection and processing are crucial to the early detection of hypothyroidism. The optimal collection time is 2 to 4 days after birth. All newborns should be screened before discharge because of the consequences of delayed diagnosis.

Nursing implications with rationale

Before

☞ Explain the procedure to the patient.
- Determine whether the patient is pregnant or taking oral contraceptives because these conditions will alter serum T_4 concentrations as a result of increased amounts of estrogen. Also, verify that the patient is not taking exogenous thyroxine medication, which will affect the results. Notify the physician of any findings that may alter the accuracy of the study.

☞ Inform the patient that no fasting is necessary.
After
- Apply pressure or a pressure dressing to the venipuncture site to prevent further bleeding. Observe the site for bleeding.

Thyroiditis

J.M.P., a 23-year-old female, has had a bout of flulike symptoms over the past few weeks. Most recently, she has become increasingly tired. She is taking birth control pills to control her menses. Her anterior neck became painful during the past few weeks. The physical examination results reveal that her thyroid is diffusely enlarged and mildly tender.

Studies	Results
Routine laboratory tests	WNL
Total T_4, p. 329	8 μg/dl (normal: 5-12 μg/dl)
Free T_4, p. 329	0.5 ng/dl (normal: 0.8-2.7 ng/dl)
Free T_4 index:, p. 329	0.4 ng/dl (normal: 0.8-2.4 ng/dl)
T_3, p. 329	52 ng/dl (normal: 70-205 ng/dl)
TBG, p. 337	12 mg/dl (normal: 1.7-3.6 mg/dl)
TSH, p. 334	32 mU/ml (normal: 2-10 mU/ml)
Radioactive iodine uptake, p. 332	2 hours: 3% (normal: 4% to 12%)
	6 hours: 4% (normal: 6% to 15%)
Thyroid scanning p. 332	Enlarged gland; normal shape, position, and function of the thyroid gland. No areas of decreased or increased uptake
Thyroid ultrasound, p. 336	Enlarged gland; normal shape and position of the thyroid gland
Thyroid antibodies, p. 328	
Antithyroglobulin antibody	1:250 (normal: titer <1:100)
Antithyroid microsomal antibody	1:500 (normal: titer <1:100)
LATS	Negative

Diagnostic Analysis

Total T_4 measures protein-bound and unbound T_4. Because J.M.P. was taking birth control pills, her TBG was elevated. Therefore, her total T_4 was normal. Free T_4 and FT_4 index tests measure unbound T_4. When the free T_4 and the FT_4 index were measured, they were found to be low, indicating that the patient was hypothyroid. The TSH level was elevated because of primary failure of the thyroid. Her radioactive iodine uptake (RAIU) results indicated reduced uptake of iodine, confirming that the patient was, indeed, hypothyroid. The thyroid antibodies were elevated, indicating that J.M.P. had Hashimoto's thyroiditis. Her LATS levels were normal, discounting Graves' disease as a cause of her diffusely enlarged thyroid. Her thyroid ultrasound and scan failed to show any localized, defined tumor.

J.M.P. was started on thyroid replacement therapy, and her TSH level returned to normal. Over the next few weeks, she felt markedly better. Her thyroid pain disappeared, as did her tiredness.

Continued

Critical Thinking Questions

1. Why were the thyroid antibodies important in J.M.P.'s diagnosis?
2. What symptoms might J.M.P. experience if too much thyroid replacement medication was administered?

Thyroid Scanning (Thyroid Scintiscan)

Radioactive Iodine Uptake (RAIU, Iodine Uptake Test, ^{131}I Uptake)

Test type Nuclear scan

Normal values
Thyroid scan:
Normal size, shape, position, and function of the thyroid gland
No areas of decreased or increased uptake
RAIU:
2 hours: 4% to 12% absorbed
6 hours: 6% to 15% absorbed
24 hours: 8% to 30% absorbed
Actual values may vary according to the laboratory

Rationale
Using radionuclear scanning, thyroid scanning determines the size, shape, position, and physiologic function of the thyroid gland. A radioactive substance, such as technetium-99m (Tc 99m), is given to the patient to visualize the thyroid gland. A scintography camera is passed over the neck area, and an image is recorded on film.

Thyroid nodules are easily detected by this technique. Nodules are classified as functioning (warm/hot) or nonfunctioning (cold), depending on the amount of radionuclide taken up by the nodule (Figure 8-7). A functioning nodule may represent a benign adenoma or a localized toxic goiter. A nonfunctioning nodule may represent a cyst, carcinoma, nonfunctioning adenoma or goiter, lymphoma, or localized area of thyroiditis.

Thyroid scanning is useful in the following clinical situations:

1. Patients with a neck or substernal mass
2. Patients with a thyroid nodule; thyroid cancers usually are nonfunctioning (cold) nodules
3. Patients with hyperthyroidism; scanning will assist in differentiating Graves' disease (diffusely enlarged, hyperfunctioning thyroid gland) from Plummer's disease (nodular, hyperfunctioning gland)

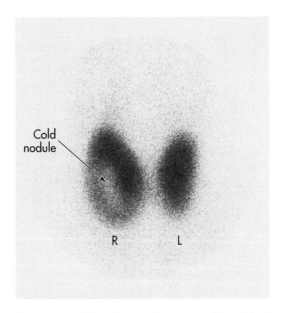

Figure 8-7 Thyroid scan. Note the cold nodule in the right (larger) lobe of the thyroid gland. This finding is consistent with tumor, cyst, or goiter.

4. Patients with metastatic tumors without a known primary site; a normal scan excludes the thyroid gland as a primary site
5. Patients with a well-differentiated form of thyroid cancer

Another form of thyroid scanning is called the *whole body thyroid scan.* This scan is performed on patients who have previously been treated for thyroid cancer. Radioactive ^{125}I is injected intravenously, and the entire body is scanned to look for metastatic thyroid tissue. A hot spot would indicate recurrent/metastatic tumor. Before this test can be performed, all of the thyroid tissue in the neck must be either surgically excised or ablated with radioactive ^{131}I. Otherwise, the thyroid tissue in the neck will take up all the iodine, and none will be available to go to any existing metastatic sites. If the patient is on thyroid replacement therapy, the thyroid medicine must be discontinued at least 6 weeks before testing. This makes any metastatic thyroid tissue particularly iodine avid. A high TSH blood level ensures that any thyroid metastatic cancer tissue will take up the administered radioactive iodine. This test is routinely performed every 1 to 2 years on patients who have had a thyroid cancer larger than 1 cm. Smaller cancers are unlikely to metastasize.

RAIU was used as a measure of thyroid function. It is rarely performed now that direct assays are available for both T_4 and T_3. However, it still is used to evaluate defects in thyroid hormone production. RAIU is based on the ability of the thyroid gland to trap and retain iodine. In this procedure, a known quantity of radioactive iodine is given orally to the patient. A gamma ray detector placed over the thyroid gland determines the quantity or percentage of radioactive iodine taken up by the gland over a specific time.

Performing the measurement at different times after the iodine is given allows several aspects of thyroid function to be evaluated. Gland visualization at 30 minutes reflects the ability of the thyroid gland to trap iodine. Visualization at 6 hours measures the ability of the thyroid gland to bind iodine organically. Maximal iodine uptake is observed within 24 hours. Determinations of iodine uptake after this time measure the ability of the gland to release iodine in the form of thyroid hormone.

Potential complication

A potential complication associated with thyroid scanning and RAIU is radiation-induced oncogenesis. Large and repeated doses of iodine can be carcinogenic to the thyroid. This complication is eliminated if Tc or low-radioactive iodine isomers are used instead of ^{131}I.

Interfering factors

Factors that interfere with thyroid scanning and RAIU include the following:

- Iodine-containing foods
  The iodine may saturate all the iodine-binding sites, and very little radioisotope will be taken up by the thyroid.
- Recent administration of radiographic contrast agents
  These agents contain large quantities of iodine.
- Diarrhea
  Decreased absorption of tracer from the GI tract will result in *decreased* RAIU levels.

Procedure
Thyroid Scan:

No patient preparation is required. The patient is taken to the nuclear medicine laboratory. A history concerning previous IV contrast radiographic studies, nuclear scanning, or intake of any thyroid suppressive or antithyroid drugs is taken. A standard dose of radioactive iodine or Tc is given by mouth. The capsule is tasteless. Scanning is performed 24 hours later. If Tc is used, scanning is performed 2 hours later. A rectilinear gamma-ray detector is passed over the thyroid area, and the radioactive counts are recorded and displayed in the image of the thyroid gland. The image is created on film.

RAIU:

The patient is asked to eat a light breakfast and report to the nuclear medicine laboratory (some laboratories prefer that the patient fasts overnight). A tasteless, standard dose of radioactive iodine (usually ^{123}I) is given by mouth. If RAIU is to be determined at 2 hours, the iodine must be administered intravenously. The patient then is asked to return to the laboratory 2 to 24 hours later (usually 24 hours). On return, the patient lies in the supine position, and a counter is placed over him or her. The amount of radioactive iodine accumulated in the thyroid is calculated. The uptake of the iodine is expressed as a percentage of the thyroid uptake compared with the total of the administered dose.

$$RAIU = \frac{\text{Neck count of patient}}{\text{Standard dose given}} \times 100\%$$

These studies are performed by a technician, and the results are interpreted by a physician. No discomfort is associated with these studies. The thyroid scan is performed in approximately 30 minutes. RAIU may take as long as 24 to 48 hours.

Contraindications

Contraindications for thyroid scanning and RAIU are as follows:

- Patients who are allergic to iodine, because iodine often is used as the radionuclide
- Patients who are pregnant, because the radionuclear tracer may cause fetal injury

Nursing implications with rationale

Before

- Explain the procedure to the patient. Confirm that the patient understands the exact time that he or she must return to the laboratory.

- Question the patient concerning his or her intake of iodine or thyroid hormones. Assess the patient's intake of large amounts of iodine in food (fish, shellfish), drugs (saturated solution of potassium iodine, Lugol's caustic solution, tolbutamide), antiseptics containing iodine, and iodinated contrast materials used in radiographic studies. Note the usage of thyroid or antithyroid drugs, TSH, estrogen, or barbiturates. These iodine and thyroid preparations should be restricted for 1 week before testing. Inform the physician of any pertinent findings.

- Instruct the patient on any food or fluid restrictions necessary before the study. Some hospitals prefer that the patient be in the fasting state before taking the tracer dose. The patient then is allowed to eat 45 minutes later.

After

- Inform the patient that the dose of radioiodine used in this test is minute and, therefore, harmless. Neither isolation nor urine precautions are needed.

Thyroid-Stimulating Hormone
(TSH, Thyrotropin)

Test type Blood

Normal values
Adult: 2-10 μU/ml or 2-10 mU/L (SI units)
Newborn: 3-18 μU/ml or 3-18 mU/L (SI units)
Cord: 3-12 μU/ml or 3-12 mU/L (SI units)
Values vary among laboratories

Rationale
The thyroid-stimulating hormone (TSH) test is used to diagnose primary hypothyroidism and differentiate it from secondary (pituitary) and tertiary (hypothalamus) hypothyroidism. Pituitary TSH secretion is stimulated by hypothalamic TRH. Low levels of triiodothyronine and thyroxine (T_3, T_4) are the underlying stimuli for TRH and TSH. Therefore a compensatory elevation of TRH and TSH occurs in patients with primary hypothyroid states (e.g., surgical or radioactive thyroid ablation); in patients with burned-out thyroiditis, thyroid agenesis, idiopathic hypothyroidism, or congenital cretinism; or in patients taking antithyroid medications.

In secondary or tertiary hypothyroidism, the function of the pituitary or hypothalamus gland, respectively, is faulty because of tumor, trauma, or infarction. Therefore TRH and TSH cannot be secreted, and plasma levels of these hormones are near zero despite the stimulation that occurs with low T_3 and T_4 levels.

TSH is used to monitor exogenous thyroid replacement or suppression. The goal of thyroid replacement therapy is to provide an adequate amount of thyroid medication so that TSH secretion is minimal, indicating a euthyroid state. The goal of thyroid suppression is to completely suppress the thyroid gland and TSH secretion by providing excessive thyroid medication. This treatment is used to diminish the size of a thyroid goiter. For replacement therapy, the dose of medication is titrated as needed to keep the TSH level less than 2.0. For suppression therapy, even lower TSH levels are preferred.

This test also is done to detect primary hypothyroidism in newborns with low screening T_4 levels. TSH and T_4 levels are frequently measured to differentiate pituitary from thyroid dysfunction. A decreased T_4 and a normal or elevated TSH level can indicate a thyroid disorder. A decreased T_4 with a decreased TSH level can indicate a pituitary disorder.

Interfering factors

Factors that interfere with determining TSH levels include the following:

- Recent radioisotope administration, because it may affect test results
- Diurnal variation in TSH levels
  Basal levels occur at approximately 10 AM and highest levels (approximately 2 to 3 times basal levels) occur at approximately 10 PM.

Procedure

Approximately 5 ml of peripheral venous blood is collected in a red-top tube. A heel stick is done on newborns.

Nursing implications with rationale

Before
☞ Explain the procedure to the patient or to the parent of the newborn. Inform the patient that no fasting is necessary.
After
- Apply pressure or a pressure dressing to the venipuncture site to prevent further bleeding. Observe the site for bleeding.

Thyroid-Stimulating Hormone Stimulation Test (TSH Stimulation Test)

Test type Blood

Normal values

Increased thyroid function with administration of exogenous TSH

Rationale

The TSH stimulation test is used to differentiate primary (thyroid) hypothyroidism from secondary (hypothalamic-pituitary) hypothyroidism. People with no thyroid disease and patients with hypothalamic-pituitary hypothyroidism are capable of increasing thyroid function when exogenous TSH is given. Patients with primary hypothyroidism, however, do not respond to the exogenous stimulation; their thyroid gland is inadequate and cannot function no matter how much stimulation it receives. Patients with less than a 10% increase in RAIU or less than a 1.5 μg/dl rise in T_4 are considered to have a primary hypothyroidism. If the hypothyroidism is caused by inadequate pituitary secretion of TSH or hypothalamic secretion of TRH, the RAIU should increase at least 10%, and the T_4 level should rise 1.5 μg/dl or more with TSH administration. These elevations are characteristic of secondary hypothyroidism.

Procedure

Baseline levels of RAIU and T_4 (or protein-bound iodine) are obtained. Five to 10 U/day of TSH is administered intramuscularly for 3 days. The RAIU or T_4 test is repeated.

Nursing implications with rationale

Before
☞ Explain the procedure to the patient. Tell the patient that no fasting is necessary.
- Attain baseline levels of RAIU or T_4 as indicated.
- Administer the TSH intramuscularly for 3 days and then obtain repeat levels of the RAIU or T_4.

After

■ Apply pressure or a pressure dressing to the venipuncture site to prevent further bleeding. Observe the site for bleeding.

Thyroid Ultrasound (Thyroid Echogram, Thyroid Sonogram)

Test type Ultrasound

Normal values

Normal size, shape, and position of the thyroid gland

Rationale

The primary purpose of thyroid ultrasound is to indicate if a thyroid nodule is a fluid-filled cyst (more likely to be benign) or a solid tumor (possibly malignant). Ultrasound also is used to monitor both the medical treatment of a thyroid nodule and the contralateral thyroid lobe when one side has been surgically removed because of cancer.

Ultrasound also can be used to guide an aspirating needle either to obtain fluid from a cyst or tissue from a solid tumor. This test also is the procedure of choice for studying the thyroid gland of pregnant patients because no radioactive material is used to visualize this organ.

Procedure

The nonfasting, unsedated patient is taken to the ultrasonography department (usually in the radiology department) and placed in the supine position. Gel is applied to the patient's neck. An ultrasound technician passes a sound transducer over the nodule. Photographs are taken of the resulting image, and these are evaluated by a physician trained in ultrasonography. No discomfort is associated with this study. It usually is performed in approximately 15 minutes by an ultrasound technician.

Nursing implications with rationale

Before

☞ Explain the procedure to the patient. Assure the patient that no discomfort is associated with this study. Inform the patient that breathing and swallowing will not be affected by the placement of a transducer on the neck.

■ Inform the patient that a liberal amount of lubricant will be applied to the neck to ensure effective transmission and reception of the sound waves.

After

■ Assist the patient in removing the lubricant from his or her neck.

Thyrotropin-Releasing Hormone Test (TRH Test, Thyrotropin-Releasing Factor Test [TRF Test])

Test type Blood

Normal values

Prompt rise in serum TSH level to approximately twice the baseline value in 30 minutes after an IV bolus of TRH

Rationale

The thyrotropin-releasing hormone (TRH) test assesses the responsiveness of the anterior pituitary gland in secreting TSH after an IV injection of TRH. After the injection, the normally functioning pituitary gland should secrete TSH (and prolactin). In hyperthyroidism, either a slight or no increase in the TSH level is seen because pituitary TSH production is suppressed by the inhibitory effect of excess circulating thyroxine and triiodothyronine (T_4 and T_3) on the pituitary gland. A normal test result is considered reliable evidence for excluding the diagnosis of thyrotoxicosis. The TRH test is one of the most reliable diagnostic procedures for hyperthyroidism; other tests are often compared with it to determine their accuracy.

In addition to assessing the responsiveness of the anterior pituitary gland, this test aids in the detection of primary, secondary, and tertiary hypothyroidism. In primary hypothyroidism (thyroid gland failure), the increase in the TSH level is 2 or more times the normal result. With secondary hypothyroidism (anterior pituitary failure), no TSH response occurs. Tertiary hypothyroidism (hypothalamic failure) may be diagnosed by a delayed rise in the TSH level. Multiple injections of TRH may be needed to induce the appropriate TSH response in this case.

Interfering factors

Factors that interfere with determining TRH levels include the following:

- Age
  The normal response may be less than expected in the elderly.
- Pregnancy, because it may increase the TSH response to TRH.

Procedure

No fasting or sedation is required. A 500-μg bolus of TRH is given intravenously. Venous blood samples are obtained at intervals and measured for TSH levels. The maximum response usually occurs in 20 minutes. The TSH concentration should return to normal within 2 hours.

Nursing implications with rationale

Before
- Explain the procedure to the patient. Check with your laboratory for the specific protocol for conducting this test.
- Indicate on the laboratory requisition slip if the patient is pregnant. The TSH response to TRH is increased during pregnancy.
- Assess the patient for medications he or she currently is taking. T_4, antithyroid drugs, estrogens, corticosteroids, or levodopa can modify the TSH response.

After
- Apply pressure or a pressure dressing to the venipuncture site to prevent further bleeding. Observe the site for bleeding.

Thyroxine-Binding Globulin (TBG)
Triiodothyronine Uptake Test (T_3 Resin Uptake Test [T_3RU], Resin Triiodothyronine Uptake Test [RT$_3$U], Thyroid Hormone-Binding Ratio [THBR])

Test type Blood

Normal values
TBG:

Age	Males (mg/dl)	Female (mg/dl)
1-5 days	2.2-4.2	2.2-4.2
1-11 months	1.6-3.6	1.7-3.7
1-9 years	1.2-2.8	1.5-2.7
10-19 years	1.4-2.6	1.4-3.0
>20 years	1.7-3.6	1.7-3.6
Oral contraceptives	—	1.5-5.5
Pregnancy (third trimester)	—	4.7-5.9

THBR:
24% to 34% or 24-34 AU (arbitrary units; SI units)

Rationale

The thyroid-binding globulin (TBG) test is a measure of TBG, the major thyroid hormone protein carrier. It is used to evaluate patients who have abnormal total T_4 and T_3 levels. When the test is done concurrently with T_4 and T_3, one can more easily interpret the T_4 and T_3 levels.

Assays of T_4 and T_3 measure total T_4/T_3 levels (i.e., they measure bound and unbound [free] thyroid hormones). Approximately 90% of T_4 and T_3 is bound to TBG. The unbound T4/T3 is the metabolically active portion of the hormone. Certain illnesses are associated with increased or decreased TBG levels. With increased TBG levels, more T_4 and T_3 is bound to that protein. Less free, metabolically active T_4/T_3 is available. TSH is stimulated to produce higher levels of T_4 and T_3 to compensate. T_4 and T_3 blood levels increase, but they do not cause hyperthyroidism because the increase is merely a compensation to the increased TBG. When total T_4/T_3 is elevated, it must be ascertained whether that elevation is due to an elevation in TBG or is a real elevation in T_4/T_3 alone (as is associated with hyperthyroidism).

The most common causes of elevated TBG are pregnancy, hormone replacement therapy, or use of oral contraceptives. Increased TBG also is present in some cases of porphyria and in infectious hepatitis. Decreased TBG is commonly associated with other causes of hypoproteinemia (e.g., nephrotic syndrome, GI malabsorption, and malnutrition).

Another indirect measurement of TBG is the *thyroid hormone-binding ratio (THBR)*, which also is known as a *T_3 resin uptake test*. This test is not to be confused with T_3 measurement. Before direct T_4 assay, THBR was used as an indirect measurement of T_4. It also is an indirect measurement of the amount of unsaturated thyroid-binding sites on protein (TBG and thyroid-binding prealbumin [TBPA]). As TBG increases, the THBR value will decrease. Conversely, as TBG decreases, THBR increases.

Interfering factors

Factors that interfere with determining TBG and THBR levels include the following:

- Radioisotope administration
  Previous administration of diagnostic radioisotopes may confound test results because TBG and THBR are measured by radioimmunoassay.
- Drugs that *increase* TBG, including estrogens and oral contraceptives.

Procedure

Approximately 5 to 7 ml of venous blood is collected in a red-top tube.

Nursing implications with rationale

Before

☞ Explain the procedure to the patient. Tell the patient that no fasting is necessary.

After

- Apply pressure or a pressure dressing to the venipuncture site to prevent further bleeding. Observe the site for bleeding.

URINE STEROIDS
17-Ketosteroids (17-KS)
17-Hydroxycorticosteroids (17-OHCS)

Test type Urine

Normal values

17-KS:
Elderly: values decrease with age
Male: 7-25 mg/24 hr or 24-88 mmol/day (SI units)
Female: 4-15 mg/24 hr or 14-52 mmol/day (SI units)
Child:
    12-15 years: 5-12 mg/24 hr
    <12 years: <5 mg/24 hr
17-OHCS:
Male:
    Elderly: values lower than for adult
    Adult: 4.5-10.0 mg/24 hr
    Child <12 years: <4.5 mg/24 hr
    Child <8 years: <1.5 mg/24 hr
Female:
    Elderly: values lower than for adult
    Adult: 2.5-10.0 mg/24 hr
    Child <12 years: <4.5 mg/24 hr
    Child <8 years: <1.5 mg/24 hr

Rationale

The urine test for 17-ketosteroids (17-KS) is used to measure adrenocortical function. 17-KS are metabolites of the testosterone and nontestosterone androgenic sex hormones that are secreted from the adrenal cortex and testes. The principal 17-KS is DHEA. In men, approximately one third of the hormone metabolites come from testosterone made in the testes, and two thirds come from nontestosterone androgens made in the adrenal cortex. In women and children, almost all the 17-KS are metabolites from nontestosterone androgenic hormones derived from the adrenal cortex. Therefore this test is very useful in diagnosing adrenocortical dysfunction. It is important to note that 17-KS are not metabolites of cortisol and do not reflect levels of cortisol production. Elevated 17-KS levels are frequently seen in patients with congenital adrenal hyperplasia and androgenic tumors of the adrenal glands. In these diseases, excess steroid synthesis is of the noncortisol, androgenic sterols. These diseases frequently cause virilization syndromes. Testicular tumors rarely cause elevations in 17-KS. Low levels of 17-KS have little clinical significance because of the inaccuracy involved in determining low levels.

Elevated levels of 17-hydroxycorticosteroids (OHCS) are seen in patients with hyperfunctioning of the adrenal gland (Cushing's syndrome), whether caused by a pituitary or adrenal tumor, bilateral adrenal hyperplasia, or ectopic tumors producing ACTH. Low levels of 17-OHCS are seen in patients who have a hypofunctioning adrenal gland (Addison's disease) caused by destruction of the adrenal glands (by hemorrhage, infarction, metastatic tumor, or autoimmunity); surgical removal of an adrenal gland without appropriate steroid replacement; congenital enzyme deficiency; hypopituitarism; or adrenal suppression after prolonged exogenous steroid ingestion.

Interfering factor

A factor that interferes with determining 17-KS and 17-OHCS levels is stress. Emotional and physical stress (e.g., infection) may cause *increased* adrenal activity, which can alter the test results. Report any evidence of stress noted in the patient to the physician. The test should be rescheduled.

Procedure

Urine is collected over a 24-hour period in a 1-gallon urine container. A preservative is necessary for the 17-KS test. Urine for the 17-OHCS test does not require a preservative. The urine specimen is refrigerated or kept on ice during the entire collection period. At the end of the collection period, the urine is sent to the chemistry laboratory.

Nursing implications with rationale

Before

- Explain the procedure to the patient. Confirm that the patient understands the collection procedure to prevent urine from being discarded. Valid interpretation of adrenal function depends on a complete 24-hour urine collection.
- List any medications the patient is taking on the laboratory requisition slip because many medications interfere with the chemical determination of the urinary steroids.
- Encourage the patient to consume foods and fluids during the 24-hour collection period,

unless they are contraindicated for medical reasons.

During

- Instruct the patient to begin the 24-hour urine collection after discarding the first morning specimen. This is the start time of the 24-hour collection.
- Collect all urine passed over the next 24 hours into a container.
- Instruct the patient to void before defecating so that the urine is not contaminated by feces.
- Remind the patient not to put toilet paper in the collection container.
- Keep the urine specimen on ice or refrigerated during the 24 hours.
- Collect the last specimen as close as possible to the end of the 24 hours.

After

- Transport the urine specimen promptly to the laboratory, preferably during the 7 AM to 3 PM shift so that it can be evaluated immediately during routine laboratory working hours.

REVIEW QUESTIONS AND ANSWERS

1. **Question:** Your 26-year-old female patient has had several episodes of hypoglycemia progressing to loss of consciousness requiring hospitalization. A thorough evaluation has been normal except for an elevated insulin assay and decreased C-peptide level. How might you approach this patient, once her condition is stabilized, in regard to her physical and psychoemotional needs?

   Answer: This patient is administering insulin to herself and deliberately causing the hypoglycemic episodes to occur. She must be thoroughly evaluated to determine whether these are suicide attempts. If not, the reason for the attention-seeking, self-destructive behavior must be elucidated. After discharge, she must be observed closely by friends or family members to prevent her from repeating any unnecessary insulin injections because such behavior could have deadly consequences.

2. **Question:** On return from adrenal venography, your patient's blood pressure is 240/130 mm Hg, heart rate is 144 beats/minute, and respiration rate is 42 breaths/minute. What might be developing, and what are the appropriate interventions from a physical, pharmacologic, and psychoemotional standpoint?

   Answer: This patient is probably experiencing adrenergic stimulation caused by a pheochromocytoma (pressor crisis). Venous access and continuous monitoring of vital signs must be initiated. Alpha-adrenergic blockade drugs should be administered immediately. Alternatively, angiotensin-converting enzyme (ACE) blockers or nitroprusside can be used. After accomplishing an adequate alpha-adrenergic blockade, beta-adrenergic blockade can be accomplished using beta blockers to reduce the heart rate. The patient should be constantly reassured that the situation is under control.

3. **Question:** Your patient is scheduled to have thyroid scanning. While obtaining a medical history of the patient, you discover that he had an IVP 1 week ago to evaluate a urologic complaint. Should thyroid scanning be cancelled?

   Answer: Yes. The iodine load that the patient received during his IVP will inhibit thyroidal uptake of any radioactive material for at least 4 weeks. Therefore the results of the scanning would be inadequate. The physician should be informed, and the test should be cancelled. Occasionally an ^{127}I urine excretion test can be performed by giving the patient a standard dose of ^{127}I by mouth. If the urine excretion of iodine is greater than 1 mg/day, excess iodine in the blood is still present and blocking the thyroid uptake of ^{127}I. The excess iodine also will block uptake of any scanning material.

4. **Question:** Your patient is scheduled to have an RAIU test to rule out hyperthyroidism. One of the symptoms of hyperthyroidism is diarrhea, and this patient is having four loose bowel movements a day. Should the test be performed?

   Answer: No. The results of this test require GI absorption of the orally administered radioactive iodine. If the patient has diarrhea, only a small portion of the iodine will be absorbed, and this will bias the results of the test. It is best not to perform the test with orally administered iodine. However, iodine may be given intravenously, and the uptake measured at 2 hours (in contrast to the 24 hours required for the orally administered iodine).

5. **Question:** On a routine evaluation for lower back pain, a 54-year-old woman is found to have hypercalcemia. Her serum PTH level is below normal. What might elucidate the cause of this patient's problems?

   Answer: The most common cause of hypercalcemia and a concomitantly low PTH level in a postmenopausal woman is bone metastasis from a primary breast cancer. Therefore mammography and a lumbosacral spinal x-ray study are indicated. (Primary and tertiary hyperparathyroidism were eliminated as causes in light of the low PTH level.)

6. **Question:** A patient is transferred to your floor 2 days after having a complete workup for an adrenal tumor. This workup included a dexamethasone suppression test, adrenal angiography, adrenal venography, and ACTH assay. You notice that over the next 24 hours this patient becomes progressively more obtunded. All laboratory tests are normal except for a low sodium level and a high potassium level. Although the physician orders appropriate IV fluids, the patient dies 48 hours after transfer to your floor. What might have been attempted to reverse the progressive deterioration of this patient?

   Answer: Adrenal gland hemorrhage and infarction are complications of adrenal venography. Autopsy of this patient did, indeed, demonstrate bilateral adrenal gland hemorrhage. These complications should have been considered, and the patient should have been given cortisone intravenously.

7. **Question:** Your patient, who is suspected of having an adrenal tumor, returns to the floor after having adrenal angiography. On physical assessment of the patient, blood pressure is 280/140 mm Hg, pulse rate is 145 beats/minute, oral temperature is 101° F, and respiration rate is 38 breaths/minute. Is this

patient having an allergic reaction to the dye?
Answer: No. Most patients having a serious allergic reaction to iodinated dye are hypotensive. Allergy also would be highlighted by urticaria and wheezing. This patient is most probably having a serious hypertensive episode caused by a pheochromocytoma and induced by the arteriography.

8. **Question:** Your patient is scheduled for a 24-hour urine collection for 17-KS. Why should creatinine also be measured in the urine specimen?
Answer: Excretion of creatinine is relatively constant. If the creatinine concentration in the 24-hour urine collection is less than normal (male, 20 to 26 mg/kg; female, 14 to 22 mg/kg), one must suspect that the specimen does not represent a complete 24-hour collection. Some of the urine may have been discarded. This will bias the results for 17-KS or other urine components. The urine collection should be repeated.

9. **Question:** Your patient is having a GTT performed. Thirty minutes after ingestion of the glucose, the patient vomits. What should be done?
Answer: After assessing the patient's vital signs, a blood glucose specimen should be obtained to ensure that the patient is not dangerously hyperglycemic or hypoglycemic. The GTT then should be cancelled because its results are based on the ingestion and digestion of the entire glucose load. Incomplete absorption of the glucose load will bias the results. If the patient cannot tolerate the ingestion of the glucose load, then an IV-GTT can be performed.

10. **Question:** Your patient is admitted to the hospital for evaluation of signs and symptoms suggesting Cushing's syndrome. The doctor has requested that you begin collecting a 24-hour urine specimen for a 17-OHCS test. In your initial assessment of the patient, you discover that she has a severe upper respiratory tract infection. Should the test be performed?
Answer: No. The ongoing, acute upper respiratory tract infection acts as a physical stress to the patient. As a result, the adrenal gland may be appropriately hyperfunctioning, and elevated urine 17-OHCS levels would be expected even in normal patients. For that reason, you should notify the physician of the upper respiratory tract infection. The physician will most probably want to cancel the planned evaluation and treat the patient's respiratory tract infection.

Bibliography

Anderson RJ: Adrenocortical insufficiency. In Rakel RE, editor: Conn's current therapy, Philadelphia, 1998, WB Saunders.

Arafah BM: Hypopituitarism. In Rakel RE, editor: Conn's current therapy, Philadelphia, 1998, WB Saunders.

Ayala A, Wartofsky L: Minimally symptomatic (subclinical) hypothyroidism, *Endocrinologist* 7:44, 1997.

Behrman RE et al, editors: Nelson textbook of pediatrics, ed 15, Philadelphia, 1996, WB Saunders.

Beierwaltes WH: Endocrine imaging: parathyroid, adrenal cortex, and medulla, and other endocrine tumors, Part II, *J Nucl Med* 32(8):1627-1639, 1991.

Biller BK, Daniels GH: Neuroendocrine regulation and diseases of the anterior pituitary and hypothalamus. In Fauci AS et al, editors: Harrison's principles of internal medicine, ed 14, New York, 1998, McGraw-Hill.

Burch HB: Evaluation and management of the solid thyroid nodule, *Endocrinol Metab Clin North Am* 24:663, 1995.

Carpenter PC: Cushing's syndrome. In Rakel RE, editor: Conn's current therapy, Philadelphia, 1998, WB Saunders.

Chopra IJ: Hypothyroidism. In Rakel RE, editor: Conn's current therapy, Philadelphia, 1998, WB Saunders.

Daniels GH: Hyperthyroidism. In Rakel RE, editor: Conn's current therapy, Philadelphia, 1998, WB Saunders.

Foster DW: Diabetes mellitus. In Fauci AS et al, editors: Harrison's principles of internal medicine, ed 14, New York, 1998, McGraw-Hill.

Gross MD et al: Scintigraphic imaging of the thyroid, parathyroid, and adrenal glands, *Curr Opin Radiol* 2(6):851-859, 1990.

Hintz RL: Disorders of growth. In Fauci AS et al, editors: Harrison's principles of internal medicine, ed 14, New York, 1998, McGraw-Hill.

Landin-Olsson M et al: Islet cell antibodies and fasting C-peptide predict insulin requirement at diagnosis of diabetes mellitus, *Diabetologia* 33(9):561-568, 1990.

Makita Z et al: Radioimmunoassay for the determination of glycated haemoglobin, *Diabetologia* 34(1):40-45, 1991.

Mallette LE: Hyperparathyroidism and hypoparathyroidism. In Rakel RE, editor: Conn's current therapy, Philadelphia, 1998, WB Saunders.

Masters PA, Simons RJ: Clinical use of sensitive assays for thyroid-stimulating hormone, *J Gen Intern Med* 11:115, 1996.

Oertel YC: Fine needle aspiration and the diagnosis of thyroid cancer, *Endocrinol Metab Clin North Am* 25:69, 1996.

Orth DN: Cushing's syndrome, *N Engl J Med* 332:791, 1995.

Taylor A, Datz FL, editors: Clinical application of nuclear medicine, New York, 1991, Churchill Livingstone.

Torrens JI, Burch HB: Serum thyroglobulin measurement: utility in clinical practice, *Endocrinologist* 6:125, 1996.

Tsang WM et al: Glycated hemoglobin measurement in uremic patients, *Ann Clin Biochem* 28(4):414-416, 1991.

Tsuji A et al: Recent progress in neonatal mass screening for congenital hypothyroidism and adrenal hyperplasia using enzyme immunoassays, *Adv Clin Chem* 28:109-143, 1990.

Wartofsky L: Diseases of the thyroid. In Fauci AS et al, editors: Harrison's principles of internal medicine, ed 14, New York, 1998, McGraw-Hill.

Williams GH, Dluhy RG: Diseases of the adrenal cortex. In Fauci AS et al, editors: Harrison's principles of internal medicine, ed 14, New York, 1998, McGraw-Hill.

Wilson JD: Approach to the patient with endocrine and metabolic disorders. In Fauci AS et al, editors: Harrison's principles of internal medicine, ed 14, New York, 1998, McGraw-Hill.

Wilson JD, Foster DW, editors: Williams textbook of endocrinology, ed 9, Philadelphia, 1997, WB Saunders.

Yalow RS: Radioimmunoassay of hormones. In Wilson JD, Foster DW, editors: Williams textbook of endocrinology, ed 8, Philadelphia, 1992, WB Saunders.

Chapter 9

Diagnostic Studies Used in the Assessment of the
Reproductive System

ANATOMY AND PHYSIOLOGY

This discussion of anatomy and physiology of the reproductive system deals only with material relevant to the diagnostic studies included in this chapter. A detailed discussion of this complex system can be found in many textbooks (see Bibliography).

Male Generative Organs

The testes (Figure 9-1) are located in the scrotum, which provides the appropriate temperature required for sperm production (spermatogenesis). The epithelial cells lining the seminiferous tubules within the testes give rise to the spermatozoa, or sperm cells. Sperm production is one of the major functions of the testes. Genital ducts, which include the epididymis, vas deferens, ejaculatory duct, seminal vesicles, and urethra (see Figure 9-1), provide a conduit for transport of the sperm cells.

The other major function of the testes is secretion of testosterone, which is the major androgen (male hormone). Testosterone is secreted by the interstitial cells of the testes. It stimulates

development of part of the genital tract, as well as development of secondary male sexual characteristics.

Female Reproductive Organs

The ovaries are the essential sex organs in the female reproductive system (Figure 9-2). Like the testes, the ovaries are multifunctional. They are responsible for ovulation (production of ova) and the secretion of the female hormones (estrogen and progesterone). The fallopian tubes (oviducts) arise from the uterus and terminate adjacent to the ovary. These oviducts transport the ovum to the uterus. Fertilization of the ovum by the sperm usually occurs within these ducts.

The uterus is a muscular organ whose inner cavity is lined with a specialized mucosa called the *endometrium*. The endometrium undergoes cyclic (menstrual) structural changes in preparation for conception and pregnancy. Events occurring in the ovary and uterus during the menstrual cycle are shown in Figure 9-3.

There are three phases of the menstrual cycle: the menstrual phase, the proliferative phase, and the secretory phase. The average menstrual cycle

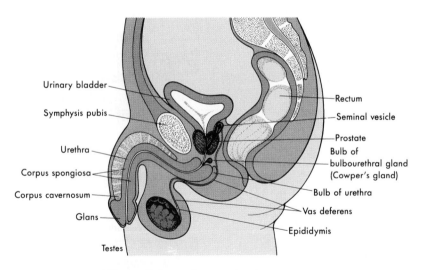

Figure 9-1 Male reproductive system.

is 28 days and begins with the first day of vaginal blood flow. During the menses (menstrual phase), the endometrium undergoes degenerative change so that the superficial layer of the endometrium sloughs and is discharged in the menstrual flow. After the blood flow ceases, a gradual growth of the endometrium occurs (proliferative phase), which is stimulated by ovarian estrogen. At approximately the fourteenth day of the cycle (see Figure 9-3), the graafian follicle within the ovary ruptures, and the ovum is expelled (ovulation) into the fallopian tubes. The ruptured ovarian follicle then is called a *corpus luteum.* Large amounts of progesterone and some estrogen are secreted by the corpus luteum and cause the endometrial glands to thicken and mature. This is called the *endometrial secretory phase.* The submucosal layers become extremely vascular and edematous. The purpose of the secretory phase is to prepare the uterine lining to receive (nidation) and nourish a fertilized ovum. If fertilization does not take place, the corpus luteum degenerates, and the endometrium sloughs, leading to vaginal bleed-ing, which occurs at approximately the twenty-eighth day of the cycle.

Pregnancy

When fertilization does occur, the zygote (fertilized ovum) moves through the fallopian tubes and into the prepared uterine cavity. On coming into contact with the endometrial mucosa, the exposed cells on the outside (trophoblast) of the developing embryonic cell mass (blastocyst) begin to digest a portion of the mucosa. This allows the trophoblast to sink into the mucosa (implant) and absorb nutrition from the uterine glands until the placenta forms. The trophoblast and, later, the placenta produce human chorionic gonadotropin (HCG), which maintains the existence of the corpus luteum. The corpus luteum continues to secrete the progesterone required to maintain the pregnancy. Through continued growth, the embryo becomes surrounded by two membranes: the amnion (inner layer of the fetal membrane) and the chorion (outer layer of the fetal membrane). The space

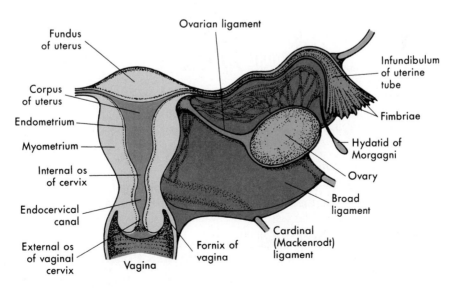

Figure 9-2   Female reproductive system. Cross section of uterus, adnexa, and upper vagina.

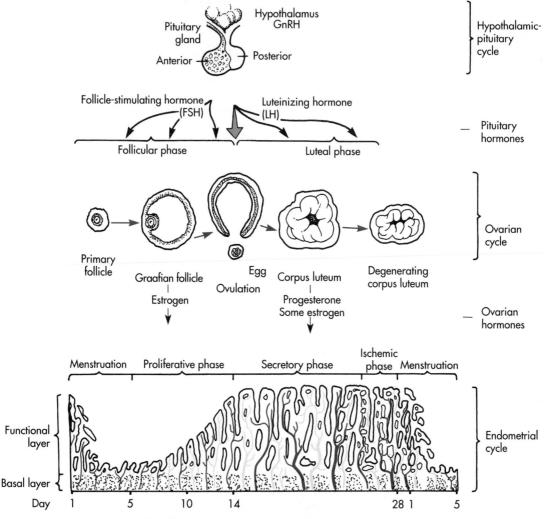

Figure 9-3   Hormonal control of menstrual cycle.

between the embryo and the amnion, the amniotic cavity, is filled with amniotic fluid.

At approximately 8 weeks from the last menstrual period, the embryo is completely developed and is called a *fetus*. For the remaining 32 weeks of gestation, the fetus develops on the nutritional support provided by the mother through the placenta. Toward the end of pregnancy, HCG and progesterone levels decrease, perhaps as a result of placental deterioration. Uterine contractions begin in an effort to expel the fetus vaginally.

High-Risk Pregnancy

Many disease states can jeopardize the normal events associated with pregnancy, labor, and delivery. When such threats are recognized beforehand, the pregnancy is considered at high risk and monitored more closely than usual. Some examples of factors in the patient's history or current health status responsible for a high-risk pregnancy include the following:

1. Advanced maternal age of 35 years or older
2. Past or current history of primary, idiopathic hypertension
3. Two or more spontaneous or induced abortions in the past
4. Previous stillbirths
5. Previous premature deliveries
6. Previous infant with rhesus (Rh) isoimmunization
7. Previous infant with genetic or familial disorders
8. Previous infant with congenital anomaly
9. Previous small-for-status infant or present small-for-status fetus (intrauterine growth retardation)
10. Multiple pregnancies
11. Genital tract anomalies (e.g., incompetent cervix, cervical malformation, or uterine malformation)
12. Medical conditions (e.g., hypertension, diabetes mellitus [DM], heart disease, renal disease, cancer, or thyroid dysfunction)
13. Social problems (e.g., teen pregnancy, drug or tobacco use, or poor nutrition)

Infertility

Infertility can be diagnosed whenever a woman is unable to conceive during at least 1 year of regular, unprotected intercourse. Ninety percent of couples are able to achieve a pregnancy within a 1-year period. Normal fertility is dependent on many factors in both the man and woman. The man must be able to produce a sufficient number of normal, motile spermatozoa that can be ejaculated through a patent pathway (vas deferens) into the vagina. The spermatozoa then must be able to survive in the cervical environment and ascend through the cervix, uterus, and fallopian tubes. The woman must be able to produce an ovum that remains in the fallopian tubes until it is fertilized by sperm. To begin normal development, the products of conception must be allowed to move into the uterus and implant themselves in an endometrium capable of sustaining life. Any defect in these processes will result in infertility.

Male infertility

Problems in male fertility are the sole factor, or an important contributing factor, in 30% to 40% of infertile couples. These problems usually involve defects in spermatogenesis or insemination. Male infertility may be caused by one or more of the following:

1. Spermatozoal abnormalities. These include reduction in the quantity of spermatozoa (<50 million/ml), reduction of the ejaculatory volume (<3.4 ml), abnormal sperm quality (e.g., too dilute), and abnormally shaped spermatozoa (e.g., two-headed or tailless).
2. Sperm antibodies (autoimmunization). Autoantibodies may be responsible for interference with normal spermatogenesis or may affect the spermatozoa and prevent pregnancy.
3. Testicular abnormalities (e.g., complete absence or inappropriate development of the testes). Infections, particularly suppurative orchitis, which may accompany mumps, can destroy the epithelium of the seminiferous tubules. Abnormal testicular location (cryptorchidism), testicular trauma, irradiation, prolonged exposure to high temperatures, or varicocele may result in inadequate spermatogenesis.
4. Abnormalities of the penis. If the penis is abnormally short, buried in fat, or malformed (as in hypospadias), semen emission may take place outside of the vagina.
5. Faulty sperm transmission. Insemination may be inhibited because of scarring that obstructs the epididymis, vas deferens, or

urethra. Postgonorrheal scarring is the most frequent cause.

6. Prostate and seminal vesicle abnormalities. The number of quality of sperm may be reduced or altered by chronic prostatitis or seminal vesiculitis.

7. Advanced nutritional deficiency. This condition alters the function of all organ systems, including the gonads.

8. Emotional factors. These may induce impotence or premature ejaculation.

Female infertility

Ovulation occurs between the twelfth and sixteenth day of most menstrual cycles. Unprotected intercourse must take place within 12 to 24 hours of ovulation. Often failure to conceive is the result of incorrect timing of ovulation. Other causes of female infertility include:

1. Cervical abnormalities. Alterations in cervical mucosa caused by either hormonal deficiency or cervicitis interfere with sperm passage. Obstructions in the cervical canal caused by polyps, fibroids (leiomyomas), atresia, or suppurative discharge impair the transit of the spermatozoa.

2. Vaginal disorders. Absence or incomplete formation of the vagina prevents vaginal penetration by the penis and sperm. Inflammation of the vagina alters the pH, which may destroy or inactivate sperm.

3. Endocrine abnormalities. The abnormal function of the hypothalamus, anterior pituitary, ovaries, thyroid, or adrenal glands can result in anovulation.

4. Uterine disorder. Scarring (after dilation and curettage [D&C]), malformation, malposition, or tumors of the uterus may prevent nidation of the fertilized ovum into the uterine mucosa or cause early abortion.

5. Tubal disorders. Partial or complete occlusion of the fallopian tubes occurs in a large number of women who fail to conceive. The most common cause of tubal obstruc-

tion is scarring (as a result of pelvic inflammatory disease [PID]). Appendicitis and other pelvic infections, along with pelvic endometriosis, may result in adhesions that subsequently can partially or completely obstruct the tubes.

6. Ovarian disorders. Ovarian agenesis or incomplete development can cause anovulation. Tumors, infections, or endometriosis also can disrupt ovarian function transiently or permanently.

7. Severe nutritional deficiencies and chronic disease states. These conditions reduce or inhibit ovulation.

8. Advancing age. Fertility in women reaches a peak at about 20 to 25 years of age and slowly declines until menopause.

9. Emotional factors. Vaginismus (painful spasm of the vagina that prevents coitus) and dyspareunia (pain during coitus) may be the result of psychologic disturbances.

10. Immunologic reactions to sperm. Unexplained infertility may be caused by female production of antisperm antibodies.

11. Drugs. Nearly all ovulating women cease to ovulate while on antineoplastic chemotherapy and many psychotropic drugs.

12. Radiation. Ovulation is permanently obliterated by exposure of the ovaries to radiation levels greater than 800 rad.

Because one or many factors may be the cause of infertility, the man and woman must both be evaluated. A systematic investigation of infertility is described after the case study entitled, "Infertility." During the diagnostic course, it is important to allow the couple the opportunity to express feelings of isolation, guilt, depression, or anger that often accompany infertility. Therapy for infertility may require correction of faulty coital techniques, attention to proper timing, surgery to correct a malfunction or anatomic anomalies, or recognition and correction of emotional factors. If the infertility persists, the condition is then referred to as *sterility.* Approximately 1 of 10 American couples is truly barren.

Amniocentesis (Amniotic Fluid Analysis)

Test type Fluid analysis

Normal values

Amniotic fluid volume:
   Full term: <1500 ml
   30-35 weeks' gestation: 1500 ml
   25 weeks' gestation: 750 ml
   15 weeks' gestation: 450 ml
Appearance of amniotic fluid: clear; pale to straw yellow
Lecithin/sphingomyelin (L/S) ratio: ≥2:1
Bilirubin: <0.2 mg/dl
No chromosomal or genetic abnormalities
Phosphatidylglycerol (PG): positive for PG
Lamellar body count: >30,000
Alpha-fetoprotein (AFP): 2 μg/ml

Rationale

Amniocentesis is performed to gather information about the fetus. Fetal maturity, fetal distress, and risk of respiratory distress syndrome (RDS) can be assessed. Genetic and chromosomal abnormalities can be identified. Maternal/fetal Rh incompatibility can be diagnosed. The sex of the child can be ascertained. This is important for mothers carrying a sex-linked gene associated with a disease. Neural tube defects also can be recognized. The test is performed on expectant mothers whose pregnancies are considered to be high risk, such as those who are diabetic, obese, or older than age 35. Amniocentesis is especially helpful if there is a family history of trisomy 21, repeated spontaneous abortions, or prior children with genetic defects, and if either the mother or father is a carrier for genetic defects. This test is also done on women who have an abnormal obstetric ultrasound.

For amniocentesis, a needle is placed through the patient's abdominal and uterine walls and into the amniotic cavity to withdraw fluid for analysis. The study of amniotic fluid is vitally important in assessing the following:

1. **Fetal maturity status,** especially pulmonary maturity (when early delivery is preferred). Fetal maturity is determined by analysis of the amniotic fluid in the following manner:

   a. *L/S ratio.* The L/S ratio measures fetal lung maturity. Lecithin is the major constituent of surfactant, an important substance required for alveolar ventilation. If surfactant is insufficient, the alveoli collapse during expiration. This results in atelectasis and RDS, which is a major cause of death in premature babies. In the immature fetal lung, the sphingomyelin concentration in amniotic fluid is higher than the lecithin concentration. At 35 weeks of gestation, the concentration of lecithin rapidly increases, whereas sphingomyelin concentration decreases. An L/S ratio of 2:1 (3:1 in mothers with diabetes) or greater is a highly reliable indication that the fetal lung, and, therefore, the fetus, are mature. In such a case, the infant would be unlikely to develop RDS after birth. As the L/S ratio decreases, the risk of RDS increases.

   b. *PG.* This is a minor component (approximately 10%) of lung surfactant phospholipids. However, because PG is almost entirely synthesized by mature lung alveolar cells, it is a good indicator of lung maturity. In healthy, pregnant women, PG appears in amniotic fluid after 35 weeks of gestation, and levels gradually increase until term. The simultaneous determination of the L/S ratio and the presence of PG is an excellent method of assessing fetal maturity based on pulmonary surfactant.

   c. *Lamellar body count.* This new test to determine fetal maturity also is based on the presence of surfactant. Lamellar bodies are concentrically layered structures produced by type II pneumocytes. On microscopic cross-section, these structures look like an onion and are called *lamellar bodies.* These lamellar bodies represent the storage form of pulmonary surfactant. Because lamellar bodies and platelets are indistinguishable to cell counters, the lamellar body count is obtained by analyzing the amniotic fluid with a cell counter and recording the platelet count. If the count is greater than 30,000, there is a 100% chance that the infant's lungs are mature enough to avoid RDS. If the lamellar body count is less than 10,000, the probability of RDS is high (67%). Lamellar body counts have several advantages. First, they are faster, more precise, and more objective, and they require less amniotic fluid than does phospholipid analysis. Second, test results are not invalidated by the presence of blood or meconium. Third, the instrumentation required for this test is readily available, thus allowing it to be performed in all laboratories.

2. **Genetic and chromosomal aberrations.** Genetic and chromosomal studies performed on cells aspirated within the amniotic fluid can indicate the gender of the fetus (important in sex-linked diseases such as hemophilia) or any of the described genetic and chromosomal aberrations (e.g., trisomy 21). Sons of mothers who are known to be carriers of X-linked recessive traits would have a 50:50 chance of inheritance. It is important to note that amniocentesis is not done merely to satisfy curiosity regarding the sex of the child.

3. **Fetal status affected by Rh isoimmunization.** Mothers with Rh isoimmunization will have a series of amniocentesis procedures during the second half of pregnancy to assess the level of bilirubin pigment in the amniotic fluid. The quantity of bilirubin is used to assess the severity of hemolytic anemia in Rh-sensitized pregnancy (Rh-positive fetus, Rh-negative mother). The higher the amount of bilirubin, the greater the red blood cell (RBC) hemolysis in the

fetus, and the lower the amount of fetal hemoglobin. Amniocentesis usually is initiated at 24 to 25 weeks' gestation to assess the severity of the disease and the status of the fetus. Early delivery and blood transfusion may be indicated.

4. **Hereditary metabolic disorders,** such as cystic fibrosis.

5. **Anatomic abnormalities,** such as neural tube closure defects (myelomeningocele, anencephaly, spina bifida). Increased levels of alpha-fetoprotein (AFP) in the amniotic fluid may indicate a neural crest abnormality. Decreased levels of AFP may be associated with an increased risk of trisomy 21.

6. **Fetal distress,** detected by meconium staining of the amniotic fluid. This is caused by relaxation of the fetal anal sphincter. In this case, the normally pale, straw-colored amniotic fluid may be tinged with green. Other color changes also may indicate fetal distress. For example, a yellow discoloration may indicate a blood incompatibility. A yellow-brown, opaque appearance may indicate intrauterine death. A red color indicates blood contamination either from the mother or the fetus.

In the past, other tests were performed on the amniotic fluid. Most of these, however, are no longer done. The shake test (also called *foam stability,* or *rapid surfactant test*) was a crude way of determining fetal maturity by identifying surfactant as an agent that prolongs the stability of an emulsifier. Creatinine was another test to determine fetal maturity based on the muscle mass of the fetus. Again, this test is too inaccurate to be useful. Staining fetal cells with Nile blue for identification of fat as a determinant of fetal maturity also has lost favor because of its inaccuracy.

The timing of the amniocentesis varies according to the clinical circumstances. With advanced maternal age and if chromosomal or genetic aberrations are suspected, the test should be done early enough (at 14 to 16 weeks of gestation when at least 150 ml of fluid exists) to allow a safe abortion. This early timing is essential because of the 2 weeks necessary for cell growth to determine the study's results. If information on fetal maturity is sought, performing the study during or after the thirty-fifth week of gestation is best. Placental localization by ultrasonography should be done before amniocentesis to avoid passing the needle into the placenta, possibly interrupting the placenta, and inducing bleeding or abortion.

Potential complications

Potential complications associated with amniocentesis are as follows:

- Miscarriage
- Fetal injury
- Leak of amniotic fluid
- Infection (amnionitis)
- Abortion
- Premature labor
- Maternal hemorrhage with possible maternal Rh isoimmunization
- Amniotic fluid embolism
- Inadvertent damage to maternal bladder or intestines

All of the above complications are the result of needle penetration during amniocentesis.

Interfering factors

Factors that interfere with amniocentesis include the following:

- Fetal blood contamination, because it can cause falsely *elevated* AFP levels
- Hemolysis of the specimen, which can alter results
- Contamination of the specimen with meconium or blood, which may give inaccurate L/S ratios

Procedure

The patient's bladder is emptied to minimize the risk of puncture; however, before 20 weeks'

gestation, the bladder is often kept full to support the uterus. Before the amniocentesis, the mother's blood pressure is assessed, and the fetal heart rate (FHR) is auscultated. The placenta should be localized by ultrasound before the study to permit selection of a site that will avoid placental puncture. Ultrasonography also aids in identification of uterine abnormalities (e.g., bicornuate uterus) that may complicate the amniocentesis procedure. The patient then is placed in a supine position, and the skin overlying the chosen site is prepared, draped, and locally anesthetized.

A 22-gauge, 5-inch spinal needle with a stylet is inserted through the midabdominal wall and directed at an angle toward the middle of the uterine cavity. The stylet then is removed, and a sterile, plastic syringe is attached (Figure 9-4). After 10 to 15 ml of amniotic fluid is withdrawn, the needle is removed. The site is covered with an adhesive bandage. If the amniotic fluid is bloody, the physician must determine whether the blood is maternal or fetal in origin.

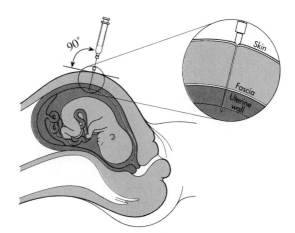

Figure 9-4 Amniocentesis. Ultrasound scanning usually is used to determine the placental site and to locate a pocket of amniotic fluid. The needle then is inserted. Three levels of resistance are felt as the needle penetrates the skin, fascia, and uterine wall. When the needle is placed within the uterine cavity, amniotic fluid is withdrawn.

The amniotic fluid is placed in a sterile, siliconized glass container and transported to a special chemistry laboratory for analysis. Sometimes the specimen may be sent by air mail to another commercial laboratory. The results usually are not available for at least 10 days. After the procedure, the mother's blood pressure is checked, and the fetal heart tone is assessed. The patient should be instructed to report any fluid loss, bleeding, cramping, dizziness, or fever following this study.

Amniocentesis should be performed by an experienced obstetrician, who is able to provide counseling and treatment based on the results of this study. The discomfort associated with this study is that of mild uterine cramping, which occurs when the needle contacts the uterus. Some women may complain of a pulling sensation as the amniotic fluid is withdrawn. Most women describe injection of the local anesthetic as being the most uncomfortable part of amniocentesis. Many women are extremely anxious during this procedure. The duration of this procedure is approximately 20 to 30 minutes.

The maternal blood type should be determined (if unknown). Women who have Rh-negative blood should receive RH_0 (D) immune globulin, (RhoGAM) because of the risk of immunization from the fetal blood, which can jeopardize the fetus.

Contraindications

Contraindications associated with amniocentesis are as follows:

- Patients with a history of premature labor (before 34 weeks of gestation, unless the patient is receiving antilabor medication)
  Amniocentesis could induce labor.
- Patients with an incompetent cervix
  Amniocentesis could induce labor.

Nursing implications with rationale
Before
- Explain the procedure to the patient. Assure the patient that precautions will be taken to minimize risk to both her and the fetus. Encourage the patient to verbalize her fears concerning this study. Most patients are very apprehensive. Relaxation techniques, such as focusing and slow breathing, can help relieve some maternal anxiety.
- Inform the patient that no food or fluid restriction is needed.
- Confirm that the physician has obtained written and informed consent from the parents before the procedure.
- Instruct the patient regarding whether she should empty her bladder. Whether to do so depends on gestational age. Before 20 weeks, the bladder may be kept full to support the uterus. After 20 weeks, the bladder may be emptied to minimize the chance of puncture.
- Assess the FHR before and after the study to detect any ill effects related to the procedure. In the event of ill effects, bed rest and fetal heart monitoring are prescribed. An immediate cesarean section may be performed if gestation is greater than 35 weeks, and signs of fetal dizziness are evident.
- Instruct the patient that the needle used in this procedure is long because it passes through layers of fat and muscle before reaching the uterus. Only a small portion of the needle passes into the uterus.

After
- If the woman feels dizzy or nauseated during the procedure, allow her to rest on her left side for several minutes before leaving the examining room.
- Administer RhoGAM for women who have Rh-negative blood, because of the risk of immunization from the fetal blood.
- Instruct the patient to observe the puncture site for bleeding or other drainage and to call her physician if she has any fluid loss or temperature elevation.
- Inform the patient about how she can obtain the results of this study from her physician. Verify that the patient knows the results will not be available for at least 2 weeks.

Antispermatozoal Antibody (Sperm Agglutination and Inhibition, Sperm Antibodies, Antisperm Antibodies, Infertility Screen)

Test type Fluid analysis, blood

Normal values
Negative

Rationale
The antispermatozoal antibody test is commonly used in the evaluation of an infertile couple. Antisperm antibodies may be found in the blood of men with blocked efferent ducts (the ducts leading to the vas deferens) exiting the testes (a common cause of low sperm counts or poor sperm mobility) and in 30% to 70% of men who have had a vasectomy. Reabsorption of sperm components from the blocked ducts results in the formation of autoantibodies to sperm as a result of sperm antigens interacting with the immune system. The immunoglobulin (Ig) A antisperm antibodies to the sperm tail are associated with poor motility and poor penetration of cervical mucus. IgG antisperm antibodies are associated with blockage of sperm to ovum fusion. High titers of IgG autoantibodies are often associated with postvasectomy degeneration of the testes, which explains why 50% of males remain infertile after successful repair of vasectomy.

In men, high serum titers of antispermatozoal antibodies are considered strong evidence of infertility. Low titers are of unknown significance because they are not an uncommon finding among fertile males. Serum antispermatozoal antibodies are found in nearly 20% of women. However, many of these women become pregnant. The significance of these antibodies in women, therefore, is uncertain.

Antispermatozoal antibodies also can be detected in the sperm of infertile males and the cervical mucus of infertile females. To thoroughly evaluate infertility, it often is necessary to identify these antibodies in these other body fluids.

Procedure
Blood is collected from both partners in a red-top tube. A semen specimen should be collected after avoiding ejaculation for at least 3 days and brought to the laboratory in a plastic cup within 2 hours after collection.

Nursing implications with rationale
Before
- Explain the procedure to the male and/or female patient. Describe the blood, sperm, and vaginal collection methods.
- Be certain that the male patient knows that a 3-day period of sexual abstinence is necessary for the sperm collection.
- Give the male patient the proper container in which to collect the sperm. He may find the collection and delivery of the semen to the laboratory embarrassing. Be matter-of-fact about specimen collection and delivery.
- If the specimen is to be obtained at home, be certain that the male patient is informed that it must be taken to the laboratory for testing within 2 hours after collection.

After
- Apply pressure or a pressure dressing to the venipuncture to prevent further bleeding. Observe the site for bleeding.
- Place a sperm, blood, or cervical specimen in a plastic vial, freeze it, pack it in dry ice, and send it to a reference laboratory.
- Instruct the patient regarding when and how to obtain the test results. Abnormal results may have a devastating effect on a patient's sexuality.

Case Study

Infertility

After 1 year of unsuccessfully trying to conceive, Mr. and Mrs. S., both age 28, were referred to an infertility specialist. The history and physical examination results were negative, and a diagnostic evaluation was performed.

Studies	Results	
Basic laboratory procedures	**Husband**	**Wife**
Urinalysis, p. 268	Within normal limits (WNL)	WNL
Complete blood count, p. 412	WNL	WNL
Serologic test for syphilis, p. 392	Negative	Negative
Culture/serology for sexually transmitted diseases (STDs), p. 388	Negative	Negative
Blood type and Rh factor, p. 406	B+	A+
Thyroid function studies, p. 329	WNL	WNL

Evaluation of semen (semen analysis), p. 386

Volume	5 ml (normal: 2-5 ml)
Sperm count	105 million/ml (normal: 20-200 million/ml)
Motility	62% actively motile (normal: 60%-80% actively motile)
Sperm morphology	75% normally shaped (normal: 70%-90% normally shaped)

Evaluation of ovulation

Endometrial biopsy, p. 362	Good proliferative and secretory endometrium
Progesterone, p. 384	Follicular phase 40 ng/dL (normal: <50 ng/dL) Luteal phase 785 ng/dL (normal: 300-2500 ng/dL)
Estrogen, p. 364	Follicular phase 60 pg/ml (normal: 20-350 pg/ml) Mid-cycle peak 425 pg/ml (normal: 150-750 pg/ml) Luteal phase 275 pg/ml (normal: 30-450 pg/ml)

Evaluation of cervical factors

Sims-Huhner test, p. 391	Normal (cervical mucus adequate for sperm survival, transmission, and penetration); four active sperm per high-power field

Antisperm antibodies, p. 353

Positive for IgA antibodies in the cervical mucus

Laparoscopy, p. 125

Normal-appearing patent fallopian tubes

Diagnostic Analysis

Because the results of most of these studies were normal, laparoscopy was performed. The decreased number of mobile sperm in the vaginal secretions led the physician to suspect that antisperm antibodies were the cause of infertility. Although the husband wore condoms during coitus for the next several months to decrease his wife's level of antisperm antibodies, a pregnancy still did not occur within the next year. The couple initiated adoption procedures.

Critical Thinking Questions

1. Why was this couple evaluated for STDs?
2. What was the significance of the IgA antisperm antibodies?

Chorionic Villus Sampling (CVS, Chorionic Villus Biopsy [CVB])

Test type Cell analysis

Normal values

No genetic or biochemical disorders

Rationale

Chorionic villus sampling (CVS) is performed on women whose unborn child may be at risk for a life-threatening or significant life-altering genetic defect. This would include women who:

1. Are over age 35 at the time of pregnancy
2. Have had frequent spontaneous abortions
3. Have had previous pregnancies with fetuses or infants with chromosomal or genetic defects (e.g. Down's syndrome)
4. Have a genetic defect in themselves (e.g., hemoglobinopathies)

The CVS test can be performed between 8 and 12 weeks of gestation for the early detection of genetic and biochemical disorders. Because CVS detects congenital defects early in pregnancies, first-trimester, therapeutic abortions can be performed if indicated and desired.

For this study, a sample of chorionic villi from the chorion frondosum, which is the trophoblastic (fetal) origin of the placenta, is obtained for analysis. These villi in the chorion frondosum are present beginning at 8 to 12 weeks of gestation and are believed to reflect fetal chromosome, enzyme, and deoxyribonucleic acid (DNA) content. This permits a much earlier diagnosis of prenatal problems than amniocentesis, which cannot be done before 14 to 16 weeks of gestation. Furthermore, the cells derived by CVS are more easily grown in tissue culture for karyotyping (determination of chromosomal/genetic abnormalities). The cells obtained during amniocentesis require a longer time to grow in culture. This further adds to the delay in obtaining answers from amniocentesis compared with CVS. Although amniocentesis is a safer procedure, the information obtained is available much later in the pregnancy. At this late point, therapeutic abortion for severe genetic defects is more difficult.

Potential complications

Potential complications associated with CVS are as follows:

■ Accidental abortion stimulated by the procedure

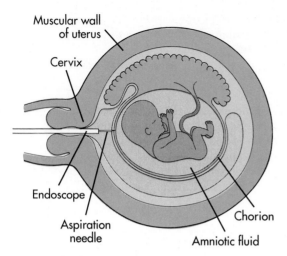

Muscular wall of uterus

Cervix

Endoscope

Aspiration needle

Chorion

Amniotic fluid

Figure 9-5 Chorionic villus sampling. Diagram of an 8-week pregnancy showing endoscopic aspiration of extraplacental villi.

- Infection introduced by the procedure
- Bleeding from the placenta or uterus caused by the procedure
- Amniotic fluid leakage from the puncture sites in the amniotic sac
- Fetal limb deformities as a result of placenta interruption

Procedure

The patient is placed in the lithotomy position. A cannula is inserted into the cervix and uterine cavity. Under ultrasonic guidance, the cannula is rotated to the site of the developing placenta. A syringe is attached, and suction is applied to obtain several samples of villi (Figure 9-5). This procedure is performed by an obstetrician in approximately 5 minutes. Discomfort associated with this study is similar to that of a Papanicolaou (Pap) smear.

After the procedure, some Rh-negative mothers may receive RhoGAM. The clients are briefly monitored for signs of bleeding and discharged shortly after the procedure because no cervical dilation is required. Ultrasound is often performed in 2 to 4 days after the procedure to determine the continued viability of the fetus. Genetic determinations require 3 to 5 weeks to obtain results.

Nursing implications with rationale

Before

- ☞ Explain the procedure to the patient. Assure the patient that precautions are taken to minimize risk to both her and the fetus. Encourage the patient to verbalize her fears concerning this study. Most patients are very apprehensive.
- ■ Verify that written and informed consent has been obtained before the procedure.

After

- ■ Administer RhoGAM, if ordered, to Rh-negative mothers. It is administered because of the risk of immunization from the fetal blood, which can jeopardize the fetus.
- ■ Carefully monitor the mother for signs of bleeding. Before discharging the patient, schedule her for ultrasound in 2 to 4 days to confirm the continued viability of the fetus.
- ☞ Instruct the mother to immediately report signs of spontaneous abortion (e.g., cramps, bleeding).
- ☞ Educate the mother regarding how to identify and report signs of endometrial infection (e.g., vaginal discharge, fever, crampy abdominal pain).
- ☞ Inform the patient how to obtain the results from her physician. Ensure that she understands the results will not be available for several weeks.

Chromosome Karyotype (Blood Chromosome Analysis, Chromosome Studies, Cytogenetics, Karyotype)

Test type Blood

Normal values

Female: 44 autosomes + 2 X chromosomes; karyotype: 46,XX
Male: 44 autosomes + 1 X, 1 Y chromosome; karyotype: 46,XY

Rationale

The term *karyotyping* refers to the arrangement of cell chromosomes in order from the largest to the smallest to analyze their number and structure. Variations in either number or structure can produce numerous developmental abnormalities and diseases. A normal karyotype of chromosomes consists of a pattern of 22 pairs of autosomal chromosomes and a pair of sex chromosomes: XY for the male and XX for the female. Chromosomal karyotype abnormalities can be congenital or acquired. These karyotype abnormalities can occur because of duplication, deletion, translocation, reciprocation, or genetic rearrangement of chromosomes.

Chromosome karyotyping is useful in evaluating congenital anomalies, mental retardation, growth retardation, delayed puberty, infertility, hypogonadism, primary amenorrhea, ambiguous genitalia, chronic myelogenous leukemia, neoplasm, recurrent miscarriage, prenatal diagnosis of serious congenital diseases (especially in situations of advanced maternal age), Turner's syndrome, Klinefelter's syndrome, Down's syndrome, and other suspected genetic disorders. The products of conception also can be studied to determine the cause of stillbirth or miscarriage.

Special chromosome studies can be done on cells grown in special medium in order to identify certain chromosome abnormalities.

Procedure

Specimens for chromosome analysis can be obtained from numerous sources. Leukocytes from a peripheral venipuncture are the most easily obtained and most often used for this study. Bone marrow biopsy specimens and surgical specimens also can sometimes be used as sources for analysis. During pregnancy, specimens can be collected by amniocentesis (see p. 349) and CVS (see p. 355). Fetal tissue or products of conception also can be studied to determine the reason for the loss of the pregnancy.

Nursing implications with rationale

Before

☞ Explain the procedure to the patient. Determine how the specimen will be collected. Many patients are fearful of the test results and require considerable emotional support.

After

■ Postprocedure care depends on how the specimen was collected.

☞ Inform the patient that results generally are not available for several months.

■ If the test results showed an abnormality, encourage the patient to verbalize his or her feelings. Provide emotional support.

Colposcopy

Test type Endoscopy

Normal values

Normal vagina and cervix

Rationale

Colposcopy provides an in situ macroscopic examination of the vagina and cervix with a colposcope, which is a macroscope with a light source and a magnifying lens. With this procedure, tiny areas of dysplasia, carcinoma in situ, and invasive cancer that would be missed by the naked eye can be visualized, and biopsy specimens can be obtained. The study is performed on patients with abnormal vaginal epithelial patterns, cervical lesions, or suspicious Pap smear results, and on those women who were exposed to diethylstilbestrol (DES) while in utero. It may be a sufficient substitute to *cone biopsy* (removal and examination of a cone of tissue from the cervix) in evaluating the cause of abnormal cervical cytologic findings.

The patient will need to have diagnostic conization if:

1. Colposcopy and endocervical curettage do not explain the problem or match the cytologic findings of the Pap smear within one grade.
2. The entire transformation zone (between squamous and columnar epithelium) is not seen. This area also is called the *endocervix*, where many cancers can initiate.
3. The lesion extends up the cervical canal beyond the vision of the colposcope.

The need for up to 90% of cone biopsies is eliminated by an experienced colposcopist. Endocervical curettage may routinely accompany colposcopy to detect unseen lesions in the endocervical canal.

Potential complication

Hemorrhage from the biopsy site is a potential complication associated with colposcopy.

Procedure

The patient is placed in the lithotomy position, and a vaginal speculum is used to expose the vagina and cervix. After the cervix is examined for cytologic findings, it is cleansed with a 3% acetic acid solution to remove excess mucus and cellular debris. The acetic acid also accentuates the difference between normal and abnormal epithelial tissues. The colposcope then is focused on the cervix (especially the squamocolumnar junction), which is then carefully examined. Usually the entire lesion can be outlined, and the most atypical areas can be selected for biopsy specimen removal.

Colposcopy is performed by a physician in approximately 5 to 10 minutes. Some patients complain of pressure pains from the vaginal speculum. Momentary discomfort may be felt when the biopsy specimens are obtained.

Contraindication

Colposcopy is contraindicated for patients with heavy menstrual flows. Heavy menses will preclude adequate visualization.

Nursing implications with rationale

Before

- ☞ Explain the procedure to the patient. The very fact that this study is required arouses anxiety in most women. Encourage verbalization of the patient's fears and provide emotional support.
- ▪ Obtain written and informed consent, if required by the institution.
- ☞ Describe the sensations that the patient may feel during this study.

After

- ☞ Inform the patient she may have some vaginal bleeding if biopsy specimens were taken. Suggest that she wear a sanitary pad.
- ☞ Instruct the patient to abstain from intercourse and not to insert anything (except a tampon) into the vagina until healing of the biopsy site is confirmed.
- ☞ Inform the patient regarding when and how to obtain the test results. The results usually are available in 2 to 3 days.

Case Study

Cervical Cancer

J.M. has been sexually active with multiple partners since she was 14 years old. She is now 28 years old, is married, and wants to have children. She has intermittent breakout of vulvar ulcers/sores but no other complaints. Her pelvic examination during a routine visit with her gynecologist was normal. She had a lump in her left breast.

Studies	Results
STDs, p. 388	
Herpes test	Positive for herpes simplex virus-2 (HSV-2) (normal: negative)
	No change in serology 4 weeks later
Cytomegalovirus	No antibodies detected

Chlamydia	No antibodies detected
Gonorrhea	Culture negative
Syphilis serology	No antibodies detected
Pap smear, p. 374	
Adequacy of specimen	Adequate
Category	Epithelial abnormality
Descriptive diagnosis	Squamous, atypical cells
Breast sonogram, p. 498	Benign fibroadenoma

Diagnostic Analysis

J.M. was informed of her test results. Her herpes titers indicated that the disease was not acute, but rather chronic. No treatment was recommended. Because of her age, mammograms were contraindicated. A breast ultrasound indicated the lesion was not cancerous. A fibroadenoma is common in this age group. Because of her suspicious Pap smear, further evaluation was recommended.

Studies	Results
Colposcopy, p. 357	Several suspicious areas
	Biopsy: Squamous cell carcinoma
Cervical cone biopsy, p. 357	Invasive squamous cell carcinoma
Hysteroscopy, p. 371	No extension to the endocervical canal or uterus
Pelvic ultrasound, p. 377	No extension of tumor beyond the cervix

J.M. was advised to have a radical hysterectomy. She refused because she wanted to have a family. She began psychologic counseling for guilt over her past promiscuity, which had increased her risk for cervical cancer. She became pregnant 1 year later and lost the pregnancy during the second trimester. One year later, she developed a large pelvic mass, which represented progressive, inoperable cervical cancer. Despite radiation therapy and chemotherapy, she died at age 31 of cervical cancer.

Critical Thinking Questions

1. Why was mammography contraindicated for J.M.?
2. How is sexual promiscuity related to the risk for cervical cancer?

Contraction Stress Test, Fetal (CST, Oxytocin Challenge Test [OCT])

Test type Electrodiagnostic

Normal values
Negative

Rationale

The contraction stress test (CST), frequently called the *oxytocin (Pitocin) challenge test* (OCT), is a relatively noninvasive test of fetoplacental adequacy used in the assessment of high-risk pregnancy. CST documents the ability of the placenta to adequately supply blood to the fetus and can be used to evaluate any high-risk pregnancy in which fetal well-being may be threatened. These risks include pregnancies marked by diabetes, hypertensive disease of pregnancy (toxemia), intrauterine growth retardation, Rh-factor sensitization, history of stillbirth, postmaturity, or low estriol levels.

For this study, a temporary stress in the form of uterine contractions is applied to the fetus after the intravenous (IV) administration of oxytocin. The fetal reaction to the contractions is assessed by an external fetal heart monitor. Uterine contractions cause transient impediment of placental blood flow. If the placental reserve is adequate, the maternal-fetal oxygen transfer is not significantly compromised during the contractions, and the FHR remains normal (a *negative* test). The fetoplacental unit then can be considered adequate for the next 7 days.

If the placental reserve is inadequate, then the fetus does not receive enough oxygen during the contraction. This results in intrauterine hypoxia and late deceleration of the FHR. The test is considered to be *positive* if consistent, persistent, late decelerations of the FHR occur with two or more uterine contractions. False-positive results caused by uterine hyperstimulation can occur in 10% to 30% of patients. Thus, positive test results warrant a complete review of other studies (e.g., amniocentesis) before the pregnancy is terminated by delivery.

Although this test can be performed reliably at 32 weeks of gestation, it usually is done after 34 weeks of gestation. CST can induce labor. Nonstress testing (see p. 374) of the fetus is the preferred test in almost every instance and can be performed more safely at 32 weeks of gestation; it can then be followed 2 weeks later by CST, if necessary.

A noninvasive, alternative method of performing the CST is called the *breast stimulation,* or *nipple stimulation,* technique. Stimulation of the nipple causes nerve impulses to the hypothalamus to trigger the release of endogenous oxytocin into the mother's bloodstream. This causes uterine contractions and may eliminate the need for IV administration of oxytocin. Advantages of this technique include ease of performing the test, shorter duration of the study, and elimination of the need to start, monitor, and stop IV infusions.

Potential complication

A potential complication associated with CST is premature labor, which may be induced by the oxytocin.

Interfering factor

A factor that interferes with CST is maternal hypotension because it may cause false-positive results.

Procedure

The CST is safely performed on an outpatient basis in the labor and delivery unit, where qualified nurses and necessary equipment are accessible. The patient should be kept NPO (*nil per os,* nothing by mouth) in case labor occurs as a result of testing. The test is performed by a nurse, with a physician available. After emptying her bladder, the patient is placed in the semi-Fowler position and tilted slightly to one side to avoid vena caval compression by the enlarged uterus. Her blood pressure is checked every 10 minutes during the procedure to avoid hypotension, which may cause diminished placental blood flow and a false-positive test result. An external fetal monitor is placed over the abdomen to record the fetal heart tones, and an external tocodynamometer is attached to the abdomen at the fundal region to monitor uterine contractions. The output of the fetal heart tones and uterine contractions is recorded on a two-channel strip recorder. Baseline FHR and uterine activity are monitored for 15 to 20 minutes. If uterine contractions are detected during this pretest period, oxytocin is withheld, and the response of the fetal heart tone to spontaneous uterine contractions is monitored. Oxytocin may not be needed.

If no spontaneous uterine contractions occur, oxytocin is administered by an IV infusion pump at 0.5 to 1.0 mU/minute. The rate of oxytocin infusion is increased every 20 minutes until the patient is having moderate-quality contractions. The FHR pattern is recorded.

The oxytocin infusion then is discontinued, although FHR monitoring is continued for another 30 minutes until the uterine activity has returned to its preoxytocin state. The woman should be informed of the test results at this time.

The discomfort associated with these procedures may consist of mild labor contractions. Breathing exercises usually control any discomfort. Analgesics are given, if needed. The duration of this study is approximately 2 hours.

Contraindications

Contraindications associated with CST are as follows:

- Patients with multiple pregnancies
  The myometrium is under greater tension and is more likely to be stimulated to premature labor.
- Patients with a prematurely ruptured membrane
  Labor may be stimulated by the CST.
- Patients with placenta previa, because vaginal delivery may be induced
- Patients with a history of abruptio placentae
  The placenta may separate from the uterus as a result of the oxytocin-induced uterine contractions.
- Patients with a previous hysterotomy
  The strong uterine contractions may cause uterine rupture.
- Patients with pregnancies of less than 32 weeks' gestation
  Early delivery may be induced by the procedure.

Nursing implications with rationale

Before

- ☞ Explain the procedure to the patient. The necessity of the test usually raises realistic fears in the mother. Encourage verbalization and provide factual information. Provide emotional support for the patient.
- Obtain written and informed consent for this procedure.
- ☞ Teach and practice breathing and relaxation exercises with the patient before the study.

During

- Administer analgesics during the study, if ordered. The need for narcotics must be carefully assessed, because these drugs may affect the FHR tracing.
- Monitor the patient's blood pressure and the FHR before, during, and after the study, as indicated. Record these signs and the oxytocin infusion rate every 15 minutes on the monitor strip.
- Administer the oxytocin by means of an infusion pump, because the infusion can be more precisely controlled than with manual drip methods.

After

- Discontinue the IV line after the study and apply an adhesive bandage to the site. Continue fetal monitoring for 30 minutes. Assess the IV site for bleeding.
- Provide emotional support to the parents. Many patients have this study repeated at weekly intervals until delivery. This regimen is tiring and produces anxiety for the parents.

Cytomegalovirus (CMV)

Test type Blood, urine, sputum

Normal values
No virus isolated

Rationale

Cytomegalovirus (CMV) is part of the viral family that includes herpes simplex, Epstein-Barr, and varicella-zoster viruses. CMV infection is widespread and common. Infections often occur in the fetus, during early childhood, and in the young adult. Certain populations are at increased risk. Male homosexuals, patients who have undergone a transplantation, and patients with acquired immunodeficiency syndrome (AIDS) are particularly susceptible. CMV infections are acquired by contact with body secretions or urine. Blood transfusions are a common transmission source for CMV. As many as 35% of patients receiving multiple transfusions become infected with CMV. Most patients with acute disease have no or very few (mononucleosis-like) symptoms. After infection, an asymptomatic incubation period lasts approximately 60 days. Acute symptoms then develop, followed by a latent phase. Reactivation can occur anytime.

CMV is the most common congenital infection. Pregnant mothers can become exposed to CMV during their pregnancy, or a previous CMV infection can become reactivated. Approximately 10% of infected newborns exhibit permanent damage, usually mental retardation and auditory damage. Fetal infection can cause microcephaly, hydrocephaly, cerebral palsy, mental retardation, or death.

CMV is evaluated as part of TORCH testing. The term *TORCH* (*t*oxoplasmosis, *o*ther, *r*ubella, *c*ytomegalovirus, *h*erpes) has been applied to infections with recognized detrimental effects on the fetus. The effects on the fetus may be direct or indirect (e.g., precipitating abortion or premature labor). Included in the category of "other" are STD infections (e.g., syphilis). All of these tests are discussed separately.

Viral culture is the most definitive method of CMV diagnosis. However, a culture cannot differentiate an acute infection from a chronic, inactive infection. Methods of identifying anti-CMV antibodies reveal much more information about the activity of the infection. CMV IgG antibody levels persist for years after infection. Identification of IgM antibodies, however, indicates a relatively recent infection. Three different CMV antigens can be detected immunologically. They are called *early, intermediate-early,* and *late antigens,* and they indicate onset of infection.

No specific therapy is known for this infection. If the diagnosis is established early by viral culture or serology, abortion may be an option. A fourfold increase in CMV titer in paired sera drawn 10 to 14 days apart is usually indicative of an acute infection.

Procedure

For culture specimens, a urine, sputum, or mouth swab is the specimen of choice. Fresh specimens are essential. The specimens are cultured in a virus laboratory in approximately 3 to 7 days.

For antibody or antigen titer, 4 to 7 ml of blood are collected in a gold- or red-top tube. A specimen is collected from the mother with suspected acute infection as early as possible. A convalescent specimen is collected 2 to 4 weeks later.

Nursing implications with rationale

Before

☞ Explain the procedure to the patient. Describe the method of specimen collection (blood, urine, sputum, or mouth swab).

After

■ Apply pressure or a pressure dressing to the venipuncture site to prevent further bleeding. Observe the site for bleeding.

☞ If indicated, instruct the patient to return for a convalescent blood test 2 to 4 weeks later.

Endometrial Biopsy

Test type Microscopic study

Normal values

No pathologic conditions
Presence of a secretory-type endometrium 3 to 5 days before normal menses

Rationale

An endometrial biopsy can determine whether ovulation has occurred. A biopsy specimen taken 3 to 5 days before normal menses should demonstrate a secretory-type endometrium on histologic examination if ovulation and corpus luteum formation have occurred. If not, only a preovulatory proliferative-type endometrium will be seen.

Occasionally an endometrial biopsy is performed to indicate the effect of estrogen (proliferative endometrium) on patients with suspected ovarian dysfunction or suspected menopause. Similarly, adequate circulating progesterone levels can be determined by identifying secretory endometrium. Another major use of endometrial biopsy is to diagnose endometrial cancer, polyps, or inflammatory conditions and to evaluate uterine bleeding.

Potential complications

Potential complications associated with endometrial biopsy are as follows:

- Perforation of the uterus from forceful advancement of the curet
- Uterine bleeding from the biopsy site
- Interference with early pregnancy caused by curettage

Procedure

This study is performed on the nonfasting and unsedated patient in the physician's office. No anesthesia is required. The patient is placed in the lithotomy position, and a bimanual pelvic examination is performed to determine the position of the uterus. The cervix is exposed and cleaned. After a tenaculum is placed on the cervix for stabilization, a sound (metal probe) is passed into the uterine cavity to determine the size of the uterus. This prevents inadvertent perforation of the uterus during biopsy specimen removal. A suction-tube curet or an endometrial biopsy curet is inserted into the uterus, and specimens are obtained from the anterior, posterior, and lateral walls. (Specimens are taken only from the lateral wall in infertility workups.) The specimens are placed in a solution containing 10% formalin and sent to the pathologist for histologic examination. This study is performed by an obstetrician-gynecologist in approximately 10 to 30 minutes. Obtaining the biopsy tissue may cause the patient momentary discomfort (mild to severe, menstrual-type cramping).

This procedure differs from a D&C in that significant cervical dilation is not required. Also, the curettage is much more extensive during a D&C. In effect, such curettage involves taking an endometrial biopsy specimen from the entire endometrium. (D&C usually requires general anesthesia with progressive cervical dilation before the curettage.) When an endometrial biopsy alone is performed to rule out endometrial cancer, it may easily miss the cancer. D&C is often therapeutic, in that endometrial polyps and other growths that may cause uterine bleeding can be removed.

Contraindications

Contraindications for endometrial biopsy are as follows:

- Patients with infections (e.g., trichomonal, candidal, or suspected gonococcal) of the cervix or vagina
  The infection may spread to the uterus.
- Patients in whom the cervix cannot be visualized
  Access to the cervix may be prevented because of abnormal position or previous surgery.

Nursing implications with rationale

Before

- ☞ Explain the procedure to the patient. Inform her that although momentary discomfort is associated with this study, analgesics are not needed. Encourage verbalization of the patient's fears.
- Ensure that written and informed consent is obtained.
- Instruct the patient that no fasting or sedation is necessary.

After

- Assess the patient's vital signs at regular intervals for the next 48 hours. Any temperature elevations (>100.4° F) should be reported to the physician because this procedure may activate PID.
- ☞ Instruct the patient to rest during the next 24 hours and avoid heavy lifting to prevent uterine hemorrhage.
- ☞ Advise the patient to wear a sanitary pad because some vaginal bleeding is to be expected. Instruct the patient to call her physician if excessive bleeding (requiring more than one pad per hour) occurs.
- ☞ Inform the patient that douching and intercourse are not permitted for 72 hours after the biopsy specimen removal.
- ☞ Inform the patient regarding how to obtain her test results. Generally, the report is available within 72 hours.

Estrogen Fractions (Estriol Excretion, Estradiol, Estrone)

Test type Blood, urine

Normal values

	Serum	Urine μg/24 Hours
Estradiol		
Child <10 years	<15 pg/ml	0-6
Adult male	10-50 pg/ml	0-6
Adult female		
Follicular phase	20-350 pg/ml	0-13
Midcycle peak	150-750 pg/ml	4-14
Luteal phase	30-450 pg/ml	4-10
Postmenopausal	<20 pg/ml	0-4
Estriol		
Male or child <10 years	N/A	1-11
Adult female		
Follicular phase	N/A	0-14
Ovulatory phase	N/A	13-54
Luteal phase	N/A	8-60
Postmenopausal	N/A	0-11
Pregant		
First trimester	<38 ng/ml	0-800
Second trimester	38-140 ng/ml	800-12,000
Third trimester	31-460 ng/ml	5000-12,000
Total Estrogen		
Male or child <10 years	N/A	4-25
Female, not pregnant	N/A	4-60
Female, pregnant		
First trimester	N/A	0-800
Second trimester	N/A	800-5000
Third trimester	N/A	5000-50,000

Rising estriol levels, indicating normal fetal growth

Possible critical values Values 40% below the average of two previous values demand immediate evaluation of fetal well-being.

Rationale

Measurement of estrogen fractions is used to evaluate sexual maturity, menstrual problems, and fertility problems in females. It also is used in the evaluation of males with gynecomastia or feminization syndromes. In pregnant women, it is used to indicate fetal-placental health. In patients with estrogen-producing tumors, it can be used as a tumor marker.

There are three major estrogens. E_1 (estrone) is predominantly produced in the ovary. This hormone is measured most often to evaluate menopausal status, sexual maturity, gynecomastia, or feminization syndromes, and as a tumor marker for patients with certain ovarian tumors. E_1 is the most active endogenous estrogen in the nonpregnant female. E_2 (estradiol-17β) and estrone production and actions are similar to E_1.

E_3 (estriol) is the major estrogen in the pregnant female. Serial urine and blood studies for estriol excretion provide an objective means of assessing placental function and fetal normality in high-risk pregnancies. Excretion of estriol increases around the eighth week of gestation and continues to rise until shortly before delivery. The measurement of excreted estriol is an index of fetal well-being. Rising values indicate an adequately functioning fetoplacental unit. Decreasing values suggest fetoplacental deterioration (failing pregnancy, dysmaturity, preeclampsia/eclampsia, complicated diabetes mellitus, encephaly, fetal death) and require prompt reassessment of the pregnancy. If the estriol levels fall, early delivery of the fetus may be indicated. Serial studies usually begin at approximately 28 to 30 weeks of gestation and then are repeated weekly.

Estriol excretion studies can be done using 24-hour urine tests or blood studies. Because urinary creatinine excretion is relatively constant, creatinine clearance is often simultaneously done to assess the adequacy of the 24-hour urine collection for estriol. Plasma estriol determinations also can be used to evaluate the fetoplacental unit. The advantage of the plasma estriol determination is that it is more easily obtained than a 24-hour urine specimen.

Unfortunately, only severe placental distress will decrease urinary estriol sufficiently to reliably predict fetoplacental stress. Because these problems create many false-positive and false-negative findings, most clinicians now use nonstress fetal monitoring (see p. 374) to indicate fetoplacental health.

Interfering factors

Factors that interfere with determining estrogen fractions include the following:

- Recent administration of radioisotopes
  Test results may be altered if they are done by radioimmunoassay (RIA) methods.
- Glycosuria and urinary tract infections, because they can *increase* urine estriol levels.

Procedure

Serial studies usually are begun around 28 to 30 weeks of gestation and repeated weekly. The frequency of these estriol determinations can be increased as needed to evaluate a high-risk pregnancy. Collections may be done daily. Although the first collection is the baseline value, all collection results are compared with previous ones. Some physicians suggest using an average of three previous values as a control value.

Urine:
A 24-hour urine specimen is collected using a preservative. The urine specimen must be refrigerated or kept on ice during the collection period. It is taken to the laboratory at the end of the collection period.

Blood:
For plasma estriol studies a venipuncture is performed, and 5 ml of venous blood is obtained in the manner specified by the laboratory. Some laboratories require a heparinized container.

Nursing implications with rationale

Before
- ☞ Explain the procedure to the patient. Allow ample time for the patient to verbalize her fears regarding the results of this study. Provide emotional support.
- ☞ Explain to the patient the importance of a complete collection. Every urine specimen must be included, or the study must be started over. The specimen requires a preservative

and must be kept on ice throughout the collection period.

- ☞ If the woman is going to collect the 24-hour urine specimen at home, give her the collection bottle (with the preservative) and instruct her to keep the urine refrigerated. Supply her with the urine collection device (which is hat-like) to fit under the toilet seat.

During
- ☞ Instruct the patient to begin the 24-hour urine collection after discarding the first morning specimen. This is the start time of the 24-hour collection.
- Using a preservative, collect all urine passed over the next 24 hours.
- ☞ Instruct the patient to void before defecating so that the urine is not contaminated by feces.
- ☞ Remind the patient not to put toilet paper in the collection container.
- Keep the urine specimen on ice or refrigerated during the 24 hours.
- Collect the last specimen as close as possible to the end of the 24 hours.
- If serum estriol studies are needed, draw the blood according to the laboratory's procedure.

After
- Transport the urine specimen promptly to the laboratory.
- Apply pressure or a pressure dressing to the venipuncture site to prevent further bleeding. Observe the site for bleeding.
- ☞ Inform the patient regarding how and when to obtain the results of this study from her physician.

Fetal Biophysical Profile
(Biophysical Profile, BPP)

Test type Ultrasound, fetal activity study

Normal values
Score of 8 to 10 points (if amniotic fluid volume is adequate)

Possible critical value Less than 4 may necessitate immediate delivery

Rationale

The biophysical profile (BPP) is a method of evaluating fetal status based on five variables originating within the fetus: FHR, fetal breathing movement, gross fetal movements, fetal muscle tone, and amniotic fluid volume. FHR reactivity is measured by the nonstress test (see p. 374), and the other four parameters are measured by ultrasound scanning.

The major premise behind the BPP is that variable assessments of fetal biophysical activity are more reliable than an examination of a single parameter (e.g., FHR). Indications for this test include factors such as postdate pregnancy (delivery is delayed 2 weeks beyond expected date), maternal hypertension, DM, vaginal bleeding, maternal Rh sensitization, maternal history of stillbirth, and premature rupture of membranes. The BPP is probably more useful in identifying a fetus that is in jeopardy than in predicting future fetal well-being. Testing usually begins around 32 weeks of gestation but can be done earlier if maternal complications exist.

The five parameters are briefly described here. Each parameter is scored as either a 2 or a 0. Therefore, 10 is the perfect total score, and 0 is the lowest total score.

1. **Fetal heart rate reactivity.** This parameter is measured and interpreted in the same way as the nonstress test (see p. 374). The FHR is considered reactive when there are movement-associated FHR accelerations of at least 15 beats/minute above baseline and 15 seconds in duration over a 20-minute period. A score of 2 is given for reactivity, and a score of 0 indicates that the FHR is nonreactive.

2. **Fetal breathing movements.** This parameter is assessed based on the assumption that fetal breathing movements indicate fetal well-being and their absence may indicate hypoxemia. Fetal breathing becomes increasingly regular in frequency and uniformity after the thirty-sixth week of gestation. To earn a score of 2, the fetus must have at least one episode of fetal breathing lasting at least 60 seconds within a 30-minute observation. Absence of this breathing pattern is scored as 0 on the BPP.

3. **Fetal body movements.** Fetal activity is a reflection of neurologic integrity and function. The presence of at least three discrete episodes of fetal movements within a 30-minute observation period is given a score of 2. A score of 0 is given with two or fewer fetal movements in this time period. It is important to note that fetal activity is greatest 1 to 3 hours after the mother has consumed a meal. For this reason, it is often suggested that this test be arranged relative to mealtime.

4. **Fetal tone.** In the uterus, the fetus is normally in a position of flexion. However, the fetus also stretches, rolls, and moves in the uterus. The arms, legs, trunk, and head may be flexed and extended. A score of 2 is earned when there is at least one episode of active extension with return to flexion. An example of this would be the opening and closing of the hand. A score of 0 is given for slow extension with a return to only partial flexion; fetal movement not followed by return to flexion; limbs or spine in extension; and an open fetal hand.

5. **Amniotic fluid volume.** Amniotic fluid volume has been demonstrated to be an effective predictor of fetal distress. Oligohydramnios (too little amniotic fluid) has been associated with fetal anomalies, uterine growth retardation, and postterm pregnancy. Immediate delivery is recommended for a postterm patient with oligohydramnios because of the high risk of associated problems such as umbilical cord compromise. A score of 2 is given for this parameter when there is at least one pocket of amniotic fluid that measures 1 cm in two perpendicular planes. A score of 0 indicates either that fluid is absent in most areas of the uterine cavity or that the largest pocket measures 1 cm or less in the vertical axis.

A total score of 8 to 10 with a normal amount of amniotic fluid indicates a healthy fetus. A score of 8 with oligohydramnios or a score of 4 to 6 is equivocal. An equivocal test result is interpreted as possibly abnormal. Some clinicians would recommend repeating the test within 24 hours. However, others may advocate extending testing after any equivocal or abnormal test result. A score of 0 or 2 is abnormal and indicates the need for assessment of immediate delivery.

Some physicians have added placental grading as a sixth parameter. Information concerning fetal size, position, and placenta location also can be obtained. Further information concerning fetal well-being can be gained by the use of Doppler ultrasound evaluations of the placenta and the umbilical artery velocity. Alterations in umbilical artery flow and direction may indicate fetal stress or illness.

Interfering factors

Factors that interfere with BPP include the following:

- Magnesium sulfate ingestion or use of nicotine, which can *decrease* fetal activity
  Other drugs that may *decrease* BPP include analgesics, anesthetics, and sedatives.
- Hypoxemia and trauma, which may *decrease* fetal biophysical activities

- Sleeping fetus
  Occasionally, no movement will be noted. If no eye movement or respiratory movement is noted, the fetus may be sleeping.

Procedure

No fasting is required. FHR reactivity is measured and interpreted from a nonstress test (see p. 374). Fetal breathing movements, fetal body movements, fetal tone, and amniotic fluid volume are determined by ultrasound imaging (see obstetric ultrasonography, p. 377). A total score is determined.

Nursing implications with rationale

Before
- Explain the procedure to the patient.
- Inform the patient that no fasting is necessary.
After
- If the test results are abnormal or equivocal, provide emotional support to the patient in the next phase of the fetal evaluation process.

Case Study

High-Risk Pregnancy

Mrs. P., a 42-year-old patient in otherwise good health, went to her obstetrician 4 weeks after missing her menstrual period. Her physical examination results were essentially normal. Positive findings on the pelvic examination included mild uterine enlargement associated with softening and cyanosis of the cervix. She had a history of prior spontaneous abortions. There is a history of hemophilia in her family.

Studies	Results
Routine laboratory studies	Blood and urine tests WNL except: fasting blood glucose: 160 mg/dl (normal: 60-120 mg/dl)
2-hour postprandial glucose, p. 309	200 mg/dl (normal: 60-120 mg/dl)
Pap smear, p. 375	No abnormal or atypical cells
Pregnancy test, p. 382	
Quantitative (whole HCG):	2750 mIU/mL (normal: 5-50 mIU/mL)
Serologic/cultures for STDs, p. 381	Negative
TORCH testing, p. 362	Negative
Blood type, p. 404	B+

The pregnancy test confirmed the clinical diagnosis of pregnancy with 80% accuracy. Although considered high risk because of her age, she was very healthy. Unfor-

Continued

Case Study

High-Risk Pregnancy–cont'd

tunately, she was found to have gestational diabetes, which increased her risks. She had no evidence of STDs that could affect her baby in utero or at birth.

The pregnancy was progressing well, and her diabetes was well-controlled with 12 units of Humulin N daily.

Studies	Results
Ultrasonography (at 24 weeks of gestation), p. 377	Biparietal diameter of the fetal skull 5 cm (baseline value); good heart rate
Amniocentesis, p. 349	Male child with no genetic or chromosomal abnormalities
CVS, p. 355	No genetic evidence of hemophilia

Mrs. P.'s pregnancy seemed to be going well. Hemophilia is a disease that is sex-linked so that males are most likely to inherit the disease. CVS indicated no evidence of that disease, much to the patient's relief.

In her thirty-eighth week of pregnancy, Mrs. P. noticed marked reduction in fetal kicking.

Studies	Results
Ultrasonography (at 36 weeks of gestation), p. 377	Normal placenta located high in fundus; biparietal diameter of the fetal skull 8.7 cm
	Larger than normal volume of amniotic fluid
Serial 24-hour urine tests for estriol, p. 364	12,000 mg/24 hours
	11,000 mg/24 hours
	7,000 mg/24 hours
	Abnormal, falling results (normal: 5,000-12,000 mg/24 hours)
Serial 24-hour urine test for pregnanediol, p. 364	110 mg/day
	102 mg/day
	84 mg/day
	Abnormal, falling results (normal: 70-100 mg/day)

The pregnancy was suspected to be compromised, and further investigation was recommended.

Studies	Results
BPP, p. 365	6; fetal activity and fetal respiration were reduced
Nonstress test, p. 374	No accelerations with fetal movement (normal: heart rate acceleration with movement)

CST, p. 359

Amniocentesis, p. 349

Positive: late decelerations of fetal heart
  rate (normal: negative)
L/S ratio: 3:1 (normal: >2:1)
Creatinine level: 2.3 mg/dl
  (normal: >2 mg/dl)
Cytologic findings: 30% of cells stained
  orange with Nile blue sulfate
  (normal: >20%)

The fetoplacental unit was threatened, and the fetus was not doing well. Amniocentesis indicated fetal maturity compatible with life outside the womb. A cesarean section was performed, and a healthy 5-pound, 8-ounce boy was delivered. While initially having low American Pediatric Gross Assessment Record (APGAR) scores, the baby improved rapidly. Mrs. P. and her healthy son were discharged 4 days after delivery.

Critical Thinking Questions
1. What is TORCH testing, and why is it done during pregnancy?
2. Why were the results of the 24-hour urine tests decreasing for estriol and pregnanediol?

Fetoscopy

Test type Endoscopy

Normal values
No fetal distress, diseases, or hematologic abnormalities noted

Rationale
Fetoscopy is an endoscopic procedure that allows direct visualization of the fetus by insertion of a tiny, telescope-like instrument through the abdominal wall and into the uterine cavity (Figure 9-6). Direct visualization may lead to diagnosis of a severe malformation, such as a neural tube defect. During the procedure, fetal blood samples to detect congenital blood disorders (e.g., hemophilia, sickle cell anemia) can be drawn from a blood vessel in the umbilical cord for biochemical analysis. Fetal skin biopsy specimens also can be removed to detect primary skin disorders. Fetoscopic surgery (e.g., placement of central nervous system (CNS) shunts) is becoming a more realistic option.

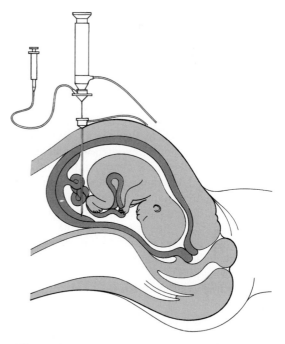

Figure 9-6 Fetoscopy for fetal blood sampling.

Fetoscopy is performed at approximately 18 weeks of gestation. At this time, the vessels of the placental surface are of adequate size, and the fetal parts are readily identifiable. A therapeutic abortion at this time would not be as hazardous as it would be if done later in the pregnancy. An ultrasound usually is performed the day after the procedure to confirm the adequacy of the amniotic fluid and fetal viability.

Potential complications

Potential complications associated with fetoscopy are as follows:

- Spontaneous abortion
- Premature delivery
- Amniotic fluid leak
- Intrauterine fetal death
- Amnionitis (infection of the amniotic fluid)

Procedure

Before this procedure, the mother may be given meperidine (Demerol) because it crosses the placenta and quiets the fetus. This prevents excessive fetal movement, which makes the procedure more difficult. For fetoscopy the woman is placed in the supine position on an examining table. The abdominal wall is anesthetized with a local anesthetic. Ultrasonography is done to locate the fetus and placenta. The endoscope then is inserted. Biopsy and blood samples may be obtained. This procedure is performed by a physician in 1 to 2 hours.

After the study, the mother and fetus are monitored for several hours for alterations in blood pressure and pulse, FHR abnormalities, uterine activity, vaginal bleeding, and loss of amniotic fluid. Rh-negative mothers are given RhoGAM unless the fetal blood is found to be Rh-negative. A repeat ultrasound often is performed the day following the procedure to confirm the adequacy of the amniotic fluid and fetal viability.

Nursing implications with rationale

Before

- Explain the procedure to the patient. Assure the patient that precautions are taken to mini-

mize risk to both her and the fetus. Encourage the patient to verbalize her fears concerning this study. Most patients are very apprehensive.
- Verify that written and informed consent is obtained before the procedure.
- Assess the FHR to serve as a baseline value.

After

- Monitor the mother and fetus very carefully for alterations in blood pressure, pulse, FHR abnormalities, uterine activity, vaginal bleeding, and loss of amniotic fluid.
- If a woman is Rh-negative and the fetus is Rh-positive, make certain that she receives RhoGAM.
- Instruct the woman to report any pain, bleeding, amniotic fluid loss, or fever after the study.
- Instruct the mother to avoid strenuous activity for 1 to 2 weeks following the procedure.
- If ordered, administer antibiotics prophylactically to prevent amnionitis.

Herpes Simplex Virus (Herpesvirus Type 2, Herpes Simplex Virus Types 1 & 2 [HSV 1 & 2], Herpes Genitalis)

Test type Blood, microscopic examination

Normal values

No virus present
No HSV antigens or antibodies present

Rationale

Herpes simplex virus (HSV) can be classified as either type 1 or type 2. Type 1 is primarily responsible for oral lesions (blisters on the lips, or "cold sores") or even corneal lesions. About half of the patients with HSV 1 develop recurrent infections. HSV 2 is a sexually transmitted viral infection of the urogenital tract. Vesicular lesions may occur on the penis, scrotum, vulva, perineum, perianal region, vagina, or cervix. Initial infections are often associated with generalized symptoms of fever and malaise.

Because most infants become infected if they pass through a birth canal containing HSV, determining its presence at delivery is necessary. Infections at birth may result in problems such as chorioretinitis and mental retardation. Disseminated neonatal HSV infections carry a high incidence of infant mortality. A vaginal delivery is possible if no virus is present, and birth by cesarean section is needed if HSV is present. Viral testing can be performed on males or females to determine the risk of sexual transmission.

Culture is still the gold standard for HSV detection and can identify HSV in 90% of infected patients. Serologic tests are more easily and conveniently available for detection of HSV 1 and HSV 2 antigen. Unfortunately, the accuracy is not great. Only approximately 85% of patients who are culture positive have positive serologies. The advantage of antigen tests is that results can be available in a day. Serologic tests for antibodies are cumbersome because they require repeated blood tests during the acute and convalescent phases of an acute viral outbreak (the phases occur approximately 2 weeks apart). A fourfold rise in titer is expected to diagnose acute initial herpes infection. Recurrent infections are far less likely to demonstrate titer elevations. Furthermore, perhaps more than 50% of people in the United States have positive herpes antibodies. Antibody testing cannot diagnose whether there is active recurrent genital herpes. Culture testing is required to diagnose recurrent active disease.

Procedure

For serologic testing, approximately 7 ml of venous blood is obtained in a red-top tube. Urethral and cervical culture procedures are described for STDs, (see page 388). For pregnant women with herpes genitalis, note that the cervix is cultured weekly for the herpesvirus beginning 4 to 6 weeks before the due date. Vaginal delivery is possible if the following criteria are met:

1. The two most recent cultures are negative.
2. The woman is not experiencing any symptoms.

3. No lesions are visible on inspection of the vagina and vulva.
4. Throughout pregnancy, the woman has not had more than one positive culture, during which she was symptom free.

Nursing implications with rationale

Before
- ☞ Explain the procedure to the patient.
- ☞ Instruct the female patient to refrain from douching and tub-bathing before the cervical culture is performed.
- ▪ Obtain the urethral specimen from the male patient before voiding because voiding washes secretions out of the urethra.

After
- ☞ Inform the patient regarding how to obtain the test results.
- ☞ If genital herpes is suspected, instruct the patient to refrain from sexual activity until the results are available.
- ☞ If the results are positive, instruct the patient to inform previous sexual partners of the newly diagnosed infection and avoid further disease transmission.

Hysteroscopy

Test type Blood, urine

Normal values
Normal structure and function of the uterus

Rationale
Hysteroscopy is an endoscopic procedure that provides direct visualization of the uterine cavity by inserting a hysteroscope (a thin, telescope-like instrument) through the vagina and dilated cervix and into the uterus. Hysteroscopy can be used to identify the cause of abnormal uterine bleeding, infertility, and repeated miscarriages. It also is used to evaluate and diagnose cancer, uterine adhesions (Asherman's syndrome), polyps, fibroids, and displaced intrauterine devices (IUDs).

In addition to diagnosing and evaluating uterine problems, hysteroscopy also can correct uterine problems. For example, uterine adhesions and small fibroids can be removed through the hysteroscope, thus avoiding open abdominal surgery. Hysteroscopy also can be used to perform endometrial ablation, which destroys the uterine lining in order to treat some cases of heavy uterine bleeding.

The hysteroscope can be used with many other instruments. For example, it may be done before a D&C or concurrently with a laparoscopy. Hysteroscopy also may confirm the results of other tests.

Potential complications

Potential complications associated with hysteroscopy are as follows:

- Uterine perforation, by forceful progression of the scope
- Infection, introduced by the instrumentation

Procedure

The patient is placed in the lithotomy position. After prepping the vagina, the cervix is dilated slightly. The hysteroscope is placed through the cervical os and into the endometrial cavity. Using carbon dioxide (CO_2) gas to insufflate the uterine cavity, the entire endometrium is examined. Areas suspicious for cancer or hyperplasia can be sampled for biopsy. Polyps can be removed, and the base ablated. The procedure takes approximately 30 minutes and is not associated with any significant postoperative pain. This test usually is performed by a gynecologist. Depending on the extent and length of surgery associated with hysteroscopy, general, spinal, or light-sedative anesthesia is used. The patient receiving local anesthesia or only light sedation may feel some cramping during the procedure.

Contraindication

Hysteroscopy is contraindicated for patients with PID because the infection could be exacerbated.

Nursing implications with rationale
Before
- Explain the procedure to the patient.
- Obtain written and informed consent for this procedure.

- Schedule the procedure after menstrual bleeding has ceased and before ovulation. This allows better visualization of the inside of the uterus and avoids damage to a newly formed pregnancy.
- Inform the patient that hysteroscopy may be performed with local, regional, or general anesthesia. Instruct the patient to remain NPO for at least 8 hours before the test, if general anesthesia will be given.
- Instruct the patient to void before the procedure because a distended bladder can be more easily perforated.

After
- Inform the patient that it is normal to have slight vaginal bleeding and cramps for a day or two after the procedure.
- Instruct the patient to report signs of fever, severe abdominal pain, or heavy vaginal discharge or bleeding to the physician.
- Inform the patient that discomfort may result from the gas inserted during the hysteroscopy or laparoscopy. This usually lasts less than 24 hours.

Luteinizing Hormone Assay (LH Assay, Lutropin)
Follicle-Stimulating Hormone (FSH)

Test type Blood, urine

Normal values

Adult	LH (IU/L)	FSH (IU/L)
Male	1.24-7.8	1.42-15.4
Female		
Follicular phase	1.68-15	1.37-9.9
Ovulatory peak	21.9-56.6	6.17-17.2
Luteal phase	0.61-16.3	1.09-9.2
Postmenopause	14.2-52.3	19.3-100.6
Child (age 1-10 yrs)		
Male	0.04-3.6	0.3-4.6
Female	0.03-3.9	0.68-6.7

Rationale

Luteinizing hormone (LH) and follicle-stimulating hormone (FSH) are glycoproteins that are produced in the anterior pituitary gland in response to stimulation by gonadotropin-releasing hormone (GnRH), previously called *luteinizing-releasing hormone*. GnRH is stimulated when circulating levels of estrogen (in the female) or testosterone (in the male) are low. Through a feedback mechanism, GnRH is stimulated by the hypothalamus, which, in turn, stimulates the production and release of LH and FSH. These two hormones then act upon the ovary or testes. In the female, FSH stimulates the development of follicles in the ovary. In the male, FSH stimulates Sertoli's cell development. In the female, LH stimulates follicular production of estrogen, ovulation, and formulation of a corpus luteum. In the male, LH (also called *interstitial cell-stimulating hormone*) stimulates Leydig's cells to produce testosterone, which, in turn, stimulates the seminiferous tubules to produce sperm. In the end, estrogen or testosterone is produced, which, in turn, inhibits FSH and LH.

In the female, these hormones are secreted differently at different times in the menstrual cycle. The midcycle peak of FSH is necessary for follicle/ovum formation. LH also must peak about that same time or a little later to stimulate ovulation and corpus luteum formation, which could potentially support an embryo if fertilization were to occur.

LH is secreted in a pulsatile manner. The variable nature of LH can be diminished by measuring LH in a 24-hour urine sample. Spot urine tests have become very useful in the evaluation and treatment of infertility. Because LH is rapidly excreted into the urine, the plasma LH surge that precedes ovulation by 24 hours can be recognized quickly and easily. This is used to indicate the period when the woman is most fertile. The best time to obtain a urine specimen is between 11 AM and 3 PM. Usually the woman begins to test her urine on the day following her menses and continues to do so daily. Home kits using a color change as an endpoint are now marketed to make this process even more convenient.

These hormones are used in the evaluation of infertility. Performing an LH assay is an easy way to determine if ovulation has occurred. An LH surge in blood levels indicates that ovulation has taken place. Under the influence of LH, the corpus luteum develops from the ruptured graafian follicle. Daily samples of serum LH around the woman's midcycle can detect the LH surge, which is believed to occur on the day of maximal fertility.

These assays also determine whether a gonadal insufficiency is primary (originating in the ovary/testicle) or secondary (caused by pituitary insufficiency resulting in reduced levels of FSH and LH). Elevated levels of FSH and LH in patients with gonadal insufficiency indicate primary gonadal failure, as may be seen in women with polycystic ovaries or menopause. In secondary gonadal failure, LH and FSH levels are low as a result of pituitary failure or some other pituitary-hypothalamic impairment, stress, malnutrition, or physiologic delay in growth and sexual development.

FSH and LH assays are often done to diagnose menopause so that hormone replacement therapy can be instituted as soon as possible. As just stated, menopause would be evident by high FSH and LH levels. LH hormones also are used to study testicular dysfunction in men and evaluate endocrine problems related to precocious puberty in children.

Interfering factor

A factor that interferes with FSH and LH assays is the recent use of radioisotopes.

Procedure

LH assays can be performed using a home urine test, a 24-hour urine test, or a blood study. A red-top tube is used for the blood study. No fluid or food restrictions apply. The date of the last menstrual period should be indicated on the laboratory requisition slip.

Nursing implications with rationale

Before

☞ Explain the procedure to the patient. Confirm that the patient understands that the peak period is the time of maximum fertility.

☞ Instruct the patient regarding how to perform the urine test and record the results.

After

■ If a blood test is drawn, apply pressure to the venipuncture site and assess the site for bleeding.

Nonstress Test, Fetal (NST, Fetal Activity Determination)

Test type Fetal activity study

Normal values

"Reactive" fetus (heart rate acceleration associated with fetal movement)

Rationale

The nonstress test (NST) evaluates fetal viability and documents the placenta's ability to adequately supply blood to the fetus. The NST can be used to evaluate any high-risk pregnancy in which fetal well-being may be threatened. These risks include pregnancies marked by diabetes, hypertensive disease of pregnancy (toxemia), intrauterine growth retardation, Rh-factor sensitization, and history of stillbirth, postmaturity, or low estriol levels.

The NST is a noninvasive study that monitors acceleration of the FHR in response to fetal movement. This FHR acceleration reflects the integrity of the CNS and fetal well-being. Fetal activity may be spontaneous, induced by uterine contraction, or induced by external manipulation. Oxytocin stimulation is not used. Fetal response is characterized as "reactive" or "nonreactive." The NST indicates a reactive fetus when, with fetal movement, two or more FHR accelerations are detected, each of which must be at least 15 beats/minute for 15 seconds or more within any 10-minute period. The test is 99% reliable in indicating fetal viability. If the test detects a nonreactive fetus (i.e., no FHR acceleration with fetal movement) within 40 minutes, the patient is a candidate for the CST (see p. 359). A 40-minute test period is used because this is the average duration of the sleep-wake cycle of the fetus. The cycle may vary considerably, however.

Procedure

The NST is performed by a nurse in the physician's office or on a hospital ward. After emptying her bladder, the patient is placed in the Sim's position. An external fetal monitor is placed on the abdomen to record the FHR. The mother can indicate the occurrence of fetal movement by pressing a button on the fetal monitor whenever she feels the fetus move. FHR and fetal movement are concomitantly recorded on a two-channel strip graph. The fetal monitor then is observed for FHR accelerations associated with fetal movement. If the baby is quiet for 20 minutes, fetal activity is stimulated by external methods, such as rubbing the mother's abdomen, compressing the abdomen, ringing a bell near the abdomen, or placing a pan on the abdomen and banging on the pan.

This study should be performed after a recent meal because the fetus frequently is more active when the maternal serum glucose level is increased. The duration of the study is approximately 20 to 40 minutes. No discomfort is associated with the NST.

Nursing implications with rationale

Before

☞ Explain the procedure to the patient. Assure the patient that no discomfort or adverse effects are associated with this study.

■ Encourage verbalization of the patient's fears. The necessity for this study usually raises realistic fears in the expectant mother. Provide emotional support.

☞ If the patient is hungry, instruct her to eat before initiating the NST. Fetal activity is enhanced with a high maternal serum glucose level.

After

■ If the results detect a nonreactive fetus, inform the patient that she is a candidate for the CST.

Papanicolaou Smear (Pap Smear, Pap Test, Cytologic Test for Cancer)

Test type Microscopic examination

Normal values
No abnormal or atypical cells

Rationale
Pap smears are the mainstay of screening for cancer of the vagina, cervix, and uterus. They are routinely performed on women over age 18, or younger if the woman is sexually active.

A Pap smear is performed to detect neoplastic cells in cervical and vaginal secretions. This test is based on the fact that normal cells and abnormal cervical and endometrial cells are shed into the cervical and vaginal secretions. By examining these secretions microscopically, one can detect early cellular changes compatible with premalignant conditions or an existing malignant condition. The Pap smear is 95% accurate in detecting cervical carcinoma; however, its accuracy in detection of endometrial carcinoma is only approximately 40%.

Pap smears can be reported in terms of cervical intraepithelial neoplasia (CIN). This is a simple designation of the spectrum of intraepithelial dysplasia, which usually occurs before invasive cervical cancer. In contrast to the rigid original classification, CIN reporting recognizes the continuum of cervical dysplasia and allows for some overlap. The subclasses of CIN are defined as follows:

CIN 1: mild and mild-to-moderate dysplasia

CIN 2: moderate and moderate-to-severe dysplasia

CIN 3: severe dysplasia and carcinoma in situ

Most recently, the Bethesda System for reporting cervical/vaginal cytologic diagnoses was developed and revised by the National Cancer Institute. This system includes the following:

Adequacy of specimen
Satisfactory for evaluation
Satisfactory for evaluation but limited by (specify disease)
Unsatisfactory for evaluation (specify reason)

General categorization (optional)
Within normal limits
Benign cellular changes: see descriptive diagnosis
Epithelial cell abnormality: see descriptive diagnosis

Descriptive diagnosis
Benign cellular changes
Infection
Reactive changes

Epithelial cell abnormalities
Squamous cell
Atypical squamous cells
Low-grade squamous intraepithelial lesion
High-grade squamous intraepithelial lesion
Squamous cell carcinoma
Glandular cell
Endometrial cells, cytologically benign
Atypical glandular cell
Endocervical adenocarcinoma
Endometrial adenocarcinoma
Extrauterine adenocarcinoma
Adenocarcinoma

A Pap smear also may be performed to determine endocrine abnormalities (e.g., infertility). An abnormal maturation index (MI) is characteristic of an estrogen-progesterone imbalance. The MI is calculated by determining the ratio of parabasal cells to intermediate cells to superficial cells. The normal ovulating adult MI is 0/70/30. The MI is not a routine part of a Pap smear but can be calculated if requested. The more superficial cells present, the greater the hormone influence (ovarian estrogen, progesterone, and adrenal sex hormones). The more parabasal cells present, the less hormonal influence on vaginal mucosa.

Pap smears should be part of the routine pelvic examination, which is usually performed once a year on women over age 18 (or even earlier when the patient is sexually active). Opinions differ regarding the necessity for annual Pap smears. The American Cancer Society recommends that a Pap smear be taken annually for two negative examinations, then repeated once every 3 years until age 65 in asymptomatic women. More frequent testing may be indicated for patients with venereal infections, patients with a family history of cervical cancer, and patients whose mothers had ingested DES during their pregnancies.

Interfering factors

Factors that interfere with a Pap smear include the following:

- A delay in fixing a specimen
  This allows the cells to dry, destroys the effectiveness of the stain, and makes cytologic interpretation difficult.
- Using lubricating jelly on the speculum, which can alter the specimen
- Douching and tub-bathing
  They may wash away cellular deposits and interfere with the test results.
- Menstrual flow
  This may alter test results. The best time to perform a Pap test is 2 weeks after the start of the last menses.

- Infections, which may interfere with hormonal cytology

Procedure

The patient should refrain from douching and tub-bathing for 24 to 48 hours before her Pap smear. She should not be menstruating. If abnormal bleeding is present, however, the Pap smear and examination should be performed because of the significant possibility that serious cervical or uterine lesions may be present. A common error is to delay Pap testing 2 to 3 months because of intermittent bleeding or continuous spotting (which may be due to disease).

The patient is placed in the lithotomy position. An examining light is positioned for visualization of the pelvic area. A nonlubricated vaginal speculum is inserted to expose the cervix. Material is collected from the cervical canal by rotating a moist, saline cotton swab or spatula within the cervical canal and in the squamocolumnar junction (Figure 9-7). The cells are immediately wiped across a clean glass slide and fixed either by immersing the slide in equal parts of 95% alcohol and ether or by using a commercial spray. Aqua Net hair spray is also an effective fixative. The secretions must be fixed before drying because drying distorts the cells and makes interpretation difficult. The slide is labeled with the patient's

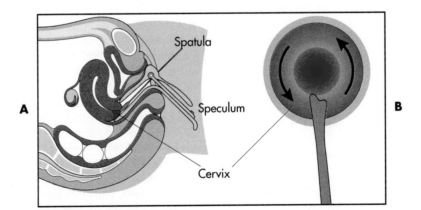

Figure 9-7 Papanicolaou (Pap) smear. **A,** Cross-sectional view of the process of obtaining a cervical specimen. **B,** Cervix is scraped with a bifid end of a spatula to obtain Pap smear.

name. The patient's name, age, parity, date of her last menstrual period, and the reason for the cytologic examination should be written on the laboratory requisition form. No discomfort other than the speculum insertion is associated with this procedure. A Pap smear is obtained in approximately 10 minutes by a physician or nurse.

Contraindications

Contraindications for Pap smears are as follows:

- Menstrual flow, which may alter test interpretation.
- Vaginal infections, which can create cellular changes that may be misinterpreted as dysplastic.

Nursing implications with rationale

Before

☞ Explain the procedure to the patient. Assure the patient that she will be appropriately draped to prevent unnecessary exposure.

☞ Inform the patient that no fasting or sedation is necessary.

- Determine if the patient has douched or tub-bathed during the 24 hours before the Pap smear. Douching and tub baths may wash away cellular deposits, which are desired in the specimen.

After

☞ Inform the patient regarding how to obtain the test results. Usually, the patient is notified by the office staff only if further evaluation is necessary. If the smears were abnormal, assure the patient that this does not necessarily mean that she has a malignancy. Many patients associate a suspicious test with malignancy and become very frightened. Provide emotional support.

- After the smear is obtained, ensure that it is fixed immediately without being allowed to dry. Fixing causes rapid killing of the cells so that they look as much as possible like they did in situ. If the cells are allowed to die slowly and dry, they will not be able to be evaluated accurately.

Pelvic Ultrasonography (Obstetric Echography, Pregnant Uterus Ultrasonography, Pelvic Ultrasonography in Pregnancy, Obstetric Ultrasonography, Vaginal Ultrasound)

Test type Ultrasound

Normal values

Normal fetal and placental size and position

Rationale

Pelvic ultrasonography is used in the obstetric patient to evaluate the pregnancy. It is especially important in high-risk pregnancies. In the nonpregnant female, it is used to evaluate the female genital tract for pathology. It is used to monitor known pelvic pathology (e.g., benign cysts of the ovary). Pelvic ultrasound in the male is discussed on page 251 (rectal ultrasound).

Ultrasound examination of the female patient is a harmless, noninvasive method of evaluating the genital tract and fetus. In real-time diagnostic ultrasound, harmless, high-frequency sound waves are emitted from the transducer and penetrate the structure (e.g., uterus, ovaries, parametria, placenta, fetus) to be studied. These sound waves are bounced back to a sensor within the transducer and arranged by electronic conversion into a pictorial image of the desired organ.

Pelvic ultrasonography can be performed with the transducer placed on the anterior abdomen or in the vagina with a specially designed vaginal probe (the latter approach provides the best view of the pelvic organs in a nonpregnant female). The anterior abdominal probe, however, provides better visualization of the upper pelvis than does the vaginal probe, especially in the pregnant female.

Pelvic ultrasonography may be useful in the obstetric patient as an aid in the following circumstances:

1. Making an early diagnosis of abnormal pregnancy (e.g., tubal pregnancy)
2. Identifying multiple pregnancies

3. Differentiating a tumor (e.g., hydatidiform mole) from a normal pregnancy
4. Determining the age of the fetus by the diameter of the head
5. Measuring the rate of fetal growth
6. Identifying placental abnormalities (e.g., abruptio placentae and placenta previa)
7. Determining the position of the placenta (ultrasound localization of the placenta is done before amniocentesis)
8. Making differential diagnoses of various uterine and ovarian enlargements (e.g., polyhydramnios, neoplasms, cysts, abscesses)
9. Determining fetal position

Pelvic ultrasound is used in the nonpregnant woman to aid in the diagnosis of:

1. Ovarian cyst
2. Ovarian tumor
3. Tubo-ovarian abscess
4. Uterine fibroid
5. Uterine cancer
6. PID
7. Endometrial cancer

Interfering factors
Factors that interfere with pelvic ultrasonography include the following:

- Recent gastrointestinal (GI) contrast studies
  Barium creates severe distortion of reflective sound waves.
- Air-filled bowels
  Gas does not transmit the sound waves well.
- Obesity and failure to fill the bladder
  These conditions may make the image uninterpretable.

Procedure
No fasting or sedation is required. The patient is given 3 to 4 glasses of water 1 hour before the study and instructed *not* to void. The full bladder provides better transmission of the sound waves and better visualization of the uterus by pushing the uterus away from the symphysis pubis and by

pushing the bowel out of the pelvis. The patient then is taken to the ultrasound room (usually in the radiology department) and placed in the supine position on the examining table. The ultrasonographer (usually a radiologist or ultrasound technician) applies a greasy, conductive paste to the abdomen. The paste enhances sound transmission and reception of the sound waves. An abdominal transducer then is passed vertically and horizontally over the skin, and the reflections are photographed (Figure 9-8). The duration of this study is approximately 20 minutes, and no discomfort is associated with it. During the ultrasound examination, the fetal structures should be pointed out to the mother. Seeing the fetus during ultrasound study may promote prenatal attachment. With the transvaginal approach, a lubricated transducer is gently inserted into the vagina with the patient in a lithotomy position.

Contraindication
Pelvic ultrasonography is contraindicated for patients with a latex allergy. Vaginal ultrasound requires placement of the probe in a latex condom-like sac. Patients with a latex allergy may react significantly to that contact.

Nursing implications with rationale
Before
☞ Explain the procedure to the patient. Assure the patient that this study has no known deleterious effect on maternal or fetal tissues even when it is repeated several times.
☞ Give the patient three or four glasses (200 to 350 ml) of water or other liquids 1 hour before the examination, and instruct her *not* to void until after ultrasonography is completed. A full bladder permits better transmission of the sound waves and enhances visualization of the uterus.
☞ Inform the patient that this study is not associated with any pain. The patient may have some discomfort because she will have a full bladder and the urge to void. Some patients may be uncomfortable lying on a hard x-ray table.
☞ Explain to the patient that a liberal amount of gel or lubricant will be applied to her skin to

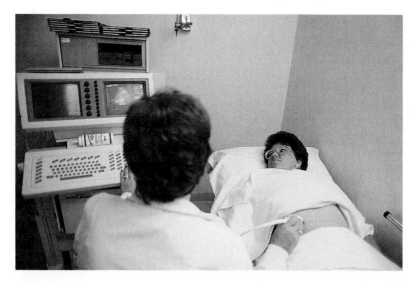

Figure 9-8   Pelvic ultrasonography is a safe, painless method of scanning a mother's abdomen with high-frequency sound waves to follow fetal growth and development. (Courtesy March of Dimes.)

enhance the transmission and reception of the sound waves. The gel will feel cold.

After

■ Remove the lubricant from the patient's skin and allow the patient an opportunity to void.

pH, Fetal Scalp

Test type Blood

Normal values
pH: 7.25-7.35
O_2 saturation: 30% to 50%
PO_2: 18-22 mm Hg
PCO_2: 40-50 mm Hg
Base excess: 0 to 10 mEq/L

Rationale
Measurement of fetal scalp blood pH provides valuable information on fetal acid-base status. This screening test is useful clinically for diagnosing fetal distress.

Although the oxygen partial pressure (PO_2), carbon dioxide partial pressure (PCO_2), and bicarbonate ion ($HCO_3{}^-$) concentration can be measured with the fetal scalp blood sample, the pH is the most useful clinical measurement. The pH normally ranges from 7.25 to 7.35 during labor; a mild decline within the normal range is noted with contractions and as labor progresses.

Fetal hypoxia causes anaerobic glycolysis, resulting in excess production of lactic acid, which, in turn, causes an increase in hydrogen ion concentration (acidosis) and a decrease in pH. Acidosis reflects the effect of hypoxia on cellular metabolism. A high correlation exists between low pH levels and low Apgar scores.

Potential complications
Potential complications associated with fetal scalp pH are as follows:

■ Continued bleeding from the puncture site
■ Hematoma of the scalp from the needle stick
■ Infection from the needle stick

Procedure
Amnioscopy is performed with the mother in the lithotomy position. Under sterile conditions, the

amnioscope (an endoscope) is introduced into the vagina and the dilated cervix. The fetal scalp is cleansed with an antiseptic and dried with a sterile cotton ball. A small amount of petroleum jelly is applied to the fetal scalp. The skin on the scalp then is pierced with a small, metal blade. The droplets of blood that result from the piercing bead because of the petroleum jelly. The beaded droplets of blood are collected in long, heparinized capillary tubes. The tube is sealed with wax and placed on ice to retard cellular respiration, which can alter the pH. The physician performing the procedure then applies firm pressure to the puncture site to retard bleeding. Scalp blood sampling can be repeated as necessary. A blood sample may be obtained simultaneously from the mother to aid in interpretation of the fetal pH and reduce the frequency of false-positive results.

Contraindications

Contraindications for fetal scalp pH are as follows:

- Patients with premature membrane rupture, because infectious organisms can be introduced into the uterus
- Patients with active cervical infection (e.g., gonorrhea), because the active infection can be spread to the fetus

Nursing implications with rationale

Before
☞ Explain the procedure to the patient.
After
- After the delivery of the infant, assess the newborn and identify and document the puncture site(s).
- Cleanse the fetal scalp puncture site with an antiseptic solution. Then apply an antibiotic ointment.

Phenylketonuria Test (PKU Test, Guthrie Test, Phenylalanine Screening)

Test type Blood, urine

Normal values

Blood: negative (<2 mg/dl) (Guthrie technique)
Urine: no green coloration

Possible critical value

Blood: >4 mg/dl (Guthrie technique)

Rationale

An autosomal-recessive inherited disease, phenylketonuria (PKU) is characterized by deficiency of the enzyme called phenylalanine hydroxylase, which converts phenylalanine to tyrosine. Phenylalanine is an essential amino acid necessary for growth and metabolism; however, any excess must be degraded by conversion to tyrosine. An infant with PKU lacks the ability to make this necessary conversion. Thus, phenylalanine accumulates in the blood. Its catabolic product, phenylpyruvic acid, builds up in the body and spills over into the urine. It is this metabolic product that is detected in the urine. If the amount of phenylalanine is not restricted in infants with PKU, progressive mental retardation results from the deposit of phenylalanine and its metabolic products in the brain. Dietary control must begin early to avoid brain damage; therefore, early diagnosis is essential.

Routine screening of newborn infants for PKU is now mandatory in the United States. It is important to note that this test is not valid until the newborn has ingested an ample amount (for 2 or 3 days) of the amino acid phenylalanine, which is a constituent of both human and cow's milk. If the infant is not eating well or does not weigh at least 5 lbs, the test should not be done because results may be invalid. The urine PKU test is done normally after 6 weeks of age if, for some reason, a blood test was not done in the hospital.

Interfering factors

Factors that interfere with determining PKU levels include the following:

- Premature infants
  False-positive results may occur because of delayed development of the liver enzymes such as phenylalanine hydroxylase.
- Ketonuria (from malnutrition or diabetes), be-

cause it can produce an altered urine color test reaction

- Testing too early
  Infants tested before 24 hours of age may have false-negative results because they have not ingested enough milk containing phenylalanine.
- Feeding problems (e.g., vomiting)
  False-negative results may occur because the infant may not have tolerated enough milk containing phenylalanine.

Procedure

Blood usually is collected on the infant's day of discharge and analyzed for increased amounts of phenylalanine. For this procedure, a few drops of blood obtained by a heel stick are placed on a filter paper for the Guthrie test. Urine tests also can be used to detect PKU in infants who are at least 4 to 6 weeks of age. These tests usually are done at the baby's first checkup. For the diaper test, 10% ferric chloride is dropped on a freshly wet diaper. A green spot indicates probable PKU. Another test, the Phenistix test, is done by pressing a test stick against a wet diaper or dipping the stick in urine. A green color reaction indicates probable PKU. PKU tests usually are performed by a nurse in less than 2 minutes. A slight amount of discomfort is associated with the heel stick.

Nursing implications with rationale

Before

- ☞ Inform the mother about the purpose of the test and the method of performance.
- Assess the infant's feeding patterns before performing the PKU test. An inadequate amount of protein before performing the test can cause false-negative results.
- Note that urine tests for PKU are commonly done on the infant's first well-baby examination. This is vitally important if the infant was not checked for PKU while in the hospital. The infant must be at least 4 to 6 weeks old for appropriate screening with the urine test.

After

- ☞ If the results of the test are positive, inform the mother that dietary control must begin immediately to prevent brain damage. This is done by substituting Lofenalac for milk. Later, strained foods low in protein are added to the diet. Monitor the dietary treatment by blood and urine testing.
- ☞ Instruct women with PKU who wish to have children to begin a low phenylalanine diet before conception and to continue it throughout the pregnancy. The risk of producing a mentally retarded infant is very high if the mother remains on a general diet.

Case Study

Routine Well-Baby Newborn Evaluation

After an 8-hour labor, Mrs. R., age 26, delivered her first child, a 7-pound, 13-ounce, 21-inch boy. The baby's APGAR scores at 1 minute and 5 minutes after birth were both 9. Because the newborn cried seconds after birth, no special procedures were necessary other than routine close observation, maintaining a clear airway, and supplying warmth. The umbilical cord was evaluated; it contained the normal two arteries and one vein. The infant's eyes received a prophylactic treatment for protection against ophthalmia neonatorum. A single dose (1 mg, 0.5 ml) of phytonadione solution (Aqua-MEPHYTON) was administered intramuscularly as a preventative measure against neonatal hemorrhagic disease.

Studies	**Results**
PKU test, p. 380	Negative (normal: negative)
T_4, TSH, p. 334	Negative for hypothyroidism

Continued

Case Study

Routine Well-Baby Newborn Evaluation—cont'd

Studies—cont'd	Results—cont'd
Hemoglobin and hematocrit, p. 412	WNL for newborn
White blood cell (WBC), p. 412	WNL for newborn

Diagnostic Analysis

The healthy infant and his mother were discharged 3 days after birth. The PKU test was done on the day of discharge. A well-baby clinic appointment was scheduled before discharge.

Critical Thinking Questions

1. What is ophthalmia neonatorum, and why is it treated prophylactically?
2. If this child had been hypothyroid, what treatment would have been indicated? What would be the implications of nondetection and no treatment?

Pregnancy Tests (Human Chorionic Gonadotropin [HCG], B [Beta] Subunit)

Test type Blood, urine

Normal values

Qualitative: negative; positive in pregnancy
Quantitative:
   Whole HCG:

Weeks of Gestation	Whole HCG (mIU/ml
<1	5-50
2	50-500
3	100-10,000
4	1000-30,000
5	3500-115,000
6-8	12,000-270,000
12	15,000-220,000
Males and nonpregnant females	<5

B subunit: normal values depend on the method and test used

Rationale

All pregnancy tests are based on the detection of human chorionic gonadotropin (HCG), which is secreted by the placental trophoblast after the ovum is fertilized. HCG will appear in the blood and urine of pregnant women as early as 10 days after conception. In the first few weeks of pregnancy, HCG markedly rises, and serum levels are higher than urine levels. After about a month, HCG is approximately the same in either specimen.

HCG is a glycoprotein very similar to the pituitary proteins. Glycoprotein hormones are made up of two fractions, alpha (A) and beta (B) subunits. The A subunit is the same for all the glycoproteins. The B subunit is unique to each. Therefore, the B subunit for HCG is specific for HCG. The whole HCG molecule is metabolized into the A and B subunits in the blood. They are then excreted by the kidneys into the urine. Testing for the whole HCG will cross-react with the pituitary hormones (especially LH). Therefore, testing for the whole HCG is less specific with a high incidence of false-positives (cross-reactions with LH).

All pregnancy studies demonstrate the presence of HCG. Methods of pregnancy testing fall into four categories: biologic, immunologic, radioimmunologic, and radioreceptor assays.

Biologic tests (urine)

Biologic (animal) tests have been used since the 1920s and are primarily of historical interest today. Urine from the patient is injected into an animal (mouse, rabbit, toad, frog). If HCG is present, a specific response (usually corpus luteum development in the ovaries) will occur in that animal. The exact response varies according to the animal used. The result is usually positive by the fortieth day after the last menses. These biologic tests have largely been replaced by less expensive, more accurate, and more rapidly performed immunologic tests.

Immunologic tests (agglutination inhibition test [AIT]) (blood and urine)

Immunologic tests are performed using commercially prepared antibodies against the whole HCG molecule and can be completed within 2 minutes or 2 hours, depending on the method used. These immunologic tests have a high false-positive rate and usually are not positive until approximately 28 days after the last menses. The high false-positive rate (lack of specificity) occurs because these antibodies were directed toward the whole HCG unit.

Immunologic testing for the B subunit of HCG, however, greatly improved accuracy and shortened the time for positive testing (18 days after the last menses). Now, with the development of monoclonal antibodies, immunoassays can identify very small levels of HCG, and pregnancy can be detected in 3 to 7 days after conception. Several immunologic tests are now commercially available to the public. In these tests, the patient's urine is tested, and its color is compared with a standard containing a known small amount of HCG. If the color matches that standard, pregnancy is present. These tests require 5 to 120 minutes to perform.

Radioimmunoassay (RIA) (serum)

The RIA is a highly sensitive and reliable blood test for the detection of the B unit of HCG. In this test, maternal serum HCG and "test" HCG, which has been radioactively bound to labeled antibody, compete for binding sites on a resin form. The

higher the concentration of maternal HCG, the fewer the number of binding sites available for the radiolabeled test HCG.

This study requires a blood sample in a red-top tube; however, RIA also may be performed with a urine test. The test can be done in 1 to 5 hours. This test is so sensitive that pregnancy can be diagnosed before the first missed menstrual period.

Radioreceptor assay (RRA) (serum)

The RRA for serum HCG measures the ability of the patient's serum to inhibit the binding of radiolabeled HCG to receptors. It is a highly sensitive and accurate test that can be performed in 1 hour. The chief advantage of this study is its reliable diagnosis of early gestation in patients requesting an early termination of pregnancy and in cases in which infertile couples are anxious to confirm pregnancy. This study is 90% to 95% accurate 6 to 8 days after conception. Even the minute amounts of HCG secreted in an ectopic pregnancy can be measured with this study. This test also is used to determine early spontaneous abortion in patients who have difficulties maintaining early pregnancy.

• • •

Normally, HCG is not present in nonpregnant women, although in a very small number of women (<5%), HCG exists in very minute levels. The presence of HCG does not necessarily indicate a normal uterine pregnancy. Ectopic pregnancy, hydatidiform mole of the uterus, and choriocarcinoma of the uterus can produce HCG. Germ cell tumors (choriocarcinoma and embryonal cell cancers) of the testes or ovaries can produce HCG in men and nonpregnant women, respectively. Primary liver cell cancers (hepatoma) also can produce HCG. In these tumors, HCG is used as a valuable tumor marker, which can help in tumor identification. HCG also is used to monitor the therapy and disease progression/regression of these tumors. When HCG levels are elevated in these patients, tumor progression must be suspected. Decreasing HCG levels indicate effective antitumor treatment.

Interfering factors

Factors that interfere with determining HCG levels include the following:

- Timing
  Tests performed too early in the pregnancy, before a significant HCG level exists, may cause false-negative results.
- Hematuria and proteinuria, which may cause false-positive results.
- Hemolysis of blood, which may interfere with test results.
- Dilution of the urine
  HCG levels may be nondetectable on a dilute urine but may be detectable on a concentrated urine.

Procedure

Urine:

Urine specimens should be collected in a standard container and taken to the laboratory. A first-voided morning specimen is preferred. Urine tests for pregnancy usually are recommended at least 2 weeks after the first missed menstrual period.

Blood:

Blood samples are obtained according to the requirements of the specific test to be performed. Hemolysis of blood may interfere with test results.

Nursing implications with rationale

Before

- ☞ Explain the procedure to the patient. Encourage verbalization of the patient's fears. Many patients are very anxious in anticipation of the results. Inform the patient regarding how and when to obtain the test results.
- If urine specimens are required, give the patient the urine container on the evening before the test so that she can provide a first-voided morning specimen. This specimen generally contains the greatest concentration of HCG.

After

- ☞ If the patient is using a home pregnancy testing kit, emphasize that she should still have antepartal health examinations.
- If a blood sample is required, obtain this as in-dicated by the laboratory. Check the site afterward for bleeding.

Progesterone and Pregnanediol

Test type Blood, urine

Normal values

Considerable variation according to method used and laboratory

Progesterone:

Situation	Progesterone ng/dl*
<9 years	<20
10-15 years	20
Adult male	10-50
Female	
Follicular phase	<50
Luteal phase	300-2500
Postmenopausal	<40
Pregnancy (trimester)	
First	725-4400
Second	1950-8250
Third	6500-22,900

Pregnanediol:

Situation	Pregnanediol mg/day
<9 years	<0.1
10-15 years	0.1-1.2
Adult male	0-1.9
Female	
Follicular phase	<2.6
Luteal phase	2.6-10.6
Pregnancy (trimester)	
First	10-35
Second	35-70
Third	70-100

Rationale

Pregnanediol is a metabolite of progesterone, which is produced by the ovaries or placenta. The main effect of progesterone is on the endometrium. It initiates the secretory phase of the endometrium in anticipation of implantation of a fertilized ovum. Normally, progesterone is secreted by the ovarian corpus luteum following ovulation.

---

*Extraction/radioimmunoassay.

Both serum progesterone levels and the urine concentration of progesterone metabolites (pregnanediol and others) are significantly increased during the latter half of an ovulatory cycle. Pregnanediol is the most easily measured metabolite of progesterone.

Because progesterone and pregnanediol levels rise rapidly after ovulation, these hormone assays are useful in documenting whether ovulation has occurred and, if so, its exact time. This is very useful information for a woman who has difficulty becoming pregnant. During pregnancy, progesterone and pregnanediol levels normally rise because of the placental production of progesterone. Repeated assays can be used to monitor the status of the placenta in cases of high-risk pregnancy.

Hormone assays for progesterone and urinary pregnanediol are primarily used today to monitor progesterone supplementation in patients with an inadequate luteal phase to maintain an early pregnancy. Plasma assays are quicker and may be more accurate.

Procedure

Progesterone determinations begin 4 to 6 days after ovulation if the patient is being followed for an inadequate luteal phase. A venous blood sample is obtained by peripheral venipuncture in a red-top tube. The laboratory requisition slip should include the date of the last menstrual period. A 24-hour urine specimen for progesterone or pregnanediol is collected in a standard specimen container and sent to the chemistry laboratory. During the entire collection, the specimen should be refrigerated. No food or fluid restrictions are necessary during the collection period.

Nursing implications with rationale

Before
- ☞ Explain the procedure to the patient. Inform the patient that no fasting is required for the blood or urine collection.

During
- ☞ Instruct the patient to begin the 24-hour urine collection after discarding the first morning

specimen. This is the start time of the 24-hour collection.
- ■ Collect all urine passed over the next 24 hours. Check with the laboratory to see if a preservative is needed.
- ☞ Instruct the patient to void before defecating so that the urine is not contaminated by feces.
- ☞ Remind the patient not to put toilet paper in the collection container.
- ■ Keep the urine specimen on ice or refrigerated during the 24 hours.
- ■ Collect the last specimen as close as possible to the end of the 24 hours.

After
- ■ Record the date of the last menstrual period or the week of gestation on the laboratory requisition slip.
- ☞ Inform the patient regarding when and how she can obtain the test results.

Rubella Antibody Test (German Measles Test, Hemagglutination Inhibition [HAI])

Test type Blood

Normal values

Method	Result	Interpretation
HAI	<1:8	No immunity to rubella
HAI	>1:20	Immune to rubella
Latex agglutination	Negative	No immunity to rubella
Enzyme-linked immunosorbent assay (ELISA) (IgM)	<0.9 IU/ml	No infection
ELISA (IgM)	>1.1	Active infection
ELISA (IgG)	<7 IU/ml	No immunity to rubella
ELISA (IgG)	>10 IU/ml	Immune to rubella

Possible critical values Evidence of susceptibility in pregnant women with recent exposure to rubella

Rationale

These tests detect the presence of IgG and/or IgM antibodies to rubella. They become elevated a few days to a few weeks (depending on what method of testing is used) after the onset of the rash. IgM tends to disappear after approximately 6 weeks. IgG, however, persists at low, but detectable, levels for years. These antibodies become elevated in patients with active rubella infection or with past infections. This test is very accurate, therefore, in determining a patient's susceptibility or immunity to the rubella virus, the causative agent for German measles. It is vitally important to identify exposure to rubella infection and susceptibility status in pregnant women because congenital rubella infection in the first trimester of pregnancy is associated with congenital abnormalities (e.g., heart defects, brain damage, deafness), spontaneous abortion, or stillbirth. All pregnant women should be screened for rubella during the first prenatal test. This test is sometimes used before pregnancy if a woman is not sure that she has had rubella. If antibodies are not present, she can be immunized before pregnancy.

If the woman's titer is greater than 1:10 to 1:20, she is not susceptible to rubella. If the woman's titer is 1:8 or less, she has little or no immunity to rubella. Pregnant women should be strongly advised to stay away from any small children, especially those with symptoms of an upper respiratory tract infection (prodromal symptoms of rubella) during pregnancy. In addition, all health care personnel associated with maternal and child care should be screened for rubella. Immunization, if required, is not done during pregnancy but should be done before or after delivery for nonimmune women.

A fourfold increase in titer from the acute to the convalescent titer indicates that the rash was caused by an active rubella infection. Alternatively, in a pregnant woman with a rash suspected to be from rubella, an IgM antibody titer could be done. If the titer is positive, recent infection has occurred. IgM titers appear 1 to 2 days after onset of the rash and disappear 5 to 6 weeks after infection.

Antirubella antibody testing also is used to diagnose congenital rubella in infants. Rubella is suspected in low-birth–weight babies. While IgG antibodies can be passed from mother to fetus, IgM antirubella antibodies cannot pass through the placenta. If an infant has IgM antibodies, acute congenital or newborn rubella is suspected. Antibody testing is often used in children with congenital abnormalities, which may have come from congenital rubella infection. This test also is recommended for any patient who presents with a rash that may be due to rubella.

Rubella testing is part of the TORCH evaluation (see p. 362). The term *TORCH* (*t*oxoplasmosis, *o*ther, *r*ubella, *c*ytomegalovirus, *h*erpes) has been applied to infections with recognized detrimental effects on the fetus. These effects may be direct or indirect (e.g., precipitating abortion or premature labor). Included in the category of "other" are STD infections (e.g., syphilis). All of these tests are discussed separately.

Procedure

A peripheral venous blood sample is obtained and sent to the laboratory for analysis.

Nursing implications with rationale

Before

☞ Explain the purpose of the test to the patient.

After

- Apply pressure or a pressure dressing to the venipuncture site to prevent further bleeding. Observe the site for bleeding.
- If indicated, instruct the patient when to return for follow-up testing titers.

Semen Analysis (Sperm Count, Sperm Examination, Seminal Cytology, Semen Examination)

Test type Fluid analysis

Normal values

Volume: 2-5 ml

Liquification time: 20 to 30 minutes after collection

pH: 7.12-8.00

Sperm count (density): 50-200 million/ml

Sperm motility: 60% to 80% actively motile

Sperm morphology: 70% to 90% normally shaped

Rationale

Semen analysis is used to evaluate the quality of sperm, evaluate an infertile couple, and document the adequacy of a vasectomy. Semen production depends on the function of the pituitary/hypothalamic tract and the testicles. GnRH is secreted by the hypothalamus in response to decreased levels of testosterone. GnRH stimulates the pituitary to produce FSH and LH (also called *interstitial cell-stimulating hormone*). The FSH stimulates Sertoli's cell growth with the seminiferous tubules (location of sperm production). LH stimulates Leydig's cells to produce testosterone, which, in turn, stimulates the seminiferous tubules to produce sperm. Semen analysis is a measure of testicular function. Inadequate sperm production can be the result of primary gonadal failure (genetic [Klinefelter's syndrome], infection, radiation, or surgical orchidectomy) or secondary gonadal failure (caused by pituitary diseases). These forms of gonadal failure can be differentiated by measuring LH and FSH levels. In the first type, LH and FSH levels are increased. In the second type, they are decreased. Stimulation tests using GnRH, clomiphene citrate, or HCG also are used in the differentiation.

Semen analysis is one of the most important aspects of the fertility workup because the cause of a couple's inability to conceive often lies with the man. Sperm is collected and examined for volume, sperm count, motility, and morphology.

The freshly collected semen is first measured for volume. Men with very low or very high volumes are likely to be infertile. After liquefaction of the white, gelatinous ejaculate, a sperm count is done. The motility of the sperm is then evaluated; at least 60% should show progressive motility. Morphology is studied by staining a semen preparation and calculating the number of normal versus abnormal sperm forms. A sperm specimen is considered abnormal if greater than 70% of the sperm has abnormal morphology.

A single sperm analysis, especially if it indicates infertility, is inconclusive because sperm count varies from day to day. A semen analysis should be done at least twice, and possibly a third time, with 3 weeks between each test. Men with aspermia (no sperm) or oligospermia (<20 million/ml) should be evaluated endocrinologically for pituitary, thyroid, adrenal, or testicular aberrations.

A normal semen analysis alone does not accurately assess the male factor unless the effect of the partner's cervical secretion on sperm survival also is determined (see Sims-Huhner test, p. 391). In addition to its value in infertility workups, semen analysis also is helpful in documenting adequate sterilization after a vasectomy. It usually is performed 6 weeks after the surgery. If any sperm are seen, the adequacy of the vasectomy must be suspect.

Procedure

After 2 to 3 days of the patient's sexual abstinence, a semen specimen is collected by ejaculation into a clean container. For best results, this specimen should be collected in the physician's office or laboratory by masturbation. Less satisfactory specimens can be obtained in the patient's home by coitus interruptus or masturbation. These home specimens must be delivered to the laboratory within 1 hour after collection. Excessive heat and cold should be avoided during transportation of the specimen.

If the couple cannot obtain a specimen by masturbation or coitus interruptus, a plastic condom can be used. Rubber condoms should not be used because the powders and lubricants used in their manufacture may be spermicidal.

Nursing implications with rationale

Before

✐ Explain the procedure to the patient. Confirm that the patient understands that 2 to 3 days of sexual abstinence are necessary. Prolonged abstinence before the collection should be discouraged because the quality of the sperm cells, and especially their motility, may diminish.

☞ Give the patient the proper container for the sperm collection. Be matter-of-fact about the specimen collection and delivery because the collection and delivery of the semen to the laboratory may be embarrassing for the patient.

☞ If the specimen is obtained at home, instruct the patient that he must bring the specimen to the laboratory for testing within 1 hour after collection, keeping it at room temperature. Exposure to heat or cold during the transportation may alter sperm cell motility.

After

■ Record the date of the previous semen emission, along with the collection time and date of the fresh specimen. The laboratory will refer to these dates.

■ Allow time for the patient to discuss any questions or fears regarding the results of this study.

☞ Instruct the patient regarding when and how to obtain the test results. Abnormal results may have a devastating effect on the patient's sexuality.

Sexually Transmitted Disease Cultures (STD Cultures, Culture of Cervix, Urethra, and Anus)

Test type Microscopic examination

Normal values

No evidence of sexually transmitted disease (STD) (gonorrhea, chlamydia, trichomonas)

Rationale

These cultures and smears are performed for patients who have a vaginal discharge, pelvic pain, urethritis, or penile discharge and are at risk for STDs. In the United States and other countries, some STDs have become epidemic, whereas others have become increasingly common. These organisms can cause urethritis, vaginitis, endometritis, PID, pharyngitis, proctitis, epididymitis, prostatitis, and salpingitis. Children born to in-

fected mothers may develop conjunctivitis, pneumonia, neonatal blindness, neonatal neurologic injury, and even death.

Cultures for STD infections are performed on men and women with suggestive symptoms. If the culture is positive, sexual partners should be evaluated and treated. Cervical cultures are usually done for women; urethral cultures are done for men. Rectal and throat cultures are performed in persons who have engaged in anal and oral intercourse. Because rectal gonorrhea accompanies genital gonorrhea in a high percentage of women, rectal cultures may be recommended in all women with suspected gonorrhea. If the STD culture is positive, treatment during pregnancy can prevent possible fetal complications (e.g., ophthalmia neonatorum) and maternal complications. Rectal and orogastric cultures should be done on the neonates of infected mothers.

STDs are identified by culture or smear of a genital lesion, tissue biopsy, serologic testing, and observation of a classic clinical lesion. Each suspected organism must be specifically requested on the laboratory requisition slip. Organisms involved in STDs include: *Neisseria gonorrhoeae*, *Chlamydia*, *Herpes genitalis*, *Treponema pallidum* (the causative agent of syphilis), the hepatitis virus, human immunodeficiency virus (HIV) (the causative agent of AIDS), *Trichomonas vaginalis* (the causative agent of trichomoniasis), *Sarcoptes scabiei* (the causative agent of scabies), molluscum, *Pediculidae* (lice), *Haemophilus* (the causative agent of chancroid), and *Gardnerella*. Many of these STDs are discussed separately in this book.

Interfering factors

Factors that interfere with STD cultures include the following:

■ Lubricants and disinfectants
Some organisms, such as *N. gonorrhoeae*, are very sensitive to these.
■ Menses, which may alter test results
■ Female douching
Fewer organisms are available for culture if

douching occurs within 24 hours of a cervical culture.

■ Male voiding within 1 hour of a urethral culture This washes secretions out of the urethra.

■ Fecal material, which may contaminate an anal culture

Procedure

For a *cervical culture,* the female patient is told to refrain from douching and tub-bathing beforehand. The patient is placed in the lithotomy position, and a moistened, nonlubricated vaginal speculum is inserted to expose the cervix. Cervical mucus is removed with a cotton ball held in a ring forceps. A sterile, cotton-tipped swab is inserted into the endocervical canal and moved from side to side to obtain the culture. The swab is placed in sterile saline or a transporting fluid obtained from the laboratory. The specimen should be plated as soon as possible, it should not be refrigerated.

Anal canal culture of the female or male patient is taken by inserting a sterile, cotton-tipped swab approximately 1 inch into the anal canal (Figure 9-9). If stool contaminates the swab, a repeat swab is taken.

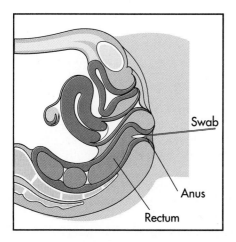

Figure 9-9 Obtaining a specimen of exudate from the rectum for sexually transmitted diseases.

The *urethral culture* specimen should be obtained from the male patient before voiding. Voiding within 1 hour of collection washes secretions out of the urethra, making fewer organisms available for culture. The best time to obtain the specimen is before the first morning micturition. A culture is taken by inserting a sterile swab gently into the anterior urethra. It is advisable to place the male patient in the supine position to prevent falling if vasovagal syncope occurs during introduction of the cotton swab or wire loop into the urethra. In the male, prostatic massage may increase the chances of obtaining positive cultures.

The *oropharyngeal culture* should be obtained in male and female patients who have engaged in oral intercourse. A throat culture is best obtained by depressing the patient's tongue with a wooden tongue blade and touching the posterior wall of the throat with a sterile, cotton-tipped swab.

STD cultures and smears are obtained by a physician or nurse in several minutes. Very little discomfort is associated with these procedures. No fasting or sedation is required.

Nursing implications with rationale

Before

☐ Explain the purpose and procedure to the patient. Use a matter-of-fact, nonjudgmental approach to reduce any patient embarrassment.

■ Handle all specimens as though they were capable of transmitting disease.

After

■ Mark the laboratory requisition slip with the collection time, date, source of specimen, patient's age, current antibiotic therapy, and clinical diagnosis.

☐ Advise the patient to avoid intercourse and all sexual contact until test results are available.

☐ If the culture results are positive, instruct the patient to receive treatment and to have sexual partners evaluated.

☐ Inform the patient that repeat cultures should be taken after completion of treatment to evaluate therapy.

Case Study

Routine Prenatal Evaluation

Mr. and Mrs. K., a 23-year-old black couple, were excited when Mrs. K's menstrual period was 3 weeks late. Mrs. K. was seen by her obstetrician, and her pregnancy was confirmed. The following routine laboratory tests were performed.

First Prenatal Visit

Studies	Results
Urinalysis, p. 268	WNL
Urine culture, p. 273	Negative (normal: negative)
Complete blood count (CBC) and platelets, p. 412	WNL
Pap smear, p. 375	Negative (normal: negative)
Serologic test for syphilis, p. 392	Negative (normal: negative)
Gonorrhea culture, p. 388	Negative (normal: negative)
Toxoplasmosis antibody titer, p. 394	1:100 (normal: 1:4 to 1:256 in general population)
Blood type and Rh factor, p. 406	B+
Rubella antibodies, p. 385	1:20 (titer >1:10 indicates immunity)
Tuberculin skin test, p. 181	Negative (normal: negative)
Sickle cell test, p. 438	Negative (normal: negative)

28-Week Checkup

Studies	Results
Hematocrit (Hct), p. 412	WNL
2-hour postprandial glucose (PPG) test, p. 309	WNL

36-Week Checkup

Studies	Results
Hct	WNL

Diagnostic Analysis

The urinalysis was done primarily to detect glucose (glycosuria), which could have suggested diabetes, and to detect albumin (proteinuria), which could have suggested preeclampsia. The urine culture results did not detect urinary tract infection or renal problems. The normal CBC and platelets ruled out anemia (the most common nutritional complication of pregnancy), infectious processes, and alterations in the blood clotting ability. The STDs of syphilis and gonorrhea were not detected. The level of the toxoplasmosis antibody titer did not indicate any problem for the mother or fetus. The blood typing and Rh factor determination studies were performed to detect a possible incompatibility disease. If the mother had been Rh-negative, checking the father would have been necessary. Antibody titer levels then would have been followed throughout the pregnancy. The rubella antibody test assured Mrs. K. that she was protected from rubella. The Pap smear was normal, and the tuberculin skin test indicated tuberculosis was not suspected. The sickle cell test, which was done because the disease occurs more frequently in blacks, was negative. Mrs. K.'s Hct was checked again at weeks 28 and 36. The 2-hour PPG test ruled out gestational diabetes.

Mr. and Mrs. K. were happy that all the studies showed good results. Mrs. K. was seen by a certified nurse-midwife (CNM) monthly until week 28, biweekly from weeks 28 through 36, and weekly from week 36 until delivery. Her urine was checked at each visit for glucose and acetone, which may have indicated gestational diabetes, and protein, which would have indicated preeclampsia. She and her husband attended Lamaze classes. With the assistance of a CNM, Mrs. K. delivered a healthy 8-pound, 2-ounce boy 4 days after her estimated date of confinement (EDC).

Critical Thinking Questions
1. What would be the concern if this couple had an Rh factor incompatibility?
2. Why is the presence of protein in the urine an indication for preeclampsia?

Sims-Huhner Test (Postcoital Test, Postcoital Cervical Mucus Test, Cervical Mucus Sperm Penetration Test)

Cervical Mucus Test

Test type Fluid analysis, microscopic examination

Normal values
Sims-Huhner:
Cervical mucus adequate for sperm transmission, survival, and penetration of 6 to 20 active sperm per high-power field
Cervical Mucus:
Arborization, or ferning, of cervical mucus during midcycle

Rationale
The **Sims-Huhner** study evaluates interaction between the sperm and the cervical mucus. It also measures the quality of the cervical mucus. This test can determine the effect of vaginal and cervical secretions on the activity of the sperm. This procedure is performed only after a previously performed semen analysis has been determined to be normal.

This test is performed during the middle of the ovulatory cycle because, at this time, the secre-

tions should be optimal for sperm penetration and survival. During ovulation, the quantity of cervical mucus is maximal, whereas the viscosity is minimal, thus facilitating sperm penetration. The postcoital endocervical mucus sample is examined for color, viscosity, and tenacity (spinnbarkeit) (Figure 9-10). The fresh specimen then is spread on a clean glass slide and examined for the presence of sperm. Estimates of the total number and of the number of motile sperm per high-power field are reported. Normally, 6 to 20 active sperm cells should be seen in each microscopic high-power field; if the sperm are present but not active, the cervical environment is unsuitable (e.g., abnormal pH) for their survival.

After the specimen has dried on the glass slide, the mucus **(cervical mucus test)** can be examined for cervical ferning to demonstrate the estrogen effect. During a normal ovulatory cycle, the ferning of cervical mucus will occur at midcycle, and no ferning will occur before menstruation. Besides its absence in anovulatory, premenopausal patients, ferning of the cervical mucus also is absent in postmenopausal, castrated, or normally pregnant women. This is due to the presence of fern-inhibiting progesterone.

The Sims-Huhner study is invaluable in fertility examinations; however, it is not a substitute for the semen analysis. If the results of the Sims-

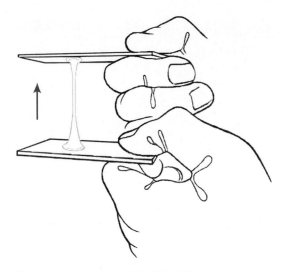

Figure 9-10 Spinnbarkeit (elasticity) of the cervical mucus increases at ovulation.

Huhner test are less than optimal, the test usually is repeated during the same or next ovulatory cycle. This analysis also is helpful in documenting cases of suspected rape by testing the vaginal and cervical secretions for sperm.

Procedure

During ovulation, the woman is instructed to report to the physician for examination of her cervical mucus within 2 hours after coitus. (Some clinics suggest 4 to 8 hours.) Precoital lubrication and postcoital douching, bathing, or voiding are not permitted. This study should be performed after 3 days of male sexual abstinence. After intercourse, the patient should rest in bed for 10 to 15 minutes to ensure cervical exposure to semen. After resting, the patient should wear a perineal pad until she is placed in the lithotomy position in the physician's office. The cervix then is exposed by an unlubricated speculum. The specimen is aspirated from the endocervix and delivered to the laboratory for analysis.

This procedure is performed by a physician in approximately 5 minutes. The specimen analysis is done in 15 minutes. The only discomfort associated with this study is the insertion of the speculum.

Nursing implications with rationale

Before

Sims-Huhner test

☞ Explain the procedure to the patient. Inform her that basal body temperature (BBT) recordings should be used to indicate ovulation.

☞ Inform the patient that no vaginal lubrication, douching, or bathing is permitted until after the vaginal cervical examination because these activities alter the cervical mucus.

☞ Instruct the patient that this test should be performed after 3 days of male sexual abstinence.

☞ Instruct the patient to rest in bed for 10 to 15 minutes after coitus to ensure cervical exposure to the semen. She should then wear a perineal pad and report to her physician within 2 hours.

☞ Encourage the patient to verbalize her feelings. Many patients are very anxious at this point in the fertility workup. They often fear that the results of this study will determine that they are infertile.

Cervical mucus test

☞ Explain the procedure to the patient. Inform her that this procedure is performed at midcycle to detect estrogen-induced ferning and is repeated approximately 7 days later to detect the progesterone inhibition of ferning.

After

☞ Inform the patient regarding how and when she may obtain the test results.

Syphilis Detection Test (Serologic Test for Syphilis [STS], Venereal Disease Research Laboratory [VDRL], Rapid Plasma Reagin Test [RPR], Fluorescent Treponemal Antibody Test [FTA])

Test type Blood

Normal values

Negative, or nonreactive

Rationale

Syphilis is caused by the spirochete, *Treponema pallidum*. The disease is divided into four stages: acute, secondary, latent, and tertiary. The acute stage is marked by the development of a chancre on the skin near the infection site (usually the genitals). The chancre develops approximately 3 to 6 weeks after inoculation and lasts approximately 4 to 6 weeks. The secondary stage is characterized by a rash (often on the soles and palms) and generalized lymphadenopathy. This stage lasts approximately 3 months. The latent stage represents a period of disease inactivity and can last as long as 5 years. Some patients experience a cure during this stage. Most go on to the tertiary stage, which is marked by CNS, cardiovascular, and ocular signs and symptoms.

The immunologic tests for syphilis detect antibodies to *T. pallidum*. Nonspecific antibodies are detected by the Wassermann test or the Venereal Disease Research Laboratory (VDRL) test. A newer, more sensitive, nonspecific test is the rapid plasma reagin (RPR) test. The VDRL and RPR tests, by virtue of their testing for a nonspecific antibody, have a high false-positive (or cross-reactive) rate. The VDRL test becomes positive approximately 2 weeks after the patient's inoculation with *T. pallidum*. The test is positive in nearly all primary and secondary stages of syphilis and in two thirds of patients with tertiary syphilis.

If the VDRL or RPR test is positive, the diagnosis must be confirmed by the more specific and more accurate *Treponema* test, such as the fluorescent treponemal antibody absorption test (FTA-ABS). The FTA-ABS test, which tests for a specific treponemal antibody, is more accurate than the VDRL and RPR tests and becomes positive approximately 4 to 6 weeks after inoculation.

If the VDRL or RPR test is positive and the FTA-ABS is negative, one must look for other diseases that can cause positive-screening, serologic syphilis tests such as malaria, leprosy, typhus, and lymphogranuloma venereum.

Screening for syphilis usually is done with the VDRL test during the first prenatal checkup for pregnant women. Syphilis, if untreated, may cause spontaneous abortion, stillbirth, and premature labor. The effects on the fetus can include CNS damage, hearing loss, and possible death.

Syphilis testing is part of TORCH testing. The term *TORCH* (*t*oxoplasmosis, *o*ther, *r*ubella, *c*ytomegalovirus, *h*erpes) has been applied to infections with recognized detrimental effects on the fetus. These effects may be direct or indirect (e.g., precipitating abortion or premature labor). Included in the category of "other" are STD infections (e.g., syphilis). All of these tests are discussed separately.

In general, serologic tests return to normal after successful treatment for syphilis. The earlier the disease is treated, the sooner the serologic tests return to normal. In the early primary stage, the serologic tests may become negative 2 to 4 months after successful antibiotic treatment. When treating later stages of the disease, it may take longer than 1 year for the patient to convert to a seronegative result. In the tertiary stage, the patient may never convert to negative. Testing should be performed routinely to document successful therapy.

Interfering factors

Factors that interfere with the syphilis detection test include the following:

- Excessive hemolysis and gross lipemia, which may cause false-positive test results.
- Excess chyle in the blood, which may cause false-positive test results. Testing should be performed after at least an 8-hour fast.
- Many diseases cause false-positive results when VDRL and RPR tests are used (Box 9-1).
- Early testing
  If the patient is tested too soon after inoculation and before antibodies have developed, the tests may be falsely negative. The test should be repeated in 2 months, or the patient should be treated despite the negative test results (if clinical suspicion is high).

Procedure

The VDRL, RPR, and FTA-ABS tests can be performed on 7 ml of peripheral venous blood collected in a red-top tube. These tests are performed

Box 9-1	*Diseases That Can Cause False-Positive VDRL/RPR Results*

Acute viral or bacterial infections
Cat-scratch fever
Hepatitis
Hypersensitivity reactions
Leprosy
Leptospirosis
Lymphogranuloma venereum
Malaria
Mononucleosis
Mycoplasmal pneumonia
Periarteritis nodosa
Recent vaccinations
Systemic lupus erythematosus
Typhus

by a technician and are not associated with any patient discomfort except for the venipuncture. Hemolysis can affect the results.

Nursing implications with rationale

Before

☞ Explain the procedure to the patient. Obtain the blood as ordered. Assess the patient for other diseases that may cause false-positive results.

After

■ Apply pressure or a pressure dressing to the venipuncture site to prevent further bleeding. Observe the venipuncture site for bleeding.

■ If the test is positive, obtain a history of the patient's recent sexual contacts so that these persons may be evaluated for syphilis.

■ If the test is positive, ensure that the patient receives appropriate antibiotic therapy.

Toxoplasmosis Antibody Titer

Test type Blood

Normal values

IgG titers <1:16 indicate no previous infection
IgG titers 1:16-1:256 usually are prevalent in the general population

IgG titers >1:256 suggest recent infection
IgM titers >1:256 indicate acute infection

Rationale

Toxoplasmosis is a protozoan disease caused by *Toxoplasma gondii,* which is found in humans and many animals, especially cats. Humans become infected by eating poorly cooked or raw meat. Exposure to feces of cats or other infected material can cause infection. Most often, humans are asymptomatic from the infection. When symptoms occur, this disease is characterized by CNS lesions, which may lead to blindness, brain damage, and death. The condition may occur congenitally or sometime afterward. Approximately 25% to 70% of the adult population has been exposed to toxoplasmosis.

The presence of antibodies before pregnancy indicates prior exposure and chronic asymptomatic infection. The presence of these antibodies probably ensures protection against congenital toxoplasmosis in the child. Fetal infection occurs if the mother acquires toxoplasmosis after conception and passes it to the fetus through the placenta. Hydrocephaly, microcephaly, chronic retinitis, and convulsions are complications of congenital toxoplasmosis. Congenital toxoplasmosis is diagnosed when the antibody levels are persistently elevated or a rising titer is found in the infant 2 to 3 months after birth.

IgM levels rise approximately 1 week after inoculation, peak in approximately 2 to 3 months, and decline to undetectable levels in approximately 1 year. IgG levels begin to rise approximately 2 weeks after inoculation, peak in approximately 2 to 3 months, and decline to low, but persistent, levels in approximately 6 months. Low titers, especially of IgG, indicate past infections and protection from passing acute infection to an unborn child. High or rapidly rising titers of either IgM or IgG indicate acute infection in the adult or newborn infant. This is often used as a screening method for pregnant women.

Elevated IgM antibodies, IgG titers of greater than 1:1000, or a fourfold rise in IgG antibodies indicate an acute toxoplasmosis infection. Low, but significant, titers of IgG indicate past infection. High, nonrising titers indicate acute infection that has occurred more than 3 to 12 months before testing.

Toxoplasmosis is part of TORCH testing. The term *TORCH* (*t*oxoplasmosis, *o*ther, *r*ubella, *c*ytomegalovirus, *h*erpes) has been applied to infections with recognized detrimental effects on the fetus. These effects may be direct or indirect (e.g., precipitating abortion or premature labor). Included in the category of "other" are STD infections (e.g., syphilis). All of these tests are discussed separately.

Interfering factors
- Rheumatoid factor or antinuclear antibodies, which can cause false-positive results
- Other active congenital infections, which can cause false-positive results

Procedure
A peripheral venipuncture is performed, and approximately 5 ml of blood is collected in a red-top tube and sent to the laboratory for analysis. Some laboratories request that the laboratory requisition slip indicate if the patient is pregnant or has been exposed to cats.

Nursing implications with rationale
Before
☞ Explain the purpose of the test to the patient.
After
- Apply pressure or a pressure dressing to the venipuncture site to prevent further bleeding. Observe the venipuncture site for bleeding.

REVIEW QUESTIONS AND ANSWERS

1. **Question:** Your 51-year-old patient indicates that she thinks she is experiencing menopausal symptoms but is not sure. What tests might she need?
   Answer: Many tests are available for indicating the menopausal state. Urine testing for pregnanediol or estriol may be performed. Serum progesterone or estradiol testing more easily indicates the menopausal state. De-

creased levels would be expected in the menopausal woman. Elevated levels of follicular-stimulating or luteinizing hormones indicate menopause. Combined with the symptoms of menstrual irregularity and hot flashes, menopause can be determined easily.

2. **Question:** A 12-year-old girl is brought to the emergency room by her mother, who alleges that her daughter was raped by her husband (the daughter's stepfather). For which tests should you prepare the child? What are the important forensic, physical, and emotional nursing interventions?
   Answer: First, an external examination would be performed. If the victim is old enough to menstruate, an internal examination is done. Cervical mucus would be obtained for a Sims-Huhner test. The cervical mucus would be examined for the presence of sperm. A Wood's light is shone on the external vagina and into the introitus. Sperm would be apparent as fluorescence. Vaginal and anal swabs would be obtained for STDs. One-time antibiotic treatment (e.g., ciprofloxcin and azithromycin) is provided to treat a possible STD. Norgestrel, a progestational agent and an ovulation suppressant, is usually provided if ovulation is expected within the next few days. This reduces the chances of pregnancy resulting from the rape. Finally, and importantly, arrangements for immediate protection and long-term counseling of the child are provided.

3. **Question:** A 59-year-old woman returns to the same-day surgery unit after having a hysteroscopy and endometrial biopsy. She complains of lower abdominal pain. After analgesics are provided, she is discharged. Three days later she returns to the emergency room with persistent and worsening pelvic pain and an elevated temperature. What are the possible complications from her diagnostic surgery that could cause these symptoms, and for what test should you prepare the patient at this point?
   Answer: An uncommon, but possible, complication from a hysteroscopy is perforation of the uterus. This could lead to a pelvic abscess, best identified by an ultrasound or computed to-

mography (CT) scan of the pelvis. Another possibility is that the patient has cystitis induced during the catheterization required for hysteroscopy. A urinalysis would be helpful in determining this diagnosis.

4. **Question:** Your patient tells you that she and her husband have been unsuccessful in conceiving a child. Her husband is angry with her because she cannot get pregnant. How might you support her, and what testing should the couple be prepared to undergo?

Answer: Your patient may feel less responsible when she learns that the most common factor associated with infertility lies with the male. Her husband should provide a sperm specimen that is tested for sperm quantity and motility. Besides a thorough examination, your patient can expect blood testing to indicate ovulation. FSH, LH, estrogen, and progesterone metabolites are measured. If ovulation is believed to occur, hysteroscopy and hysterosalpingography may be performed. Your patient and her husband may be tested for antisperm antibodies.

5. **Question:** Your patient has not had a Pap smear in 5 years and asks you how often she should have this test done. What should you recommend?

Answer: The American Cancer Society recommends that all asymptomatic women age 20 and older and those under 20 who are sexually active have a Pap test annually for two negative examinations and then one every 3 years until age 65. However, this recommendation is not supported by many gynecologists, who recommend yearly Pap smears.

6. **Question:** Your neighbor calls and asks for your advice. She has just been told that her Pap smear contains cells that "do not appear to be too good." What should you tell her?

Answer: Explain to your neighbor that many possible causes exist for the type of cells reported as being "not too good." These include inflammation, as well as benign and malignant tumors. Tell her that her physician will most probably recommend colposcopy or cervical cone biopsy. Briefly and optimistically describe both procedures. Provide support for your neighbor during this very anxious time.

7. **Question:** Your patient has been trying unsuccessfully to get pregnant for 6 months. She says she would like to have a laparoscopy to elucidate the cause of her infertility. How might she best be advised?

   Answer: The patient should be helped to understand that to be considered for an infertility evaluation, she should have been trying to get pregnant for at least 1 year. Furthermore, she should be told that laparoscopy is not the first step of the evaluation. She also should be reminded that because nearly 40% of all cases of infertility are caused by a male factor, her husband should undergo concomitant evaluation.

   The patient should be advised to have coitus around the time of expected ovulation for another 6 months. If she still does not become pregnant, she and her husband then should return for an infertility workup.

8. **Question:** While you are working on the night shift, a patient who is 36 weeks pregnant calls and states that she had a CST that morning. She is now having vaginal bleeding and thinks her "water may have broken." How should you advise this patient?

   Answer: Labor may have been unexpectedly induced by the CST. Her condition certainly warrants a physical evaluation. Recommend that she call her physician immediately to arrange for such an examination.

9. **Question:** Your pregnant patient has been instructed to collect a 24-hour urine specimen for estriol determination to evaluate fetal viability. Because she was out at a party during the evening, she voided once without collecting the urine. Should the specimen be sent for the analysis?

   Answer: No. The collection must be complete. An incomplete specimen may artificially lower the estriol value. Because a low estriol level is indicative of fetal distress, the consequences of an incomplete specimen analysis are grave. Therefore, the patient should be instructed to repeat the 24-hour urine collection.

Bibliography

Bernsleen IM et al: Ultrasonographic estimation of fetal body composition for children of diabetic mothers, *Invest Radiol* 26(8):722-726, 1991.

Brent RL et al: Medical sonography: reproductive effects and risks, *Teratology* 44(2):123-146, 1991.

Catanzarite VA: Antepartal care. In Rakel RE (editor): Conn's current therapy, Philadelphia, 1998, WB Saunders.

Chauhan SP et al: Limitations of clinical and sonographic estimates of birth weight: experience with 1034 parturients, *Obstet Gynecol* 91(1):72-77, 1998.

Chu DC et al: Insulin-like growth factor binding factor protein-3 in the detection of fetal Down syndrome pregnancies, *Obstet Gynecol* 91(2):192-195, 1998.

Creasy RK, Resnik R: Maternal-fetal medicine: principles and practice, ed 3, Philadelphia, 1994, WB Saunders.

Dalence CR et al: Amniotic fluid lamellar body count: a rapid and reliable fetal lung maturity test, *Obstet Gynecol* 86(2):235-239, 1995.

De Veciana M et al: Postprandial versus preprandial blood glucose monitoring in women with gestational diabetes mellitus requiring insulin therapy, *N Engl J Med* 333(19):1239-1241, 1995.

Dolinger MB, Donnenfeld AE: Therapeutic amniocentesis using a vacuum bottle aspiration system, *Obstet Gynecol* 91(1):143-144, 1998.

Eschenbach DA: Pelvic infections and sexually transmitted diseases. In Scott JR et al, editors: Danforth's obstetrics and gynecology, ed 7, Philadelphia, 1994, JB Lippincott.

Faro S: *Chlamydia trachomatis.* In Rakel RE, editor: Conn's current therapy, Philadelphia, 1998, WB Saunders.

Greenberg LR, Moore TR, Murphy H: Gestational diabetes mellitus: antenatal variables as predictors of postpartum glucose intolerance, *Gest Diabetes* 86(1):97-101, 1995.

Gregor CL: Antepartum fetal assessment techniques: an update for today's perinatal nurse, *J Perinatol Neonatol Nurs* 5(4):1-15, 1992.

Guzick DS: Amenorrhea. In Rakel RE, editor: Conn's current therapy, Philadelphia, 1998, WB Saunders.

Hammond CB: Infertility. In Scott JR et al, editors: Danforth's obstetrics and gynecology, ed 7, Philadelphia, 1994, JB Lippincott.

Hogge JS, Hogge WA, Golbus MS: Chorionic villus sampling, *J Obstet Gynecol Neonatol Nurs* 15:24, 1986.

Hohlfeld RE et al: Cytomegalovirus fetal infection: prenatal diagnosis, *Obstet Gynecol* 78(4):6158, 1991.

Jaffe SB et al: The basic infertility investigation, *Fertil Steril* 56(4):599-613, 1991.

Keye WR: Gynecologic history, examination, and diagnostic procedures. In Scott JR et al, editors: Danforth's obstetrics and gynecology, ed 7, Philadelphia, 1994, JB Lippincott.

Kochenour NK: Normal pregnancy and prenatal care. In Scott JR et al, editors: Danforth's obstetrics and gynecology, ed 7, Philadelphia, 1994, JB Lippincott.

Langer B et al: Plasma active renin, angiotensin I, and angiotensin II during pregnancy and in preclampsia, *Obstet Gynecol* 91(2):196-202, 1998.

Millard S: Emotional responses to infertility: understanding patients' needs, *AORN J* 54(2):301-305, 1991.

Miller KE: Sexually transmitted diseases, *Prim Care* 24(1):179-193, 1997.

Morell V: Basic infertility assessment, *Prim Care* 24(1):195-204, 1997.

Murtha AP et al: Maternal serum interleukin-6 concentration as a marker for impending preterm delivery, *Obstet Gynecol* 91(2):161-164, 1998.

Reed KL: Ultrasound during pregnancy. In Scott JR et al, editors: Danforth's obstetrics and gynecology, ed 7, Philadelphia, 1994, JB Lippincott.

Ryan KJ, Berkowitz R, Barbieri R, editors: Kistner's gynecology: principles and practice, ed 5, St Louis, 1990, Mosby.

Shushan A, Samueloff A: Correlation between fasting glucose in the first trimester and glucose challenge test in the second, *Obstet Gynecol* 91(4):596-599, 1998.

Soffici AR, Eden RD: Assessment of fetal well-being. In Scott JR et al, editors: Danforth's obstetrics and gynecology, ed 7, Philadelphia, 1994, JB Lippincott.

Spellacy WN: Diabetes mellitus and pregnancy. In Scott JR et al, editors: Danforth's obstetrics and gynecology, ed 7, Philadelphia, 1994, JB Lippincott.

Tracker HL: Menopause, *Prim Care* 24(1):205-221, 1997.

Vintzileos AM et al: A cost-effectiveness analysis of prenatal carrier screening for cystic fibrosis, *Obstet Gynecol* 91(4):529-34, 1998.

Vintzileos AM et al: An economic evaluation of first-trimester genetic sonography for prenatal detection of Down's syndrome, *Obstet Gynecol* 91(4):535-539, 1998.

Zeitune M et al: Screening for Down's syndrome in older women based on maternal serum alpha-fetoprotein levels and age: preliminary results, *Prenat Diagn* 11(6):393-398, 1991.

Zilianti M et al: Transperineal sonography in second trimester to term pregnancy and early labor, *J Ultrasound Med* 10(9):481-485, 1991.

Chapter 10

Diagnostic Studies Used in the Assessment of the
Hematologic System

ANATOMY AND PHYSIOLOGY

The hematologic system is responsible for the production of red blood cells (RBCs), white blood cells (WBCs), and platelets and for hemostasis (i.e., the blood's ability to clot following vascular injury). The bone marrow within the central bones (e.g., the ilium, sternum, and proximal long bones) is the site of blood cell production (hematopoiesis). The primary function of the RBCs is to transport oxygen (O_2) from the lungs to the tissues. Carbon dioxide (CO_2) is transported in the opposite direction. WBCs are primarily a defense against infection, foreign particles, and foreign tissues. Blood clotting (coagulation) is the primary function of the platelets.

Red Blood Cells (Erythrocytes)

Pluripotent stem cells within the bone marrow are capable of differentiating into either the RBC line or the WBC line (Figure 10-1). A proerythroblast is formed during RBC differentiation. With further cell division and differentiation, the proerythroblast becomes a normoblast. As the cell matures, it accumulates hemoglobin (Hgb) and gradually loses its nucleus. These cells are called *reticulocytes* and are deposited into the circulating blood. They further differentiate into mature RBCs (erythrocytes). This process is stimulated by

many factors (e.g., hypoxia, catecholamines, and growth hormone); however, the major stimulating factor is erythropoietin, a hormone produced primarily by the kidney.

Packed within each RBC are molecules of Hgb that permit the transport and exchange of O_2 and CO_2. Four polypeptide chains (two alpha and two beta) make up the normal Hgb protein, called *Hgb A_1*. Hgb A_2, a normal variant, is composed of two alpha and two delta chains. Hgb F is the main Hgb component in the fetus and infant and consists of two alpha and two gamma chains. Hgb F is capable of transporting O_2 even when very little O_2 is available. Hemoglobinopathies (e.g., sickle cell disease, Hgb C disease, and thalassemia) are a result of genetically induced abnormalities in the normal alpha and beta polypeptide Hgb chains.

Iron is the major inorganic component of Hgb and is essential for Hgb synthesis. When the patient is iron deficient, Hgb synthesis is markedly diminished, which results in small (microcytic), pale (hypochromic) RBCs.

Normally the RBCs exist in the peripheral blood for approximately 120 days. Toward the end of the RBC's life, the cell membrane becomes less pliable, and the aged RBC is hemolyzed and extracted from the circulation by the spleen. Abnormal RBCs have a shorter life span and are extracted earlier. Intravascular RBC trauma (e.g., that caused by artificial heart valves or peripheral vascular atherosclerotic plaques) also shortens the RBC's life. An enlarged spleen (e.g., that caused by portal hypertension or leukemias) may inappropriately destroy and remove normal RBCs from the circulation.

With RBC destruction, the heme molecule of Hgb is broken down and metabolized into bilirubin. Bilirubin is then excreted by the normal liver into bile. Liver disease, bile duct obstruction, or increased hemolysis can result in hyperbilirubinemia and jaundice (see Figure 4-2, p. 103).

White Blood Cells (Leukocytes)

The major function of the WBCs is to fight infection and react against foreign bodies or tissues. Five types of WBCs can easily be identified on a routine blood smear. These cells, in order of fre-

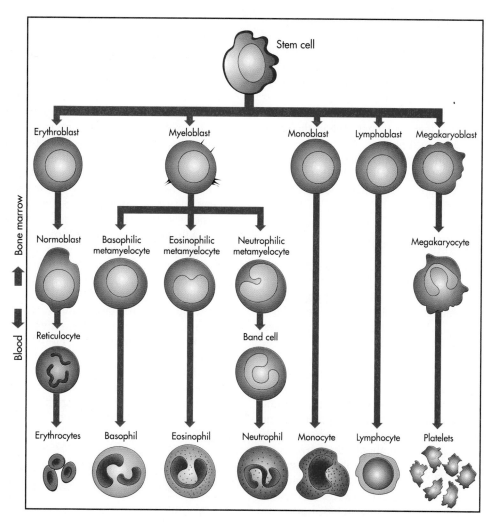

Figure 10-1   Development of blood cells.

quency, include neutrophils, lymphocytes, monocytes, eosinophils, and basophils. All of these
WBCs arise from the same pluripotent stem cell
within the bone marrow that the RBCs do. Beyond
this origin, however, each cell line differentiates
separately. The mature WBC then is deposited
into the circulating blood.

Polymorphonuclear (PMN) neutrophils are
produced in 7 to 14 days and exist in the circulation for only 6 hours. The primary function of the
neutrophil is phagocytosis (killing and digestion
of bacterial microorganisms). Acute bacterial in-

fections and trauma stimulate neutrophil production, resulting in an increased WBC count. Often
when neutrophil production is stimulated, early,
immature forms of neutrophils enter the circulation. These immature forms are called *band,* or
stab, cells. This process, called a *shift to the left* in
WBC production, is indicative of an ongoing,
acute bacterial infection.

Lymphocytes are divided into two types:
thymus-derived cells (T cells) and bone marrow–
derived cells (B cells). T cells are primarily
involved with cellular-type immune reactions,

whereas B cells participate in humoral immunity (antibody production). The primary function of the lymphocytes is fighting chronic bacterial and acute viral infections.

Monocytes are phagocytic cells capable of fighting bacteria in a way similar to that of the neutrophil. However, they can be produced more rapidly and can spend a longer time in the circulation than the neutrophils.

Basophils, and especially eosinophils, are involved in the allergic reaction. Parasitic infestations also are capable of stimulating the production of these cells.

Platelets (Thrombocytes)

Platelets are formed in the bone marrow, the lungs, and, to some extent, the spleen. Platelets play a vital role in hemostasis and blood clotting. The pluripotent stem cell differentiates into a megakaryocyte. When this cell fragmentizes, platelets are formed and discharged into the circulation.

Physiologic hemostasis is an ongoing response to vascular injury to avoid excessive loss of blood. The process involves platelet aggregation around the site of the injury, thereby creating an early and temporary plug over the injury site. The presence of the platelets and thromboplastin activates serial clotting factors, resulting in fibrin production. The fibrin strengthens the platelet plug into a fibrin clot. Vascular repair is followed by a dissolution of the fibrin clot. This fibrin clot lysis is accomplished by the fibrinolytic (or plasmin) system (Figure 10-2).

Abnormalities in any part of this normal physiologic process can result in bleeding tendencies or hypercoagulable states. The balance of hemostasis and fibrinolysis must be maintained, otherwise bleeding tendencies or hypercoagulation results.

Hemostasis

Hemostasis (see Figure 10-2) is a multiphasic process that involves:

1. Platelet aggregation and plugging of the hole in the injured vessel

2. Fibrin formation to strengthen the platelet plug
3. Vessel repair and lysis of the fibrin clot (fibrinolysis)

Platelet aggregation, although quickly initiated, offers only transient interruption of active blood loss. The platelet aggregate (red clot) must be strengthened and supported by fibrin strands (white clot). Fibrin is the result of a process in which the clotting factors are sequentially activated by chemical enzymes. Two mechanisms are capable of producing fibrin. The first is the intrinsic system, which includes activation of factors XII, XI, IX, and VIII. Injury of the vessel surface is the stimulus for this system. Tissue damage, on the other hand, is capable of stimulating the extrinsic system of clot formation, which includes factors VII and III. Both the intrinsic and extrinsic systems activate the common pathway, which involves activation of factors X, V, II, and I (fibrinogen). Fibrin is the final result.

Fibrinolysis, through the action of plasmin (an activated form of plasminogen), is necessary to monitor and appropriately restrict the clotting system by dissolving fibrin clots after vascular repair.

Bleeding Time (Ivy Bleeding Time)

Test type Blood

Normal values
1-9 minutes (Ivy method)

Possible critical values >15 minutes on repeated evaluation

Rationale
The bleeding time test is used to evaluate the vascular and platelet factors associated with hemostasis. It frequently is performed on preoperative patients to ensure adequate hemostasis.

When vascular injury occurs, the first hemostatic response is a spastic contraction of the lacerated microvessels. Next, platelets adhere to the

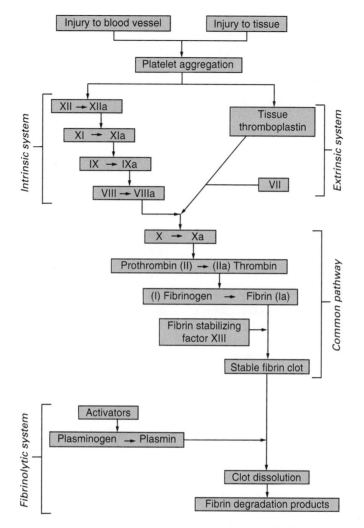

Figure 10-2 Process of hemostasis and fibrinolysis. Injury to a blood vessel surface or tissue initiates platelet aggregation. The intrinsic or extrinsic system is activated, subsequently activating the common pathway of fibrin formation. Finally, fibrin is physiologically dissolved by the fibrinolytic system.

wall of the vessel at the area of laceration in an attempt to plug the hole. Failure of either process results in a prolonged bleeding time.

For this study a small, standard, superficial incision is made in the forearm, and the time required for the bleeding to stop is recorded. This is called *the bleeding time.* Normal values vary according to the method used; the method most often used today is the Ivy bleeding time test. Be-

cause vessel constriction and platelet adherence are not affected by coagulation (intrinsic and extrinsic system), defects in this part of hemostasis will not affect the bleeding time. Therefore this test only evaluates platelet function and quantity and vascular constriction capability.

A single prolonged bleeding time does not prove that an abnormality exists. A larger vessel could potentially have been lacerated during the test, thereby prolonging the bleeding time, not because of a defect in hemostasis but because the caliber of the vessel is too large to stop bleeding without pressure. Because of this and the fact that test performance may vary among technicians, abnormal bleeding times should be repeated to ensure accuracy. Prolonged values occur in the following:

1. Patients with decreased platelet counts (see p. 431) or function
2. Patients with disseminated intravascular coagulation (DIC) resulting from consumption of platelets
3. Patients with uremia, because the platelets are reduced in number and function
4. Patients with warfarin (Coumadin, Panwarfin) overdosage
5. Patients with increased capillary fragility secondary to collagen vascular disease, Cushing's disease, or Henoch-Schönlein syndrome (purpura)
6. Patients ingesting antiinflammatory drugs (e.g., aspirin, indomethacin)

Potential complications

Potential complications associated with bleeding time tests are as follows:

■ Skin infection
■ Excessive bleeding from test site

Interfering factors

Factors that interfere with determining bleeding time values include the following:

■ Aggressively wiping the site of laceration, which can prolong the test results.
■ Extremes in body temperatures
  High temperatures can prolong results; low body temperatures can factitiously shorten results.
■ Drugs that may cause *increased* bleeding times include alcohol, anticoagulants, dextran, indomethacin, nonsteroidal antiinflammatory drugs (NSAIDs) salicylates, streptokinase, urokinase, and warfarin.

Procedure

The bleeding time test usually is performed at the patient's bedside. The skin of the inner forearm is cleansed with alcohol or povidone-iodine (Betadine). A blood pressure cuff (tourniquet) is placed on the arm above the elbow, inflated to 40 mm Hg, and maintained at this pressure during the study. A small laceration is then made 3 mm deep into the skin, and the time is recorded. Bleeding ensues, and the blood is blotted clean at 30-second intervals. When no new bleeding occurs, the time is again recorded. The time interval (from the beginning to the end of bleeding) is calculated and called *the bleeding time*. The blood pressure cuff is removed, and an adhesive bandage is applied to the patient's arm.

If the bleeding persists for more than 10 minutes, the test is stopped, and a pressure dressing is applied. If the patient has a factor deficiency, the bleeding time may be normal, but subsequent oozing of blood from the test site may occur 20 minutes after the original bleeding has stopped. Pressure should be applied to the wound. A minor amount of discomfort occurs with this test because of the skin laceration.

Contraindications

Contraindications for bleeding time tests are as follows:

■ Patients with known low platelet counts
■ Patients with a history of keloid formation
  They must be informed of the potential for scars.
■ Patients with senile skin changes
  Their capillaries are fragile, and vessel constriction is inadequate.

Nursing implications with rationale

Before

☞ Explain the procedure to the patient. Tell the patient that no fasting is necessary.

■ Assess the patient for aspirin ingestion or other NSAIDs, such as ibuprofen (Motrin), during the week preceding the test. These medications prolong bleeding time.

After

- If the patient is taking anticoagulants, indicate this on the laboratory requisition slip.
- Apply a dressing to the patient's forearm after the study. Assess the arm for subsequent bleeding. Apply a pressure dressing if oozing of blood is noted.

Blood Smear (Peripheral Blood Smear, Red Blood Cell Morphology, RBC Smear)

Test type Blood

Normal values
Normal quantity of RBCs, WBCs, and platelets
Normal size, shape, and color of RBCs
Normal WBC differential count

Rationale
Examination of the peripheral blood smear can provide information concerning drugs and diseases that affect RBCs and WBCs. Furthermore, other congenital and acquired diseases can be diagnosed by an examination of the peripheral blood smear. When special stains are applied to the blood smear, leukemia, infection, infestation, and other diseases can be identified.

When adequately prepared and examined microscopically by an experienced technologist and pathologist, a smear of peripheral blood is the most informative hematologic test. All three hematologic cell lines (erythrocytes [RBCs], platelets, and leukocytes [WBCs]) can be examined. In the peripheral blood, five different types of leukocytes can routinely be identified: neutrophils, eosinophils, basophils, lymphocytes, and monocytes. The first three also are referred to as *granulocytes.* See the discussion of complete blood count (CBC), page 412, for more information concerning the various elements of blood.

Microscopic examination of the RBCs can reveal variations in RBC size (anisocytosis), shape (poikilocytosis), color, or intracellular content. Classification of RBCs according to these variables is most helpful in identifying the causes of anemia and the presence of other diseases.

RBC size abnormalities
Microcytes (small RBCs)

Iron deficiency
Hereditary spherocytosis
Thalassemia

Macrocytes (large RBCs)

Vitamin B_{12} or folic acid deficiency
Reticulocytosis secondary to increased erythropoiesis (RBC production)
Occasional liver disorder
Postsplenectomy anemia

RBC shape abnormalities
Spherocytes (small and round RBCs)

Hereditary spherocytosis
Acquired immunohemolytic anemia

Elliptocytes (crescent- or sickle-shaped RBCs)

Hereditary elliptocytosis
Sickle cell anemia

Leptocytes, or "target cells" (thin cells with less Hgb)

Hemoglobinopathies
Thalassemia

Spicule cell (needlelike cell)

Uremia
Liver disease
Bleeding ulcer

RBC color abnormalities
Hypochromic (pale)

Iron deficiency
Thalassemia
Cardiac disease

Hyperchromatic (intensely colored)

Concentrated Hgb, usually caused by dehydration

RBC intracellular structure
Nucleus: In normal RBC maturation, the nucleus is lost. When increased RBC production is required (e.g., in anemia or chronic hypoxemia), the bone marrow floods the peripheral

blood with immature, nucleated forms of RBCs called *normoblasts.*

Basophilic stippling: This term refers to bodies enclosed or included in the cytoplasm of the RBCs. This often occurs with lead poisoning or reticulocytosis.

Howell-Jolly bodies: Small, round remnants of nuclear material remaining within the RBC. These occur after a surgical splenectomy or with hemolytic or megaloblastic anemia.

Heinz bodies: Small, irregular particles of Hgb. These occur with hemoglobinopathies or hemolytic anemia.

The WBCs are examined for total quantity, differential count, and degree of maturity. An increased number of immature WBCs may indicate leukemia. A decreased WBC count indicates failure of the bone marrow to produce WBCs, resulting from drugs, chronic disease, neoplasia, or fibrosis (see CBC, page 412). Finally, an experienced cell examiner also can estimate platelet number on a peripheral blood smear.

Procedure

This procedure is usually performed in the hematology department. The patient's finger is prepared with alcohol, and a fingerstick is performed. A drop of blood is spread on a slide; a second slide is used to smear the drop across the first slide. The slide is then colored with a polychromatic stain (usually Wright's or Giemsa) and examined under a microscope. The slide is prepared by a technician and should be examined by an experienced physician. The only discomfort associated with the study is that of the fingerstick. Often the blood can be taken from a CBC specimen.

Nursing implications with rationale

Before

☞ Explain the procedure to the patient. Tell the patient that no fasting is necessary.

■ Note that many laboratories prefer to have the patient sent to the hematology department for the fingerstick.

After

■ Apply pressure or a pressure dressing to the venipuncture site to prevent further bleeding. Observe the site for bleeding.

Blood Typing

Test type Blood

Normal values

Compatibility

Rationale

This test is used to determine the blood type of the patient before he or she donates or receives blood. This test also is used to determine the blood type of expectant mothers to determine the risks of Rh incompatibility between mother and newborn.

A description of the ABO system, rhesus (Rh) factors, and blood crossmatching is reviewed below.

ABO system

The two major antigens, A and B, form the basis of the ABO grouping system. The surface membrane of group A RBCs contain A antigens; group B RBCs contain B antigens; group AB RBCs have both A and B antigens; and group O RBCs have neither A nor B antigens. In general, a person will not have antibodies in their serum to match the surface antigens on their RBCs. That is, a person with group A antigens (type A) blood will not have anti-A antibodies. However, that person may have anti-B antibodies. The same is true for someone with group B antigens, who may have anti-A antibodies. Group O blood may have both anti-A and anti-B antibodies (Table 10-1).

Blood transfusions are actually transplantations of tissue (blood) from one person to another. The recipient must not have antibodies to the donor's RBCs, therefore, or a hypersensitivity reaction, which can vary from mild fever to anaphylaxis with severe intravascular hemolysis, could occur. If donor ABO antibodies are present against the recipient antigens, usually only minimal reactions occur, unless the recipient is immunocompromised.

Persons with group O blood are considered universal donors because they have no antigens on their RBCs that could cause an immunogenic reaction. People with group AB blood are consid-

TABLE 10-1	Blood Types		
Blood Type (ABO, Rh)	Antigens Present	Antibodies Possibly Present	Percent of General Population
O, +	Rh	A, B	35
O, −*	None	A, B, Rh	7
A, +	A, Rh	B	35
A, −	A	B, Rh	7
B, +	B, Rh	A	8
B, −	B	A, Rh	2
AB, +†	A, B, Rh	None	4
AB, −	A, B	Rh	2

*Universal donor.
†Universal recipient.

ered universal recipients because they have no antibodies that could react to the transfused blood. Group O blood is often transfused in emergency situations in which crossmatching is contraindicated because it requires approximately 20 minutes to complete and rapid, life-threatening blood loss requires an immediate transfusion. The chance of a transfusion reaction is least with type O blood.

Rh factors
The presence or absence of Rh antigens on the RBC's surface determines the classification of Rh positive (Rh+) or Rh negative (Rh−). After ABO compatibility, Rh factor is the next most important antigen associated with a blood transfusion. The major Rh factor is Rh_0 (D). There are several minor Rh factors. If Rh_0 (D) is absent, the minor Rh antigens are tested. If these are also absent, the patient is considered Rh negative.

Rh negative persons may develop antibodies to Rh antigens if exposed to Rh positive blood by prior transfusions or by fetal-maternal blood mixing. All pregnant women should have a blood typing and Rh factor determination. If the mother's blood is Rh negative, the father's blood also should be typed. If his blood is Rh positive, the woman's blood should be examined for the presence of Rh antibodies (see the Coombs' test, p. 420).

Blood crossmatching
Typing for the major ABO and Rh antigens does not guarantee that no reaction will occur, but it does greatly reduce the possibility of such a reaction. Many potential minor antigens are not routinely detected during blood typing. If unrecognized, these minor antigens also can initiate a blood transfusion reaction. Therefore, blood not only is typed but also crossmatched to identify a mismatch caused by minor antigens. Crossmatching involves mixing the recipient's serum with the donor's RBCs in saline solution followed by the addition of Coombs' serum (see Coombs' test, p. 420). Only blood products containing RBCs need to be crossmatched.

Homologous (recipient and donor are different people) and directed (recipient chooses the donor) blood donation must be rigorously tested before transfusion. Autologous (recipient and donor are the same person) blood transfusions, however, are not subject to that same testing. It is important to note, however, that autologous blood transfusion is not 100% safe. As a result of the additives used for blood banking purposes, blood and hypersensitivity reactions can still occur.

Interfering factors
Factors that can interfere with blood typing are non-ABO or non-Rh (D) minor antibodies, which can interfere with obtaining an adequate crossmatch.

Procedure
Usually 7 to 14 ml of peripheral venous blood is obtained in one or two red-top tubes and sent to the blood bank. The RBCs are diluted and suspended in saline solution divided into many quanta. Antisera A, B, and Rh_0 are each added to a quantum and mixed. The blood is typed by RBC agglutination in one or more of the antisera as listed in Table 10-2.

Next, crossmatching is performed by placing a small quantum of the patient's serum and a quantum of the proposed donor's blood in saline solution. The solution is assessed for agglutination.

TABLE 10-2	Blood Typing by RBC Agglutination
Agglutination in	**Blood Type**
A only	A−
B only	B−
A and B only	AB−
A and Rh$_O$ only	A+
B and Rh$_O$ only	B+
A, B, and Rh$_O$	AB+
None	O−
Rh$_O$ only	O+

The indirect Coombs' test (see p. 420) is then performed. If no agglutination occurs, the blood can be given safely with a minimal chance of an in vivo blood reaction. The type and crossmatch is done in the blood bank in approximately 45 minutes.

Nursing implications with rationale

Before

☞ Explain the procedure to the patient. Assess the patient for a previous allergic reaction to transfused blood products.

During

■ Collect the blood as indicated. Label the blood tubes appropriately with a stamped nameplate sticker. Label the blood requisition slips appropriately and deliver the blood specimens to the blood bank.

After

■ Apply pressure or a pressure dressing to the venipuncture site to prevent further bleeding. Observe the site for bleeding.

Bone Marrow Biopsy (Bone Marrow Examination, Bone Marrow Aspiration)

Test type Microscopic examination

Normal values

Active erythroid, myeloid, and lymphoid cell lines and megakaryocyte (platelet) production:

Cell Type	Range (%)
Myeloblasts	<5
Promyelocytes	1-8
Myelocytes	
Neutrophilic	5-15
Eosinophilic	0.5-3.0
Basophilic	<1
Metamyelocytes	
Neutrophilic	15-25
Eosinophilic	<1
Basophilic	<1
Mature myelocytes	
Neutrophilic	10-30
Eosinophilic	<5
Basophilic	<5
Mononuclear	
Monocytes	<5
Lymphocytes	3-20
Plasma cells	<1
Megakaryocytes	<5
Myeloid/erythroid (M/E) ratio	<4
Normoblasts	25-50

Normal iron content demonstrated by staining with Prussian blue

Rationale

Bone marrow examination is an important part of the evaluation of patients with hematologic diseases. Indications for bone marrow examination include the following:

1. To confirm the diagnosis of megaloblastic anemias
2. To diagnose leukemia or myeloma
3. To determine if the marrow is the cause of reduced blood cells in the peripheral bloodstream
4. To document deficient iron stores
5. To document bone marrow infiltrative diseases (neoplasm or fibrosis)
6. To stage lymphomas

The bone marrow is located in the central fatty core of cancellous bone (sternum, rib, and pelvis) and the long bones (femur, tibia, and humerus). There, the stem cells produce the blood cells and release them into the circulation.

By examination of a bone marrow specimen, the hematologist can fully evaluate hematopoiesis. Examination of the bone marrow reveals the number, size, and shape of the RBCs, WBCs, and megakaryocytes (platelet precursors) as these cells develop in the bone marrow. Samples of the bone marrow can be obtained by either aspiration or surgical removal. Microscopic examination includes estimation of cellularity, determination of the presence of fibrotic tissue or neoplasms (both primary and metastatic), and estimation of iron storage.

For the estimation of cellularity, the specimen is examined, and the relative quantity of each cell type is determined. Leukemias or leukemoid reactions (nonmalignant, extremely elevated levels of WBCs) are suspected when increased numbers of leukocyte precursors are present. Physiologic marrow WBC compensation for infection also will be recognized by finding an increased number of leukocyte precursors. Decreased numbers of marrow leukocyte precursors occur in patients with myelofibrosis, metastatic neoplasia, or agranulocytosis; in elderly patients; and following radiation therapy or chemotherapy.

Increased numbers of marrow RBC precursors occur with polycythemia vera or as physiologic compensation to greater O_2 demands or anemias. Decreased numbers of marrow RBC precursors occur with erythroid hypoplasia following chemotherapy, radiation therapy, administration of other toxic drugs, iron deficiency, or marrow replacement by fibrotic tissue or neoplasms.

Increased numbers of platelet precursors (megakaryocytes) are seen in the marrow of patients who are compensating after an episode of acute hemorrhage or decreased platelet survival. They also are seen in some forms of chronic myeloid leukemia. Decreased numbers of megakaryocytes occur in patients who have had radiation therapy, chemotherapy, or other drug therapy and in patients with neoplastic or fibrotic marrow infiltrative diseases. Patients with aplastic anemia also have decreased numbers of megakaryocytes.

Increased numbers of lymphocyte precursors occur in chronic, viral, or mycoplasmal infections (e.g., mononucleosis), lymphocytic leukemia, and lymphoma. Plasma cells (plasmocytes) are increased in patients with multiple myelomas, Hodgkin's disease, hypersensitivity states, rheu-

matic fever, and other chronic inflammatory diseases.

Estimation of cellularity also can be expressed as a ratio of myeloid (WBC) to erythroid (RBC) cells (M/E ratio). The normal M/E ratio is approximately 3:1. The M/E ratio is greater than normal in those diseases previously mentioned in which increased leukocyte precursors are present or erythroid precursors are decreased.

Myelofibrosis (fibrosis of the bone marrow) can be detected by examination of the bone marrow. Using special stains, one can estimate iron stores with a marrow biopsy. Although fibrosis or neoplasia occasionally can be detected in aspiration studies, biopsy is the best method. Leukemias, multiple myelomas, and polycythemia vera can easily be detected in biopsy specimens. Similarly, lymphomas and other metastatic tumors (e.g., cancers of the breast, kidney, and lung) can be seen. Bone marrow biopsy is an important part of staging for lymphomas and Hodgkin's disease.

Potential complications

Potential complications associated with bone marrow biopsy are as follows:

- Hemorrhage, especially if the patient has a coagulopathy
- Infection, especially if the patient is leukopenic
- Sternal fracture
  This can occur when too much pressure is applied to the sternum at the time of the biopsy.
- Inadvertent puncture of the heart or great vessels by the biopsy needle

Procedure

Bone marrow aspiration is performed on the sternum, iliac crest (Figure 10-3), anterior or posterior iliac spines, and proximal tibia (in children). The removal of specimens for bone marrow biopsy is done on the iliac spines or wherever tumor is suspected. Bone marrow aspiration is usually performed at the patient's bedside using a local anesthetic. The preferred site is the posterior iliac crest, with the patient placed in a prone or side-lying position. The area overlying the bone is prepared and draped in a sterile manner. The overlying skin and soft tissue, along with the periosteum, is infiltrated with lidocaine (Xylocaine). If aspiration is to be done, a large-bore (14-gauge) needle containing a stylus is slowly advanced through the soft tissues and into the outer table of the bone. Once inside the marrow, the stylus is removed, and a syringe is attached. A total of 0.5 to 2 ml of bone marrow is aspirated, smeared on slides, and allowed to dry. The slides are then sprayed with a preservative and taken to the pathology laboratory, where some of the slides are stained with Wright's stain and others with a supravital stain.

If bone marrow biopsy is to be performed, the skin and soft tissues overlying the bone are incised, and a core biopsy instrument is screwed into the bone. The biopsy specimen is obtained and sent to the pathology laboratory for analysis.

Aspiration is performed by a trained nurse or physician. Bone marrow biopsy specimen removal is performed only by a physician. The duration of either procedure is approximately 10 to 20 minutes. After the needle or core biopsy instrument is removed, pressure is applied to the site, and a sterile dressing is applied. The patient usually feels pain during the lidocaine infiltration and pressure when the syringe plunger is pulled back for aspiration. The patient may experience some apprehension when pressure is applied to the bone for outer table puncture during biopsy specimen removal or aspiration.

Contraindications

Contraindications for bone marrow biopsy are as follows:

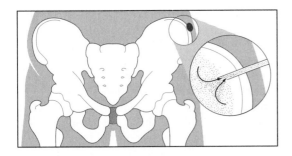

Figure 10-3 Aspiration of bone marrow.

- Patients with acute coagulation disorders, because of the risk of excessive bleeding
- Patients who cannot cooperate and remain still during the procedure

Nursing implications with rationale
Before
✏ Explain the procedure to the patient. Describe the purpose of the study. Encourage the patient to verbalize fears because many patients are anxious about this procedure.
- Verify that the physician has obtained written and informed consent before the study.
- Assess the coagulation studies performed on the patient before the study. Report any evidence of coagulopathy to the physician.
- Obtain an order for sedatives if the patient appears extremely apprehensive before the study.

During
- Assist the physician or nurse in obtaining the specimen. During the study remind the patient to remain very still. If the patient moves, the needle could accidentally puncture a vital organ.
- Label the slides appropriately with the patient's name, date, and room number.

After
- After the needle is removed, apply pressure to the puncture site to arrest the scant amount of bleeding from the puncture site. Apply an adhesive bandage. Ice packs may be used to help control bleeding. Uncontrolled hemorrhage can lead to hematoma formation, which can be very uncomfortable.
- Observe the puncture site for bleeding. Tenderness and erythema may indicate infection and should be reported to the physician.
- Assess the patient for signs of shock (increased pulse rate, decreased blood pressure) and pain. Normally, bed rest is prescribed for 30 to 60 minutes after the study. After that time, allow the patient to resume normal activity.
- Some patients complain of tenderness at the puncture site for several days after the study. Administer mild analgesics as ordered.

Coagulating Factors Concentration (Factor Assay, Coagulating Factors, Blood-Clotting Factors)

Test type Blood

Normal values

Factor	Normal Value (% of Normal)
II	80-120
V	50-150
VII	65-140
VIII	55-145
IX	60-140
X	45-155
XI	65-135
XII	50-150

Rationale

Coagulating factors concentration tests measure the quantity of each specific factor suspected to be responsible for defects in hemostasis. When these factors exist in concentrations below their minimal hemostatic level, clotting will be impaired.

The hemostasis and coagulation system normally functions in a homeostatic balance between factors encouraging clotting and factors encouraging clot dissolution. The coagulation mechanism is shown in Figure 10-2, p. 403. Factors were assigned Roman numerals based on the order in which they were identified, not by their functional order in the hemostatic mechanism. See Table 10-3 for a list of factor names and coagulation test abnormalities associated with factor deficiencies.

Deficiencies of these factors may be a result of inherited genetic defects, acquired diseases, or drug therapy. Common medical conditions associated with decreased factor concentrations are listed in Table 10-4. It is important to identify the exact factor or factors involved in the coagulating defect so that appropriate blood component replacement can be administered as listed in Table 10-5.

TABLE 10-3   Coagulation Factors

Factor	Name	Quantitation Available	Abnormal Coagulation Tests Associated with Deficiency
I	Fibrinogen	Yes	
II	Prothrombin	Yes	Prothrombin time
III	Tissue factor or thromboplastin	No	Prothrombin time
IV	Calcium	Yes	
V	Proaccelerin	Yes	Prothrombin time, activated partial thromboplastin time
VII	Stable factor	Yes	Prothrombin time
VIII	Antihemophilic factor	Yes	Activated partial thromboplastin time
IX	Christmas factor	Yes	Activated partial thromboplastin time
X	Stuart factor	Yes	Prothrombin time, activated partial thromboplastin time
XI	Plasma thromboplastin antecedent	Yes	Activated partial thromboplastin time
XII	Hageman factor	Yes	Activated partial thromboplastin time, whole-blood clotting
XIII	Fibrin-stabilizing factor	No	

TABLE 10-4	Conditions that May Result in Coagulation Factor Deficiency

Condition	Diminished Factors
Autoimmune disease	VIII
Congenital deficiency	I, II, V, VII, VIII, IX, X, XI, XII
Disseminated intravascular coagulation	I, V, VIII
Fibrinolysis	I, V, VIII
Heparin administration	II
Liver disease	I, II, V, VII, IX, X, XI
Vitamin K deficiency or maldigestion	II, VII, IX, X, XI
Warfarin ingestion	II, VII, IX, X, XI

TABLE 10-5	Minimum Concentration of Coagulation Factors Required for Adequate Fibrin Production

Factor	Minimal Hemostatic Level (mg/dl)	Blood Components*
I	60-100	C, FFP, FWB
II	10-15	P, WB, FFP, FWB
V	5-10	FFP, FWB
VII	5-20	P, WB, FFP, FWB
VIII	30	C, FFP, VIII CONC
IX	30	FFP, FWB
X	8-10	P, WB, FFP, FWB
XI	25	P, WB, FFP, FWB

*Blood components capable of providing specific factor: *C*, cryoprecipitate; *FFP*, fresh frozen plasma; *FWB*, fresh whole blood (<24 hours old); *P*, unfrozen banked plasma; *WB*, banked whole blood; *VIII CONC*, factor VIII concentrate.

Interfering factors

Factors that interfere with determining coagulating factors concentration include the following:

- Temperature
  Many of these proteins are heat sensitive, and their levels will be *decreased* the longer the specimen is kept at room temperature.
- Pregnancy or the use of contraceptive medication
  These situations can *increase* levels of several of these factors, especially VIII and IX, and a mild deficiency could be masked.
- Acute illness, stress, exercise, or inflammation
  Many of these protein coagulation factors are "acute reactant" proteins, and levels could be raised by these stressors.

Procedure

Peripheral venous blood (7 to 10 ml) is collected in a blue-top tube. The blood is then sent to the hematology laboratory for bioassay of the desired coagulation factor. The test results usually require 1 to 7 days to be reported, depending on whether the specimen has to be sent to a commercial laboratory or can be tested in the hospital.

Nursing implications with rationale

Before

- Explain the procedure to the patient. Tell the patient that no fasting is necessary.

After

- Apply pressure or a pressure dressing to the venipuncture site to prevent further bleeding. Observe the site for bleeding, especially if the patient has had other episodes of clotting deficiency.

COMPLETE BLOOD COUNT (CBC)

Red Blood Cell Count (RBC Count, Erythrocyte Count)

Red Blood Cell Indices (RBC Indices, MCV, MCH, MCHC, Blood Indices, Erythrocyte Indices, Red Blood Cell Distribution Width [RDW])

Hemoglobin (Hb, Hgb)

Hematocrit (Hct, Packed Red Blood Cell Volume, Packed Cell Volume [PCV])

White Blood Cell Count and Differential Count (WBC and Differential, Leukocyte Count, Neutrophil Count, Lymphocyte Count, Monocyte Count, Eosinophil Count, Basophil Count)

Test type Blood

Normal values
RBC count:

Adult/Elderly	(Million/mm³ or Million/UL)
Male	4.7-6.1
Female	4.2-5.4

Children	(Million/mm³ or Million/UL)
6-18 years	4.0-5.5
1-6 years	4.0-5.5
6 months-1 year	3.5-5.2
2-6 months	3.5-5.5
2-8 weeks	4.0-6.0
Newborn	4.8-7.1

RBC indices:
Mean corpuscular volume (MCV)
  Adult/elderly/child: 80-95 mm³
  Newborn: 96-108 mm³
Mean corpuscular hemoglobin (MCH)
  Adult/elderly/child: 27-31 pg
  Newborn: 32-34 pg
Mean corpuscular hemoglobin concentration (MCHC)
  Adult/elderly/child: 32-36 g/dl
    (or 32% to 36%)
  Newborn: 32-33 g/dl (or 32% to 33%)
Red blood cell distribution (RDW)
  Adult: variation = 11% to 14.5%
Hgb:
Elderly: values are slightly decreased
Male: 14-18 g/dl or 8.7-11.2 mmol/L (SI units)
Female: 12-16 g/dl or 7.4-9.9 mmol/L (SI units)
Pregnant female: >11 g/dl

Children:
  16-18 years: 10.0-15.5 g/dl
  1-6 years: 9.5-14.0 g/dl
  6 months-1 year: 9.5-14.0 g/dl
  2-6 months: 10-17 g/dl
  0-2 weeks: 12-20 g/dl
  Newborn: 14-24 g/dl
Hct:
Elderly: values may be slightly decreased
Male: 42%-52% or 0.42-0.52 volume fraction
  (SI units)
Female: 37%-47% or 0.37-0.47 volume fraction
  (SI units)
Pregnant female: >33%
Children (%):
  6-18 years: 32-44
  1-6 years: 30-40
  6 months-1 year: 29-43
  2-6 months: 35-50
  2-8 weeks: 39-59
  Newborn: 44 to 64
WBC and differential:
Total WBCs:
  Adult/child >2 years: 5000-10,000/mm³ or
    5-10 10⁹/L (SI units)
  Child <2 years: 6200-17,000/mm³
  Newborn: 9000-30,000/mm³
Differential count

Cell Type	(%)	Absolute (per mm³)
Neutrophils	55-70	2500-8000
Lymphocytes	20-40	1000-4000
Monocytes	2-8	100-700
Eosinophils	1-4	50-500
Basophils	0.5-1.0	25-100

Possible critical values
Hgb: <5.0 g/dl or >20 g/dl
Hct: <15% or >60%
WBCs: <2500 or >30,000/mm³

Rationale
The CBC and differential count are a series of tests of the peripheral blood that provide a tremendous amount of information about the hematologic system and many other organ systems. They are inexpensively, easily, and rapidly performed as a

screening test on almost every patient who enters the hospital. Each test included in the series is discussed below.

RBC count

This test is a count of the number of circulating RBCs in 1 mm^3 of peripheral venous blood. Within each RBC are molecules of Hgb, which permit the transport and exchange of O_2 to and CO_2 from the tissues. RBCs are produced by the erythroid elements in the bone marrow. Under the stimulation of erythropoietin, RBC production is increased. Normally, RBCs survive in the peripheral blood for approximately 120 days. During that time, the RBC is transported through the bloodstream. In the smallest of capillaries, the RBC must fold and bend to conform to the size of these tiny vessels. Toward the end of the RBC's life, the cell membrane becomes less pliable and the aged RBC is lysed and extracted from the circulation by the spleen. Abnormal RBCs have a shorter life span and are extracted earlier (see RBC survival studies p. 436). Intravascular RBC trauma (e.g., that caused by artificial heart valves or peripheral vascular atherosclerotic plaques) also shortens the RBC's life. An enlarged spleen (e.g., that caused by portal hypertension or leukemia) may inappropriately destroy and remove normal RBCs from the circulation.

When the RBC value is decreased by more than 10% of the expected normal value, the patient is said to be anemic. Low RBC values are caused by many factors, including:

1. Hemorrhage (as in gastrointestinal [GI] bleeding or trauma)
2. Hemolysis (as in glucose-6-phosphate dehydrogenase [G6PD] deficiency, spherocytosis, or secondary splenomegaly)
3. Dietary deficiency (as of iron or vitamin B_{12})
4. Genetic aberrations (as in sickle cell anemia or thalassemia)
5. Drug ingestion (as of chloramphenicol, hydantoins, or quinidine)
6. Marrow failure (as in fibrosis, leukemia, or antineoplastic chemotherapy)

7. Chronic illness (as in tumor or sepsis)
8. Other organ failure (as in renal disease)

RBC counts greater than normal can be physiologically induced as a result of the body's requirements for greater oxygen-carrying capacity (e.g., at high altitudes). Diseases that produce chronic hypoxia (e.g., congenital heart disease) also provoke this physiologic increase in RBCs. Polycythemia vera is a neoplastic condition involving uncontrolled production of RBCs.

Like the Hgb and Hct values, the RBC count can be altered by many factors other than RBC production. For instance, in dehydrated patients the total blood volume is decreased. The RBCs will be more concentrated, and the RBC count will be falsely high. Likewise, in overhydrated patients the RBCs are diluted, and the RBC count/mm^3 will be falsely low.

RBC indices

When investigating anemia, it is helpful to categorize the anemia according to the RBC indices, as shown in Box 10-1. Cell size is indicated by the terms *normocytic, microcytic,* and *macrocytic.* Hgb content is indicated by the terms *normochromic, hypochromic,* and *hyperchromic.* Additional information about RBC size, shape, color, and intracellular structure is described in the blood smear study (see p. 405). Normal values for all the RBC indices vary considerably. Each laboratory must develop its own normal values indices.

MCV The MCV is a measure of the average volume, or size, of a single RBC and is used in classifying anemias. When the MCV value is increased, the RBC is said to be abnormally large, or macrocytic. This is most frequently seen in megaloblastic anemias (e.g., vitamin B_{12} or folic acid deficiency). When the MCV value is decreased, the RBC is said to be abnormally small, or microcytic. This is associated with iron deficiency anemia or thalassemia.

MCH The MCH is a measure of the average amount (weight) of Hgb within an RBC. Because macrocytic cells generally have more Hgb and microcytic cells have less Hgb, the causes for these values are similar to those for the MCV value. The

Box 10-1	*Categorization of Anemia According to RBC Indices*

Normocytic,[1] Normochromic[2] Anemia

Acquired hemolytic anemias (e.g., from a prosthetic cardiac valve)
Acute blood loss
Aplastic anemia (e.g., chloramphenicol toxicosis)
Chronic illness (e.g., sepsis, tumor)
Iron deficiency (detected early)

Microcytic,[3] Hypochromic[4] Anemia

Iron deficiency (detected late)
Lead poisoning
Thalassemia

Microcytic, Normochromic Anemia

Renal disease (because of the loss of erythropoietin)

Macrocytic,[5] Normochromic Anemia

Chemotherapy
Hydantoin ingestion
Vitamin B_{12} or folic acid deficiency

[1]Normal RBC size.
[2]Normal color (normal hemoglobin content).
[3]Smaller than normal RBC size.
[4]Less than normal color (decreased hemoglobin content).
[5]Larger than normal RBC size.

MCH adds very little information to the other indices.

MCHC The MCHC is a measure of the average concentration or percentage of Hgb within a single RBC. When values are decreased, the cell has a deficiency of Hgb and is said to be hypochromic (frequently seen in iron deficiency anemia and thalassemia). When values are normal, the anemia is said to be normocytic (e.g., hemolytic anemia). RBCs cannot be considered hyperchromic.

RDW The RDW is an indication of the variation in RBC size. It is calculated by a machine that generates a histogram using the MCV and RBC values. Variations in the width of the RBCs may be helpful when classifying certain types of anemia.

The RDW is essentially an indicator of the degree of anisocytosis, a blood condition characterized by RBCs of variable and abnormal size.

Normally, RBCs are approximately the same size, showing little variation. This characteristic is represented on the histogram as a single narrowed peak. Certain diseases change the size of some of the RBCs, with less abnormal RBCs being less affected. For example, with folic acid deficiency or iron deficiency, newer RBCs are more significantly affected than older cells and therefore the size of the newer cells will differ significantly from that of the older cells. This is represented on the histogram as multiple peaks, indicating many cells of various sizes.

Hgb

The Hgb concentration is a measure of the total amount of Hgb in the peripheral blood. Hgb serves as a vehicle for O_2 and CO_2 transport. The oxygen-carrying capacity of the blood is determined by the Hgb concentration. Hgb also acts as an important acid/base buffer system.

As with the RBC count, normal Hgb values vary according to gender and age. Women tend to have lower values than do men, and values tend to decrease with age. Hgb values closely reflect the Hct and RBC values. The Hct in percentage points usually is approximately three times the Hgb concentration in grams per deciliter when RBCs are of normal size and contain normal amounts of Hgb.

Abnormal Hgb values indicate the same pathologic states as do abnormal RBC counts and Hct concentrations. Decreased levels indicate anemia (reduced number of RBCs). Increased levels can indicate erythrocytosis. In addition, however, plasma volume changes are more accurately reflected by the Hgb concentration. Dilutional overhydration decreases the concentration, whereas dehydration tends to cause an artificially high value. Slight decreases in the values of Hgb and Hct during pregnancy are a result of expanded blood volume caused by chronic overhydration. Hgb usually is measured by an automated cell counter. There is very little variability (2% to 3%) among most well-maintained machines.

Hgb is composed of heme (iron surrounded by protoporphyrin) and globin, which consists of an alpha and beta polypeptide chain. Abnormalities in the globin structure are called *hemoglobinopathies* (e.g., sickle cell disease, Hgb C disease). Some diseases are caused by abnormalities in globin-chain synthesis (e.g., thalassemia). In these diseases, RBC counts can be low, RBC survival diminished, and RBC-carrying capacity reduced.

Too little Hgb puts a strain on the cardiopulmonary system to maintain good oxygen-carrying capacity. With critically low Hgb levels, patients are at great risk for angina, heart attack, congestive heart failure, and stroke. When Hgb levels are too high because of increased numbers of RBCs, intravascular sludging occurs, leading to stroke and other organ infarction. Decisions concerning the need for blood transfusion are usually based on the Hgb level or the Hct. In an otherwise healthy person, transfusion is not considered if the Hgb level is above 8 g/dl or the Hct is above 24. In younger people, who can safely and significantly increase their cardiac output, a Hgb level of 6 g/dl may be acceptable. The Hgb level can be expected to rise 1 gram for every unit of packed RBCs that is transfused.

Hct

The Hct is an indirect measurement of the RBC number and volume. It is used as a rapid measurement of RBC count and is expressed as the percentage of the total blood volume that consists of RBCs. The height of the RBC column is measured after centrifugation. It is compared with the height of the column of the total whole blood. The ratio of the RBC column height compared with the total blood column height is multiplied by 100%, resulting in the Hct value. The Hct closely reflects the Hgb and RBC values, as described in the previous section.

WBC

The WBC count comprises two components. The first is a count of the total number of WBCs (leukocytes) in 1 mm³ of peripheral venous blood. The second is the differential count, which measures the percentage of each type of leukocyte

present in the same specimen. An increase in the percentage of one type of leukocyte means a decrease in the percentage of another. Neutrophils and lymphocytes compose 75% to 90% of the total number of leukocytes. These leukocyte types may be identified easily by their morphology (see Figure 10-1, p. 401) on a peripheral blood smear (see p. 405) or by automated counters. An increased total WBC count (leukocytosis: WBC > 10,000) usually indicates infection, inflammation, tissue necrosis, or leukemic neoplasia. Trauma or stress, either emotional or physical, may increase the WBC count. In some instances of infection, especially sepsis, the WBC count may be extremely high, similar to the levels associated with leukemia. This is called a *leukemoid reaction* and quickly resolves as the infection is successfully treated.

A decreased total WBC count (leukopenia: WBC < 4000) occurs in many forms of bone marrow failure (e.g., following antineoplastic chemotherapy or radiation therapy, marrow infiltrative diseases, overwhelming infections, dietary deficiencies, and autoimmune diseases).

The major functions of the WBCs are to fight infection and react against foreign bodies or tissues. Five types of WBCs may be identified easily on a routine blood smear. These cells, in order of descending frequency, include neutrophils, lymphocytes, monocytes, eosinophils, and basophils. These WBCs arise from the same pluripotent stem cells within the bone marrow as do the RBCs. Beyond this shared origin, however, each cell line differentiates separately. Most mature WBCs are then deposited into the circulating blood.

WBCs are divided into granulocytes and nongranulocytes. Granulocytes have granules visible in their cytoplasm when stained and examined on a routine smear. Granulocytes include neutrophils, basophils, and eosinophils. Granulocytes have multilobed nuclei and are sometimes referred to as *polymorphonuclear leukocytes (PMNs or "polys")*.

Neutrophils are the most common PMNs. They are produced in 7 to 14 days and exist in the circulation for only 6 hours. The primary function of the neutrophil is phagocytosis (killing and digestion of bacterial microorganisms). Acute bacterial infections and trauma stimulate neutrophil production, resulting in an increased WBC count. Often, when neutrophil production is significantly stimulated, early, immature forms of neutrophils enter the circulation. These immature forms are called *band,* or *stab, cells.* This occurrence is referred to as a *shift to the left* in WBC production and is indicative of an ongoing, acute bacterial infection.

Basophils (also called *mast cells*), and especially *eosinophils,* are involved in the allergic reaction. They are capable of phagocytosis of antigen-antibody complexes. As the allergic response diminishes, the eosinophil count decreases. These cells infiltrate the tissue involved in the allergic reaction (e.g., hives, in the skin) and promote the inflammatory reaction. Parasitic infestations also are capable of stimulating the production of these cells.

Nongranulocytes (agranulocytes) include lymphocytes and monocytes (the count also includes histiocytes). They have no cytoplasmic granules and possess small, single, rounded nuclei. *Lymphocytes* are divided into two types: T cells (mature in the thymus) and B cells (mature in the bone marrow). T cells are primarily involved with cellular-type immune reactions, whereas B cells participate in humoral immunity (antibody production). The T cells are the killer cells, suppressor cells, and the T4 helper cells (see lymphocyte immunophenotyping, p. 483). *Monocytes* are phagocytic cells capable of fighting bacteria in a way similar to that of the neutrophil. Through phagocytosis, they remove necrotic debris and microorganisms from the blood. The monocytes produce interferon, which is the body's endogenous immunostimulant.

The WBC and differential count are routinely measured as part of the CBC. Serial WBC and differential counts have both diagnostic and prognostic value. For example, a persistent increase in the WBC count may indicate a worsening of an infection (e.g., appendicitis). A reduction of an elevated WBC to normal range indicates resolution of an infection. A dramatic decrease in the WBC count below the normal range may indicate marrow failure. In patients receiving chemotherapy, a reduced WBC may be a contraindication to further chemotherapy.

Interfering factors

Factors that interfere with determining CBC values include the following:

- Normal decreases in the RBCs during pregnancy
  This *decreased* value is due to normal body fluid increases, which dilute the RBCs. Also, the nutritional deficiency often associated with pregnancy may play a role in the anemia of pregnancy.
- Living in high altitudes
  This causes *increased* RBC, Hgb, and Hct values as a result of a physiologic response to the decreased O_2 available at these high altitudes.
- Extremely elevated WBC counts (>50,000)
  These may *increase* the MCV and MCH indices when performed by automated counters.
- Large RBC precursors (e.g., reticulocytes [see p. 437])
  These can cause an abnormally *increased* MCV value and commonly occur in response to anemias in which the bone marrow is not pathologic.
- The presence of cold agglutinins, which can falsely *elevate* MCHC, MCH, and MCV
- Abnormalities in RBC size may alter Hct values
  Larger RBCs are associated with *increased* Hct levels because the larger RBCs take up a greater percentage of the total blood volume.
- Blood fluid volume
  Hbg and Hct values may not be reliable immediately after hemorrhage because the percentage of total blood volume taken up by the RBCs has not changed. Not until the total blood volume is replaced with fluids will the Hct decrease.
- Postsplenectomy
  These patients have a persistent, mild to moderate *elevation* of WBC counts.
- Time of day
  WBCs tend to be decreased in the morning and *increased* in the late afternoon.
- Age
  The WBC count tends to be age-related. Newborns and infants normally have higher levels

of WBCs than do adults. It is common for the elderly to experience diminished leukocytosis, even in the face of a severe bacterial infection.

Procedure

A peripheral venipuncture using at least a 20-gauge needle to prevent hemolysis is performed, and 5 to 7 ml of blood is collected in a lavender-top tube containing ethylenediamine tetraacetic acid (EDTA), an anticoagulant. The tube is tilted up and down several times to ensure adequate mixture of the EDTA with the blood. The specimen is then sent to the hematology laboratory for analysis.

The only discomfort associated with this study is that of the peripheral venipuncture. Finger sticks may be performed for some of these tests.

Most modern clinical hospital laboratories have a machine that automatically measures the WBC, RBC, Hgb, MCV, and MCHC and calculates the Hct and MCH values. With some reliability, a machine can provide a WBC differential. The dif-

ferential count alternatively may be performed by a technician, who examines a cubic millimeter of a blood smear under a microscope. Each type of WBC is counted, and the percentages are recorded.

Nursing implications with rationale

Before

☞ Explain the procedure to the patient. Tell the patient that no fasting is necessary. If serial determinations are necessary, explain the rationale.

During

■ Obtain the specimen and immediately transfer the blood to the appropriate container. Thoroughly mix the blood with the anticoagulant by tilting the tube.

After

■ Apply pressure or a pressure dressing to the venipuncture site to prevent further bleeding. Observe the site for bleeding.

Case Study

Iron Deficiency Anemia

Mr. R.S., 72 years old, developed chest pain whenever he was physically active. The pain ceased on stopping his activity. He has no history of heart or lung disease. His physical examination was normal except for notable pallor.

Studies	Result
Electrocardiogram (EKG), p. 34	Ischemia noted in anterior leads
Chest x-ray study, p. 155	No active disease
CBC, p 412	
RBC count	2.1 million/mm (normal: 4.7-6.1 million/mm)
RBC indices	
MCV	72 mm^3 (normal: 80-95 mm^3)
MCH	22 pg (normal: 27-31 pg)
MCHC	21 pg (normal: 27-31 pg)
RDW	9% (normal: 11%-14.5%)
Hgb	5.4 g/dl (normal: 14-18 g/dl)
Hct	18% (normal: 42%-52%)
WBC count	7800/mm^3 (normal: 5000-10,000/mm^3)
Differential count	Normal differential

Platelet count (thrombocyte count)	*Within normal limits (WNL)* *(normal: 150,000-400,000/mm³)*
RBC survival study, p. 436	
Half-life of RBC	26-30 days (normal value)
Spleen/liver ratio	1:1 (normal value)
Spleen/pericardium ratio	<2:1 (normal value)
Reticulocyte count, p. 437	3.0% (normal: 0.5% to 2.0%)
Haptoglobin, p. 423	122 mg/dl (normal: 100-150 mg/dl)
Blood typing, p. 406	O positive
Iron level studies, p. 425	
Iron	42 (normal: 65-175 µg/dl)
Total iron-binding capacity (TIBC)	500 (normal: 250-420 µg/dl)
Transferrin (siderophilin)	200 (normal: 215-365 mg/dl)
Transferrin saturation	15% (normal: 20%-50%)
Ferritin	8 ng/ml (normal: 12-300 ng/ml)
B_{12}, p. 441	140 pg/ml (normal: 100-700 pg/ml)
Folic acid, p. 441	12 mg/ml (normal: 5-20 mg/ml or 14-34 mmol/L)

Diagnostic Analysis

Mr. R.S. was found to be significantly anemic. His angina was related to his anemia. His normal RBC survival studies and normal haptoglobin eliminated the possibility of hemolysis. His B_{12} and folate levels eliminated the possibility of vitamin deficiencies. His RBCs were small and hypochromic. His iron studies were compatible with iron deficiency. His marrow was inadequate for the degree of anemia because his iron level was reduced.

On transfusion of O-positive blood, his angina disappeared. While receiving his third unit of packed RBCs, he developed an elevated temperature to 38.5° C, muscle aches, and back pain. The transfusion was stopped, and the following studies were performed.

Studies	Results
Hgb	7.6 g/dl
Hct	24%
Direct Coombs' test	Positive; agglutination (normal: negative)
Platelet count	85,000/mm³
Platelet antibody	Positive (normal: negative)
Haptoglobin	78 mg/dl

Diagnostic Analysis

Mr. R.S. was experiencing a blood transfusion incompatibility reaction. His direct Coombs' test and haptoglobin studies indicated some hemolysis as a result of the reaction. His platelet count dropped because of antiplatelet antibodies, probably the same ABO antibodies that caused the RBC reaction.

Continued

Iron Deficiency Anemia–cont'd

He was given iron orally over the next 3 weeks, and his Hgb level improved. A rectal examination indicated that his stool was positive for occult blood. Colonoscopy indicated a right colon cancer, which was removed 4 weeks after his initial presentation. He tolerated the surgery well.

Critical Thinking Questions
1. What was the cause of Mr. R.S.'s iron deficiency anemia?
2. Explain the relationship between anemia and angina.

Coombs' Test, Direct (Direct Antiglobulin Test)

Coombs' Test, Indirect (Indirect Antiglobulin Test, Blood Antibody Screening)

Test type Blood

Normal values

Negative; no agglutination

Rationale

Direct Coombs' test: This test is performed to identify hemolysis (lysis of RBCs) or investigate hemolytic transfusion reactions. Most of the antibodies to RBCs are directed against the ABO/Rh blood grouping antigens, such as that which occurs in hemolytic anemia of the newborn (erythroblastosis fetalis) or blood transfusion reaction. When blood incompatibility occurs, the direct Coombs' test can detect the patient's antibodies coating the foreign RBCs.

Some drugs can cause nonblood-grouping antigens to develop on the RBC membrane and stimulate formation of antibodies. Also, in some diseases, antibodies not originally directed against the patient's RBCs can attach to the RBCs and cause hemolysis, which can be detected by the direct Coomb's test. Frequently, the production of these autoantibodies against RBCs is not associated with any identifiable disease, and the resulting hemolytic anemia is, therefore, called *idiopathic anemia.*

Indirect Coombs' test: This test is used to detect circulating antibodies against RBCs in the serum and is used most commonly for screening potential blood recipients. The major purpose of this test is to determine if the patient has minor serum antibodies (other than the major ABO/Rh system) to RBCs that he or she is about to receive by transfusion. Therefore this test is the screening portion of the "type and screen" routinely performed for blood compatibility testing (crossmatching in the blood bank). This test also is used to detect other agglutinins (e.g., cold agglutinins associated with mycoplasmal infections). Circulating antibodies against RBCs also may occur in an Rh-negative pregnant woman who is carrying an Rh-positive fetus.

If antibodies exist in the patient's serum, agglutination of the RBCs intended to be transfused occurs. In blood transfusion screening, visible agglutination indicates that the recipient has antibodies to the donor's RBCs. If the recipient has no antibodies against the donor's RBCs, agglutination will not occur; transfusion should then proceed safely and without any transfusion reaction.

Procedure

Direct Coombs' test: Coombs' serum is produced by injecting human serum antibodies into a rabbit, which then makes antibodies to the human serum antibodies. The rabbit's serum contains antibodies against human serum (Coombs' serum). Approximately 5 to 7 ml of the patient's blood is collected in a red-top tube and transported to the blood bank. (Venous blood from the umbilical cord is used to detect the presence of antibodies in the newborn.) The patient's RBCs are mixed with the Coombs' serum. Agglutination indicates a positive test, and the patient is said to have an autogenous production of antibodies against RBCs that causes RBC hemolysis. No agglutination indicates a negative study.

Indirect Coombs' test: Seven milliliters of peripheral venous blood is obtained from the proposed recipient in a red-top tube (without an anticoagulant) and transported to the blood bank. The proposed recipient's serum is mixed with the donor's RBCs, and Coombs' serum is subsequently added. Agglutination, or clumping, indicates a positive test. The degree of agglutination is an indication of the quantity of antibodies against RBCs present in the recipient's serum. Positive results vary from trace to +4. No agglutination indicates a negative result.

No food or fluid restrictions are associated with either test.

Nursing implications with rationale

Before

☞ Explain the procedure to the patient. Tell the patient that no fasting is necessary.

During

■ Obtain the blood specimen as ordered. Verify that the blood specimen is correctly labeled with a stamped patient nameplate sticker.

After

■ Transport the blood specimen to the laboratory as soon as possible.

■ Apply pressure or a pressure dressing to the venipuncture site to prevent further bleeding. Observe the site for bleeding.

Disseminated Intravascular Coagulation Screening (DIC Screening)

Test type Blood

Normal values
No evidence of DIC

Rationale

Disseminated intravascular coagulation (DIC) screening tests are indicated for patients suspected to have DIC (demonstrate a coagulopathy). Many pathologic conditions can instigate or are associated with DIC. The more common ones include bacterial sepsis, amniotic fluid embolism, retention of a dead fetus, malignant neoplasia, liver cirrhosis, extensive surgery (especially on the prostate or liver), postextracorporeal heart bypass, extensive trauma, severe burns, and transfusion reactions.

In DIC, the entire clotting mechanism is triggered inappropriately (Figure 10-4), resulting in significant systemic or localized intravascular formation of fibrin clots. This futile clotting results in intravascular slugging and excessive bleeding from consumption of the platelets and clotting factors used in intravascular clotting. The fibrinolytic system also is activated to break down the clot formation and the fibrin involved in the intravascular coagulation. This fibrinolysis results in the formation of fibrin degradation products (FDPs), which, by themselves, act as anticoagulants; these FDPs only serve to enhance the bleeding tendency.

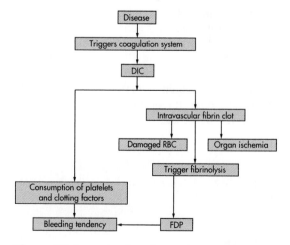

Figure 10-4 Pathophysiology of disseminated intravascular coagulation *(DIC)*, which may result in bleeding tendency, organ ischemia, and hemolytic anemia. *FDP*, Fibrin degradation product; *RBC*, red blood cell.

		Reference
Test	**Result**	**Page**
Bleeding time	Prolonged	402
Coagulation factors	I, II, V, VIII, X, XIII decreased	411
D-dimer	Increased	
Euglobulin lysis time	Normal or prolonged	
Fibrin degradation products	Increased	422
Partial thromboplastin time	Prolonged	427
Platelet count	Decreased	431
Prothrombin time	Prolonged	434
Red blood smear	Damaged RBC	405
Thrombin time	Prolonged	

TABLE 10-6 DIC Blood Tests

Organ injury can occur as a result of the intravascular clots, which cause microvascular occlusion in various organs. This may cause serious anoxic injury in affected organs. Also, RBCs passing through partly plugged vessels are injured and subsequently hemolyzed.

When a patient with a bleeding tendency is suspected to have DIC, a series of routine laboratory tests are done (prothrombin time [PT], partial thromboplastin time [PTT], bleeding time, and platelet count). If the results are abnormal, further testing should be performed (Table 10-6). With these tests, the hematologist can make the appropriate diagnosis.

Fibrin Degradation Products (FDPs, Fibrin Split Products [FSPs], Fibrin Breakdown Products)

Test type Blood

Normal values
<10 mg/ml or dilution <1:4

Possible critical values >40 mg/ml

Rationale
Measurement of fibrin degradation products (FDPs) provides a direct indication of the activity of the fibrinolytic (clot dissolution) system. The fibrinolytic system is an important part of the balance that exists between clot formation and clot dissolution. Clot formation stimulates the three major activators of the fibrinolytic system. When the fibrin clot breaks up, fragments called *FDPs* (X, D, E, and Y) are formed. If present in increased quantities, FDPs can have an anticoagulant effect.

When present in large amounts, FDPs indicate increased fibrinolysis, as occurs in DIC and other secondary fibrinolytic disorders. This test is one of the DIC screening tests. FDPs are also present in thrombotic (clot-forming) states (e.g., venous thrombosis) in which the thrombosis stimulates activation of the fibrinolytic system. Other diseases can potentially cause activation of the fibrinolytic system and elevate FDP levels. These may include extensive malignancy, tissue necrosis, and gram-negative sepsis. Thrombolytic therapy used, for example, in myocardial infarction also is associated with increased FDPs. Streptokinase or urokinase stimulates clot dissolution, and FDPs are formed, as previously discussed.

Procedure
Peripheral venous blood (usually 2 ml) is collected in a blue-top tube and immediately taken on ice to the hematology laboratory. Avoid excessive agitation of the blood sample.

Nursing implications with rationale
Before
☞ Explain the procedure to the patient. Tell the patient that no fasting is necessary.
After
■ Apply pressure or a pressure dressing to the venipuncture site to prevent further bleeding. Observe the site for bleeding, especially if the patient has had other episodes of clotting deficiency.

Glucose-6-Phosphate Dehydrogenase (G6PD Screen)

Test type Blood

Normal values

Negative (screening test) or 8.0-8.6 U/g of Hgb

Rationale

This test is used to identify G6PD deficiency in patients who have developed hemolysis because of exposure to oxidizing agents. Glucose-6-phosphate dehydrogenase (G6PD) is an enzyme used in glucose metabolism. In the RBC, a G6PD deficiency causes precipitation of Hgb and cellular membrane changes. This may result in hemolysis of variable severity. This disease is caused by a sex-linked, recessive trait carried on the X chromosome. The full effect of this genetic defect is not seen if the normal gene is present on a second X chromosome, which opposes the genetic defect. In males, because there is no second X chromosome, the genetic defect is unopposed. Women who are carriers of the gene have variable disease severity. In the United States, G6PD is found mainly in blacks.

In patients with G6PD deficiency, oxidizing drugs can cause RBC destruction and hemolysis. Susceptible persons do not experience hemolysis before exposure to the oxidizing drugs. After the oxidizing drug is administered, however, hemolysis can begin as early as the first day of exposure and usually by the fourth day. The most common oxidizing drugs known to precipitate hemolysis and anemia in G6PD are antimalarials, sulfonamides, nitrofurantoins, aspirin, and phenacetin. Infections or acidosis can also precipitate a hemolytic process in these patients. Certain foods (e.g., fava beans) are oxidizing and are, therefore, harmful to the G6PD-deficient patient.

Procedure

No food or fluid restrictions are associated with this test. Venipuncture is performed according to the laboratory guidelines.

Nursing implications with rationale

Before

☞ Explain the procedure to the patient. Tell the patient that no fasting is necessary.

After

■ Apply pressure or a pressure dressing to the venipuncture site to prevent further bleeding. Observe the site for bleeding, especially if the patient has had other episodes of clotting deficiency.

☞ If the test indicates that a lack of G6PD exists, give the patient a list of drugs that can precipitate hemolysis. Fava beans should not be eaten by patients with the Mediterranean variant of this disease. Teach the patient to read the labels on any over-the-counter drugs for the presence of products (e.g., aspirin and phenacetin) that may cause hemolytic anemia.

Haptoglobin

Test type Blood

Normal values

Adult: 100-150 mg/dl or 16-31 mmol/L (SI units)
Newborn: 0-10 mg/dl

Possible critical values <40 mg/dl

Rationale

The serum haptoglobin test is used to detect intravascular hemolysis of RBCs. Haptoglobins are powerful, free, hemoglobin-binding glycoproteins produced by the liver. In hemolytic anemias the released Hgb is quickly bound to haptoglobin, and the new complex is quickly catabolized, resulting in a diminished amount of free haptoglobin in the serum. This decrease cannot be quickly compensated for by normal liver production. As a result, the patient demonstrates a transient, reduced level of haptoglobin in the serum.

Haptoglobins also are decreased in patients with primary liver disease not associated with hemolytic anemias. This occurs because the diseased liver is unable to produce these glycoproteins. Hematoma can reduce haptoglobin levels by absorbing Hgb into the blood and binding with haptoglobin.

Elevated haptoglobin concentrations are found in many inflammatory diseases and, therefore, can be used as a nonspecific, acute-phase, protein in much the same way as a sedimentation rate test (see p. 476).

Procedure

At least 2 ml of peripheral venous blood is collected from the nonfasting patient in a red-top tube (containing no anticoagulant). The blood is sent to the chemistry laboratory for analysis.

Interfering factor

A factor that interferes with determining haptoglobin levels is ongoing infection, which can *increase* test results.

Nursing implications with rationale

Before

☞ Explain the procedure to the patient. Tell the patient that no fasting is necessary.

■ Assess the patient for signs of ongoing infection, which could falsely elevate the results. Notify the physician of any significant findings.

After

■ Apply pressure or a pressure dressing to the venipuncture site to prevent further bleeding. Observe the site for bleeding, especially if the patient has had other episodes of clotting deficiency.

Hemoglobin Electrophoresis (Hgb Electrophoresis)

Test type Blood

Normal values

Adult/elderly:
Hgb A_1: 95% to 98%
Hgb A_2: 2% to 3%
Hgb F: 0.8% to 2.0%
Hgb S: 0%
Hgb C: 0%

Children: Hgb F
>6 months: 1% to 2%
<6 months: <8%
Newborn: 50% to 80%

Rationale

Hgb electrophoresis detects abnormal forms of Hgb (hemoglobinopathies). This test is used to diagnose sickle cell anemia, thalassemia, and other hemoglobinopathies.

Although many different Hgb variations have been described, the more common types are A_1, A_2, F, S, and C. Each major Hgb type is electrically charged to varying degrees. When the Hgb from lysed RBCs is placed in an electromagnetic field, the Hgb variants spread apart. Each electrophoretic band represents a different form of Hgb, which can be quantitated as a percentage of the total Hgb.

Hgb A_1 constitutes the major component of Hgb in the normal RBC. Hgb A_2 is only a minor component (2% to 3%) of the normal Hgb total. Hgb F is the major hemoglobin component in the fetus but normally exists in only minimal quantities in the adult. Levels of Hgb F greater than 2% in patients older than age 3 years are considered abnormal. Hgb F is able to transport O_2 when only small amounts of O_2 are available (e.g., in fetal life). In patients requiring compensation for prolonged chronic hypoxia (e.g., in congenital cardiac abnormalities), Hgb F may be found in increased levels later in life to assist in the transport of the available O_2.

Hgb S is an abnormal form of Hgb associated with sickle cell anemia, which occurs predominantly in blacks. When little O_2 is available, Hgb S assumes a crescent (sickle) shape that greatly distorts the RBC morphology. Vascular sludging results from the localized sickling and may lead to organ infarction. The Hgb C variant is another that exists in blacks. RBCs containing Hgb C have a decreased life span and are more readily lysed than are normal RBCs. Mild to severe hemolytic anemia may result.

The Hgb content of some common hemoglobinopathies, as determined by electrophoresis, are as follows:

Sickle cell disease (homozygous sickle cell [SS])
Hgb S: 80% to 100%
Hgb A$_1$: 0%
Hgb A$_2$: 2% to 3%
Hgb F: 2%

Sickle cell trait (heterozygous SA)
Hgb S: 20% to 40%
Hgb A$_1$: 60% to 80%
Hgb A$_2$: 2% to 3%
Hgb F: 2%

Hgb C disease (homozygous)
Hgb C: 90% to 100%
Hgb A$_1$: 0%
Hgb A$_2$: 2% to 3%
Hgb F: 2%

Hgb H disease
Hgb A$_1$: 65% to 90%
Hgb A$_2$: 2% to 3%
Hgb H: 5% to 30%

Thalassemia major (homozygous)
Hgb A$_1$: 5% to 20%
Hgb A$_2$: 2% to 3%
Hgb F: 65% to 100%

Thalassemia minor (heterozygous)
Hgb A$_1$: 50% to 85%
Hgb A$_2$: 4% to 6%
Hgb F: 1% to 3%

Interfering factor

A factor that interferes with Hgb electrophoresis is blood transfusions within the previous 12 weeks, which may alter test results.

Procedure

Approximately 7 ml of peripheral venous blood is collected in a lavender-top tube, or any EDTA-containing tube, and sent to the hematology laboratory as soon as possible. There, a small quantity of the blood is placed on a starch gel or cellulose acetate medium. Electrophoresis ensues within an electromagnetic field, and the Hgb variants are separated and quantified by spectrophotometry.

Nursing implications with rationale

Before
☞ Explain the procedure to the patient. Tell the patient that no fasting is necessary.

■ Assess whether the patient has had any recent blood transfusions, which could alter the test results.

After
■ Apply pressure or a pressure dressing to the venipuncture site to prevent further bleeding. Observe the site for bleeding, especially if the patient has had other episodes of clotting deficiency.

■ Transport the blood specimen to the laboratory as soon as possible to avoid hemoglobin dilution, which could alter the results.

IRON STUDIES
Iron Level (Fe)
Total Iron-binding Capacity (TIBC)
Transferrin (Siderophilin)
Transferrin Saturation (TS)
Ferritin

Normal values

Iron:
Males: 65-175 μg/dl or 11.6-31.3 μmol/L (SI units)
Females: 50-170 μg/dl or 9.0-30.4 μmol/L (SI units)
Child: 50-120 μg/dl
Newborn: 100-250 μg/dl

TIBC: 250-420 μg/dl or 45-73 mmol/L (SI units)

Transferrin:
Adult male: 215-365 mg/dl
Adult female: 250-380 mg/dl
Child: 203-360 mg/dl
Newborn: 130-275 mg/dl

TS:
Males: 20%-50%
Females: 15%-50%

Ferritin:
Male: 12-300 ng/ml or 12-300 mg/L (SI units)
Female: 10-150 ng/ml or 10-150 mg/L (SI units)
Children:
6 months-15 years: 7-142 ng/ml
2-5 months: 50-200 ng/ml

1 month: 50-200 ng/ml
Newborn: 25-200 ng/ml

Rationale

Iron studies are used to evaluate iron metabolism in patients who are suspected to have iron deficiency, overload, or poisoning.

Serum iron

Abnormal levels of iron are characteristic of many diseases, including iron deficiency anemia and iron overload (acquired or genetic hemochromatosis). In the body, 70% of the iron is found in the Hgb of the RBCs. The other 30% is stored iron in the form of ferritin and hemosiderin. Iron is supplied by the diet. Approximately 10% of the ingested iron is absorbed in the small intestine and transported to the plasma. There, the iron is bound to a globulin protein called *transferrin* and carried to the bone marrow for incorporation into Hgb. The serum iron determination is a measurement of the quantity of iron bound to transferrin. Ferritin is a storage protein. Transferrin is a carrier protein.

Loss of blood (e.g., from menstruation, bleeding peptic ulcer, and colon neoplasm) is the most common cause of iron deficiency. Iron deficiency anemia is a result of reduced serum iron, resulting in a decreased production of Hgb, which, in turn, results in a small, pale (microcytic, hypochromic) RBC.

Iron overload or poisoning is called *hemochromatosis* or *hemosiderosis*. Excess iron is usually deposited in the brain, liver, and heart, where it causes organ dysfunction. Massive blood transfusions also may cause elevated serum iron levels, although only transiently.

TIBC and transferrin

TIBC is a measurement of all proteins available for binding mobile iron. Transferrin represents the largest quantity of iron-binding proteins. Therefore TIBC is an indirect, yet accurate, measurement of transferrin. Ferritin is not included in TIBC because it binds only stored iron. In most patients, TIBC increases in response to iron deficiency.

Transferrin also is diminished in the face of chronic illnesses (e.g., malignancy, collagen vascular diseases, or liver diseases). Hypoproteinemia also is associated with reduced transferrin levels.

TIBC usually is measured by adding excess iron to the patient's serum, which saturates all the transferrin. The excess iron is then removed. The remaining iron is measured and provides a direct measurement of TIBC and, indirectly, transferrin. In many laboratories, TIBC is not performed. Instead, transferrin is directly measured.

TIBC varies minimally according to iron intake. TIBC is more indicative of liver function (transferrin is produced by the liver) and nutrition than of iron metabolism. Transferrin values often are used to monitor the success of hyperalimentation.

TIBC saturation or TS

The percentage of transferrin and other mobile iron-binding proteins saturated with iron is calculated by dividing the serum iron level by the TIBC (transferrin):

$$TS\ (\%) = \frac{Serum\ iron\ level \times 100\%}{TIBC}$$

The normal value for TS is 20% to 50%. Calculation of TS is helpful in determining the cause of abnormal iron and transferrin levels. TS is decreased to less than 15% in patients with iron deficiency anemia. TS is increased in patients with iron overload or poisoning.

Chronic illness (e.g., infections, neoplasia, cirrhosis) is characterized by a low serum iron level, decreased TIBC, and normal TS. Pregnancy is marked by high levels of protein, including transferrin. Because iron requirements are high, it is not unusual to find low serum iron levels, high TIBC, and a low percentage of TS in late pregnancy.

Ferritin

The serum ferritin study is a good indicator of available iron stores in the body. This is the most sensitive test to determine iron deficiency anemia. Ferritin, the major iron storage protein, is normally present in the serum in concentrations directly related to iron storage. In normal patients, 1 ng/ml of serum ferritin corresponds to approximately 8 mg of stored iron. Decreases in ferritin levels indicate a decrease in iron storage associated with iron deficiency anemia. A ferritin level of less than 10 ng/100 ml is diagnostic of iron deficiency anemia. Only when protein depletion is severe can ferritin be decreased by malnutrition. Increased levels are a sign of iron excess.

A limitation of this study is that ferritin also can act as an acute-phase reactant protein, and levels may be elevated in conditions not reflecting iron stores (e.g., acute inflammatory diseases, infections, metastatic cancer, lymphomas).

Interfering factors

Factors that interfere with determining iron study values include the following:

- Recent blood transfusions, which may *increase* serum iron and transferrin
- Recent ingestion of a meal containing high iron content
  This may *increase* serum iron and ferritin.
- Hemolytic diseases, which may be associated with an artificially *increased* iron content
- Time of day
  Serum iron levels may vary significantly during the day. The blood specimen should be drawn in the morning, especially when the results are used to monitor iron replacement therapy.
- Pregnancy and estrogen therapy
  Female hormones are associated with *increased* transferrin levels.

Procedure

The patient should fast, except for water, for at least 12 hours before the study. Approximately 7 ml of peripheral venous blood is obtained in a red-top tube. Some laboratories require the use of iron-free needles and iron-free plastic containers for the blood collection. The specimens always should be obtained using a 20-gauge or larger needle. Smaller needles may traumatize the RBC during collection, resulting in hemolysis. With hemolysis, the iron usually contained in the RBC

pours into the serum and causes artificially high iron levels.

Nursing implications with rationale

Before

- Explain the procedure to the patient. Instruct the patient to remain fasting, except for water, for 12 hours before the blood test.
- Assess the patient for a history of blood transfusions and recent meals high in iron content.

During

- Perform a peripheral venipuncture, using at least a 20-gauge needle. Blood usually is drawn in the morning.

After

- Apply pressure or a pressure dressing to the site to prevent bleeding. Observe for bleeding.

Partial Thromboplastin Time, Activated (APTT, Partial Thromboplastin Time [PTT])

Test type Blood

Normal values

APTT: 30-40 seconds
PTT: 60-70 seconds
Patients receiving anticoagulant therapy: 1.5-2.5 times control value in seconds

Possible critical values

APTT: >70 seconds
PTT: >100 seconds

Rationale

The hemostasis and coagulation system normally functions in a homeostatic balance between factors encouraging clotting and factors encouraging clot dissolution. Blood vessel constriction is the first bodily reaction to active bleeding. In small-vessel injury, this may stop bleeding. In large-vessel injury, however, hemostasis is required to form a clot that will plug the hole until healing can occur. The primary phase of the hemostatic mechanism involves platelet aggregation to the injured blood vessel. Next, secondary hemostasis occurs. Two pathways of hemostasis exist. The first phase of reactions is called the *intrinsic system;* the second is the *extrinsic system* (see Figure 10-2, p. 403).

The PTT test is used to assess the intrinsic system and the common pathway of clot formation. The PTT also is used to monitor heparin therapy. The PTT evaluates factors I (fibrinogen), II (prothrombin), V, VIII, IX, X, XI, and XII. When the PTT is combined with the PT, nearly all the hemostatic abnormalities can be recognized. When any clotting factor exists in an inadequate quantity (e.g., in hemophilia A and B or consumptive coagulopathy), the PTT is prolonged. Because factors II, IX, and X are vitamin K-dependent factors, biliary obstruction, which precludes GI absorption of fat and fat-soluble vitamins (e.g., vitamin K), can reduce their concentration and thus prolong the PTT. Because coagulation factors are made in the liver, hepatocellular diseases also will prolong the PTT.

Heparin inactivates prothrombin (factor II) and prevents the formation of thromboplastin. These actions prolong the intrinsic clotting pathway for approximately 4 to 6 hours after each dose of heparin. As a result, heparin is capable of providing therapeutic anticoagulation. The appropriate dose of heparin can be monitored by the PTT. PTT test results are given in seconds along with a control value, which may vary slightly from day to day because of the reagents used.

Recently, activators have been added to the PTT test reagents to shorten normal clotting time and provide a narrow normal range. This shortened time is called the activated PTT (APTT). The normal APTT is 30 to 40 seconds. Desired ranges for therapeutic anticoagulation are 1.5 to 2.5 times normal (e.g., 70 seconds). The APTT specimen should be drawn 30 to 60 minutes before the patient's next heparin dose is given. If the APTT is less than 50 seconds, the patient may not be receiving therapeutic anticoagulation and needs more heparin. Most hospitals have a nomogram or schedule by which the heparin is adjusted based on the APTT. An APTT greater than 100 seconds indicates that too much heparin is being given; the risk of serious, spontaneous bleeding

exists when the APTT is this high. The effects of heparin can be reversed by the administration of 1 mg of protamine sulfate for every 100 units of the heparin dose.

Often, small doses of heparin (5000 U subcutaneously every 12 hours) are given to prevent thromboembolism in high-risk patients. This dose alters the PTT very little, and the risk of spontaneous bleeding is minimal.

Interfering factors

Factors that interfere with determining PTT values include the following:

- Drugs (e.g., antihistamines, ascorbic acid, chlorpromazine, heparin, and salicylates) may prolong PTT test values.

Procedure

Peripheral venipuncture is performed, and a blue-top tube (containing sodium citrate) is filled with blood. The tube must be filled to capacity; otherwise the PTT value may be incorrect because of the extra citrate within the tube. PTT levels are now being determined from fingerstick specimens using a machine similar to a glucometer. This is generally done in critical care units. Nurses vary the heparin dose based on sliding-scale heparin orders.

Nursing implications with rationale

Before

- Explain the procedure to the patient. Tell the patient that no fasting is necessary.
- If the patient is receiving heparin by intermittent injection, draw the APTT blood specimen 30 minutes to 1 hour before the next dose of heparin is scheduled to be administered.
- If the patient is receiving a continuous heparin infusion, draw the blood at any time.

After

- Apply pressure or a pressure dressing to the venipuncture site.
- Assess the venipuncture site for bleeding. If the patient is receiving anticoagulants or has coagulopathies, the bleeding time will be increased.
- Assess the patient to detect any other possible

bleeding. Check for blood in the urine and other excretions and assess the patient for bruises, petechiae (small hemorrhages in the skin), and bleeding gums.

- If severe bleeding occurs, administer protamine sulfate, as ordered, to reverse the anticoagulant effect of heparin.

Case Study

Hemophilia

K.D., a 10-year-old boy, fell and lacerated his lower leg while climbing a fence. In the emergency department, no signs of neurovascular damage were detected, and the wound was closed. One hour later, the dressings were saturated with blood. K.D. was taken to the operating room, and the wound was explored. No arterial lacerations were seen; however, there was diffuse oozing of blood from the wound's edges. In a review of K.D.'s bleeding history, a tendency to bleed larger quantities and for a greater duration than normal was found.

Studies	Results
Routine laboratory studies	Within normal limits (WNL)
PT, p. 434	Patient/control: 11 seconds/12 seconds; 85% (normal: 11-12.5 seconds; 85%-100%)
APTT, p. 427	62 seconds (normal: 30-40 seconds)
Platelet count, p. 431	200,000/mm^3 (normal: 150,000-400,000/mm^3)
Ivy bleeding time, p. 402	8.5 minutes (normal: 1-9 minutes)
Platelet aggregation, p. 430	Normal
Factor VIII concentration, p. 411	10% of normal concentration (absolute normal value varies according to the laboratory performing the test)
DIC screening test, p. 421	No evidence of DIC (normal: negative)

Diagnostic Analysis

The abnormal APTT result indicated a defect in the intrinsic system, or common pathway, of clot formation (see p. 403). The normal PT results indicated that the extrinsic pathway of clot formation was adequate. The normal bleeding time, platelet count, and blood clot retraction test eliminated insufficient platelet quantity or function as a cause of the coagulopathy. The factor VIII concentration was well below normal and caused the clot failure. Hemophilia A was diagnosed, and K.D. was given factor VIII concentration. All obvious bleeding ceased, and the leg wound healed.

After discharge, the patient returned to the hospital at regular intervals for factor VIII concentration (e.g., cryoprecipitate). He had no further bleeding difficulties.

Critical Thinking Questions

1. What clinical manifestations were suggestive of hemophilia?
2. What part of the hemostatic mechanism involves factor VIII?

Platelet Aggregation Test

Test type Blood

Normal values
Values depend on the platelet agonist used

Rationale
The platelet aggregation test is a measure of platelet function and aids in the evaluation of bleeding disorders. Platelet aggregation is an important first part of hemostasis. A clump of platelets surrounds an area of acute blood vessel endothelial injury. Normal platelets adhere to this area of injury, and through a series of chemical reactions, attract other platelets to the area. After this step, the normal coagulation factor waterfall occurs. Certain diseases that affect either platelet number or function can inhibit platelet aggregation and thereby prolong bleeding times. Congenital syndromes, uremia, myeloproliferative disorders, and some drugs are associated with abnormal platelet aggregation. If blood is passed through a heart-lung or dialysis pump, platelet injury can occur and aggregation capability can be reduced.

Interfering factors
Factors that interfere with determining platelet aggregation values include the following:

- Blood storage temperature, hyperlipidemia, and high platelet count
  These factors can *increase* platelet aggregation
- Drugs that may cause *decreased* platelet aggregation include aspirin, clofibrate, dextran, ethanol, heparin, NSAIDS, sodium warfarin, and heparin.

Procedure
No fasting is required. Approximately 5 to 7 ml of venous blood is collected in a blue-top tube and sent to the hematology laboratory.

Nursing implications with rationale
Before
- Explain the procedure to the patient. Tell the patient that no fasting is necessary.

After
- Apply pressure or a pressure dressing to the venipuncture site to prevent further bleeding. Observe the venipuncture site for bleeding.
- Note that abnormalities in platelet aggregation can prolong bleeding time, and a significant hematoma at the venipuncture site may occur.

Platelet Antibody (Antiplatelet Antibody Detection)

Test type Blood

Normal values
No antiplatelet antibodies identified

Rationale
The platelet antibody test is used in the evaluation of thrombocytopenia to identify an immune-associated etiology. Immune-mediated destruction of platelets may be caused either by autoantibodies directed against a person's own antigens or alloantibodies, which develop after exposure to transfused platelets received from a donor. These antibodies usually are directed to an antigen on the platelet membrane, such as human leukocyte antigen (HLA) (see p. 478) or platelet specific antigen (e.g., PLA_1, PLA_2).

Antibodies directed to platelets will cause early destruction of the platelets and subsequent thrombocytopenia. Immunologic thrombocytopenia occurs in the following conditions:

1. *Idiopathic thrombocytopenia purpura (ITP)* is a term that describes a group of disorders characterized by immune-mediated destruction of the platelets within the spleen or other reticuloendothelial organs. Platelet-associated IgG antibodies are detected in 90% of these patients.
2. Posttransfusion purpura is a rare syndrome characterized by the sudden onset of severe thrombocytopenia a few hours to a few days after transfusion of RBCs or platelets. This is usually associated with an antibody to ABO, HLA, or PLA antigens on the RBC. In most situations, the blood recipient has

been sensitized previously to a PLA$_1$ antigen during previous transfusions or a previous pregnancy.

3. Maternal-fetal platelet antigen incompatability (neonatal thrombocytopenia) occurs when the fetal platelet contains a PLA$_1$ antigen that is absent in the mother. Just like Rh RBC incompatibility, the mother creates anti-PLA$_1$ antibodies, which cross the placenta and destroy the fetal platelets. The mother is not thrombocytopenic. Neonatal thrombocytopenia also can occur if the mother has ITP autoantibodies that are passed through the placenta and also destroy the fetal platelets.

4. Drug-induced thrombocytopenia usually is caused by platelet-associated IgG antibodies. These antibodies are the result of a hypersensitivity reaction to certain drugs. A host of drugs are known to induce autoimmune-mediated thrombocytopenia. They include cimetidine, sulfonamides, quinidine-like drugs, and heparin.

Procedure

No fasting is required for this test. A peripheral venipuncture is performed, and approximately 7 to 30 ml of blood is collected in a red-top tube. The amount of blood required depends on the initial platelet count. The blood is sent to the laboratory, where radioimmunoassay is performed to identify the antiplatelet antibodies.

Nursing implications with rationale

Before

☞ Explain the procedure to the patient. Tell the patient that no fasting is necessary.

After

■ Apply pressure or a pressure dressing to the venipuncture site to prevent further bleeding.

■ Ensure adequate hemostasis in all patients suspected to have thrombocytopenia.

■ Note that a platelet count usually is done 1 to 2 hours after platelet transfusion. This not only documents the posttransfusion platelet count but also detects a large proportion of posttransfusion immune thrombocytopenia reactions.

Platelet Count (Thrombocyte Count)

Test type Blood

Normal values

Adult/elderly: 150,000-400,000/mm^3 or 150-400 $\times$ 10^9/L (SI units)

Children:

Child: 150,000-400,000/mm^3

Infant: 200,000-475,000 mm^3

Newborn: 150,000-300,000/mm^3

Premature infant: 100,000-300,000/mm^3

Possible critical values

<50,000 or >1 million/mm^3

Rationale

The platelet count is an actual count of the number of platelets (thrombocytes) per cubic milliliter of blood. It is performed on all patients who develop petechiae, spontaneous bleeding, increasingly heavy menses, or thrombocytopenia. It is used to monitor the course of the disease or therapy for thrombocytopenia or bone marrow failure.

Platelets are formed in the bone marrow from megakaryocytes. They are small, round, nonnucleated cells whose main role is maintenance of vascular integrity. The primary phase of the hemostatic mechanism involves platelet aggregation. After that phase, the platelets help initiate the coagulation factor waterfall (see Figure 10-2, p. 403). Most of the platelets exist in the bloodstream. A smaller percentage (25%) exists in the liver and spleen.

Platelet counts of 150,000 to 400,000/mm^3 are considered normal. Counts less than 100,000/mm^3 indicate thrombocytopenia; thrombocytosis exists when counts are greater than 400,000/mm^3. *Thrombocythemia* is a term used to indicate a platelet count in excess of 1 million/mm^3. Vascular thrombosis with tissue or organ infarction is the major complication of thrombocythemia. The disease most commonly associated with spontaneous thrombocytosis is malignancy (leukemia, lymphoma, or solid tumors such as colon). Thrombocytosis may also occur with polycythemia vera and postsplenectomy syndromes.

Spontaneous hemorrhage may occur with thrombocytopenia. If thrombocytopenia is severe, the platelets are often hand-counted. Spontaneous bleeding is a serious danger when platelet counts fall below 20,000/mm^3. Petechiae and ecchymosis also will occur at that level of thrombocytopenia. With counts above 40,000/mm^3, spontaneous bleeding rarely occurs, but prolonged bleeding from trauma or surgery may occur at this level.

Causes of thrombocytopenia include:

1. Reduced production of platelets (secondary to bone marrow failure, infiltration of fibrosis, tumor)
2. Sequestration of platelets (secondary to hypersplenism)
3. Accelerated destruction of platelets (secondary to antibodies [see antiplatelet antibodies, p. 430], infections, drugs, prosthetic heart valves)
4. Consumption of platelets (secondary to DIC)
5. Platelet loss from hemorrhage
6. Dilution, occurring with a large volume of blood transfusions, which contain very few, if any, platelets

Interfering factors

Factors that interfere with determining platelet count values include the following:

- Platelet clumping
  Because platelets can clump together, automated counting is subject to at least a 10% to 15% error.
- Strenuous exercise, which may cause *increased* levels
- Menstruation
  Decreased levels may be seen prior to menstruation.

Procedure

Approximately 5 to 7 ml of peripheral venous blood is obtained in a lavender-top tube and sent to the hematology laboratory. A small quantity of blood then is analyzed by an automatic counter simultaneously with the CBC.

Nursing implications with rationale

Before

- Explain the procedure to the patient. Tell the patient that no fasting is necessary.

After

- Apply pressure or a pressure dressing to the venipuncture site to prevent further bleeding. Observe the site for bleeding.

Platelet Volume, Mean (MPV)

Test type Blood

Normal values

25 μm in diameter

Rationale

The mean platelet volume is a measure, determined by an automated analyzer, of the volume of many platelets. MPV is to platelets what MCV (see p. 414) is to RBCs. This test is helpful in the evaluation of platelet disorders, especially thrombocytopenia.

The MPV varies with total platelet production. In cases of thrombocytopenia despite a normal reactive bone marrow (e.g., hypersplenism), the marrow releases immature platelets in an attempt to maintain a normal platelet count. These immature platelets are larger, and, as a result, the MPV is increased. When bone marrow production of platelets is inadequate, the platelets that are released are smaller and the MVP is decreased. In this way, the MPV is very useful in the differential diagnosis of thrombocytopenic disorders.

Interfering factor

A factor that interferes with determining MPV is the collection tube additive, EDTA, which can create a variation of as much as 25% in the size of the platelets.

Procedure

No fasting is required. Approximately 5 to 7 ml of venous blood is collected in a lavender-top tube and sent to the hematology laboratory.

Nursing implications with rationale

Before

☞ Explain the procedure to the patient. Tell the patient that no fasting is necessary.

After

■ Apply pressure or a pressure dressing to the venipuncture site to prevent further bleeding. Observe the venipuncture site for bleeding.

■ If the patient is known to have a low platelet count, observe the patient for signs and symptoms of bleeding; check for blood in the urine and all excretions; and assess the patient for bruises, petechiae, bleeding of the gums, epistaxis, and low back pain.

Porphyrins
Porphobilinogens
Uroporphyrinogen-1-Synthase
Delta-aminolevulinic Acid
(Aminolevulinic Acid [ALA], DALA)

Test type Urine

Normal values

Porphyrins	Male (μg/24 hrs)	Female (μg/24 hrs)
Total porphyrins	8-149	3-78
Uroporphyrin	4-46	3-22
Coproporphyrin	<96	<60

Porphobilinogens: 0-2.0 mg/24 hr or 0-8.8 mmol/day (SI units)

Uroporphyrinogen-1-synthase: 1.27-2.00 mU/g of Hgb or 81.9-129.6 U/mol of Hgb (SI units)

DALA: 1-7 mg/24 hr or 11.1-57.2 mmol/24 hr (SI units)

Possible critical value DALA: >20 mg/24 hr

Rationale

Porphyria is a collective name for a group of genetic disorders associated with deficiencies of enzymes involved with porphyrin synthesis. Porphyrins, such as uroporphyrin and coproporphyrin, and porphobilinogens are important building

blocks in heme synthesis. Heme is incorporated into Hgb within the RBCs. Porphyrias are classified according to the location of the accumulation of the porphyrin precursors. In most forms of porphyria, increased levels of porphyrins and porphobilinogen are found in the urine.

Variable symptoms are associated with the different types of porphyrias. Intermittent porphyria, the most common type, is associated with bouts of abdominal pain and neurologic symptoms. Intermittent porphyria is caused by a deficiency of uroporphyrinogen-1-synthase. This enzyme can be measured in the blood to identify patients with this disease. Heavy metal (lead) intoxication is also associated with increased porphyrins in the urine. Certain drugs (e.g., barbiturates, amphetamines, sulfonamides, estrogens, and theophylline) can induce porphyria and cause elevated porphyrins in the urine. This test is a quantitative analysis of urinary porphyrins and porphobilinogens. If porphyrins are present, the urine may be colored amber-red or burgundy; the urine specimen may turn even darker after exposure to light.

Urine tests for porphyrins are not as accurate as plasma measurements. However, the urine tests are an accurate screening method for porphyria, especially the intermittent variety. Although the test also can be done on a fresh stool specimen, random and 24-hour urine collections are more accurate.

DALA is a basic building block of porphyrin. In patients with porphyria, DALA will be elevated in the urine. In lead intoxication, heme synthesis is similarly diminished, and DALA accumulates in the blood and urine.

Procedure

Most of the porphobilinogen studies just described require a 24-hour urine specimen, which is collected in a light-resistant specimen bottle with a preservative to prevent degradation of the light-sensitive porphyrin. The specimen is kept on ice or refrigerated during the 24 hours. Porphobilinogens usually are elevated with the 24-hour urine porphyrin test or can be detected in a single, fresh-voided, random urine specimen. The specimen should be protected from light and sent immediately to the laboratory for analysis.

For uroporphyrinogen-1-synthase, 7 ml of peripheral venous blood is collected in a purple-top tube. Because this test is based on the Hgb measurement, a Hgb level is concurrently obtained. The blood samples should be stored on ice during laboratory transfer to avoid a false decrease in synthase levels.

Nursing implications with rationale

Before

☞ Explain the procedure to the patient and assist the patient as needed with the urine collection. Tell the patient that food and fluids are permitted during the 24-hour urine collection.

During

☞ Instruct the patient to begin the 24-hour urine collection after discarding the first morning specimen. This is the start time of the 24-hour collection.

■ Collect all urine passed over the next 24 hours.

☞ Instruct the patient to void before defecating so that the urine is not contaminated by feces.

☞ Remind the patient not to put toilet paper in the collection container.

■ Keep the urine specimen on ice or refrigerated during the 24 hours.

■ Collect the last specimen as close as possible to the end of the 24 hours.

After

■ Transport the urine specimen promptly to the laboratory.

Prothrombin Time (PT, Pro-time, International Normalized Ratio [INR])

Test type Blood

Normal values

PT: 11.0-12.5 seconds; 85%-100%
Full anticoagulant therapy: >1.5-2.0 times control value; 20%-30%
INR: 0.7-1.8

Possible critical values

PT: >20 seconds
INR: >3.5

Rationale

The hemostatic and coagulation system normally maintains a homeostatic balance between factors encouraging clotting and factors encouraging clot dissolution. Blood vessel constriction is the first bodily reaction to active bleeding. In small-vessel injury, this may stop bleeding. In large-vessel injury, however, hemostasis is required to form a clot, which will plug the hole until healing can occur. The primary phase of the hemostatic mechanism involves platelet aggregation to the injured blood vessel. Next, secondary hemostasis occurs. Two pathways of hemostasis exist. As previously described, the first phase of reactions is the intrinsic system; the second is the extrinsic system (see Figure 10-2, p. 403).

The PT measures the clotting ability of factors I (fibrinogen), II (prothrombin), V, VII, and X, (i.e., the extrinsic system and common pathway). When these clotting factors are deficient, the PT is prolonged. Many diseases and drugs are associated with decreased levels of these factors. These include the following:

1. Hepatocellular liver disease (e.g., cirrhosis, hepatitis, neoplastic invasive processes). Factors I, II, V, VII, IX, and X are produced in the liver. With severe hepatocellular dysfunction, synthesis of these factors will not occur, and their serum concentration will be decreased. Even a small decrease in factor VII will result in marked prolongation of the PT.

2. Obstructive biliary disease (e.g., bile duct obstruction secondary to tumor or gallstones; intrahepatic cholestasis secondary to sepsis or drugs). As a result of the biliary obstruction, the bile necessary for fat absorption fails to enter the gut, and fat malabsorption results. Vitamins A, D, E, and K are fat soluble and also are not absorbed. Because the synthesis of factors II, VII, IX, and X depends on vitamin K, these factors will not be adequately produced, and serum concentrations will fall. Parenchymal (hepatocellular) liver disease can be differentiated from obstructive biliary disease by

determination of the patient's response to parenteral vitamin K administration. If the PT returns to normal after 1 to 3 days of vitamin K administration (10 mg intramuscularly [IM] twice a day), one can safely assume that the patient has obstructive biliary disease that is causing vitamin K malabsorption. If, on the other hand, the PT does not return to normal with the vitamin K injections, one can assume that severe hepatocellular disease exists and that the liver cells are incapable of synthesizing the clotting factors regardless of how much vitamin K is available.

3. Coumarin ingestion. The coumarin derivatives, dicumarol and warfarin, are used to prevent coagulation in patients with thromboembolic disease (e.g., pulmonary embolism, thrombophlebitis, arterial embolism). These drugs interfere with the production of vitamin K-dependent clotting factors, which results in a prolongation of the PT, as already described. The adequacy of coumarin therapy can be monitored with PT tests. Appropriate coumarin therapy for full anticoagulation should prolong the PT by 1.5 to 2 times the control value (or 20% to 30% of the normal value if percentages are used).

The World Health Organization has recommended that PT results now include the use of the *INR value.* Many hospitals are now reporting PT times in both absolute numbers and INR numbers. Therapeutic INR is usually considered to be 2.0 to 3.5 in most institutions, depending on the clinical situation.

PT test results may also be given in seconds along with a control value. The control value usually varies somewhat from day to day because the reagents used may vary. The patient's PT should be approximately equal to the control value. Some laboratories report PT values as percentages of normal activity because the patient's results are compared with a curve representing normal clotting time. Normally, the patient's PT is 85% to 100%.

Interfering factors

Factors that interfere with determining PT values include the following:

- Alcohol intake
  Alcohol diminishes liver function. Because many clotting factors are made in the liver, lesser quantities of these factors result in a *prolonged* PT time.
- A diet high in fat or leafy vegetables
  Such a diet enhances absorption of vitamin K. Vitamin-K–dependent factors are made at increased levels, thereby *shortening* PT times.
- Diarrhea or malabsorption syndromes
  In these conditions, vitamin K is malabsorbed, and, as a result, factors II, VII, IX, and X are not made. This can *prolong* PT times.

Procedure

Peripheral venipuncture is performed, and a blue-top tube (containing sodium citrate) is filled with blood. The tube must be filled to capacity, otherwise the PT results may be artificially prolonged because of the extra citrate in the tube. In the laboratory, tissue thromboplastin is added, thereby circumventing the intrinsic system of clotting. The time required for clotting is then noted.

Nursing implications with rationale

Before

☞ Explain the procedure to the patient. Tell the patient that no fasting is necessary.

During

- Completely fill the blue-top tubes with blood. Deliver the blood specimen to the laboratory immediately after venipuncture.
- If the patient is receiving warfarin, the PT specimen should be drawn before the patient is given his or her daily dose. The daily dose may be increased, decreased, or kept the same, depending on the PT test results for that day. Maintain a flow chart indicating the PT test results, control value, and dose of anticoagulant.

After

- Observe the site for bleeding after the venipuncture. Apply pressure to the site until the bleeding stops. The bleeding time will be prolonged if the patient is taking warfarin or if the patient has any coagulopathies.

- If the PT is markedly prolonged, evaluate the patient for bleeding tendencies (i.e., check for blood in the urine and all excreta and assess the patient for bruises, petechiae, and low back pain).

- If severe bleeding occurs, the anticoagulant effect of warfarin can be reversed by the slow parenteral administration of vitamin K (phytonadione).

- ☞ If the patient is taking warfarin, instruct the patient not to take any medication because of drug interactions, unless it is specifically ordered by the physician.

Red Blood Cell Survival Study
(RBC Survival Study, Splenic Sequestration Study)

Test type Blood

Normal values
Half-life of RBC: 26-30 days
Spleen/liver ratio: 1:1
Spleen/pericardium ratio: <2:1

Rationale
The RBC survival study is a nuclear test used to identify reduced RBC survival as a result of hemolysis. It is used in the evaluation of hemolytic anemia. It also is helpful in the determination of RBC survival in patients with splenomegaly and anemia.

In patients with hemolytic anemia, the RBCs are destroyed and sequestered in the spleen. As a result of this ongoing RBC destruction, the RBC life span will be significantly reduced. This reduction in RBC survival indicates that active hemolysis is occurring and is the cause of the patient's anemia.

The determination of the RBC life span by nuclear studies can provide a semiquantitative measurement of the degree of hemolysis. This quantitation can best be performed by determining the half-life of the RBC within the circulation.

This portion of the test is performed by extracting some of the patient's RBCs, labeling them with chromium 51 (Cr 51), and reinjecting them into the patient. Subsequent blood levels of Cr 51 indicate the half-life of the labeled RBCs. As RBC survival decreases, more labeled RBCs are sequestered by the spleen. As a result, the amount of Cr 51 activity in the blood decreases.

The second portion of the test is the imaging of the spleen, liver, and pericardium. In patients with hemolytic anemia associated with abnormal splenic sequestration, the spleen/liver ratio is in excess of 1:1. However, this same abnormally high ratio also can occur without hemolysis in patients who have splenomegaly caused by a disease other than hemolytic anemia. To eliminate that confusion, the spleen/pericardium ratios are performed; those ratios greater than 2:1 indicate abnormal splenic sequestration of hemolyzed RBCs. A normal spleen/pericardium ratio with an increased spleen/liver ratio indicates splenomegaly caused by portal hypertension, for example.

This second portion of the splenic sequestration study is also helpful in determining which patients with hemolytic anemia will benefit from splenectomy. Patients with increased splenic sequestration can be expected to improve after splenectomy.

Interfering factors
Factors that interfere with the RBC survival study include the following:

- Recent RBC transfusion, increased RBC production, active bleeding, high WBC counts in excess of 25,000, and high platelet counts greater than 500,000
  These factors can *decrease* RBC survival.
- Splenomegaly, which can *increase* spleen/pericardium ratios

Procedure
Approximately 20 ml of blood is withdrawn from the patient, and the RBCs are labeled with Cr 51. The RBCs are immediately reinjected into the patient. On the first day of testing, 10 ml of blood is withdrawn by peripheral venipuncture in a red-

top tube. The RBCs are quantitated for Cr 51 counts per minute. Nuclear imaging of the spleen, liver, and pericardium is carried out. This process is repeated 3 times a week for about 3 weeks. The peripheral venous blood Cr 51 counts are plotted on a graph, and a half-life is determined. The spleen/liver and spleen/pericardium ratios and nuclear counts are determined.

This test takes place over a 2- to 3-week period. The results are available on the day after the test is completed. The study is performed by a nuclear medicine technologist or physician. No discomfort is associated with this test other than the frequent venipuncture. The patient must lie still during the nuclear imaging portion of the test.

Contraindication

RBC survival study is contraindicated in patients who are pregnant because of the risk of fetal damage caused by the radiation exposure.

Nursing implications with rationale

Before

☞ Explain the procedure to the patient. Tell the patient that no fasting or sedation is necessary.

☞ Assure the patient that he or she will not be exposed to large amounts of radioactivity because only tracer doses of the isotope are used. No precautions need to be taken against radioactive exposure.

■ Notify the nuclear medicine technologist or physician if blood transfusion or hemorrhage has occurred shortly before or during the test.

After

■ Apply pressure or a pressure dressing to the venipuncture site. Observe the venipuncture site for bleeding.

Reticulocyte Count (Retic Count)

Test type Blood

Normal values

Reticulocyte count:
Adult/elderly/child: 0.5%-2% of total number of RBCs

Infant: 0.5%-3.1% of total number of RBCs
Newborn: 2.5%-6.5% of total number of RBCs
Reticulocyte index: 1.0

Rationale

The reticulocyte count is a test for determining bone marrow function and evaluating erythropoietic activity. This test is also useful in classifying anemias. A reticulocyte (Figure 10-1, p. 401) is an immature RBC. It can be identified readily with a microscope by staining the peripheral blood smear with Wright's or Giemsa stains. A reticulocyte is an RBC that still has some microsomal and ribosomal material left in the cytoplasm. It sometimes requires a few days for that material to be cleared from the cell. Normally, a small number of reticulocytes exists in the bloodstream.

The reticulocyte count indicates RBC production by the bone marrow. Increased reticulocyte counts indicate the marrow is putting more RBCs into the bloodstream, usually in response to anemia. A normal or low reticulocyte count in a patient with anemia indicates that the marrow response to the anemia (production of RBCs) is inadequate and may be contributing to or causing the anemia (as in aplastic anemia, iron deficiency, vitamin B_{12} deficiency, or depletion of iron stores). An elevated reticulocyte count found in patients with a normal hemogram indicates increased RBC production compensating for an ongoing loss of RBCS (hemolysis or hemorrhage) or increased O_2 requirements.

Because the reticulocyte count is a percentage of the total number of RBCs, a normal to low number of reticulocytes can still appear normal in the anemic patient because the total number of mature RBCs is low. To determine if a reticulocyte count indicates an appropriate erythropoietic (RBC marrow) response in patients with anemia, one should calculate the reticulocyte index:

Reticulocyte index =

$$\text{Reticulocyte count (\%)} \times \frac{\text{Patient's Hct}}{\text{Normal Hct}}$$

The reticulocyte index in a patient with a good marrow response to the anemia should be 1.0. If it is less than 1.0, even though the reticulocyte count is elevated, the bone marrow response is inadequate in its ability to compensate (as seen in iron deficiency, vitamin B_{12} deficiency, or marrow failure).

Interfering factors

Factors that interfere with determining the reticulocyte count include Howell-Jolly bodies, which are blue stippling material in the RBC that occurs in severe anemia or hemolytic anemia. The RBCs containing these Howell-Jolly bodies look like reticulocytes and are miscounted by the automated counter machines, giving a falsely high number of reticulocytes.

Procedure

Blood is obtained for a CBC (see p. 412) and sent to the hematology laboratory. A technician applies a supravital stain to a peripheral blood smear and examines the slide under a microscope. The reticulocytes exhibit a network of purple strands. The reticulocytes are counted, and their percentage of the total RBCs is determined.

Nursing implications with rationale

Before

☞ Explain the procedure to the patient. Tell the patient that no fasting is necessary.

After

■ Apply pressure or a pressure dressing to the venipuncture site to prevent further bleeding. Observe the site for bleeding.

Sickle Cell Test (Sickle Cell Prep, Sickledex, Hgb S Test)

Test type Blood

Normal values

No sickle cells present

Rationale

The sickle cell test is used to screen for sickle cell disease or trait. Both sickle cell disease (homozygous for Hgb S) and sickle cell trait (heterozygous for Hgb S) can be detected by this study. Sickle cell anemia results from a genetic homozygous defect and is caused by the presence of Hgb S instead of Hgb A. In the United States, 5% to 10% of blacks have sickle cell trait and less than 1% have sickle cell anemia. When Hgb S becomes deoxygenated, it tends to precipitate in a way that causes the RBC to assume a sickle shape, which causes plugging of the microvascular tree (Figure 10-5). This may compromise the blood supply to various organs.

The routine peripheral blood smear of patients with sickle cell disease does not contain sickled RBCs unless hypoxemia is present. In the sickle cell preparation test, a deoxygenating agent (e.g., 2% sodium metabisulfite) is added to the patient's blood. If 25% or more of the patient's Hgb is of the S variation, the cells will assume the crescent (sickle) shape, and the test is positive. If no sickling occurs, the test is negative. In the solubility tests (e.g., Sickledex), a dithionate is added to the patient's blood. Hgb S will precipitate. A negative test indicates that the patient has no or very little Hgb S. These tests cannot differentiate between sickle cell disease and trait.

The sickle cell test is only a screening test, and its sensitivity varies according to the method used by the laboratory. The definitive diagnosis of sickle cell disease or trait is made by Hgb electrophoresis (see p. 424), in which Hgb S can be identified and quantified.

Interfering factors

Factors that interfere with the sickle cell test include the following:

■ Blood transfusions within 3 to 4 months
  False-negative results may occur because the donor's normal Hgb may dilute the recipient's abnormal Hgb S.
■ Infants younger than 3 months of age
  False-negative results may occur because of the significant amount of Hgb F in the RBCs at that age. Hgb F will not cause sickling.

Procedure

Approximately 7 ml of peripheral venous blood is obtained in a lavender-top tube and sent to the

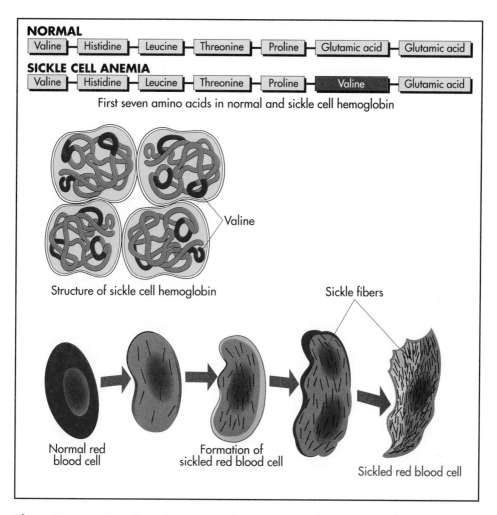

Figure 10-5 Sickle cell anemia. Sickle cell Hgb is produced by a recessive allele of the gene encoding the beta chain of Hgb. It represents a single amino acid change from a glutamic acid to valine at the sixth position in the chain. In the folded beta chain the sixth position contacts the alpha chain, and the amino acid change causes the Hgbs to aggregrate into long chains, altering the shape of the cell.

hematology laboratory. In the laboratory, a technician mixes a small quantity of blood with a bisulfite solution and then examines a peripheral blood smear for crescent-shaped RBCs. The sickling procedure takes less than 30 minutes. The only discomfort associated with this study is the venipuncture.

Nursing implications with rationale

Before

☞ Explain the procedure to the patient. Tell the patient that no fasting is necessary.

■ Assess the patient for recent blood transfusions.

After

■ Note that positive results should be confirmed by Hgb electrophoresis.

☞ If the test is positive, offer the family genetic counseling. A patient with one recessive gene (heterozygous) is said to have sickle cell trait. A patient with two recessive genes (homozygous) has sickle cell anemia.

☞ Inform patients with sickle cell anemia that they should avoid situations in which hypoxia may occur (e.g., strenuous exercise, air travel in unpressurized aircraft, and travel to high-altitude regions).

Case Study

Sickle Cell Anemia

B.J., a 10-year-old black boy, experienced sudden abdominal, chest, and diffuse joint pain while playing ice hockey. Both his parents had a family history of sickle cell disease. The results of physical examination were negative except for conjunctival pallor.

Studies	Results
CBC, p. 412	
RBC count	3.8 million/mm^3 (normal: 3.8-5.5 million/mm^3)
Hgb concentration	9.4 g/dl (normal: 11-16 g/dl)
Hct	28% (normal: 31%-43%)
MCV	83 mm^3 (normal: 80-95 mm^3)
MCH	28 pg (normal: 27-31 pg)
MCHC	34 g/dl (normal: 32-36 g/dl)
WBC and differential counts, p. 413	
Total WBC	6500/mm^3 (normal: 5000-10,000/mm^3)
Neutrophils	60% (normal: 55%-70%)
Lymphocytes	29% (normal: 20%-40%)
Monocytes	8% (normal: 2%-8%)
Eosinophils	2% (normal: 1%-4%)
Basophils	1% (normal: 0.5%-1%)
Peripheral blood smear, p. 405	Sickled forms of RBCs (normal: normocytic, normochromic RBCs)
Reticulocyte count, p. 437	4% (normal: 0.5%-2%)
Serum haptoglobin level, p. 423	74 mg/dl (normal: 100-150 mg/dl)
Bone marrow aspiration, p. 408	Erythroid hyperplasia M:E ratio 2:1 (normal: 3:1)
G6PD, p. 423	Negative (screening test)
Hgb electrophoresis, p. 424	
Hgb F	20% (normal: <1%)
Hgb A$_2$	3% (normal: approximately 2%)
Hgb S	77% (normal: 0)
Hgb A$_1$	0 (normal: 95%-98%)
Sickle cell test, p. 438	Positive (normal: negative)
Coombs' test, direct, p. 420	Negative (normal: negative)
Blood type, p. 406	O+

Diagnostic Analysis

B.J.'s physician suspected that the child had sickle cell anemia. The CBC indicated that B.J. had a normochromic, normocytic anemia. The increased reticulocyte count and erythroplasia seen on bone marrow aspiration indicated that his marrow was attempting to compensate for the anemia. His decreased serum haptoglobin level indicated that hemolysis was occurring. A negative direct Coombs' test eliminated an autoimmune cause of the hemolysis. The negative G6PD screen eliminated that deficiency, which is common in the black population. The peripheral blood smear, sickle cell test, and Hgb electrophoresis confirmed the diagnosis of sickle cell anemia.

B.J. was treated for his sickle cell crisis and released from the hospital. He continued to experience many sickle cell crises and frequently required transfusion of O+ blood. He died at the age of 18 from pneumonia.

Critical Thinking Questions

1. Explain the relationship, if any, between B.J.'s physical activity and the onset of his symptoms.
2. Why was the reticulocyte count increased?

Vitamin B_{12} (Cyanocobalamin)
Folic Acid (Folate)

Test type Blood

Normal values

Vitamin B_{12}: 100-700 pg/ml or 74-517 pmol/L
Folic acid: 5-20 mg/ml or 14-34 mmol/L (SI units)

Rationale

Vitamin B_{12} is measured to identify the cause of megaloblastic anemia and evaluate malnourished patients. Vitamin B_{12} is necessary for conversion of the inactive form of folate to the active form. This reaction is vital in the synthesis of nucleic acids and amino acids. This reaction is vital in the synthesis of nucleic and amino acids, such as that which occurs in the formation and function of RBCs. Vitamin B_{12} deficiency, like folic acid deficiency, causes anemia. The RBCs formed as a result of these deficiencies are large, megaloblastic RBCs, which cannot conform to the size of small capillaries. Instead, they fracture and hemolyze. The shortened life span ultimately leads to anemia. Other marrow cells also are affected, causing giant, segmented neutrophils and large, nucleated platelets.

Meats, eggs, and dairy products are the main sources of vitamin B_{12}. In the stomach, gastric acid detaches vitamin B_{12} from its binding proteins. Intrinsic factor (IF), necessary for vitamin B_{12} absorption in the small intestine, is made in the stomach mucosa. Without IF, vitamin B_{12} cannot be absorbed. Deficiency of IF is the most common cause of vitamin B_{12} deficiency (pernicious anemia). Another cause of vitamin B_{12} deficiency is malabsorption caused by diseases of the small terminal ileum. The causes of vitamin B_{12} deficiency can be determined by the Schilling test (see p. 85).

As with vitamin B_{12}, the folate level is dependent on adequate dietary ingestion and normal intestinal absorption. The main causes of folic acid deficiency include dietary deficiency (usually in the alcoholic patient) and malabsorption syndrome. Like vitamin B_{12} deficiency, decreased folic acid levels cause megaloblastic anemia.

Elevated levels of folic acid may be seen in patients with pernicious anemia. Because the amount of vitamin B_{12} is inadequate to metabolize folic acid, levels of folic acid rise in pernicious anemia. The folic acid test should be done in conjunction with tests for vitamin B_{12} levels.

Folate is often tested in the laboratory workup for alcoholic patients to assess nutritional status. Folate must be depleted for at least 5 months before megaloblastic anemia occurs.

Interfering factor

A factor that interferes with determining folic acid levels is recent nuclear scans. Because radioimmunoassay is the method of choice for folic acid determination, radionuclide administration should be avoided for at least 24 hours.

Procedure

Fasting usually is not required before this test; however, patients should not consume alcoholic beverages beforehand. Approximately 7 to 10 ml of blood is collected in a red-top tube and sent to the laboratory.

Nursing implications with rationale

Before
- ☞ Explain the procedure to the patient. Tell the patient that fasting usually is not necessary. (However, some laboratories prefer an 8-hour fast.)
- ☞ Instruct the patient not to consume alcoholic beverages before the test because alcohol can cause results to be falsely decreased.
- ■ Obtain the specimen before beginning vitamin therapy.

During
- ■ Prevent hemolysis of the blood sample. Hemolysis can cause false-negative results.

After
- ■ Apply pressure or a pressure dressing to the venipuncture site. Observe the venipuncture site for bleeding and hematoma formation.

REVIEW QUESTIONS AND ANSWERS

1. **Question:** Your patient with cirrhosis was scheduled for a liver biopsy. His blood work showed a marked elevation of his PT. How could this be elevated if the patient was not on coumadin therapy?

Answer: Many clotting factors are produced in the liver. With cirrhosis or any other hepatocellular dysfunction, synthesis of certain clotting factors will not occur, and serum levels decrease. This can result in a prolonged PT.

2. **Question:** Your patient is having blood drawn and banked for autologous transfusion after cardiac surgery. He said he has been referred to as a "universal donor" and asks you to explain this term.

Answer: Persons with group O blood are considered universal donors because they do not have antigens on the RBCs to create an immunogenic reaction. Group O blood is often transfused in emergency situations, when there is insufficient time for crossmatching, because the chance of a transfusion reaction is least with type O blood.

3. **Question:** Your male patient, who has a long history of peptic ulcer disease, has a Hct of 24% (normal: 52%) on routine laboratory testing. His reticulocyte count is 1.5% (WNL). Does this reticulocyte count represent adequate marrow response in light of this patient's low Hct?

Answer: No. Although the reticulocyte count is WNL according to normal values, it is actually low when one considers the fact that the appropriate marrow response in this anemic patient should raise the reticulocyte count well *above* normal. This situation is more accurately demonstrated by a determination of the reticulocyte index, which should be 1 or greater in all patients regardless of the Hct level.

$$\text{Reticulocyte index} = \text{Reticulocyte count} \times \frac{\text{Patient's Hct}}{\text{Normal Hct}}$$

In this case:

$$\text{Reticulocyte index} = 1.5 \times \frac{24}{52} = 0.69$$

This represents an inadequate marrow response most probably caused by iron deficiency resulting from the chronic blood loss. The anemia, therefore, is caused by a combination of chronic blood loss and inadequate marrow response.

4. **Question:** Your 72-year-old patient is suspected of having acute appendicitis. The WBC count is 3800. Can an infectious process, such as appendicitis, still be considered a possibility without the normally suspected leukocytosis?
Answer: Yes. Although the expected normal response to infection is elevation of the WBC count, this may not occur in the geriatric and pediatric population. Leukopenia may actually occur in response to sepsis in these two groups of patients.

5. **Question:** Your patient has been receiving intravenous (IV) heparin therapy (6000 units) every 4 hours. A PTT specimen is drawn at 4 PM (1 hour before the next heparin dose). The results indicate that the PTT is greater than 100 seconds. At 5 PM bleeding develops from the patient's gums while she is eating dinner. Shortly thereafter, she voids grossly bloody urine. Epistaxis (nosebleed) follows. What should you do for this patient?
Answer:
a. Place the patient in bed in the supine position. She may become hypovolemic and hypotensive from the blood loss. Monitor her vital signs every 15 minutes.
b. Instruct the patient to pinch her nasal alae closed to attempt to stop the epistaxis.
c. Notify the physician, who will probably order protamine sulfate as an antidote to the heparin. One milligram of protamine sulfate equilibrates 100 units of heparin. The physician needs to know when the last dose of heparin was given because 2 hours after administration 50% of the heparin will have been metabolized and after 4 hours almost all of the heparin will have metabolized. By knowing when the last dose of heparin was given, the physician can determine how much heparin is present in the blood and can calculate the appropriate amount of protamine sulfate.

6. **Question:** A male construction worker is brought to the emergency room with a severe laceration of the leg. He is bleeding profusely and is in shock. After pressure is applied to the bleeding site, blood is obtained for a CBC and crossmatch. IV access is obtained with several large-bore IV needles, and vigorous fluid replacement is begun. The Hgb concentration and Hct results return at 14 g/dl and 52%, respectively. Can these values be correct in light of the apparent severe hemorrhage?
Answer: Yes, because of the time at which the blood was drawn. One of the major physiologic responses to hemorrhage is complete conservation of all free body water. This, combined with vigorous IV fluid therapy, tends to dilute the RBC count and results in the decrease in Hgb associated with the hemorrhagic state. However, these physiologic responses take time to occur. This patient's CBC specimen was drawn before these physiologic responses became effective and before IV fluids were administered. Therefore there was no time for dilution of the RBC count and Hgb to occur. A repeat CBC performed 4 to 8 hours later will probably more accurately reflect the severity of the patient's bleeding.

7. **Question:** Your 2-year-old (12-kg) patient is admitted for lower GI bleeding. The patient's Hgb concentration is 7.8 g/dl. How much blood is required to transfuse the patient to a Hgb concentration of 10 g/dl? How much blood would be required to transfuse an adult patient (70 kg) to the same Hgb concentration?
Answer: In general, a useful guide to blood replacement in infants and children is to consider that 10 ml/kg of whole blood or 5 ml/kg of packed cells will raise the Hgb 1 g/dl. Therefore the 12-kg child requires 264 ml of whole blood or 132 ml of packed cells to raise the Hgb concentration from 7.8 to 10 g/dl.

   In adults 1 unit of packed cells or whole blood can be expected to raise the Hgb concentration 1 g/dl. Therefore, slightly more than 2 units of packed cells or whole blood is required to raise the adult's Hgb concentration from 7.8 to 10 g/dl.

8. **Question:** During blood administration, your patient suddenly suffers fever, chills, flushing of the face, shortness of breath, tachycardia, and pain along the vein into which the blood is being transfused. How should you intervene,

and what laboratory studies should be performed to elucidate the cause of the acute problem?

Answer: Your patient is most probably having a transfusion reaction. The appropriate nursing interventions include:

a. Stop the transfusion and run saline solution through the IV line.

b. Record the patient's vital signs and notify the physician immediately.

c. Administer an antihistamine, steroids, or both (e.g., diphenhydramine, 50 mg intramuscularly; hydrocortisone sodium succinate, 100 mg intravenously; or both) as ordered. Epinephrine, administered subcutaneously, may also be indicated.

d. Return the blood pack and tubing to the blood bank along with a completed transfusion reaction report.

e. Obtain 20 ml of peripheral venous blood in one lavender-top and two red-top tubes and send them to the blood bank for testing.

f. Collect a urine specimen immediately and again 24 hours after the transfusion.

g. Do not administer any more blood until the cause of the reaction is established. The following tests are helpful in determining the cause of the reaction:

(1) Repeated blood typing of the patient's blood and the donor pack

(2) Repeated crossmatching

(3) Direct and indirect Coombs' tests

(4) Free Hgb, haptoglobin, and bilirubin level determinations (which indicate hemolysis)

(5) Serum Hgb level determination

(6) Urine tests for free Hgb and bilirubin

(7) Culture and sensitivity study of donor's packed cells to detect bacterial contamination

9. **Question:** A patient is being transferred to the intensive care unit after surgery following a severe motor vehicle accident. In receiving the patient, you are told that the patient has required 23 units of blood. To replace clotting factors not present in banked blood, one pack of fresh frozen plasma (FFP) has been given appropriately for every five units of blood. In the ensuing hours you notice that the patient seems to be oozing blood from all wound and venipuncture sites. You also detect cutaneous petechiae. What would be helpful in elucidating the cause of this patient's bleeding tendency?

Answer: A common problem with multiple transfusions is dilution of the patient's platelets. Banked blood contains very few functioning platelets, and no platelets are contained in FFP. A low platelet count and a normal PT and PTT would document the cause of this patient's bleeding tendency. The patient would need platelet transfusions to correct the bleeding.

Bibliography

Applebaum FR et al: Bone marrow transplantation for chronic myelogenous leukemia, *Semin Oncol* 22:405, 1995.

Babior BM, Bunn HF: Megaloblastic anemias. In Fauci AS et al, editors: Harrison's principles of internal medicine, ed 14, New York, 1998, McGraw-Hill.

Bachner RL: Neutropenia. In Rakel RE, editor: Conn's current therapy, Philadelphia, 1998, WB Saunders.

Bagby GC: Leukocytosis and leukemoid reaction. In Wyngaarden JB et al, editors: Cecil textbook of medicine, ed 19, Philadelphia, 1992, WB Saunders.

Bagby GC: Leukopenia. In Wyngaarden JB et al, editors: Cecil textbook of medicine, ed 19, Philadelphia, 1992, WB Saunders.

Betts RF: Mononucleosis syndromes. In Beutler E, editor: Williams hematology, ed 5, New York, 1995, McGraw-Hill.

Beutler E: Disorders of hemoglobin. In Fauci AS et al, editors: Harrison's principles of internal medicine, ed 14, New York, 1998, McGraw-Hill.

Brauverman PE: Disseminated intravascular coagulation. In Rakel RE, editor: Conn's current therapy, Philadelphia, 1998, WB Saunders.

Cook JD: Iron deficiency anemias. In Rakel RE, editor: Conn's current therapy, Philadelphia, 1998, WB Saunders.

Coulter JS: Red blood cell distribution width and mean corpuscular volume: clinical applications, *Adv Clin Care* 6(6):13, 1991.

Dale DC: Neutropenia. In Beutler E, editor: Williams hematology, ed 5, New York, 1995, McGraw-Hill.

Erslev AJ: Anemia of chronic disease. In Beutler E, editor: Williams hematology, ed 5, New York, 1995, McGraw-Hill.

Hancock RD: Venipuncture vs. arterial catheter activated partial thromboplastin times in heparinized patients, *DCCN* 12(5):238-245, 1993.

Handin RI: Anticoagulant, fibrinolytic, and antiplatelet disorders. In Fauci AS et al, editors: Harrison's principles of internal medicine, ed 14, New York, 1998, McGraw-Hill.

Handin RI: Disorders of coagulation and thrombosis. In Fauci AS et al, editors: Harrison's principles of internal medicine, ed 14, New York, 1998, McGraw-Hill.

Handin RI: Disorders of the platelet and vessel wall. In Fauci AS et al, editors: Harrison's principles of internal medicine, ed 14, New York, 1998, McGraw-Hill.

Koepke JA: Practical laboratory hematology, New York, 1991, Churchill Livingstone.

Lindenbaum J: An approach to the anemias. In Wyngaarden JB et al, editors: Cecil textbook of medicine, ed 19, Philadelphia, 1992, WB Saunders.

Martinelli AM: Sickle cell disease: etiology, symptoms, and patient care, *AORN J* 53(3):716-724, 1991.

McMillan R: Platelet-mediated bleeding disorders. In Rakel RE, editor: Conn's current therapy, Philadelphia, 1998, WB Saunders.

Menitove JE: Blood transfusion. In Wyngaarden JB et al, editors: Cecil textbook of medicine, ed 19, Philadelphia, 1992, WB Saunders.

Nathan DG: Introduction to hematologic diseases. In Wyngaarden JB et al, editors: Cecil textbook of medicine, ed 19, Philadelphia, 1992, WB Saunders.

Norris MKG: Assessing fibrin-split products, *Nursing* 22(6):29, 1992.

Pagana KD, Pagana TJ: Mosby's Manual of Diagnostic and Laboratory Tests, St. Louis, 1998, Mosby.

Sassa S: The porphyrias. In Beutler E, editor: Williams hematology, ed 5, New York, 1995, McGraw-Hill.

Tsevat J et al: Neonatal screening for sickle cell disease: a cost effectiveness analysis, *J Pediatr* 118(4):546-554, 1991.

Walters MC et al: Bone marrow transplantation for sickle cell disease, *N Engl J Med* 335:369, 1996.

Chapter 11

Diagnostic Studies Used in the Assessment of the
Skeletal System

ANATOMY AND PHYSIOLOGY

The skeletal system (Figure 11-1) consists of a
framework of bones whose main purpose is to
support the tissues of the body, protect delicate
internal organs, and facilitate movement. Bones
also serve as a reservoir for calcium, magnesium,
phosphorus, sodium, and other ions necessary for
various homeostatic functions. Hematopoiesis,
which is the production of blood cells (see Chapter 10), is another important function of the bone.

Bones are classified according to the following
shapes:

1. Long bones. Long bones are found in the
   extremities. Examples include the bones of
   the upper and lower arm (humerus and
   ulna, respectively); bones of the thigh and
   leg (femur, tibia, and fibula); and bones of
   the fingers and toes (phalanges). They are
   called *long bones* because their length is
   greater than their breadth.
2. Short bones. Examples include the wrist
   and ankle bones (carpals and tarsals, respectively).
3. Flat bones. These bones have a large surface area and provide protection for soft
   body parts. Examples include the frontal

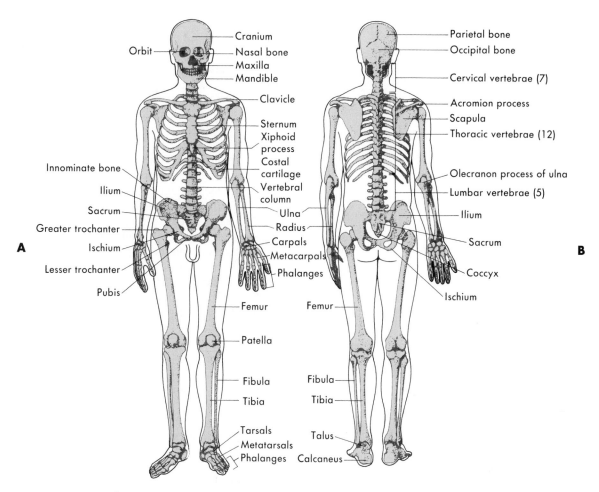

A

B

Figure 11-1   Musculoskeletal system. **A,** Anterior view. **B,** Posterior view.

and parietal bones of the cranium, ribs, sternum, scapulae, ilium, and pubis.

4. Irregular bones. These bones are of various shapes and compositions and include the bones of the spinal column (e.g., the vertebrae, sacrum, coccyx) and certain skull bones (e.g., the mandible).

Histologically, bones are composed of cancellous (spongy) and compact (dense) bone. Red marrow, which produces blood cells, occupies the spaces of cancellous bone. Compact bone is strong and dense, with many networks of interconnecting canals called *haversian systems*. A haversian canal runs centrally through each system, parallel to the bone's long axis, and contains one or two blood vessels, which supply most of the bone's blood. Bones have an intergenerative membrane called the *marrow cavity*. Yellow marrow is present in the shafts of the long bones and extends into the haversian system. Yellow marrow is composed of adipose cells and can change to red marrow, if necessary, to produce blood cells.

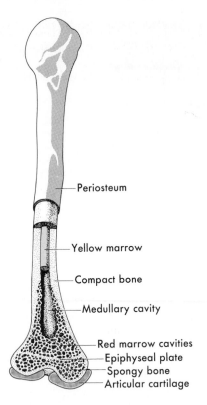

Periosteum

Yellow marrow

Compact bone

Medullary cavity

Red marrow cavities
Epiphyseal plate
Spongy bone
Articular cartilage

Figure 11-2   Anatomic structure of a typical long bone.

A typical long bone consists of the following structures: periosteum, diaphysis, epiphyses, articular cartilage, medullary (or marrow) cavity, and endosteum (Figure 11-2).

The periosteum is the dense, white, fibrous membrane that covers the bone except at the joint surface where the articular cartilage forms a covering. The periosteum contains many blood vessels and osteoblasts, which are bone-forming cells. In children the periosteum produces new bone easily. Because the periosteum regenerates slowly in adults, fractures heal more slowly than in children.

The diaphysis is the main shaftlike portion of the bone.

The epiphyses are cancellous portions with a bulbous shape at the end of the bone.

The articular cartilage covers the articular, or joint, surface of the epiphyses. The resiliency of this cartilage material cushions the bone.

The medullary (marrow) cavity is tubelike and contains marrow.

The endosteum is the membrane that lines the medullary cavity. In long bones the cancellous portions (epiphyses) are found in the ends of the bones. Short bones, flat bones, and irregular bones have an inner portion of cancellous bone covered by an outer portion of compact bone.

Although the size and shape of the 208 bones in the human body vary greatly, bones are all subject to the same disease processes. Fractures, infections (osteomyelitis), tumors (osteogenic sarcoma), congenital defects (ranging from complete absence to extra limbs), demineralization (osteoporosis and osteomalacia), and acquired diseases (e.g., hyperparathyroidism and vitamin D insufficiency or deficiency) may involve and affect any of these bones.

A joint (articulation) exists at the connection of two or more bones. Joints hold the bones firmly to each other and permit movement between them. The three kinds of joints are classified according to their characteristic structural features. The fibrous joints are those in which the articular surface of two bones are joined by fibrous connective tissue, which binds them closely and tightly. They allow only minute motion and provide stability when tight union is necessary (e.g., the sutures joining the skull's cranial bones). Cartilaginous joints are those in which cartilage joins one bone to another. They allow limited movement, such as between the vertebrae. The majority of the body's articulations are synovial, or diarthrodial, joints, which provide free movement between two bones.

Diarthrodial joints have a complex structure to provide mobility (Figure 11-3). Each synovial joint contains a small space called a joint cavity, or *synovial cavity*, between the articulating surfaces of the bones that constitute the joint. The joint capsule completely encases the epiphyses and binds them to each other. Because no tissue grows between the articulating surfaces of the bones, the bones are free to move against each other. For this

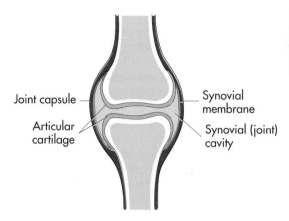

Joint capsule

Articular
cartilage

Synovial
membrane

Synovial (joint)
cavity

Figure 11-3   Structure of a diarthrotic joint.

reason, synovial joints are freely movable joints. The joint capsule is lined with a synovial membrane, which is a moist, slippery membrane that binds the inner surface of the joint capsule. The synovial membrane attaches to the margins of the articular cartilage and secretes synovial fluid, which lubricates and nourishes the inner joint surfaces. The articular cartilage is the hyaline cartilage that covers and cushions the articulating ends of the bones.

Ligaments are strong cords of dense, white, fibrous connective tissue that are present in some synovial joints to provide internal stability. Menisci are small pieces of dense cartilage that may be interposed between the articulating surfaces of two joints. The meniscus of the knee is the most clinically significant cartilage because it is the most frequently injured in athletics.

The synovial membrane may become inflamed, granular, and eventually destroyed by ongoing arthritis. Common forms of arthritis include degenerative, which usually occurs in older age; rheumatoid, which can occur at any age; or infectious, which occurs as a result of direct bacterial contact. Similarly, the components of a joint can be involved in tumors (e.g., synovial cell sarcomas). Because the joints are supported by a series of fibrous ligaments, they can become partially or completely torn (minor or major sprains) when stressed.

Arthrocentesis with Synovial Fluid Analysis (Synovial Fluid Analysis, Joint Aspiration)

Test type Fluid analysis

Normal values
Synovial fluid: clear and straw colored with few white blood cells (WBCs), no crystals, and a good mucin clot
Chemical test values (e.g., glucose determination): approximating those found in the bloodstream

Rationale
Arthrocentesis is performed to diagnose joint infection, arthritis, crystal-induced arthritis (gout and pseudogout), synovitis, or neoplasms involving the joint. This procedure also is used to identify the cause of joint inflammation or effusion, to monitor chronic arthritic diseases, and to inject antiinflammatory medications (usually corticosteroids) into a joint space.

Arthrocentesis is performed by inserting a sterile needle into the joint space of the involved joint to obtain synovial fluid for analysis. Synovial fluid is a liquid found in small amounts within the joints. Aspiration (withdrawal of the fluid) may be performed on any major joint (e.g., the knee, shoulder, hip, elbow, wrist, or ankle).

The fluid sample is examined microscopically and chemically. A culture of the fluid usually is performed. Normal joint fluid is clear, straw-colored, and viscous because of hyaluronic acid, which acts as a lubricant. Viscosity is reduced in patients with inflammatory arthritis. Viscosity can be roughly estimated by forcing some synovial fluid from a syringe. Fluid of high viscosity forms a string several inches long; fluid of low viscosity drips similarly to water. The *mucin clot test* correlates with the viscosity. This test is performed by adding acetic acid to joint fluid. The formation of a tight, ropy clot indicates qualitatively good mucin and the presence of adequate molecules of intact hyaluronic acid.

The synovial fluid glucose value is usually within 10 ml/dl of the serum glucose value. The synovial fluid glucose level decreases with inflammatory or infectious arthritis. Synovial fluid also is tested for protein, uric acid, and lactate levels. Increased uric acid levels indicate gout. Increased protein and lactate levels indicate bacterial infection.

Cell counts also are performed on synovial fluid. Normally, the joint fluid contains less than 200 WBCs/mm^3 and 2000 red blood cells (RBCs)/mm^3. An increased WBC count with a high percentage of neutrophils (greater than 75%) supports the diagnosis of acute bacterial infectious arthritis. Leukocytes also can be present in other conditions (e.g., acute gouty arthritis and rheumatoid arthritis); however, the differential WBC count will indicate monocytosis or lymphocytosis with these diseases.

Bacterial and fungal cultures are usually performed when infection is suspected. Synovial fluid is examined under polarized light for the presence of crystals, permitting differential diagnosis between gout and pseudogout.

The synovial fluid also is analyzed for complement levels (see p. 472). Complement levels are decreased in patients with systemic lupus erythematosus, rheumatoid arthritis, or other immunologic arthritis. These decreased joint complement levels are due to consumption of the complement induced by the antigen-antibody immune complexes within the joint cavity.

One of the most important tests routinely performed on synovial fluid is microscopic examination for crystals. Urate crystals indicate gouty arthritis. Calcium pyrophosphate crystals are found in pseudogout. Cholesterol crystals occur in rheumatoid arthritis.

Potential complications

Potential complications associated with arthrocentesis are as follows:

- Joint infection introduced by the aspirating needle
- Hemorrhage in the joint area from the aspirating needle

Procedure

It is recommended that the patient fast for 6 hours before this test. If the patient does not fast, however, the procedure can still be done, although some of the chemical evaluations (e.g., glucose) may be altered by the food intake.

For an arthrocentesis of the knee, the patient is placed in a supine position, with the knee to be examined fully extended. The knee is locally anesthetized to minimize pain. The area is meticulously cleansed because this procedure requires strict sterile technique. A needle is then inserted through the skin and into the joint space. Fluid is obtained for analysis. Sometimes the joint area may be wrapped with an elastic bandage to compress free fluid into a certain area, enhancing the maximal collection of fluid. If a corticosteroid is to be injected, a syringe containing the steroid preparation is attached to the needle and injected. The needle is then removed. Pressure or a pressure dressing is applied to the site. Sometimes a peripheral venous blood sample is taken after the study to compare chemical tests of the blood with chemical studies of the synovial fluid.

A physician performs this procedure in the office in approximately 10 minutes. The only discomfort is that associated with injection of the local anesthetic.

Contraindications

Arthrocentesis is contraindicated in patients with skin or wound infections in the area of the needle puncture because of the risk of sepsis.

Nursing implications with rationale

Before
- ☞ Explain the procedure to the patient.
- Ensure that written and informed consent for this procedure is obtained.
- ☞ Instruct the patient to remain NPO (*nil per os*, nothing by mouth) from midnight on the day of the test. This prevents alterations of the chemical determinations (e.g., glucose) that may be performed with the study.

After
- Assess the joint for pain, increased warmth, or swelling, which may indicate infection. Apply

ice to decrease pain and swelling. Keep a pressure dressing on the joint.

☞ Instruct the patient that he or she can resume usual activity. Inform the patient, however, to avoid strenuous use of the joint for the next several days.

■ Collect all specimens in the appropriate containers. Send the specimen to the laboratory immediately after the procedure is completed.

Case Study

Knee Injury

M.R., a 15-year-old gymnast, has noted knee pain that has become progressively worse during the past several months of intensive training for a statewide meet. Her physical examination indicated swelling in and around the left knee. She had some decreased range of motion and a clicking sound on flexion of the knee. The knee was otherwise stable.

Studies	Results
Routine laboratory values	Within normal limits (WNL)
Long bone (femur, fibula, and tibia) x-ray, p. 457	No fracture
Arthrocentesis with synovial fluid analysis, p. 449	
Appearance	Bloody (normal: clear and straw-colored)
Mucin clot	Good (normal: good)
Fibrin clot	Small (normal: none)
WBC	<200 WBC/mm^3 (normal: <200 WBC/mm^3)
Neutrophils	$<25\%$ (WNL)
Glucose	100 mg/dl (normal: within 10 mg/dl of serum glucose level)
Magnetic resonance imaging (MRI) of the knee, p. 459	Blood in the joint space. Tear in the posterior aspect of the medial meniscus. No cruciate or other ligament tears
Arthrography, p. 452	Small tear in medial meniscus of left knee
Arthroscopy, p. 453	Tear in posterior aspect of medial meniscus

Diagnostic Analysis

The radiographic studies of the long bones eliminated any possibility of fracture. Arthrocentesis indicated a bloody effusion, which was probably a result of trauma. The fibrin clot was further evidence of bleeding within the joint. Arthrography indicated a tear of the medial meniscus of the knee, a common injury for gymnasts. Arthroscopy corroborated that finding. Transarthroscopic medial meniscectomy was performed. Her postoperative course was uneventful.

Continued

Case Study

Knee Injury—cont'd

Critical Thinking Questions

1. One of the potential complications of arthroscopy is infection. What signs and symptoms of joint infection would you emphasize in your patient teaching?
2. Why is glucose evaluated in the synovial fluid analysis?

Arthrography (Arthrogram)

Test type X-ray

Normal values

Normal bursae, menisci, ligaments, and articular cartilage of the joint

Rationale

Arthrography affords radiographic visualization of a joint after the injection of a radiopaque substance, air, or both into the joint cavity to outline the soft tissue structures not normally seen on routine radiographic films.

Arthrography usually is performed on the knee, hip, and shoulder, as well as many other joints. Bones, menisci, cartilage, and ligaments are clearly visualized with this procedure. Joint derangement and synovial cysts also are diagnosed with arthrography. This procedure is usually performed on patients with persistent, unexplained joint pain, swelling, or dysfunction.

Potential complications

Potential complications associated with arthrography are as follows:

- Infection at the puncture site
- Allergic reaction to the iodinated dye
  This rarely occurs because the dye is not administered intravenously.

Procedure

No fasting or sedation is required for this procedure. It is performed using local anesthesia and sterile technique. The patient is placed in the supine position on an examining table. The skin overlying the desired joint is aseptically cleansed and anesthetized. The needle is then inserted into the joint space, and fluid is aspirated to prevent dilution of the contrast agent and diminished quality of the radiographic films. With the needle still in place, the aspirating syringe is removed and replaced with a syringe containing dye. The contrast agent or agents are then injected. The needle is removed, and the joint is manipulated to distribute the contrast material. (The patient may be asked to walk a few steps or move the joint through a range-of-motion exercise.) Radiographic films are then taken with the joint held in various positions.

A physician usually performs this procedure in approximately 30 minutes. The patient may feel pressure or a tingling sensation as the contrast medium is injected. Some joint inflammation may occur a few days after the procedure.

Contraindications

Contraindications for arthrography are as follows:

- Patients with active arthritis, because the injection may worsen the arthritis
- Patients with joint infection, because the injection may worsen or spread the infection

Nursing implications with rationale

Before
- Explain the procedure to the patient. Tell the patient that no fasting or sedation is necessary.
- Obtain written and informed consent for this procedure.
- Assess the patient for an allergy to iodinated dye.

After
- Inform the patient that the joint is usually rested for at least 12 hours. Apply an elastic

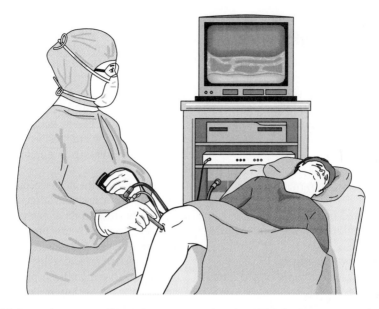

Figure 11-4   Arthroscopy. The arthroscope is placed within the joint space of the knee. Video arthroscopy requires the availability of a water source to distend the joint space, a light source to see the contents of the joint, and a television monitor to project the image. Other trocars are used to access the joint space for insertion of other operative instruments.

bandage to the involved joint and leave it in place for several days.
- If swelling occurs, apply ice to the joint. Administer a mild analgesic (e.g., aspirin or acetaminophen [Tylenol]), if the patient has minor discomfort. Report any increase in pain or swelling to the physician.
- Inform the patient that crepitant noises in the joint may be heard after the test. This is normal and usually stops in 1 to 2 days. The noise is a result of the air that was injected into the joint during the procedure.

Arthroscopy

Test type Endoscopy

Normal values
Normal ligaments, menisci, and articular surfaces of the joint

Rationale
Arthroscopy is an endoscopic procedure that allows examination of a joint space with a specially designed endoscope. Arthroscopy is a highly accurate test because it allows direct visualization of an anatomic site. Although this technique can visualize many joints of the body, it is most often used to evaluate the knee for meniscus cartilage or ligament injury (Figure 11-4). It also is used in the differential diagnosis of acute and chronic disorders of the knee (e.g., arthritic inflammation versus injury).

Physicians can now perform corrective surgery on the knee through the endoscope. Meniscus removal, spur removal, ligamentous repair, and biopsy are only a few of the procedures being done through the arthroscope. Arthroscopy provides a safe, convenient alternative to open surgery (arthrotomy) because surgery is done through small trocars placed into the joint. Surgical maneuvers are carried out under direct vision of a camera, which is attached to the arthroscope. Because a large incision is avoided, recovery is faster and more comfortable.

Arthroscopy also is used to monitor the progression of disease and the effectiveness of therapy. Joints that can be evaluated by the arthroscope include the tarsal, ankle, knee, hip, carpal, wrist, shoulder, and temporomandibular joints.

Potential complications

Potential complications associated with arthroscopy are as follows:

- Infection, introduced by the procedure
- Hemarthrosis (bleeding into the joint), caused by the aspirating needle
- Swelling, induced by the surgery
- Thrombophlebitis, caused by prolonged immobilization
- Joint injury, caused by unsuccessful surgery
- Synovial rupture at the site of trocar placement

Procedure

The patient should be kept NPO after midnight on the day of the procedure. It commonly is performed using spinal or general anesthesia, especially when knee surgery is anticipated. Knee arthroscopy will be described as a typical arthroscopic procedure.

Before knee arthroscopy, the patient's body hair is removed 6 inches above and below the joint, either by shaving or using a depilatory creme. The patient is placed in a supine position on an operating table. The patient's leg is surgically scrubbed, elevated, and wrapped with an elastic bandage from the toes to the lower thigh to drain as much blood from the leg as possible. A tourniquet is then placed on the patient's leg. If a tourniquet is not used, a solution may be instilled into the patient's knee immediately before insertion of the arthroscope to distend the knee and help reduce bleeding.

The foot of the table is lowered so that the patient's knee is approximately at a 45-degree angle. The elastic bandage is opened. A small skin incision is made, and the arthroscope is inserted in the joint space to visualize the inside of the knee

joint. Although the entire joint can be viewed from one puncture site, making additional punctures for better visualization often is necessary. The accessory trocars are also used for placement of operative instruments. After the area is examined and surgery is performed, the arthroscope is removed. The joint is then irrigated. Pressure is applied to the knee to remove the irrigating solution. After a few stitches are placed into the skin, a pressure dressing is applied over the incision site.

This procedure is performed in an operating room by an orthopedic surgeon in approximately 30 minutes to 2 hours. If extensive orthopedic surgery is performed, the procedure could take as long as 4 hours. Patients receiving local anesthesia experience transient discomfort from injection of the anesthetic and the pressure of the tourniquet on the leg. A thumping sensation may be felt as the arthroscope is inserted into the joint. There is moderate joint pain postoperatively, depending on what procedure was done.

Contraindications

Contraindications for arthroscopy are as follows:

- Patients with ankylosis, because it is almost impossible to maneuver the instrument into a joint stiffened by adhesions
- Patients with local skin or wound infections, because of the risk of sepsis
- Patients who have recently had an arthrogram, because they will have some residual inflammation subsequent to injection of the contrast dye

Nursing implications with rationale

Before

- Explain this procedure to the patient. Follow the routine preoperative procedure. Instruct the patient to remain NPO after midnight on the day of the procedure.
- Ensure that the physician has obtained written and informed consent.
- Instruct the patient regarding how to perform the appropriate crutch gait, if ordered by the surgeon.

Crutches usually should be used after arthroscopy until the patient can walk without limping. Whether the patient can walk with crutches, however, depends on the extent of the procedure and the physician's protocol.

After

- Assess the vital signs frequently according to hospital routine. Assess the neurovascular status of the affected leg by checking pulses, color, temperature, and sensation.
- Observe the patient for signs of infection, which include fever, swelling, increased pain, and redness or drainage at the incision site. Administer a mild analgesic (e.g., aspirin or acetaminophen), if needed.
- Instruct the patient to elevate the knee when sitting and to avoid twisting the knee.
- Instruct the patient to avoid excessive use of the joint for several days. Also, instruct the patient to perform isometric quadriceps exercises according to the physician's protocol.
- Examine the incision site for bleeding; apply ice to reduce pain and swelling.
- Inform the patient that the sutures will be removed in approximately 7 days.

Bone Densitometry (Bone Mineral Content [BMC], Bone Absorptiometry, Bone Mineral Density [BMD])

Test type X-ray

Normal values
Normal: <1.0 standard deviation below normal (>−1.0)
Osteopenia: 1.0-2.5 standard deviations below normal (−1.0 to −2.5)
Osteoporosis: >2.5 standard deviations below normal (<−2.5)

Rationale
Bone densitometry studies determine bone mineral content (BMC) and density in order to diagnose osteoporosis. *Osteoporosis* and *osteopenia* are terms used to describe bone that becomes weakened and fractures easily. This most commonly occurs in postmenopausal women. However, other diseases are associated with osteoporosis (e.g., renal failure, hyperparathyroidism, prolonged immobility.) Vertebral and hip fractures are consequences of osteoporosis. Approximately 20% of patients over age 65 will die within 1 year of their hip fracture.

Methods to identify the early stages of osteoporosis have become available. The earlier osteoporosis is recognized, the more effective the treatment will be. If the diagnosis of osteoporosis is delayed until fractures occur or plain film x-rays identify "thin" bones, the success of treatment is less likely.

The diagnosis of osteoporosis should lead to aggressive medical therapy, which can be expensive and not without risks. Therefore the diagnosis of osteoporosis must be made based on accurate data. Bone densitometry was developed to provide accurate and precise measurement of bone strength based on bone density. Several groups of bones are routinely evaluated because they accurately represent the entire skeleton. The lumbar spine is the most representative of cancellous bone. The radius is the most easily studied cortical bone. The proximal hip (neck of the femur) is the most representative of cancellous/cortical-mixed bone.

The two methods of determining bone density are single-photon densitometry (absorptiometry) and dual-energy densitometry (absorptiometry). With these techniques, one or two radioactive radionuclides (photon emitters) are placed in a tube and passed over the bony area to be studied. A photon detector is placed on the opposite side of the bone. The greater the density of the bone, the fewer the number of photons that reach the detector. The relative absorption is calibrated to express bone mineral and mass per unit length of bone (gm/cm). Dual-energy x-ray absorptiometry (DEXA) uses x-rays in place of the radionuclide to provide two different x-ray energies that produce dual photons in the x-ray spectrum.

Patients whose values are between 0.8 and 0.99 g/cm^2 have a 20% or less chance of developing a spontaneous fracture, whereas patients with a value of less than 0.62 g/cm^2 have nearly a 100% chance of developing a spontaneous fracture. Usually, bone density is reported in terms of standard deviations (SDs) from mean values. T scores compare the patient's results to a group of healthy young adults. Z scores compare the patient's results to a group of age-matched controls. T scores are probably more accurate in predictive value of fracture risk. The World Health Organization has defined osteopenia as bone density value greater than 1 SD below peak bone mass levels of young women and osteoporosis as a value of greater than 2.5 SDs below that same measurement scale. Most clinicians believe that therapeutic intervention should occur in patients with osteopenia to prevent its progression to osteoporosis.

Interfering factors

Factors that interfere with bone densitometry studies include the following:

- Barium, which may falsely *increase* the density of the lumbar spine
  Bone density measurements should not be performed for approximately 10 days after barium studies.
- Posterior vertebral calcific, arthritic sclerosis, which can falsely *increase* bone density of the spine
- Calcified abdominal aortic aneurysm, which may falsely *increase* bone density of the spine
- Overlying metal jewelry or other objects, which may falsely *increase* bone density
- Previous bone fractures
  Healed fracture sites can falsely *increase* bone density.
- Patients who have had previous abdominal surgery
  The metallic clips placed in the vertebral plane can falsely *increase* bone density.
- Recent bone scans, which can falsely *decrease* bone density
  The photons generated from the bone (as a result of the previously administered bone scan radionuclide) will be detected by the scintillator detector.

Procedure

The machine is usually calibrated by the x-ray or nuclear medicine technician before the patient's arrival. No fasting or sedation is required. The patient lies on an imaging table, with his or her legs supported on a padded box to flatten the pelvis and lumbar spine. A photon generator located beneath the table is slowly passed under the lumbar spine. A gamma or x-ray detector/camera located above the table is passed over the patient in a manner parallel to the generator. An image of the lumbar and hip bone is obtained by the scintillator camera and projected via a computer monitor.

Next, the foot is inserted into a brace that internally rotates the nondominant hip, and the imaging procedure is repeated over the hip. A similar procedure is performed for evaluation of the radius. When the radius is examined, the nondominant arm is preferred, unless there is a history of fracture to that bone. On the computer screen, a small window of the lumbar spine, femoral neck, or distal radius is drawn. The computer calculates the amount of photons not absorbed by the bone. This is called the *bone mineral content (BMC)*. Bone mineral density (BMD) is computed as follows:

$$BMD = \frac{BMC(gm/cm^2)}{\text{Surface area of the bone}}$$

The data are interpreted by a radiologist or a physician trained in nuclear medicine. Bone density studies require approximately 30 to 45 minutes to perform and cause no discomfort. Minimal radiation exposure (less than that of a chest x-ray) occurs with this procedure. Future advances in bone densitometry will be directed toward reducing the time involved to perform the study.

Nursing implications with rationale

Before

- Explain the procedure to the patient. Tell the patient that no fasting or sedation is necessary.
- Instruct the patient to remove all metallic objects (e.g., belt buckles, zippers, coins, keys) that might be in the scanning path.

Case Study

Osteoporosis

J.K. is a 60-year-old, thin woman who, while walking, experienced sudden pain in her right hip and fell to the ground. On admission to the emergency room, her only abnormality on physical examination was pain with motion of the right hip and an internally rotated and shortened right leg.

Studies	Result
Routine laboratory values	WNL
X-ray of the right hip, p. 457	Fracture of the neck of the hip. Significant bone thinning noted.

Diagnostic Analysis

J.K. had a hip fracture, based on her clinical findings and x-rays. Her hip did not fracture because of the fall, but rather she fell as a result of her hip fracture. Her bones were very weak. In light of her thin body habitus and postmenopausal state, she probably had osteoporosis. J.K. underwent an open reduction and fixation of the hip. She recovered well and later underwent an evaluation for her bone thinning.

Studies	Result
Bone densitometry, p. 455	Bone density is <2.5 SDs below normal (normal: <1.0 SD below normal)
Parathyroid hormone assay, p. 324	22 pg/ml (normal: 10-65 pg/ml)

Diagnostic Analysis

J.K. had osteoporosis. She had no evidence of hyperparathyroidism, renal failure, or other problems. She was started on hormone replacement therapy (estrogen/progesterone) and alendronate (Fosamax). J.K. had no further bone fractures.

Critical Thinking Questions

1. How does the parathyroid hormone assay relate to the differential diagnosis of J.K.'s problem?
2. Why was renal failure a consideration in this case situation?

Bone, X-rays

Test type X-ray

Normal values

No evidence of fracture, tumor, infection, or congenital abnormalities

Rationale

This x-ray is performed on any bone to evaluate a patient for fracture, bone infection, arthritis, tendinitis, or bone spurs. Bone age can be determined in children in order to evaluate growth and development. Tumors (primary and metastatic) can be identified. Osteoporosis in the advanced stage also can be detected.

Radiographic films of the long bones are usually taken when the patient has complaints about a particular body area. Fractures or tumors are readily detected by radiographic studies (Figure 11-5). A severe or chronic infection overlying a bone (osteomyelitis) may be detected by a radiographic film. Radiographic studies of the long bones also can detect joint destruction and bone spurring as a result of persistent arthritis. Growth patterns can be followed by serial radiographic studies of long bones, usually the wrists and hands. Healing of a fracture also can be documented and monitored. Radiographic films of the joints can reveal the presence of joint effusions and soft tissue swelling. Calcifications in the soft tissue indicate chronic inflammatory changes of the nearby bursae or tendons. Because the cartilage and tendons are not directly visualized by radiographic films, cartilage fractures, sprains, or ligamentous injuries cannot be seen.

At least two x-rays at 90-degree angles are required so that the bone region being studied can

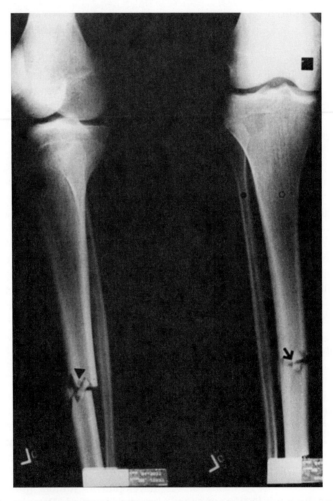

Figure 11-5 X-ray film of tibia and fibula. Left side of photograph is lateral view of tibia and fibula. Solid pointer indicates fracture. Right side of photograph indicates the same patient with a posteroanterior view. Solid square indicates distal femur. Solid circle indicates fibula. Circle outline indicates tibia. Arrow indicates anteroposterior view of tibial fracture.

be visualized from two different angles (usually anterior to posterior and lateral). Some bone studies (e.g., skull, spine, hip) require oblique views to visualize all the parts that need to be seen.

Interfering factors

Factors that interfere with bone x-rays include the following:

■ Jewelry or clothing, which can obstruct radiographic visualization of part of the bone to be evaluated
■ Prior barium studies
These can diminish the full radiographic visualization of some of the bones surrounding the abdomen (e.g., spine and pelvis).

Procedure

No fasting or sedation is required before radiographic examination of the long bones. This test is routinely performed in the radiology department by an x-ray technician in several minutes. The patient is asked to place the involved extremity in several positions; an x-ray image is taken in each position. No discomfort or complications are associated with this test.

Nursing implications with rationale

Before

☞ Explain the procedure to the patient. Tell the patient that no fasting or sedation is necessary.
■ Handle carefully any injured parts of the body.
☞ Instruct the patient to hold the extremity still while the radiographic films are being taken. This can be difficult if the patient has severe pain associated with a recent injury.
■ Shield the patient's testes, ovaries, or pregnant abdomen during the procedure to avoid exposure from scattered radiation.
☞ Inform the patient that although no pain is associated with these radiographic examinations, many patients (especially those with arthritis) are extremely uncomfortable lying on the hard x-ray table.
■ Note that young children requiring radiographic examinations are usually frightened by the large equipment and the practice of be-

ing isolated from their parents. Check the radiology department's policy on allowing parents (protected with lead shielding) to accompany the child during the procedure.

After

■ No special aftercare is necessary. Provide pain relief if indicated.

Magnetic Resonance Imaging (MRI) of Bones and Joints

Test type Magnetic field study

Normal values

No evidence of bone or joint pathology

Rationale

The indications for MRI scanning continue to expand as this relatively new technique evolves (see discussion of central nervous system [CNS] MRI on p. 213). Patients with neck and back pain can be evaluated with MRI for disk herniation. The bones and joints (especially of the knees) can be evaluated with MRI after traumatic injury or for chronic pain.

MRI is a noninvasive diagnostic scanning technique that provides valuable information about the bones and joints by placing the patient in a magnetic field. The unique feature of MRI is that it does not require exposure to ionizing radiation.

An important advantage of MRI is that serial studies can be performed on the patient without risk of radiation exposure. Abnormalities of the bones, cartilage, ligaments, and tendons can be recognized. MRI is useful in assessing the response to corrective orthopedic surgery. It also is helpful in monitoring arthritic joint deterioration. The increased use of MRI in orthopedics has replaced the need for arthrography, in most instances, and diagnostic arthroscopy, in some instances.

Procedure

No fluid or food restrictions are necessary before MRI. The patient lies on a platform that slides into a tube containing the doughnut-shaped magnet.

To visualize an extremity, only that extremity needs to be inside the MRI tube; the rest of the patient's body can remain outside the tube. The patient is instructed to be very still during the procedure.

MRI is performed by a qualified radiologic technologist in approximately 30 to 90 minutes. The only discomfort associated with this procedure may be that of lying still on a hard surface and a possible tingling sensation in teeth containing metal fillings. Some patients may experience claustrophobia while they are in the tubelike MRI unit. This claustrophobia is minimized with the newer, more open machines.

Contraindications

Contraindications for MRI are as follows:

- Patients who are extremely obese (weighing more than 300 pounds), because the table will not support the weight
- Patients with implanted metal objects (e.g., pacemakers, infusion pumps, aneurysm clips, inner ear implants, and metal fragments in one or both eyes), because the magnet may move the object within the body and injure the patient. Patients with orthopedic screws and plates are not affected by MRI.

Nursing implications with rationale

Before

- ☞ Explain the procedure to the patient. Inform the patient that no radiation exposure occurs.
- Obtain written and informed consent, if required by the institution.
- Assess the patient for any contraindications for testing (e.g., aneurysm clips).
- ☞ Instruct the patient to remove all metal objects (e.g., dental bridges, jewelry, hair clips, belts, credit cards) because they will create artifacts on the scan. The magnetic field can damage watches and credit cards.
- ☞ Inform the patient that he or she will be required to remain motionless during this study. Any movement can distort the scan. Young children are often sedated for this procedure.
- ☞ Inform the patient that he or she may hear a

thumping sound during the test. Earplugs and music are available.
- ☞ For comfort, instruct the patient to empty his or her bladder before this test.

Uric Acid

Test type Blood

Normal values
Blood:
Elderly: values may be slightly increased
  Adult:
    Male: 2.1-8.5 mg/dl or 0.15-0.48 mmol/L
    Female: 2.0-6.6 mg/dl or 0.09-0.36 mmol/L
Child: 2.5-5.5 mg/dl or 0.12-0.32 mmol/L
Newborn: 2.0-6.2 mg/dl
Urine: 250-750 mg/day or 1.48-4.43 mmol/day (SI units)

Possible critical values Blood: >12 mg/dl

Rationale

Uric acid levels can be measured in both the blood and urine. Uric acid is a nitrogenous compound that is the final breakdown product of purine (a deoxyribonucleic acid [DNA] building block) catabolism. Seventy-five percent of uric acid is excreted by the kidney and 25% by the intestinal tract. When uric acid levels are elevated (hyperuricemia), the patient may have gout. Gout is associated with arthritis caused by deposition of uric acid crystals in periarticular tissue. Soft tissue deposits of uric acid also can occur and are called *tophi.* Uric acid can become supersaturated in the urine and crystalizes to form kidney stones, which can block the ureters.

Uric acid is mostly produced in the liver. The uric acid blood level reflects the rate of synthesis by the liver combined with the rate of excretion by the kidney. Causes of hyperuricemia can be overproduction or decreased excretion of uric acid (e.g., kidney failure). Overproduction of uric acid may occur in patients with a catabolic enzyme deficiency that promotes purine catabolism or in patients with cancer, in whom purine and DNA turnover is great. Many causes of hyperuricemia are undefined and therefore labeled as *idiopathic*.

Interfering factor

A factor that interferes with determining uric acid levels includes high protein infusion (especially glycine) related to total parenteral nutrition. This may *increase* uric acid because it is a breakdown product of glycine.

Procedure

The blood test is usually included in any multiphasic, automated systems analysis of the blood. Some laboratories require that the patient be fasting. Usually for these multiphasic analysis studies, two red-top tubes of blood are obtained from a peripheral vein. Urine studies require the collection of a 24-hour urine specimen.

Nursing implications with rationale

Before

☞ Explain the procedure to the patient. Follow the laboratory requirements regarding fasting.

During

■ The **blood** test requires approximately 5 to 7 ml of venous blood. Prevent hemolysis of the blood sample.

☞ Instruct the patient to begin the 24-hour **urine** collection after discarding the first morning specimen. This is the start time of the 24-hour collection.

■ Collect all urine passed over the next 24 hours.

☞ Instruct the patient to void before defecating so that the urine is not contaminated by feces.

■ Remind the patient not to put toilet paper in the urine collection container.

■ Keep the urine specimen on ice or refrigerated during the 24-hour collection period.

■ Collect the last urine specimen as close as possible to the end of the 24 hours.

After

■ Apply pressure or a pressure dressing to the venipuncture site to prevent further bleeding. Observe the site for further bleeding.

■ Transport the urine specimen promptly to the laboratory.

☞ If the uric acid levels are high, instruct the patient to avoid foods high in purine (e.g., liver, kidney, heart, brain, sweetbreads, sardines, anchovies, and mincemeat). Foods that contain a moderate amount of purine nitrogens include poultry, fish, asparagus, mushrooms, peas, and spinach.

☞ Instruct patients with elevated uric acid levels to decrease their alcohol intake because alcohol causes renal retention of urate.

REVIEW QUESTIONS AND ANSWERS

1. **Question:** Mr. and Mrs. P. brought their crying 3-year-old daughter into the emergency room because she fell off a seesaw and landed on her shoulder. Because of the child's complaints of pain in the clavicular area, a fractured clavicle was the suspected diagnosis. The child was extremely frightened by the thought of a radiographic examination, and Mrs. P. insisted on accompanying her daughter during the procedure. What is the appropriate intervention in this situation?

   Answer: Because of exposure from scattered radiation during the radiographic procedure, you should first assess whether Mrs. P. is pregnant. If she is not currently menstruating, you should suggest that Mr. P. don a lead apron and accompany his daughter during this procedure.

2. **Question:** Your 17-year-old male patient is scheduled for a knee arthroscopy in the morning. When you go into his room to shave the knee 6 inches above and below the joint, you note that the knee is red and swollen. Should the arthroscopy be canceled?

   Answer: Notify the physician. The procedure may be canceled because of the possibility of infection in the knee, which is a contraindication to arthroscopy because of the possibility of sepsis.

3. **Question:** Your 62-year-old female patient underwent an arthrocentesis of her right knee

and an injection of steroids 2 days ago. She now complains of pain in the right knee, which she describes as worse than the initial symptoms. What is the appropriate nursing intervention?

Answer: Severe pain 48 hours after arthrocentesis is unusual. With the injection of steroids, however, a temporary chemical arthritis frequently occurs. This often lasts 1 to 3 days. The patient should be reassured of this possibility, and the physician should be contacted to prescribe an appropriate pain medication.

4. **Question:** Your 55-year-old male patient was admitted to the hospital with complaints of a fever of unknown etiology. Initial physician orders called for blood, urine, and sputum cultures. During your nursing history, you detected that the patient had an arthrogram 3 days ago because of complaints of unexplained shoulder pain. What is the appropriate intervention?

Answer: Septic arthritis is a known complication of arthrography. Notify the physician of the patient's recent arthrogram. The physician will probably order an arthrocentesis to identify the causative agent. The infection is then treated with the appropriate antibiotic.

5. **Question:** Your 5-year-old patient fell during play therapy and injured his right arm. You notify the physician, who requests a radiographic examination of both arms. Why should both arms be included in the radiographic examination?

Answer: Fracture lines of the long bones in children are often difficult to distinguish from normal growth lines in radiographic film. If the suspicious line is seen in the film of both arms, one can be confident that a fracture did not occur. However, if the suspicious line is unilateral, a fracture is strongly suspected.

Bibliography

Abbott AV: Common sports injuries. In Rakel RE, editor: Conn's current therapy, Philadelphia, 1998, WB Saunders.

Arnett FC: Rheumatoid arthritis. In Wyngaarden JB et al, editors: Cecil textbook of medicine, ed 19, Philadelphia, 1992, WB Saunders.

Aspelin P: Ultrasound examination of soft tissue injury of the lower limb in athletes, Am J Sports Med 20(5):601-603, 1992.

Baum J, Morris Z: Laboratory findings in rheumatoid arthritis. In McCarty DJ, editor: Arthritis and allied conditions: a textbook of rheumatology, ed 11, Philadelphia, 1989, Lea and Febiger.

Bellamy N, Buchanan W: Clinical evaluation in rheumatic diseases. In McCarty DJ: Arthritis and allied conditions: a textbook of rheumatology, ed 11, Philadelphia, 1989, Lea and Febiger.

Brandt KD: Osteomyelitis. In Fauci AS et al, editors: Harrison's principles of internal medicine, ed 14, New York, 1998, McGraw-Hill.

Brower AC: Septic arthritis, Radiol Clin North Am 34:293, 1996.

Cush JJ, Lipsky PE: Approaches to articular and musculoskeletal disorders. In Fauci AS et al, editors: Harrison's principles of internal medicine, ed 14, New York, 1998, McGraw-Hill.

Eustace SJ et al: Lyme arthropathy, Radiol Clin North Am 34:454, 1996.

Evans J: Lyme disease, Curr Opin Rheumatol 7:322, 1995.

Fries JF: Approach to the patient with musculoskeletal disease. In Wyngaarden JB et al, editors: Cecil textbook of medicine, ed 19, Philadelphia, 1992, WB Saunders.

Gentry LO: Osteomyelitis. In Rakel RE, editor: Conn's current therapy, Philadelphia, 1998, WB Saunders.

Goldenberg DL: Bacterial arthritis, Curr Opin Rheumatol 7:310, 1995.

Hahn BH: Osteopenic bone diseases. In Koopman WJ, editor: Arthritis and allied conditions, ed 13, Baltimore, 1997, Williams and Wilkins.

Jenkins DB: Hollinshead's functional anatomy of the limbs and back, ed 6, Philadelphia, 1991, WB Saunders.

Kalunian KC et al: Arthroscopy. In Koopman WJ, editor: Arthritis and allied conditions, ed 13, Baltimore, 1997, Williams and Wilkins.

Kelly WN: Textbook of rheumatology, ed 5, Philadelphia, 1997, WB Saunders.

Koopman WJ: Arthritis and allied conditions, ed 13, Baltimore, 1997, Williams and Wilkins.

Krane SM, Holic MF: Metabolic bone disease. In Fauci AS et al, editors: Harrison's principles of internal medicine, ed 14, New York, 1998, McGraw-Hill.

Macfarlane DG et al: Comparison of clinical, radionuclide, and radiographic features of osteoarthritis of the hands, Ann Rheum Dis 50(9):623-626, 1991.

Malawista SE: Lyme disease. In McCarty DJ: Arthritis and allied conditions: a textbook of rheumatology, ed 11, Philadelphia, 1989, Lea and Febiger.

Marino C et al: Osteoarthritis and rheumatoid arthritis in elderly patients: differentiation and treatment, Postgrad Med 90(5):237-243, 1991.

Maskowitz RW: Clinical and laboratory findings in osteoarthritis. In McCarty DJ: Arthritis and allied conditions: a textbook of rheumatology, ed 11, Philadelphia, 1989, Lea and Febiger.

McCarty DJ: Differential diagnosis of arthritis: analysis of signs and symptoms. In Koopman WJ, editor: Arthritis and allied conditions, ed 13, Baltimore, 1997, Williams and Wilkins.

McCarty DJ: Synovial fluid. In Koopman WJ, editor: Arthritis and allied conditions, ed 13, Baltimore, 1997, Williams and Wilkins.

Miller PD et al: Clinical utility of bone mass measurements in adults: consensus of an international panel, *Semin Arthritis Rheum* 25(6):361-372, 1996.

Mitlak BH, Nussbaum SR: Diagnosis and treatment of osteoporosis, *Annu Rev Med* 44:265-277, 1993.

Mussolino ME et al: Phalangeal bone density and hip fracture risk, *Arch Intern Med* 157(4):433-438, 1997.

Neustadt DH: Osteoarthritis. In Rakel RE, editor: Conn's current therapy, Philadelphia, 1998, WB Saunders.

Pagana KD, Pagana TJ: Mosby's manual of diagnostic and laboratory tests, St. Louis, 1998, Mosby.

Sharp JT: Rheumatoid arthritis. In Rakel RE, editor: Conn's current therapy, Philadelphia, 1998, WB Saunders.

Stalberg E: The value to the clinical neurologist of electromyography in the 1990s, *Clin Exp Neurol* 27:1-28, 1990.

Stoller DW, Genant HK: Magnetic resonance imaging of the joints. In McCarty DJ, editor: Arthritis and allied conditions: a textbook of rheumatology, ed 11, Philadelphia, 1989, Lea and Febiger.

Swezey RL et al: Bone densitometry: comparison of dual energy x-ray absorptiometry to radiographic absorptiometry, *J Rheumatol* 23(10):1734-38, 1996.

Chapter 12

Diagnostic Studies Used in the Assessment of the
Immune System

ANATOMY AND PHYSIOLOGY

The immune system comprises the various physiologic mechanisms involved in recognizing antigens as foreign bodies and eliminating or neutralizing them. Serologic tests are used to diagnose and monitor immune system diseases, all of which are associated with the production of antibodies directed against body components. The diseases associated with antibodies directed against connective tissue are called *connective tissue* or *collagen vascular diseases.* They also are referred to as *rheumatic diseases* because musculoskeletal pain is a frequent symptom manifestation.

Rheumatology is the study of joints and periarticular structures. Immunology is the study of the processes involved in the recognition and protection of the body from foreign, noxious elements. The immunologic system includes cells such as thymus-derived (T) and bone marrow-derived (B) lymphocytes, plasma cells, and other white blood cells (WBCs). Noncellular components (e.g., antibodies and the complement enzymatic system) are vitally important in the immunologic response. Systemic lupus erythematosus (SLE) and rheumatoid arthritis (RA) are the more common types of rheumatologic/immunologic diseases and are discussed in the case studies. Many other diseases exist that are marked by the presence of antibodies, which may cause false-positive serologic tests. These other diseases must be evaluated by other appropriate diagnostic testing. Many variations occur in the normal immunologic processes. Descriptions of these are beyond the scope of this text.

Agglutinins, Febrile/Cold

Test type Blood

Normal values
Febrile (warm) agglutinins: no agglutination in titers $\leq 1:80$
Cold agglutinins: no agglutination in titers $\leq 1:16$

Rationale
Febrile and cold agglutinins are antibodies that cause red blood cells (RBCs) to aggregate at high or low temperatures, respectively. It is believed they are caused by infectious organisms having antigenic groups similar to some of those found on the RBCs. Normally, agglutination may occur in concentrated serum (less than $1:32$ dilution).

Febrile agglutinin serologic studies are used to diagnose infectious diseases such as salmonellosis, rickettsiosis, brucellosis, and tularemia. Neoplastic diseases, such as leukemia, are also associated with febrile agglutinins. Appropriate antibiotic treatment of the infectious agent is associated with a drop in the titer activity of febrile agglutinins. *Cold agglutinins* occur in patients who are infected by other agents, most notably *Mycoplasma pneumoniae.* Influenza, mononucleosis, RA, lymphoma, and hemolytic anemia are also associated with cold agglutinins.

Agglutination occurring at titers greater than $1:16$ for cold agglutinins and $1:80$ for febrile agglutinins is considered abnormal and diagnostic of the infectious agent or disease with which the agglutinins are associated. When agglutinins exist in high titers, they can attack RBCs and cause hemolytic anemias. Cold agglutinins often are obtained during the suspected acute phase of the disease and are repeated during the convalescence phase (7 to 10 days later). A fourfold or higher increase in antibody titer is considered diagnostic for the associated infectious disease. Titer elevation is directly related to severity of infection.

Interfering factors
Factors that interfere with determining agglutinin titers include some antibiotics (penicillin and cephalosporins), which can interfere with the development of cold agglutinins.

Procedure
Venipuncture is performed, and 7 ml of blood is collected in a red-top tube. Before obtaining the cold-agglutinin specimen, the red-top tube is warmed to a temperature above 37° C; for the febrile-agglutinin specimen, the red-top tube is cooled. The specimen is taken immediately to the

laboratory to prevent hemolysis. Before arrival in the laboratory, the cold-agglutinin specimen should not be refrigerated; the febrile-agglutinin specimen should not be heated.

Once in the laboratory, the cold-agglutinin specimen is chilled and then evaluated for agglutination. The febrile-agglutinin specimen is heated and inspected for agglutination. Serial dilutions are performed to detect agglutination titers.

The only discomfort associated with this test is that of the venipuncture.

Nursing implications with rationale

Before

☞ Explain the procedure to the patient. Tell the patient that no fasting is required.

■ Note that temperature regulation is important for performing these tests. For cold-agglutinin testing, the red-top tube is warmed to above 37° C before obtaining the specimen; for febrile-agglutinin testing, the red-top tube is cooled.

After

■ Apply pressure or a pressure dressing to the venipuncture site to prevent further bleeding. Observe the site for bleeding.

■ Ensure that the specimen is taken immediately to the laboratory so that no hemolysis will occur. Avoid refrigeration of the cold-agglutinin specimen or warming of the febrile-agglutinin specimen. Ensure that the patient has not been exposed to marked abnormalities in temperature, which may affect the agglutination testing.

Acquired Immunodeficiency Syndrome Serology (AIDS Serology, AIDS Screen, Human Immunodeficiency Virus [HIV] Antibody Test, Western Blot Test for HIV and Antibody, Enzyme-linked Immunosorbent Assay [ELISA] for HIV and Antibody)

Test type Blood

Normal values

No evidence of HIV antigen or antibodies

Rationale

Acquired immunodeficiency syndrome (AIDS) serology tests are used to detect the antibody to HIV, the virus that causes AIDS. HIV is also known as *human T-lymphotrophic virus, type III (HTLV-III)*, or *lymphadenopathy-associated virus (LAV)*. There are two types of HIV. Type 1 is most prevalent in the United States and western Europe; type 2 is primarily limited to western African nations.

Persons at high risk for AIDS include sexually active male homosexuals and bisexual men and women with multiple partners, intravenous (IV) drug abusers, persons receiving blood products containing HIV, and infants exposed to the virus during gestation and delivery.

Because of the medical and social significance of a positive test for HIV antibody, test results and interpretation must be accurate. Therefore the United States Public Health Service has emphasized that an individual is considered to have serologic evidence of HIV infection only after an enzyme immunoassay (EIA) screening test is repeatedly reactive, and another test (e.g., Western blot or immunofluorescence assay) validates the results. However, a positive EIA result that is not confirmed by Western blot or immunofluorescence assay should not be considered negative. Repeat testing is required in 3 to 6 months. A person with a positive HIV test result does not have AIDS until the clinical criteria for that disease syndrome are fulfilled.

The enzyme-linked immunosorbent assay (ELISA) tests for antibodies to HIV in serum or plasma. Because it does not detect viral antigens, it cannot detect infection in its earliest stage, before antibodies are formed.

The sensitivity (i.e., the probability that the test result will be reactive if the specimen is a true positive) of the ELISA test is approximately 99% for blood from persons infected with HIV for 12 weeks or longer. The probability of a false-negative test is remote, except during the first few weeks after infection, before detectable antibodies appear.

The ELISA test detects HIV infection based on demonstration of antibodies to HIV. Recently it has become possible to diagnose HIV infection by direct detection of HIV or one of its components. The simplest of these tests is the *p24 antigen* capture assay. The p24 antigen may be detectable as early as 2 to 6 weeks after infection.

HIV home testing kits are now available. Advantages of home testing include specimen collection done in the privacy of one's home, anonymous test registration, laboratory processing, and pre- and posttest counseling, which is available via a toll-free telephone call.

Interfering factors

Factors that interfere with determining AIDS serology results include the following:

- Autoimmune disease, lymphoproliferative disease, leukemia, lymphoma, syphilis, or alcoholism
  False-positive results can occur in these diseases.
- Early incubation stage or end-stage AIDS
  Because false-negative results can occur, tests for HIV antigens should be performed at this stage.

Procedure

Many states have requirements for preserving the confidentiality of tests results. Informed patient consent also is required. No food or fluid restrictions are necessary. Peripheral venipuncture is performed, and 7 ml of blood is collected in a red-top tube. If the ELISA results are repeatedly reactive (two consecutive positive results), the Western blot test is performed on the same blood sample. If the ELISA results have been repeatedly reactive and the Western blot result is equivocal, a second serum specimen should be collected and tested in 2 to 4 months.

Nursing implications with rationale

Before

- ☞ Explain the procedure to the patient. Tell the patient that no fasting is required.
- Follow institution guidelines concerning confidentiality and informed consent.
- Most patients are extremely anxious regarding the need for the test. Maintain a nonjudgmental demeanor and allow the patient ample time to express his or her feelings.
- Observe universal blood and body precautions. Gloves should be worn when handling blood products. Cuts on the hands can serve as sites for entry of the virus.

After

- Apply pressure or a pressure dressing to the venipuncture site to prevent further bleeding. Observe the site for bleeding.
- Follow institution policy regarding test results. Results are not given over the telephone. Positive results for many patients may jeopardize employment and medical insurance coverage.
- ☞ If test results are positive, explain to the patient that this implies exposure to and probably presence of the virus in the body. Positive results do not indicate the patient has AIDS because not all patients with positive antibodies acquire the disease.
- Assess the patient for symptoms of AIDS, which include fever, fatigue, weight loss, anorexia, diarrhea, swollen neck glands, and night sweats.
- ☞ Encourage a patient with positive HIV results to identify all sexual contacts so they can be informed and tested. Confirm that the patient understands unprotected sexual contact puts sexual partners at high risk for contracting HIV.

Case Study

AIDS

S.Z., a 30-year-old homosexual man, complained of unexplained weight loss, chronic diarrhea, and respiratory congestion during the past 6 months. Physical examination revealed no evidence of Kaposi's sarcoma. The following studies were performed:

Continued

Case Study

AIDS—cont'd

Studies	Results
Complete blood count (CBC), p. 412	
Hemoglobin	12 g/dl (normal: 14-18 g/dl)
Hematocrit	36% (normal: 42%-52%)
Bronchoscopy, p. 71	*Pneumocystis carinii* pneumonia (PCP)
Stool culture, p. 89	*Cryptosporidium muris*
AIDS serology, p. 466	
p24 antigen	Positive
ELISA	Positive
Western blot	Positive
Lymphocyte immunophenotyping, p. 483	
Total CD4	280 (normal: 600-1500 cells/μl)
CD4%	18% (normal: 60%-75%)
CD4/CD8 ratio	0.58 (normal: >1.0)

Diagnostic Analysis

The bronchoscopic detection of *Pneumocystis carinii* pneumonia (PCP) confirmed the suspected diagnosis of AIDS. PCP is an opportunistic infection occurring only in immunocompromised patients and is the most common infection in persons with AIDS. S.Z.'s diarrhea was caused by *Cryptosporidium muris,* an enteric pathogen, which occurs frequently with AIDS and can be identified on a stool culture. The AIDS serology tests supported the diagnoses.

S.Z. was hospitalized for a short time for treatment of PCP. Several months after he was discharged, he developed Kaposi's sarcoma. He eventually developed psychoneurologic problems and died 18 months after the AIDS diagnosis.

Critical Thinking Questions

1. What is the relationship between levels of CD4 lymphocytes and the likelihood of clinical complications from AIDS?
2. Why does the United States Public Health Service recommend monitoring CD4 counts every 3 to 6 months in patients infected with HIV?

Aldolase

Test type Blood

Normal values
Adult: 3.0-8.2 Sibley-Lehninger U/dl or 22-59 mU at 37° C (SI units)
Child: approximately two times the adult values

Newborn: approximately four times the adult values

Rationale
Aldolase is an enzyme used in the glycolytic breakdown of glucose and is similar to the enzymes aspartate aminotransferase (AST) and creatine phosphokinase (CPK) (see pp. 15 and 28, respectively). As with AST and CPK, aldolase

exists in most body tissues. The serum aldolase test is most useful in indicating muscular or hepatic cellular injury or destruction. The serum aldolase level is elevated in patients with muscular dystrophies, dermatomyositis, and polymyositis. Levels also are increased in patients with gangrenous processes, muscular trauma, and muscular infectious diseases (e.g., trichinosis). Elevated levels also are noted in chronic hepatitis, obstructive jaundice, and liver cirrhosis. This test can differentiate between neurologic and muscular causes of weakness. Normal aldolase values are seen in patients with neurologic diseases such as poliomyelitis, myasthenia gravis, and multiple sclerosis. Elevated levels are seen in the primary muscular disorders.

Interfering factors

Factors that can interfere with determining aldolase levels include previous intramuscular injections, which may cause *elevated* levels.

Procedure

Venipuncture is performed, and 7 ml of blood is obtained in a red-top tube. The blood is taken to the laboratory, where it is analyzed for levels of aldolase.

Nursing implications with rationale

Before

- ☞ Explain the procedure to the patient. Tell the patient that no fasting is required.
- ■ Avoid giving intramuscular injections because they can increase serum aldolase levels.

After

- ■ Apply pressure or a pressure dressing to the venipuncture site to prevent further bleeding. Observe the site for bleeding.

Anticardiolipin Antibodies (aCL Antibodies, ACA)

Test type Blood

Normal values

Immunoglobulin G (IgG) anticardiolipin antibodies: <23 g/L

Immunoglobulin M (IgM) anticardiolipin antibodies: <11 mg/L

Rationale

Antiphospholipid antibodies include anticardiolipin antibodies (ACAs) and the lupus anticoagulant. ACAs (IgG and IgM) are found in approximately 40% of patients with SLE. The lupus anticoagulant received its name because it is present in 50% of patients with SLE and can act as an anticoagulant to prolong the phospholipid-dependent coagulation test (e.g., partial thromboplastin time [PTT]). Despite its name, it is not associated with bleeding tendencies.

Patients with SLE who are positive for ACAs and the lupus anticoagulant are at higher risk for the development of antiphospholipid antibody syndrome. Clinical features of this syndrome include venous and arterial thrombosis, neuropsychiatric disorders, recurrent spontaneous abortion, and thrombocytopenia. Strokes in young adults have been associated with elevated levels of these antibodies. Both antibodies may be found in drug-induced lupus, in nonautoimmune diseases (e.g., syphilis and acute infection), and in the normal elderly person.

Interfering factors

Factors that interfere with determining ACAs are:

- ■ Patients who have or have had syphilis infections
  False-positive results can occur from crossreactions with the radiolabeled antibody used in radioimmunoassay (RIA) or the antibody used in ELISA.
- ■ Patients with infections, AIDS, inflammation, autoimmune diseases, or cancer
  The transient presence of ACAs can occur in these patients.

Procedure

No fasting is required. Approximately 5 to 7 ml of venous blood is collected according to laboratory protocol.

Nursing implications with rationale
Before
☑ Explain the procedure to the patient. Tell the patient that no fasting is necessary.
After
■ Apply pressure or a pressure dressing to the venipuncture site to prevent further bleeding. Observe the venipuncture site for bleeding.

Antimyocardial Antibody (AMA)

Test type Blood

Normal values
Negative (if positive, serum will be titrated)

Rationale
The antimyocardial antibody (AMA) test is used to detect an autoimmune source of myocardial injury and disease. AMAs may be detected in rheumatic heart disease, cardiomyopathy, postthoracotomy syndrome, and postmyocardial infarction. This test is used not only to detect an autoimmune cause for these conditions but also to monitor treatment response.

AMA may be detected before clinical symptoms of heart disease develop. An immunologic cause for rheumatic heart disease has been suspected for a long time. Research now has documented the presence of serum antibodies against myocardial components and deposits of immunoglobulin and complement in lesional areas. Antimyocardial antibodies also are found in 20% to 40% of postcardiac surgery patients and in a smaller number of postmyocardial infarction patients. These antibodies usually are associated with cardiac surgery, pericarditis following myocardial injury, or myocardial infarction (Dressler's syndrome). AMA also has been detected with cardiomyopathy; however, its role in this latter disease is unknown.

Procedure
No fasting or special preparation is necessary. Venipuncture is performed, and blood is collected in a red-top tube.

Nursing implications with rationale
Before
☑ Explain the procedure to the patient. Tell the patient that no fasting is required.
After
■ Apply pressure or a pressure dressing to the venipuncture site to prevent further bleeding. Observe the site for bleeding.

Antinuclear Antibodies (ANAs)

Test type Blood

Normal values
Negative (titer <1:20)

Rationale
Autoantibodies are directed against either cellular nuclear material (antinuclear antibodies [ANAs]) or cytoplasmic material (anticytoplasmic antibodies). The ANA test is used to diagnose various autoimmune diseases but is primarily a screening test for SLE. Positive ANA results occur in 95% of patients with SLE; other corroborative serologic tests must be done to confirm the diagnosis because other rheumatic diseases (e.g., Sjögren's syndrome, scleroderma, and RA) also are associated with ANAs. False-negative results occur in 5% of patients with SLE. Tables 12-1 and 12-2, respectively, list ANAs and anticytoplasmic antibodies and the diseases with which they are associated. None of the ANA subtypes, however, are exclusive for any one autoimmune disease.

The relationship between ANA titer elevation and disease presence and severity is directly proportional. In general, the higher the titer of an ANA associated with a particular disease is, the greater the likelihood of disease presence and severity. ANA titer also reflects disease treatment; the titer can be expected to decrease as the disease becomes less active.

Interfering factors
Factors that interfere with determining ANA levels include the following:

TABLE 12-1	**Common Antinuclear Antibodies and Diseases They Cause**

Common Antinuclear Antibodies	Diseases
Anticentromere	CREST syndrome
Anti-ENA	SLE, MCTD
Anti-Jo-1	Polymyositis, dermato-myositis
Antinucleolar	PSS, SLE
Anti-RNP	MCTD, SLE, PSS
Anti-scleroderma-70	PSS
Anti-Smith	SLE
Anti-sNP	SLE
Anti-ss-A (Ro) and Anti-ss-B (La)	Sjögren's syndrome, SLE
Rheumatoid arthritis precipitin	RA, Sjögren's syndrome

SLE, Systemic lupus erythematosus; *MCTD,* mixed connective tissue disease; *PSS,* progressive systemic sclerosis (scleroderma); *CREST,* calcinosis, Raynaud's phenomenon, esophageal dysfunction, sclerodactyly, telangiectasia; *RA,* rheumatoid arthritis.

- Chlorothiazides, griseofulvin, hydralazine, penicillin, procainamide, and other drugs, which may cause a false-positive ANA result
- Steroids, which may cause a false-negative result

Procedure

No fasting or preparation is required for the test. Venipuncture is performed, and 7 ml of blood is collected in a red-top tube. The serum is serially diluted, and the ANA test is performed on each dilution. The most dilute serum in which ANA is detected is called the *titer.* The test result is considered positive if ANA is found in a titer with a dilution of greater than 1:32.

TABLE 12-2	**Common Anticytoplasmic Antibodies and Diseases They Cause**

Common Anticytoplasmic Antibodies	Diseases
Antimicrosomal	Chronic active hepatitis
Antimitochondrial	Primary biliary cirrhosis
Antineutrophil cytoplasmic	Wegener's granulomatosis
Antiribosomal	SLE

Nursing implications with rationale

Before

☞ Explain the procedure to the patient. Tell the patient that no fasting is required.

After

- Apply pressure or a pressure dressing to the venipuncture site to prevent further bleeding. Observe the site for bleeding.
- Indicate on the laboratory test requisition slip any drugs that may affect the results.

☞ Because they are usually immunocompromised, instruct patients with an autoimmune disease to check for signs of infection at the venipuncture site.

Case Study

Systemic Lupus Erythematosus

Mrs. R.D., 24 years old, had been complaining of multiple joint and muscular pains and stiffness in the morning. She also noted some hair loss and increased skin sensitivity to light. Her physical examination showed slight erythema around the cheek bones and some swelling in the joints of her hands.

Continued

Case Study

Systemic Lupus Erythematosus—cont'd

Studies	Results
Routine laboratory work	Within normal limits (WNL), except for mild anemia
Urinalysis, p. 268	Profuse proteinuria and cellular casts
ANAs, p. 470	*1:256 (normal: <1:20)*
Anti-DNA	398 U (normal: <70 U)
Anti-ENA	Positive (normal: negative)
ACAs, p. 469	
IgG	96 g/L (normal: <23 g/L)
IgM	78 mg/L (normal: <11 mg/L)
Erythrocyte sedimentation rate (ESR), p. 476	75 mm/hour (normal: up to 20 mm/hour)
Immunoglobulin electrophoresis, p. 479	
IgG	1910 mg/dl (normal: 565-1765 mg/dl)
IgA	450 mg/dl (normal: 85-385 mg/dl)
IgM	475 mg/dl (normal: 55-375 mg/dl)
Total complement assay, p. 472	22 hemolytic U/ml (normal: 41-90 hemolytic U/ml)

Diagnostic Analysis

The positive ANA and ACA tests strongly supported the diagnosis of SLE. Mrs. R.D. also had a facial rash suggestive of SLE. The elevated ESR indicated a systemic inflammatory process. The immunoelectrophoresis results were compatible with either RA or SLE. However, a decreased complement assay is commonly associated with SLE. The abnormal urinalysis indicated that the kidneys also were involved with the disease process. Mrs. R.D. was treated with steroids and did well for 7 years. Unfortunately, her renal function deteriorated, and she required chronic renal dialysis.

Critical Thinking Questions

1. Explain the significance of the urinalysis results as they relate to renal involvement with SLE.
2. Why is the ESR increased in inflammatory conditions?

Complement Assay

Test type Blood

Normal values

Total complement: 75-160 U/ml or 75-160 U/L (SI units)

C3: 55-120 mg/dl or 0.55-1.20 g/L (SI units)
C4: 20-50 mg/dl or 0.20-0.50 g/L (SI units)

Rationale

Measurements of complement are used primarily to diagnose angioedema and monitor disease activity in patients with SLE nephritis, membranoproliferative nephritis, poststreptococcal nephritis, and other immune-mediated diseases.

Serum complement is a group of globulin proteins that act as enzymes. These enzymes facilitate the immunologic and inflammatory response. The complement system destroys foreign cells and isolates foreign antigens. The total complement, sometimes labeled CH_{50}, is made up of nine major components: C1 through C9. Classic complement activation starts when an IgM or IgG antibody binds with the C1q subcomponent of C1. C1 activates C4, which activates C2, and so on to C9. There are also alternative pathways to the activation of this system.

Once activated, complement increases vascular permeability, allowing antibodies and WBCs to be delivered from the blood to the area of the immune/antigen complex. Complement also acts to increase chemotaxis (attracting WBCs to the area), phagocytosis, and immune adherence of antibody to antigen. These processes are vitally important in the normal inflammatory response.

Specimens for complement assays usually must be sent out to reference laboratories. These tests assess the overall function of the entire complement system. The C3 and C4 components can be quantitated by direct immunologic measurement. These subcomponents are measured when total complement has been found to be reduced. C3 makes up the majority of the total complement.

Reduced complement levels can be congenital, as in hereditary angioedema. Diseases associated with increased antibody/antigen complexes (e.g., serum sickness, SLE, renal transplant rejection, some forms of glomerulonephritis) may reduce complement levels by stimulating the complement system, which then uses up or consumes complement components, and serum complement levels fall. As these diseases are treated successfully, complement levels can be expected to return to normal.

Complement components are increased following the onset of various acute or chronic inflammatory diseases or acute tissue damage. This is similar to an acute-phase reactant protein (see ESR, p. 476).

Interfering factors

A factor that interferes with determining C3 levels is room temperature. If the specimen is left standing at room temperature for more than 1 hour, complement levels could be falsely low. When the specimen arrives at the laboratory, the serum should be separated and frozen immediately.

Procedure

Venipuncture is performed, and 7 ml of blood is collected in a red-top tube and sent to the laboratory. No pretest preparation is needed. No complications are associated with this test.

Nursing implications with rationale

Before
- 🖍 Explain the procedure to the patient. Tell the patient that no fasting is required.

After
- ■ Apply pressure or a pressure dressing to the venipuncture site to prevent further bleeding. Observe the site for bleeding.

C-reactive Protein (CRP)

Test type Blood

Normal values

<0.8 mg/dl

Rationale

C-reactive protein (CRP) is a nonspecific, acute-phase reactant used to diagnose bacterial infectious diseases and inflammatory disorders (e.g., acute rheumatic fever and RA). It also is elevated when tissue necrosis is present. CRP levels do not rise consistently with viral infections. CRP is an abnormal protein produced primarily by the liver during an acute inflammatory process. A positive test result indicates the presence, but not the cause, of an acute inflammatory reaction. The synthesis of CRP is initiated by antigen-immune complexes, bacteria, fungi, and trauma. CRP is functionally analogous to IgG, except that it is not antigen specific. CRP interacts with the complement system.

The CRP test is a more sensitive and rapidly responding indicator than the ESR (see p. 476). In an acute inflammatory change, CRP shows an earlier and more intense increase than ESR; with recovery, the disappearance of CRP precedes the return of ESR to normal. The CRP disappears when the inflammatory process is suppressed by antiinflammatory agents, salicylates, or steroids. Therefore CRP is not a good monitor of disease status.

This test also is useful in evaluating patients with an acute myocardial infarction. The level of CRP correlates with peak levels of the MB isoenzyme of creatine kinase (see p. 28), but CRP peaks occur 18 to 72 hours later. Failure of CRP to normalize may indicate ongoing damage to the heart tissue. Levels are not elevated in patients with angina.

This test also may be used postoperatively to detect wound infections. CRP levels increase within 4 to 6 hours after surgery and generally begin to decrease after the third postoperative day. Failure of the levels to fall is an indicator of complications (e.g., infection or pulmonary infarction).

Interfering factor

A factor that interferes with determining CRP levels is an intrauterine device, which may cause false-positive test results because of tissue inflammation.

Procedure

Peripheral venipuncture is performed, and 7 ml of blood is collected in one red-top tube. Fasting usually is not required.

Nursing implications with rationale

Before

☞ Explain the procedure to the patient. Tell the patient that no fasting is required.

After

■ Apply pressure or a pressure dressing to the venipuncture site to prevent further bleeding. Observe the site for bleeding.

Cryoglobulin

Test type Blood

Normal values

No cryoglobulins detected

Rationale

Cryoglobulins are abnormal serum immunoglobulins that precipitate at low temperatures and redissolve with rewarming. Cryoglobulins can precipitate within blood vessels of the fingers when exposed to cold temperatures. This precipitation causes sludging of the blood within those vessels. Patients in whom this occurs may exhibit purpura, arthralgia, or Raynaud's phenomenon (pain, cyanosis, coldness of the fingers).

Cryoglobulins exist in varying degrees depending on the disease entity with which they are associated. Serum cryoglobulin levels greater than 5 mg/ml are associated with multiple myeloma, macroglobulinemia, and leukemia. Cryoglobulin levels between 1 and 5 mg/ml are associated with rheumatoid arthritis. Levels less than 1 mg/ml can be associated with SLE, RA, infectious mononucleosis (IM), viral hepatitis, endocarditis, cirrhosis, and glomerulonephritis. Idiopathic or primary cryoglobulinemia is not associated with any primary disease.

Procedure

Peripheral venipuncture is performed, and 10 ml of blood is collected in a red-top tube prewarmed to body temperature. The sample is sent to the chemistry laboratory, where it is refrigerated for 72 hours and then evaluated for precipitation. If precipitation is identified, the tube is rewarmed, and the specimen is examined for dissolution of that precipitation. If precipitation of the refrigerated specimen is identified and dissolved on rewarming, cryoglobulins are present. An 8-hour fast may be required to minimize serum turbidity caused by the ingestion of a recent meal. Turbidity may interfere with detection of precipitation. Cryoglobulins also can be identified by immunoelectrophoresis.

Nursing implications with rationale

Before

☞ Explain the procedure to the patient. Instruct the patient to fast for 8 hours before obtaining the specimen, if indicated by the laboratory.

After

■ Apply pressure or a pressure dressing to the venipuncture site to prevent further bleeding. Cryoglobulins may be caused by diseases that are associated with coagulation defects. Observe the venipuncture site for a possible hematoma.

☞ If cryoglobulins are present, instruct the patient to avoid cold temperatures to minimize symptoms of Raynaud's phenomenon.

Epstein-Barr Virus Titer (EBV)

Test type Blood

Normal values

Titers ≤ 1:10 are nondiagnostic

Titers of 1:10 to 1:60 indicate infection at an undetermined time

Titers ≥ 1:320 suggest active infection

A fourfold increase in titer in paired sera drawn 10 to 14 days apart usually indicates acute infection

Rationale

Epstein-Barr virus (EBV) infects 80% of the United States population. After infection, the virus becomes dormant but can be reactivated. EBV infection can produce infectious mononucleosis (IM), which is seen most often in children, adolescents, and young adults. Clinical features include acute fatigue, fever, sore throat, lymphadenopathy, and splenomegaly. Laboratory findings of lymphocytosis, atypical lymphocytes, and transient serum heterophil antibodies are present in patients with acute EBV infection. Most patients with IM recover uneventfully and return to normal activity within 4 to 6 weeks. In Africa, EBV has been associated with Burkitt's lymphoma. In China, EBV infection has been associated with nasopharyngeal carcinoma.

After recovery from primary EBV infection, a lifelong, latent EBV-carrier status is established. In the past several years, specific immunologic tests for EBV activity indicate that latent EBV can reactivate and become associated with a constellation of chronic signs and symptoms resembling IM.

Serologic testing is the only method for diagnosing EBV. The heterophil agglutination slide test (monospot test) (see p. 484) is one such test. Other more specific immunologic tests indicate precisely the timing of infection (Table 12-3).

The viral capsid antigen (VCA) can be IgG or IgM. The EBV nuclear antigen (EBNA) is located in the nucleus of the infected lymphocyte. An-

TABLE 12-3 Serologic Studies and the Timing of Infections

Serologic Study	Appears/Disappears	Clinical Significance
Monospot heterophil	5 days/2 wk	Acute or convalescent infection
VCA-IgM	7 days/3 mos	Acute or convalescent infection
VCA-IgG	7 days/exists for life	Acute, convalescent, or old infection
EBNA-IgG	3 wk/exists for life	Old infection
EA-D	7 days/2 wk	Acute or convalescent infection

VCA, Viral capsid antigen; *EBNA,* Epstein-Barr virus–associated nuclear antigen; *EA-D,* early antigen-D.

other EBV antigen is the early antigen (EA). There are two types of EAs. The first type, EA-D, is spread diffusely throughout the cytoplasm of the lymphocyte. The second type, EA-R, is restricted to one area of the cytoplasm. EA-D is commonly found in patients with nasopharyngeal cancer. EA-R is commonly found in patients with Burkitt's lymphoma.

Interpretation of EBV antibody tests is based on the following assumptions:

1. After infection with EBV, the anti-VCA antibodies appear first.
2. Anti-EA antibodies follow or are present with anti-VCA antibodies early in the course of illness. An anti-EA antibody titer greater than 80 present 2 years after acute IM indicates chronic EBV syndrome.
3. During recovery, anti-VCA and anti-EA antibodies decrease, and anti-EBNA antibodies appear. Anti-EBNA antibodies persist for life and reflect a previous infection.
4. After recovery, anti-VCA and anti-EBNA antibodies are persistently present but at lower ranges. Occasionally, anti-EA antibodies also may be present.

If an acute infection is suspected to have occurred more than a few weeks before testing, the monospot test may be negative. Detecting anti-VCA-IgG or anti-EBNA antibodies is not helpful because their presence indicates that an EBV infection has occurred at some time in the patient's life but not necessarily at the time of the most recent complaint. Detection of anti-VCA-IgM antibodies, however, indicates that the recent complaint was caused by EBV.

Procedure

Peripheral venipuncture is performed, and approximately 5 to 10 ml of blood is collected in a red-top tube. The date of illness onset should be recorded on the laboratory requisition slip. Serum samples should be obtained as soon as possible after the onset of illness. A second specimen should be obtained 14 to 21 days later.

Nursing implications with rationale

Before
☞ Explain the procedure to the patient. Tell the patient that no fasting is required.

After
■ Apply pressure or a pressure dressing to the venipuncture site to prevent further bleeding. Observe the site for bleeding.
☞ Instruct the patient with IM regarding the following aspects of self-care: bed rest during febrile periods, use of analgesics (e.g., aspirin) for general discomfort and fever, and use of throat lozenges and gargling with warm water to relieve a sore throat.

Erythrocyte Sedimentation Rate
(ESR, Sed Rate Test)

Test type Blood

Normal values
Westergren method:
Male: ≤15 mm/hr
Female: ≤20 mm/hr
Child: ≤10 mm/hr
Newborn: 0-2 mm/hr

Rationale

The erythrocyte sedimentation rate (ESR) is a nonspecific test used to detect illnesses associated with acute and chronic infection, inflammation (collagen vascular diseases), advanced neoplasm, and tissue necrosis or infarction. Because the test is nonspecific, it is not diagnostic for any particular organ disease or injury.

ESR measures the rate of RBC settlement in saline solution or plasma during a specific period. Because inflammatory, neoplastic, infectious, and necrotic diseases increase the protein (mainly fibrinogen) content of plasma, RBCs tend to stack up on one another, which increases their weight and causes them to descend faster. Therefore, in these diseases the ESR will be increased. ESR provides the same information as an acute phase, or reactant, protein. That is to say that it occurs as a reaction to acute illnesses as just described.

The ESR test can be used to detect occult disease. Many physicians use the ESR test in routine patient evaluation for vague symptoms. Other physicians believe the test's lack of specificity makes it useless as a routine study.

The ESR is a fairly reliable indicator of the course of disease and therefore can be used to monitor therapy, especially for inflammatory autoimmune diseases (e.g., temporal arteritis or polymyalgia rheumatica). In general, as the disease worsens, the ESR increases; as the disease improves, the ESR decreases. If the results of the ESR are equivocal or inconsistent with the clinical impressions, the C-reactive protein test (see p. 473) is often performed.

Interfering factors

Factors that interfere with determining the ESR include the following:

- Delays in testing
  Artificially low results can occur when the specimen is allowed to stand longer than 3 hours before testing.
- Pregnancy (second and third trimester), which can cause *elevated* levels
- Menstruation, which can cause *elevated* levels
- Some anemias, which can falsely *increase* the ESR

Correction nomograms are available for variations in RBC count.

- Polycythemia, which is associated with a *decreased* ESR
- Diseases associated with increased proteins (e.g., macroglobulinemia), which can falsely *increase* the ESR

Procedure

Peripheral venous blood (5 to 10 ml) is obtained and placed in a lavender-top tube (containing ethylenediaminetetraacetic acid [EDTA]). The blood is taken to the hematology laboratory where the ESR is measured. If the specimen is allowed to stand before the test is performed, the ESR may be retarded, which causes artificially low results. Therefore the study should be performed within 3 hours after the specimen has been obtained. The only discomfort associated with this test is that of the venipuncture.

Nursing implications with rationale

Before

- Explain the procedure to the patient. Tell the patient that no fasting is required.

After

- Apply pressure or a pressure dressing to the venipuncture site to prevent further bleeding. Observe the site for bleeding.

Case Study

Chronic Fatigue Syndrome

Ms. A.M., 35 years old, complained of persistent, debilitating fatigue for more than 4 months with no history of similar symptoms. Her history and physical examination noted the following: mild fever, enlarged cervical and axillary lymph nodes, muscle weakness, generalized weakness, insomnia, confusion, and inability to concentrate. A thorough evaluation was done.

Studies	Results
CBC and differential count, p. 412	WNL
Electrolytes, p. 518	WNL
Glucose, p. 305	80 mg/dl (normal value: 70-105 mg/dl)
Creatinine, p. 237	0.8 mg/dl (normal value: 0.5-1.1 mg/dl)

Continued

Case Study

Chronic Fatigue Syndrome—cont'd

Blood urea nitrogen (BUN), p. 266	13 mg/dl (normal value: 10-20 mg/dl)
Calcium, p. 299	9.4 mg/dl (normal value: 9.0-10.5 mg/dl)
Phosphorus, p. 326	3.8 mg/dl (normal value: 3.0-4.5 mg/dl)
Bilirubin (total), p. 111	0.8 mg/dl (normal value: 0.1-1.0 mg/dl)
Alkaline phosphatase (ALP), p. 108	64 ImU/ml (normal value: 30-85 ImU/ml)
Alanine aminotransferase (ALT), p. 106	22 IU/L (normal value: 5-35 IU/L)
AST, p. 15	8 U/L (normal value: 8-20 U/L)
CPK, p. 28	29 U/ml (normal value: 10-55 U/ml)
Aldolase, p. 468	4.9 U/dl (normal value: 3-8.2 U/dl)
Urinalysis, p. 268	WNL
Chest x-ray study, p. 155	Normal
ESR, p. 476	15 mm/hr (normal value: ≤20 mm/hr)
ANA, p. 470	None (normal value: none)
Thyroid stimulating hormone (TSH), p. 334	8 μU/ml (normal value: 2-10 μU/ml)
HIV, p. 466	Negative (normal value: negative)
PPD (tuberculin test), p. 181	Negative (normal value: negative)
Lyme disease test, p. 481	Negative (normal value: negative)

Diagnostic Analysis

All test results in the recommended evaluation were normal. If any test results had been abnormal, the physician would have had to investigate which conditions could have caused such a result. Based on the history, physical examination, and laboratory test evaluation, chronic fatigue syndrome was diagnosed. Ms. A.M. eventually had to quit her job because of her overwhelming fatigue and numerous symptoms. After 2½ years, she was able to resume working part-time.

Critical Thinking Questions

1. Why were the BUN and creatinine tests indicated based on Ms. A.M.'s symptoms?
2. Why was the TSH test ordered?

Human Lymphocyte Antigen B27

(HLA-B27, Human Leukocyte A Antigen, White Blood Cell Antigen, Histocompatibility Leukocyte A Antigen)

Test type Blood

Normal values
Negative

Rationale

Human lymphocyte antigens (HLAs) exist on the surface of WBCs and all nucleated cells in other tissues. HLAs, however, are detected most easily on the surface of lymphocytes. The presence or absence of these antigens is determined by the four genes on chromosome 6. Each gene controls the presence or absence of HLA-A, B, C, or D.

The HLA system of antigens has been used to indicate tissue compatibility with tissue transplantation. If the HLA antigens of the donor are not compatible with the recipient, the recipient will make antibodies to those antigens and accelerate rejection. Survival of the transplant tissue is increased if HLA matching is good. Prior HLA sensitization causes antibodies to form in the recipient's blood, which may shorten the survival of blood cells (RBCs or platelets) when transfused.

The HLA system also has been used to assist in diagnosing certain diseases. For example, HLA-B27 is present in 80% of patients with Reiter's syndrome. When a patient presents with recurrent and multiple arthritic complaints, the presence of HLA-B27 supports the diagnosis of Reiter's syndrome. HLA-B27 is found in 5% to 7% of normal patients.

Because HLAs are genetically determined, they are useful in paternity investigations, particularly when the child or the man alleged to be the father share an unusual HLA genotype. Conversely, the presence of a common HLA genotype in either the man or the child reduces the likelihood of that man being the child's father.

Procedure
Although HLA testing can be done on almost any human cell, RBCs are the most easily accessible. A venous sample of at least 10 ml is obtained in a heparinized solution and transported to the laboratory. Usually the test is performed at a referral laboratory. No prestudy preparations are necessary. The only discomfort associated with the test is that of the venipuncture.

Nursing implications with rationale
Before
☞ Explain the procedure to the patient. Tell the patient that no fasting is required.
After
■ Apply pressure or a pressure dressing to the venipuncture site to prevent further bleeding. Observe the site for bleeding.

Human T-cell Lymphotrophic Virus (HTLV) I/II Antibody

Test type Blood

Normal values
Negative

Rationale
Several types of the human T-cell lymphotrophic virus (HTLV), a retrovirus, affect humans. The virus is endemic in southern Japan, the Caribbean islands, South America, and portions of Africa. HTLV-I is associated with adult T-cell leukemia/lymphoma and neurologic disorders such as tropical spastic paraparesis. HTLV-II is associated with adult hairy cell leukemia. Humans can be infected with these viruses, however, and not develop any malignancy or diseases.

Although both HTLV and HIV, the causative agent of AIDS, are retroviruses, HTLV infection is not associated with AIDS. HTLV transmission is similar, however, to HIV transmission (e.g., body fluid contamination, IV drug use, sexual contact, breast-feeding).

Procedure
No fasting is required. Approximately 7 ml of venous blood is collected in a red-top tube.

Nursing implications with rationale
Before
☞ Explain the procedure to the patient. Tell the patient that no fasting is required.
After
■ Apply pressure or a pressure dressing to the venipuncture site to prevent further bleeding. Observe the site for bleeding.

Immunoglobulin Electrophoresis
(Gamma Globulin Electrophoresis)

Test type Blood

Normal values
IgG:
Adults: 565-1765 mg/dl
Children:
   4-12 years: 460-1600 mg/dl
   2-3 years: 420-1200 mg/dl
   1 year: 340-1200 mg/dl
   6-9 months: 220-900 mg/dl

2-5 months: 200-700 mg/dl

1 month: 250-900 mg/dl

IgA:

Adults: 85-385 mg/dl

Children:

4-12 years: 25-350 mg/dl

2-3 years: 18-150 mg/dl

1 year: 15-110 mg/dl

6-9 months: 8-80 mg/dl

2-5 months: 4-80 mg/dl

1 month: 1-4 mg/dl

IgM:

Adult: 55-375 mg/dl

Children:

9-12 years: 50-250 mg/dl

1-8 years: 45-200 mg/dl

6-9 months: 35-125 mg/dl

2-5 months: 25-100 mg/dl

1 month: 20-80 mg/dl

IgD and IgE: minimal

Rationale

Serum proteins are composed of albumin and globulin. Several types of globulin exist, one of which is gamma globulin. Antibodies composed of gamma globulin protein are called *immunoglobulins*. There are many types of immunoglobulins (antibodies). IgG constitutes approximately 75% of the serum immunoglobulins; therefore it constitutes the majority of circulating serum antibodies. IgA constitutes approximately 15% of the immunoglobulins within the body and is present primarily in saliva, colostrum, tears and the secretions of the respiratory and gastrointestinal tract. IgA is also present, to a smaller degree, in the blood. IgM is an immunoglobulin primarily responsible for ABO blood grouping and rheumatoid factor, yet it is involved in the immunologic reaction to many other infections. IgM does not cross the placenta so that an elevation of IgM in the newborn indicates intrauterine infection (e.g., rubella, cytomegalovirus, or sexually transmitted diseases). IgE often mediates an allergic response and is measured to detect allergic diseases. IgD, which constitutes the smallest portion of the immunoglobulins, is rarely evaluated or detected.

Serum immunoelectrophoresis is used to detect and monitor the course of diseases, including hypersensitivity diseases, immune deficiencies, autoimmune diseases, chronic infections, multiple myeloma, chronic viral infections, and intrauterine fetal infections. It is often ordered if a serum protein electrophoresis (see p. 135) indicates a spike at the immunoglobulin (antibody) level.

Procedure

Venipuncture is performed, and 7 ml of blood is collected in a red-top tube. The serum is placed on a slide containing agar gel, and an electric current is passed through the gel. The immunoglobulins then separate according to the quantity and difference in electric charges. Specific antisera are placed alongside the slide to identify the specific type of immunoglobulin. In some laboratories the patient is asked to refrain from eating 12 hours before the blood sample is obtained.

Nursing implications with rationale

Before

☞ Explain the procedure to the patient. Tell the patient that no fasting is required.

After

■ Apply pressure or a pressure dressing to the venipuncture site to prevent further bleeding. Observe the site for bleeding.

Legionnaires' Disease Antibody

Test type Blood

Normal values

No *Legionella* antibody titer

Rationale

Legionnaires' disease was originally described as a fulminating pneumonia caused by *Legionella pneumophila,* a tiny, gram-negative, rod-shaped bacterium. Nearly half of the clinical cases have been caused by serogroup type 1. This organism also can cause an influenza type of illness called *Pontiac fever.*

The diagnosis of legionnaires' disease can be made by culturing *Legionella* from blood, sputum, lung tissue, or pleural fluid. Sputum for this test is best obtained by transtracheal aspiration or from bronchial washings. However, growth of this organism in culture medium is difficult. A negative culture does not rule out legionnaires' disease. Another method of diagnosis is to identify the organism in a microscopic smear of infected fluid with the use of direct fluorescent antibody (FA) methods. A positive result allows for a rapid diagnosis of *Legionella*. However, this method also is difficult because the bacterial concentration may not be high enough to reveal the bacterium in the specimen.

The most common and easiest method for diagnosis is detection of the serum antibody directed against the *Legionella* bacterium. The antibody test is performed if the culture or direct fluorescent tests are negative. A presumptive diagnosis of legionnaires' disease can be made in a symptomatic patient when a single antibody titer is 1:256 or greater. Another way to make the diagnosis is to perform the antibody test 1 and 3 weeks after the onset of symptoms. A fourfold rise in titer to at least 1:128 between the acute (1-week) and the convalescent (3-week) phase is diagnostic. Unfortunately, it may take 4 to 6 weeks for serologic tests to be positive. The identification of *Legionella* antigens in the urine may be present in a few days after the onset of the clinical symptoms. Unfortunately, the sensitivity is very low (approximately 30%).

Procedure

Legionnaires' disease can be diagnosed by either a blood test or by a direct FA microscopic examination of a specimen smear. For the blood test, venipuncture is performed, and one red-top tube of blood is collected. A convalescent sample should be drawn 2 to 3 weeks after the acute sample.

Organisms also may be cultured on special media from pleural fluid, lung biopsy specimens, bronchial washings, transtracheal or bronchial aspirates, or other body fluids. Direct FA staining may demonstrate the organism in sputum, lung tissue, or pleural fluid within 2 to 3 days after the onset of clinical disease. This direct FA

method is more specific compared with the blood test.

Nursing implications with rationale

Before

✒ Explain the procedure to the patient. Tell the patient that no fasting is required.

After

■ Apply pressure or a pressure dressing to the venipuncture site to prevent further bleeding. Observe the site for bleeding.

Lyme Disease Test

Test type Blood

Normal values

Negative (low titers of IgM and IgG antibodies)

Rationale

Lyme disease was first recognized in Lyme, Connecticut, in 1975. It is caused by a spirochete called *Borrelia burgdorferi*. The disease usually begins in the summer with a skin lesion called *erythema chronicum migrans (ECM)*, which occurs at the site of a bite by a deer tick, usually *Ixodes dammini* or *pacificus*. Ticks are the best documented vectors of this spirochete.

Weeks to months after the insect bite, some patients develop fatigue, meningoencephalitis, cranial or peripheral neuropathies, myocarditis, atrioventricular nodal block, or arthritis. The last manifestation is joint involvement, which often occurs intermittently in a few large joints for several years.

Cultures of the ECM can isolate the spirochete in half of the cases. However, it is hard to culture the spirochete, and it is a slow-growing organism. Cultures of the blood or cerebrospinal fluid (CSF) are even less helpful. Currently, serologic studies are the most sensitive and specific tests for detection of Lyme disease.

Early in the illness, the diagnosis usually can be determined from the gross appearance of ECM and known exposure to an endemic area (e.g., woods, where large populations of deer exist). Affected patients do not require antibody determination. In the absence of ECM lesions, however, Lyme disease can be confused with various viral infections. In such patients, a single titer of specific IgM antibody may suggest the correct diagnosis. Acute and convalescent sera can be tested to confirm the presence of the disease. The diagnosis of Lyme disease can be made with certainty only when the clinical picture of the acute disease and the serology both support the diagnosis. Without the clinical picture, the serology often is falsely positive, and the diagnosis is incorrectly made.

Because of the high incidence of false-positive ELISA test results for Lyme disease, it is now recommended that patients who have positive serologies for Lyme disease using the ELISA test method be tested by a Western blot specific Lyme disease test to confirm the diagnosis.

Interfering factors

Factors that interfere with determining Lyme disease test results include the following:

- Previous infection with *B. burgdorferi*
  This can cause positive serologic testing although the patient no longer has Lyme disease.
- Other spirochete diseases (syphilis or leptospirosis), which can cause false-positive results

Procedure

No food or fluid restrictions are needed. Peripheral venipuncture is performed to collect 7 to 10 ml of venous blood in a red-topped tube.

Nursing implications with rationale

Before

☞ Explain the procedure to the patient. Tell the patient that no fasting is required.

After

- Apply pressure or a pressure dressing to the venipuncture site to prevent further bleeding. Observe the site for bleeding.

Case Study

Lyme Disease

Mr. J.W., 38 years old, had a 3-week history of fatigue and lethargy with intermittent complaints of headache, fever, chills, myalgia, and arthralgia. According to the history, the patient's symptoms began shortly after a camping vacation. The patient recalled a bug bite and rash on his thigh immediately after the trip. The following studies were ordered:

Studies	Results
Lyme disease test, p. 481	Elevated IgM antibody titers against *B. burgdorferi* (normal value: low)
ESR, p. 476	30 mm/hr (normal value: ≤15 mm/hr)
AST, p. 15	32 U/L (normal value: 8-20 U/L)
Hemoglobin, p. 415	12 g/dl (normal value: 14-18 g/dl)
Hematocrit, p. 416	36% (normal value: 42%-52%)
Rheumatoid factor, p. 485	Negative (normal value: negative)
Antinuclear antibodies, p. 470	Negative (normal value: negative)

Diagnostic Analysis

Based on Mr. J.W.'s history of camping in the woods and an insect bite and rash on the thigh, Lyme disease was suspected. Early in the course of this disease, testing for specific IgM antibodies against *B. burgdorferi* is the most helpful in diagnosing Lyme disease. An elevated ESR, increased AST levels, and mild anemia are frequently seen early in this disease. Rheumatoid factor and antinuclear antibodies are usually absent.

The therapeutic goal for Lyme disease is to eradicate the causative organism. Lyme disease, like other spirochetal diseases, is most responsive to antibiotics early in its course. Mr. J.W. was placed on oral doxycycline, 100 mg twice a day, for 21 days. His symptoms resolved completely, and he had no further problems.

Critical Thinking Questions

1. At what stages of Lyme disease are the IgG and IgM antibodies elevated?
2. Why was the ESR elevated?

Lymphocyte Immunophenotyping
(AIDS T-lymphocyte Cell Markers, CD4 Marker, CD4/CD8 Ratio, CD4 Percentage)

Test type Blood

Normal values

Cells	Percentage (%)	Number of Cells/μl
T cells	60-95	800-2500
T helper (CD4) cells	60-75	600-1500
T suppressor (CD8) cells	25-30	300-1000
B cells	4-25	100-450
Natural killer cells	4-30	75-500
CD4/CD8 ratio	>1.0	

Rationale

All lymphocytes originate from stem cells in the bone marrow (see Figure 10-1, p. 401). Lymphocytes that mature in the bone marrow are called *B lymphocytes.* These lymphocytes provide humoral immunity (produce antibodies). Lymphocytes that mature in the thymus are called *T lymphocytes,* and they are responsible for cellular immunity. CD4 helper cells and CD8 suppressor cells are examples of T lymphocytes. Finally, lymphocytes that have neither T or B markers are called *natural killer cells* and chemically attack foreign or cancer cells without prior sensitization. Monoclonal antibodies against cell surface markers are used to identify the various forms of lymphocytes. The absolute numbers and percentages of antibodies are then counted.

There are three related measurements of CD4 T lymphocytes. The first measurement is the *total CD4 cell count.* This is measured in a whole-blood sample and is the product of the WBC count, the lymphocyte differential count, and the percentage of lymphocytes that are CD4 T cells. The second measurement, the *CD4 percentage,* is a more accurate prognostic marker. It directly measures the percentage of CD4 lymphocytes in the whole-blood sample. The third prognostic marker, which is also more reliable than the total CD4 count, is the *ratio of CD4 cells to CD8 (T-suppressor) cells.*

Of the three T-cell measurements, the total CD4 count is subject to substantial diurnal variation. Very little diurnal variation and laboratory error occurs with the CD4 percentage and CD4/CD8 ratio. The Multicenter AIDS Cohort Study suggests that the latter two measurements are more accurate than the total CD4 count. However, because the total CD4 cell count originally was thought to be the best marker, it was used in many of the studies that now form the basis for practice recommendations. It will take time before the more accurate measurements find clinical pertinence in practice recommendations.

The pathogenesis of AIDS is largely attributed to a decrease in the T lymphocyte that bears the CD4 receptor. Progressive depletion of CD4 T lymphocytes is associated with an increased likelihood of clinical complications from AIDS. The United States Public Health Service has recommended that CD4 prognostic markers be monitored every 3 to 6 months in all persons infected with HIV.

As the CD4 cell measurements decrease, the

percentage of patients developing AIDS increases. Forty-eight percent of patients can be expected to develop AIDS within 6 months when their CD4 count is 100 cells/mm^3. It is recommended that antiviral therapy be started in patients whose CD4 count is less than 500 to 600 cells/mm^3. *Pneumocystis carinii* pneumonia prophylaxis should start when the CD4 count is less than 200 to 300 cells/mm^3.

Immunodeficiency associated with organ transplant also is monitored with lymphocyte immunophenotyping. Lymphomas and other lymphoproliferative diseases are now classified and treated according to the predominant lymphocyte type identified. In some instances, prognosis of these diseases depends on lymphocyte immunophenotyping.

Interfering factors

Factors that interfere with determining lymphocyte immunophenotyping include the following:

- Diurnal variation
  Although this is usually of no significance, it may have some impact when lymphocyte counts are low. Higher counts can be expected in the late morning hours.
- A recent viral illness, which can *decrease* total T lymphocyte counts
- Nicotine and very strenuous exercise
  These factors have been shown to *decrease* lymphocyte counts. However, the data are now being questioned.
- Steroids, which can *increase* lymphocyte counts
- Immunosuppressive drugs, which will *decrease* lymphocyte counts

Procedure

No fasting or preparation is required. The time of day when the blood specimen is being obtained should be recorded on the laboratory requisition slip. While observing universal precautions, venipuncture is performed, and 10 ml of venous blood is obtained in a large green-top tube (containing sodium heparin). Approximately 5 ml of venous blood also is collected in a small purple-top tube (containing EDTA). The specimens must be kept at room temperature. Do not refrigerate. Most specimens are sent to a reference laboratory.

Contraindications

Lymphocyte immunophenotyping is contraindicated for patients who are not emotionally prepared for the prognosis that the results may indicate.

Nursing implications with rationale

Before

- ☞ Explain the procedure to the patient. Tell the patient that no fasting is required.
- ■ Maintain a nonjudgmental attitude toward the patient's sexual practices.
- ■ Allow the patient ample time to express his or her concerns regarding the possible test results.

After

- ■ Apply pressure or a pressure dressing to the venipuncture site to prevent further bleeding. Observe the site for bleeding.
- ☞ Instruct the patient to observe the venipuncture site for infection. Patients with AIDS or organ recipients are immunocompromised and susceptible to infection.
- ■ Encourage the patient to discuss his or her concerns regarding the prognostic information that may be obtained by these results.

Mononucleosis Spot Test
(Mononuclear Heterophil Test, Heterophil Antibody Test, Monospot Test)

Test type Blood

Normal values
Negative (1:28 titer)

Rationale

The mononucleosis spot test aids in the diagnosis of infectious mononucleosis (IM), a disease caused by EBV. Usually, young adults are affected by mononucleosis. The clinical presentation is fever, pharyngitis, lymphadenopathy, and splenomegaly. Approximately 2 weeks after the onset of the disease, many patients are found to have IgM heterophil antibodies in their serum that react against warm RBCs. When these antibodies are present in serial dilutions of greater than 1:56, IM can be strongly considered. However, false-positive results can occur in patients with other diseases that cause elevation of heterophil antibodies (e.g., lymphoma and SLE). Burkitt's lymphoma is strongly associated with EBV.

Heterophil antibodies normally present in most individuals are increased in patients with IM. These antibodies strongly and readily agglutinate equine RBCs. The monospot test is performed by adding the patient's serum to equine RBCs on a slide. If agglutination occurs, heterophil antibodies are present in the patient's serum, indicating an EBV infection. Approximately 30% of IM cases are heterophil antibody negative. When the diagnosis of IM is still suspected, a repeat monospot test or EBV serology is performed (see p. 484).

Procedure

No pretest preparations are required. Venipuncture is performed, and 7 ml of blood is collected in a red-top tube. The specimen is sent to the laboratory for testing, and the results are available within an hour.

Nursing implications with rationale

Before
- ☞ Explain the procedure to the patient. Tell the patient that no fasting is required.

After
- ■ Apply pressure or a pressure dressing to the venipuncture site to prevent further bleeding. Observe the site for bleeding or ecchymosis.

Rabies-neutralizing Antibody

Test type Blood

Normal values
<1:16

Rationale

Identification and documentation of the rabies-neutralizing antibody is important for veterinary health care workers and others who are at risk

for or may have been exposed to the rabies virus. This test is performed on persons at great risk for animal bites (veterinarians and their staff, zoo workers, and laboratory staff who work with animals) and on those who have received the human diploid cell vaccine (HDCV). A rabies titer of greater than 1:16 is considered to be protective.

Rabies antibody also is used to diagnose rabies in patients suspected to have been exposed to the virus. A fourfold rise in antibody titer over several weeks in a person not previously exposed to the HDCV indicates rabies exposure. If the patient has received HDCV and has been bitten by an animal suspected of having rabies infection, a very high antibody titer may support the diagnosis. The presence of antibodies in the CSF also supports the diagnosis because antibodies are not usually present in the CSF after the HDCV vaccine but are present after a bite from a rabies-infected animal. In patients who may have been exposed to rabies, human rabies immunoglobulin (HRIG) is given after the antibody titers have been obtained.

Procedure

No fasting or special preparation is required. Approximately 7 to 10 ml of venous blood is collected in a red-top tube.

Nursing implications with rationale

Before
- ☞ Explain the procedure to the patient. Tell the patient that no fasting is necessary.

After
- ■ Apply pressure or a pressure dressing to the venipuncture site to prevent further bleeding. Observe the venipuncture site for bleeding.

Rheumatoid Factor (RF, Rheumatoid Arthritis Factor [RAF])

Test type Blood

Normal values

Negative (<60 U/ml by nephelometric testing)
Elderly patients may have slightly increased values

Rationale

The rheumatoid factor (RF) test is useful in the diagnosis of RA, a chronic inflammatory disease that affects most joints. In this disease, abnormal IgG antibodies produced by lymphocytes in the synovial membranes act as antigens. Other IgG and IgM antibodies in the patient's serum react with these antigens to produce immune complexes. These immune complexes activate the complement system and other inflammatory systems to cause joint damage. The reactive IgM and, occasionally, IgG and IgA make up the RF. Tissues other than the joints, including blood vessels, lungs, nerves, and heart, also may be involved in the autoimmune inflammation.

The RF test identifies IgM antibodies. Approximately 80% of patients with RA have positive RF titers. To be considered positive, RF must be found in a dilution greater than 1:80. If RF is found in titers less than 1:80, other autoimmune diseases (e.g., SLE, scleroderma) should be considered. The RF test is not a useful disease marker because its presence does not disappear in patients experiencing a remission from disease symptoms. In addition, a small number of normal patients will have RF present at a very low titer. Furthermore, a negative titer does not exclude the diagnosis of RA. Other autoimmune diseases, such as SLE or Sjögren's syndrome, may also cause a positive RF test. RF is occasionally seen in patients with tuberculosis, chronic hepatitis, IM, and subacute bacterial endocarditis. Elderly patients often have false-positive results.

Procedure

Venipuncture is performed, and 7 ml of blood is collected in a red-top tube.

Nursing implications with rationale

Before

☞ Explain the procedure to the patient. Tell the patient that no fasting is required.

After

■ Apply pressure or a pressure dressing to the venipuncture site to prevent further bleeding. Observe the site for bleeding.

Case Study

Rheumatoid Arthritis

Mrs. J.D., 46 years old, complained of bilateral knee and hand pain that had become progressively worse during the past 2 years. She also noted subcutaneous nodules in her elbow and knees. Her physical examination showed some ulnar deviation of the digits and swelling of the metacarpal, phalangeal, and proximal interphalangeal joints. Signs of acute inflammation and some instability of both knees also were present. The right knee was in worse condition than the left.

Studies	Results
Routine laboratory studies	WNL, except for mild anemia
RF, p. 485	320 U/mL (normal: <60 U/mL)
CRP, p. 473	4 mg/dl (normal value: <0.8 mg/dl)
HLA-B27 antigen, p. 478	Negative
X-ray examination of the knee, p. 457	Marked destruction of both knees with joint narrowing
Synovial fluid analysis, p. 449	
Appearance	Turbid (normal value: clear)
Fibrin clot	Large (normal value: none)

Mucin clot	Fair to poor (normal value: good)
WBCs	8000/mm^3 (normal value: <200)
Polymorphonuclear lymphocytes	80% (normal value: <25%)
Glucose level	60% (normal value: within 10 mg/dl of serum glucose)

Diagnostic Analysis

Mrs. J.D.'s presenting symptoms were physical findings compatible with RA. The radiographic films of the knee joint confirmed the significant joint destruction. Her RF and CRP results were markedly positive. Synovial fluid analysis corroborated the findings of RA. The HLA antigen was negative, thereby eliminating ankylosing spondylitis or Reiter's syndrome. Mrs. J.D. was given an aggressive antiarthritic medication regimen and physical therapy. She improved markedly and was able to enjoy a relatively normal life.

Critical Thinking Questions

1. Explain the reason for the results of the radiographic examination of the knee.
2. Why is the synovial fluid glucose level decreased in this patient?

REVIEW QUESTIONS AND ANSWERS

1. **Question:** Your patient presents with acute swelling and tenderness of the knee joint. How might an ESR be helpful in this situation?
   Answer: The ESR would not be helpful in this situation for several reasons. ESRs often are normal despite the presence of acute disease. Furthermore, the ESR cannot differentiate the possible causes of this patient's joint swelling. Septic, autoimmune, or degenerative arthritis could, in time, cause elevation of the ESR.

2. **Question:** Your patient is HIV positive and free of any signs or symptoms of AIDS. How does monitoring the CD4 and CD8 counts contribute to the care of this patient? Review some of the important psychoemotional aspects associated with this testing.
   Answer: CD4 counts and the CD4/CD8 ratio are accurate prognosticators of AIDS. The lower these values, the greater the risks of AIDS. When CD4 counts are less than 200 to 500 cells/mm^3, antiviral and *Pneumocystis carinii* treatment is usually begun. These tests are associated with much anxiety for patients

infected with HIV. The nurse should demonstrate nonjudgmental support and understanding of the significance of the test results to the patient.

3. **Question:** A student tells the school nurse that she has had significant fatigue, intermittent sore throat, and anorexia for 2 months. "Do I have mono?" she asks. What would be the most appropriate test to assist in this diagnosis?
   Answer: A monospot test, if positive, may be helpful in diagnosing infectious mononucleosis, an EBV infection. However, in more than 30% of cases the monospot test will be falsely negative this late in the course of the disease. Testing for the anti-VCA IgM antibody will be much more accurate at this time.

4. **Question:** The physician has requested an RF test for your young female patient. She is terribly frightened that the physician suspects rheumatoid arthritis (RA) and that she will soon be paralyzed by incapacity and joint pain. What are the appropriate nursing interventions?
   Answer: Remind the patient that many diseases are associated with a positive RF. Some of these diseases are self-limiting viral infec-

tions. The RF is merely a part of an immunologic workup to document a pattern associated with the disease that may explain her complaints. Also, assist her in verbalizing her fears and frustrations concerning this workup.

5. **Question:** Your patient has undergone antimitochondrial antibody and antismooth–muscle antibody testing. Several hours later you notice an enlarged hematoma around the venipuncture site. What might be the cause of that hematoma, and what is the appropriate nursing intervention?

   Answer: The antimitochondrial antibody and antismooth muscle antibody tests were performed to diagnose and distinguish forms of liver disease. These liver diseases are often associated with inadequate levels of coagulation factors. Your patient most probably has a coagulopathy and does not have the normal capability to form a clot at the venipuncture site. You should:

   1. Ensure that the hematoma has not caused compression of the arterial supply to the hand. Check the pulses.
   2. Ensure that there is no compression on the nerves of the hand. Check for muscular capability and pinprick sensation.
   3. Elevate the arm.
   4. Place cold compresses over the hematoma site.
   5. Notify the physician to document and determine the cause of the coagulopathy more accurately.

Bibliography

Barrick B, Vogel S: Application of laboratory diagnostics in HIV testing, *Nurs Clin North Am* 31(1):41-45, 1996.

Carson D: Rheumatoid factor. In Kelley WN et al, editors: Textbook of rheumatology, ed 3, Philadelphia, 1989, WB Saunders.

Cooper MD, Lawton AR: Primary immune deficiency diseases. In Fauci AS et al, editors: Harrison's principles of internal medicine, ed 14, New York, 1998, McGraw-Hill.

Croft JE, Grodzicki RL, Steere AC: Antibody response to Lyme disease evaluation of diagnostic tests, *J Infect Dis* 149(5):789-795, 1984.

Dearborn JT, Jergesen HE: The evaluation and initial management of arthritis, *Prim Care* 23(2):215-240, 1996.

Densen P: Complement. In Mandell G et al, editors: Principles and practices of infectious diseases, ed 3, New York, 1990, Churchill Livingstone.

Dominquez A et al: Inclusion of laboratory test results in the surveillance of infectious diseases, *Int J Epidemiol* 20(1):290-292, 1991.

Fauci AS, Lane HC: Human immunodeficiency virus (HIV) disease: AIDS and related disorders. In Fauci AS et al, editors: Harrison's principles of internal medicine, ed 14, New York, 1998, McGraw-Hill.

Frank AP et al: Anonymous HIV testing using home collection and telemedicine counseling, *Arch Intern Med* 157(3):309-313, 1997.

Fries JF: Assessment of the patient with rheumatic diseases. In Kelley WN et al, editors: Textbook of rheumatology, ed 3, Philadelphia, 1989, WB Saunders.

Gawlikowski J: White cells at war, *Am J Nurs* 92(3):44-51, 1992.

Gerberding JL: Management of occupational exposure to blood-borne viruses, *N Engl J Med* 322:444, 1995.

Hahn BH: Systemic lupus erythematosus. In Fauci AS et al, editors: Harrison's principles of internal medicine, ed 14, New York, 1998, McGraw-Hill.

Haynes BF et al: Toward an understanding of the correlates of protective immunity to HIV infection, *Science* 271:324, 1996.

Holmes GP et al: Chronic fatigue syndrome: a working case definition, *Ann Intern Med* 108(3):387-389, 1988.

Jenkins SR: Rabies. In Rakel RE, editor: Conn's current therapy, Philadelphia, 1998, WB Saunders.

Katz W: Diagnosis and management of rheumatic disease, Philadelphia, 1988, JB Lippincott.

Kieff ED: Infectious mononucleosis (Epstein-Barr virus infection). In Wyngaarden JB et al, editors: Cecil textbook of medicine, ed 19, Philadelphia, 1992, WB Saunders.

Komaroff AL: Chronic fatigue syndrome. In Rakel RE, editor: Conn's current therapy, Philadelphia, 1998, WB Saunders.

Kristoferitsch W: Neurological manifestation of Lyme borreliosis, *Infection* 19(4):268-272, 1991.

Lackritz EM et al: Estimated risk of HIV transmission by screened blood in the United States, *N Engl J Med* 333:1721, 1995.

Lipski PE: Rheumatoid arthritis. In Fauci AS et al, editors: Harrison's principles of internal medicine, ed 14, New York, 1998, McGraw-Hill.

Malawista SE: Lyme disease. In Wyngaarden JB et al, editors: Cecil textbook of medicine, ed 19, Philadelphia, 1992, WB Saunders.

Mellors JW et al: Prognosis of HIV-1 infection predicted by the quantity of virus in plasma, *Science* 272:1167, 1996.

Metcalf RW: Arthroscopy. In Kelley WN et al, editors: Textbook of rheumatology, ed 3, Philadelphia, 1989, WB Saunders.

Milton JD et al: Immune responsiveness in chronic fatigue syndrome, *Postgrad Med J* 67(788):532-537, 1991.

O'Brien WA et al: Changes in plasma HIV-1 RNA and CD4+ lymphocyte count and the risk of progression to AIDS, *N Engl J Med* 334:426, 1996.

Pagana KD, Pagana TJ: Mosby's manual of diagnostic and laboratory tests, St. Louis, 1998, Mosby.

Polsky B: Human immunodeficiency virus and its complications. In Rakel RE, editor: Conn's current therapy, Philadelphia, 1998, WB Saunders.

Rao JK et al: The role of antineutrophil cytoplasmic antibody (c-ANCA) testing in the diagnosis of Wegener granulomatosis, *Ann Intern Med* 123(12):925-932, 1995.

Reichlin M: Antinuclear antibodies. In Kelley WN et al, editors: Textbook of rheumatology, ed 3, Philadelphia, 1989, WB Saunders.

Ruddy S: Complement. In Kelley WN et al, editors: Textbook of rheumatology, ed 3, Philadelphia, 1989, WB Saunders.

Schleupner CJ: Detection of HIV-1 infection. In Mandell G et al, editors: Principles and practices of infectious diseases, ed 3, New York, 1990, Churchill Livingstone.

Stanek G: Laboratory and seroepidemiology of Lyme borreliosis, *Infection* 19(4):263-267, 1991.

Steere AC: Lyme disease. In Rakel RE, editor: Conn's current therapy, Philadelphia, 1998, WB Saunders.

Straus SE: Chronic fatigue syndrome. In Fauci AS et al, editors: Harrison's principles of internal medicine, ed 14, New York, 1998, McGraw-Hill.

Sumaya CV: Infectious mononucleosis. In Rakel RE, editor: Conn's current therapy, Philadelphia, 1991, WB Saunders.

Tavris DE: Criteria for chronic fatigue syndrome, *Penn Med* 94(7):34, 1991.

Willis D: Lyme disease, *J Neurosci Nurs* 23(4):211-217, 1991.

Chapter 13

Diagnostic Studies Used in the Assessment of
Cancer

ANATOMY AND PHYSIOLOGY

Cancer is characterized by abnormal cell division and metastasis. Because of its variability and complexity, cancer has no single cause or treatment. Early detection of cancer usually offers the best prognosis for the patient.

The studies described in this chapter are commonly performed to detect primary and metastatic tumors. The test results assist in accurate staging of the tumor. When performed at appropriately timed intervals during the course of anticancer treatment, these studies can be used to determine whether the tumor is becoming smaller (regressing) or getting larger (progressing). Metastasis is a form of progression.

Some types of tumors more commonly involve certain organs in their pattern of metastasis. Because the lymph nodes, bone, brain, liver, and lungs are commonly involved with metastatic cancer, these organs are evaluated during diagnostic staging studies. If the staging studies indicate tumor progression, the physician may elect to change or reinstitute anticancer therapy. If, on the other hand, the staging studies indicate tumor regression, the present anticancer therapy would be continued. Therefore, accurate patient preparation and test results are vitally important because they may significantly affect the clinical course of the patient.

Alpha-fetoprotein (AFP, α_1-Fetoprotein)

Test type Blood

Normal values

Adult: <40 ng/ml or <40 mg/L (SI units)
Child (<1 yr): <30 ng/ml
Ranges are stratified by weeks of gestation and vary according to different laboratories.

Rationale

Alpha-fetoprotein (AFP) is an oncofetal protein normally produced by the fetal liver and yolk sac. It is the dominant fetal serum protein in the first trimester of life and diminishes to very low levels by age 1. Normally it is found in very low levels in the adult. Increased serum levels of AFP are found in as many as 90% of patients with hepatomas. The higher the AFP level, the greater the tumor burden. A decrease in the AFP level would be seen if the patient were experiencing a response to antineoplastic therapy. AFP is not specific for hepatoma, although extremely high levels (greater than 500 ng/ml) are diagnostic for hepatoma. Other neoplastic conditions, such as nonseminomatous germ cell tumors and teratomas of the testes; yolk sac and germ cell tumors of the ovaries; and, to a lesser extent, Hodgkin's disease, lymphoma, and renal cell carcinoma, also are associated with elevated AFP levels. Noncancerous causes of elevated AFP levels occur in patients with cirrhosis or chronic active hepatitis.

AFP also is helpful in the diagnosis of fetal body wall defects. The most notable of these is neural tube defects (NTDs) relative to spinal defects, which can vary from a small myelomeningocele to anencephaly. Although not widely used in the United States, AFP can be used for widespread screening for NTDs.

If a fetus has an open body wall defect, fetal serum AFP leaks into the amniotic fluid and is picked up by the maternal serum. Normally AFP from fetal sources can be detected in the amniotic fluid or the mother's blood after 10 weeks of gestation. Peak levels occur between 16 and 18 weeks. Maternal serum levels reflect the change in amniotic AFP levels. When elevated maternal serum AFP levels are identified, further evaluation with repeat serum AFP levels, amniotic fluid AFP levels, and ultrasound is warranted. Other examples of fetal body wall defects include omphalocele and gastroschisis (abdominal wall defects). Elevated serum AFP levels in pregnancy also may indicate multiple pregnancy, fetal distress, fetal congenital abnormalities, or intrauterine death. Low AFP levels after correction as to age of gestation, maternal weight, race, and presence of diabetes are found in mothers carrying offspring with trisomy 21 (Down syndrome).

Interfering factors

Factors that interfere with determining AFP levels include the following:

- Fetal blood contamination
  This may occur during amniocentesis and can cause *increased* AFP levels.
- Recent administration of radioisotopes
  These can affect values because results are determined by radioimmunoassay.

Procedure

If an AFP test is to be performed on amniotic fluid, see amniocentesis, p. 349. For a blood test, peripheral venipuncture is performed, and approximately 10 ml of blood is collected in a red-top tube. No food or fluid restrictions are necessary. For the AFP triple screen profile, maternal age, weight, race, presence of diabetes, and gestational age of the fetus also must be provided.

Nursing implications with rationale
Before
- ☞ Explain the purpose of this test to the patient. Tell the patient that no fasting is necessary.
- ■ Anticipate parental anxiety. Provide opportunities for verbalization of fears.

After
- ■ Apply pressure or a pressure dressing to the venipuncture site to prevent further bleeding. Observe the site for bleeding.
- ■ Indicate the gestational age of the fetus on the laboratory requisition slip.
- ☞ If the AFP level is elevated, refer the patient for further testing. Explain the normal evaluation procedure.

Bence Jones Protein

Test type Urine

Normal value
No Bence Jones protein present in urine

Rationale
The Bence Jones protein is a lightweight immunoglobulin commonly found in a patient with multiple myeloma. It also may be associated with tumor metastasis to the bone, chronic lymphocytic leukemia, and amyloidosis. This protein is most notably made by plasma cells in a patient with multiple myeloma. The Bence Jones protein is rapidly cleared by the kidney and excreted in the urine. Because the Bence Jones protein is rapidly cleared from the blood by the kidney, it is difficult to detect in the blood; therefore, only urine is used for this study. Normally the urine should contain no Bence Jones proteins.

Interfering factors
A factor that interferes with determining Bence Jones protein levels is dilute urine, which may yield a false-negative result.

Procedure
An early-morning specimen of at least 50 ml of uncontaminated urine is collected in a container. It is sent to the laboratory where immunoelectrophoresis is performed on the specimen. Less accurate thermal coagulation methods also are used. It is important to avoid contamination of the specimen with stool, menstrual blood, prostatic excretions, or semen. If the specimen cannot be taken immediately to the laboratory, it should be refrigerated because heat-coagulable proteins can decompose and cause a false-positive test.

Nursing implications with rationale
Before
- ☞ Explain the procedure to the patient. Tell the patient that no fasting is necessary.
- ☞ Verify that the patient understands how to obtain a noncontaminated urine specimen. Assist the patient as needed.

After
- ■ Ensure that the specimen is taken to the laboratory as soon as possible; if there is any delay, refrigerate the specimen.

Bone Scan

Test type Nuclear scan

Normal value
No evidence of abnormality

Rationale
The bone scan is a test that examines the skeleton with a scanning camera after intravenous injection of a radioactive material. The degree of radionuclide uptake is related to bone metabolism. Normally a uniform radionuclide concentration should be seen throughout the bones. An increased uptake of isotope is abnormal and may represent tumor (Figure 13-1), arthritis, fracture, or degenerative disorders. These areas of concentrated radionuclide uptake are often called *hot spots* and are detectable months before an ordinary radiographic film can reveal a lesion.

A bone scan can detect primary and metastatic

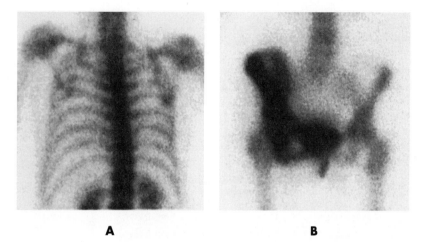

A   **B**

Figure 13-1 Bone scan. **A,** Upper body. **B,** Lower body. There is normal uptake of radionuclide in the bones of the upper body. In the lower body view, the right iliac, ischial, and pubic bones are associated with diffuse increased uptake of radionuclide, consistent with Paget's disease.

tumor. All malignancies capable of metastasis may reach the bone, especially those of the prostate, breast, lung, kidney, urinary bladder, and thyroid. Bone scanning may be repeated to detect the patient's response to radiation or chemotherapy treatment.

Bone scanning also provides valuable information in the evaluation of patients with trauma or unexplained pain. Detection of hot spots can incriminate the bone or periosteum as a source of the pain. Bone scanning is especially important in areas where fractures are not immediately seen on radiographic film (e.g., the spine, ribs, face, and small bones of the extremities). With routine radiographic examinations the radiologist may not be able to detect secondary changes produced by healing until 10 to 14 days after trauma. In contrast, with bone scans many fracture sites are revealed 3 days after the trauma. A fracture site that is revealed on a radiographic film but not on a bone scan at least 7 days after the trauma usually represents an old, healed injury.

Bone scanning also is valuable in the evaluation of patients with osteomyelitis. Routine radiographic examination changes usually do not appear until 10 to 14 days after the onset of the disease. However, bone scan abnormalities are evident days or weeks before detection on radiographic film.

The major disadvantage of bone scanning is that it is nonspecific. Many conditions (e.g., fractures, osteomyelitis, osteoarthritis, area bone necrosis, renal osteodystrophy, and Paget's disease) produce similar abnormal scans. No complications are associated with bone scanning.

Procedure

No fasting or sedation is required before bone scanning. The patient receives an intravenous injection of an isotope (e.g., sodium pertechnetate technetium [Tc] 99m) in a vein in the arm. The patient then is encouraged to drink several glasses of water between the injection of the radioisotope and the actual scanning to facilitate renal clearance of the circulating tracer not picked up by the bone. The waiting period before scanning is approximately 1 to 3 hours. The patient is instructed to urinate and then is positioned on a scanning table in the radiology department (Figure 13-2). A scanning machine moves back and forth over the patient's body and detects radiation emitted by the skeleton. This information then is translated

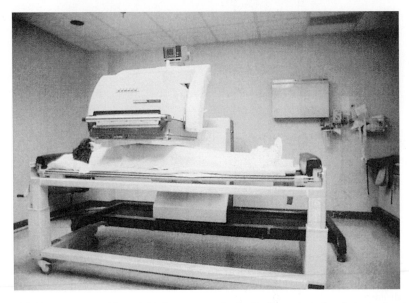

Figure 13-2 Patient positioned for bone scan. Patient's feet are tied to help maintain hips in position for maximal scanning uptake.

into radiographic film, thereby showing a two-dimensional view of the skeleton. Many radiographic films are taken; the patient may have to be repositioned several times during the test.

The only discomfort associated with this study is that of the injection of the radioisotope. This test is performed by a physician or a nuclear medicine technician in 30 to 60 minutes. Sedatives may be given if a patient has difficulty remaining still during the scanning period.

Contraindications
Contraindications associated with a bone scan are as follows:

- Pregnancy, because of the risk of fetal injury
- Lactation, because of the risk of contaminating maternal milk

Nursing implications with rationale
Before
- Explain the procedure and assure the patient that the dose of radiation received is less than the amount he or she would receive from regular diagnostic x-rays.

- Inform the patient that the injected radionuclide will not affect family, visitors, or hospital staff members. The radioactive substance usually is excreted via the urine in 6 to 24 hours.
- Inform the patient that during the scanning the patient is not exposed to any radiation. The scanning machine detects the radiation emitted from the patient, as opposed to a regular x-ray machine, in which radiation is emitted from the machine to the body. Therefore, even though the patient may be scanned for 1 hour, the amount of exposure does not cause the same radiation effects that exposure of this length to an x-ray machine would. Tell the patient that the scanning machine makes a clicking sound as it detects radioactivity.
- Instruct the patient to remove jewelry or any metal objects that may obscure radiographic visualization of the bones.
- Tell the patient that no fasting or sedation is necessary.
- After the patient receives the intravenous injection of the radioisotope, give him or her the exact time at which scanning will be done.

The patient's activities are not restricted during this waiting period. However, encourage the patient to drink several glasses of water to facilitate renal clearance of the circulating radioisotope not picked up by the bone. The patient should void before scanning because a full bladder will mask the pelvic bones.

After

- Check the injection site of the radioisotope for redness or swelling. If a hematoma forms, apply warm compresses to the area to relieve pain.   .
- Encourage the patient to drink fluids to aid in the excretion of the radioactive substance.

Case Study

Breast Cancer

Mrs. M.W. was a 48-year-old woman with an asymptomatic lump in her breast. Her physical examination indicated a 2-cm lump in the upper outer quadrant of her left breast.

Studies	Results
Routine laboratory studies	Within normal limits (WNL)
Mammography, p. 507	Poorly defined density in the upper outer quadrant of the left breast with microcalcifications strongly suspicious for cancer
Carcinoembryonic antigen (CEA), p. 65	5.8 ng/ml (normal: <2 ng/ml)
CA 27-29, p. 499	33 U/ml (normal: <38 U/ml)
Computed tomography (CT) scan of liver (see CT of abdomen, p. 113)	No evidence of metastatic tumor
Liver/spleen scan, p. 131	No evidence of metastatic tumor
Bone scan, p. 492	Mild arthritis in the lumbosacral (LS) spine
Estrogen receptor assay, p. 502	2 fmol/mg (normal: ≤3 fmol/mg)
Progesterone receptor assay, p. 509	4 fmol/mg (normal: ≤5 fmol/mg)
CT scan of the brain, p. 196	No metastasis
LS spinal x-ray examination, p. 222	Arthritis

Diagnostic Analysis

The mammography results were highly suspicious for cancer. Other possibilities included cystic breast disease and benign tumors (e.g., fibroneuroma). The CEA level was mildly elevated, which is compatible with breast cancer. Other abnormalities, however, can mildly and transiently elevate the CEA level. The CA 27-29 level was normal, as would be expected with benign disease or with nonmetastatic breast cancer. CT scans of the liver and brain, a liver/spleen scan, and bone scan were performed to detect metastasis of breast cancer. No metastasis was seen. The bone scan did "light up" in the LS spinal area; however, this is compatible with arthritis. The LS spinal x-ray examination also showed arthritis, not bone destruction by tumor.

Mrs. M.W. underwent a breast biopsy, which indicated cancer. The tumor estrogen and progesterone receptor assays were negative, indicating an aggressive tumor. After the alternatives to primary treatment for breast cancer were explained, Mrs. M.W.

Continued

Case Study

Breast Cancer—cont'd

chose lumpectomy, axillary lymph node dissection, and primary radiation with preservation of her breast. She received chemotherapy for 6 months. Yearly chest x-ray examinations, bone scans, liver scans, CEA, CA 27-29 tests, and mammograms have all been negative, indicating no evidence of recurrent tumor.

Critical Thinking Questions
1. Would Mrs. M.W.'s treatment have been different had the estrogen and progesterone assays been positive?
2. What other conditions could have resulted in an elevated CEA level?

Breast Cancer Genetic Screening
(BRCA Genetic Testing)

Test type Blood

Normal values
No genetic mutation in the BRCA 1 or 2 gene

Rationale
BRCA (BR = breast, CA = cancer) genes are the first major genes that have been recognized to indicate an increased susceptibility for development of breast cancer. BRCA 1 and 2 have been identified. The BRCA 1 gene exists on chromosome 17. BRCA 2 is on chromosome 13. More than half the women with mutations of this gene will develop breast cancer by age 50.

BRCA 1 also confers an increased susceptibility for ovarian cancer. In the normal population, only 1% of women develop ovarian cancer by age 70. However, 44% of women with mutations of the BRCA gene develop ovarian cancer.

Testing a select group of women who may be at high risk for BRCA genetic mutations offers the following benefits:

1. Identification of women at high risk for developing breast or ovarian cancer
2. Consideration of interventions for women who test positive for BRCA mutations (e.g., prophylactic mastectomy/oophorectomy)
3. Adoption of risk-management screening testing
4. Estimation of potential for passing the mutated BRCA gene to offspring

Potential complication
A potential complication associated with BRCA genetic testing is psychologic distress. Positive test results may significantly affect the psychoemotional stability of the patient or family members who also may have the BRCA gene.

Procedure
No fasting is required. It is recommended that all patients who undergo testing should receive genetic counseling before and after testing. Written and informed consent should be obtained. Venous blood is collected in the special collecting tube provided by the reference laboratory. The specimen then is sent to the laboratory by mail.

Contraindication
BRCA genetic testing is contraindicated for patients who are not emotionally able to deal with the results.

Nursing implications with rationale
Before
- Explain the procedure to the patient. Tell the patient that no fasting is necessary.
- Be aware of the ethical problems and disad-

vantages posed by genetic testing. Patients may face financial discrimination for health or life insurance or employment if the results are positive.

After

■ Apply pressure or a pressure dressing to the venipuncture site to prevent further bleeding. Observe the site for bleeding.

Breast Scintigraphy (Breast Scan, Sestamibi Scan, Scintimammography)

Test type Nuclear scan

Normal values

Negative: minimal, symmetrical, bilateral, and uniform breast uptake equal to soft tissue uptake

Rationale

Nuclear scans of the breast, using Tc 99m sestamibi, are used to identify breast cancer in patients whose dense breast tissue precludes accurate evaluation by conventional mammography. This test has been used as an adjunct in patients with indeterminate mammograms and in women with lumpy breasts. However, this scan may miss as many as 10% to 15% of cancers. Furthermore, the false-positive rate is approximately 15%. Breast cancer takes up sestamibi, causing an increased uptake of radiotracer at the site of a cancer. Areas of benign cellular hyperplasia, however, also trap the radiotracer. Because cellular breast hyperplasia is a common finding just before menses, imaging at this time in the menstrual cycle should be avoided.

Breast nuclear scans will not replace mammography's role in breast imaging. Nor will they ever be an effective screening tool for the early detection of breast cancer among large populations. However, their role as a second-line imaging modality is growing.

Breast scintigraphy also is used to identify the lymphatic drainage of a certain area of the breast. This allows a more directed approach to lymph node staging for breast cancer. The radiotracer often goes directly to the axillary lymph node (sentinel lymph node) most likely to drain that specific area of the breast. If there is a metastatic tumor in the lymph nodes, it would be found in the sentinel lymph node.

Procedure

The patient may be positioned in the supine, prone, or sitting position. Twenty mCi of Tc 99m sestamibi is injected intravenously into the arm contralateral to the suspicious breast. Imaging begins 10 minutes after injection. A scintillator camera is placed over the breast and records the radiation emitted. This information is translated into a two-dimensional view of the skeleton, which then is visualized on film. These images are compared with surrounding soft tissue readings.

Contraindications

Contraindications for breast scintigraphy are as follows:

■ Pregnancy, because of the risk of fetal injury
■ Lactation, because of the risk of contaminating maternal milk

Nursing implications with rationale

Before

☞ Explain the procedure to the patient. Tell the patient that no fasting or sedation is required.
☞ Inform the patient that she will not be exposed to large amounts of radioactivity because only tracer doses of the isotope are used. No precautions are necessary to prevent radioactive exposure to personnel or family.
☞ Assure the patient that the radioactive substance is usually excreted from the body within 6 to 24 hours.

After

☞ Encourage the patient to drink fluids to aid in the excretion of the radioactive substance.
■ Observe the injection site for redness or swelling.

Breast Sonogram (Ultrasound Mammography, Ultrasound of the Breast)

Test type Ultrasound

Normal values
No evidence of cyst or tumor

Rationale
In diagnostic real-time ultrasound, harmless high-frequency sound waves are emitted and penetrate the breast. The sound waves are bounced back to a sensor and arranged in a pictorial image by electronic conversion. Ultrasound of the breast is a useful test for differentiating cystic (fluid-filled) from solid breast lesions. It is helpful in identifying a mass in breast tissue that is too dense for accurate mammography. It can be used to monitor a cyst to determine if it enlarges or disappears. Ultrasound also can be used to locate a nonpalpable breast abnormality for biopsy or aspiration. In addition, ultrasound of the breast is useful in the examination of symptomatic women for whom the radiation of mammography is potentially harmful. These include:

1. Pregnant women. Radiation may be harmful to the fetus.
2. Women under the age of 25. These women may experience a greater oncologic risk from the radiation of mammography.
3. Women who have silicone-augmented breasts. The prosthesis can be penetrated by the ultrasound beam. Ordinarily these prostheses would obscure residual tissue on physical examination and x-ray mammography.
4. Women who refuse to have x-ray mammography because of fear of diagnostic radiation.

Procedure
No fasting or sedation is required before the test. The patient lies in the prone position on the examining table, which contains a tank that holds heated and chlorinated water. The transducer that produces the ultrasound waves and detects their echoes is positioned at the bottom of the water tank. One breast at a time is immersed in the water. Alternatively, and now more frequently, the patient is placed in the supine position, and the transducer is directly

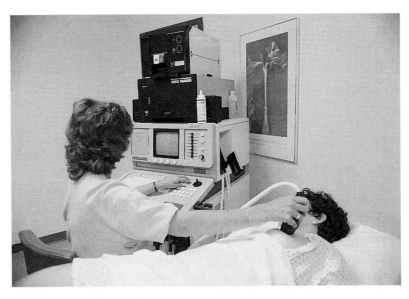

Figure 13-3 Ultrasonography of the breast.

applied to the breast using contact gel to improve sound transmission (Figure 13-3). This test is performed by an ultrasound technician in approximately 15 minutes.

Nursing implications with rationale
Before
- ☞ Explain the procedure to the patient. Inform the patient that no discomfort is associated with this study and that no fasting or sedation is necessary.
- ▪ Instruct the patient not to apply any lotions or powders to her breasts on the examination day.

After
- ▪ Assist the patient with drying her breasts and removing the conductive paste.

Cancer 19-9 Tumor Marker (CA 19-9)

Test type Blood

Normal values
<37 U/ml

Rationale
Cancer antigen (CA) 19-9 is a tumor marker used in diagnosis, evaluation of response to treatment, and surveillance of patients with pancreatic or hepatobiliary cancer. It is used primarily in the diagnosis of pancreatic carcinoma. For example, in a patient whose presenting symptom is pancreatic mass or biliary obstruction, markedly elevated levels of CA 19-9 would confirm that pancreatic cancer exists. Likewise, a patient whose presenting symptoms are ascites, jaundice, and an elevated CA 19-9 level may have hepatobiliary cancer. CA 19-9 levels, however, may not be elevated in all patients with pancreatic carcinoma. Approximately 70% of patients with pancreatic carcinoma and 65% of patients with hepatobiliary cancer have elevated CA 19-9 levels.

CA 19-9 serum tumor marker also is used to determine response to treatment. In the few patients with pancreatobiliary cancer who have a good tumor response to surgery, chemotherapy, or radiation therapy a decline in serum levels of CA 19-9 confirms this response. CA 19-9 levels are used in the posttreatment surveillance of patients who have had pancreatohepatobiliary cancers. A rapid rise in CA 19-9 levels can be associated with a recurrent or progressive tumor growth. Mildly elevated levels may exist in patients with gastric or colorectal cancer and even in 6% to 7% of patients with nongastrointestinal malignancies (e.g., of the lung). Patients who have pancreatitis, gallstones, cirrhosis, and cystic fibrosis may have minimally elevated levels of CA 19-9. Because of its lack of sensitivity and specificity, CA 19-9 is not effective in screening for pancreatobiliary tumors in the general population.

Procedure
CA 19-9 testing is performed on the serum of a patient with suspected hepatobiliary neoplasms. No pretesting preparation is required. Venipuncture is performed, and 7 to 10 ml of blood is collected in a red-top tube. The blood is usually sent to a reference laboratory that frequently performs this test. The results are available in 3 to 5 days.

Nursing implications with rationale
Before
- ☞ Explain the procedure to the patient. Tell the patient that no fasting is required.

After
- ▪ Apply pressure or a pressure dressing to the venipuncture site to prevent further bleeding. Observe the site for bleeding.

Cancer 27.29 and Cancer 15-3 Tumor Markers (CA 27.29 and CA 15-3)

Test type Blood

Normal values
CA 27.29: <38 U/mL
CA 15-3: <22 U/ml

Rationale
The cancer antigens (CAs) 15-3 and 27.29 are tumor-associated serum markers available for staging breast cancer and monitoring its treat-

ment. Carcinoembryonic antigen (CEA, see p. 65), the most widely used tumor marker, is limited by poor sensitivity and specificity for patients with breast cancer. Recently, monoclonal antibody technology has permitted the development of CA 15-3 and CA 27.29 testing. However, these antigens are not as sensitive in the diagnosis of primary breast cancer as other tumor markers are for their respective tumors. CA 15-3 and CA 27.29 levels are high in only 50% of patients who have a localized breast cancer or a small tumor burden. Eighty percent of patients with metastatic breast cancer do have elevated CA 15-3 levels, and 65% have elevated CA 27.29 levels; therefore the usefulness of these antigen tests as a screening technique in early breast cancers (the most common cancer in women) is limited.

Benign breast disease and nonbreast malignancies (e.g., lung, pancreas, ovary, and prostate) also can cause elevation of these antigen levels. These antigens are useful in monitoring the patient's response to therapy for metastatic breast cancer. A partial or complete response to treatment will be confirmed by declining levels. Likewise, a persistent rise in these antigen levels, despite therapy, strongly suggests progressive disease.

Interfering factors

Factors that interfere with determining CA 27.29 and CA 15-3 levels include other benign and malignant diseases that may be associated with elevations of these antigens (e.g., cancer of the lung, ovary, pancreas, prostate, and colon; fibrocystic disease of the breast; cirrhosis; and hepatitis).

Procedure

No fasting is required. Approximately 7 to 10 ml of venous blood is collected in a red-top tube. The blood sample is sent to a reference laboratory for testing.

Nursing implications with rationale

Before
- Explain the procedure to the patient. Tell the patient that no fasting is required.

After
- Apply pressure or a pressure dressing to the venipuncture site to prevent further bleeding. Observe the site for bleeding.
- Note that results are available in 7 to 10 days.

Cancer Antigen-125 Tumor Marker (CA-125)

Test type Blood

Normal values
0-35 U/ml

Rationale

The detection, extent of disease, and response to the treatment of ovarian cancer can be determined by cancer antigen (CA)-125 testing. This tumor marker has a high degree of sensitivity and specificity for ovarian cancer and has proved to be of great benefit for clinicians. Although AFP and human chorionic gonadotropin (HCG) are accurate tumor markers for germ cell tumors of the ovary, CA-125 is an extremely accurate tumor marker for epithelial tumors of the ovary.

CA-125 can be used in many ways. It is helpful in making the diagnosis of ovarian cancer. For example, CA-125 can be used in patients whose presenting symptoms are sudden onset of abdominal distention, ascites, and palpable pelvic masses. In these patients, a markedly elevated CA-125 is strong confirmatory evidence that the underlying etiology represents epithelial ovarian malignancy.

CA-125 also is used to determine response to therapy. Serial comparative testing shows a progressive decline in CA-125 levels for patients having a response to treatment. CA-125 tumor markers also can predict whether a second-look diagnostic laparotomy will be positive. In 97% of patients whose CA-125 level is greater than 35 U/ml, a residual tumor is detected at a second-look laparotomy, whereas only 56% of ovarian cancer patients whose CA-125 level is less than 35 U/ml have a positive second-look laparotomy.

Finally, CA-125 determinations can be used in posttreatment surveillance of patients with ovarian cancer. If a patient has had complete tumor response as a result of radiation therapy, chemotherapy, or surgery, a delayed rise in CA-125 levels may be an early predictor of a recurrent tumor. CA-125 has not yet been used as a screening test for the asymptomatic population; however, it currently is being studied in high-risk patients.

Other tumors and benign processes can cause elevation of CA-125 levels. In 20% of patients with colon cancer and 60% of patients with upper gastrointestinal cancers, CA-125 levels exceed 35 U/ml. Endometrial, fallopian tube, lung, and breast cancers also can cause elevations of CA-125. It is interesting to note that patients with benign peritoneal diseases (e.g., cirrhosis and endometriosis) have mild CA-125 elevations. Pregnancy and normal menstruation also may cause mild elevations of CA-125. Increased levels occur in 2% of healthy people and 6% of patients with nonmalignant diseases.

Procedure

Serum from the female patient is obtained in a red-top tube by a laboratory technician. No fasting or other preparatory steps are required. Although the blood can be drawn in any local hospital, it is usually sent to one of the few reference laboratories for determination of the CA-125 level.

Nursing implications with rationale

Before

✒ Explain the procedure to the patient. Tell the patient that no fasting is required.

After

■ Apply pressure or a pressure dressing to the venipuncture site to prevent further bleeding. Observe the site for bleeding.

Case Study

Serum Tumor Markers

Ms. T.G., 52 years old, had a 2-week history of abdominal discomfort associated with rapid onset of abdominal distention, weight gain, anorexia, and mild nausea. She also noted marked shortness of breath and weakness. Her physical examination indicated that she had decreased breath sounds bilaterally. Her abdomen was distended and obviously ascitic. She was mildly edematous in both lower extremities.

Studies

Chest x-ray examination, p. 155
Routine laboratory studies
CT scan of the abdomen, p. 113

Serum tumor markers
   CA 27.29, p. 499
   CA-125, p. 500
   CA-19-9, p. 499
   CEA, p. 65

Results

Bilateral effusion
WNL
Diffuse ascites and nodular peritoneal
   tumor implantation

20 U/ml (normal: <38 U/ml)
859 U/ml (normal: 0-35 U/ml)
18 units/ml (normal: <37 U/ml)
1 ng/ml (normal: <2 ng/ml)

Diagnostic Analysis

Ms. T.G.'s test results supported the clinical findings of diffuse ascites and a pleural effusion apparently resulting from a neoplastic cause. Neoplasms that might have caused

Continued

Serum Tumor Markers—cont'd

the above findings included metastatic bowel cancer, pancreatic cancer, breast cancer, or ovarian cancer. The normal CEA level did not suggest the bowel as a primary cancer site. Likewise, the normal CA 19-9 level excluded pancreatic cancer, and the normal CA 27.29 level made it unlikely that the primary cancer site was the breast. The markedly elevated CA-125 level provided strong supportive evidence that the primary site of cancer was the ovaries. The results reflect the typical tumor marker profile of a patient with ovarian cancer. Ms. T.G. underwent a diagnostic laparotomy and tumor debulking. She subsequently underwent chemotherapy, and on a second-look operation 1 year later she was found to be free of disease.

Critical Thinking Questions

1. How does the diagnosis of ovarian cancer relate to Ms. T.G.'s presenting symptoms?
2. Which tumor markers would be evaluated in the follow-up of this patient?

Estrogen Receptor Assay (ERA, ER, Estradiol Receptor)

Test type Microscopic examination

Normal values

Negative: ≤10 fmol/mg of protein
Positive: >10 fmol/mg of protein

Rationale

Estrogen receptor (ER) assays are useful in the prognosis and treatment of breast carcinoma. They are used to determine whether a tumor is likely to respond to endocrine medicinal therapy or to removal of the ovaries or adrenal gland. Hormone receptor assays should be done for all patients with primary or recurrent breast carcinomas. Levels tend to be higher in postmenopausal women. In general, ER-positive tumors have a better prognosis than ER-negative tumors.

Slightly more than half of patients with breast carcinoma who are ER-positive respond to endocrine therapy (e.g., tamoxifen [Nolvadex], estrogens, androgens, oophorectomy, or adrenalectomy). The response is greater when progesterone receptors (see p. 509) also are positive. Patients whose breast cancers lack these hormone receptors (ER-negative) have a much lower chance of tumor response to hormone therapy and may not be candidates for endocrine therapy.

Specimens are collected during surgery according to the protocol of the pathologist. Usually the paraffin-embedded tissue is stained with a monoclonal antibody that stains the ER-positive sites. Usually, if greater than 5% to 10% of the tumor takes up stain, the ER is considered positive. This is usually done at a reference laboratory. Hormones should be discontinued before the breast biopsy procedure.

Interfering factors

Factors that interfere with determining ER assays include the following:

- Delay in tissue fixation, which may cause deterioration of receptor proteins and produce lower values
- Antiestrogen preparations (e.g., tamoxifen) during the past 2 months, because they may cause false-negative ER assays
- Exogenous hormones, which are taken for contraception or menopausal hormone replacement therapy, which may produce lower receptor values

Procedure

Before the biopsy procedure, a gynecologic history is obtained, including menopausal status and exogenous hormone use. The surgeon removes at least 1 g of tumor tissue. This is placed on ice and immediately transferred to the pathology department. Part of the tissue is used for routine histology, and at least 1 g is frozen. The frozen specimen is packed in dry ice and sent to a reference laboratory for ER analysis. Results are usually available in 2 weeks. Immunohistochemical methods of ER assay are available on specimens weighing less than 1 g.

Nursing implications with rationale

Before

☞ Explain the procedure to the patient. Answer any questions that she may have.

☞ Provide emotional support because women are usually very anxious regarding breast surgery.

After

☞ Tell the patient that results are usually available in 2 weeks.

Gallium Scan

Test type Nuclear scan

Normal values

Gallium uptake in the liver, spleen, bone, and colon; no other concentration noted

Rationale

Gallium scan is a total body scan usually performed 24, 48, and 72 hours after an intravenous injection of radioactive gallium (Ga 67 citrate). Gallium is a radionuclide that is concentrated by areas of inflammation, infection, abscess, and benign and malignant tumors. However, not all types of tumors concentrate gallium. Tumors that can be detected by gallium scans include sarcomas, lymphomas, hepatomas, and carcinomas of the colon, kidney, uterus, stomach, and testicle.

This test is useful in detecting primary or meta-static tumors when cancer is suspected but cannot be located by other diagnostic techniques. It also is very useful in demonstrating the source of infection in patients who have fever of unknown origin. Unfortunately, this test is not capable of differentiating tumor from infection, inflammation, or abscess.

The radionuclide is normally taken up by the liver, spleen, bone, and large bowel. As a result, the uniformity of uptake by the liver and spleen can be determined in a way similar to that described by a technetium liver scan (see p. 131). A normal total body gallium scan study would demonstrate some uptake of gallium in the liver, spleen, bone, and colon; no marked concentration of gallium would occur elsewhere.

Procedure

The unsedated patient is injected with gallium citrate. A total body scan may be performed 4 to 6 hours later by slowly passing a radionuclide detector over the body. Additional scans are taken 24, 48, and 72 hours later. During the scanning process, the patient is positioned in the supine, prone, and lateral positions. Because the bowel can take up the gallium, suppositories or enemas are sometimes given a few hours before scanning. This is especially important when accurate imaging of the abdomen or pelvis is required. The patient is asked to lie very still during the actual scanning, which takes about 30 to 60 minutes each time. It usually is performed in the nuclear medicine department by a nuclear medicine technician and interpreted by a nuclear medicine physician.

Contraindication

A contraindication for gallium scan is pregnancy because of the risk of fetal injury.

Nursing implications with rationale

Before

☞ Explain the procedure to the patient. Reassure the patient that the test is painless and the dose of radionuclide is safe.

■ Administer enemas or suppositories as ordered before scanning is performed to wash out the gallium secreted in the bowel. This eliminates the possibility that increased uptake in the sigmoid colon could be misread as a pathologic process.

☑ Instruct the patient to return for subsequent scanning.

After

☑ Assure the patient that only tracer doses of radioisotopes have been used and that no precautions against radioactive exposure to others are necessary.

Human Chorionic Gonadotropin
(HCG)

Test type Blood, urine

Normal value
Negative

Rationale
Human chorionic gonadotropin (HCG) can be used to determine fetal or placental function. However, it also is useful in determining the clinical course of patients with germ cell tumors.

HCG is produced by trophoblastic cells in the fetoplacental unit. HCG provides the basis for all pregnancy tests (see p. 382). Gestational tumors (e.g., hydatidiform moles and uterine choriocarcinomas) and gonadal tumors can be detected by increased levels of HCG in patients who have clinical pictures suspicious for those tumors. Once these tumors have been diagnosed, HCG measurements can act as guidelines for evaluation of the success of therapy. Elevated HCG levels are suspicious for tumor progression; decreased levels indicate effective antitumor treatment. Cancers of the gastrointestinal tract, lung, and liver also are occasionally associated with elevated HCG levels.

Interfering factors
A factor that interferes with determining HCG levels is urine dilution. HCG levels may be nondetectable in dilute urine but may be detectable in concentrated urine.

Procedure
Urine:
Urine specimens should be collected in a standard container and taken to the laboratory. A first-voided morning specimen is preferred.

Blood:
Blood samples are obtained according to the requirements of the specific test to be performed. Hemolysis of blood may interfere with test results.

Nursing implications with rationale
☑ Explain the procedure to the patient. Encourage verbalization of the patient's fears. Many patients are very anxious in anticipation of the results.

■ If a urine specimen is required, give the patient a urine container on the evening before the test so that she can provide a first-voided morning specimen. This specimen generally contains the greatest concentration of HCG.

☑ Inform the patient regarding how and when to obtain the test results.

5-Hydroxyindoleacetic Acid
(5-HIAA)

Test type Urine

Normal values
2-6 mg/24 hours or 10.4-31.2 mmol/day (SI units)
Women's levels are lower than men's

Rationale
Qualitative analysis of urine levels of 5-hydroxyindoleacetic acid (5-HIAA) is used to detect and follow the clinical course of patients with carcinoid tumors. Carcinoid tumors are serotonin-secreting tumors and may grow in the appendix, intestine, pancreas, ovaries, or lungs or are derived from the neuroectoderm. These tumors contain argentaffin cells, which produce serotonin and other powerful vasopressors that are metabolized by the liver to 5-HIAA and excreted in the urine. These powerful vasopressors are responsible for the clinical presentation of the carci-

noid syndrome (bronchospasm, flushing, and diarrhea).

This test is used to evaluate the possibility of carcinoid tumor in patients who present with bronchospasm, diarrhea, and flushing. Also, patients with known carcinoid tumor may be evaluated by serial levels of urinary 5-HIAA. Rising levels of 5-HIAA indicate worsening of tumor; falling levels of 5-HIAA indicate a response to antineoplastic therapy.

Interfering factors
Factors that interfere with determining 5-HIAA levels include bananas, plantains, pineapples, kiwi, walnuts, plums, pecans, and avocados, which can factitiously elevate 5-HIAA levels.

Procedure
Urine is collected for 24 hours in a large container with a preservative to keep the specimen at an appropriate pH level. The specimen is kept refrigerated during the collection period. After the 24-hour collection has been completed, the specimen is taken to the chemistry laboratory.

Nursing implications with rationale
Before
- ☞ Explain to the patient the procedure for collecting a 24-hour urine sample.
- ☞ Tell the patient that no fasting is necessary.
- ☞ Instruct the patient regarding medication restrictions. Many medications affect test results.
- ☞ Instruct the patient to refrain from eating foods containing serotonin (e.g., plums, pineapples, bananas, eggplants, tomatoes, avocados, walnuts) for several days (usually 3) before and during the testing period.

During
- ☞ Instruct the patient to begin the 24-hour urine collection after discarding the first morning specimen. This is the start time of the 24-hour collection.
- ▪ Collect all urine passed over the next 24 hours.
- ☞ Instruct the patient to void before defecating so that the urine is not contaminated by feces.

- ☞ Remind the patient not to put toilet paper in the collection container.
- ▪ Keep the urine specimen on ice or refrigerated during the 24 hours. A preservative is needed to maintain an appropriate pH.
- ▪ Collect the last specimen as close as possible to the end of the 24 hours. Add this specimen to the container.

After
- ▪ Transport the urine specimen promptly to the laboratory.
- ▪ List all medications on the laboratory requisition slip because many drugs can affect test results.

Lymphangiography
(Lymphangiogram, Lymphography)

Test type X-ray with contrast dye

Normal values
Normal lymph nodes and vessels

Rationale
Lymphangiography provides a radiographic examination of the lymphatic system after the injection of contrast medium into a lymphatic vessel in each foot or hand. The lymphatic system consists of lymph vessels and nodes. Assessment of this system is important because cancer often spreads via the lymphatic system. When the lymph vessels become obstructed, edema usually results. Lymphangiography aids in evaluating unexplained swelling of an extremity.

Lymphangiography is indicated in patients with edema or signs of tumor (e.g., unexplained fever, weight loss, or enlarged lymph nodes) or to evaluate the spread of cancer within the body. Lymphangiography is useful in staging a lymphoma to determine appropriate therapy and in evaluating the results of chemotherapy or radiation therapy. Because the contrast medium remains in the lymph nodes for 6 months to 1 year, repeat plain film x-ray examinations may be done for follow-up evaluation of disease progression or response to treatment.

Potential complications

Potential complications associated with lymphangiography are as follows:

- Lipoid (lipid) pneumonia
  This occurs if the contrast medium flows into the thoracic duct and causes micropulmonary emboli. These small emboli usually disappear after several weeks or months.
- Allergic reaction or allergy to iodine dye
  Allergic reactions vary from flushing, itching, and urticaria to life-threatening anaphylaxis (evidenced by respiratory distress, drop in blood pressure, shock).

Procedure

No fasting or sedation is usually required for lymphangiography. This procedure is performed in the radiology department with the patient in the supine position. A blue dye is injected between each of the first three toes of each foot to outline the lymphatic vessels (Figure 13-4). (The dye can also be injected into the web of skin between the fingers.) A local anesthetic then is injected before a small incision is made in each foot. A lymphatic vessel is identified, and a cannula is inserted to infuse the iodine contrast agent. The dye is infused into the vessels, usually with an infusion pump, which injects the dye at a slow, continuous rate for approximately 1½ hours. The patient must lie very still during the dye injection. The flow of iodine dye throughout the body is followed by fluoroscopy (moving x-ray pictures on a television monitor). When the contrast medium reaches a certain level of the lumbar vertebrae, the dye is discontinued. Films of the stomach, pelvis, and upper body are then taken to demonstrate the filling of the lymphatic vessels. The patient must return in 24 hours to have additional radiographic studies taken to visualize the lymph nodes. When the injection is given in the hand, the axillary and supraclavicular lymph nodes are evaluated. When the injection is completed, the cannula is removed, and the incision is sutured.

This procedure is performed by a radiologist in approximately 3 hours. Additional radiographic films must be taken again at 24 hours, but these take less than 30 minutes to perform. Discomfort

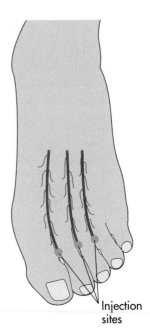

Figure 13-4 Lymphangiogram. Sites for dye injection.

may be felt when the toes are locally anesthetized. Injection of the dye between the toes or fingers causes transient discomfort. However, the most uncomfortable part of this procedure may be that associated with lying still on the hard x-ray table.

Contraindications

Contraindications for lymphangiography are as follows:

- Patients with an allergy to iodine dye or shellfish
- Patients with severe chronic lung disease or cardiac, kidney, or liver disease, because the lipid-containing radiopaque dye may further injure these organs

Nursing implications with rationale

Before
- Explain the procedure to the patient. Inform the patient that remaining still during the test is essential.
- Ensure that the patient has signed a consent form.

■ Assess the patient for allergies to iodine, seafood, or dyes used in diagnostic studies (e.g., intravenous pyelography).

☞ Inform the patient that the blue dye gives the skin a bluish tinge and may discolor the urine and stool for 2 days.

After

■ Assess the patient for signs of shortness of breath, chest pain, fever, or hypotension, which could be caused by microemboli from spillage of the contrast dye into the thoracic duct.

■ Note that bed rest usually is prescribed for approximately 24 hours after this test.

■ Elevate the patient's affected extremity to help prevent edema.

☞ Inform the patient that the incision site may be sore for several days. Administer mild analgesics for pain after the local anesthetic wears off. Apply warm compresses as ordered to reduce discomfort from inflammation.

☞ Tell the patient that the sutures are removed in approximately 1 week. Until this time keep the incision site clean and dry. Examine the site for signs of infection (e.g., redness, swelling, and oozing). Because of the possibility of nerve damage, immediately report any numbness in the extremity to the physician.

Mammography (Mammogram)

Test type X-ray

Normal values
Category I: Negative
Category II: Benign findings

Rationale
A mammogram is able to detect breast cancers, benign tumors, and cysts before they are palpable. Mammography can be performed for screening or diagnostic purposes. For *screening* purposes, all women between ages 50 and 80 should have a two-view mammogram annually. (Some controversy exists about screening women between ages 40 and 50.) Annual screening mammograms should be done on women with

(1) a personal history of breast cancer, (2) lumpy or dense breasts, (3) genetic susceptibility to breast cancer, (4) more than four first- or second-degree relatives with breast cancer, especially breast cancer or ovarian cancer in each generation, (5) a close relative with breast cancer, or (6) first pregnancy after age 30. A two-view *diagnostic* mammogram is recommended for women older than age 25 if they have breast symptoms (e.g., a palpable nodule or lump, breast skin thickening or indentation, nipple discharge or retraction, erosive sore of the nipple, breast pain).

Radiographic signs of breast cancer include fine, stippled, clustered calcifications (white specks on the breast radiographic films); a poorly defined, spiculated mass; asymmetric density; and skin thickening (Figure 13-5). The accuracy of breast cancer detection with mammography is approximately 85%; 15% of breast cancers are missed by mammography. Almost 35% of breast cancers are not palpable and are detected only by mammography. Therefore, the combination of mammography and close physical examination provides the best approach to detect breast cancer at its earliest stage.

Mammography also can detect other diseases of the breast, including acute suppurative mastitis, abscess, fibrocystic changes, cysts, benign tumors (e.g., fibroadenoma), and intraglandular lymph nodes. Mammography also can be used to locate a mammographically identifiable lesion (i.e., not palpable) for biopsy. The most common method is called *preoperative mammogram localization* of the mammogram abnormality followed by an open biopsy procedure.

In the past, radiation exposure was significant with mammography. Today, however, because of fast-speed film, little radiation (0.25 rads) is required to expose mammogram film.

The American College of Radiology (ACR) has recommended standardization of mammogram reports as follows:

Class I: Negative
Class II: Benign
Class III: Benign; short-term follow-up suggested

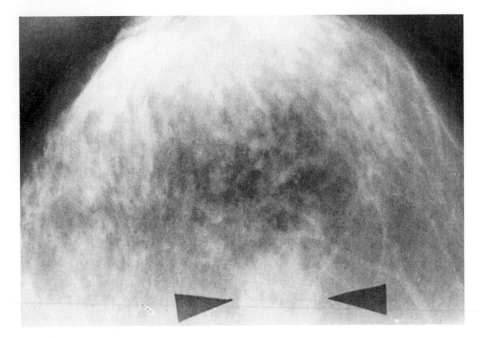

Figure 13-5 Mammogram. Craniocaudal view of breast. Pointers indicate typical breast cancer. Note poorly defined margins.

Class IV: Suspicious for cancer; further evaluation suggested

Class V: Cancer highly suspected

Interfering factors

Factors that interfere with mammography include the following:

- Talc powder, which can give the impression of calcification within the breast
- Jewelry worn around the neck, because it can preclude total visualization of the breast
- Breast augmentation implants, because they prevent total visualization of the breast
- Previous breast surgery, because it can distort the mammogram

Procedure

The nonfasting, unsedated patient is taken to the breast imaging center and placed in front of the mammographic x-ray machine (Figure 13-6). One breast is placed on an x-ray plate, and the x-ray cone is brought down on top of the breast to compress it gently between the broadened cone and the x-ray film plate. A radiographic film is taken. This is called the *craniocaudal view*. Next, the x-ray plate is turned perpendicular to the floor and placed laterally on the outer aspect of the breast. The broadened cone then is brought in medially, again gently compressing the breast. This creates the *mediolateral view*. Other views also are performed.

Discomfort associated with mammography varies. Some women report pain caused by the pressure, which is required to flatten the breast tissue on the x-ray plate. Mammography is performed by a radiologic technician in approximately 10 minutes. The x-ray films are viewed and interpreted by a skilled radiologist.

Contraindications

Contraindications associated with mammography are as follows:

- Patients who are pregnant, because of the risk of fetal damage
- Women under age 25
  These women are particularly susceptible to

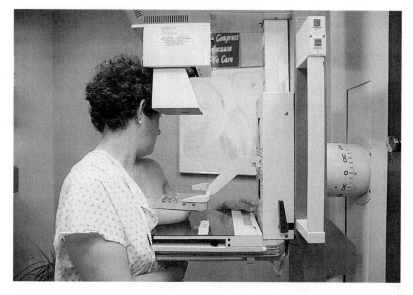

Figure 13-6   Mammography procedure.

the neoplastic effects of ionizing radiation associated with mammography.

Nursing implications with rationale

Before

☞ Explain the procedure to the patient. Inform the patient of the recent advances in mammography and of the minimal risk associated with this study.

☞ Tell the patient that no fasting or sedation is necessary.

■ Some patients may be embarrassed by this procedure. Allow them to verbalize their feelings.

■ Some patients are very anxious regarding breast mammography. Provide emotional support.

☞ Inform the patient that some discomfort may be experienced during breast compression. Compression allows better visualization of the breast tissue. Assure the patient that the breast will not be harmed by compression.

After

■ Support the patient in her concerns if additional views are required. Usually these views include *spot magnified views*, which allow the radiologist to better visualize an area of the breast.

☞ Tell the patient how and when she can get the results of this study. Usually the results are available 1 day after the test.

☞ Instruct the patient to perform a breast self-examination after each menstrual period. Teach the patient this procedure, if necessary.

Progesterone Receptor Assay
(PRA, PgR assay)

Test type Microscopic examination

Normal values
Negative: ≤10 fmol/mg
Positive: >10 fmol/mg

Rationale
Progesterone receptor (PR) assays are useful in the prognosis and treatment of breast cancer. They determine whether a tumor is likely to respond to endocrine medical therapy or removal of the ovaries or adrenal glands. Hormone receptor assays should be done on all patients with primary or recurrent breast carcinomas. This test is used in conjunction with ER assays (see p. 502) to increase predictability of tumor

response to hormonal therapy in patients with breast carcinoma. PR levels tend to be higher in postmenopausal women. PR-positive tumors usually have a better prognosis than do PR-negative tumors.

Tumor response rate to medical or surgical hormonal manipulation is potentiated if the ER assay also is positive. Response rates are as follows:

ER-positive; PR-positive = 75%
ER-negative; PR-positive = 60%
ER-positive; PR-negative = 35%
ER-negative; PR-negative = 25%

Exogenous hormones should be discontinued before breast tumor biopsy.

Interfering factor

A factor that interferes with determining PR assays includes the use of hormones (e.g., progesterone or estrogen), which may cause false-negative results.

Procedure

Before biopsy, a gynecologic history, including menopausal status and exogenous hormone use, is obtained. The surgeon removes at least 1 g of tumor tissue. This is placed on ice and immediately transferred to the pathology department. Part of the tissue is used for routine histology, and at least 1 g is frozen. The frozen specimen then is packed in dry ice and sent to a reference laboratory for PR analysis. Results usually are available in 2 weeks. Immunohistochemical methods of PR assay are available on specimens weighing less than 1 g.

Nursing implications with rationale

Before
☞ Explain the procedure to the patient.
■ Record the menstrual status of the patient and note if the patient was or is undergoing hormonal therapy.
■ Provide emotional support. Women are usually very anxious regarding breast surgery.
After
☞ Inform the patient that results usually are available in 2 weeks.

REVIEW QUESTIONS AND ANSWERS

1. **Question:** Your 36-year-old patient indicates that she wants both of her breasts removed because of a strong family history of breast cancer. Her mother developed breast cancer at age 45 and died of that disease at age 50. Her older sister is now dying of breast cancer at age 44. She has two young daughters and does not want to risk the chance of dying before her children grow up. What advice might you give her?

   Answer: This woman does have a significant family history of breast cancer. Depending on a more thorough evaluation of the family, she may have a 25% or greater chance of having a genetic defect in a BRCA gene. Rather than blindly proceeding with bilateral mastectomies, you may suggest genetic counseling. If appropriate, the patient and her sister could be tested for the BRCA gene. If negative, the patient would not be at any increased risk of breast cancer, and mastectomy would not be helpful. Furthermore, her two daughters would be free of an increased risk for the future. It is important to indicate to the BRCA-negative patient that her risk is not zero. She still has a risk similar to the general public for the development of breast cancer.

2. **Question:** Your postmenopausal patient had breast cancer several years ago and is complaining of hot flashes and vaginal dryness. Her lipid profile is abnormal. She would like to take hormone replacement therapy. Her original tumor was ER- and PR-positive. Should this information have any impact on her decision?

   Answer: Estrogen and progesterone receptors merely indicate the likelihood that the breast cancer would respond to hormonal manipulation were it to return. They in no way can indicate the risks of hormone replacement therapy in a previously treated breast cancer patient. As larger numbers of younger women are being diagnosed with breast cancer, the question of the risk and benefits of hormone replacement therapy is being increasingly discussed. The ER/PR status of the original tumor should not affect that discussion.

3. **Question:** Your 48-year-old patient is concerned about the radiation exposure risk associated with mammography. She would like to undergo a new breast scintigraphy instead. How might you advise her?

   Answer: Mammography is associated with less than 0.25 rads per study. At most the patient receives less than 1 rad per year. The minimum radiation exposure to present a 1% increased risk in a woman over age 30 is 100 rads. Therefore, mammography is very safe to have annually after age 40. Breast scintigraphy probably equals mammography in radiation exposure but is much less sensitive and less specific than mammography. Breast scintigraphy is not an appropriate screening tool for the diagnosis of breast cancer.

4. **Question:** Your patient, who is having a routine evaluation, is found to have a suspicious lesion during mammography. Her physical examination results are negative, and she has no palpable masses. Should a biopsy of this mass be performed?

   Answer: With the widespread routine use of mammography, early, nonpalpable cancers are being found more often. It is not unusual for a small cancer to be clinically undetectable. Therefore, if the mammography is suspicious, a biopsy should be performed so that the cancer can be treated at the earliest stage if the results are positive.

5. **Question:** Your patient is a 56-year-old woman who had a colon cancer removed 2 years ago. Her CEA level is now 4.2. Is this significant?

   Answer: This patient's CEA level (see Chapter 3) is clearly elevated. However, without knowing previous CEA levels, one cannot say with certainty that the level is representative of recurrent disease. Some patients persistently have a mildly elevated CEA level without evidence of recurrent disease. A rising CEA level is of clinical significance. If the CEA level is found to be rising monthly on three successive tests, one should strongly consider the possi-

bility of recurrent colon cancer in this patient. Remember, however, that many causes other than recurrent cancer can produce an elevated CEA level. These are listed in Chapter 3.

6. **Question:** Your 62-year-old patient is admitted to the hospital for melanoma. During his staging workup a bone scan is performed. The bone scan is normal except for a "hot spot" in the right rib. What might cause this abnormality?

   Answer: Increased uptake on a bone scan ("hot spot") can be caused by many factors. Obviously, metastatic tumor to the bone is one. Other possibilities include an old, healed fracture; arthritis; or benign bone disease. In this case an x-ray examination of the rib was performed, and an old, healed rib fracture was identified. On obtaining a more accurate history from the patient, it was noted that he fell several years ago and had severe pain in that area for more than 2 weeks. This history is compatible with a previous fractured rib.

7. **Question:** Your 22-year-old female patient has been complaining of right upper quadrant abdominal pain. A gallbladder series and upper gastrointestinal study have been performed and were found to be negative. A liver-spleen scan has indicated a filling defect in the anterior surface of the liver. Does this indicate a liver tumor?

   Answer: No. Many diseases can produce an abnormal liver scan such as this. Benign tumors (e.g., adenomas, cysts, or congenital abnormalities) can cause such an appearance. A CT scan should be performed to eliminate the possibility of a cyst. CT-guided liver biopsies also can be performed to elucidate more clearly the cause of this abnormal liver scan. If these fail to resolve the problem, peritonoscopy with actual visualization of that portion of the liver can be performed.

8. **Question:** Your patient has recently been admitted to the hospital with a rapid onset of ascites. She is extremely uncomfortable and very anxious to institute treatment for this symptom. You are aware that tumor markers have been performed. The patient's family is frus-

trated with the delay in her diagnosis and treatment. What explanation can you give the family for the delay?

Answer: The nurse must explain to the family that because many of the serum tumor markers require radioimmunoassay testing for accurate results, they must be sent to a major diagnostic laboratory. Therefore, the test results may take 7 to 10 days. If these results are required before the institution of therapy, indicate that all efforts will be made to provide comfort to the patient until this information is available.

Bibliography

Bischof P et al: Peripheral CA 125 levels in patients with uterine fibroids, *Hum Reprod* 7(1):35-38, 1992.

Carnaille B et al: Scintiscans and carcinoid tumors, *Surgery* 116(6):1118-1122, 1994.

Casperson DS: Focus on oncology: prostatic specific antigen testing, *Urol Nurs* 11(1):31-34, 1992.

Collins FS, Trent JM: Cancer genetics. In Fauci AS et al, editors: Harrison's principles of internal medicine, ed 14, New York, 1998, McGraw-Hill.

Cruickshank DJ et al: An independent evaluation of the potential clinical usefulness of proposed CA-125 indices previously shown to be of prognostic significance in epithelial ovarian cancer, *Br J Cancer* 65(4):597-600, 1992.

Cruickshank DJ et al: CA 125-response assessment in epithelial ovarian cancer, *Int J Cancer* 51(1):58-61, 1992.

Cupp MR, Oesterling JE: Prostate-specific antigen, digital rectal examination, and transrectal ultrasonography: their role in diagnosing early prostate cancer, *Mayo Clin Proc* 68:297-306, 1993.

Glenn J et al: Evaluation of the utility of a radioimmunoassay for serum CA 19-9 levels in patients before and after treatment of carcinoma of the pancreas, *J Clin Oncol* 6(3):462-468, 1988.

Grover S et al: Factors influencing serum CA 125 levels in normal women, *Obstet Gynecol* 79(4):511-514, 1992.

Kvols LK et al: Evaluation of a radiolabeled somatostatin analog (1-123 octreotide) in the detection and localization of carcinoid and islet cell tumors, *Radiology* 187(1):129-133, 1993.

Lancaster LE: Immunogenetic basis of tissue and organ transplantation and rejection, *Crit Care Nurs Clin North Am* 4(1):1-24, 1992.

Lavin J: Anergy testing: a vital weapon, *RN* 56(9):31-33, 1993.

Lippman ME: Breast cancer. In Fauci AS et al, editors: Harrison's principles of internal medicine, ed 14, New York, 1998, McGraw-Hill.

Littrup PJ, Goodman AC, Mettlin CJ: The benefit and cost of prostate cancer early detection, *Cancer* 43(3):134-149, 1993.

Liu L et al: Evaluation of second-look laparotomy for ovarian cancer: second-look versus serum CA 125, *Clin Med Sci J* 6(2):96-99, 1991.

Lowry WS: Tumor suppressor genes and risk of metastasis in ovarian cancer, *BMJ* 307(6903):542, 1993.

Mija J et al: Analysis of cytosel CA 15-3, carcinoembryonic antigen, estrogens, and progesterone receptors in breast cancer tissues, *Jpn J Cancer Res* 83(2):171-177, 1992.

Minna JD: Neoplasms of the lung. In Fauci AS et al, editors: *Harrison's principles of internal medicine*, ed 14, New York, 1998, McGraw-Hill.

Moore S: Screening for prostate cancer: PSA blood test, rectal examination, and ultrasounds, *Urol Nurs* 12(3):106-107, 1992.

Motzer RJ, Bosl GT: Testicular cancer. In Fauci AS et al, editors: *Harrison's principles of internal medicine*, ed 14, New York, 1998, McGraw-Hill.

Pagana KD, Pagana TJ: Mosby's manual of diagnostic and laboratory tests, St. Louis, 1998, Mosby.

Parker SL et al: Cancer statistics, *CA Cancer J Clin* 46:5, 1996.

Rainwater LM et al: Prostate-specific antigen testing in untreated and treated prostatic adenocarcinoma, *Mayo Clin Proc* 65(8):1118-1126, 1990.

Salmon SE: Principles of cancer therapy. In Wyngaarden JB et al, editors: *Cecil textbook of medicine*, ed 19, Philadelphia, 1992, WB Saunders.

Tian F et al: Prognostic value of serum CA 19-9 levels in pancreatic adenocarcinoma, *Ann Surg* 215(4):350-355, 1992.

Woolf SH: Screening for prostate cancer with prostate-specific antigen. *N Engl J Med* 333:1401, 1995.

Wozniak-Petrofsky J: Prostate specific antigen in prostate cancer, *J Urol Nurs* 12(3):104-105, 1992.

Chapter 14

Diagnostic Studies Used in

Routine Laboratory Testing and Miscellaneous Testing

ROUTINE LABORATORY TESTING

Although a complete and thorough history and physical examination are essential to adequate patient evaluation, they cannot detect many serious imbalances that may afflict a patient. Today with the availability of multiphasic laboratory testing machines the patient can be more completely screened for the presence of disease. Nearly every hospital clinical laboratory has multiphasic, serum-screening machines capable of rapidly and inexpensively measuring calcium, phosphorus, triglycerides, protein, bilirubin, transaminases, alkaline phosphatase, lactic dehydrogenase (LDH), blood urea nitrogen (BUN), creatinine, electrolytes, and glucose. Also, the complete blood count (CBC) can be performed easily with the help of automation. Because many unsuspected diseases can be detected by the use of chest radiographic studies and electrocardiography (EKG), these tests also have been standardized so that they, too, can be performed rapidly and easily. All these studies are essential components of a complete medical evaluation of most patients.

Because multiple, simultaneous testing techniques permit an easily performed and inexpensive evaluation of numerous patient samples at the same time, coagulation studies have become part of routine testing. Furthermore, the development of multiple dipstick testing (e.g., Multistix) has greatly increased the ease and availability of routine urine evaluation.

Routine testing, coupled with a thorough history and physical examination, provides screening for a large number of diseases that might otherwise go undetected. Also, many diseases can be detected at an early stage before symptoms become apparent and can therefore be treated more easily and effectively. The cost of routine testing is relatively small in comparison with its effectiveness.

When serum evaluations are performed singly, they are both costly and time-consuming and, as a result, cannot be performed frequently (e.g., for monitoring therapy). However, multiphasic automation has made these single serum tests inexpensive and easily available. An inexpensive and practical method for effectively monitoring electrolyte abnormalities and diseases such as gout and diabetes is thus available. Examples of multiphasic testing include the sequential multiple analysis (SMA) 6, SMA 12, and Astra 7. The numeral indicates the number of different laboratory tests performed in that series. Many combinations are available and can be obtained from the laboratory in one's institution.

Routine laboratory admission testing usually is done at a designated admission center in the hospital or in the patient's room by a technician or nurse. Collecting the blood in the appropriate color-coded test tube is important. The rubber stoppers of the test tubes are coded by color to indicate the presence or absence of different additives in the collection tube. The most common additives are preservatives, which prevent chemical or physical changes in the specimen, and anticoagulants, which inhibit clot formation. Institutional procedure manuals should be consulted to determine the appropriate number and color of the specimen tubes that are required.

In addition to collecting the correct number of properly color-coded tubes of blood, the nurse or technician should prevent hemolysis of the blood sample. A hemolyzed sample is unsuitable for many tests and usually necessitates repeated venipuncture. Hemolysis can be prevented by avoiding the use of a small venipuncture needle. Usually a 20-, 21-, or 22-gauge needle is used. If a syringe is used in contrast to a Vacutainer holder, the plunger should not be pulled back too forcefully. After the needle is removed, the blood should be slowly injected into the side of the glass test tube. The collected specimens should not be agitated. Gentle inversion of the tube is sufficient to allow mixture of the additive with the blood.

The following section describes routine and miscellaneous tests not discussed in previous chapters.

Anion Gap (AG, R Factor)

Test type Blood

Normal values
8-16 mEq/L (if potassium is used in the calculation)
8-12 mEq/L (if potassium is not used in the calculation)

Rationale
The calculation of the anion gap (AG) assists in the evaluation of patients with acid/base disorders by indicating the potential cause of the electrolyte or acid/base disorders and monitoring the therapy for acid/base abnormalities.

The AG is the difference between the cations and anions in the extracellular space.

$$\text{Anion gap} = (\text{Sodium} + \text{Potassium}) - (\text{Chloride} + \text{Bicarbonate})$$

In some laboratories the potassium is not measured. The normal value is adjusted downward if potassium is eliminated from the equation. Normally the AG is created by the small amounts of anions in the blood (e.g., lactate, phosphates, sulfates, and proteins).

This calculation can help identify the cause of metabolic acidosis. When acids (e.g., lactic acid [from shock] or ketoacids [from uncontrolled diabetes]) accumulate in the bloodstream, bicarbonate levels diminish in order to regulate the pH within the blood. The bicarbonate mixes with the hydrogen in the blood to form water and carbon dioxide (CO_2). The acid anion combines with sodium to form a new salt that is excreted in the urine. Mathematically, when bicarbonate decreases, the AG increases. If bicarbonate is lost from the extracellular space through diarrhea or increased excretion by a diseased kidney, the AG will increase.

Diseases that increase bicarbonate within the bloodstream will decrease the AG. Metabolic alkalosis due to excessive loss of acid from the gastrointestinal tract or excessive resorption of bicarbonate by the kidneys will increase bicarbonate and decrease AG.

Interfering factors

Factors that interfere with determining the AG include carbonic anhydrase inhibitors (e.g., acetazolamide), which can increase the AG.

Procedure

Approximately 5 to 10 ml of venous blood is collected in a red- or green-top tube. If the patient is receiving an intravenous (IV) infusion, obtain the blood from the opposite arm. The sodium, potassium, chloride, and bicarbonate levels are determined by an automated multichannel analyzer. The AG then is calculated as previously described.

Nursing implications with rationale

Before

☞ Explain the procedure to the patient. Tell the patient that no food or fluid is restricted.

After

■ Apply pressure or a pressure dressing to the venipuncture site. Observe the venipuncture site for bleeding.

Culture and Sensitivity Testing
(C & S of the Throat, Sputum, Urine, Stool, Blood, Wound, Cervix, and Urethra)

Test type Microscopic examination

Normal values Negative (for all cultures)

Rationale

When a patient develops a fever of unknown origin (FUO), all the potential causes of infection must be investigated. This investigation includes a thorough history and physical examination along with obtaining the appropriate specimens for culture and sensitivity (C & S) testing. When a patient has an obvious site of infection this, too, should be cultured to identify the infectious agent. Knowledge about the organism's sensitivity to commonly used antibiotics allows the physician to accurately determine the appropriate antibiotic therapy. If the organisms are not sensitive to an antibiotic being administered, no improvement in the disease occurs. In addition, when more than one organism is causing the infection, the sensitivity report assists the physician in choosing one drug to which all of the involved organisms will be sensitive. In cases of epidemics of a particular type of infection, the sensitivity report can be used as a rough guide to the common source. All similar organisms should have the same degree of sensitivity to the same antibiotics.

Culture media may vary according to the type of organism suspected to be causing the infection. Blood agar is used to grow most routine aerobic organisms (e.g., *Staphylococcus* and *Escherichia coli*). Anaerobic bacteria (e.g., *Bacteroides* and *Clostridium* organisms) do not grow in the presence of oxygen and thus require an anoxic environment. Chocolate (denatured blood) agar is the best medium for *Neisseria gonorrhoeae* growth. Fungi grow best on Sabouraud dextrose agar.

All cultures should be performed before antibiotic therapy is initiated; otherwise, the antibiotic may interrupt the growth of the organism in the laboratory. More often than not, however, the physician wants to institute antibiotic therapy before the culture results are reported. In these instances a Gram stain of the specimen smeared on a slide is helpful and can be reported in less than 10 minutes. All forms of bacteria are grossly classified as gram-positive (blue-staining) or gram-negative (red-staining). Knowledge of the shape of the organism (e.g., spherical or rod-shaped) also can be helpful in the tentative identification of the infectious organism. With knowledge of the Gram-stain results the physician can institute a reasonable antibiotic regimen based on past experience as to what the organism might be. Most organisms take approximately 24 hours to grow in the laboratory, and a preliminary report can be given at that time. Occasionally 48 to 72 hours are required for growth and identification of the organism. Cultures may be repeated after appropriate antibiotic therapy to assess for complete resolution of the infection (especially in urinary tract infections).

Procedure

In general all culture specimens should be delivered to the microbiology (bacteriology) laboratory and cultured as soon as they are obtained; otherwise, overgrowth of the bacteria occurs. If the specimen is obtained at night or on weekends and the bacteriology laboratory is closed, the specimen should be refrigerated until it can be placed on the culture medium. When an anaerobic infection is suspected the specimen should be aspirated into a sterile syringe and "topped" until it can be cultured in anaerobic conditions.

Throat culture

See discussion on throat culture and streptococcal screen (p. 180).

Sputum culture

See discussion on sputum culture (p. 173).

Urine culture

The urine culture specimen must be a clean-catch, midstream collection. The patient is instructed to wipe the distal urethra with an antiseptic in a front-to-back direction. Voiding is initiated. During midstream the sterile container is placed into the urine stream to collect 5 to 50 ml of urine. The container is removed from the stream, and voiding is completed. The urine also can be collected by suprapubic aspiration or directly from an indwelling catheter. The specimen container is covered, labeled, and transported to the bacteriology laboratory as soon as possible.

Frequently it is beneficial to culture the urine of a patient who has an indwelling Foley catheter immediately before the removal of the catheter. This procedure is called a *terminal urine for C & S* and usually is more accurate than culturing the tip of the catheter.

Stool culture

See discussion on stool culture (p. 89).

Blood culture

Bacteremia (bacteria in the blood) usually is intermittent and transient except in endocarditis or suppurative thrombophlebitis. Because bacteremia usually is marked by chills and fever, a blood culture specimen should be drawn at the time the patient manifests chills and fever. At least two culture specimens should be obtained from two different sites. The two culture specimens are important because if one produces bacteria and the other does not, it is safe to assume that the bacteria in the first culture is a contaminant and not the infecting agent. When both cultures produce the infecting agent, bacteremia exists. If the patient is receiving antibiotics, the laboratory should be notified, and the blood culture specimen should be obtained shortly before the next antibiotic dose is administered.

To obtain the blood specimens, two different peripheral venous sites are carefully prepared with povidone-iodine (Betadine). The tops of the vacutainer tubes or culture bottles are cleaned with povidone-iodine and allowed to dry. The venipuncture is performed aseptically, and enough blood (approximately 8 ml) is aspirated to allow a dilution ratio of blood to culture broth of approximately 1:10. The culture bottles should be transported immediately to the laboratory. Culture specimens drawn through an intravenous catheter are frequently contaminated and should not be used unless catheter sepsis is suspected. In these situations blood culture specimens drawn through the catheter indicate the causative agent more accurately than a culture specimen from the catheter tip.

Wound culture

Wound infections are most commonly caused by pus-forming organisms. The specimen for a wound culture can best be obtained by aseptically placing a sterile cotton swab into the pus and then putting the swab into a sterile, covered test tube. The specimen is transported to the laboratory as soon as possible. Culturing specimens taken from the skin edge is much less accurate than culturing the suppurative material. If an anaerobic organism is suspected, obtain an anaerobic culture tube from the microbiology laboratory. Routine wound cultures also are done at the same time.

Cervical culture

Cervical cultures are most commonly done to detect gonorrhea (see p. 389) or other sexually transmitted diseases (STDs). The female patient should refrain from douching and tub-bathing before a cervical culture is performed. The patient is placed in the lithotomy position, and a nonlubricated vaginal speculum is inserted to expose the cervix (see Figure 9-7, *A*, p. 376). Cervical mucus is removed with a cotton ball held in ring forceps. A sterile-tipped swab then is inserted into the endocervical canal and moved from side to side.

Urethral culture

Urethral cultures are most commonly performed on men in whom gonorrhea or other STDs are suspected (see p. 389). The urethral specimen should be obtained before voiding. This is done by inserting a sterile swab gently into the anterior urethra (Figure 14-1).

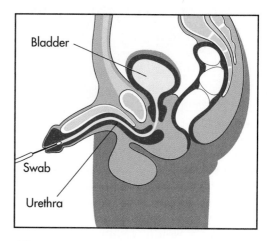

Figure 14-1 Obtaining a urethral specimen.

Nursing implications with rationale

Before

☞ Explain the purpose and procedure to the patient. Thoroughly explain the instructions if the patient is to obtain the specimen. Provide the patient with the appropriate cleansing agents and sterile supplies. If the patient cannot obtain the specimen, provide nursing assistance. Drape the patient appropriately during the procedure to prevent unnecessary exposure.

During

- Obtain the specimens in a sterile manner. Handle all specimens as though they were capable of transmitting disease. Specimens should be transported to the laboratory immediately (at least within 30 minutes).
- Obtain the specimens before initiating the prescribed antibiotic therapy. Antibiotics alter the growth of organisms in culture media.
- If wound cultures are to be obtained from a patient requiring wound irrigation, obtain the culture before the wound is irrigated.

After

- Carefully label all the specimens. Include the precise time at which the specimen was collected. Indicate any medications the patient may be taking that could affect the reults.
- Notify the physician of any positive results so that appropriate antibiotic therapy can be initiated.

ELECTROLYTES, SERUM
Sodium (Na)
Potassium (K)
Chloride (Cl)
Carbon Dioxide (CO₂)

Test type Blood

Sodium (Na)
Normal values
Adult/elderly: 136-145 mEq/L or 136-145 mmol/L
(SI units)
Child: 136-145 mEq/L
Infant: 134-150 mEq/L
Newborn: 134-144 mEq/L

Possible critical values
<120 or >160 mEq/L

Potassium (K)
Normal values
Adults/elderly: 3.5-5.0 mEq/L, or 3.5-5.0 mmol/L
(SI units)
Children: 3.4-4.7 mEq/L
Infants: 4.1-5.3 mEq/L
Newborns: 3.9-5.9 mEq/L

Possible critical values
Adults: <2.5 or >6.5 mEq/L
Newborns: <2.5 or >8.0 mEq/L

Chloride (Cl)
Normal values
Adults/elderly: 90-110 mEq/L, or 90-110 mmol/L
(SI units)
Children: 90-110 mEq/L
Newborns: 96-106 mEq/L
Premature infants: 95-110 mEq/L

Possible critical values
<80 or >115 mEq/L

Carbon dioxide (CO₂)
Normal values
Adults/elderly: 23-30 mEq/L, or 23-30 mmol/L
(SI units)

Children: 20-28 mEq/L
Infants: 20-28 mEq/L
Newborns: 13-22 mEq/L

Possible critical values
≤6 mEq/L

Rationale
Sodium
The sodium content of the blood is a result of a balance between dietary sodium intake and renal excretion. In the healthy individual nonrenal sodium losses are minimal. Many factors assist in this homeostatic sodium balance. The role of aldosterone is described on p. 229 (see Figure 7-4). Aldosterone tends to conserve sodium by decreasing renal losses. Natriuretic hormone tends to encourage renal losses of sodium. Water and sodium are physiologically very closely interrelated. As free body water is increased, serum sodium is diluted, and the concentration may decrease. The kidney compensates by conserving sodium and excreting water. If free body water were to decrease, the serum sodium concentration would rise. The kidney then would respond by conserving free water.

Sodium is the major cation in the extracellular space, where serum levels of approximately 140 mEq/L exist. The intracellular concentration of sodium is only 5 mEq/L. Sodium salts therefore are the major determinants of extracellular osmolality.

The following outline shows the causes of hypernatremia (increased serum sodium concentration) and hyponatremia (decreased serum sodium concentration).

A. Hypernatremia
  1. Increased sodium intake (without access to water)
     a. Excessive dietary intake
     b. Excessive sodium in IV fluid
  2. Decreased sodium loss
     a. Cushing's syndrome
     b. Hyperaldosteronism
  3. Excessive free body water loss (hypernatremic dehydration)
     a. Excessive sweating

b. Extensive thermal burns

c. Diabetes insipidus

d. Osmotic diuresis (as in glycosuria and overzealous mannitol administration)

e. Prolonged hyperpnea

f. Severe water loss from diarrhea or vomiting

4. Inadequate water intake

5. Drugs such as steroids, carbenicillin, diazoxide, and sodium bicarbonate

B. Hyponatremia

1. Decreased sodium intake

a. Deficient dietary intake

b. Deficient sodium in IV fluid

2. Increased sodium loss

a. Addison's disease

b. Diarrhea

c. Vomiting or nasogastric aspiration

d. Diuretic administration

e. Chronic renal insufficiency (inadequate tubular resorption of sodium)

3. Increased free body water (dilutional)

a. Excessive oral water intake

b. Excessive IV water intake

c. Congestive heart failure

d. Inappropriate secretion of antidiuretic hormone

e. Osmotic dilution (as in hyperglycemia and hyperproteinemia)

4. Third-space losses of sodium

a. Ascites

b. Peripheral edema

c. Pleural effusion

d. Intraluminal bowel loss (ileus or mechanical obstruction)

5. Drugs such as captopril, amitriptyline, diuretics, and antiinflammatory agents

Symptoms of hypernatremia may include dry mucous membranes, thirst, agitation, restlessness, hyperreflexia, mania, and convulsions. Symptoms of hyponatremia are weakness, confusion, lethargy, stupor, and coma.

Potassium

Potassium is the major cation within the cell. The intracellular potassium concentration is approximately 150 mEq/L, whereas normal serum potassium concentration is about 4 mEq/L. This ratio is the most important determinant in maintaining membrane potential in excitable neuromuscular tissue. Because the serum concentration of potassium is so small, minor changes in concentration have significant consequences.

Serum potassium concentration is dependent on many factors, including:

1. Aldosterone. This hormone tends to increase renal loss of potassium.

2. Sodium resorption. As sodium is reabsorbed, potassium is lost.

3. Acid-base balance. Alkaline states tend to lower serum potassium levels, causing a shift of potassium into the cell. Acidotic states tend to raise serum potassium levels by reversing the shift.

The following outline shows the causes of hyperkalemia (increased serum potassium concentration) and hypokalemia (decreased serum potassium concentration).

A. Hyperkalemia

1. Increased potassium intake

a. Excessive dietary intake

b. Excessive IV intake

2. Decreased potassium loss

a. Acute or chronic renal failure

b. Addison's disease

c. Hypoaldosteronism

d. Aldosterone-inhibiting diuretics (e.g., spironolactone and triamterene)

3. Shift from intracellular space

a. Acidosis

b. Infection

c. Crushing injury to tissues

d. Malignant hyperthermia

4. Pseudohyperkalemia

a. Poor venipuncture technique

b. Transfusion of hemolyzed blood

5. Drugs such as arginine, ibuprofen, indomethacin

B. Hypokalemia

1. Decreased potassium intake

a. Deficient dietary intake

b. Deficient IV intake

2. Excessive potassium loss
   a. Gastrointestinal disorders (diarrhea, vomiting, and villous adenomas)
   b. Diuretics
   c. Hyperaldosteronism
   d. Cushing's syndrome
   e. Renal tubular acidosis
   f. Licorice ingestion
3. Shift to intracellular space
   a. Alkalosis
   b. Insulin or glucose administration
   c. Calcium administration
4. Drugs such as albuterol, bisacodyl, steroids, and diuretics

Symptoms of hyperkalemia include irritability, nausea, vomiting, intestinal colic, and diarrhea. The EKG may demonstrate peaked T waves, a widened QRS complex, and depressed S-T segments. Signs of hypokalemia are related to a decrease in contractility of smooth, skeletal, and cardiac muscles, which results in weakness, paralysis, hyporeflexia, ileus, increased cardiac sensitivity to digoxin, cardiac arrhythmias, flattened T waves, and prominent U waves.

Chloride

Chloride is the major extracellular anion, whose primary purpose is to maintain electrical neutrality, mostly as a salt with sodium. Chloride follows sodium losses and accompanies sodium excesses. Chloride also serves as a buffer to assist in acid-base balance. As CO_2 increases, bicarbonate moves from intracellular space to the extracellular space. To maintain electrical neutrality, chloride shifts back into the cell.

Hypochloremia and hyperchloremia rarely occur by themselves and usually parallel shifts in sodium levels, the causes of which are listed in the outline under the discussion of sodium.

Carbon dioxide content

As discussed in Chapter 5 (see p. 146), CO_2 content is a measure of the bicarbonate ion (HCO_3^-) that exists in the serum. This anion is of secondary importance in electrical neutrality of extracellular and intracellular fluid. Its major role is in acid-base balance (see p. 146). Increases occur with alkalosis, and decreases occur with acidosis.

Procedure

Venipuncture is performed, and 7 ml of peripheral venous blood is obtained in a red-top tube (without any anticoagulants). It is important to use at least a 20-gauge needle to obtain the blood to prevent hemolysis, which may cause pseudohyperkalemia. If the patient has an IV line, the venipuncture should be performed in the contralateral extremity to avoid artificial results caused by the fluid infusion.

The blood is sent to the chemistry laboratory, where a multiphasic machine performs the electrolyte concentration determinations. Results can frequently be reported in approximately 30 minutes. The only discomfort associated with this study is that of the venipuncture.

Nursing implications with rationale

Before

☞ Explain the procedure to the patient. Tell the patient that no fasting is necessary.

During

■ Obtain the blood by peripheral venipuncture. Avoid hemolysis by using a 20-gauge needle. Do not aspirate very strongly or push the plunger into the vacutainer tube too forcefully. Either action can cause hemolysis, which affects results.

After

■ If the patient is receiving an IV infusion, obtain the blood from the opposite arm.

■ Apply a pressure dressing to the site. Assess the site for bleeding.

■ Because this study is usually performed with a glucose level determination, mark on the laboratory requisition slip the time that the test was performed to avoid confusion in the glucose reading.

■ If the results are abnormal, notify the physician. If the results are unexpectedly abnormal, the physician may repeat the test because the chance of laboratory error is great since many specimens are tested simultaneously, and the machine that performs the determinations may malfunction.

Case Study

Routine Admission Workup

Mrs. A., 51 years old, developed an umbilical hernia after her last pregnancy at age 41. She had no other medical problems, and the results of her physical examination were normal. She was admitted to the hospital for repair of her hernia.

Studies	Results
CBC, p. 412	
Hemoglobin concentration	14 g/dl (normal: 12-16 g/dl)
Hematocrit	43% (normal: 37%-47%)
White blood cells (WBCs)	5300 (normal: 5000-10,000)
Differential count	
Neutrophils	60% (normal: 55%-70%)
Lymphocytes	30% (normal: 20%-40%)
Monocytes	7% (normal: 2%-8%)
Eosinophils	2% (normal: 1%-4%)
Basophils	1% (normal: 0.5%-1%)
Red blood cells (RBCs)	4.8 million/mm^3 (normal: 4.2-5.4 million/mm^3)
Mean corpuscular volume (MCV)	88μ^3 (normal: 80-95 μ^3)
Mean corpuscular hemoglobin concentration (MCHC)	34 g/dl (normal: 32-36 g/dl)
Mean corpuscular hemoglobin (MCH)	30 pg (normal: 27-31 pg)
Platelet count	350,000/mm^3 (normal: 150,000-400,000/mm^3)
SMA 12	
Calcium, p. 298	9.9 mg/dl (normal: 9-10.5 mg/dl)
Phosphorus, p. 326	3.2 mg/dl (normal: 2.5-4.5 mg/dl)
Triglycerides, p. 51	100 mg/dl (normal: 40-150 mg/dl)
Uric acid, p. 460	6.1 mg/dl (normal: 2.5-8.5 mg/dl)
Creatinine, p. 237	1 mg/dl (normal: 0.7-1.5 mg/dl)
BUN, p. 266	9 mg/dl (normal: 5-20 mg/dl)
Total bilirubin, p. 111	0.8 mg/dl (normal: 0.1-1.0 mg/dl)
Alkaline phosphate, p. 108	45 ImU/ml (normal: 30-85 ImU/ml)
AST, p. 15	15 U/L (normal: 8-20 U/L)
Lactate dehydrogenase, p. 42	125 ImU/ml (normal: 90-200 ImU/ml)
Total protein, p. 135	7.2 mg/dl (normal: 6-8 mg/dl)
Albumin, p. 135	3.8 g/dl (normal: 3.2-4.5 g/dl)
Serologic test for syphilis (VDRL), p. 392	Negative, nonreactive (normal: negative, nonreactive)
SMA 6	
Sodium, p. 520	138 mEq/L (normal: 136-145 mEq/L)
Potassium, p. 521	4.1 mEq/L (normal: 3.5-5.0 mEq/L)

Continued

Case Study

Routine Admission Workup—cont'd

SMA 6—cont'd

Chloride, p. 520	103 mEq/L (normal: 90-110 mEq/L)
Total CO$_2$, p. 520	24 mEq/L (normal: 23-30 mEq/L)
Glucose, p. 305	90 mg/dl (normal: 60-120 mg/dl)
BUN, p. 266	9 mg/dl (normal: 5-20 mg/dl)
Erythrocyte sedimentation rate (sed rate), p. 476	14 mm/hour (normal: up to 20mm/hour)

Urinalysis, p. 268

pH	6.2 (normal: 4.6-8.0)
Specific gravity	1.020 (normal: 1.010-1.025)
Color	Yellow (normal: amber-yellow)
Glucose	0 (normal: negative)
Protein	0 (normal: negative)
Blood	0 (normal: ≤2 RBCs)
Casts	
RBC	0-1 (normal: negative)
WBC	0-1 (normal: negative)
Crystals	0 (normal: negative)

Coagulation profile

Prothrombin time (PT), p. 434	90% (normal: 11-12.5 seconds or 85%-100%)
Activated partial thromboplastin time (APTT), p. 427	32 seconds (normal: 30-40 seconds)
EKG, p. 34	Normal sinus rhythm: no ischemic changes
Chest x-ray study, p. 155	No active disease seen
Tuberculin skin test, p. 181	Negative
Mammography, p. 507	Negative

Diagnostic Analysis

In light of the completely negative routine laboratory evaluation, Mrs. A. underwent herniorrhaphy. Unfortunately, she developed a high fever 4 days after the operation. Specimens were obtained for culture and sensitivity testing.

Studies	**Results**
Throat culture, p. 180	Negative
Sputum culture, p. 173	Normal throat flora
Urine culture, p. 516	No bacteria
Blood culture, p. 516	No bacteria
Wound culture, p. 517	*Staphylococcus aureus;* resistant to penicillin, sensitive to oxacillin

Diagnostic Analysis

The wound was drained, and Mrs. A. was treated with oxacillin for a 10-day period. She did well with no further problems.

Critical Thinking Questions

1. If the results of the glucose test had been 150 mg/dl, what factors would you need to consider?
2. If the wound culture had revealed methicillin-resistant *Staphylococcus aureus* (MRSA), what precautions would have been needed?

Ethanol (Ethyl Alcohol, Blood Alcohol, Blood EtOH)

Test type Blood

Normal values
0

Possible critical values >300 mg/dl

Rationale

The ethanol test measures alcohol blood. It is used to diagnose alcohol intoxication and overdose. Ethanol depresses the central nervous system and may lead to coma and death. This test is usually performed to evaluate alcohol-impaired driving or overdose. Proper collection, handling, and storage of the blood alcohol specimen are important for medical/legal cases involving sobriety. The blood test is the specimen of choice. Blood is taken from a peripheral vein in living patients and from the aorta in cadavers. Ethanol also can be detected in the urine, gastric contents, or breath.

Blood alcohol levels between 50 to 100 mg/dl (0.05% to 0.10% weight/volume) may cause flushing, slowing of reflexes, and impaired visual activity. Most courts do not consider this clinical level of impairment definite proof of intoxication. Persons with alcohol levels less than 0.05% are not considered under the influence of alcohol. Levels greater than 0.10% are considered in most states to be illegal and definite evidence of intoxication. Depression of the central nervous system occurs with levels greater than 100 mg/dl, and fa-

talities are reported with levels greater than 400 mg/dl. Blood alcohol levels greater than 100 mg/dl can cause hypotension. This is especially important to recognize in the trauma patient in shock.

Interfering factors

Factors that interfere with determining ethanol levels include the following:

- Elevated blood ketones (as with diabetic ketoacidosis), which can cause false elevation of blood and breath test results
- Alcohols other than ethanol (e.g., isopropyl [rubbing] alcohol or methanol [grain]), which also will be detected by this test
- The use of large amounts of isopropyl alcohol in skin cleansing for the needle stick, because it can falsely elevate the test results

Procedure

A povidone-iodine wipe or peroxide (instead of an alcohol wipe) is used to cleanse the skin at the venipuncture site. A venous blood sample is collected in a gray- or red-top tube, according to the agency's protocol. If a gastric or urine specimen is indicated, approximately 20 to 50 ml of fluid is necessary. A breath specimen is analyzed at the end of expiration after a deep inspiration.

Nursing implications with rationale

Before

- Explain the procedure to the patient. Tell the patient that no fasting is necessary.
- Follow the institution's protocol if the specimen will be used for legal purposes. Patients

should be advised of their legal rights. Sometimes this is best done by a law enforcement officer. The alcohol level may be used as evidence for later court proceedings.

After

- Apply pressure or a pressure dressing to the venipuncture site. Observe the venipuncture site for bleeding.
- Follow the agency's protocol regarding specimen collection. The exact time of specimen collection should be indicated on the laboratory requisition slip. In some instances signatures of the collector and a witness may be needed for legal evidence.

Magnesium (Mg)

Test type Blood

Normal values
Adults: 1.2-2.0 mEq/L
Child: 1.4-1.7 mEq/L
Newborn: 1.4-2.0 mEq/L

Possible critical values <0.5 mEq/L or >3.0 mEq/L

Rationale
Most of the magnesium (Mg) found within the body exists intracellularly with approximately half found in the bone. Most of the Mg is bound to an adenosine triphosphate (ATP) molecule and is important in phosphorylation of ATP (the main source of energy for the body). Therefore Mg is critical in nearly all metabolic processes. Furthermore, Mg acts as a cofactor that modifies the activity of many enzymes. Carbohydrate, protein, and nucleic acid synthesis and metabolism depend on Mg.

Most organ functions, including those of neuromuscular tissue, also depend on Mg. It is important to monitor Mg levels in cardiac patients because low Mg may increase cardiac irritability and aggravate cardiac arrhythmias. Hypermagnesemia retards neuromuscular conduction and is demonstrated as cardiac conduction slowing (widened P-R and Q-T intervals with a wide QRS

complex), diminished deep-tendon reflexes, and respiratory depression.

The intracellular elements, potassium, Mg, calcium, (in order of quantity) are intimately tied together in their body levels. Intracellular electrical charges must be maintained. When one of these positively charged elements is low, another positively charged element is driven into the intracellular space to maintain electrical neutrality. Extracellular and blood levels of the other positive ion therefore also decrease.

Mg deficiency occurs in patients who are malnourished because of malabsorption or maldigestion or lack of food intake. This becomes especially significant in the postoperative patient who may not eat for 5 to 7 days and whose metabolism (and therefore the need for Mg) is accelerated. Toxemia of pregnancy also is believed to be associated with reduced Mg levels. Symptoms of Mg depletion are mostly neuromuscular (e.g., weakness, irritability, tetany, electrocardiographic changes, delirium, and convulsions).

Because most of the serum Mg is excreted by the kidney, chronic renal diseases cause elevated Mg levels. Increased Mg levels are most commonly associated with ingestion of Mg-containing antacids. Symptoms of increased Mg include lethargy, nausea and vomiting, and slurred speech.

Interfering factors
- Hemolysis
  Mg is an intracellular ion, and RBC lysis will release great quantities of Mg into the blood, causing falsely *elevated* results.
- Mg-containing antacids or laxatives, because they can falsely *elevate* Mg levels

Procedure
Approximately 5 to 7 ml of venous blood is collected in a red- or green-top tube. Hemolysis must be avoided to prevent a factitious increase in Mg levels.

Nursing implications with rationale
Before
- Explain the procedure to the patient. Tell the patient that no special diet or fasting is required.

After

■ Apply pressure or a pressure dressing to the venipuncture site to prevent further bleeding. Observe the site for bleeding.

Positron Emission Tomography (PET)

Test type Nuclear scan, x-ray

Normal values
Normal patterns of tissue metabolism

Rationale
This new generation of imaging scans is not routinely used outside large medical institutions. Positron emission tomography (PET) techniques have been used to identify pathophysiologic conditions of the brain, heart, lungs, and other tissues and organs.

PET is a unique technique that combines the early biochemical assessment of pathology achieved by nuclear medicine with the precise localization achieved by computerized tomography (CT). PET is able to penetrate the body's metabolism by recording tracers of nuclear annihilations in body tissue. The dose of radioactive material given either by gas or injection to the patient produces a radiation exposure comparable to that of other nuclear medicine studies. The selected tracers are chemically designed to measure body processes (e.g., blood flow and volume, protein metabolism). See Table 14-1 for a list of radionuclides used in PET scanning.

A chemical compound with the desired biologic activity is labeled with a radioactive isotope that decays by emitting a positron (positive electron). The positron combines with an electron, and the two are mutually annihilated with emission of two gamma rays. The gamma rays penetrate the surrounding tissue and are recorded outside the body by a circular array of detectors. A computer reconstructs the spatial distribution of the radioactivity and creates an image.

PET technology is now well developed, and both its capabilities and limitations are being increasingly understood. Many PET studies provide results that cannot be obtained by other techniques. These results include the following:

1. Determination of regional metabolism in the heart and brain (e.g., radioactive glucose used to map biochemical activity in the brain)
2. Studies of tissue permeability
3. Measurement of the size of cardiac infarcts from a coronary occlusion
4. Investigation into the physiology of psychosis
5. Assessment of drug effects on diseased or malfunctioning tissues
6. Evaluation of cancer treatment by measuring changes in malignant tissues and biochemical reactions in surrounding normal tissues

Interfering factors
Factors that interfere with determining PET scans include the following:

■ Recent use (within 24 hours) of caffeine, alcohol, or tobacco, which may affect test results
■ Excessive anxiety, because it may affect brain function evaluation

TABLE 14-1	**Radionuclides Used in PET Scanning**
Radionuclide	**Application**
Carbon-11	Cerebral, cardiac, pulmonary perfusion
	Detection of myocardial infarction
	Cerebral function
Fluorine-18	Cerebral function and glucose metabolism
Gallium-68	Cerebral perfusion
	Lymphoreticular function
Nitrogen-13	Cerebral and cardiac perfusion
	Pulmonary inhalation
	Liver function
Oxygen-15	Cerebral perfusion and oxygen utilization

- Drugs (e.g., tranquilizers and sedatives), which may influence results

Procedure

No food or fluids are restricted on the day of the test; however, the patient should refrain from alcohol, caffeine, and tobacco for 24 hours. Patients with diabetes should administer their pretest dose of insulin at a meal 3 to 4 hours before the test.

The patient is positioned in a comfortable, reclining chair. Two IV lines are inserted. The radioactive material can be infused through an IV line or inhaled as a radioactive gas. The gamma rays that penetrate the tissues are recorded outside the body by a circular array of detectors and displayed by a computer. If the brain is being scanned, the patient may be asked to perform different cognitive activities (e.g., reciting the Pledge of Allegiance) to measure changes in brain activity during reasoning or remembering. Extraneous auditory and visual stimuli are minimized by a blindfold and ear plugs.

This procedure is performed by a physician or trained technologist in approximately 60 to 90 minutes. The only discomfort associated with this procedure is the insertion of the two IV lines.

Nursing implications with rationale

Before

- Explain the procedure to the patient. Because most patients are not familiar this study, they are often anxious and require emotional support.
- Obtain written and informed consent, if required by the institution.
- Inform the patient that two IV lines may be inserted, one for infusion of the radioisotope and the other for serial blood samples.
- Tell the patient that no sedatives or tranquilizers should be taken because he or she may need to perform certain mental activities during the test.
- Tell the patient to empty the bladder before the test for comfort.

After

- Instruct the patient to change slowly from a lying to standing position to avoid postural hypotension.

- Encourage the patient to drink fluids and urinate frequently to aid removal of the radioisotope from the bladder.

Sialography

Test type X-ray

Normal values

No evidence of pathology in salivary ducts and related structures

Rationale

Sialography is a radiographic procedure used to examine the salivary ducts (parotid, submaxillary, submandibular, and sublingual) and related glandular structures after the injection of a contrast medium into the desired duct. This procedure is used to detect calculi, strictures, tumors, or inflammatory disease in patients who complain of pain, tenderness, or swelling in these areas.

Potential complications

A potential complication associated with sialography is infection of the salivary gland. This may occur in patients with mouth infections (e.g., yeast), which may be spread to the salivary glands.

Procedure

No special preparation is required before sialography. However, the patient is instructed to rinse his or her mouth with an antiseptic solution before the dye is injected. Radiographic studies are performed before the injection is administered to ensure that stones are not present in the salivary ducts, which could prevent the contrast material from entering the ducts. After the patient is placed in a supine position on an x-ray table, the contrast medium is injected directly into the desired orifice via a cannula or a special catheter. Radiographic films are taken with the patient in various positions.

The patient then is given orally a sour substance (e.g., lemon juice) to stimulate salivary excretion. Another set of radiographic studies are performed to evaluate ductal drainage. A radiologist performs this procedure in less than 30 minutes. The patient may feel slight pressure as the contrast medium is injected into the ducts.

Nursing implications with rationale

Before

☞ Explain the procedure to the patient. Instruct the patient to remove jewelry, hairpins, and dentures, which could obscure radiographic visualization.

☞ Instruct the patient to rinse his or her mouth with an antiseptic solution before the procedure to reduce the possibility of introducing bacteria into the ductal structures.

■ Obtain written and informed consent, if required by the institution.

After

☞ Instruct and encourage the patient to drink fluids to eliminate the dye.

Therapeutic Drug Monitoring

Test type Blood

Normal values

See Table 14-2

Rationale

Therapeutic drug monitoring measures serum drug levels to determine effective drug dosages and prevent toxicity. Drug monitoring is especially important for patients taking medications (e.g., antiarrhythmics, bronchodilators, antibiotics, anticonvulsants, and cardiotonics) that have a narrow margin of safety between therapeutic and toxic levels.

Table 14-2 lists the therapeutic and toxic ranges for most patients. One should note, however, that these ranges may not apply to all patients because clinical response is influenced by many factors (e.g., noncompliance; concurrent drug use; other clinical conditions; age; weight; drug absorption, metabolism, and excretion). One also should be aware that different laboratories use different units for reporting test results and normal ranges. It is important that a sufficient amount of time pass between the ad-

ministration of the medication and the collection of the blood sample to allow for therapeutic levels to occur.

Blood samples can be taken at the drug's *peak* level (the highest concentration) or at the *trough* level (the lowest concentration). Peak levels are useful when testing for toxicity; trough levels are useful for demonstrating a satisfactory therapeutic level. (Trough levels are often referred to as *residual levels.*)

Procedure

No fluid or food restrictions are needed for therapeutic drug monitoring. A peripheral venipuncture is performed, and a blood specimen is collected in a tube as designated by the laboratory. The blood samples can be taken at the drug's peak level or at the trough (residual) level; one of the most significant laboratory problems with drug monitoring is obtaining the specimen at the proper time. Serum drug levels should have reached a steady state, or equilibrium, which as a rule of thumb takes five drug half-lives. *Half-life* (biologic half-life) refers to the time required to decrease the serum drug concentration by 50% and is usually measured after absorption has been completed. *Steady state* refers to serum drug level equilibrium between drug intake and elimination. Loading doses can decrease this time span considerably. Also, the blood level should be drawn at the true peak or residual level. Peak levels are usually obtained approximately 1 to 2 hours after oral intake, 1 hour after intramuscular administration, and 30 minutes after IV administration. Residual levels are usually obtained shortly before (0 to 15 minutes) the next scheduled dose.

All blood samples should be marked clearly with the following information: patient's name, diagnosis, name of drug, time of last drug ingestion, time of sample collection, and any other medications the patient is currently taking. The specimen should be sent to the laboratory immediately after the venipuncture.

Nursing implications with rationale

Before

☞ Explain the purpose of therapeutic drug monitoring to the patient. Tell the patient that monitoring ensures appropriate drug levels in the blood, thereby preventing toxicity from overdosage.

☞ Tell the patient that no fluid or food restrictions are necessary.

During

■ Ensure that the serum drug level is drawn at the appropriate peak or trough level. If a peak level is needed, record the exact time at which the drug was administered and then either draw the blood at the appropriate time or notify the laboratory technologist to obtain the specimen. If a residual level is needed, the next dose of the drug is usually held until the blood specimen is drawn, approximately 15 minutes before the scheduled dose. After the blood is drawn, the dose then can be administered. Unless the exact times that the specimen

TABLE 14-2 Therapeutic Drug Monitoring Data

Drug	Use	Therapeutic Level*	Toxic Level*
Acetaminophen	Analgesic, antipyretic	Depends on use	>250 μg/ml
Amikacin	Antibiotic	15-25 μg/ml	>25 μg/ml
Aminophylline	Bronchodilator	10-20 μg/ml	>20 μg/ml
Amitriptyline	Antidepressant	120-150 ng/ml	>500 ng/ml
Carbamazepine	Anticonvulsant	5-12 μg/ml	>12 μg/ml
Chloramphenicol	Antiinfective	10-20 μg/ml	>25 μg/ml
Desipramine	Antidepressant	150-300 ng/ml	>500 ng/ml
Digitoxin	Cardiac glycoside	15-25 ng/ml	>25 ng/ml
Digoxin	Cardiac glycoside	0.8-2.0 ng/ml	>2.4 ng/ml
Disopyramide	Antiarrhythmic	2-5 μg/ml	>5 μg/ml
Ethosuximide	Anticonvulsant	40-100 μg/ml	>100 μg/ml
Gentamicin	Antibiotic	5-10 μg/ml	>12 μg/ml
Imipramine	Antidepressant	150-300 ng/ml	>500 ng/ml
Kanamycin	Antibiotic	20-25 μg/ml	>35 μg/ml
Lidocaine	Antiarrhythmic	1.5-5.0 μg/ml	>5 μg/ml
Lithium	Manic episodes of manic-depression psychosis	0.8-1.2 mEq/L	>2.0 mEq/L
Methrotrexate	Antitumor agent	>0.01 μmol	>10 μmol/24 hr
Nortriptyline	Antidepressant	50-150 ng/ml	>500 ng/ml
Phenobarbital	Anticonvulsant	10-30 μg/ml	>40 μg/ml
Phenytoin	Anticonvulsant	10-20 μg/ml	>30 μg/ml
Primidone	Anticonvulsant	5-12 μg/ml	>15 μg/ml
Procainamide	Antiarrhythmic	4-10 μg/ml	>16 μg/ml
Propranolol	Antiarrhythmic	50-100 ng/ml	>150 ng/ml
Quinidine	Antiarrhythmic	2-5 μg/ml	>10 μg/ml
Salicylate	Antipyretic, antiinflammatory, analgesic	100-250 μg/ml	>300 μg/ml
Theophylline	Bronchodilator	10-20 μg/ml	>20 μg/ml
Tobramycin	Antibiotic	5-10 μg/ml	>12 μg/ml
Valproic acid	Anticonvulsant	50-100 μg/ml	>100 μg/ml

*Levels vary according to the laboratory performing the test.

was obtained and the last dose was given are known, serum drug levels cannot be properly interpreted and may be grossly misleading.

■ Confirm that appropriate blood concentrations have been reached. This can be determined by consulting with the pharmacist regarding the half-life of the drug.

After

■ Observe the patient for signs of toxicity related to the appropriate drug. Record all observations and notify the physician as needed.

■ After the venipuncture has been obtained, assess the site for bleeding and hematoma formation.

■ Promptly send the specimen to the laboratory.

Toxicology Screening

Test type Blood, urine

Normal values
See Tables 14-3 and 14-4

Rationale
Toxicology screening is done to determine the cause of acute drug toxicity, monitor drug dependency, and detect the presence of narcotics in the body for medical-legal purposes. Toxicology screening is especially important in patients with a drug overdose or poisoning.

TABLE 14-3   Blood Toxicology Screening

Drug	Type	Therapeutic Level*	Toxic Level*
Acetaminophen	Analgesic, antipyretic	Depends on use	>250 µg/ml
Alcohol	—	None	80-200 mg/dl (mild to moderate intoxication)
			250-400 mg/dl (marked intoxication)
			>400 mg/dl (severe intoxication)
Amobarbital	Sedative, hypnotic	0.5-3.0 µg/ml	>10 µg/ml
Butabarbital	Sedative, hypnotic	0.5-3.0 µg/ml	>10 µg/ml
Carboxyhemoglobin (COHb, carbon monoxide)	Gas	None	>30% CoHb (beginning of coma)
Glutethimide	Sedative	0.5-3.0 µg/ml	>10 µg/ml
Lead	—	None	>40 µg/dl
Lithium	Manic episodes of manic-depression psychosis	0.8-1.2 mEq/L	>2.0 mEq/L
Meprobamate	Antianxiolytic	0.5-3.0 µg/ml	>10 µg/ml
Methyprylon	Hypnotic	0.5-3.0 µg/ml	>10 µg/ml
Phenobarbital	Anticonvulsant	15-30 µg/ml	>40 µg/ml
Phenytoin (Dilantin)	Anticonvulsant	10-20 µg/ml	>20 µg/ml
Salicylate	Antipyretic, antiinflammatory, analgesic	100-250 µg/ml	>300 µg/ml

*Varies according to institution performing the test.

TABLE 14-4   Urine Toxicology Screening for Amphetamines

Drug	Therapeutic Level*	Toxic Level*
Amphetamine	2-3 μg/ml	>3 μg/ml
Dextroamphetamine	0.1-1.5 μg/ml	>15 μg/ml
Methamphetamine	3-5 μg/ml	>40 μg/ml
Phenmetrazine	5-30 μg/ml	>50 μg/ml

*Varies according to institution performing the test.

Procedure

Peripheral venipuncture is performed, and the blood is collected in a tube as designated by the laboratory. The blood usually is drawn immediately after admission to the emergency room. Random urine specimens can be collected, and gastric contents can be aspirated for analysis. The hair and nails are used for detecting or documenting long-term exposure to arsenic or mercury.

Nursing implications with rationale

Before

☞ Explain the procedure to the patient's significant others. Obtain as much information as possible about the type, amount, and ingestion time of the consumed drug.

■ Carefully assess the patient for respiratory distress, which is a common side effect of drug overdosage.

During

■ Collect blood or urine specimens as indicated. Urine specimens are collected in the presence of a trained health care professional.

■ Note that hair and nail samples may be used to detect or document exposure to arsenic or mercury.

■ If the specimen is obtained for medical-legal testing, ensure that the patient or the family member has signed a consent form.

■ Perform gastric lavage as indicated.

After

■ Apply pressure or a pressure dressing to the venipuncture site to prevent bleeding. Observe for further bleeding.

■ Approach the patient in a nonjudgmental fashion. Refer the patient for appropriate drug or psychiatric counseling.

■ Follow the predetermined chain of specimen transfer to the laboratory. Each person involved in handling the specimen must document his or her role in its handling.

White Blood Cell (WBC) Scan
(Inflammatory Scan)

Test type Nuclear scan

Normal values

No signs of white blood cell localization outside the liver or spleen

Rationale

The white blood cell (WBC) scan is based on the fact that WBCs are attracted to areas of infection or inflammation. When a patient is suspected to have an infection or inflammation, but the site cannot be localized, the injection of radiolabeled WBCs may identify and localize the area of inflammation or infection. Appropriate treatment then can be performed. This is especially helpful in patients who have an FUO, suspected occult intraabdominal infection, or suspected (but radiographically unapparent) osteomyelitis. WBC scan is used to indicate whether an abnormal mass (e.g., a pancreatic pseudocyst) is infected. Areas of noninfectious inflammation (e.g., inflammatory bowel disease) also take up the radiolabeled WBCs.

This scan requires drawing approximately 40 to 50 ml of blood from the patient, separating the WBCs, labeling the WBCs with technetium (Tc) or indium (In), and reinjecting the WBCs into the patient. In 4 to 24 hours, imaging of the body may show an area of increased radioactivity suggestive of accumulation of the radiolabeled WBCs in an area of infection or inflammation.

Interfering factor

A factor that interferes with determining WBC scan is the reticuloendothelial system (liver, spleen, and bone marrow), which tends to accumulate these radiolabeled cells normally.

Procedure

No preparation or sedation is required. Approximately 40 to 50 ml of blood is withdrawn from the patient, and the WBCs are extracted from the rest of the blood cells. This usually is done by centrifugation. If the patient has leukopenia (reduced WBCs), the WBC count is so low that separating them from the other blood cellular components is very difficult. In this instance donor WBCs are used instead of autologous WBCs. Donor WBCs also are used for human immunodeficiency virus (HIV)-positive patients in order to minimize the risk to laboratory workers.

The WBCs are suspended in saline and tagged with a Tc 99m- or In 111-lipid-soluble product. Tc 99m is preferable to In 111 because its half-life is longer. Therefore it is cheaper and more readily available for the infrequent times that this scan is requested. The tagged WBCs are reinjected into the patient. In 4, 24, and 48 hours after injection, a gamma ray detector/camera is placed over the body. The patient is placed in the supine, lateral, and prone positions in order to visualize all the body surfaces. The radionuclide image is recorded on film.

The imaging procedure is performed by a trained technologist in approximately $1/2$ an hour. A physician trained in nuclear medicine interprets the results. The only discomfort associated with this procedure is the IV injection of the radionuclide.

Nursing implications with rationale

Before

☞ Explain the procedure to the patient. Tell the patient that no fasting is necessary.

☞ Assure the patient that he or she will not be exposed to large amounts of radioactivity because only tracer doses of the isotope are used.

After

☞ Inform the patient that because only tracer doses of radioisotopes are used, no precautions need to be taken against radioactive exposure.

REVIEW QUESTIONS AND ANSWERS

1. **Question:** Your patient is admitted to the hospital for routine surgery. On routine admission testing, her potassium level was found to be 7 (normal: 3.5 to 5.0). Should the surgery be canceled?

   Answer: The elevated potassium level is probably the result of RBC hemolysis caused by poor venipuncture technique in obtaining the specimen. Therefore the electrolytes test should be repeated using good technique. (The repeat potassium level in this patient was 4.)

2. **Question:** Your patient is suspected of having a urinary tract infection. The urine culture report indicates that three bacterial species are present. Should antibiotic therapy be initiated based on the culture results?

   Answer: No. It is very rare for any nongastrointestinal infection to involve more than one bacterial species. Culture reports with more than one species usually indicate contamination of the specimen. Therefore the specimen should be carefully obtained a second time, and the culture should be repeated.

3. **Question:** Your patient has been admitted for eye surgery and is found to have a positive VDRL test result on routine testing. Should this patient be given antibiotic therapy?

   Answer: Because of the high incidence of false-positive results (20%) associated with the VDRL test, a positive result does not necessarily indicate syphilitic infection. A more accurate and specific test, such as the fluorescent treponemal antibody (FTA) test, should be performed. If the FTA test result is positive, appropriate antibiotic therapy should be given (4.8 million U of procaine penicillin administered intramuscularly). If the FTA test is negative, the patient does not have syphilis, and therapy is not indicated.

4. **Question:** Your 48-year-old patient was admitted for a delayed repair of a nerve laceration. Eight weeks earlier, at the time of the original injury, a complete routine laboratory evaluation was performed, and its results were negative. Should the routine testing be repeated?

   Answer: The final decision rests with the attending anesthesiologist. However, as a rule, most anesthesiology departments request that all tests be performed not less than 14 days before the day of surgery. During longer time intervals, much can happen to the patient that could possibly increase the risk of general anesthesia. Therefore the workup should be repeated.

5. **Question:** Your 28-year-old patient was admitted for incision and drainage of an infected pilonidal cyst. Should the routine evaluation include a chest x-ray study and EKG?

   Answer: A chest x-ray study should be included because serious pulmonary disease, which increases the risk of anesthesia, can occur at any age. The chance that EKG will demonstrate unsuspected cardiac disease is minimal. Therefore in this age group routine performance of EKG would not be worthwhile for clinical purposes or from a cost-benefit standpoint.

Bibliography

Dillon WP: Neuroimaging in neurologic disorders. In Fauci AS et al, editors: Harrison's principles of internal medicine, ed 14, New York, 1998, McGraw-Hill.

Ellenhorn MJ, Barceloux DG: Medical toxicology: diagnosis and treatment of human poisoning, New York, 1988, Elsevier.

Hu H: Heavy metal poisoning. In Fauci AS et al, editors: Harrison's principles of internal medicine, ed 14, New York, 1998, McGraw-Hill.

Koepke JA: Practical laboratory hematology, New York, 1991, Churchill-Livingstone.

Linden CH, Lovejoy FH: Poisoning and drug overdose. In Fauci AS et al, editors: Harrison's principles of internal medicine, ed 14, New York, 1998, McGraw-Hill.

Margulis AR: Overview of imaging techniques and projection for the future. In Wyngaarden JB et al, editors: Cecil textbook of medicine, ed 19, Philadelphia, 1992, WB Saunders.

Pagana KD, Pagana TJ: Mosby's manual of diagnostic and laboratory tests, St. Louis, 1998, Mosby.

Perkins A: An approach to diagnosing the acute sore throat, *Am Fam Physician* 55(1):131-138, 1997.

Wyngaarden JB: The use and interpretation of laboratory derived data. In Wyngaarden JB et al, editors: Cecil textbook of medicine, ed 19, Philadelphia, 1992, WB Saunders.

Comprehensive Practice Test

QUESTIONS

1. Which of these instructions should a nurse give an elderly, dehydrated patient after a computed tomography (CT) scan of the kidney utilizing intravenous (IV) iodine contrast?
   a. Drink plenty of fluids for 24 hours.
   b. Do not perform any heavy lifting for 2 days.
   c. Use a laxative to clear the contrast from the bowel.
   d. None of the above.

2. With severe bone destruction from tumor or osteomalacia, what serum laboratory results would the nurse expect to assess?
   a. Decreased serum alkaline phosphatase (ALP)
   b. Increased serum ALP
   c. Decreased erythrocyte sedimentation rate
   d. Increased red blood cell (RBC) count

3. Your patient's laboratory reports indicate the presence of Bence Jones proteins. These are increased in the urine of patients who have:
   a. Multiple myeloma
   b. Carcinoid syndrome
   c. Breast cancer
   d. Colorectal cancer

4. Your patient is admitted for evaluation of a perforated diverticulitis. Which of the following tests would be indicated?
   a. CT of the abdomen
   b. Barium enema
   c. Colonoscopy
   d. All of the above

5. Abnormally low blood urea nitrogen (BUN) levels may be detected in which patients:
   a. Overly hydrated patients
   b. Patients with liver disease
   c. Malnourished patients in negative nitrogen balance
   d. All of the above

6. An elevated serum creatinine level is usually seen in patients with:
   a. Renal disease
   b. Liver disease
   c. Lung disease
   d. Muscular diseases

7. Your patient presents with upper gastrointestinal (GI) bleeding from a suspected peptic ulcer. Which test is most appropriate?
   a. Upper GI x-ray study
   b. Gastric bleeding scan

c. Esophagogastroduodenoscopy (EGD)

d. None of the above

8. Your patient is admitted with abdominal pain. An ultrasound of the abdomen, CT scan of the abdomen, and barium enema have been ordered. In what order should these tests be performed?

a. Ultrasound first, barium enema second, CT scan third

b. Ultrasound first, CT scan second, barium enema third

c. Barium enema first, CT scan second, ultrasound third

d. CT scan first, barium enema second, ultrasound third

9. Ferning of the cervical mucus at midcycle of menses indicates which of the following?

a. Increased estrogen activity

b. Decreased estrogen activity

c. Increased progesterone activity

d. Decreased progesterone activity

10. Your patient is scheduled for a cardiac exercise stress test to evaluate chest pain. While obtaining the patient history, you note that the patient has intermittent claudication when walking two blocks. Based on your finding, which of the following is indicated?

a. The test will be performed as scheduled.

b. The test is contraindicated because of the intermittent claudication.

c. The test will be rescheduled after resolution of the claudication.

d. The patient will most likely be a candidate for the dipyridamole-thallium stress test.

11. M.C. is scheduled for a cardiac catheterization. Which of the following activities is a postprocedure nursing priority?

a. Ambulating the patient

b. Encouraging coughing and deep-breathing exercises

c. Keeping the patient NPO (*nil per os*, nothing by mouth)

d. Keeping the involved extremity immobilized

12. One of the blood studies used to detect a myocardial infarction (MI) is creatine phosphokinase (CPK, CK). Which value is most helpful for diagnosing an MI?

a. The total CPK value

b. The isoenzyme CPK-MM

c. The isoenzyme CPK-MB

d. The isoenzyme CPK-BB

13. During your patient's exercise stress test, his blood pressure dropped. Which of the following activities should be avoided in the 2-hour period after the test?

a. Walking

b. Taking a hot shower

c. Eating a light meal

d. Resting in his bed

14. Your neighbor had a lipid profile done and asked you about her results. Which of the following is considered the ideal high-density lipoprotein (HDL)/total cholesterol ratio?

a. 1:2

b. 1:3

c. 1:4

d. 1:5

15. J.P. had a tuberculin skin test 48 hours ago. He has returned to the clinic for the nurse to read the test results. Which of the following is considered a positive result?

a. A reddened area measuring 20 mm

b. A flat, red area measuring 10 mm

c. An indurated area measuring 8 mm

d. An indurated area measuring 12 mm

16. T.J., a patient with diabetes, was brought to the emergency room. His arterial blood gas results were as follows:

pH: 7.25

pCO_2: 38 mm Hg

HCO_3^-: 19 mEq/L

pO_2: 95 mm Hg

These results indicate:

a. Respiratory acidosis

b. Respiratory alkalosis

c. Metabolic acidosis

d. Metabolic alkalosis

17. M.R. just returned from the endoscopy suite where he had a bronchoscopy. Which of the following is *not* a nursing priority after the procedure?

a. Observing the sputum for hemorrhage

b. Monitoring the vital signs frequently

c. Observing the patient closely for laryngospasm

d. Encouraging cool fluids to comfort his throat

18. What is the best time of the day for obtaining a sputum specimen?

a. Early morning

b. After breakfast

c. Evening

d. The time does not matter

19. R.J. is scheduled for a magnetic resonance imaging (MRI) scan. Which of the following factors is a contraindication for this procedure?

a. An iodine allergy

b. A severe visual impairment

c. A cardiac pacemaker

d. None of the above

20. Which of the following activities should be *avoided* before an electroencephalogram (EEG)?

a. Washing the hair the night before the procedure

b. Taking anticonvulsant medications

c. Drinking coffee, tea, or cola

d. None of the above

21. After a lumbar puncture, a nursing priority is to prevent a spinal headache. Which of the following activities is to be avoided?

a. Ambulating the patient in the room

b. Drinking fluids through a straw

c. Keeping the patient on bed rest

d. Keeping the patient's head flat

22. Your patient is scheduled for a lumbar puncture. Which of the following is a contraindication for this procedure?

a. The patient with meningitis

b. The patient with neurosyphilis

c. The patient with multiple sclerosis

d. The patient with increased intracranial pressure (ICP)

23. Which of the following statements regarding a glycosylated hemoglobin test is *false*?

a. The test provides an accurate long-term index of the patient's average blood glucose.

b. The test aids in determining the duration of hyperglycemia in a patient with newly diagnosed diabetes.

c. No fasting is required for this test.

d. Short-term variations (e.g., food intake, exercise, and stress) affect the test result.

24. You are concerned about M.A.'s elevated glucose level. Which of the following factors in his history may cause hyperglycemia?

a. Insulinoma

b. Corticosteriod therapy

c. Hypothyroidism

d. Addison's disease

25. Cortisol levels normally rise and fall during the day. This is referred to as the *diurnal variation*. At which time of the day are levels the highest?

a. 8 AM

b. Noon

c. 4 PM

d. Midnight

26. Symptoms that may indicate hypocalcemia include which of the following?

a. Nausea, vomiting, and anorexia

b. Polyuria and dehydration

c. Muscle weakness and coma

d. Tetany and carpal pedal spasms

27. Your patient has been diagnosed with primary hypothyroidism. Her triiodothyronine (T_3) and thyroxine (T_4) levels are decreased. What would you expect the thyroid-stimulating hormone (TSH) levels to be?

a. Normal

b. Increased

c. Decreased

d. Near zero

28. Often during a nonstress test (fetal activity determination test) fetal activity must be stimulated. Which of the following activities is *not* part of this test?

a. Rubbing the mother's abdomen

b. Administering IV oxytocin

c. Ringing a bell near the abdomen

d. Compressing the mother's abdomen

29. Which of the following statements best describes the Sims-Huhner test?

a. This test evaluates the quality of cervical mucus.

b. This test examines cervical mucus for color, viscosity, and tenacity.

c. This test assesses the number of motile sperm per high-power microscopic field.

d. This test evaluates the interaction between the sperm and cervical mucus.

30. Which of the following tests is used to screen blood for antibody compatibility before a blood transfusion?
    a. Direct Coombs' test
    b. Indirect Coombs' test
    c. Complete blood count (CBC)
    d. Serum haptoglobin test

31. Which of the following statements is *false* regarding the semen analysis test?
    a. A single sperm analysis can be conclusive evidence of male infertility.
    b. Men with little or no sperm should be evaluated for pituitary, thyroid, adrenal, or testicular aberrations.
    c. A 2- to 3-day period of sexual abstinence is necessary before collection of the semen specimen.
    d. For best results a semen collection should be collected in the physician's office or laboratory by masturbation.

32. Which of the following tests is used to monitor coumadin administration?
    a. Activated partial thromboplastin (APTT)
    b. Platelet count
    c. Bleeding time
    d. International normalized ratio (INR)

33. Which of the following factors may cause an increase in hematocrit (Hct) concentration?
    a. Hemorrhage
    b. Bone marrow failure
    c. Pregnancy
    d. Dehydration

34. A "shift to the left" in the white blood cell (WBC) production indicates an acute bacterial infection. Which of the following cells are increased in this situation?
    a. Mature neutrophils
    b. Monocytes
    c. Lymphocytes
    d. Band, or stab, cells

35. The physician orders a blood culture for your patient with suspected bacteremia. Which of the following statements is *incorrect* regarding the collection of this specimen?
    a. Blood culture specimens should be drawn at the time the patient has a fever or chills.
    b. If the patient is receiving antibiotics already, the laboratory should be notified, and the blood culture specimen should be collected shortly before the next dose of antibiotics is administered.
    c. Two culture specimens should be obtained from two different sites.
    d. The culture specimen can be drawn at any time without regard to medications and vital signs.

36. Which of the following is a possible cause of hyperkalemia?
    a. Diarrhea and vomiting
    b. Diuretic drug therapy
    c. Cushing's syndrome
    d. Acidosis

37. After returning from an EGD and dilation of an esophageal stricture, D.K. began to complain of fever and chest pain. The nurse should suspect:
    a. MI and obtain an electrocardiogram (EKG) immediately
    b. Gastroesophageal reflux and administer an antacid
    c. Esophageal perforation and notify the physician immediately
    d. Dyspepsia from not eating before the procedure and allow the patient to eat a bland diet

38. After having a barium enema, patients should be instructed to:
    a. Take an oral laxative to completely evacuate the barium.
    b. Try to retain the barium in case additional radiographic studies are needed the same or following day.
    c. Await normal bowel function.
    d. None of the above.

39. After returning from colonoscopy, T.P. complains of increasing abdominal pain. Appropriate nursing interventions would include:
    a. Limiting T.P.'s diet to clear liquids
    b. Assisting T.P. with a warm bath to soothe the anal-rectal area
    c. Administering a gentle enema to assist in evacuation of colon contents and air
    d. Administering a laxative to assist in evacuation of excess colon contents
    e. None of the above

40. A woman in her first trimester of pregnancy develops pain consistent with gallbladder disease. The most appropriate diagnostic test to perform is:
    a. Gallbladder ultrasound
    b. Gallbladder radioscintography scan
    c. Oral cholecystogram
    d. CT scan

41. After a liver biopsy, the patient should:
    a. Ambulate to maintain mobility
    b. Lie on the left side
    c. Lie on the right side
    d. Lie prone

42. A nurse has been stuck by a needle from a patient being treated for hepatitis. The appropriate actions would include:
    a. Immediate enteric and blood product precautions to isolate the involved nurse
    b. Immediately obtaining hepatitis viral studies on the affected nurse
    c. Hospitalizing the nurse for bed rest
    d. All of the above
    e. None of the above

43. J.M. has developed a swollen leg 1 week after arthroscopy. J.M. should be evaluated for:
    a. Hemarthrosis
    b. Joint stiffness after prolonged immobilization
    c. Postoperative thrombophlebitis
    d. Joint dislocation

44. A 5-year-old patient has fallen and injured the right arm during play therapy. The physician is notified and orders an x-ray of both arms because:

a. The noninjured arm could have been injured in the fall.
b. Fracture lines of long bones in children are difficult to distinguish from normal growth lines, which make comparison films necessary.
c. The battered child syndrome can be diagnosed by documenting multiple fractures.
d. All of the above.

45. B.K. has just had a diagnostic arthroscopy and has mild discomfort. Which of the following interventions is most appropriate?
    a. Ambulate the patient.
    b. Notify the physician.
    c. Administer a mild analgesic (e.g., acetominophen).
    d. Administer an intramuscular (IM) narcotic.

46. What drug should be discontinued before obtaining a serum gastrin level?
    a. Hydrochlorothiazide
    b. Propranolol (Inderal)
    c. Cimetidine (Tagamet)
    d. All of the above

47. Which of the following instructions should the nurse give the client after an upper GI study?
    a. Expect your stools to be chalky white for at least a day.
    b. Take a cathartic (e.g., Milk of Magnesia).
    c. Drink plenty of fluids when you get home.
    d. All of the above.

48. After having a percutaneous transhepatic cholangiogram (PTHC), F.M. returned to the floor. Which is the most appropriate nursing intervention?
    a. Maintain bed rest.
    b. Mobilize the patient as soon as possible.
    c. Provide systemic pain medication for severe pain.
    d. All of the above.

49. After returning from an endoscopic retrograde cholangiopancreatography (ERCP), which of the following test results would indicate a complication of this procedure?
    a. RBC in the urine
    b. Elevated serum amylase

c. Elevated serum calcium

d. All of the above

50. Carcinoembryonic antigen (CEA) is used to monitor patients with:

a. Colon cancer

b. Breast cancer

c. Gastric cancer

d. All of the above

51. Specific gravity in the urine is increased in patients with:

a. Dehydration

b. Diabetes insipidus

c. Chronic renal failure

d. All of the above

52. An intravenous pyelogram (IVP) may be contraindicated in:

a. Patients who are allergic to shellfish

b. Patients who are severely dehydrated

c. Patients with renal insufficiency

d. All of the above

53. Immediately after a kidney biopsy, your patient noticed gross hematuria. Appropriate nursing interventions would include:

a. Collecting serial urine specimens

b. Dehydrating the patient to diminish urine output and bleeding

c. Notifying the physician immediately and obtaining a specimen for blood typing and crossmatching

d. All of the above

54. Foods that may interfere in determining the results of urinary vanillylmandelic acid (VMA) or catecholamines include:

a. Potatoes and red meat

b. Coffee and licorice

c. Beer and salted pretzels

d. All of the above

55. A "no added salt" diet is necessary for patients before which of the following studies?

a. Urine specific gravity

b. IVP

c. Plasma renin assay

d. Renal scan

56. The most specific test for identifying recurrent prostate cancer is:

a. Prostatic acid phosphatase (PAP)

b. Prostate-specific antigen (PSA)

c. Digital rectal examination

d. Transrectal ultrasound

57. The nurse should ask the patient which of the following questions before scheduling an IVP:

a. Are you allergic to shellfish or iodine?

b. Have you ever had an IVP before?

c. Are you able to drink a lot of fluids?

d. All of the above.

58. Appropriate teaching information before mammography should include:

a. Mammograms utilize a low dose of radiation and therefore can safely be performed annually.

b. Mammograms can detect breast cancer 1 to 2 years before the tumor is clinically palpable.

c. Although mammography is an accurate means of detecting breast cancer, it is only 85% accurate.

d. All of the above.

59. The most accurate method of screening for breast cancer is:

a. Thermography

b. Mammography

c. Ultrasound of the breast

d. Physical examination

60. Which of the following tumor markers is associated with breast cancer:

a. Alpha-fetoprotein (AFP)

b. Human chorionic gonadotropin (HCG)

c. CA 15-3

d. CA-125

ANSWERS

1. a

Rationale: Elderly patients often are chronically dehydrated and therefore especially susceptible to renal impairment after receiving IV iodine contrast. Not only is the use of laxatives unnecessary to eliminate the contrast material, but also it will further dehydrate the patient. No physical limitations are required.

2. b

Rationale: Patients with destructive bone diseases commonly have elevated ALP levels as a result of bone cell destruction and regeneration.

3. a

Rationale: Bence Jones proteins are immunoglobulins that are commonly excreted in the urine of patients with multiple myeloma.

4. a

Rationale: CT is very accurate in identifying an abdominal abscess. Colonoscopy and barium enema are contraindicated in patients with suspected perforated viscus.

5. d

Rationale: Decreased BUN levels can occur normally in patients who are well hydrated. Because adequate liver function is required to make urea, severe liver dysfunction will be associated with decreased BUN levels. Because BUN also is a measure of protein nutrition, this level can be diminished in starving patients.

6. a

Rationale: An elevated serum creatinine level indicates renal disease. No other diseased organ will primarily cause elevation of the serum creatinine level.

7. c

Rationale: EGD is the most accurate diagnostic test. Furthermore, with EGD transendoscopic coagulation of active bleeding can be performed.

8. b

Rationale: Ultrasound should be performed first because intraabdominal barium will distort the sound waves and decrease the accuracy. Likewise, barium within the bowel will distort the CT scan image. Therefore ultrasound should be done first, CT scan second, and barium enema last.

9. a

Rationale: During a normal ovulatory cycle, ferning is the result of increased estrogen levels, which occur at midcycle.

10. d

Rationale: The patient's peripheral vascular disease will cause calf pain. This pain probably will precede exercise-induced chest pain

and cause the test to be terminated prematurely.

11. d

Rationale: The extremity in which the catheter was placed must be kept straight and immobilized for several hours after catherization to prevent bleeding.

12. c

Rationale: The isoenzyme CPK-MB provides a unique marker for damaged myocardial cells.

13. b

Rationale: A hot shower may cause an increase in cutaneous vasodilation and lead to orthostatic hypotension.

14. b

Rationale: The ideal ratio of HDL/total cholesterol is 1:3. An acceptable ratio should be at least 1:5.

15. d

Rationale: An indurated (hardened) area measuring more than 10 mm indicates a positive result. This means that the patient has been exposed to tuberculosis.

16. c

Rationale: The pH indicates acidosis. The lower bicarbonate value indicates a metabolic problem.

17. d

Rationale: The patient is kept NPO until the tracheobronchial anesthesia has worn off and the gag reflex has returned. This usually occurs within 2 hours. A patient who drinks or eats before this time could aspirate and develop pneumonia.

18. a

Rationale: Obtaining an early-morning specimen is best because secretions pool and collect in the lungs during sleep. The early-morning specimen is likely to be the most productive.

19. c

Rationale: An implantable metal pacemaker is a contraindication for this procedure because the magnet may move the object within the body and cause damage.

20. c

Rationale: Coffee, tea, or cola are not permitted on the morning of the study because of their stimulating effect.

21. a

Rationale: Walking may induce a headache.

22. d

Rationale: Patients with increased ICP cannot have a lumbar puncture because the lumbar puncture may induce cerebral or cerebellar herniation.

23. d

Rationale: An advantage of this test is that the blood sample can be drawn at any time because it is not affected by short-term variations.

24. b

Rationale: Corticosteriod therapy causes a chemically induced diabetes.

25. a

Rationale: Cortisol levels are highest around 6 AM to 8 AM and gradually fall during the day to their lowest point around midnight.

26. d

Rationale: Symptoms such as tetany and carpal pedal spasms indicate the need for a calcium level test to rule out hypocalcemia.

27. b

Rationale: Low levels of T_3 and T_4 are the underlying stimuli for TSH. Therefore in primary hypothyroidism a compensatory elevation of TSH occurs.

28. b

Rationale: Oxytocin administration is not used in the nonstress test. It is part of the contraction stress test (oxytocin challenge test).

29. d

Rationale: Options a, b, and c are all performed as part of this test. However, this test is mainly used as a postcoital examination of the cervical mucus to determine the ability of the sperm to penetrate the mucus and maintain mobility.

30. b

Rationale: The indirect Coombs' test is used to determine if the patient has antibodies to the RBCs that he or she is about to receive by blood transfusion.

31. a

Rationale: Because the sperm count varies from day to day, a single sperm analysis is inconclusive, especially if it indicates infertility.

32. d

Rationale: To have uniform prothrombin time (PT) results throughout the world, PT results now include the INR value.

33. d

Rationale: Dehydration causes an artificially high Hct value.

34. d

Rationale: Band, or stab, cells are immature forms of neutrophils that occur in the circulation during an acute bacterial infection.

35. d

Rationale: Specimens should be collected as indicated in options a, b, and c.

36. d

Rationale: Acidotic states tend to raise serum potassium levels by causing a shift of potassium out of the cell. All the other options (a, b, and c) are causes of hypokalemia.

37. c

Rationale: Esophageal perforation is a complication associated with EGD, especially when esophageal dilation has been performed. The nurse should notify the physician immediately, keep the patient NPO, maintain IV access, and record the vital signs.

38. a

Rationale: A laxative should be provided to the patient to evacuate retained barium, which may cause an impaction. Stool will be light in color until all the barium has been expelled.

39. e

Rationale: Bowel perforation should be suspected. The patient should be kept NPO, and IV access maintained. The physician should be notified immediately, and vital signs monitored.

40. a

Rationale: This is the only test that does not expose potentially harmful radiation to the fetus.

41. **c**
Rationale: In this position, the liver capsule is compressed against the chest wall, creating a tamponade for any hemorrhage or bile leak that may occur.

42. **e**
Rationale: Enteric precautions isolating the nurse will not help because the hepatitis B and C virus are bloodborne. Hepatitis viral tests do not become positive for at least 2 to 12 weeks. Hospitalization and bed rest are not required for cases of hepatitis exposure.

43. **c**
Rationale: Thrombophlebitis is a complication associated with arthroscopy and usually occurs 5 to 10 days after surgery.

44. **b**
Rationale: Fracture lines of long bones in children often are difficult to distinguish on radiographic film from normal growth lines. Any line suspicious for a fracture that is seen on both arms is not a fracture. It merely represents a normal growth pattern in the young child. However, unilateral suspicious lines are considered fractures until proven otherwise.

45. **c**
Rationale: For the mild discomfort following diagnostic arthroscopy, a mild analgesic usually controls the pain.

46. **c**
Rationale: Cimetidine is a histamine antagonist, which diminishes gastric acid secretion. The normal physiologic feedback mechanism creates factitiously elevated serum gastrin levels.

47. **d**
Rationale: After any barium contrast study, the nurse should recommend that the client use a laxative and drink plenty of fluids to help eliminate barium.

48. **a**
Rationale: After a PTHC, the patient is placed on bed rest for several hours to diminish any blood or bile leak from the liver. Early mobilization is contraindicated. Administration of systemic narcotics may blunt any abdominal signs associated with hemorrhage or bile extravasation.

49. **b**
Rationale: A known complication of ERCP is pancreatitis following injection of contrast material into the pancreatic duct. An elevated amylase level is diagnostic.

50. **d**
Rationale: Abnormal levels of CEA can exist in patients with various carcinomas (e.g., GI and breast carcinomas). Also, many benign diseases (e.g., diverticulitis, ulcerative colitis, and cirrhosis) may be associated with moderate CEA elevations.

51. **a**
Rationale: Because the kidneys are reabsorbing all available free water, the excreted urine will be very concentrated. The urine is very dilute in patients with diabetes insipidus and chronic renal failure.

52. **d**
Rationale: Patients who are allergic to shellfish also can be allergic to iodine. Severely dehydrated patients can go into renal failure with iodine injection. Kidney function, when already diminished, can deteriorate with iodine injection.

53. **a**
Rationale: After a kidney biopsy, it is not unusual for the patient to develop hematuria for the first 24 hours. Urine samples may be collected in consecutive chronologic order to facilitate comparison for evaluation of hematuria. This is referred to as *rack*, or *serial*, urines.

54. **b**
Rationale: The foods that generally should be restricted for patients collecting a 24-hour urine specimen for VMA or catecholamines include coffee, tea, bananas, chocolate, licorice, citrus fruits, vanilla, and aspirin.

55. **c**
Rationale: A high intake of sodium can cause decreased levels of plasma renin.

56. b
   Rationale: PSA is more sensitive and more specific for recurrent prostate cancer than other tumor markers. Because recurrence may develop outside the pelvis, digital rectal examination and transrectal ultrasound would not identify recurrences in other locations.

57. d
   Rationale: Patients who are allergic to shellfish or iodine will have an allergic reaction to the contrast material used during an IVP. Having had an IVP previously without a reaction eliminates serious anaphylactic reaction to the dye. Patients must be able to adequately hydrate themselves before and after administration of IV iodine to avoid subsequent renal impairment.

58. d
   Rationale: All of the above remarks concerning mammography are accurate.

59. b
   Rationale: Thermogram, ultrasound, and physical examination have an accuracy level inferior to mammography.

60. c
   Rationale: CA 15-3 is specific to breast cancer.

Appendix A

Alphabetical List of Tests

A

Abdominal ultrasound, p. 105
Acid-fast bacilli (AFB), p. 184
Acid phosphatase, p. 230
Acquired immunodeficiency syndrome (AIDS) serology, p. 466
Acquired immunodeficiency syndrome (AIDS) T-lymphocyte cell markers, p. 483
Activated partial thromboplastin time (APTT), p. 427
Adenosine stress test, p. 24
Adrenal venography, p. 292
Adrenocorticotropic hormone (ACTH), p. 293
Adrenocorticotropic hormone (ACTH) stimulation test, p. 296
Adrenocorticotropic hormone (ACTH) suppression test, p. 303
Agglutinins, febrile/cold, p. 465
Agranulocyte cell count, p. 417
Alanine aminotransferase (ALT), p. 106
Albumin, p. 135
Aldolase, p. 468
Aldosterone, blood, p. 231
Aldosterone, urine, p. 231
Alkaline phosphatase (ALP), p. 108
Alpha-fetoprotein (AFP), p. 491
Alpha$_1$-globulin, p. 135
Alpha$_2$-globulin, p. 135
Ambulatory monitoring, p. 40

δ-Aminolevulinic acid, p. 433
Aminopeptidase cytosol, p. 127
Ammonia, p. 109
Amniocentesis, p. 349
Amylase, blood, p. 110
Amylase, urine, p. 110
Anal culture, p. 89
Angiocardiography, p. 16
Anion gap, p. 514
Anoscopy, p. 86
Antegrade pyelography, p. 233
Antibiotic-associated colitis assay, p. 66
Anticardiolipin antibodies, p. 469
Anticentromere antibody, p. 471
Antideoxyribonuclease-B titer, p. 234
Antidiuretic hormone (ADH), p. 297
Antiextractable nuclear antigens (Anti-ENA), p. 471
Antimitochondrial antibody, p. 471
Antimyocardial antibody, p. 470
Antinuclear antibodies (ANA), p. 470
Antiribonucleoprotein (anti-RNP) antibody, p. 471
Antiscleroderma antibody, p. 471
Antispermatozoal antibody, p. 353
Anti-SS-A/Anti-SS B, p. 471
Antistreptococcal antibodies, p. 234
Antistreptolysin O (ASO) titer, p. 234
Antithyroglobulin antibody, p. 328
Antithyroid microsomal antibody, p. 328

543

K

Karyotype, p. 356
Ketones, urine, p. 313
17-Ketosteroids (17-KS), p. 338
Kidney, ureter, bladder (KUB) x-ray study, p. 249

L

Lactic acid, p. 41
Lactic dehydrogenase (LDH), p. 42
Lactose tolerance test, p. 77
Lamellar body count, p. 349
Laparoscopy, p. 125
Lecithin/sphingomyelin (L/S ratio), p. 349
Legionnaires' disease antibody, p. 480
Leucine aminopeptidase (LAP), p. 127
Leukocyte count, p. 413
Leukocyte esterase, p. 270
Lipase, p. 127
Lipids, p. 43
Lipoprotein (a), p. 43
Lipoproteins, p. 43
Liver biopsy, p. 128
Liver enzyme tests, p. 106
Liver/spleen scanning, p. 131
Long bone x-rays, p. 457
Long-acting thyroid stimulator (LATS), p. 321
Low-density lipoprotein (LDL), p. 43
Lower extremity arteriography, p. 12
Lumbar puncture and cerebrospinal fluid (CSF) examination, p. 208
Lumbar sacral (LS) spine x-ray, p. 222
Lung biopsy, p. 159
Lung scan, p. 160
Luteinizing hormone (LH), p. 372
Lyme disease test, p. 481
Lymphangiography, p. 505
Lymphocyte count, p. 413
Lymphocyte immunophenotyping, p. 483

M

Magnesium, p. 524
Magnetic resonance imaging (MRI), p. 215
Magnetic resonance imaging (MRI) of bones and joints, p. 459
Mammography, p. 507
Mantoux test, p. 181

Maximal midexpiratory flow (MMEF), p. 169
Maximal volume ventilation (MVV), p. 169
Mean corpuscular hemoglobin (MCH), p. 414
Mean corpuscular hemoglobin concentration (MCHC), p. 415
Mean corpuscular volume (MCV), p. 414
Mean platelet volume (MPV), p. 432
Meckel's diverticulum nuclear scan, p. 79
Mediastinoscopy, p. 164
Metanephrine, p. 277
Metyrapone, p. 321
Minute volume (MV), p. 170
Monocyte count, p. 413
Mononucleosis spot test, p. 484
Multiple gated acquisition (MUGA) cardiac scan, p. 21
Myelography, p. 216

N

Nerve conduction studies, p. 202
Neutrophil count, p. 413
Nitrite test, p. 271
Nonstress test, fetal, p. 374
Norepinephrine, p. 277
Normetanephrine, p. 277
5'-nucleotidase, p. 132

O

Obstetric ultrasonography, p. 377
Obstruction series, p. 80
Ocular pressures, p. 219
Oculoplethysmography (OPG), p. 219
Oculovestibular reflex study, p. 192
Osmolality, blood, p. 323
Osmolality, urine, p. 323
Oximetry, p. 164
Oxygen content, p. 147
Oxygen saturation, p. 147
Oxytocin challenge test (OCT), p. 359

P

Packed cell volume (PCV), p. 413
Pancreatic enzymes, p. 137
Pancreozymin enzyme, p. 137
Papanicolaou (PAP) smear, p. 375
Paracentesis, p. 81
Parathyroid hormone, p. 324

List of Tests by Type

Tests in this list are grouped by the following types: blood, electrodiagnostic, endoscopy, fluid analysis, manometric, microscopic examination, nuclear scan, other studies, sputum, stool, ultrasound, urine, and x-ray.

BLOOD TESTS

Acid phosphatase, p. 230
Acquired immunodeficiency syndrome (AIDS) serology, p. 466
Acquired immunodeficiency syndrome (AIDS) T-lymphocyte markers, p. 483
Activated partial thromboplastin time, p. 427
Adrenocorticotropic hormone, p. 293
    stimulation test, p. 296
    suppression test, p. 305
Agglutinins, febrile/cold, p. 465
Agranulocyte cell count, p. 417
Alanine aminotransferase, p. 106
Albumin, p. 135
Aldolase, p. 468
Aldosterone assay, p. 231
Alkaline phosphatase, p. 108
Alpha-fetoprotein, p. 491
Ammonia, p. 109
Amylase, p. 110
Anion gap, p. 514
Anticardiolipin antibodies, p. 469

Anticentromere antibody, p. 471
Antideoxyribonuclease-B titer, p. 234
Antidiuretic hormone, p. 297
Antiextractable nuclear antigens, p. 471
Antimitochondrial antibody, p. 471
Antimyocardial antibodies, p. 470
Antinuclear antibody test, p. 470
Antiribonucleoprotein antibody, p. 471
Antiscleroderma antibody, p. 471
Anti-Smith antibody, p. 471
Antispermatozoal antibody, p. 353
Anti-SS-A and anti-SS-B, p. 471
Antistreptolysin O titer, p. 234
Antithyroglobulin antibody, p. 328
Antithyroid microsomal antibody, p. 328
Apolipoproteins, p. 11
Aspartate aminotransferase, p. 15
Australian antigen, p. 123
Band cell, p. 417
Bicarbonate, p. 146
Bilirubin, p. 111
Bleeding time, p. 402
Blood culture and sensitivity, p. 516
Blood gases, arterial, p. 145
Blood smear, p. 405
Blood sugar, p. 305
Blood typing, p. 406
Breast cancer genetic screening, p. 496

ELECTRODIAGNOSTIC TESTS

Isonitrile scan, p. 21
Liver/spleen scanning, p. 131
Lung scan, p. 160
Meckel's diverticulum nuclear scan, p. 79
Multiple gated acquisition (MUGA) scan, p. 21
Positron emission tomography, p. 525
Radioactive iodine uptake, p. 332
Red blood cell liver scan, p. 131
Red blood cell survival study, p. 436
Renal scanning, p. 258
Scrotal nuclear imaging, p. 264
Testicular imaging, p. 264
Thallium scan, p. 21
Thyroid scanning, p. 332
Ventilation scan, p. 160
White blood cell scan, p. 530

OTHER STUDIES

Chorionic villus sampling, p. 355
Colposcopy, p. 357
Fetal nonstress test, p. 374
Magnetic resonance imaging, p. 213
Mantoux test, p. 181
Oximetry, p. 164
Pulmonary function tests, p. 168
Sleep apnea studies, p. 171
Tuberculin test, p. 181

SPUTUM TESTS

Acid-fast bacilli, p. 184
Culture and sensitivity, p. 173
Cytology, p. 173

STOOL TESTS

Clostridial toxin assay, p. 66
Culture, p. 89
Fecal fat, p. 120
Occult blood testing, p. 90
Ova and parasites, p. 89

ULTRASOUND TESTS

Abdominal ultrasound, p. 105
Biophysical fetal profile, p. 365
Breast sonogram, p. 498
Carotid duplex scanning, p. 26
Doppler studies, p. 26

Echocardiography, p. 32
Gallbladder ultrasound, p. 105
Kidney sonogram, p. 105
Liver and pancreatobiliary system ultrasonography, p. 105
Obstetric ultrasonography, p. 377
Prostate/rectal sonogram, p. 251
Scrotal ultrasound, p. 266
Testicular ultrasound, p. 266
Thyroid ultrasound, p. 336
Transesophageal echocardiography, p. 49
Transrectal ultrasonography, p. 251

URINE TESTS

Aldosterone assay, p. 231
Amylase, p. 110
Appearance and color, p. 269
Casts, p. 271
Cortisol, p. 301
Creatinine clearance, p. 237
Crystals, p. 271
Culture and sensitivity, p. 273
δ-aminolevulinic acid, p. 433
Dexamethasone suppression test, p. 303
Dopamine, p. 277
Epinephrine, p. 276
Epithelial casts, p. 271
Estriol excretion, p. 364
Ethanol, p. 523
Fatty casts, p. 271
Flow studies, p. 274
Glucose, p. 313
Glucose tolerance test, p. 310
Granular casts, p. 271
Hyaline casts, p. 271
17-Hydroxycorticosteroids, p. 338
5-Hydroxyindoleacetic acid, p. 504
Ketones, p. 313
17-Ketosteroids, p. 338
Leucine aminopeptidase, p. 127
Leukocyte esterase, p. 270
Metanephrine, p. 277
Metyrapone, p. 321
Nitrites, p. 271
Normetanephrine, p. 277

Odor, p. 269
Osmolality, p. 323
pH, p. 270
Phenistix test, p. 381
Phenylketonuria test, p. 380
Porphyrins and porphobilinogens, p. 433
Pregnancy, p. 382
Pregnanediol, p. 384
Protein, p. 270
Red blood cells and casts, p. 272
Schilling test, p. 85
Specific gravity, p. 270
Toxicology screening, p. 529
Uric acid, p. 460
Urinalysis, p. 268
Vanillylmandelic acid and catecholamines, p. 276
Waxy casts, p. 271
White blood cells and casts, p. 272
D-xylose absorption test, p. 98

X-RAY EXAMINATIONS

Adrenal venography, p. 292
Angiocardiography, p. 16
Antegrade pyelography, p. 233
Arteriography, p. 12
Arthrography, p. 452
Barium enema, p. 60
Barium swallow, p. 62
Bone densitometry, p. 455
Bone x-rays, p. 457
Cardiac catheterization, p. 46

Cerebral angiography, p. 193
Chest x-ray, p. 155
Computed tomography
    of abdomen, p. 113
    of adrenal glands, p. 113
    of brain, p. 196
    of chest, p. 157
    of kidney, p. 113
Computed tomography portogram, p. 117
Cystography, p. 239
Intravenous pyelogram, p. 245
Kidney, ureter, and bladder x-ray study, p. 249
Lymphangiography, p. 505
Magnetic resonance imaging, p. 213
Mammography, p. 507
Myelography, p. 216
Obstruction series, p. 80
Percutaneous transhepatic cholangiography, p. 133
Positron emission tomography, p. 525
Pulmonary angiography, p. 167
Renal angiography, p. 253
Retrograde pyelography, p. 262
Scout abdominal film, p. 249
Sialography, p. 526
Skull x-rays, p. 220
Spinal x-rays, p. 222
Upper gastrointestinal x-ray study, p. 92
Venography of lower extremities, p. 53
Videofluoroscopy, p. 91

Appendix C

Abbreviations for Diagnostic and Laboratory Tests

A

ABGs	Arterial blood gases
ACE	Angiotensin-converting enzyme
ACTH	Adrenocorticotropic hormone
ADH	Antidiuretic hormone
AFB	Acid-fast bacilli
AFP	Alpha-fetoprotein
A/G ratio	Albumin/globulin ratio
ALP	Alkaline phosphatase
ALT	Alanine aminotransferase
AMA	Antimitochondrial antibody
ANA	Antinuclear antibody
APTT	Activated partial thromboplastin time
ASO	Antistreptolysin O titer
AST	Aspartate aminotransferase

B

BE	Barium enema
BMD	Bone marrow density
BRCA	Breast cancer
BUN	Blood urea nitrogen

C

Ca	Calcium
C&S	Culture and sensitivity
CAT	Computed axial tomography
CBC	Complete blood count
CEA	Carcinoembryonic antigen
CK	Creatine kinase
Cl	Chloride
CMV	Cytomegalovirus
CO	Carbon monoxide
CO_2	Carbon dioxide
COHb	Carboxyhemoglobin
CPK, CP	Creatine phosphokinase
CRP	C-reactive protein
CSF	Cerebrospinal fluid
CST	Contraction stress test
CT	Computed tomography
CVB	Chorionic villi biopsy
CVS	Chorionic villi sampling
CXR	Chest x-ray

D

D&C	Dilation and curettage
DIC	Disseminated intravascular coagulation
DMSA	Disodium monomethanearsonate renal scan
DSA	Digital subtraction angiography
DST	Dexamethasone suppression test

E

EBV	Epstein-Barr virus
ECG, EKG	Electrocardiogram
ECHO	Echocardiography
EEG	Electroencephalogram
EGD	Esophagogastroduodenoscopy
ELISA	Enzyme-linked immunosorbent assay
EMG	Electromyography
ENeG	Electroneurography
ENG	Electronystagmography
EP	Evoked potential
EPS	Electrophysiologic study
ER	Estrogen receptor
ERCP	Endoscopic retrograde cholangiopancreatography
ESR	Erythrocyte sedimentation rate
EUG	Excretory urography

F

FBG	Fasting blood glucose
FDPs	Fibrin degradation products
Fe	Iron
FSH	Follicle-stimulating hormone
FSPs	Fibrin split products
FTA-ABS	Fluorescent treponemal antibody absorbed test
FTI	Free thyroxine index

G

G-6-PD	Glucose-6-phosphate dehydrogenase
GB	Gallbladder
GER	Gastroesophageal reflux
GGT	Gamma-glutamyl transferase
GGTP	Gamma-glutamyl transpeptidase
GH	Growth hormone

GHb, GHB	Glycosylated hemoglobin
GI	Gastrointestinal
GTT	Glucose tolerance test

H

HAA	Hepatitis-associated antigen
HAI	Hemagglutination inhibition
HAV	Hepatitis A virus
Hb, Hgb	Hemoglobin
HB_cAb	Hepatitis B core antibody
HB_cAg	Hepatitis B core antigen
HBV	Hepatitis B virus
HCG	Human chorionic gonadotropin
HCO_3^-	Bicarbonate
Hct	Hematocrit
HDL	High-density lipoprotein
5-HIAA	5-hydroxyindoleacetic acid
HIDA	Hepato-iminodiacetic acid
HIV	Human immunodeficiency virus
HLA-B27	Human lymphocyte antigen B27
HSV-2	Herpes simplex virus, type 2
HTLV	Human T-cell lymphotropic virus

I

Ig	Immunoglobulin
INR	International normalized ratio
IVP	Intravenous pyelography
IVU, IUG	Intravenous urography

K

K	Potassium
KS	Ketosteroid
KUB	Kidney, ureter, and bladder x-ray study

L

LAP	Leucine aminopeptidase
LATS	Long-acting thyroid stimulator
LDH	Lactate dehydrogenase
LDL	Low-density lipoprotein
LE	Lupus erythematosus
LFTs	Liver function tests
LH	Luteinizing hormone
LP	Lumbar puncture
L/S ratio	Lecithin/sphingomyelin ratio
LS spine	Lumbosacral spine

M

MCH	Mean corpuscular hemoglobin
MCHC	Mean corpuscular hemoglobin concentration
MCV	Mean corpuscular volume
Mg	Magnesium
MRI	Magnetic resonance imaging
MUGA	Multiple gated acquisition cardic scan

N

Na	Sodium
NMR	Nuclear magnetic resonance
NST	Nonstress test

O

O&P	Ova and parasites
OB	Occult blood
OCT	Oxytocin challenge test
OGTT	Oral glucose tolerance test
OHCS	Hydroxycorticosteroid
OPG	Ocular pneumoplethysmography

P

P	Phosphorus
PAP	Prostatic acid phosphatase
Pb	Lead
P_{CO_2}	Partial pressure of carbon dioxide
PET	Positron emission tomography
PFTs	Pulmonary function tests
pH	Hydrogen ion concentration
PKU	Phenylketonuria
PMN	Polymorphonuclear
PNH	Paroxysmal nocturnal hemoglobinuria
P_{O_2}	Partial pressure of oxygen
PO_4	Phosphate
PPBS	Postprandial blood sugar
PPD	Purified protein derivative
PPG	Postprandial glucose
PR	Progesterone receptor
PRA	Plasma renin assay
PSA	Prostate-specific antigen
PT	Prothrombin time

PTH	Parathormone, parathyroid hormone
PTHC, PTC	Percutaneous transhepatic cholangiography
PTT	Partial thromboplastin time

R

RAIU	Radioactive iodine uptake
RBC	Red blood cell
RDW	Red cell distribution width
RF	Rheumatoid factor
RIA	Radioimmunoassay
RPR	Rapid plasma reagin test

S

S&A	Sugar and acetone
SBFT	Small bowel follow-through
SGOT	Serum glutamate oxaloacetate transaminase
SGPT	Serum glutamate pyruvate transaminase
SLE	Systemic lupus erythematosus
SPECT	Single photon emission computed tomography
STS	Serologic test for syphilis

T

T_3	Triiodothyronine
T_4	Thyroxine
T&C	Type and crossmatch
T&S	Type and screen
TB	Tuberculosis
TBG	Thyroxine-binding globulin
TBPA	Thyroxine-binding prealbumin
TEE	Transesophageal echocardiography
TG	Triglyceride
TIBC	Total iron-binding capacity
TRF	Thyrotropin-releasing factor
TRH	Thyrotropin-releasing hormone
TRP	Tubular reabsorption of phosphate
TSH	Thyroid-stimulating hormone
TTE	Transthoracic echocardiography

U

UA	Urinalysis
UGI series	Upper gastrointestinal series
UPP	Urethral pressure profile
US	Ultrasound

V

VDRL	Venereal Disease Research Laboratory

VLDL Very-low-density lipoprotein
VMA Vanillylmandelic acid
VPS Ventilation/perfusion scanning

W

WBC White blood cell (count)

Values of Commonly Performed Blood Tests

Test	Conventional values*
Activated partial thromboplastin time (APTT)	30-40 seconds
Alanine aminotransferase (ALT)	5-35 IU/L or 8-20 U/L (SI units)
Albumin	3.5-5.5 g/dl
Alcohol (ethanol)	0; >0.10% indicates intoxication
Alkaline phosphatase (ALP)	30-85 ImU/ml or 42-128 U/L (SI units)
Amylase	56-190 IU/L, 80-150 Somogyi units/dl, or 25-125 U/L (SI units)
Aspartate aminotransferase (AST, SGOT)	8-20 U/L or 5-40 IU/L (SI units)
Bilirubin, total	0.1-1.0 mg/dl or 5.1-17.0 mmol/L (SI units)
Indirect bilirubin	0.2-0.8 mg/dl or 3.4-12.0 mmol/L (SI units)
Direct bilirubin	0.1-0.3 mg/dl or 1.7-5.1 mmol/L (SI units)
Bleeding time	1-9 minutes (Ivy method)
Blood gases (arterial)	
pH	7.35-7.45
Pco_2	35-45 mm Hg
HCO_3^-	21-28 mEq/L
Po_2	80-100 mm
O_2 saturation	95%-100%
O_2 content	15-22 vol%
Blood urea nitrogen (BUN)	10-20 mg/dl
Calcium (Ca)	9.0-10.5 mg/dl

*Test results may vary among different laboratories. Investigate the normal values for the specific laboratory where the test is performed.

Continued

Carbon dioxide (CO_2) content	23-30 mEq/L or 23-30 mmol/L (SI units)
Chloride (Cl)	90-110 mEq/L or 98-106 mmol/L (SI units)
Cholesterol	<200 mg/dl
Creatine phosphokinase (CPK)	Male: 12-70 U/ml or 55-170 U/L (SI units)
	Female: 10-55 U/ml or 30-135 U/L (SI units)
Digoxin	0.8-2.10 ng/ml
Erythrocyte sedimentation rate (ESR)	<15-20 mm/hr
Glucose	
Fasting (FBS)	70-105 mg/dl
2-hour post postprandial (2-hour PPG)	<140 mg/dl
Hematocrit (Hct)	Male: 42%-52% or 0.42-0.52 vol fraction (SI units)
	Female: 37%-47% or 0.37-0.47 vol fraction (SI units)
Hemoglobin (Hgb)	Male: 14-18 g/dl or 8.7-11.2 mmol/L (SI units)
	Female: 12-16 g/dl or 7.4-9.9 mmol/L (SI units)
Magnesium (Mg)	1.2-2.0 mEq/L
Platelet count	150,000-400,000/mm^3
Potassium (K)	3.5-5.0 mEq/L
Prothrombin time (PT)	11.0-12.5 seconds
Red blood cell (RBC) count	Male: 4.7-6.1 million/mm^3
	Female: 4.2-5.4 million/mm^3
Reticulocyte count	0.5%-2% of RBCs
Sodium (Na)	136-145 mEq/L
Uric acid	Male: 2.1-8.5 mg/dl
	Female: 2.0-6.6 mg/dl
White blood cell (WBC) count	5000-10,000/mm^3
Differential	
Neutrophils	55%-70%
Lymphocytes	20%-40%
Monocytes	2%-8%
Eosinophils	1%-4%
Basophils	0.5%-1.0%

Credits

CHAPTER 1

Figures: 1-1, Grimes DE: Infectious Diseases, St. Louis, 1991, Mosby; 1-2, Wilson SF, Thompson JM: Respiratory Disorders, St. Louis, 1990, Mosby.

Box 1-1, Centers for Disease Control and Prevention, Atlanta, 1987.

CHAPTER 2

Figures: 2-1 and 2-2, Beare PG, Myers JL: Principles and Practice of Adult Health Nursing, ed 2, St. Louis, 1994, Mosby; 2-3, Pagana KD, Pagana TJ: Mosby's Manual of Diagnostic and Laboratory Tests, St. Louis, 1998, Mosby; 2-5, 2-6, and 2-10, Canobbio MM: Cardiovascular Disorders, St. Louis, 1990, Mosby; 2-7, 2-11, and 2-13, Pagana KD, Pagana TJ: Mosby's Diagnostic and Laboratory Test Reference, ed 4, St. Louis, 1999, Mosby.

Tables: 2-1, 2-3, 2-4, and 2-5, Pagana KD, Pagana TJ: Mosby's Manual of Diagnostic and Laboratory Tests, St. Louis, 1998, Mosby; 2-2, Pagana KD, Pagana TJ: Mosby's Diagnostic and Laboratory Test Reference, ed 4, St. Louis, 1999.

CHAPTER 3

Figures: 3-1, Beare PG, Myers JL: Principles and Practice of Adult Health Nursing, ed 2, St. Louis, 1994, Mosby; 3-2, Doughty D: Gastrointestinal Disorders, St. Louis, 1993, Mosby; 3-4 and 3-5, Pagana KD, Pagana TJ: Mosby's Diagnostic and Laboratory Test Reference, ed 4, St. Louis, 1999, Mosby.

Table 3-1, Pagana KD, Pagana TJ: Mosby's Manual of Diagnostic and Laboratory Tests, St. Louis, 1998, Mosby.

CHAPTER 4

Figures: 4-1, Beare PG, Myers JL: Principles and Practice of Adult Health Nursing, ed 2, St. Louis, 1994, Mosby; 4-2, 4-4, 4-7, 4-9, and 4-11, Pagana KD, Pagana TJ: Mosby's Diagnostic and Laboratory Test Reference, ed 4, St. Louis, 1999, Mosby; 4-3 and 4-5, Pagana KD, Pagana TJ: Mosby's Manual of Diagnostic and Laboratory Tests, St. Louis, 1998, Mosby; 4-6, Brundage DJ: Renal Disorders, St. Louis, 1992, Mosby; 4-10, Mourad LA: Orthopedic Disorders, St. Louis, 1991, Mosby; 4-12, Wilson SF,

Thompson JM: Respiratory Disorders, St. Louis, 1990, Mosby.

CHAPTER 5

Figures: 5-1 and 5-11, Beare PG, Myers JL: Principles and Practice of Adult Health Nursing, ed 2, St. Louis, 1994, Mosby; 5-2, 5-6, 5-8, and 5-13, Wilson SF, Thompson JM: Respiratory Disorders, St. Louis, 1990, Mosby; 5-3, 5-5, 5-7, Pagana KD, Pagana TJ: Mosby's Manual of Diagnostic and Laboratory Tests, St. Louis, 1998, Mosby; 5-4, 5-9, and 5-10, Pagana KD, Pagana TJ: Mosby's Diagnostic and Laboratory Test Reference, ed 4, St. Louis, 1999, Mosby; 5-12, Grimes DE: Infectious Diseases, St. Louis, 1991, Mosby.

Tables: 5-1 and 5-2, Pagana KD, Pagana TJ: Mosby's Diagnostic and Laboratory Test Reference, ed 4, St. Louis, 1999, Mosby; 5-3, Pagana KD, Pagana TJ: Mosby's Manual of Diagnostic and Laboratory Tests, St. Louis, 1998, Mosby.

CHAPTER 6

Figures: 6-1, Beare PG, Myers JL: Principles and Practice of Adult Health Nursing, ed 2, St. Louis, 1994, Mosby; 6-4, 6-6, 6-7, Chipps E, Clanin N, Campbell V: Neurologic Disorders, St. Louis, 1992, Mosby; 6-10, Pagana KD, Pagana TJ: Mosby's Diagnostic and Laboratory Test Reference, ed 4, St. Louis, 1999, Mosby; 6-11, Lewis SM, Collier IC, Heitkemper MH: Medical-Surgical Nursing: Assessment and Management of Clinical Problems, ed 4, St. Louis, 1996, Mosby; 6-12, Brundage DJ: Renal Disorders, St. Louis, 1992, Mosby.

CHAPTER 7

Figures: 7-1, 7-2, 7-3, and 7-6, Beare PG, Myers JL: Principles and Practice of Adult Health Nursing, ed 2, St. Louis, 1994, Mosby; 7-4, 7-7, 7-10, and 7-11, Pagana KD, Pagana TJ: Mosby's

Diagnostic and Laboratory Test Reference, ed 4, St. Louis, 1999, Mosby; 7-8, Pagana KD, Pagana TJ: Mosby's Manual of Diagnostic and Laboratory Tests, St. Louis, 1998, Mosby; 7-9, Doughty D: Gastrointestinal Disorders, St. Louis, 1993, Mosby; 7-12, Brundage DJ: Renal Disorders, St. Louis, 1992, Mosby.

CHAPTER 8

Figures: 8-1, 8-2, and 8-3, Beare PG, Myers JL: Principles and Practice of Adult Health Nursing, ed 2, St. Louis, 1994, Mosby; 8-6, Pagana KD, Pagana TJ: Mosby's Diagnostic and Laboratory Test Reference, ed 4, St. Louis, 1999, Mosby; 8-7, Pagana KD, Pagana TJ: Mosby's Manual of Diagnostic and Laboratory Tests, St. Louis, 1998, Mosby.

Tables: 8-3 and 8-4, Pagana KD, Pagana TJ: Mosby's Manual of Diagnostic and Laboratory Tests, St. Louis, 1998, Mosby.

CHAPTER 9

Figures: 9-1 and 9-2, Beare PG, Myers JL: Principles and Practice of Adult Health Nursing, ed 2, St. Louis, 1994, Mosby; 9-3, Lowdermilk DL, Perry SE, Bobak IM: Maternity and Women's Health Care, ed 6, St. Louis, 1996, Mosby; 9-4, 9-5, 9-6, and 9-10, Pagana KD, Pagana TJ: Mosby's Diagnostic and Laboratory Test Reference, ed 4, St. Louis, 1999, Mosby; 9-7 and 9-9, Pagana KD, Pagana TJ: Mosby's Manual of Diagnostic and Laboratory Tests, St. Louis, 1998, Mosby; 9-8, Brundage DJ: Renal Disorders, St. Louis, 1992, Mosby.

Box 9-1, Pagana KD, Pagana TJ: Mosby's Manual of Diagnostic and Laboratory Tests, St. Louis, 1998, Mosby.

CHAPTER 10

Figures: 10-1, 10-3, and 10-5, Pagana KD, Pagana TJ: Mosby's Manual of Diagnostic and Laboratory Tests, St. Louis, 1998, Mosby; 10-2 and 10-4, Pagana KD, Pagana TJ: Mosby's Diagnostic and Laboratory Test Reference, ed 4, St. Louis, 1999, Mosby.

Tables: 10-1, 10-3, 10-4, 10-5, and 10-6, Pagana KD, Pagana TJ: Mosby's Manual of Diagnostic and Laboratory Tests, St. Louis, 1998, Mosby; 10-4, 10-5, and 10-6, Pagana KD, Pagana TJ: Mosby's Diagnostic and Laboratory Test Reference, ed 4, St. Louis, 1999, Mosby.

Box 10-1, Pagana KD, Pagana TJ: Mosby's Manual of Diagnostic and Laboratory Tests, St. Louis, 1998, Mosby.

CHAPTER 11

Figures: 11-1 and 11-2, Beare PG, Myers JL: Principles and Practice of Adult Health Nursing, ed 2, St. Louis, 1994, Mosby; 11-4, Pagana KD, Pagana TJ: Mosby's Diagnostic and Laboratory Test Reference, ed 4, St. Louis, 1999, Mosby.

CHAPTER 12

Tables: 12-1 and 12-2, Pagana KD, Pagana TJ: Mosby's Manual of Diagnostic and Laboratory

Tests, St. Louis, 1998, Mosby; 12-3, Pagana KD, Pagana TJ: Mosby's Diagnostic and Laboratory Test Reference, ed 4, St. Louis, 1999, Mosby.

CHAPTER 13

Figures: 13-1 and 13-4, Pagana KD, Pagana TJ: Mosby's Manual of Diagnostic and Laboratory Tests, St. Louis, 1998, Mosby; 13-2, Mourad LA: Orthopedic Disorders, St. Louis, 1991, Mosby; 13-3 and 13-6, Belcher AE: Cancer Nursing, St. Louis, 1992, Mosby.

CHAPTER 14

Figure 14-1, Pagana KD, Pagana TJ: Mosby's Manual of Diagnostic and Laboratory Tests, St. Louis, 1998, Mosby.

Tables: 14-1, Pagana KD, Pagana TJ: Mosby's Manual of Diagnostic and Laboratory Tests, St. Louis, 1998, Mosby; 14-2, 14-3, and 14-4, Pagana KD, Pagana TJ: Mosby's Diagnostic and Laboratory Test Reference, ed 4, St. Louis, 1999, Mosby.

Index

Multicultural Education in a Pluralistic Society

Third Edition

Donna M. Gollnick

National Council for Accreditation of Teacher Education
Washington, DC

Philip C. Chinn

California State University at Los Angeles

Merrill Publishing Company
Columbus London Toronto Melbourne

To Willard C. Loftis
D.M.G.

To Stanley E. Jackson
P.C.C.

Cover Photo: Background: Mark Antman/The Image Works. Upper left: Tony Freeman/Photo Edit. Upper right: Richard Hutchings/Photo Edit. Bottom left: Alan Carey/The Image Works. Bottom right: Michael Okoniewski/The Image Works.

Published by Merrill Publishing Company
Columbus, Ohio 43216

This book was set in Palatino

Administrative Editor: David Faherty
Production Editor: Ben Ko
Art Coordinator: Lorraine Woost
Cover Designer: Russ Maselli
Photo Editor: Terry L. Tietz

Library of Congress Catalog Card Number: 89-63629
International Standard Book Number: 0-675-21125-5
Printed in the United States of America
1 2 3 4 5 6 7 8 9—94 93 92 91 90

Preface

The United States is a multicultural nation of persons of different ethnic backgrounds, classes, religions, and native languages. In addition, there are natural differences based on sex, age, and physical and mental abilities. Every day, educators and their students are exposed to a social curriculum that makes positive and negative statements about these differences through radio, television, and newspapers, as well as through family attitudes. Often, distorted messages about people who are ethnically or religiously different from oneself are portrayed in the social curriculum. We learn that Italian-Americans control organized crime, African-Americans are on welfare, old people are useless, females are helpless, hard hats are racist, and handicapped individuals must be taken care of. These stereotypes about groups of people are broad generalizations that totally neglect the majority of individuals within each of these groups. Decisions made by employers, educators, politicians, and neighbors are often based on such misconceptions. As educators, we must help students interpret and analyze the cultural cues that are forced on them daily.

An overall goal of multicultural education is to help all students develop their potential for academic, social, and vocational success. Educational and vocational options should not be limited by sex, age, ethnicity, native language, religion, class, or exceptionality. Educators are given the responsibility to help students contribute to and benefit from our democratic society. Within our pluralistic society, multicultural education values the existing diversity, positively portrays that diversity, and uses that diversity in the development of effective instructional strategies for students in the classroom. In addition, multicultural education should help students think critically about institutionalized racism, classism, and sexism. Ideally, educators will begin to develop individual and group strategies for overcoming the debilitating effects of these societal scourges.

Our approach to multicultural education is based on a broad definition of the concept. By using culture as the basis for understanding multicultural education, we have presented descriptions of seven microcultures to which Americans belong. Of course, these are not the only microcultures to which individuals belong, but in our view these are the most critical in understanding pluralism and multicultural education at this time. Not limiting the approach to ethnicity, as many authors have, we focus on the complex nature of pluralism in this country. An individual's cultural identity is based not only on ethnicity but also on such factors as class, religion, and gender. To further complicate matters, the degree of identification with one's ethnic origins, religion, and other microcultural memberships varies greatly from individual to individual. For example, we are not men and women alone with our separate cultural patterns; we are women and men within the context of our ethnic, religious, and class background. The complexity of pluralism in the United States makes it difficult for the educator to develop expectations of students based on their group memberships. This text is designed to examine these group memberships and ways in which the educator can develop educational programs to meet the needs of those groups and the nation.

Multicultural Education in a Pluralistic Society provides an overview of the different microcultures to which students belong. The first chapter examines the pervasive influence of culture and the importance of understanding our own cultural background and experiences as well as those of our students. The following seven chapters examine the microcultures of class, ethnicity and race, gender, exceptionality, religion, language, and age. The final chapter describes how the educator can portray and use this pluralism in the implementation of multicultural education.

All of the chapters in this edition have been revised to reflect current thinking and research in the area. The chapters on exceptionality and language have been rewritten to reflect more of a cultural perspective than was presented in past editions. Topics addressed in this edition that have not been included before are the underclass and the homeless, homosexuality, sign language, and equality issues. The section entitled "Critical Incidents in Teaching" at the end of the book is also a new feature. The purpose is to help readers apply their knowledge about microcultural memberships to classroom and school situations. We believe that you will find these examples challenging.

The reader should be aware of several caveats related to the language used in this text. First, both male and female pronouns are used sparingly throughout the text. Second, although we realize that the term American includes populations beyond the boundaries of the United States, it has been used here to refer to the U.S. population. We have limited our use of the term minority in the text and have focused more on the subordinate and dominant relationships that exist between groups in this country. We realize that not all members of subordinate/minority groups are equally affected by these power relationships, but the impact on the groups as a whole is extremely important in these discussions.

Students in undergraduate, graduate and in-service courses should find this text helpful in examining social and cultural conditions that influence education. It is designed to assist them in understanding pluralism and how to use it effectively in the classroom and schools. Other professionals in the social services will find it helpful in understanding the complexity of cultural backgrounds and experiences as they work with their clients.

The preparation of any book involves the contributions of many individuals in addition to those whose names are found on the cover. We thank our colleagues who reacted to our ideas as the book originally was conceptualized, particularly Gwendolyn C. Baker, James A. Banks, Carl A. Grant, and the many individuals at all educational levels who have been developing and implementing multicultural education programs across the nation. We also thank our reviewers—Sandra De Costa, West Virginia University; Herbert Hendricks, Humboldt State University; and Lavon Gappa, University of Nebraska-Lincoln—and are especially indebted to Christine E. Sleeter, who provided insights that are reflected in this edition of the book. A special thanks is extended to Teresa Uland for her assistance in conducting some of the necessary preliminary work. The patience shown by our editors, David Faherty and Ben Ko, throughout the preparation of this edition is sincerely appreciated. For typing of parts of the manuscript, we thank Juanita Butler. Finally, we thank our children— Michele, Kelleth, and Kristin—for their continued support throughout this revision.

Donna M. Gollnick

Philip C. Chinn

Contents

CHAPTER 1
Tenets of Multicultural Education: Culture, Pluralism, and Equality

Local, state, and national reports on education that were issued in the 1980s called on educators, parents, and students to push for excellence in the nation's schools. State legislators and local school boards responded by requiring more rigorous curricula and standards for student achievement. However, teachers have been provided with little direction or assistance to ensure that *all* students are able to realize that excellence or gain the rewards provided by such an educational opportunity. Thus, educators today are faced with an overwhelming challenge to prepare students from diverse cultural backgrounds to live in a rapidly changing society and world in which some groups have greater societal benefits than others because of their race, sex, socioeconomic level, religion, lack of disability, or age.

Students who will make up our future schools will represent much greater cultural diversity than is currently seen. Harold Hodgkinson's (1986) examination of demographic data on birthrates and immigration in the mid-1980s indicates that children will be inexorably more Asian-American, more Hispanic (but not more Cuban-American), more African-American, and less white. By the end of this century, over 30 percent of the school population will be composed of students of color. They already make up over 50 percent of the student population in two states, California and Texas. Nearly 25 percent of our children currently live below the poverty line. Although the national data are still sketchy, it appears that there may be an increase in the number of children with physical and emotional handicaps.

To work effectively with the heterogeneous student populations found in our schools, educators need to understand and feel comfortable with their own cultural backgrounds. They also must understand the cultural setting in which the school is located to develop effective instructional strategies and to assist students in becoming aware of cultural diversity in the nation and world. An educational goal is to help students value cultural differences while realizing that individuals across cultures have many similarities.

Although prospective teachers may have in mind the type of school or community in which they would like to teach after they have been licensed, jobs are not always available in those areas. A look at four different school settings will show the diversity of student populations with which one may work.

School 1.   Until ten years ago, this suburban community had been made up of primarily white middle-class families and several dozen African-American and Japanese-American families. Within the past ten years, there has been an influx of Vietnamese students with limited English skills. Although their names reflect an ethnic identity, there are not observable differences among most of the white students. Most parents are professionals (e.g., lawyers, teachers, and engineers) and managers or employees of several large corporations located in the city. About 10 percent of the students live with single parents. Mothers of nearly half the students work outside the home as professionals, secretaries, or salespersons. Students come from Catholic, Jewish, Buddhist, and Protestant families. Most students seldom venture into the major city, which is within thirty miles of their homes.

School 2.   Spanish is the first language of nearly half the students in this inner-city school. Students identify themselves as African-American, Puerto Rican, and Mexican-American. Children from Central America also have entered the school recently. Many students live with their families in small private apartments; others live in housing projects that stretch for blocks. About

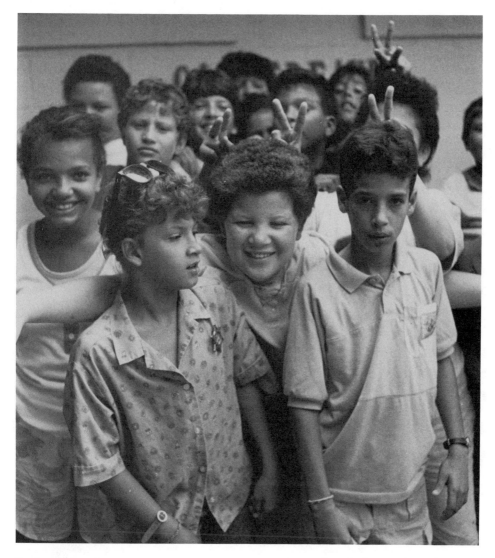

Students in rural areas are sometimes representative of a number of ethnic and racial groups, as in this southern Alabama school.

(Photo by Susan Tucker).

30 percent live in households headed by women who work outside of the home when work is available. A disproportionately large number of parents are unemployed, and those that work primarily hold unskilled jobs. Many students are Catholic, and some of the Protestant students attend charismatic churches. Most students have never been beyond the area in which they live; most have never been outside the city or interacted with individuals outside of the few blocks that surround their apartment.

School 3.   All students are white with a German or English surname in this rural area. Parents are self-employed farmers, farm laborers, or employees at factories in the area. Most families have lived in this community for over a century, and much of the community's social activities are centered around the one Catholic and three Protestant churches. The only recent

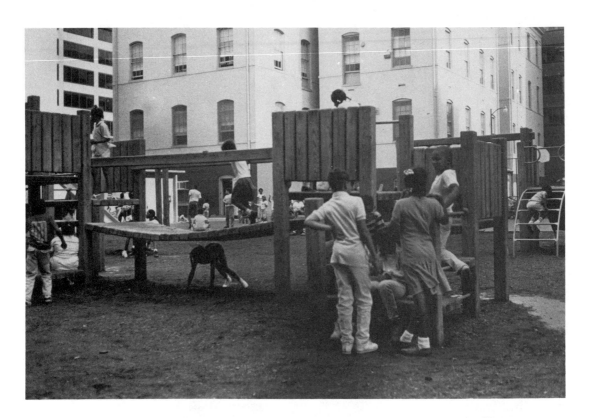

Some urban schools are squeezed between office buildings and housing units, leaving small playgrounds that differ greatly from those in suburban and rural areas.

(Photo by Susan Tucker).

migration to this community occurred about fifteen years ago when an Amish community purchased farmland in the area and settled there. About one-fourth of the students' mothers work outside the home as teachers, secretaries, salespersons, or factory workers. Only a few students live with a single mother or father. Most students are familiar with the small town that is the county seat, where they shop and occasionally see movies. The nearest large city is the state capital, which they sometimes visit for a special activity such as the state 4-H fair. Few, if any, have ever interacted directly with members of minority groups, and they remain puzzled about the Amish culture.

School 4.   The student body of this urban school is 55 percent African-American, 30 percent white, 7 percent Hispanic, 4 percent Asian-American, and 2 percent American Indian. Students from several foreign countries also attend the school. There are students who speak no English when they enter the classroom; twenty languages other than English are used by students. Parents are government officials from the United States and other countries, professionals, business managers, small business owners, skilled and unskilled workers, and unemployed. The mothers of 80 percent of the students work in jobs ranging from unskilled to professional positions. Students come from homes of wide religious diversity, including the Catholic, Protestant, Jewish, Black Muslim, and Islamic faiths. Students travel from all over the city to attend school. Many students are very cosmopolitan, but others interact only in their primary cultural communities.

Teachers who enter a classroom with thirty students will find that students have individual differences even though they may appear to be from the same cultural group. These differences extend far beyond intellectual and physical abilities. Students bring to class different historical backgrounds, religious experiences, and day-to-day living experiences. These experiences direct the way the students behave in school. The cultural background of some students will be mirrored in the school culture. For others, the difference between the home and school cultures will cause dissonance unless the teacher can use the cultural backgrounds of the students to develop a supportive environment. If the teacher fails to understand the cultural factors in addition to the intellectual and physical factors that affect student learning and behavior, it will be impossible to teach all thirty students effectively.

Multicultural education is the educational strategy in which students' cultural backgrounds are viewed as positive and essential in developing classroom instruction and school environments. It is designed to support and extend the concepts of culture, cultural pluralism, and equality into the formal school setting. An examination of the theoretical precepts of these concepts will lead to an understanding of the development and practice of multicultural education.

CULTURE

Everyone has culture. Unfortunately, many individuals believe that persons who are culturally different from themselves have an inferior culture. Until early this century, the term *culture* was used to indicate groups of people who were more developed in the ways of the Western world and less *primitive* than tribal groups in many parts of the world. Individuals who were knowledgeable in the areas of history, literature, and the fine arts were said to possess culture.

No longer is culture viewed so narrowly. Anthropologists define culture as a way of perceiving, believing, evaluating, and behaving (Goodenough, 1987) or as "a shared organization of ideas that includes the intellectual, moral, and aesthetic standards prevalent in a community and the meanings of communicative actions" (LeVine, 1984, p. 67). Culture provides the blueprint that determines the way an individual thinks, feels, and behaves in society. At the same time, culture develops within "unequal and dialectical relations that different groups establish in a given society at a particular historical point" (Giroux, 1988, p. 116). These differing and unequal power relations have a great impact on "the ability of individuals and groups to define and achieve their goals" (Giroux, 1988, p. 117). The dynamics of those power relationships and the effect they have on the development of groups must also be an integral part of the study of culture.

Thus, in a classroom of thirty students, each student has culture. Parts of the culture are shared by all of the class members, whereas other aspects of the culture are shared only with family members or the community. All of the students belong to the same age cohort and as such share membership in an age group. All live in the same country, state, and community and as such are subject to the basic values, rules, and regulations that govern the shared national culture. Students with English as their first language may differ in the dialect spoken, and other students will be learning English as a second or third language. In most classes, there will be both boys and girls, and within both groups, aspects of being either a boy or a girl are shared with others of the same sex.

In one elementary classroom, a number of ethnic backgrounds might be identified. Even when the class is composed totally of white students, ethnic identities could include Swedish-Americans, German-Americans, Irish-Americans, and Polish-Americans. Students within each ethnic group might share the same religion, lifestyles, and values, and these may be somewhat different from those of classmates with a different ethnic background. Black students may identify themselves ethnically as Jamaican-American, Puerto Rican, Panamanian-American, Nigerian-American, or African-American.

Unless the school is parochial and limits attendance to children of a specific religion, several religious affiliations will be represented in the classroom. Some rural or small-town communities will be composed primarily of liberal and fundamentalist Protestant families. Large urban schools may include students who identify themselves as Protestant, Roman Catholic, Greek Orthodox, Latter-Day Saint (Mormon), Jewish, Buddhist, or Islamic in addition to those who claim no religious affiliation. Other cultural differences will result from the socioeconomic status of students's families and from the geographical areas from which the families may have recently moved.

To understand the different cultural experiences brought to the classroom by students, it is necessary first to examine culture itself. All people have the same psychological and biological needs that must be met to survive. How they fulfill these needs varies greatly. These variations depend in part on the resources available and on the climatic conditions of the region. More importantly, they depend on the group's relationship to the dominant society.

All human groups undergo the same poignant life experiences of birth, marriage, helplessness, illness, old age, and death. We even share many of the same institutions, such as marriage ceremonies and incest taboos. However, the ways in which we use our biological characteristics, handle the same poignant life experiences, and create the same institutions are limitless. These differences are not innate, but are culturally determined. A traditional Greek-American may show a great outpouring of emotion at the funeral of a family member. On the other hand, a third-generation Greek-American who has been acculturated is likely to be more emotionally restrained at the public funeral. None of the events, reactions, or habits of a group of people can be understood without understanding the context of the culture of which they are a part.

Culture is so much a part of us that we do not realize that we might behave differently from others. Most of us do not think that sitting at a table to eat, eating three meals a day, having different foods for breakfast and dinner, brushing our teeth, or sleeping in a bed are culturally determined behaviors. We know these habits and customs as the only way to behave. These ways of doing things have become the accepted and patterned ways of behavior for people who live in the Western part of the world, particularly the United States. As a matter of fact, we must know and use these patterns to be acceptable to other members of the culture. Culture gives us our identity through acceptable words; through our actions, postures, gestures, and tones of voice; through our facial expressions; through our handling of time, space, and materials; and through the way we work, play, express our emotions, and defend ourselves (Hall, 1977).

Generally accepted and patterned ways of behavior are necessary for a group of people to live together. Culture imposes order and meaning on all our experiences. It allows us to predict how others will behave in certain situations. On the other hand, it prevents us from predicting how people from a different culture will behave in the same situation.

Culture gives us a certain life-style that is peculiarly our own. It becomes so peculiar to us that someone from a different culture can easily identify us as Americans. A traveler from our country who goes overseas will usually be identified as American by the people of the country being visited, whether the individual is African-, Native, European-, Hispanic-, or Asian-American.

Culture is not only reflected in our behavior. It also determines the way we think and feel. It makes assumptions about the ends and purposes of human existence, about what humans have a right to expect from each other and from God (gods), and about what constitutes fulfillment or frustration (Hall, 1977).

Characteristics of Culture

We all have culture, but how did we get it? It is learned, and the learning starts at birth. Most individuals born in the United States first saw the world in a hospital delivery room, where attendants were dressed in white or aqua green uniforms. The first days of life were characterized by cleanliness—sterile sheets and gowns, sterile bottles or nipples, and a sterile environment behind glass, except during nursing hours. The way the baby was held, fed, bathed, and dressed was culturally determined. Parents and hospital personnel knew this procedure as the only way, or at least the best way, to care for a baby in the first days because it had been the acceptable pattern in this country.

A person learns how to become a functioning adult within a specific society through culture. Two similar processes interact as one learns how to act in society: *enculturation* and *socialization*. Enculturation is the process of acquiring the characteristics of a given culture and generally becoming competent in its language. Socialization is the general process of learning to function as a member of the society by learning social roles, such as mother, husband, student, or child, and occupational roles, such as teacher, banker, plumber, custodian, or politician (Miller, 1979). Enculturation and socialization are processes initiated at birth by others, including parents, siblings, nurses, physicians, teachers, and neighbors. These varied instructors may not identify these processes as enculturation or socialization, but they demonstrate and reward one for acceptable behaviors. All people learn how to behave by observation of and participation in their society and culture. Thus, individuals will be socialized and enculturated according to the patterns of the culture in which they are raised. The culture in which one is born becomes unimportant unless one is also socialized in the same culture, as Kluckhohn (1949) illustrated:

> I met in New York City a young man who did not speak a word of English and was obviously bewildered by American ways. By "blood" he was as American as you or I, for his parents had gone from Indiana to China as missionaries. Orphaned in infancy, he was reared by a Chinese family in a remote village. All who met him found him more Chinese than American. The facts of his blue eyes and light hair were less impressive than a Chinese style of gait, Chinese arm and hand movements, Chinese facial expressions, and Chinese modes of thought. The biological heritage was American, but the cultural training had been Chinese. He returned to China. (p. 19)

Because culture is so much a part of us, we often tend to mix up biological and cultural heritage. Our cultural heritage is learned. It is not innately based on the culture in which we are born, as shown by Kluckhohn's example of the American man raised in China. Vietnamese infants adopted by Italian-American, Catholic, middle-class parents will share a cultural heritage with middle-class Italian-American Catholics, rather than with Vietnamese in Vietnam. Observers, however, may continue to identify these individuals as Asian-Americans because of physical characteristics and a lack of knowledge about their cultural experiences.

A second characteristic of culture is that it is shared. Shared cultural patterns and customs bind people together as an identifiable group and make it possible for them to live together and function with ease. An individual in the shared culture is provided the context for identifying with the group that shares the same culture. Although there may be some disagreement about certain aspects of the culture, there is a common acceptance and agreement about most aspects. Actually, most points of agreement are outside our realm of awareness. We do not even realize their existence as culture; eating three meals a day or sleeping on a bed are examples of this.

Culture is an adaptation. Cultures have developed to accommodate certain environmental conditions and available natural and technological resources. Thus, the Eskimo who lives with extreme cold, snow, ice, seals, and the sea has developed a culture different from the Pacific Islander, who has limited land, unlimited seas, and few mineral resources. The culture of urban residents differs from rural residents, in part because of the resources available in the different settings. The culture of subordinate groups differs from that of the dominant group because of power relationships within society.

Finally, culture is a dynamic system that changes continuously. Some cultures undergo constant and rapid change, while others are very slow to change. Some changes, such as a new word or new hairstyle, may be relatively small and have little impact on the culture as a whole. Other changes will have a dramatic impact on the culture. The introduction of technology into a culture has often produced changes far broader than the technology itself. For example, the replacement of industrial workers by robots is changing the culture of many working-class communities. Such changes may also alter traditional customs and beliefs.

Manifestations of Culture

The cultural patterns of a group of people are determined by how they organize and view the various components of culture. Culture itself is manifested in an infinite number of ways through societal institutions, daily habits of living, and the individual's fulfillment of psychological and basic needs. To understand how extensively our lives are affected by culture, let's examine a few of these manifestations.

Our values are determined initially by our culture. Values are conceptions of what is desirable and important to us or the group. Our values influence such factors as prestige, status, pride, family loyalty, love of country, religious belief, and honor. In many cultures, family loyalty is extremely important; it is so important that a relative is supported whenever possible. This support may include giving relatives a job regardless of their qualifications; it may also mean sharing all of one's money and resources with relatives if they need help. Such values are not reinforced in the dominant American culture. Status symbols differ across cultures. In the United States, accumulation of material possessions appears to be a desirable status symbol for many cultural groups. These factors, as well as what is decent or indecent, what is moral or immoral, and how punishment and reward are provided, are determined by the value system of the culture.

Culture also manifests itself in the nonverbal communication used by individuals within various cultures. The meaning of the same act or expression must be viewed in its cultural context. Raising the eyebrow is an example: "To most Americans this means surprise; to a person from the Marshall Islands in the Pacific it signals an affirmative answer; for Greeks, it is a sign of disagreement. The difference is not so much in how the eyebrows are raised but in the cultural meaning of the act" (Spradley & Rynkiewich, 1975, p. 7). We must be careful not to interpret acts and expressions of people from a different cultural background as having the same meaning as our own. Culture also determines the manner of walking, sitting, standing, reclining, and gesturing.

Language itself is a reflection of culture and provides a special way of looking at the world and organizing experiences that is often ignored in translating words from one language to another. There are many different sounds and combinations of sounds used in the languages of different cultures. Those of us who have tried to learn a second language probably have experienced difficulty in verbalizing the sounds that were not part of our first language.

Although we have discussed only a few of our daily patterns determined by culture, the patterns are limitless. Among them are weaning children, toilet training, rites of passage, forming kinship bonds, choosing a spouse, sexual relations, and division of labor. These patterns are shared by members of the culture and often seem strange and improper to nonmembers.

Ethnocentrism

Because culture helps determine the way we think, feel, and act, it becomes the lens through which we judge the world. As such, it can become an unconscious blinder to other ways of thinking, feeling, and acting. Our own culture is automatically treated as innate. It becomes the only natural way to function in the world. Even common sense in our own culture is naturally translated to common sense for the world. The rest of the world is viewed through our cultural lens. Other cultures are compared with ours and evaluated by our cultural standards. It becomes difficult, if not impossible, to view another culture as separate from our own—a task that anthropologists attempt when studying another culture.

This inability to view other cultures as equally viable alternatives for organizing reality is known as *ethnocentrism*. It is a common characteristic of cultures, whereby one's own cultural traits are viewed as natural, correct, and superior to those of another culture, whose traits are perceived as odd, amusing, inferior, or immoral (Yetman, 1985).

It is an asset for the culture to be viewed by its members as the natural and correct way of thinking, acting, and behaving. At the same time, it often solicits feelings of superiority over any other culture. The inability to view another culture through its cultural lens rather than through one's own cultural lens prevents an understanding of the second culture. This inability usually makes it impossible to function effectively in a second culture. By overcoming one's ethnocentric view of the world, one can begin to respect other cultures and even learn to function comfortably in more than one cultural group.

Cultural Relativism

There is a North American Indian proverb that says, "Never judge another man until you have walked a mile in his moccasins." This proverb suggests the importance of understanding the cultural background and experiences of other persons rather than judging them by our own standards. The principle of *cultural relativism* is an attempt "to understand other cultural systems in their own terms, not in terms of one's own cultural beliefs" (Miller, 1979, p. 44). This ability becomes more essential than ever in the world today, where various countries and cultures are becoming more dependent on the resources of others. In an effort to maintain positive relationships with the numerous cultural groups in the world, the United States can no longer afford to ignore other cultures or to relegate them to a status inferior to its own.

Within our own boundaries are many cultural groups that have been historically viewed and treated as inferior to the dominant western European culture that has been the basis for most of our institutions. Hall (1977) has found that intercultural misunderstandings occur even when there is no language barrier and large components of the major culture are shared by the people involved. These misunderstandings often occur because one cultural group is largely ignorant about the culture of another group. In addition, the members of one group are, for the most part, unable to describe their own cultural system (Hall, 1977). These misunderstandings are common among the various cultural groups in this country.

Cultural relativism would first have people learn more about their own culture than is commonly required. Then they would need to learn much more about other cultural groups. This intercultural process would involve learning and experiencing another culture so that one would know what it is like to be a member of the second culture and to view the world from that point of view. To function effectively and comfortably within a second culture, we must learn that culture.

CULTURE IN THE UNITED STATES

It is difficult to study our own culture because we are too close to it to identify traits that are characteristic of the culture (Spradley & Rynkiewich, 1975). Many individuals who have lived overseas for an extended period of time find it easier to identify American traits than those individuals who have never experienced a different culture. Often we are able to identify differences among subordinate groups and differences between subordinate and dominant groups but are unable to recognize the cultural patterns that have become uniquely American and thus shared voluntarily or under protest by group members.

A problem in studying the culture of the United States in particular is its complexity. Conflicting forces related to values, life-styles, and societal impediments within and between cultural groups are integral to this complexity and the resulting cultural adaptations. The complexity and rapid change of culture from generation to generation make inevitable the lack of harmony between cultural elements. The U.S. culture, like all others, is constantly undergoing change. Nevertheless, some of its current characteristics are described in the remainder of this chapter.

The U.S. *macroculture* is the national culture that is shared by most of the nation's citizens. In addition, numerous cultural groups exist with distinct cultural patterns that are not common to all Americans. These cultural groups are called *microcultures* or *subcultures* and will be described briefly in this section and in greater detail in Chapters 2 through 8. Finally, there are also *group cultures* that have been studied by sociologists. These cultures include occupational groups, gangs, drug cultures, peer groups, and other smaller, identifiable units of society.

The Macroculture

Historically, U.S. political and social institutions have developed from a western European tradition. The English language itself is a polyglot of languages spoken by the various conquerors and rulers of Great Britain throughout history. Our legal system is derived from English common law. The political system of democratic elections comes from France and England. The middle-class value system has been modified from a European system (Arensberg & Niehoff, 1975). Even our way of thinking, at least the way that it is rewarded in school, is based on Socrates' linear system of logic (Hall, 1977).

Our formal institutions, including government, schools, social welfare, banks, business, and laws, affect many aspects of our lives. Because of the strong Anglo-Saxon influence on these institutions, the dominant cultural influence on the United States also has been identified as Anglo-Saxon, or west European. More specifically, the major cultural influence on the United States, particularly on its institutions, has been white, Anglo-Saxon, and Protestant (WASP). But no longer is the dominant group composed only of WASPs. Instead, most members of the middle class have adopted these traditionally WASP institutions which provide the framework for the traits and values of the U.S. culture. Although most of our institutions still function under the strong influence of their WASP roots, many other aspects of American life have been greatly influenced by the numerous cultural groups that make up the U.S. population.

As members of the U.S. macroculture, we share core cultural traits. Not all members of the macroculture value these cultural traits or accept them as the most desirable traits for the culture. The traits, however, are recognized patterns around which our lives are organized. What are the characteristics, or traits, that most Americans share?

Although we have an agrarian tradition, the population now is primarily located in metropolitan areas and small towns. The country has mineral and soil wealth, elaborate technology, and a wealth of manufactured goods. Mass education and mass communication are ways of life. We are regulated by clocks and calendars rather than by seas and the sun. Time is used to organize most activities of life. Individuals are employees whose salaries or wages are paid by large, complex, interpersonal institutions. Work is done regularly, purposefully, and sometimes grimly. On the other hand, play is fun—an outlet from work. Money is the denominator of exchange.

Necessities of life are purchased rather than produced. Achievement and success are measured by the quantity of material goods purchased. Religious beliefs are concerned with general morality. Informality and equality are necessary ingredients in social relations (Arensberg & Niehoff, 1975; Stewart, 1977). Values that appear inherent in the macroculture include the following:

☐ Status based on occupation, education, and financial worth

☐ Achievement valued above inheritance

☐ Work ethic

☐ Comforts and rights to such amenities

☐ Cleanliness as an absolute value

☐ Achievement and success measured by the quantity of material goods purchased

☐ Egalitarianism as shown in the demand for political, economic, and social equality

☐ Inalienable and God-given rights for every individual that includes an equal right to self-governance or choice of representatives

☐ Humanitarianism that is usually highly organized and often impersonal

☐ New and modern perceived as better than old and traditional (Arensberg & Niehoff, 1975)

Although these traits and values may not be equally shared by the individuals that make up the United States, they are shared to some degree by all members of the macroculture. Let us examine additional traits and values that are often characterized as shared by the macroculture but that are actually shared primarily by members of the dominant cultural groups that support the country's institutions.

The overpowering value of the dominant group is individualism that is characterized by the belief that every individual is his or her own master, is in control of his or her own destiny, and will advance and regress in society only according to his or her own efforts (Bellah, Madsen, Sullivan, Swidler, & Tipton, 1985; Hsu, 1975). Traits that emphasize this core value include industriousness, ambition, competitiveness, self-reliance, independence, appreciation of the good life, and the perception of humans as separate and superior to nature. The acquisition of possessions, such as televisions, cars, boats, and homes, measures success and achievement.

Another core value is freedom. However, freedom is defined by the dominant group as "being left alone by others, not having other people's values, ideas, or styles of life forced upon one, being free of arbitrary authority in work, family, and political life" (Bellah et al., 1985, p. 23). As a result, impersonality in relations with others is common. Communication is often direct or confrontive. Most members of the dominant group rely more on associations of common interest than on strong kinship ties. The nuclear family is the basic kinship unit. Values tend to be absolute (e.g., right or wrong, moral or immoral) rather than ranging along a continuum that includes degrees of right and wrong. Personal life and community affairs are based on principles of right and wrong rather than on shame, dishonor, or ridicule, and there is an emphasis on youthfulness (Arensberg & Niehoff, 1975).

Many Americans, especially middle-class Americans, share these traits and values to some degree. The degree may depend in great part on the microcultures of which an individual is a member. The degree may also depend on how much an individual must interact with our formal institutions for economic support and subsistence. The more dependence on formal institutions, the greater the degree of sharing the common traits and values of the United States.

Microcultures in the United States

Subsocieties within the United States contain cultural elements, institutions, and groups in which cultural patterns not common to the U.S. microculture are shared. Traditionally, these groups have been called subsocieties or subcultures by sociologists and anthropologists because they exist within the context of a larger society and share political and social institutions as well as some of the traits and values of the macroculture. These cultural groups are also called microcultures to indicate that they have distinctive cultural patterns while sharing some cultural patterns with all members of the U.S. macroculture. People who belong to the same microcultures share traits and values that bind them together as a group.

Numerous microcultures exist in most nations, but the United States is exceptionally rich in the many distinct cultural groups that make up the population. Cultural identity is based on traits and values learned as part of our ethnic origin, religion, gender, age, socioeconomic level, primary language, geographical region, place of residence (e.g., rural or urban), and handicapping or exceptional conditions, as shown in Figure 1–1. Each of these groups has distinct cultural patterns shared with others who identify themselves as members of that particular group. Although sharing certain characteristics of the macroculture with most of the U.S. population, members of these various microcultures also have learned cultural traits, discourse patterns, ways of learning, values, and behaviors characteristic of the microcultures to which they belong. Unless a person is a member of the dominant group (i.e., a white, middle-class, nondisabled male), the cultural content of that person's learned experiences will be different from the cultural content of the schools. Radical critics of education argue that

> the dominant culture in the school is characterized by a selective ordering and legitimating of privileged language forms, modes of reasoning, social relations, and lived experiences. . . . School culture . . . functions not only to confirm and privilege students from the dominant classes, but also through exclusion and insult to disconfirm the histories, experiences, and dreams of subordinate groups. (Giroux, 1988, pp. xxx–xxxi)

A member of the macroculture is also a member of many microcultures. Individuals sharing one microculture may not share other microcultures. For example, all men are members of the male microculture, but not all males belong to the same ethnic, religious, or socioeconomic group. On the other hand, an ethnic group is com-

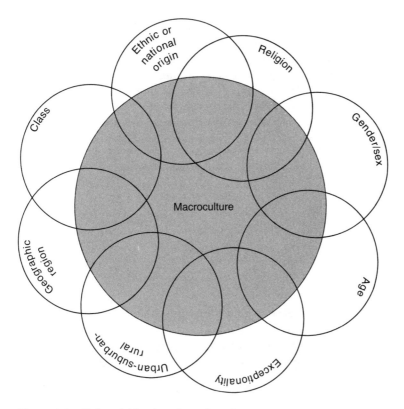

Figure 1-1   Cultural identity of an American

posed of both males and females with different religious and socioeconomic backgrounds.

The interaction of these various microcultures within the macroculture begins to determine an individual's cultural identity. Membership in one microculture often greatly influences the characteristics and values of membership in other microcultures. For instance, some fundamentalist religions have strictly defined expectations for women and men. Thus, membership in the religious group influences to a great extent the way a female behaves as a young girl, teenager, bride, and wife. One's socioeconomic level will impact greatly on the quality of life for families, especially for children and the elderly in that group. The cultural patterns of an ethnic or religious group often influence one's behavior in the other microcultures of which one is a member.

This interaction is most dynamic across race, class, and gender relations. Hicks (1981) has found that "individuals (or groups) in their relation to their economic and political systems do not share similar consciousness or similar needs at the same point in time" (p. 221). The feminist movement, for example, has been influenced primarily by white, middle-class women. The labor movement had an early history of excluding minorities, women, and their causes; in some areas this antagonism continues. Membership in one microculture often conflicts with the interests of another.

One microculture may have a greater influence on an individual than others. For example, one middle-class, Catholic, Italian-American, thirty-year-old woman in New York City may identify more strongly with being Catholic and Italian-American than with the other microcultures to which she belongs. Another woman who belongs to the same microcultures may identify more strongly with her female microculture than with the others. The degree that individuals identify with the various microcultures to which they belong and share their common cultural characteristics determines to a great extent their individual cultural identities, as illustrated in Figure 1–2.

The interaction of these microcultures within the macroculture is also very important. Most political, business, educational, and social institutions (e.g., the courts, the welfare system, and the city government) have been developed and controlled by the dominant group. The values and practices that have been internalized by the dominant group also are inherent within these institutions. Subordinate or minority groups are usually beholden to the dominant group to share in that power. These groups "possess imperfect access to positions of equal power, prestige, and privilege in a society" (Yetman, 1985, p. 2).

Members of subordinate groups are affected by the status accorded them by the dominant group. "Different ways of thinking and behaving become differentially

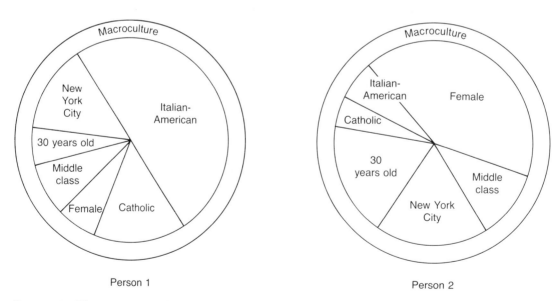

Figure 1–2 The importance of one's microcultural memberships varies from individual to individual and from microculture to microculture. The interaction of membership in these microcultures helps determine our own individual cultural identity.

rewarded in the society at large, and membership in particular racial, ethnic, class, and gender groups has traditionally entailed the ascription of particular roles and statuses within a broader system of relations" (Lubeck, 1988, p. 55). African-Americans, Hispanics, Asian-Americans, and other racially distinguished groups generally experience institutional discrimination and are not allowed to share equally in societal benefits. Women, non-Protestants, the poor, non–English speakers, the handicapped, children, and the elderly also are not able to share equally in power and societal benefits with the dominant group. This relationship with the dominant group can impact greatly on one's own cultural identity.

Thus, the interaction of these microcultures within the macroculture begins to answer the questions, Who am I? and Who are my students? The various microcultures that educators are likely to confront in a classroom will be examined in detail in Chapters 2 through 8.

Multiculturalism

Individuals who have competencies in and can operate successfully in two or more different cultures are *bicultural* or *multicultural.* Biculturalism and multiculturalism are "states in which one has mastered the knowledge and developed the skills necessary to feel comfortable and communicate effectively (1) with people of the culture encountered and (2) in any situation involving groups of people of diverse cultural backgrounds" (Hoopes, 1979, p. 21). Often individuals are multilingual as well as multicultural. Having proficiencies in multiple cultures does not lead to rejection of the primary cultural identification. It does allow a broad range of abilities on which one can draw at any given occasion as determined by the particular situation (Gibson, 1976).

Goodenough (1987) defines multiculturalism as the *normal human experience.* All Americans participate in more than one cultural group or microculture, as described earlier. Thus, most persons have already become proficient in multiple systems for perceiving, evaluating, believing, and acting according to the patterns of the various microcultures in which they participate. Individuals with competencies in several microcultures develop a fuller appreciation of the range of cultural competencies available to all individuals. Banks (1988) has suggested that multiethnic and multicultural education programs can help students expand their cultural competencies to include those required to function effectively in microcultures in which they are not members.

PLURALISM

There are a number of theories describing the pluralistic nature of the United States. The most prevailing theory espoused by sociologists, politicians, and educators has been *assimilation.* A second popular theory is that of *cultural pluralism,* in which cultural groups, particularly ethnic groups, maintain separate and distinct identities from the dominant group. This section will include a discussion of these two theories and an ideology that bridges the two.

Assimilation

Assimilation is the process by which subordinate groups adopt the dominant culture. Either cultural patterns that distinguished the subordinate from the dominant group have disappeared, or their distinctive cultural patterns have become part of the dominant culture, or a combination of the two has occurred. In the United States, the middle-class microculture reflects this process. In fact, the values and traits of this cultural group are often defined as the national culture or macroculture. As indicated in the previous section, however, many of the values and traits of the dominant middle-class microculture are not universally accepted by all members of the macroculture.

According to Gordon (1964), the assimilation process should develop through stages in which the new cultural group would (1) change its cultural patterns to those of the dominant group; (2) develop large-scale primary-group relationships with the dominant group; (3) intermarry fully with the dominant group; (4) lose its sense of peoplehood as separate from the dominant group; (5) encounter no discrimination; (6) encounter no prejudiced attitudes; and (7) not raise any issues that would involve value and power conflict with the dominant group. Each of these stages also represents a degree of assimilation. *Cultural* or *behavioral assimilation* is the first stage in which the new cultural group has continuous and first-hand contact with the dominant cultural group with subsequent changes in the original cultural patterns of either or both groups. *Structural assimilation* has occurred when the two groups share primary-group relationships that would include membership in the same cliques or social clubs.

In his examination of the degree of assimilation of several cultural groups in the United States, Gordon (1964) found that only limited structural assimilation had occurred for any of the groups except white Protestant immigrants from northern and western Europe. He found that *acculturation* (i.e., cultural assimilation in which cultural patterns of the dominant group have been adopted by the subordinate group) had occurred for most groups that had been here for at least one generation and was proceeding for first-generation immigrants. However, this acculturation success had neither eliminated prejudice and discrimination nor led to large-scale intermarriage with the dominant cultural group. The rapidity and success of the acculturation process depends on several factors, including location and discrimination. If a minority group is spatially isolated and segregated (whether voluntarily or not) in a rural area, as is the case with the American Indians still on reservations, the acculturation process will be very slow. Unusually marked discrimination, such as that faced by minority groups, especially African- and Mexican-Americans, deprives vast numbers of the minority group of educational and occupational opportunities and may retard indefinitely the acculturation process for the group (Gordon, 1964). Twenty-six years after Gordon's study, the amount of structural assimilation remains about the same.

It is important to note that cultural assimilation, or acculturation, is determined in part by the individual. That is, the individual can decide how much he or she wants to dress, speak, and behave like members of the dominant group. However, the extent of structural assimilation is determined by the dominant group. Those in power determine the extent of access that will be permitted at different periods.

If the assimilation process is effective, it leads to the disappearance of a cultural group that is distinct from the dominant culture. Thus, structural assimilation rather than acculturation is the key to complete assimilation. Two different theories of assimilation have been developed to describe the United States: Anglo-conformity and the melting pot.

Anglo-Conformity Theory.   "The 'Anglo-conformity' theory demanded the complete renunciation of the immigrant's ancestral culture in favor of the behavior and values of the Anglo-Saxon core group" (Gordon, 1964, p. 85). The central assumption in this theory is the "desirability of maintaining English institutions (as modified by the American Revolution), the English language, and English-oriented cultural patterns as dominant and standard in American life" (Gordon, 1964, p. 88). This ideology has received the most consistent support in federal policies throughout U.S. history. Through the public schools, television, and other mass communication, most children of immigrants have been thoroughly acculturated into the American macroculture, which has been influenced primarily by WASPs. Exceptions include the visible minority groups, for whom prejudice and discrimination have retarded the acculturation process. Nevertheless, even members of these groups have been expected to conform to the Anglo traditions and culture in order to move into the middle class.

Thus, members of immigrant and colonized groups were acculturated, either voluntarily or forcibly, through the Anglo-conformity process. However, acculturation did not ensure the next stage of assimilation—structural assimilation. Gordon (1964) reported that primary-group contacts have been maintained within the individual cultural groups rather than across cultural groups as required in structural assimilation. Cross-cultural contacts appear to occur "in considerable part only at the secondary group level of employment and the political and civic processes" (p. 111).

Melting Pot Theory.   Another popular assimilation theory, the melting pot, or amalgamation, was more generous and appealing to the immigrant population. It predicted the evolution of a new, unique American culture to which all cultural groups would contribute. Early this century, an English Jewish writer with strong social convictions, Israel Zangwill, captured this ideal in his drama, *The Melting Pot*. The protagonist, David Quixano, was a Russian Jewish immigrant who was composing a symphony to express his belief that America was a "divinely inspired crucible in which all the ethnic divisions of mankind will divest themselves of their ancient animosities and differences and become fused into one group signifying the brotherhood of man" (Gordon, 1964, p. 120).

Although some very light-skinned African-Americans "passed" into the white group and interracial marriages have occurred, the numbers have been, and remain, very small. Sociologists who have described the successful amalgamation of African-Americans have focused on their intermarriages with mulattoes, and the projections have fallen far short of amalgamation (Williamson, 1980). Until 1967, African-Americans, Hispanics, Asian-Americans, and American Indians were prevented by miscegenation laws in many states from intermarrying with persons of European descent. They were not expected to melt.

Although many cultural groups have made tremendous contributions to American civilization, the cultural patterns from the various groups have not melted with the patterns of the native WASPs. Instead, the specific cultural contributions of other groups have been transformed into the dominant core culture. The United States may be composed of a number of separate melting pots. One of those may be based on religious divisions within which whites have melted. Another may include racial groups who are not allowed to melt structurally. Still others may include certain ethnic communities composed primarily of the first generation or those that choose to remain within ethnic enclaves (Gordon, 1964).

Most writers today no longer think that either of the assimilation theories characterizes the contemporary U.S. scene. Nevertheless, the impact of these theories has been felt, and often remains, in political, social, and educational policies and practices.

Cultural Pluralism

Refusing, or not being permitted, to assimilate into the dominant American culture, many immigrants and visible minority groups maintained ethnic communities and enclaves. They developed within-group institutions, agencies, and power structures for services within their ethnic communities. These communities included Little Italy, Chinatown, Harlem, and East Los Angeles.

As early as 1915, a few philosophers and writers began to question the validity of assimilation theories. They described a nation in which the various ethnic groups would preserve their identities and cultures within an American culture (Gordon, 1964). The classic statement of the cultural pluralist position was written by Horace Kallen and appeared in *The Nation* in early 1915. He rejected both the Anglo-conformity and melting pot theories as useless in describing what was occurring or in providing worthy ideals for the future.

Kallen's cultural pluralism was based on a philosophical examination of the past and on three propositions: (1) No one chooses his or her ancestry; (2) each minority culture has something positive to contribute to American society; and (3) the idea of democracy and equality carries an implicit assumption that there are differences between individuals and groups that can be viewed as "equal" (Newman, 1973). One of the criticisms of Kallen's model was that his emphasis on an individual's ethnic membership fails to allow the individual a choice of participation.

Today's advocates of cultural pluralism often call for the maintenance of "enough subsocietal separation to guarantee the continuance of the ethnic cultural tradition and the existence of the group, without at the same time interfering with the carrying out of standard responsibilities to the general American civic life" (Gordon, 1964, p. 158). To implement this strategy effectively requires minimizing primary-group contacts across cultural groups "while cooperating with other groups and individuals in the secondary relations areas of political action, economic life, and civic responsibility" (Gordon, 1964, p. 158). However, there is some disagreement about the degree to which this implementation strategy should be employed and whether an "individual should be allowed to choose freely whether to remain within the confines of his birthright community enclave" (Pratte, 1979, p. 142).

Pratte (1979) identifies stringent criteria for the application of cultural pluralism to a society. He suggests that it applies only when

1. cultural diversity, in the form of a number of groups—be they political, racial, ethnic, religious, economic, or age—is exhibited in the society
2. the coexisting groups approximate equal political, economic, and educational opportunity
3. there is a behavioral commitment to the values of cultural pluralism as a basis for a viable system of social organization (p. 141)

Most observers of U.S. society would agree that the condition of cultural diversity is met. Data on the income inequities that exist between men and women or between blacks and whites indicate that the condition for relative parity and equality between groups is not met. The commitment to or perceived values of cultural pluralism appears not to be supported broadly by various individuals and groups in society, as documented by legislation and attacks from the political right over the past few years. Further, the values that undergird cultural pluralism may not be subscribed to in a behavioral sense by a majority of Americans.

Many educational writers today have not applied Pratte's criteria to determining the existence of cultural pluralism. They emphasize the existence of ethnic and cultural diversity in the United States and the right of individuals to maintain their ethnic identity while sharing a common culture with Americans from many different national backgrounds.

The Ideology of Voluntary Cultural Choice

Neither of the two preceding theories seem to adequately address the cultural diversity that exists in this country or the ideal that might be desirable. While many of the advocates of cultural pluralism have treated pluralism and democracy as complements, critics have charged that it does not meet one of the key democratic values—that of calling for free choice for individuals as well as groups. For instance, Patterson (1977) believes that pluralism tends to see individuals in need of group and cultural indentity, that it promotes ethnicity and parochialism, and that it views individuals in terms of their ethnicity rather than as unique, autonomous persons. Further, he worries that by drawing attention to and giving credibility to cultural distinctions, pluralism sharpens racial conflict, prejudice, and discrimination.

Within the concept of democracy and pluralism, there are two distinct aspects. One is the right of individuals to choose

whether to remain within the boundaries of communality created by his [her] birthright ethnic group, to branch out into multiple interethnic contacts, or even to change affiliation to that of another ethnic group should he [she] wish to do so as a result of religious conversion, intermarriage, or simply private wish. (Gordon, 1964, p. 263)

The second aspect is the freedom for diverse social-cultural groups to form and flourish free from the oppression of other groups (Appleton, 1983).

This ideology of voluntary cultural choice is implied by Newman (1973) in his sociological examination of American pluralism. He states that "the essential meaning of social pluralism is choice both for the society and for the groups and individuals in the society. The challenge is to create a social environment in which groups and individuals may choose voluntarily the identities they wish to play out" (p. 292). This ideology would allow the individual to choose the importance of her or his ascribed statuses such as gender, ethnicity, and age in determining who they are. In U.S. society, however, visible minority group members may become totally acculturated, but may not be allowed to structurally assimilate by the majority group, no matter how much the minority individual desires to assimilate. On the other hand, many minority group members, as well as some members of white ethnic groups, choose to preserve and maintain their cultural identity and to develop that identity for individual and group advantages.

As individual choice and mobility across cultural groups increases, social and cultural barriers are likely to decrease. Increasingly, we will move toward an open society in which cultural background may influence who an individual is, but become irrelevant in public interactions, especially as the reason for institutional discrimination.

EQUALITY IN THE UNITED STATES

The single theory of cultural pluralism does not adequately support the goals of multicultural education. Too often it overlooks the social realities of race, gender, and class inequalities. When the emphasis of cultural pluralism is on culture rather than just ethnicity, it comes closer to dealing with the impact of one's race, sex, socioeconomic status, age, geographical region, and physical and mental abilities on one's participation in society's benefits. Even though egalitarianism is an often espoused goal of democracy in this country, the inequities that actually exist in society are continually overlooked. Thus, equality must be an essential tenet of multicultural education.

Traditionally, minority groups and women have been recipients of institutional discrimination. As a result, they often exhibit anger at, dissatisfaction with, and alienation from the system. Racism, sexism, and class inequality characterize societies in which there are great disparities of income, wealth, and power. Competition over scarce resources increases conflicts between the various groups. Thus, fundamental changes in the structure of society must accompany changes in attitudes if voluntary cultural choice is to become a reality. Addressing the issue of equality is a key to such changes.

Webster's dictionary (1983) defines equity as "justice; impartiality; the giving or desiring to give to each man his due" and defines equality as "the state of being equal; likeness in magnitude or dimensions, values, qualities, degree, and the like; the state of being neither superior nor inferior." Equity is set in the context of jurisprudence and does not guarantee equality. The meaning of equality within our society varies according to one's assumptions about humankind and human existence. At least two sets of beliefs govern the ideologies of equality and inequality. The first accepts inequality as inevitable and promotes meritocracy. It stresses the right of access to society's resources as a necessary condition for equal rights to life, liberty, and happiness. The focus is on individualism and the individual's right to pursue happiness and obtain personal resources. The second set of beliefs is optimistic that a much greater degree of equality in society can be obtained and ought to be sought than exists today.

Individualism and Meritocracy

Schools and the mass media teach that the United States was founded by persons dedicated to building a nation and a society for the good of all its citizens. A constitution was fashioned with a coherent set of "checks and balances," making the systematic abuse of power virtually impossible. The principles of egalitarianism that are so widely praised suggest that while the United States is a nation of many different ethnic, regional, social, and economic groups, every group has a voice and no one group forever dominates the economic, political, social, and cultural life of the country. Finally, society and government, while not perfect, are promoted as allowing mass participation and steady advancement toward a more prosperous multicultural, egalitarian society.

It is generally accepted that different socioeconomic levels exist in society. In fact, inequalities must exist. Proponents of this ideology accept the theories of sociobiology and/or functionalism, in which inequalities are viewed as natural outcomes of individual differences. Deprived groups usually are seen as inferior, and their hardships are blamed on their personal characteristics.

A society based on meritocracy ensures that the ablest and most meritorious, ambitious, hardworking, and talented individuals will acquire the most, achieve the most, and become society's leaders (Ryan, 1981). The resulting inequalities are tolerable, fair, and just. They are viewed as a necessary consequence of equality of opportunity and roughly in proportion to inequalities of merit.

The belief system that undergirds meritocracy has at least three dimensions (Ryan, 1981). First, the individual is valued over the group. It is the individual who has the qualities, ambitions, and talent to achieve at the highest levels in society. Popular stories expound this ideology as they describe the poor immigrant who arrived on our shores with nothing, set up a vegetable stand to eke out a living, and became a millionaire owner of a chain grocery store.

The second dimension stresses differences rather than similarities between individuals. IQ and achievement tests are used throughout one's schooling to help measure those differences. Students and adults are rewarded for outstanding grades, athletic ability, and artistic accomplishment. The third dimension emphasizes internal characteristics such as motivation, intuition, and character that have been internalized by the individual. External conditions, such as racism and poverty, are to be overcome by the individual; they are not accepted as the reason for an individual not to succeed.

Both individualism and equality have long been central themes of American demagogues. The problem, of course, is that the two are not complementary. Meritocracy places the individual as supreme. Individuals should have the right to pursue happiness and obtain as many resources as their ability will allow. "In liberal societies people generally get what they deserve, or if they don't they should, and that's all they should get; and what they deserve is purely and simply a consequence of their own individual character and actions, nothing else" (Green, 1981, p. 167).

This dilemma forces supporters to promote, on the one hand, some equality while preventing any real equality from occurring. Affirmative action, for example, is viewed as evidence of group welfare gaining precedence over individual achievement. Glazer (1975) warns that "this new course threatens the abandonment of our concern for individual claims to consideration on the basis of justice and equity, now to be replaced with a concern for rights for publicly determined and delimited racial and ethnic groups" (p. 197). The outcry against reverse discrimination suggests that racism no longer exists and that decisions about employment, promotion, and so forth, are no longer influenced by racism (Dreyfuss & Lawrence, 1979).

In a system of meritocracy, equality is to be achieved through equality of opportunity rather than equality of results. "The ideology of the open or equal-opportunity society holds that individuals may obtain social position and social rewards on the basis of merit: mental ability, ambition and motivation, diligent study, hard work, or loyal performance on the job" (Matras, 1984, p. 215). However, Jencks et al. (1972) found that "neither genetic inequality nor disparities in family background dictate anything like the degree of economic inequality now found in American society" (p. 262).

Family background was found to account for a large part of the variation in educational and occupational attainment (Jencks et al., 1972). Thus, the opportunity to achieve equally is thwarted before one is born. Individuals born into a wealthy family are likely to achieve wealth; individuals born into a poor family will have difficulty in achieving wealth no matter how hard they work. Nevertheless, this ideology places the onus of responsibility on the individual alone, even though inequalities that exist in society most commonly lead to the perpetuation of inequalities in families.

Equal educational opportunity, or equal access to schooling, applies this principle to education. All students are to be provided equal educational opportunities that supposedly will give them similar chances for success or failure. Proponents of this approach believe that it is the individual's responsibility to use those opportunities to his or her advantage in obtaining life's resources and benefits. Critics find that "equal opportunity provides a rationale for discriminating against those who are poor risks. In the land of equal opportunity, poverty must be due to the deficient character and motivation of those who are poor. Thus, self-interest, social pressure, and ideology combine to perpetuate the victimization of those who are poor risks" (Deutsch, 1985, p. 60).

However, students enter this competition with different advantages and disadvantages from birth. The opportunities available in schools differ greatly from school to school; thus, students receive neither equal resources nor equal treatment. In his study of the national reports on education released in 1983, Shor (1986) found that the themes for careerism, back-to-basics, and excellence justified inequality through testing and language regimes; disguised inequality as excellence; promoted standard English and a core curriculum based on the values of the dominant society (without providing an opportunity to critically analyze that society); discredited bilingual, bidialectical, interdisciplinary, women's, and minority studies; and used licensing exams to screen out minority candidates from the teaching force.

Equality

With the persistence of racism, poverty, unemployment, chronic crisis, and inequality in major social systems such as education and health, many persons have found it difficult to reconcile daily realities with the publicized egalitarianism that characterizes the rhetoric of our nation's leaders. These persons view U.S. society as characterized by economic and noneconomic institutions representing the interests of the privileged few rather than the pluralistic majority. Elections, the two-party system, freedom of speech and assembly, and the other democratic institutions are seldom effective measures against the dominant levers of economic power that is concentrated in the hands of corporate control, which in turn dominates and controls the power of government. Even where institutions, laws, and processes have the appearance of equal access, benefit, and protection, they are almost always enforced in highly discriminatory ways. Finally, these patterns of inequality are not the product of corrupt individuals as such, but a reflection of how resources of economics, political power, and cultural and social dominance are built into the entire politico-economic system.

Even in the optimistic view that some degree of equality can be achieved, inequality is also expected. Not all resources can be redistributed so that every individual would have an equal amount, nor should all individuals expect equal compensation for the work that they do. However, the underlying belief is that there need not be the huge disparities of income, wealth, and power among individuals that currently exists (Ryan, 1981). Deutsch (1985) defines equality as distributive justice that "centers on the *fairness of the distribution* of the conditions and goods that affect individual well-being" (p. 1). Further, he believes that "we need economic policies that will foster full employment and substantially increase the share of the total income that is received by those in the bottom third of the income distribution" (p. 62).

Critics decry the proposed socialism as being against the democratic foundations that undergird the nation. They believe that equality of resources and societal benefits would undermine the capitalist system that allows a few individuals to acquire the great majority of those resources. They warn that equality of results would limit freedom and liberty for individuals. Ryan (1981) counters that "the only freedom threatened by economic equality is the freedom of one individual to oppress and exploit another by virtue of his or her specific talent for oppression or exploitation" (p. 92).

Deutsch (1985) has found that advocates of equality and egalitarianism primarily oppose

> invidious distinctions among people but do not assume that all distinctions are invidious. Invidious distinctions are ones that promote (1) generalized or irrelevant feelings of superiority-inferiority (if I am a better tennis player or more good-looking than you, I am superior to you as a person); (2) generalized or irrelevant status differences (if I am a manager and you are a worker in a factory, I should have a higher standard of living than you); (3) generalized or irrelevant superordinate-subordinate relations (if I am a captain and you are a private, I can order you to shine my shoes); or (4) the view that the legitimate needs and interests of some people are not as important or do not warrant as much consideration as those of other people (this may be because of my sex, race, age, national or family origin, religion, political affiliation, occupation, or physical handicap, or because of special talents or lack of talent). (pp. 41–42)

Further,

> equality does not imply identical treatment of everyone without regard to particular circumstance. . . . The insistence on treating people identically, without regard to circumstance, is a pseudoegalitarianism, which often masks basic doubts or ambivalence about one's commitment to egalitarian values." (Deutsch, 1985, p. 45)

Equality should mean more than just providing subordinate group members an equal chance. One proposal is the equal-results argument that is consistent with an optimistic projection of equality. Arciniega (1979) applied this equal-benefits approach to education. "The equal-benefits view . . . focuses on the distribution of the benefits derived from the system. . . . Equality of results can best be achieved by shifting full responsibility for student success to the school" (pp. 114–115). Equal educational results might be reflected in equal achievement of minority and nonminority populations or in a similarity in the dropout rate, college attendance, and college completion of different ethnic/racial, gender, and class populations. As Bourdieu (1982) explains,

> A rational and really universal pedagogy would take [no cultural capital] for granted initially, would not count as acquired what [cultural knowledge and skills] some, and only some, of the pupils in question had inherited, would do all things for all and would be organized with the explicit aim of providing all with the means of *acquiring* that which, although apparently a natural gift, is only *given* to the children of the educated classes. (p. 391)

Shor (1986) proposes an agenda for educational equality that incudes special funding for bilingual and bidialectical programs; support for students' rights to their own language; an end to tracking students out of the college-bound curriculum and the nonacademic students in general; and students' and teachers' rights to free access to all books, materials, and ideas and unhindered discussions of all subjects. He also recommends open admissions to colleges, free tuition for higher education, vigorous affirmative action in college admissions and faculty hiring, adequate financing of poor schools, raising teachers' salaries, and involvement of students and community in governance.

Traditionally, we have believed that education could help overcome the inequalities that exist in society. However, the role of education in reducing the amount of occupation and income inequality appears to be limited. School reform cannot be expected to bring about significant social changes outside of the schools. Equalizing educational opportunity has very little to do with making adults more equal. Providing equal educational opportunity for all students will not guarantee equal results at the end of a specific number of years in school. Nevertheless, Gintis (1989) believes that "education can play an important role in attacking the roots of inequality" (p. 57). Education does help people "affirm their dignity as human beings and develop the skills and resources to control their lives in the larger society" (p. 57). It also is important that resources for providing quality instruction in environments that are conducive to learning be expended equally.

In her extensive work on the tracking of students, Oakes (1988) concluded that

> evidence of unequal participation and outcomes is, in itself, insufficient to establish schooling inequities as their cause. However, the existence of these discrepancies *does* document that schools have been considerably less successful with *some groups* of students than others. Moreover, such substantially unequal participation and achievement among groups and the significant increases in outcome discrepancies over time in school provide noteworthy signals that schooling factors may contribute to them. (p. 108)

Further,

> considerable evidence suggests that these day-to-day classroom experiences are likely to differ both between schools and between students within the same school. This evidence suggests that the distribution of actual classroom experiences, resources, and opportunities to students with different race, class, and ability characteristics may be an important schooling contribution to unequal outcomes. (p. 117)

To establish equality, major changes in society must take place. This process is very difficult when power is held by those who believe in a meritocratic system. "Its proponents turn their principle into a defense of the status quo, that is, of unequal privileges already won in the past" (Green, 1981, p. 167). On the other hand, the advocates for equality support the dictum, "from each according to his [her] ability, to each according to his [her] needs."

MULTICULTURAL EDUCATION

Multicultural education is not a new concept. It is merely a relatively new name for concepts that have existed since the 1920s, when educators began writing about and training others in intercultural education and ethnic studies. The movement during the first two decades had an international emphasis with antecedents in the pacifist movement. Some textbooks were rewritten with an international point of view. Proponents encouraged teachers to make their disciplines more relevant to the modern world by being more issue oriented. The goal was to make the dominant majority populations more tolerant and accepting toward first- and second-generation immigrants in order to maintain national unity and social control (Montalto, 1978).

In 1933, the Service Bureau for Intercultural Education developed in-service programs and school assemblies to intensify ethnic consciousness for minority and immigrant children. General support for the separate ethnic approach of the early Service Bureau was limited (Montalto, 1978). By 1947, the emphasis in intercultural education was on prejudice and discrimination.

During the remainder of that decade and into the sixties, organizational support for intercultural education and intergroup relations waned. Although individual teachers and professors probably continued to incorporate these concepts into their courses and programs, such ideas were not institutionalized in most schools and universities.

In the 1960s, desegregation was being enforced in the nation's schools. At the same time, students of color were being described as culturally deprived of the background required to attend schools based on the cultural content of the dominant society. Programs like Head Start and compensatory education and special education were developed to compensate for these shortcomings. Not surprisingly, those classes were filled with students of color, in poverty, or with disabilities. Soon these groups were described as *culturally different* to acknowledge that these students came from different cultural backgrounds but that those cultures were not deficient. The goal of the approach to teach the exceptional and culturally different was to develop the cultural patterns of the dominant society so that they could "fit into the mainstream of American society" (Sleeter & Grant, 1988, p. 37).

The civil rights movement brought a renewed interest in ethnic studies, discrimination, and intergroup relations. Racial and ethnic pride emerged from subordinate groups, creating a demand for African-American and other ethnic studies programs in colleges and universities across the country. Later, similar programs were established in secondary schools.

Students and participants in ethnic studies programs of the 1960s and early 1970s were primarily members of the group being studied. Programs focused on the various ethnic histories and cultures, with the main objectives of providing students with insight and instilling pride in their own racial/ethnic backgrounds. Most of these programs were ethnic-specific: Only one ethnic group was studied. Sometimes the objectives included an understanding of the relationship and conflict between the ethnic group and the dominant or majority population, but seldom was a program's scope multiethnic.

Concurrent with the civil rights movement and growth of ethnic studies, emphasis on intergroup or human relations again emerged. Often these programs accompanied ethnic studies content for teachers. The objectives were again to promote intergroup, and especially interracial, understanding and to reduce or eliminate stereotypes. This approach emphasized the affective level—attitudes and feelings about themselves and others (Sleeter & Grant, 1988).

With the growth and development of ethnic studies came a realization that those programs alone would not guarantee support for the promotion of cultural diversity in this country. Students from the dominant culture also needed to learn about the history, culture, and contributions of subordinate groups. Thus, ethnic studies expanded into multiethnic studies. Teachers were encouraged to develop curricula that included the contributions of subordinate groups along with those of the dominant group. Textbooks were to be rewritten to represent more accurately the multiethnic nature of the United States. Students were to be exposed to perspectives of subordinate groups through literature, history, music, and other disciplines integrated throughout the regular school program.

As part of the civil rights movement, other groups that had suffered from institutional discrimination called their needs to the attention of the public. These groups included the poor, the women, the disabled, the bilingual, and the aged. Educators responded by expanding multiethnic education to a more encompassing concept— multicultural education. This broader concept focused on the various microcultures to which individuals belong, with an emphasis on the interaction of membership in those microcultures, especially race, class, and gender.

Still, after six decades of concern for civil and human rights in education, few real changes have occurred in the management of cultural diversity and provision of equality in our schools. Classrooms may be desegregated and mainstreamed, and both boys and girls may now participate in athletic activities, and yet the following gaps still exist between groups in the United States:

☐ Students of color score below white students on national standardized tests.

☐ Beginning at puberty and continuing through adulthood, females do not achieve as well as males in mathematics (Skolnick, Langbort, & Day, 1982).

☐ The income gap between white families and families of color continues to be great. In 1986, the median income of a white family was $30,809; a black family, $17,604 (i.e., 57 percent of a white family's income); and a Hispanic family, $19,995 (i.e., 65 percent of a white family's income) (U.S. Bureau of the Census, 1988).

☐ In 1986, 55 percent of all women over sixteen years of age were in the work force; on an average, a full-time working woman earned 65 cents for every $1 earned by a full-time working man (U.S. Bureau of the Census, 1988).

☐ Whites make up nearly 85 percent of the U.S. population, but they hold 90.8 percent of the managerial/professional jobs; blacks hold 16.9 percent of all service jobs, although they are 12.2 percent of the total population (U.S. Bureau of the Census, 1988).

☐ The percentage of the population below the poverty level increased from 11.4 percent in 1978 to 13.6 percent in 1986, with 31.1 percent of black families and 27.39 percent of Hispanic families below the poverty level. In 1986, 34.2 percent of families headed by a single mother were in poverty. In 1986, one-fifth of all children under eighteen years old lived in families below the poverty level. (U.S. Bureau of the Census, 1988).

☐ The National Coalition for the Homeless estimated that in 1988, there were between 500,00 and 750,000 school-age homeless children in this country and that only about 43 percent of them attended school regularly.

The United States is a multicultural nation where cultural diversity continues to increase and members of subordinate groups do not share equally in sociopolitical power. The women's movement, the Gray Panthers, and coalitions for mainstreaming the disabled into society have influenced federal funding and public concern for additional civil rights groups. The size of the minority population is increasing. Shortly after the year 2000, one-third of the population will be people of color (Hodgkinson, 1986). While immigrants early in this century were primarily from Europe, 80 percent of the current immigrants are equally from South America and Asia. Because these groups "have less power to shape the terms of classroom interaction means that their likelihood of school success is reduced and the prospects of alienation and lowered aspirations are increased" (O'Connor, 1988, p. 2).

In a country that champions equal rights and the opportunity for an individual to improve his or her conditions, we must be concerned with helping all students achieve academically, socially, and politically. After conducting a major study of the American high school, the president of the Carnegie Foundation stated that "Opportunity remains unequal. And this failure to educate *every* young person to his or her full potential threatens the nation's social and economic health" (Boyer, 1983, p. 5). It will no longer be possible to teach all students in the classroom equally, because they are not the same. They have different needs and skills that must be recognized in developing educational programs. Each student is different because of physical and mental abilities, sex, ethnicity or national origin, religion, socioeconomic level, and age. Students behave differently in school and toward authority because of cultural factors and their relationship to the dominant society. As educators, we behave certain ways toward students because of our own cultural experiences within the power structure of the country.

When educators are given the responsibilities of a classroom, they need the knowledge and skills for working effectively in our culturally diverse society. An educational concept that addresses cultural diversity and equality in schools is multicultural education. This concept is based on the following fundamental beliefs and assumptions:

☐ The U.S. culture has been fashioned by the contributions of many diverse cultural groups into an interrelated whole.

☐ Cultural diversity and the interaction among different groups strengthen the fiber of U.S. society.

☐ Social justice and equal opportunity for all people are inalienable rights of all citizens.

☐ Power should be distributed equitably among members of all ethnic groups.

☐ The education system provides the critical function of molding attitudes and values necessary for continuation of a democratic society.

☐ Teachers and other professional educators must assume a leadership role in creating an environment that is supportive of multiculturalism. (Bidol, Baptiste, Baptiste, Holmes, & Ramierz, 1977)

Regardless of the level of formal schooling, multicultural education should permeate the total school environment. It is directed to all students, those from dominant and subordinate groups alike. The goals of multicultural education are:

1. To promote the strength and value of cultural diversity

2. To promote human rights and respect for those who are different from oneself

3. To promote alternative life choices for people

4. To promote social justice and equality for all people

5. To promote equity in the distribution of power and income among groups

Several concepts undergird multicultural education. Concepts that describe the relationships and interactions among individuals and groups are essential to understanding and working effectively with different cultural groups. These concepts include an understanding of racism, sexism, prejudice, discrimination, oppression, powerlessness, power, inequality, equality, and stereotypes. Multicultural education includes various components that often manifest themselves in courses, units of courses, or degree programs. These components include ethnic studies, minority studies, bilingual education, women's studies, human relations, values clarification, special education, and urban education.

For multicultural education to become a reality in the formal school situation, the total environment must reflect a commitment to multicultural education. Sleeter and Grant (1988) refer to this commitment as "education that is multicultural"—a goal that all schools should be striving to reach. What would be the characteristics of a school that is multicultural? The composition of the faculty, administration, and staff would accurately reflect the pluralistic nature of the United States. The academic achievement levels of students would increase, and differences would disappear between males and females, dominant and subordinate group members, and classes. The school curriculum would be unbiased and would incorporate the contributions of all cultural groups. Instructional materials would be free of biases, omissions, and stereotypes. Cultural differences would be treated as differences rather than deficiencies that must be addressed in compensatory programs. Students would be able to use their own cultural resources and voices to develop new skills and critically explore the subject matter. Students would learn "to take risks, to struggle with ongoing relations of power, to critically appropriate forms of knowlege that exist outside of their immediate experience, and to envisage versions of a world which is 'not yet'—in order to be able to alter the grounds upon which life is lived" (Simon, 1989, p. 140). The faculty, administrators, and staff would see themselves as learners enhanced and changed by understanding, appreciating, and reflecting cultural diversity. Teachers and administrators would be able to deal with questions of race and intergroup relations and controversial realities on an objective, frank, and professional basis.

As educators, we face a tremendous challenge in the next decade to effectively teach all students. Every subject area can be taught to reflect the reality of cultural differences in this nation. Skills to function effectively in different cultural settings can also be taught. For students to function effectively in a democratic society, they must learn about the inequities that currently exist. As teachers, counselors, and principals throughout the remainder of this century, we will serve as the transmitters of our culture to children and youth. It is hoped that we will have the courage to try new methods and techniques, the courage to challenge ineffective procedures and policies, and the strength to change schools to ensure better learning and equity for all students.

SUMMARY

Culture provides the blueprint that determines the way an individual thinks, feels, and behaves in society. We are not born with culture, but learn it through enculturation and socialization. It is manifested through societal institutions, daily habits of living, and the individual's fulfillment of psychological and basic needs.

The U.S. macroculture is the "universal" or national culture that is shared by most of the nation's citizens. Historically, U.S. political and social institutions have developed from a western European tradition and still function under the strong influence of that tradition. Nevertheless, many other aspects of American life have been greatly influenced by the numerous cultural groups that make up the U.S. population.

In addition to participating in the macroculture, individuals belong to a number of microcultures with cultural patterns that may not be common to the macroculture. Cultural identity comes from traits and values learned through membership in microcultures based on national or ethnic origin, religion, gender, age, socioeconomic level, primary language, geographical region, place of residence (e.g., rural or urban), and handicapping or exceptional conditions. The interaction of these various microcultures within the macroculture and dominant society begins to determine an individual's cultural identity. Membership in one microculture often greatly influences characteristics and values of other microcultures, especially of race, gender, and class.

Assimilation, the process by which microcultures adopt the macroculture, has been the most prevailing theory used to describe the nature of pluralism in the United States. Two theories have been espoused during this century to describe the process and degree of assimilation: Anglo-conformity and the melting pot. The theory of cultural pluralism describes the distinct differences among cultural groups and promotes the maintenance of those differences. However, the ideal of voluntary cultural choice may better describe the direction in which we would like to move. This ideal allows individuals to maintain their cultural identity or develop new ones.

Multicultural education is an educational concept that addresses cultural diversity and the provision of equality in schools. For it to become a reality in the formal school situation, the total environment must reflect a commitment to multicultural education. The cultural backgrounds of students are as important in developing effective instructional strategies as are their physical and mental capabilities. Educators need to understand the cultural backgrounds and use those cultural advantages to develop effective instructional strategies. They also must understand the influence of racism, sexism, and classism on the lives of their students.

QUESTIONS FOR REVIEW

1. What is culture? How is culture determined?

2. What are the differences between the U.S. macroculture and microcultures? Give examples of microcultural memberships that have greatly influenced your life.

3. What are the three most prominent theories that have been used to describe pluralism in the United States during this century? What are the weaknesses of the theory of cultural pluralism in describing society today? How does the ideal of voluntary cultural choice differ from cultural pluralism?

4. What are the differences between dominant and subordinate cultural groups?

5. How are meritocracy and individualism in conflict with the ideal of equality?

6. How is multicultural education more than an addition to the curriculum used in schools? How does it differ from multiethnic studies and intercultural education?

7. What is the danger of stereotyping students based on their membership in only one microculture?

8. Why is multicultural education essential to "good" education for all students?

REFERENCES

Appleton, N. (1983). *Cultural pluralism in education: Theoretical foundations.* New York: Longman.

Arciniega, T. (1979). The challenge of multicultural education for teacher educators. In N. Colangelo, C. H. Foxley, & D. Dustin (Eds.), *Multicultural nonsexist education* (pp. 112–130). Dubuque, IA: Kendall/Hunt.

Arensberg, C. M., & Niehoff, A. H. (1975). American cultural values. In J. P. Spradley & M. A. Rynkiewich (Eds.), *The nacirema: Readings on American culture* (pp. 363–378). Boston: Little, Brown.

Banks, J. A. (1988). *Multiethnic education: Theory and practice* (2nd ed.). Boston: Allyn and Bacon.

Bellah, R. N., Madsen, R., Sullivan, W. M., Swidler, A., Tipton, S. M. (1985). *Habits of the heart: Individualism and commitment in American life.* New York: Harper & Row.

Bidol, P., Baptiste, H. P., Baptiste, M. L., Holmes, E. A., & Ramierz, M., III. (1977). *Incorporating a multicultural perspective: NCATE's revised standards for curriculum.* Unpublished manuscript, American Association of Colleges for Teacher Education, Washington, DC.

Bourdieu, P. (1982). The school as a conservative force. In E. Bredo & W. Feinberg (Eds.), *Knowledge and values in social and educational research.* Philadelphia: Temple University Press.

Boyer, E. L. (1983). *High school: A report on secondary education in America.* New York: Harper & Row.

Deutsch, M. (1985). *Distributive justice: A social-psychological perspective.* New Haven, CT: Yale University Press.

Dreyfuss, J., & Lawrence, C., III. (1979). *The Bakke case: The politics of inequality.* New York: Harcourt Brace Jovanovich.

Gibson, M. A. (1976, November). Approaches to multicultural education in the United States: Some concepts and assumptions. *Anthropology and Education Quarterly, 7,* 7–18.

Gintis, H. (1989). Education, personal development, and human dignity. In H. Holtz, I. Marcus, J. Dougherty, J. Michaels, & R. Peduzzi, *Education and the American Dream: Conservatives, liberals and radicals debate the future of education* (pp. 50–60). Granby, MA: Bergin & Garvey.

Giroux, H. A. (1988). *Teachers as intellectuals: Toward a critical pedagogy of learning.* Granby, MA: Bergin & Garvey.

Giroux, H. A. (1989). Introduction: Education, politics, and ideology. In H. Holtz, I. Marcus, J. Dougherty, J. Michaels, & R. Peduzzi (Eds.), *Education and the American Dream: Conservatives, liberals and radicals debate the future of education* (pp. 1–17). Granby, MA: Bergin & Garvey.

Glazer, N. (1975). *Affirmative discrimination: Ethnic inequality and public policy.* New York: Basic Books.

Goodenough, W. (1987). Multi-culturalism as the normal human experience. In E. M. Eddy & W. L. Partridge (Eds.), *Applied anthropology in America* (2nd ed.). New York: Columbia University Press.

Gordon, M. M. (1964). *Assimilation in American life: The role of race, religion, and national origins.* New York: Oxford University Press.

Green, P. (1981). *The pursuit of inequality.* New York: Pantheon Books.

Hall, E. T. (1977). *Beyond culture.* Garden City, NY: Anchor Press.

Hicks, E. (1981). Cultural Marxism: Nonsynchrony and feminist practice. In L. Sargent (Ed.), *Women and revolution.* Boston: South End Press.

Hodgkinson, H. (1986). *The schools we need for the kids we've got.* Paper presented at the 1987 annual meeting of the American Association of Colleges for Teacher Education, Washington, DC.

Hoopes, D. S. (1979). Intercultural communication concepts and the psychology of intercultural experience. In M. D. Pusch (Ed.), *Multicultural education: A cross-cultural training approach* (pp. 9–38). LaGrange Park, IL: Intercultural Network.

Hsu, F. L. K. (1975). American core value and national character. In J. P. Spradley & M. A. Rynkiewich (Eds.), *The nacirema: Readings on American culture* (pp. 378–394). Boston: Little, Brown.

Jencks, C., Smith, M., Acland, H., Bane, M. J., Cohen, D., Gintis, H., Heyns, B., & Michelson, S. (1972). *Inequality: A reassessment of the effect of family and schooling in America.* New York: Harper & Row.

Kluckhohn, C. (1949). *Mirror for man: The relation of anthropology to modern life.* New York: McGraw-Hill.

LeVine, R. A. (1984). Properties of culture: An ethnographic view. In R. A. Shweder and R. A. LeVine, *Culture theory: Essays on mind, self, and emotion* (pp. 67–87). New York: Cambridge University Press.

Lubeck, S. (1988). Nested contexts. In L. Weis (Ed.), *Class, race, and gender in American education.* Albany, NY: State University of New York Press.

Matras, J. (1984). *Social inequality, stratification, and mobility.* Englewood Cliffs, NJ: Prentice-Hall.

Miller, E. S. (1979). *Introduction to cultural anthropology.* Englewood Cliffs, NJ: Prentice-Hall.

Montalto, N. V. (1978). The forgotten dream: A history of the intercultural education movement, 1924–1941. *Dissertation Abstracts International, 39A,* 1061. (University Microfilms No. 78-13436)

Newman, W. M. (1973). *American pluralism: A study of minority groups and social theory.* New York: Harper & Row.

Oakes, J. (1988). Tracking in mathematics and science education: A structural contribution to unequal schooling. In L. Weis (Ed.), *Class, race, and gender in American education* (pp. 106–125). Albany, NY: State University of New York Press.

O'Connor, T. (1988, November). *Cultural voice and strategies for multicultural education.* Paper presented at the annual meeting of the American Educational Studies Association, Montreal, Canada.

Patterson, O. (1977). *Ethnic chauvinism: The reactionary impulse.* New York: Stein & Day.

Pratte, R. (1979). *Pluralism in education: Conflict, clarity, and commitment.* Springfield, IL: Thomas.

Ryan, W. (1981). *Equality.* New York: Vintage Books.

Shor, I. (1986). *Culture wars: School and society in the conservative restoration 1969–1984.* Boston: Routledge & Kegan Paul.

Simon, R. I. (1989). Empowerment as a pedagogy of possibility. In H. Holtz, I. Marcus, J. Dougherty, J. Michaels, & R. Peduzzi, *Education and the American dream: Conservatives, liberals and radicals debate the future of education* (pp. 134–146). Granby, MA: Bergin & Garvey.

Skolnick, J., Langbort, C., & Day, L. (1982). *How to encourage girls in math and science.* Englewood Cliffs, NJ: Prentice-Hall.

Sleeter, C. E., & Grant, C. A. (1988). *Making choices for multicultural education: Five approaches to race, class, and gender.* Columbus, OH: Merrill.

Spradley, J. P., & Rynkiewich, M. A. (Eds.). (1975). *The nacirema: Readings on American culture.* Boston: Little, Brown.

Stewart, E. C. (1977). *American cultural patterns: A cross-cultural perspective.* Washington, DC: Society for Intercultural Education, Training, and Research.

U.S. Bureau of the Census. (1988). *Statistical abstract of the United States: 1988* (109th ed.). Washington, DC: Government Printing Office.

Webster's new twentieth century dictionary (2nd ed.) (1983). New York: Simon & Schuster.

Williamson, J. (1980). *New people: Miscegenation and mulattoes in the United States.* New York: New York University Press.

Yetman, N. R. (Ed.) (1985). *Majority and minority: The dynamics of race and ethnicity in American life* (4th ed.). Boston: Allyn and Bacon.

SUGGESTED READINGS

Appleton, N. (1983). *Cultural pluralism in education: Theoretical foundations.* New York: Longman.

> *An analysis of theories and ideologies of cultural pluralism. Discusses related court cases and cultural conflict and presents suggestions for incorporating cultural pluralism in the schools.*

Cowan, P. (1979). *The tribes of America.* Garden City, NY: Doubleday.

> *A journalistic account of Americans and their microcultures. Explores issues accentuated by ethnic, religious, and socioeconomic experiences.*

Hall, E. T. (1977). *Beyond culture.* Garden City, NY: Anchor Press.

> *An emphasis on those aspects of culture that are so innate that they are not easily recognized as culturally determined. Describes the need for an understanding of culture and how behavior is completely determined by culture.*

Holtz, H., Marcus, I., Dougherty, J., Michaels, J., & Peduzzi, R. (1989). *Education and the American dream: Conservatives, liberals and radicals debate the future of education.* Granby, MA: Bergin & Garvey.

> *Papers presented at a symposium on how conservatives, liberals, and radicals view education today and in the future. Deals with values, society, inequality, computers, gender, race, class, excellence, and reform. Provides an excellent overview of conservative, liberal, and radical perspectives on education.*

Pratte, R. (1979). *Pluralism in education: Conflict, clarity, and commitment.* Springfield, IL: Thomas.

> *A theoretical examination of the concept of cultural pluralism and its application to education. Provides a careful analysis of theories and ideologies.*

Spradley, J. P., & Rynkiewich, M. A. (Eds.) (1975). *The nacirema: Readings on American culture.* Boston: Little, Brown.

An anthropological perspective of aspects of American culture that are often overlooked as traits and institutions unique to U.S. culture. Provides an amusing and informative discussion of the Nacirema.

Weis, L. (Ed.). *Class, race, and gender in American education.* Albany, NY: State University of New York Press.

A collection of articles that examines class, race, and gender issues in U.S. schools. The overview discusses the distinctions between cultural and structural approaches to the study of schooling. The first section of the book focuses on different knowledge, unequal structures, and unequal outcomes; the second section examines cultural forms in schools.

CHAPTER 2
Class

The two views of equality in U.S. society that were outlined in Chapter 1 suggest different class structures in the country. One view accepts the objective existence of different socioeconomic levels or classes in society. It also strongly supports the notion that one can be socially mobile and move to a higher class if one works hard enough. Deprived groups in this view are usually seen as inferior, and their hardships are blamed on their lack of middle-class values and behaviors.

In the second view of U.S. society, distinct class divisions are recognized. Those individuals and families who own and control corporations, banks, and other means of production compose the privileged upper class. Persons who earn a living primarily by selling their labor power make up other classes. Another class includes those persons who are unable to work or who can find work only sporadically. Although some individuals are able to move from one class to another, cases are rare. Most people are caught in the socioeconomic strata to which they are born, and the politico-economic system ensures that they will remain there.

"While having to recognize the existence of unequal outcomes—inequalities in the possession of wealth, power, and prestige—Americans have characteristically emphasized the *equal chance*: in reality, the equal chance for individuals to wind up unequal" (M. Lewis, 1978, p. 4). Many Americans believe that the United States is a model of egalitarianism. It is a value that is highly regarded and viewed as uniquely American. However, it is misleading. There are "real limitations on what most of us can achieve—limitations which have very little to do with our willingness to work or the quality of our effort" (M. Lewis, 1978, p. 17). This chapter will explore inequalities related to the class structure in this country and some of the limitations or advantages that may result.

SOCIAL STRATIFICATION

Social stratification is possible because consistent and recurring relationships exist between people who occupy different levels of the social structure. Many individuals accept and follow socially defined positions based on occupation, race, sex, or socioeconomic status, for which patterns of behavior have been institutionalized. Civil rights and women's organizations are trying to combat that institutionalized acceptance and expectation of behavior for certain groups of people.

What are the key elements that promote social stratification in this country? Beeghley (1978) identifies three elements: (1) division of labor, (2) inequality as measured by differences in rewards and evaluations, and (3) restrictions on people's access to positions. The division of labor requires that workers complete small, very specific tasks. Thus, the work force becomes very specialized, and seldom is an employee involved in the development of the product from its initiation to its completion. Such a division of labor calls for a hierarchical arrangement in which some individuals give orders and others follow orders. Those who give the orders are accorded a higher rank in the stratification system. Such distinct divisions of jobs lead to patterns of interaction between people at different job levels that are formally or informally understood by all employees. These patterns help maintain social stratification.

Inequality results, in part, from differential rankings within the division of labor. Different occupations are evaluated and rewarded unequally. Some jobs are viewed as more worthy, more important, more popular, and more preferable than others. Finally, the rewards and evaluations of higher-ranking positions produce common interests among those who hold those positions. They then restrict the chances of others to obtain the same status—the key to establishing and maintaining a system of stratification.

Many persons in the United States receive high or low rankings in the social stratification system based on characteristics over which they have no control. Women, handicapped persons, elderly persons, children, and persons whose skin color is not white often receive a low prestige ranking. Ascribed status affects who is allowed entrance into the higher-ranking socioeconomic positions. On the other hand, ascribed status does not ensure that all white, nonhandicapped men will achieve a high-ranking position. They are found at all levels of the continuum, from a very low socioeconomic status to the highest socioeconomic status, but they and their families are overrepresented at the highest level. People of color, women, the young, the elderly, and handicapped individuals have a disproportionately high representation at the low end of the continuum. At the same time, members of these groups can be found at all levels of the continuum, with a few at the top of the socioeconomic status scale.

Such inequities are in large part a result of historical discrimination against certain groups of people, as described in other chapters of this book. One's ascribed status affects one's socioeconomic status from birth. It influences one's ability to choose alternative courses of action, to control one's own behavior, and to achieve one's goals (Rothman, 1978). How socioeconomic status is affected by ascribed statuses for which individuals suffer the most, namely, ethnicity, gender, and age, will be examined later in this chapter.

SOCIOECONOMIC STATUS

Socioeconomic level influences many aspects of the lives of students and their parents. Historically, the American way has emphasized the necessity for an individual and family to want and to achieve the "good life." The first immigrants subscribed to the belief that everyone had the opportunity to be successful by utilizing the fullest extent of his or her talents. As a matter of fact, today many Americans believe that it is an individual's birthright to desire and aspire to reach that potential.

How is the economic success or achievement of Americans measured? The U.S. Bureau of the Census measures the economic condition of individuals with a criterion called *socioeconomic status (SES)*. It serves as a composite of the economic status of a family or unrelated individuals based on occupation, educational attainment, and income. Related to the three factors used by the Census Bureau are wealth and power, which also help determine an individual's socioeconomic status but are more difficult to measure through census data.

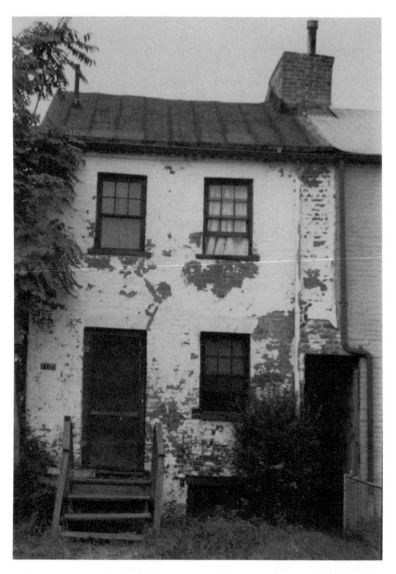

The conditions under which students live are greatly affected by the class position of their families.

These five determinants of socioeconomic status are interrelated. Although there are many forms of inequality, these factors are probably the most salient for the individual because they affect how one lives (Rothman, 1978). A family's socioeconomic status usually is observable—in what size house and what part of town they live, what schools the children attend, or to what clubs the parents belong. Many educators place their students at specific socioeconomic status levels based on similar observations.

Income

Income is the amount of money earned in wages or salaries throughout a year. Economists look at the income distribution of the population by dividing the population into fifths; the lowest fifth earns the least income, and the highest fifth earns the highest income. Figure 2–1 shows what percentage of the total income earned in 1986 was earned by each fifth of the population. The top 20 percent of the population earned 43.7 percent of the total income, while the bottom 20 percent earned 4.6 percent of the total income. The 5 percent of the population who received the highest income earned 17.0 percent of the total income (U.S. Bureau of the Census, 1988).

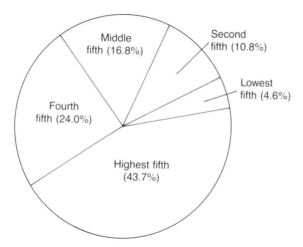

Figure 2–1   The distribution of total income in fifths of the population

Many Americans view this income inequity as a natural outcome of the American way. Because some people have achieved at a much higher level than much of the population, many people believe that they deserve to be paid more for their effort. Persons at the lower end of the continuum are either unemployed or work in unskilled jobs and thus are not expected to receive the same economic rewards. However, the degree of difference is quite large. The president of a large corporation can earn over $2 million annually, whereas persons earning the minimum wage receive less than $10,000 annually.

Between World War II and 1973, the growth of the American economy allowed incomes of workers at all levels to increase at a faster rate than expenditures. Many middle-income families were able to purchase homes, cars, boats, and luxuries for the home; often there was money left over for savings. Between 1947 and 1973, the annual median income of all persons fourteen years old and older nearly tripled, from $1,787 to $5,004. The standard of living for most of the population was markedly better in 1973 than in 1940. Beginning in 1973, however, the cost of living rose so rapidly that the cost of housing, utilities, food, and other essentials began to increase faster than income. Except for the rich, all families felt the financial pressure. No longer did they have extra income to purchase nonessentials. No longer was one full-time worker in a family enough to maintain the same standard of living. In 1986, the median annual income of a family was $29,458. In constant dollars, the median income in 1986 was less than that in 1973 (U.S. Bureau of the Census, 1988). Of those families with incomes above $25,000, nearly half had paychecks from two full-time workers.

The family income sets limits on the general life-style of a family, as well as on its general welfare. It controls the consumption patterns of a family—the amount and quality of material possessions, housing, consumer goods, luxuries, savings, and diet. The house, the paint, the furnishings, the food, the clothes, and the entertainment portrayed in many television advertisements reflect an accepted pattern of living well. According to our American mythology, almost every American lives this way, and the few who do not expect to as soon as they "get on their feet." But according to statistics, only about two-fifths of our families come close to the ideal (Gilbert & Kahl, 1982).

Wealth

Although the difference in income between families is great, an examination of income alone does not indicate the vast differences in the way families live. Income figures show the amount of money earned by a family for their labors during a year, but it neglects the amount of money earned from investments, land, and other holdings. It does not present the net worth of a family. (Net worth is the amount of money remaining if all owned property were converted to cash and all debts paid.) The wealth of a family includes savings accounts, insurance, corporate stock ownership, and property. Wealth provides a partial guarantee of future income and has the potential of producing additional income and wealth.

Whereas incomes can be determined from data gathered on federal income tax forms by the Internal Revenue Service, wealth is difficult to determine from these or any other standard forms. It is known, however, that the distribution of wealth is concentrated in a small percentage of the population. "Ten percent of American households own over 86 percent of the stocks, bonds, savings, property, and other financial assets. The top 0.5 percent owns more than 45 percent of the privately held wealth, while 90 percent of the American people have little or no net financial assets" (Parenti, 1988, p. 10).

Wealth ensures some economic security for its holders, even though the amount of security depends on the amount of wealth accumulated. It also enhances the power and prestige of those who own it. Great wealth accrues power, provides an income that allows luxury, and creates values and life-styles that are very different from those of persons without great wealth.

Occupation

For most Americans, income is determined by their occupation. Generally speaking, Americans believe that income is a fair measure of occupational success—both of the importance of the occupation to the society and of one's individual skill at the job (Gilbert & Kahl, 1982). In addition to providing an income, a person's occupation is an activity that Americans consider important. Those individuals who are unemployed often are characterized as noncontributing members of society who cannot take care of themselves. Even individuals with great wealth usually work, although additional income is unnecessary. "Work is a powerful and pervasive factor in behavior, and its demands are given precedence over almost all other institutional obligations" (Rossides, 1976, p. 134).

In the United States, there is an extreme specialization of labor that contributes to a hierarchical structure ranging from the unskilled worker to the medical doctor. The *Dictionary of Occupational Titles* (U.S. Employment Service, 1977) lists over twenty-one thousand separate occupations. These varied occupations have been classified by the U.S. Bureau of Labor Statistics (1988) in the following categories:

1. Managerial and professional specialties
2. Technical, sales, and administrative support, including secretaries and clerks
3. Service occupations, including private household work and protective service
4. Precision production, craft, and repair, including mechanics, repairers, and construction trades
5. Operators, fabricators, and laborers, including machine operators, assemblers, inspectors, transportation and material-moving occupations, handlers, equipment cleaners, and helpers
6. Farming, forestry, and fishing

Just over half of today's work force is composed of white-collar workers, that is, individuals who do mental rather than manual work. The percentage of service workers is growing, although the percentage of service workers who are private household workers continues to decline. In the last decade of this century, the job market will be expanding for medical assistants, home health aides, computer systems analysts, computer programmers, radiological technologists and technicians, legal assistants and technicians, dental assistants, guards, electrical and electronics engineers, computer operators, restaurant cooks, dining room and cafeteria attendants, and barroom helpers.

Within the working classes, the type of job one holds is the primary determinant of the income received. The job provides a relatively objective indicator of an individual's socioeconomic status. It often indicates one's education, suggests the types of associates with whom one will interact, and determines the degree of authority and responsibility one has over others. It gives individuals both differing amounts of compensation in income and differing degrees of prestige in the society.

Occupational prestige is often determined by the requirements for the job and by the characteristics of the job. The requirements for an occupation with prestige may include more education and training. Job characteristics that add to the prestige of an occupation are rooted in the division between mental and manual labor. When the prestige of an occupation is high, fewer people gain entry into that occupation. When the prestige of an occupation is low, employees are allotted less security, income, and prestige, and there is greater accessibility to that occupation. Those occupations with the highest prestige generally receive the highest salary. In most cases, an individual's occupation will determine his or her socioeconomic status.

Education

The best predictor of occupational prestige is the amount of education that one acquires (Beeghley, 1978), and the amount and quality of education one acquires is generally determined by one's "place" within society. In general, occupations require less education and less training as their prestige decreases. A college degree increases the number of job options available for an individual, but today those options are growing fewer.

The financial compensation is usually greater for occupations that require more years of education. For example, medical doctors and lawyers remain in school for several years beyond the bachelor's degree program. Many professionals and other white-collar workers have completed at least an undergraduate program at a college or university. Craft workers are an exception in that they often earn more money than many white-collar workers. At the same time, their positions require specialized training that often takes as long to complete as a college degree. There continues to be a great discrepancy in the income of persons who have less than a high school education and those who have completed professional training after college.

The job one has and the income received is strongly related to the amount of education obtained (Jencks et al., 1972). For example, the mean income of a white family in which the head of the household had not completed the eighth grade was $14,470 in 1985; it was $47,175 when the householder had completed at least four years of college. The differential for blacks was $11,612 to $35,141 and for Hispanics $15,247 to $38,278 (U.S. Bureau of the Census, 1988).

Many Americans still view education as a way to enhance economic status (Rossides, 1976). The sale of one's labor power in the U.S. labor market usually is enhanced by years of education. The credentials obtained through education are important in determining one's socioeconomic status. However, some people end up with more impressive educational credentials than others, and there are reasons for this. Jencks et al. (1972) found that the most important determinant of educational attainment is family background. The impact of family background is accounted for partly by measurable economic differences between families and partly by more elusive noneconomic differences.

The higher the socioeconomic status of students' families, the greater their chances of finishing high school and college. The conditions under which poor students live often make it difficult for them to go to school instead of work. The greater the income of families, the greater are the chances that students will have available books, magazines, and newspapers in the home; will have attended plays or concerts; and will have traveled beyond the region in which they live. Even the colleges that students attend are influenced more by the socioeconomic status of the family than by the academic ability of the student. Many students simply cannot afford to attend private colleges and choose instead state colleges or universities or community colleges. Thus, a student's socioeconomic origins have a substantial influence on the amount and type of schooling received and the type of job obtained.

Education is one of the main ways in which families pass on their class positions to their children. One's class position determines, in great part, the material conditions that affect one's life-style. Thus, educational level is a strong determinant of the future occupation and income of a family's children.

Power

Individuals and families who are at the upper socioeconomic status levels exert more power than those at any other level. These individuals are more likely to sit on boards that determine state and local policies, on boards for colleges and universities, and on boards of corporations. They determine who receives benefits and rewards in governmental, occupational, and community affairs. Parenti (1978) describes this control:

> The resources of power are not randomly scattered among the population to be used in autonomous ways but are distributed within a social system, and the way the system is organized has a decisive effect on what resources are available to whom. Any listing of the resources of power would include property, wealth, organization, social prestige, social legitimacy, number of adherents, various kinds of knowledgeability and leadership skills, technological skills, control of jobs, control of information, ability to manipulate the symbolic environment and ability to apply force and violence. (p. 63)

Groups and individuals with power control resources that influence their lives and the lives of others. Groups or individuals with little power do not have the means to get what they need or want or the access to others who could influence their interests. Powerless groups continually obtain fewer of the good things in life because they lack accessibility to power sources (Parenti, 1978). The sphere of education is not exempt from these relationships.

CLASS DIFFERENCES

Many Americans identify themselves as middle class. It is an amorphous category that often includes everyone who works steadily and who is not accepted as a member of the upper class. It ranges from well-paid professionals to service workers. Most white-collar workers, no matter what their salary, see themselves as middle class. Manual workers, on the other hand, often view themselves as working class rather than middle class. Nevertheless, for the most part their incomes and cultural values are similar to those of most white-collar workers.

Despite the popular myth, most people in America are not affluent. The U.S. Bureau of Labor Statistics (1979) figured a moderate budget that represented what might be a reasonably comfortable life in America today. In 1976, that budget, which was for $16,266, was far above the poverty level. While only 13.6 percent of the population is considered poor by federal poverty standards, 30.1 percent of the households earned less than $15,000 in 1986 (U.S. Bureau of the Census, 1988). Many of these persons identify themselves as middle class, but are unable to obtain the material goods and necessities to live comfortably.

The so-called middle class is certainly not homogeneous. The differences in education, occupation, prestige, income, and the ability to accumulate wealth vary widely among persons who identify themselves in this group.

There are two prevailing theories of class differences. In one view, "class divides society into two conflicting camps that contend for control: workers and bosses, labor and capital, proletariat and bourgeoise" (Vanneman & Cannon, 1987, p. 39). These dichotomous groups struggle for control of society. Thus, conflict between the two is inherent in this explanation. In the second view, society is hierarchical, and classes are rankings of economic success and prestige (Vanneman & Cannon, 1987). It is believed that individuals and families can move from a lower to a higher class, and examples of upward mobility can be cited. Although inequality is acknowledged, it is not explained in terms of class differences and conflict between classes. Instead, it is explained in terms of one's lack of motivation and ability. Thus, it is the individual's fault for not moving up the class ladder—a phenomenon called *blaming the victim.*

This section will provide a broad sketch of classes often categorized in describing Americans: the underclass, the working class, the middle class, and the upper class.

Underclass

The term *underclass* is sometimes viewed as negative and an inappropriate label for the portion of the population who suffer the most from the lack of a stable income or other economic resources. It usually does not include those individuals who are temporarily poor because of a job loss or family illness. It does include the long-term poor. W.J. Wilson (1987) reported that "the long-term poor constitute about 60 percent of those in poverty at any given point in time and are in a poverty spell that will last eight or more years" (p. 10).

Auletta (1982) grouped the underclass into the following four distinct groups:

1. The *passive poor,* usually long-term welfare recipients
2. The *hostile* street criminals who terrorize most cities, and who are often school dropouts and drug addicts
3. The *hustlers,* who, like street criminals, may not be poor and who earn their livelihood in an underground economy, but rarely commit violent crimes

4. The *traumatized* drunks, drifters, homeless shopping-bag ladies and released mental patients who frequently roam or collapse on city streets (p. xvi)

The underclass includes the hard-core unemployed—those who have seldom, if ever, worked and who lack the skills to find and maintain a job. It also includes many discouraged workers who have given up looking for work and who are no longer included in the federal government's report of the unemployed. Disproportionately, these families are headed by single mothers, often teenagers who have had to drop out of school. The number of persons included in this group is not found in the census data. Researchers suggest that it varies from two to fifteen million (Auletta, 1982).

Members of the underclass have become socially isolated from the dominant society. They usually are not integrated into, nor wanted in, the communities of the other classes. Recommendations to build low-income housing or halfway houses in middle- or working-class communities often result in vocal outrage from the residents of these communities. Some analysts think that the lack of integration has exacerbated the differences in behavior between members of the underclass and those of other classes. In a study of the inner city, W.J. Wilson (1987) concluded that

> the exodus of middle- and working-class families from many ghetto neighborhoods removes an important "social buffer" that could deflect the full impact of the kind of prolonged and increasing joblessness that plagued inner-city neighborhoods in the 1970s and early 1980s, joblessness created by uneven economic growth and periodic recessions. This argument is based on the assumption that even if the truly disadvantaged segments of an inner-city area experience a significant increase in long-term spells of joblessness, the basic institutions in that area (churches, schools, stores, recreational facilities, etc.) would remain viable if much of the base of their support comes from the more economically stable and secure families. Moreover, the very presence of these families during such periods provides mainstream role models that help keep alive the perception that education is meaningful, that steady employment is a viable alternative to welfare, and that family stability is the norm, not the exception. (p. 56)

Over the past decade, the number of homeless persons and families has increased dramatically. Again, the estimates of the number of homeless differ, depending on who reports the figures, from 250,000 to three million, or 1 percent of the population. Half of the homeless are now families; about one-third are persons who have been released from mental institutions; the remainder are runaway teenagers and other single persons. Many work, but at such low wages they are unable to afford housing. Half of the homeless have graduated from high school; 20 percent have attended college; and 5 percent have college degrees (Gorder, 1988).

"Contrary to popular belief, most of the people who are homeless actually do not choose to be homeless" (Gorder, 1988, p. 23). In many communities now, the homeless can be observed sleeping in parks or on grates. However, only 5 percent choose to live on the streets; most use shelters when available. In some areas, tent cities have been established by homeless persons and families (Gorder, 1988).

Who are the homeless families? Gorder (1988) reports that the following characteristics were found for homeless families in Atlanta:

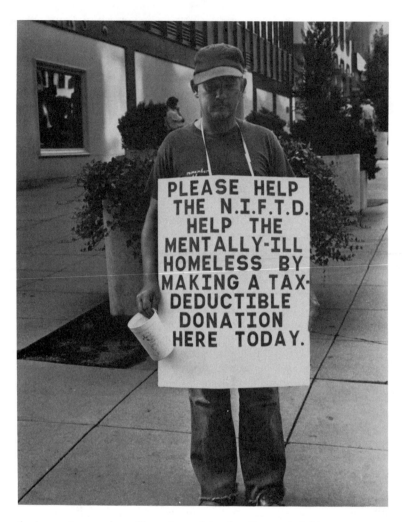

An increasing number of homeless adults, families, and children are found in communities around the country.

(Photo by Willard Loftis).

☐ Eighty-three percent were headed by single females.
☐ Forty-three percent were employed but not able to make it on their salaries.
☐ Sixty percent of the children were under the age of five.
☐ The average number of children was two.
☐ Parents' average age was twenty-nine.
☐ Only 36 percent had been on welfare programs previously. (p. 68)

What happens to the children in these families? In a number of school districts, they cannot be registered for school because they do not have an address. Therefore, many do not attend school for extended periods of time. They suffer more from illnesses, including hypothermia, and are often hungry. Further, they are more likely to be abused or neglected by parents and other adults.

The underclass suffer from economic insecurity and social, political, and economic deprivation. When they hold full-time jobs, their jobs are those of the lowest prestige and income. The jobs are often those that are eliminated as economic conditions tighten, resulting in their being unemployed again. The work for which they are hired is often the dirty work—not only physically dirty, but also often dangerous, menial, undignified, and degrading. The jobs are the least desirable ones in society, and they are performed by persons with no other options if they are going to work (Rothman, 1978).

Too often, the underclass is blamed for its own condition. The members are generally unnoticed when they remain isolated from the majority and work sporadically. However, those who are on welfare are subjected to the pejorative and inaccurate opinions of many Americans. "To be poor in America is to be stigmatized" (Beeghley, 1978, p. 139). Other persons often attribute personal qualities of dishonesty and loose morals to the poor. They are stereotyped as lazy and unwilling to work. The implication of such stereotypes is that they as individuals must not be working hard enough; otherwise, they would not be poor.

Many stereotypical notions about the underclass need to be overcome for teachers to effectively serve students who come from this background. Such students should not be blamed if they show acceptance, resignation, and even accommodation to their poverty as they learn to live with their economic disabilities. Should they be blamed for lethargy when their diets are inadequate to sustain vigor, or for family instability when they are under torturing financial stress, or for low standardized test scores when their education has been poor, or for loose work force attachments when they are in dead-end jobs that cannot lift them out of poverty anyway (Perlman, 1976)?

Anthropologists and sociologists have studied the relationship between cultural values and poverty status. Some have proposed a thesis called *culture of poverty* that asserts that the poor have a unique way of life that developed as a reaction to their impoverished environment (O. Lewis, 1969). This thesis suggests that those people who are poor have a different value system and life-style that are perpetuated as a microculture in American society.

Critics of the culture of poverty thesis believe that the cultural values of the poor are much like those of the rest of the population but have been modified in practice because of situational stresses (Valentine, 1968). In a classic study of street-corner men, Liebow (1967) suggested the following about a poor person's behavior:

> Behavior appears not so much as a way of realizing the distinctive goals and values of his own microculture, or of conforming to its models, but rather as his way of trying to achieve many of the goals and values of the larger society, of failing to do

this, and of concealing his failure from others and from himself as best he can. (p. 222)

This explanation suggests that the differences in values and life-styles of the poor are not passed from one generation to the next, but are the adaptations by the poor to the experience of living in poverty.

The Working Class

The occupations pursued by the working class are those that require manual work for which remuneration varies widely, depending on the skill required in the specific job. The factor that is most important in the description of the working class is the subordination of members to the capitalist control of production. These workers do not have control of their work. They do not give orders; they take orders from others, usually members of the middle class. Included in the working class are craft and kindred workers, transport equipment operatives, other operatives, and nonfarm laborers. When farm laborers and service workers are added to this group, the working class comprises 44.4 percent of the employed population (U.S. Bureau of the Census, 1988).

The median income of these workers, sometimes called blue-collar workers, varied from $6,292 for private household workers to $21,528 for craft and kindred workers in 1986 (U.S. Bureau of the Census, 1988). Although the income of many blue-collar workers is equal to or higher than that of nonprofessional white-collar workers, there is less job security. Work is more sporadic and unemployment is unpredictably affected by the economy. Jobs are uncertain because of displacement as a result of technology and more stringent educational requirements. Fringe benefits available to these workers are often not as good as those offered other workers. Vacation time is usually shorter, and health insurance is available less often (Beeghley, 1978).

The education required for most blue-collar jobs is not as high as for white-collar jobs. However, the better-paying, skilled jobs require specialized training and apprenticeships. Without additional training, it becomes difficult to move into a higher-level position. Many factory workers earn little more after twenty years on the job than someone who just begins, and within a few years the new worker is earning the same pay as the worker with seniority.

Except for the skilled jobs and some of the service and farm jobs that allow autonomy to the worker, most jobs at this level are routine. The jobs are often perceived as not very meaningful or satisfying to the worker. Other studies report that blue-collar workers are more likely to separate work and social activities than workers at other levels (Rothman, 1978). They tend not to socialize with co-workers to the same degree as other workers, but maintain strong kinship ties with parents and siblings for social life.

The blue-collar workers perceive themselves as hard working, honest, and performing decent and important work for society. They want to be successful, and often they hope that their children will not have to spend their lives in a factory. Mistakenly, they are often perceived by others as authoritarian and intolerant of civil rights—an

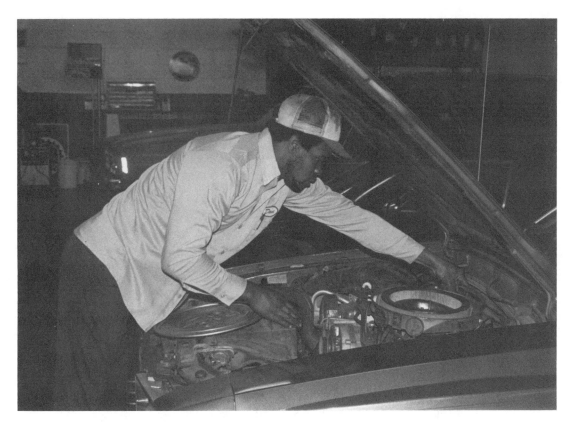

Individuals involved in manual work and classified as blue-collar workers make up nearly half of the population.

image portrayed by the term *hard hat* during the 1960s. This image, however, has not proved accurate. Blue-collar workers are no more intolerant or prejudiced than members of other classes.

The Middle Class

The media and some historians and sociologists have developed an image of middle-class Americans as a couple with two or three children in a suburban house with a double garage, a color television, and the latest household gadgets; the father is almost always the primary breadwinner. In reality, only 4 percent of all American families fit the middle-class myth (Hodgkinson, 1986).

The incomes of those Americans who are popularly considered middle class vary greatly. Contrary to myths about affluent workers, the average annual pay for full-time employees in all domestic industries was $21,935 in 1986 (U.S. Bureau of the Census, 1988). While some members of this supposed middle class have comfortable incomes, they have virtually no wealth. They have little cushion against the loss of earning power through catastrophe, recession, layoffs, wage cuts, or old age (Parenti, 1988). At various periods in the life cycle, many members of this middle class fall into poverty for brief periods of time. Many famies have found it necessary for both the husband and wife to work to make ends meet. For discussion, the middle class will be divided into two distinct groups: white-collar workers and professionals/managers.

White-collar workers also perform nonmanual labor, but professionals, managers, and administrators are accorded higher prestige in society. A major difference between these two groups is the amount of control they have over their work and the work of others. White-collar clerical workers, technicians, and salespersons are usually supervised by the professionals, managers, or administrators.

Sales workers make up 12.1 percent of employed persons in the United States; clerical and kindred workers make up 16.2 percent; registered nurses and other health assessment and treatment occupations make up 1.8 percent; teachers in preschool through secondary schools make up 3.2 percent; college and university teachers make up 0.6 percent; and executives, managers, and administrators make up 11.5 percent of the employed population.

Overall, these middle-class workers earn a median income above that of most blue-collar workers except for skilled workers and many operatives. The median income of sales workers was $18,252 in 1986; clerical workers earned less, with a median income of $15,600. The median income of the professional category was $26,260, with administrators earning more than the professionals (U.S. Bureau of the Census, 1988). As a group, these workers have greater job security and better fringe benefits than many blue-collar workers.

Many of the professional jobs are currently saturated, and their past rapid growth has now leveled off. Many college graduates who in the past would have sought and found professional positions are expected to begin to fill the lower-level white-collar jobs (J.O. Wilson, 1980). Whereas the formal education required for these jobs varies, more formal education is usually expected than for blue-collar jobs.

As white-collar jobs expanded over the past four decades, many people believed that such jobs were more meaningful and satisfying than jobs in blue-collar occupations. How meaningful and satisfying the jobs are, however, depends on the particular job. Certainly, many are as routine and boring as many blue-collar jobs. Others are highly interesting and challenging. Still others are extremely alienating in that employees cannot control their environment. The employees experience their work as meaningless, are socially isolated from co-workers, and develop low levels of self-esteem. The type of job and the environment in which it is performed vary greatly for the 60.9 million workers with white-collar jobs.

Members of this class appear to believe strongly in the Protestant work ethic. They see themselves as respectable and adhering to a specific set of beliefs and values that are inherent in the American way of life (Rothman, 1978). While they are only slightly better off economically than their blue-collar counterparts, they live or try to live a more affluent life.

Professionals, managers, and administrators are the elite of the middle class. They represent the status that many Americans who are concerned with upward mobility are trying to reach. Their income level allows them to lead a life that is in many cases quite different from that of other white-collar and blue-collar workers. They are the group that seems to have benefited the most from the nation's economic growth since the 1940s. Although at a level far below the upper class, they are the affluent middle class. They reflect the middle-class myth more accurately than any of the other middle-class groups described.

The professionals who best fit this category include those persons who must receive professional or advanced degrees and credentials to practice their profession. Judges, lawyers, physicians, college professors, teachers, and scientists are the professionals. Excluding teachers, most professionals earn far above the median income of $26,260 reported for this category.

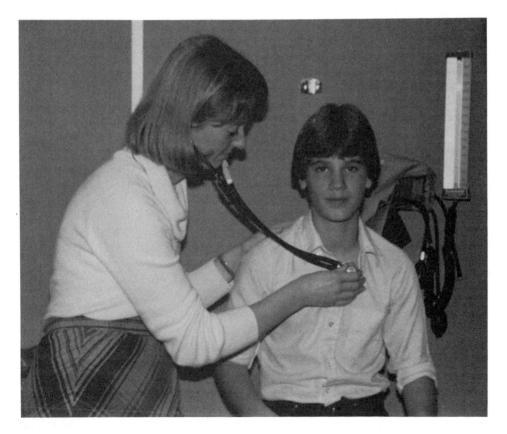

Physicians are one of the professional groups usually included in the middle class. However, their income and prestige are usually greater than the white-collar workers who are also included in the middle class.

This group also includes managers and administrators, who make up 11.5 percent of the employed populations. These persons are the successful business people and executives. They range from the chief executive officers of a major corporation to the president of a college to the owner and manager of a local nursing home. Those who are the most affluent make up the middle and upper management in financing, marketing, and production. Although the median salary of this census category was $26,260, the administrators of large corporations earn salaries far above this level—salaries and fringe benefits place them in the upper class instead of the middle class (Parenti, 1988).

Educational credentials are more important for persons at this level than at any other class level. For most of these occupations, knowlege is gained through formal education; a college degree, often an advanced degree, is a prerequisite for most of these occupations. The prospect of gaining the necessary qualifications to enter this level is severely restricted in that children of parents with college degrees are much more likely to attend and graduate from college than are children of parents who did not attend college (Parker, 1972). Thus, position in this status level most often becomes a part of one's inheritance as a result of the advantages that prestige and income bring to members of the upper middle class.

The incomes and opportunities to accumulate wealth are high for this group in comparison with the bulk of the population. Members of this class play an active role in civic and voluntary organizations. Their occupations and incomes give them access to policy-making roles within these organizations. They are active participants in political processes and thus are major recipients of public benefits. Of all the groups studied so far, this one holds the greatest power.

Their occupations play a central role in their lives, often determining their social friends as well as their business and professional associates. Their jobs allow more autonomy than jobs at any of the levels previously discussed. For the most part, they are allowed a high amount of self-direction (Beeghley, 1978). Members of this group tend to view their affluence, advantages, and comforts as universal rather than unique. They believe that their class includes almost everyone (Parker, 1972). They believe in the American dream of success because they have been successful.

The Upper Class

Whereas there is an abundance of studies about the working and middle classes in the United States, there is a dearth of information about the upper class. "The rich are defined mainly in terms of their possession of a great deal of money or economically important assets" (Beeghley, 1978, p. 203). High income and wealth are necessary characteristics for entering the upper class as well as for acceptance by those persons who are already members. However, within the upper class there are great variations in the amount of wealth held by a family.

The upper class comprises two groups. One group includes the individuals and families who control great inherited wealth; the other group includes the top-level administrators and professionals. Prestige positions, rather than great wealth, allow some families to enter or maintain their status at this level. The upper class includes persons with top-level and highly paid positions in large banks, entertainment corporations, trade unions, state and large city governments, Congress and the executive branch, the military, and industrial corporations. It also includes those who serve as primary advisors to these leaders, for example, corporate lawyers.

A study of elite boarding schools attended by the upper class identified some characteristics that confirm the differences between this and the other classes. In 1985, nearly half of the students were from families with an annual income of over $100,000; this figure is income only and does not include earnings from wealth. The wealthiest students are from Jewish, Presbyterian, Episcopalian, and Catholic backgrounds. Fifty percent of the fathers were professionals, and 40 percent were managers. Over three-fourths of the parents had finished college. "Nearly two-thirds of the fathers have attended graduate or professional school, compared to less than one-tenth of the fathers of high school seniors nationally. One-third of boarding school mothers have attended graduate or professional schools, while nationally less than one in twenty mothers of high school students have attended graduate school" (Cookson & Persell, 1985, p. 59). Families travel with their children; 69 percent of the students had traveled abroad. Books abound in the home; 51 percent had over five hundred books at home. Graduates of these schools attend elite colleges and universities at a higher rate than other students (Cookson & Persell, 1985).

Wealth and income ensure power. The extremely small proportion of the population who holds a vastly disproportionate share of the wealth also benefits disproportionately when resources are distributed. Their power allows them to protect their wealth. The only progressive tax in this country is the federal income tax, in which a greater percentage of the income is taxed as the income increases. Loopholes in the tax laws provide benefits to those whose unearned income is based on assets (Beeghley, 1978). What does this mean in terms of advantage to the rich? Beeghley reported the following:

> In 1972 there were some six million families in the United States with incomes (from all sources) of less than $3,000. These poor families received tax deductions—of "tax welfare"—totaling $92 million, or about $16 per family. At the other extreme, there were about three thousand families with incomes greater than $1 million in 1972. These rich families received deductions of $2.2 billion, or about $720,490 per family. (p. 228)

Power is also an important element in terms of civic and voluntary organizational involvement of the rich. They serve primarily in policy-making roles as members of boards for various organizations, colleges and universities, and corporations. "Nearly 90 percent of all U.S. cabinet officers between 1897 and 1973 were members of either the business or social elite" (Cookson & Persell, 1985, p. 200).

While the families with inherited wealth do not represent a completely closed status group, the group has an overrepresentation of Anglo, native-born, and Protestant members (Beeghley, 1978). They tend to intermarry with other members of the upper class. They are well educated, although a college degree is not essential. The educational mark of prestige is attendance at the elite private prep schools. For example, less than 10 percent of U.S. high school students attend private schools. Less than 1 percent of the high school population attends the elite prep schools, and these students are overwhelmingly the children of the upper class. In a study of America's elite boarding schools, Cookson and Persell (1985) found that "where a person goes to school may have little to do with his and her technical abilities, but it may have a lot to do with social abilities . . . . Where individuals go to school determines with whom they associate" (p. 16). Thus, President George Bush attended Phillips Andover, Secretary of State James Baker attended Hill School, and John F. Kennedy attended Choate.

The upper class probably represents the most distinct and closed microcultural group of all of those studied. Cookson and Persell (1985) report that

> the founding of boarding schools in the United States was part of an upper-class "enclosure movement" that took place in the late nineteenth century. In order to insulate themselves from the rest of society, the American upper class established their own neighborhoods, churches, suburban and rural recreational retreats, and a number of social and sporting clubs. It was during this period that the *Social Register* was first published and, in lavish displays of conspicuous consumption, the social season was highlighted by debutante balls and charity benefits. (p. 23)

Greater assimilation of life-styles and values has occurred within this class than for any other class. Although diversity exists within the group, members of the upper class may be the most homogeneous group, and they are likely to remain so as long as their cross-cultural and cross-class interactions are limited.

THE IMPACT OF CLASS ON OTHER MICROCULTURES

Poverty is most likely to be a condition of the young and the old, minorities, women, full-time workers in the lowest-paying jobs, and the illiterate. In 1986, the federal government's poverty level was $5,572 for a one-person family and $8,737 for a four-person family. Based on this poverty threshold, there were 32.4 million poor persons in the United States, or 13.6 percent of the total population; many of these individuals were members of poor families, of which there were 5.7 million, or 9.6 percent of all families (U.S. Bureau of the Census, 1988). "An additional forty million or more live on incomes estimated as below a 'low standard adequacy' by the Department of Labor" (Parenti, 1988, p.30). The poor include the following groups:

White poor	22.2 million persons	11.0% of all whites
Black poor	9.0 million persons	31.1% of all blacks
Hispanic poor	5.1 million persons	27.3% of all Hispanics
Older than 65 years	3.5 million persons	12.4% of all such persons
Younger than 16 years	11.7 million persons	21.0% of all such persons
Female-headed families without husband	16.9 million families	34.2% of all such families
All other families	15.4 million families	8.2% of all such families

Many poor persons do have full-time, year-round jobs but are not paid wages high enough to move their families out of poverty. "Some two million people work full time year round but live in poverty and another seven million poor individuals work full time for part of the year or in part-time jobs" (Levitan & Shapiro, 1987, p. vii). The working poor can be found in all occupational groups, but they are disproportionately located in service and agricultural occupations. "Sixteen percent of food service workers and 31 percent of farm operators and managers worked full time year round but lived in poverty" (Levitan & Shapiro, 1987, p. 29).

Although the ceiling for poverty level is supposed to indicate an income level necessary to maintain an adequate, not comfortable, living, it is misleading to assume that any family above this level can live adequately or comfortably. Many families who have incomes above this level find it difficult to pay even for essential food, housing, and clothing, let alone live comfortably by the American standard. Thus, there are probably more than fifty million persons in this country who are economically poor in the sense that they do not have enough money to purchase the necessary essentials for their families to live adequately (Harrington, 1984).

The poor are a very heterogeneous group. They do not all have the same values or life-styles. They cannot be expected to react alike to the conditions of poverty. To many, their ethnicity or religion is the more important determinant of the way that they live within the economic constraints of poverty. To others, the effect of poverty is the greatest influence in determining their values and life-styles. No matter what aspects of the various microcultures have the greatest impact on the lives of individuals or families, their life-styles are limited severely by the economic constraints that keep them poor. Individual choice is more limited for persons who are poor than for any other microcultural group studied in this book.

Ethnic Inequality

African-Americans, Hispanics, and Native Americans experience the most severe economic deprivation of all ethnic groups in this country. Although the census data on consumer income are not broken down for American Indians, Eskimos, and Aleuts, Rothman (1978) projects that they probably suffer more from economic inequity than any other group. Harrington (1984) describes the plight of American Indians: "Their poverty is extreme. Life expectancy is roughly twenty years less than whites; unemployment rates are stratospheric, and the 1970 census found that, on the twenty-four largest Indian reservations, 55.1 percent of the people were below the poverty line" (p. 221).

The median income of most European groups who immigrated early this century now nearly equals or has surpassed that of the dominant group. In 1986, the median income of white families was $30,809; of black families, $17,604; and of Hispanic families, $19,995. Thus, black families have a median income that is 57.1 percent that of whites; Hispanics earn 64.9 percent of the median income of whites (U.S. Bureau of the Census, 1988).

In 1985, when husband-wife families were compared, blacks earned 78 percent and Hispanics earned 70.6 percent of the median income of whites. When both wife and husband worked, the gap narrowed even more to 82 percent for blacks and 77.5 percent for Hispanics (U.S. Bureau of the Census, 1988). When age, education, experience, and other factors were equal to those of white men, the earnings of minorities and whites became more similar, but the income ratios between the groups still favored whites.

People of color make up a disproportionately high percentage of persons in poverty. Of the white population, 11 percent fall below the poverty level compared with 31.1 percent of the black population and 27.3 percent of the Hispanic population (U.S. Bureau of the Census, 1988). Beeghley (1978) suggests that racial discrimination causes much of the difference in income between blacks and whites. With the same level of education, blacks earn less than whites.

Persons of color are more likely to be unemployed and more likely to be concentrated in lower-paying jobs. Figure 2-2 shows the occupational levels of blacks and whites in 1988. The percentage of blacks in the higher-paying and higher-status jobs is much less than that of whites, especially for men. While both absolute and relative gains in the occupational status of blacks have been made over the past thirty years, blacks are still heavily overrepresented in the semiskilled and unskilled positions. Institutional racism has contributed to occupational inequities (Perlman, 1976).

> Most blacks do not qualify for management training opportunities because they do not have business degrees, because they cannot afford to obtain them and have been unprepared for college by poor prior schooling, because of their unfavorable environment for successful schooling and the sparse funding of their schooling, because they lived in poor districts, because they (in this case their families) did not hold high-paying jobs since they did not qualify for them. (p. 70)

This inequitable condition is perpetuated by a number of factors. Students of color drop out of school in greater proportions—39 percent for blacks and 54 percent for Hispanics, compared with a dropout rate of 22 percent for whites (Boyer, 1983). This situation is even more dire in central-city poverty areas, where more than half of all black household heads have not finished high school (Levy, 1986). Less education results in lower-paying jobs in lower-status occupations. It often means unemployment, because such jobs offer less security than higher-status positions. Unemployment for people of color is higher than for whites; at the end of 1986, 6 percent of the white population was unemployed, compared with 14.5 percent of the black population and 10.6 percent of the Hispanic population. For sixteen- to nineteen-year-olds, the differences are even greater, with 15.6 percent of white youth and 39.3 of black youth unemployed (U.S. Bureau of the Census, 1988).

The historical experiences of ethnic groups have had a great impact on a group's gains in socioeconomic status. For example, the absolute class position (income, occupation, rate of employment) of African-Americans improved as a result of their migration to America's large cities during the first half of this century, and especially during the 1940s, despite their lack of marketable skills. Since then, their educational attainments have narrowed the formerly enormous gap between blacks and whites with

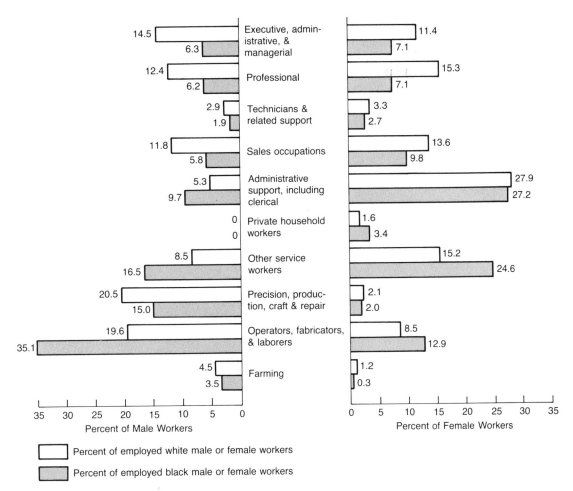

Figure 2–2 Occupation of the labor force by sex and race: 1988.

regard to completion of high school, median number of school years completed, and, to a lesser degree, prevalence of college education. However, for African-Americans, increased education has not paid off directly in terms of income or occupation, and their relative gains in education should not be seen as automatically producing relative gains in economic status (Rossides, 1976).

Since the 1960s, the number of African-American families who have entered the middle class has increased significantly. However, the gap between the middle class and the poor has also grown. Levy (1986) found that black "men at the top of the distribution [i.e., above $25,000] were doing progressively better while blacks at the bottom [i.e., under $5,000]—between a fifth and a quarter of all black men ages twenty-five to sixty-six—were doing progressively worse" (p. 19). As a part of the move into the middle class, African-Americans have increasingly moved from the inner city. "Accompanying the black middle-class exodus has been a growing movement of stable working-class blacks from ghetto neighborhoods to higher-income neighborhoods in other parts of the city and to the suburbs." These moves have left the inner city "populated almost exclusively by the most disadvantaged segments of the black urban community" (W. J. Wilson, 1987, p. 7–8).

The other subordinate groups with a disproportionately low socioeconomic status have different historical experiences from those of blacks, but suffer similarly from discrimination. Mexican-Americans are highly overrepresented as farm laborers, one of the lowest-status occupations. Many American Indians have been isolated on reservations away from all occupations except those lowest in prestige, and the numbers of such positions are limited. Thus, a highly disproportionate number of persons of color remain with a low socioeconomic status. Asian-Americans, who as a group have a high educational level and a relatively high socioeconomic status, often reach middle management positions but are seldom allowed to move into upper management positions. Although the most powerful class in the United States contains all ages and both sexes, it does not include all ethnic, religious, and racial groups at a level equal to their representation in the population.

Sexual Inequality

As a group, women earn less and are more likely to suffer from poverty than any other group, with women of color suffering the greatest oppression. The reasons for such inequality, however, have very different origins from that based on ethnicity. Institutional discrimination based on sex is a result of "accepted traditions, myths, and encrusted habits which assign women to roles and status which retard their labor force participation, channel them into a narrow range of occupations, and consequently keep their earnings low" (Perlman, 1976, p. 88). Overt discrimination against women results in the use of sex to determine wages, hiring, and promotion of individuals. Similar mechanisms that promote this inequality operate in regard to minorities.

The median income of men and women who have year-round and full-time jobs differs substantially. In 1986, the median income was $25,894 for men and $16,843 for women (U.S. Bureau of the Census, 1988). Thus, women who worked full time earned 65 cents for every $1 that a man earned—a ratio that has risen from 59 cents, where it had been for two decades.

Women, especially those who are the heads of households, are more likely to fall below the poverty level than men. Families maintained by women with no husband present are the most likely group to be in poverty; 34.2 percent of all persons in such families are below the official poverty level. The total number of poor families maintained by women has increased from 10.4 million in 1969 to 16.9 million in 1986 (U.S. Bureau of the Census, 1988). In 1984, 20 percent of all poor white families were headed by women; 70 percent of poor black families had a female head, as did almost 50 percent of the Hispanic households. This increase is primarily a result of an in-

crease in divorces, separations, and out-of-wedlock births, all leading to the formation of more female-headed households (Rodgers, 1986).

The number of women in the work force has increased dramatically over the
past two decades. By 1995, it is projected that 59.8 percent of all women will be working in the civilian work force as compared with 75.3 percent of all men. Almost 61
percent of all black women will be in the work force, as will 59.7 percent of white
women and 54.7 percent of Hispanic women (U.S. Bureau of the Census, 1988). To
maintain an adequate or desirable standard of living today, both the husband and
wife in many families must work. The difference that two incomes make on the family
income is obvious. Although the percentages in the work force of women who are
single, widowed, divorced, separated, and/or black have increased over the past fifteen years, the percentages of married women and white women in the work force
have increased dramatically since 1940. In 1940, only 16.7 percent of all married
women worked outside the home; by 1987, 56.1 pecent of them did. Only 31 percent
of all white women worked outside the home in 1947, but 55 percent of them did
by 1986. These figures reveal the stagnation of groups most likely to suffer poverty
(i.e., unmarried persons and persons of color), with the increases concentrated in
those groups least susceptible to poverty (i.e., married and white women) (Perlman,
1976).

What are the sources of low earnings for women? Perlman (1976) indicates that
there are four sources: (1) large nonparticipation of women in the work force; (2) employment in low-paying jobs; (3) low rate of pay; and (4) involvement in part-time
and sporadic work.

Below graduate and professional school levels, the percentages of graduates at
the various levels of education are similar for men and women. In 1983, 50.2 percent
of all high school graduates and 50.5 percent of all college graduates were women.
By 1985, women received 38.5 percent of all law degrees, 30.4 percent of all medical
degrees, and 12.5 percent of all engineering degrees (U.S. Bureau of the Census, 1988).
Compared with the earnings of men with the same education, women still earn less.

Historically, there has been a fairly rigid sexual division of labor. The roles of
women were limited to reproduction, child rearing, and homemaking. When they
did work outside the home, the jobs often were similar to roles in the home, that
is, caring for children or the sick. Jobs were stereotyped by sex. As late as 1986, women
composed over 85 percent of the work force in the following occupations (U.S. Bureau
of the Census, 1988):

Secretaries	99.0%
Prekindergarten and kindergarten teachers	98.5%
Licensed practical nurses	97.5%
Child-care workers	97.4%
Receptionists	97.1%
Cleaners and servants	95.3%
Typists	95.2%
Registered nurses	94.3%

Teachers' aides	94.2%
Bookkeepers, accounting and audit clerks	91.8%
Bank tellers	91.8%
Data entry keyers	91.1%
Sewing and stitching workers	90.6%
Dental assistants	90.5%
Information clerks	89.7%
Hairdressers and cosmetologists	88.8%
Telephone operators	87.9%
Librarians	85.9%
Health assessment and treatment workers	85.3%
Elementary school teachers	85.2%

These jobs are accompanied by neither high prestige nor high income. Those that fall in the category of professional (i.e., librarians, teachers, and nurses) do not compete in income or prestige with architects and engineers. Figure 2–2 outlined the job categories in which women participate. Note that women continue to be over-represented as clerical and service workers and underrepresented as managers and skilled workers.

Women as individuals are assigned a lower status than men in the stratification system of this country. The occupations most open to women are the low-status and low-paying ones. Over one-third of the women who maintain their own households without a husband are below the official poverty level. Many women, particularly nonworking married women, are economically dependent on men. They are powerless in that they do not hold direct power over their own lives. Even with the same education and occupation as men, women typically do not receive the same income or prestige as their male counterparts.

Age Inequality

The highest incidence of poverty occurs at both ends of the life span. Children and persons over sixty-five years old are at ages that society has determined to be non-working periods. The poverty rate for persons at both ends of the life span is much greater than for all other ages. The percentages of the population suffering from poverty at different ages are shown in Figure 2–3.

Men between the ages of forty-five and fifty-four earn more than at any other period in their lives; women earn their maximum between the ages of thirty-five and forty-four. The median income of persons who are fourteen to nineteen years old is lower than for any other group, primarily because most of these persons are just beginning to enter the work force at the end of this period and may not enter for several more years, especially if they attend college. Income then increases steadily for most persons until after they reach fifty-five years of age. The income of women remains fairly constant throughout much of their working life, whereas the income for a large percentage of men increases dramatically during their lifetime.

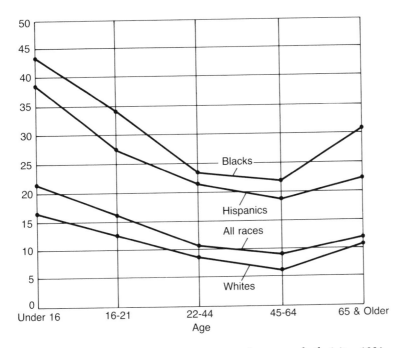

Figure 2–3 Percentage of persons in poverty by age and ethnicity: 1986.

Children "constitute one of the largest and most vulnerable low-power groups in society" (Parenti, 1978, p. 67). Their socioeconomic status depends on their family, and they have little or no control over their destiny during those early years. Parenti (1978) states:

> But if all children risk the injustices of the adult world, the offspring of the lower classes are the most victimized of all, a disproportionately high number of battered and abused youngsters coming from homes plagued by poverty, unemployment, and overcrowding. To be conceived in poverty is to suffer risks while still inside the womb. Insufficient prenatal care, poor diet, and difficult working conditions for lower-class women leave them more likely to produce miscarriages, premature births, and mentally and physically damaged infants. Once born, the lower-class child faces conditions of malnutrition, infection, and inadequate health care that may lead to maldevelopment of the central nervous system and mental retardation. (pp. 67–68)

Children born in poor families will be disadvantaged in developing their adult earning power by inferior schooling, an oppressive financial environment, and poor health as described by Parenti. Once they enter the adult world, they may be able to earn an adequate income to keep themselves and their children out of poverty, or their own children may also grow up in poverty (Perlman, 1976).

The presence of children in families headed by women is the basis of high poverty rates among women and children in such families. The poverty rate rises as the number of children in a low-income family increases. Contrary to popular belief, however, there is no tendency for low-income families to have more children than those families higher on the income scale.

To prevent poverty after sixty-five years of age, individuals must plan throughout their working life to defer or save income that can be used for support once they stop earning a regular income. Social Security benefits provide some support to the elderly, and often these may be the only support available. Some workers participate in pension plans that provide an income after a lifetime of work, but many employees, especially blue-collar and low-level white-collar workers, still do not have the opportunity to participate in such programs. Over 12 percent of all persons older than sixty-five have an income under the poverty level (U.S. Bureau of the Census, 1988). More than half of all Americans who live below the poverty level are elderly (Parenti, 1988).

In a society in which high ranking is given individuals who either control wealth or are productive in the labor force, persons who do not contribute to this production are assigned a low status. Many elderly persons receive financial and medical support from the government, making them nonproductive drawers of the nation's wealth. Often they are accorded little deference and instead face impatience, patronization, and neglect by persons still in the work force.

SOCIOECONOMIC IDENTIFICATION

Most Americans, if asked, could identify themselves by class. Whereas they do not strongly vocalize their identity with a specific class, they participate socially and occupationally within a class structure. Their behavior and value system may be based on a strong ethnic or religious identification, but that specific identification is greatly influenced by class level. For example, although the professional Italian-American family may share the ethnic ethos of the blue-collar Italian-American family, the professional family will interact primarily with other professional families of Italian-American descent and of other ethnic origins instead of interacting with Italian-Americans at a different class level. Many of their primary relationships may be with other Italian-Americans, but these will be developed at the same socioeconomic level. The first generation of a group that has moved to the middle class may continue to interact at a primary level with friends and relatives who are in the working class and underclass. However, time and differences in circumstances often lead to the reduction of those cross-class ties.

Most Americans exhibit and articulate less concern about class consciousness than many of their European counterparts. Nevertheless, many have participated in class actions like strikes or work stoppages to further interests of the class to which they belong (Vanneman & Cannon, 1987). Class consciousness, or solidarity with others at the same socioeconomic level, may not be so pronounced here because there has been overall improvement in the standard of living at all levels, especially during the period from 1940 to the early 1970s. In addition, American cultural values and belief systems emphasize the individual's personal responsibility for his or her class position (Rothman, 1978).

Class consciousness is probably strongest and most developed among the upper class. They may represent the only group that sees the value of solidarity in the protection and maintenance of their power and privilege. Fissures within all other classes in terms of income, occupation, ethnicity, race, and gender prevent coalition around socioeconomic concerns.

In the classroom, teachers are likely to find students from diverse socioeconomic backgrounds. Unless one teaches in a private preparatory school, the teacher is unlikely to find children of the upper class in the classroom. Students may not identify themselves as members of a specific class, but they can identify the factors that determine their socioeconomic status. They usually know the occupation of their parents, the area of the city in which they live, the amount of education of their parents, the amount of education that they plan to seek, and their parents' involvement or noninvolvement in civic and other organizations. Even more important in determining class status are ethnicity, age, and sex. These factors will continue to influence unequal socioeconomic outcomes until institutional discrimination is overcome.

Students, like everyone else, tend to interact most with other students with whom they feel most comfortable. In most instances, the significant peer group will include students from the same socioeconomic level and the same or similar ethnic background. They share the same cultural values and patterns and have been influenced similarly by socioeconomic conditions and environments beyond their control. They have learned to react to the environment in a similar way.

EDUCATIONAL IMPLICATIONS

Many social reformers, educators, and parents view education as a powerful device for achieving social change and the elimination of poverty. From the beginning of the public school movement in the early nineteenth century, low incomes of the poor were believed to result from inadequate education. Discrimination in employment and housing was blamed on the lack of education in other segments of the population. This view was still pervasive in the 1960s as the federal government attempted to eliminate poverty through the establishment and funding of Head Start, Title I (compensatory education), Job Corps, Neighborhood Youth Corps, and other educational programs. However, test scores of disadvantaged students have not appeared to improve, racial segregation has increased, and inner-city and rural schools have made few changes (Carnoy & Levin, 1976).

This lack of progress in overcoming the effects of poverty on students should not suggest that educational reforms are not worthwhile. Some changes make schooling more attractive to students and even increase the achievement of many individual students; educational resources also become more equitably distributed. Nevertheless, the intended goal of increasing income equity and eliminating poverty is never realized. Different sociohistorical interpretations of education explain the role of schools in society and the degree to which this goal and others are met. Two views are prevalent. One "assumes that the schools exist as an agent of social reform and that the limits of their ability to change society are conditioned only by the limits of our imagination and the difficulties of obtaining consensus" (Carnoy & Levin, 1976, p. 24). The second view assumes that schools exist as an agent of the larger social, economic, and political context, with the goal of inculcating the values necessary to maintain the current socioeconomic and political systems.

Supporters of the first view are much more benign in their description of the role of schools in helping students become socially mobile. They are optimistic that social reform can be achieved by providing poor students with more and better schools. Others see schools as preparing students to work efficiently at appropriate levels in corporate organizations. The needs of business and industry are met "by developing lower-class children to be better workers and middle-class ones to be better managers in the corporate economy and by reproducing the social relations of production in the schools to inculcate children with values and norms supportive of capitalist work organizations" (Carnoy & Levin, 1976, p. 10). Students are tracked in courses for either college or vocational preparation. The curriculum sorts and selects children so that children of blue-collar or unemployed workers and children of the elite will be socialized for jobs that they later will hold. Thus, rather than providing equal educational opportunity, schools perpetuate existing social and economic inequities in society.

Teacher Expectations

Students in most classrooms are likely to represent a number of socioeconomic statuses or classes except for the upper class. In addition, they are likely to be heterogeneous in terms of ethnicity, religious background, and conditions of exceptionality. Thus, the teacher may not be able to easily identify from which class or socioeconomic level a student comes. Too often, however, teachers do classify their students by class and assign certain expectations to students based on perceived class status. Students at the lower ranges of socioeconomic status often are expected to be academically inferior and to exhibit disruptive behavior. Many of these students are hampered academically by such expectations. Students with a high socioeconomic status usually benefit from a teacher's judgments because they are expected to perform better in school, are treated more favorably, and do perform at a higher level in many cases.

"Patterns of lower achievement and underparticipation for minorities and poor children begin early in the educational process. And perhaps most troublesome is that the discrepancies among groups grow larger the longer children remain in school" (Oakes, 1987, p. 3). Differences in mathematics and science achievement based on class and race are found by age nine, but are clearly in place by age thirteen. In junior high school, students in subordinate groups typically take fewer courses in mathematics and science, which contributes to later differences in college enrollments and vocational choices. In many schools with large minority and poor populations, advanced courses in these subjects are often not even offered. Thus, even those students who are achieving at a level equal to students from the dominant group are further stifled in their attempts to achieve equitably. "The existence of these discrepancies does document that schools have been considerably less successful with some groups of students than with others" (Oakes, 1987, p. 3).

In an ethnographic study of an inner-city school, Rist (1970) documented how students are classified, segregated, and taught differently starting with their first days in school. Most teachers can identify those personal characteristics of students that will lead to academic success; they then develop instruction and interaction with their students that ensure that the students will, in fact, behave as the teachers expect—a phenomenon called the *self-fulfilling prophecy*. Rist found that the kindergarten teacher was able to divide students into three reading and mathematics groups as early as the eighth day of school. While such groupings may be helpful in providing the most effective instruction to students who enter the classroom with different skills, the researcher found that the groups were organized by nonacademic factors. Students in the highest group were all dressed in clean clothes that were relatively new and well pressed; they interacted well with the teacher and other students; they were quite verbal and used standard English; and they came from "better families." Students in the lower two groupings were poorly dressed and often in dirty clothes; they frequently carried the odor of urine; they used black dialect; and their families were less stable than those of students in the highest group. Throughout the year, the teacher interacted more with the students in the highest group than with either of the other groups. This division of students and the teacher's differing degrees of involvement with the three groups continued through the second grade, at which time the study ended. Students in the highest group continually performed better academically and behaved in a more acceptable manner than students in the other two groups. As the kindergarten teacher had projected, these students were more successful in school than the students from lower socioeconomic levels.

When teachers make such judgments about students, they may be preventing individuals from reaching their fullest potential. Rather than ensuring that students have access to an egalitarian system, such classification and subsequent treatment of students ensure the maintenance of an inequitable system. "This, of course, is in contrast to the formal doctrine of education in this country to ameliorate rather than aggravate the conditions of the poor" (Rist, 1970, p. 106). Rist further states:

> When a teacher bases her [his] expectations of performance on the social status of the student and assumes that the higher the social status, the higher the potential of the child, those children of low status suffer a stigmatization outside of their own choice or will. Yet there is a greater tragedy than being labeled as a slow learner, and that is being treated as one. (p. 107)

Educational researchers continue to find that simply being in the low-ability group diminishes students' achievement. Students are provided fewer and poorer opportunities to learn than other students. Critical thinking tasks are reserved for the high-ability groups. Oral recitation and structured written work are common in low-ability groups. Students are exposed to low-status knowledge at a slower pace than their peers in higher-ability groups, helping them fall further behind in subjects like mathematics, foreign languages, and sciences (Gamoran & Berends, 1987).

Teachers in low-ability classrooms spend more time on administration and discipline and less time actually teaching. As one might expect, student behavior in low tracks is more disruptive than in higher-level groups, but this probably happens in part because students and teachers have developed behavioral standards more tolerant of inattention rather than because of the students' individual ability (Peterson, Wilkinson, & Hallinan, 1984). To compound the problem, the more experienced and more successful teachers are disproportionately assigned to the higher-ability groups. Further, teachers generally view high-track students positively and low-track students negatively (Gamoran & Berends, 1987).

Disproportionately large numbers of students from lower socioeconomic levels are assigned to low-ability groups beginning very early in their school careers. The long-term effects are similar to those Rist found in the 1960s. These students are seen by teachers as less able academically, classed where they belong, and perhaps condemned to that level for the rest of their academic lives (Peterson et al., 1984). Even more tragic is the fact that the number of students from low socioeconomic levels classified as mentally retarded is disproportionately high. This type of classification causes double jeopardy for students of color because they are disproportionately in poverty or at the low end of the economic scale.

How can we prevent the development of negative and harmful expectations for students? Teachers, counselors, and administrators must be aware that they can easily fall into such behavior. They must consciously review their expectations. It is helpful to systematically evaluate interactions with students. Such evaluations should indicate whether certain students are receiving more of the teacher's attention or are being encouraged to participate in the learning process to a greater degree. Necessary corrections in instructional methods and student-teacher interactions can then be made to ensure that all students in the classroom have access to one's best teaching skills.

Seeing students as individuals rather than members of a specific socioeconomic group also may assist the educator in overcoming class biases that may exist in the school and community. Information about a student's family background must not be used to rationalize stereotypes and label students. It can be used to understand the power of environment on a student's expression of self (Lightfoot, 1983). Educators must be aware of any prejudices that they themselves hold against members of lower socioeconomic groups. Otherwise, discriminatory practices will surface in the classroom in the form of self-fulfilling prophecies that harm students and perpetuate societal inequities.

Finally, in inner-city schools, the educator will face large numbers of poor and working-class students whose environment outside the school is very dissimilar from that of students in most suburban schools. Isolated rural areas require families to respond to their nonschool environment much differently than families in other areas. Educators should not expect to be able to teach every student effectively in the same way. Equal education does not mean that the same instructional strategies must be used to teach all students. While it is essential to ensure that all students learn the basic skills, how the educator teaches these skills may vary, depending on the environment in which students live—a factor greatly dependent on the family's socioeconomic status.

Curriculum and Instruction

The discussion so far has focused on teachers' expectations for students based on socioeconomic status. However, that is not the only area of the instructional program that needs to be changed to teach all students effectively regardless of the class position of their families. The curriculum should also reflect accurately the socioeconomic structure and inequities that exist in the United States.

The most common strategy for working with economically disadvantaged students has been *compensatory education.* In this program, extra resources are made available to schools to help overcome the educational deficiencies of poor students and increase their academic achievement. It is based, in part, on the belief that students from the lower socioeconomic levels do not learn as quickly or as well as other students and that their families have been unable to provide an intellectually stimulating environment that will assist them in school. Compensatory programs are most often remedial in nature to help students catch up with their middle-class counterparts.

Carnoy and Levin (1976) recommend a positive alternative to current compensatory education programs. Their strategy contradicts the theory of poor and good learners and instead assumes that learning is conditional:

> All groups of children can learn equally well but under different conditions. We may find that children's motivation is affected much more by the structure of the learning environment than by the number of years of teacher's academic preparation. The low probability of success of compensatory programs within the existing framework points to the need for new educational strategies for ethnic and racial minorities if equality is to be achieved. The solution may be to change schooling for all children and to create an educational process that does not preconceive social roles or even clearly define what or how a child must learn. This process would require new kinds of tests to measure results and a different kind of teacher to produce them. Education of this type could allow a child's own stereotypes of himself [herself] and others to be destroyed and be replaced by personal relationships. The alternative strategy, then, creates equality among groups of children, by building an educational structure that allows children to express themselves in various ways, all equally acceptable. (pp. 215–216)

Often overlooked are the experiences brought to the classroom by students. School is definitely not the only place in which students learn about life. Differences in school behavior and knowledge among students from dissimilar socioeconomic levels are strongly dependent on the knowledge and skills needed to survive appropriately in their community environments. Most poor students, especially those in urban areas, have learned how to live in a world that is not imaginable to most middle-class students. Yet the knowledge and skills that they bring to school are not valued by teachers and a system with a middle-class orientation. Educators must recognize the value of the community's informal education in sustaining its own culture and realize that formal education is often viewed as undermining that culture (Lightfoot, 1983).

The curriculum does not serve students well if it reflects only the perspective of middle-class America. Students need to see some of their own cultural values reflected in the curriculum. They need to be helped to see themselves as desirable and integral members of the school community rather than as second-class citizens who must learn the ways of the more economically advantaged to succeed even in school.

Educators should become cognizant of the materials, films, and books used in class. If students never see their communities in these instructional materials, their motivation and acceptance are likely to be limited. All students should be encouraged to read novels and short stories about people from different socioeconomic levels. When studying historical or current events, they should examine the event from the perspective of those in poverty as well as from the perspective of our country's leaders. Teaching can be enhanced by drawing examples from experiences with which students are familiar, even if they are different from the teacher's own experiences.

Instruction should show that not all persons share equally in material things in this country, but that all persons have potential to be developed. All students, no matter what their level of socioeconomic status, must be helped to develop strong and positive self-concepts. Many students do not realize the diversity that exists in this country, let alone understand the reasons for the diversity. Most middle-class children, especially those of white-collar and professional levels, believe that most persons are as well off as they are. As educators, we are expected to expand our students' knowledge of the world, not to hide from them the realities that exist because of class differences.

SUMMARY

Socioeconomic status (SES) is a composite of the economic status of a family or unrelated individuals based on income, wealth, occupation, educational attainment, and power. It is a means of measuring inequalities based on economic differences and the manner in which families live as a result of their economic well-being. Families' socioeconomic statuses range from the indigent poor to the very rich. Where a family falls along this continuum affects the manner in which its members live, how they think and act, and the way in which others react to them (Rothman, 1978). Persons who share the same class form a microculture. Although a family may participate actively in other microcultural groups centered around ethnicity, religion, gender, exceptionality, language, or age, the class to which the family belongs is probably the strongest factor in determining differences among groups.

Social stratification is possible because consistent and recurring relationships exist between people who occupy different levels of the social structure. Minorities, women, young and old people, and handicapped individuals are disproportionately represented at the low end of our social stratification system.

Americans can be divided into a number of classes based on their income and occupation. In this chapter, the following classes were described: underclass, working class, middle class, and upper class. The income and wealth that keeps families at one of these levels vary greatly. Individual choice is most limited for those persons who are poor and who often can barely meet essential needs. Whereas ethnic and religious diversity exists at all levels, the upper class is the most homogeneous. Minorities and women who head families are overly represented in the underclass, working class, and lower middle class.

One's socioeconomic level has a dramatic influence on how one is able to live, but Americans exhibit and articulate less concern about class consciousness than their European counterparts. Although they may not verbalize their class identification, most of their primary relations are conducted within the same class. Class consciousness is strongest among the upper classes, whose members know the value of solidarity in the protection and maintenance of their power and privilege.

Disproportionately large numbers of students from lower levels of socioeconomic status are assigned to low-ability groups in their early school years. Educators must consciously review their expectations for students and their behavior toward students from different levels of socioeconomic status to ensure that they are not discriminating. Instructional methods and teaching strategies may vary greatly, depending on the environment in which students live. What is essential is that all students be provided a quality education.

Educators also need to pay attention to the curriculum. Too often, poor students are placed in remedial programs because of discriminatory testing and placement. In addition, the curriculum does not serve students well if it reflects only the perspective of middle-class America. Students need to see some of their own cultural values reflected in the curriculum in addition to learning about the cultural values of others.

QUESTIONS FOR REVIEW

1. What factors promote social stratification, and how do they do it?

2. Describe the different social stratification and class theories discussed in this chapter, indicating how they differ from each other.

3. Explain why the United States is not the model of egalitarianism that many believe it to be.

4. Develop an argument against the statement, "Social mobility is possible for anyone who works hard enough."

5. Describe the mythical middle class, and explain why it does not match reality.

6. Why are blue-collar workers often called the working class?

7. What socioeconomic factors make it difficult for members of the underclass to improve their conditions?

8. Why did the authors separate the middle class into two distinct categories?

9. Contrast the two perspectives on why the schools have not been able to eliminate poverty.

10. Define the self-fulfilling prophecy, and explain why it is appropriately addressed in a chapter on class.

REFERENCES

Auletta, K. (1982). *The Underclass.* New York: Random House.

Beeghley, L. (1978). *Social stratification in America: A critical analysis of theory and research.* Santa Monica, CA: Goodyear.

Boyer, E. (1983). *High school: A report on secondary education in America.* New York: Harper & Row.

Carnoy, M., & Levin, H. M. (1976). *The limits of educational reform.* New York: McKay.

Cookson, P. W., & Persell, C. H. (1985). *Preparing for power: America's elite boarding schools.* New York: Basic Books.

Gamoran, A., & Berends, M. (1987, Winter). The effects of stratification in secondary schools: Synthesis of survey and ethnographic research. *Review of Educational Research, 57*(4), 415–435.

Gilbert, D., & Kahl, J. A. (1982). *The American class structure: A new synthesis.* Homewood, IL: Dorsey Press.

Gorder, C. (1988). *Homeless!: Without addresses in America: The social crisis of the decade.* Tempe, AZ: Blue Bird.

Harrington, M. (1984). *The new American poverty.* New York: Holt, Rinehart & Winston.

Hodgkinson, H. (1986). *The schools we need for the kids we've got.* Paper presented at the 1987 annual meeting of the American Association of Colleges for Teacher Education.

Jencks, C., Smith, M., Acland, H., Bane, M. J., Cohen, D., Gintis, H., Heyns, B., & Michelson, S. (1972). *Inequality: A reassessment of the effect of family and schooling in America.* New York: Harper & Row.

Levitan, S. A., & Shapiro, I. (1987). *Working but poor.* Baltimore: The Johns Hopkins University Press.

Levy, F. (1986). Poverty and economic growth. Unpublished manuscript, University of Maryland, School of Public Affairs, College Park, MD.

Lewis, M. (1978). *The culture of inequality.* Amherst, MA: University of Massachusetts Press.

Lewis, O. (1969). *A death in the Sanchez family.* New York: Random House.

Liebow, E. (1967). *Tally's corner: A study of Negro street corner men.* Boston: Little, Brown.

Lightfoot, S. L. (1983). *The good high school: Portraits of character and culture.* New York: Basic Books.

Oakes, J. (1987, April). *Race, class, and school responses to "ability": Interactive influences on math and science outcomes.* Paper presented at the annual meeting of the American Educational Research Association, Washington, DC.

Parenti, M. (1978). *Power and the powerless.* New York: St. Martin's Press.

Parenti, M. (1988). *Democracy for the few* (5th ed.). New York: St. Martin's Press.

Parker, R. (1972). *The myth of the middle class: Notes on affluence and equality.* New York: Liveright.

Perlman, R. (1976). *The economics of poverty.* New York: McGraw-Hill.

Peterson, P., Wilkinson, L. C., & Hallinan, M. (Eds.). (1984). *The social context of instruction: Group organization and group processes.* New York: Academic Press.

Rist, R. C. (1970). Student social class and teacher expectations: The self-fulfilling prophecy in ghetto education. *Harvard Educational Review, 40*(3), 70–110.

Rodgers, H. R. (1986). *Poor women, poor families.* Armonk, NY: Sharpe.

Rossides, D. W. (1976). *The American class system: An introduction to social stratification.* Boston: Houghton Mifflin.

Rothman, R. A. (1978). *Inequality and stratification in the United States.* Englewood Cliffs, NJ: Prentice-Hall.

U.S. Bureau of Labor Statistics. (1979). *Handbook of labor statistics* (Bulletin 2000). Washington, D.C.: Government Printing Office.

U.S. Bureau of Labor Statistics. (1988, December). *Employment and earnings.* Washington, DC: Government Printing Office.

U.S. Bureau of the Census. (1988). *Statistical Abstract of the United States, 1988* (108th ed.). Washington, DC: Government Printing Office.

U.S. Employment Service. (1977). *Dictionary of occupational titles* (4th ed.). Washington, DC: Government Printing Office.

Valentine, C. A. (1968). *Culture and poverty: Critique and counter-proposals.* Chicago: The University of Chicago Press.

Vanneman, R., & Cannon, L. W. (1987). *The American perception of class.* Philadelphia: Temple University Press.

Wilson, J. O. (1980). *After affluence: Economics to meet human needs.* New York: Harper & Row.

Wilson, W. J. (1987). *The truly disadvantaged: The inner city, the underclass, and public policy.* Chicago: The University of Chicago Press.

SUGGESTED READINGS

Carnoy, M., & Levin, H. M. (1976). *The limits of educational reform.* New York: McKay.

An analysis of educational reforms that have been designed to overcome poverty and inequality, particularly compensatory education. Questions the premise that educational reform can resolve social dilemmas that arise out of the basic nature of the economic, political, and social system.

Kozol, J. (1988). *Rachel and her children: Homeless families in America.* New York: Crown.

A chronicle of the lives of homeless families headed by women. Provides descriptions of life in emergency shelters and welfare hotels and the humiliation felt by these women and their children.

Lightfoot, S. L. (1978). *Worlds apart: Relationships between families and schools.* New York: Basic Books.

An investigation of the interaction of family and school on children. Explores the conflict between the home and teachers, especially for black and working-class students. Provides insightful examples of different types of teacher reactions and strategies to working with students from different cultural backgrounds.

Lightfoot, S. L. (1983). *The good high school: Portraits of character and culture.* New York: Basic Books.

> *Portraits of six exemplary U.S. high schools, including two inner-city schools, two upper-middle-class suburban schools, and two elite prep schools. Describes personalities of principals, teachers, and students; teaching styles; curricula; and school climate.*

Parenti, M. (1988). *Democracy for the few* (5th ed.). New York: St. Martin's Press.

> *An analysis of socioeconomic differences, class, and inequality in the United States. Describes the role of politics and government in maintaining inequalities.*

Peterson, P., Wilkinson, L. C., & Hallinan, M. (Eds.). (1984). *The social context of instruction: Group organization and group processes.* New York: Academic Press.

> *A collection of research papers that discuss ability grouping, tracking of students, influence of group culture on student behavior, independent and group learning, peer interaction in the learning process, and teacher expectations. Questions the value of tracking and ability groups for so-called low-ability students.*

Vanneman, R., & Cannon, L. W. (1987). *The American perception of class.* Philadelphia: Temple University Press.

> *An analysis of class consciousness in the United States that empirically refutes the myth that Americans are not class conscious. Examines class theory, the social psychology of stratification, and the interaction of class with gender and race.*

CHAPTER 3
Ethnicity and Race

In the United States, the indigenous Native American people make up less than 1 percent of the total population. The majority of Americans are recent immigrants or have ancestors who were immigrants. According to the *Harvard Encyclopedia of American Ethnic Groups*, this nation is composed of at least 276 different ethnic groups, including 170 different Native American groups. All of us could trace our ancestry to one or more nations that existed at one time in history.

For those of us whose families emigrated here over the past four hundred years, the reasons for coming have varied greatly. Most Africans originally were imported involuntarily to this country to provide labor for an expanding Southern agricultural economy. Many immigrants in the nineteenth and twentieth centuries voluntarily came to the United States to escape oppressive political, religious, or economic conditions. At the same time, they were encouraged to immigrate by the dominant group to meet the expanding labor needs of a developing industrial nation. Some of today's immigrants come to join family members who have already settled here. Others are fleeing oppressive conditions in their native countries, and still others are seeking the perceived advantages of U.S. citizenship.

Many of us forget that the United States was already populated by the time Europeans arrived on its shores. As more and more foreigners arrived, the native population became the enemy of the newcomers. Government policies did not treat Native Americans as equal citizens in the formation of a new nation; at best, the policies were patronizing. Eventually, these Native Americans were forced into segregation from the dominant group and, in many cases, moved from their geographical homeland to reservations in other parts of the country—a phenomenon that still exists today for many Native Americans.

Although most of the first European settlers were English, the French, Dutch, and Spanish also established early settlements. After the consolidation and development of the United States as an independent state, successive waves of western Europeans immigrated. These included the Irish, Swedes, and Germans. The primary reasons for immigration were internal economic impoverishment and political repression in the countries of origin and the demands of a vigorous U.S. economy that required an expanded labor force.

People of African descent have been a part of the American experience from the early days of colonization. The thousands of Africans who were kidnapped and sold into bondage underwent a unique process that was quite different from that of the Asian and European immigrants who voluntarily emigrated. Separated from their families and homelands, robbed of their freedom and culture, they developed a new culture out of their different African heritages and unique experiences in this country.

Initially, the majority of Africans lived in the South. Because their labor power was essential in the production of cotton needed for northern industries after the Civil War, they remained the majority population in many counties across the southern states. However, in the past century, sizable communities of African-Americans have developed outside the historical areas of concentration in the Black Belt South. Today, black communities can be found in numerous northern, eastern, and western cities. The migration of African-Americans to northern cities generally has been fueled by the same mechanisms that brought eastern and southern Europeans to the United States. Once immigrant labor was halted after World War I and additional labor was needed in northern cities, African-Americans migrated in large numbers to urban areas to obtain the industrial jobs that had become available.

Racism and political terror in the Black Belt South, along with jobs and broader political rights in other parts of the country, helped initiate the migration to the North and West. Nevertheless, the racial ideology of the dominant majority continues to block significant assimilation of the masses of African-Americans into the dominant society. The civil rights movement of the 1960s reduced the political barriers that prevented most African-Americans from enjoying the advantages of the middle class. In the past twenty-five years, the number of families and individuals who have been able to join the ranks of the middle class has increased dramatically. At the same time, the number of African-Americans who remain in poverty is disproportionately high.

Mexican-Americans also occupy a unique role in the formation of the United States. Spain was the first European country to colonize Mexico and the North American West and Southwest. In 1848, the U.S. government annexed the northern sections of Mexican Territory, including Texas, Arizona, New Mexico, and southern California. The Mexican population and various Native American peoples living within that territory became an oppressed minority within the area in which they had previously been the dominant population. Dominant supremacy theories based on color and language also were used against these ethnic groups in a way that prevents them even today from assimilating fully into the dominant culture.

Later immigrants came from the relatively more impoverished eastern and southern European countries. At the end of the nineteenth and beginning of the twentieth centuries, large numbers of immigrants arrived from nations such as Poland, Hungary, Italy, Russia, and Greece. The reasons for immigration were the same as for earlier immigrants—devastating economic and political hardships in the homeland and demand for labor in the United States. The industrial opening of the West in the nineteenth century signaled the need for labor that could be met through immigration from Asia. Thus, Chinese, Japanese, and Filipino workers were encouraged to enter the country to provide the labor needed on the West Coast.

Many of these immigrants came to the United States with the hope of sharing the better wages and living conditions that they thought existed here. Many found conditions much worse than they had expected. Most were forced to live in run-down housing near the business and manufacturing districts where they worked. Most lived in urban ghettos that grew into ethnic enclaves in which others from the same country continued to use the native language; ethnic institutions were developed to support the immigrants' social and welfare needs.

Just as dominant racist policies had been used against African-Americans and Native Americans earlier, they came to be used against these immigrants. At various times, Congress prohibited the immigration of different national or ethnic groups on the basis of racial superiority of the older, established immigrant groups that had colonized the nation. As early as 1729, immigration was being discouraged. In that

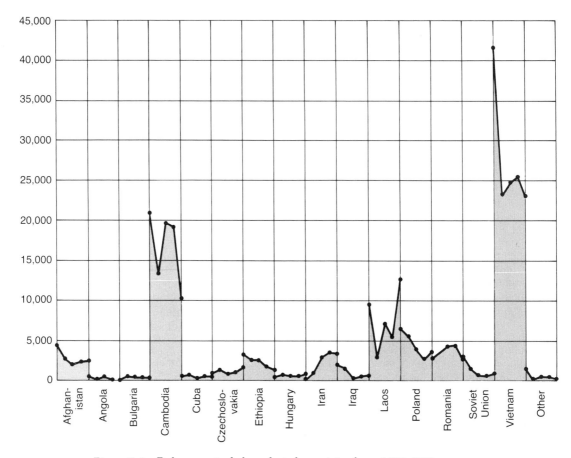

Figure 3-1   Refugee arrivals by selected countries form 1982–1986.

year, Pennsylvania passed a statute that increased the head tax on foreigners in that colony. Later that century, Congress passed the Alien and Sedition Acts, which lengthened the time required to become a citizen from five years to fourteen years. In the nineteenth century, native-born Americans began to worry about their majority and superiority status over entering immigrant groups. This movement, nativism, was designed to restrict immigration and protect the interests of the native-born Americans. It was an extreme form of nationalism and ethnocentrism.

In 1881, Congress passed the Chinese Exclusion Act, which halted all immigration from China. The Dillingham Commission reported in 1917 that all immigrants should be able to pass a literacy test. The nativists received further support for their views when Congress passed the Johnson-Reed Act in 1924, which discriminated against southern and eastern Europeans and nonwhite nations; the act also stopped all immigration from Japan. The act was written so that the annual immigrant quotas were disproportionately large for citizens from western European countries.

The Johnson-Reed Act was not abolished until 1965, when a new quota system was established that allowed 170,000 persons from the eastern hemisphere and 120,000 from the western hemisphere to immigrate annually. This change in the immigration law has allowed the influx of immigrants from nations that formerly were restricted or excluded. Thus, the nation continues to become even more multiethnic with the larger number of immigrants now from non-European nations.

Refugees are also sometimes admitted under special acts of Congress. Favoritism is granted to refugees who are fleeing Communist regimes like Vietnam, Cuba, and Afghanistan. Refugees from countries supported by the United States, no matter how oppressive the government may be, are often refused entry. Haitians and most Central Americans are usually turned away. Figure 3-1 shows the number of refugees from different countries who have been admitted between 1982 and 1986. As a result of government immigration and refugee policies, the composition of the U.S. population from various national and ethnic groups has been controlled.

Thus, persons from all over the globe joined Native Americans in populating this nation, bringing with them different cultural experiences. The conditions they encountered, the reasons they came, and their expectations about life here differed greatly, causing each ethnic group to view itself as distinct from other ethnic groups. Although we all share a common history, our experiences in that history have varied greatly from group to group.

ETHNIC AND RACIAL GROUPS

The identification with others who have the same ancestral background is called *ethnicity*. It is a sense of peoplehood, and it comes from the Greek word *ethnos*, meaning "people" or "nation." Members of an ethnic group "feel themselves bound together by a common history, values, attitudes, and behaviors—in its broadest sense, a sense of peoplehood" (Yetman, 1985, p. 6). This feeling of peoplehood is commonly developed through family, friends, and neighbors with whom we share the same intimate characteristics of living. These are the people invited to baptisms, marriages, funerals, and family reunions. These are the people with whom we feel the most comfortable. They know the meaning of our behavior; they perform the same rituals and patterns regarding such things as eating, grooming, marrying, flirting, and raising children.

There is a uniqueness about an individual, a family, and sometimes a neighborhood that can be identified as clearly ethnic by an outsider. Often this distinction is made because of the physical characteristics of individuals or the distinct language and shops in a neighborhood. Other times the distinction is based on observed behaviors.

Ethnicity is defined by the boundaries established by the group, and membership in the group is dependent on the nation from which one's ancestors came. Individuals in an ethnic group share a history, a language (whether or not they can speak the language), a value system and structure, customs and traditions, an economic life, and former geographical area. Some groups choose, or have been forced, to acculturate or assimilate quickly into the dominant society upon entry in the United States. Other groups try to maintain their ethnic origins. To maintain the group identity from generation to generation, the attitudes, values, behaviors, and rituals are practiced in the family, church, and social clubs. In many cases, families fight the assimilative aspects of schooling that draw children into adopting the dress, language, music, and values of their peers from the dominant culture. Endogamy, segregated residential areas, and restriction of activities with the dominant group are means of trying to preserve ethnic cohesiveness across generations.

Often the group identity is reinforced by the political and economic barriers established by the dominant society to prevent the assimilation of subordinate groups. Ethnicity is strongest within groups that develop group solidarity through similar life-styles, common social and economic interests, a high degree of interpersonal associations developed through working relationships, and common residential areas (Yancey, Ericksen & Juliani, 1985). Historically, oppressed groups have often been segregated from the dominant group and have developed enclaves in cities and suburbs that help members maintain a strong ethnic identity.

However, a person does not have to live in the same community with other members of the ethnic group to continue to identify with the group. The boundaries are maintained by ascription from within the group as well as from external sources that place persons in a specific group because of the way they look, the color of their skin, the location of their home, or their name. Although many individuals are several generations removed from an immigrant status, some continue to choose consciously to emphasize their ethnicity as a meaningful basis of their identity. In this case, whether to maintain one's identity with an ethnic group becomes a choice and is no longer ascriptive. Gans (1985) labels this identification as symbolic ethnicity that is "characterized by a nostalgic allegiance to the culture of the immigrant generation, or that of the old country; a love for and a pride in a tradition that can be felt without having to be incorporated into everyday behavior" (p. 435). As the dominant society views a particular ethnic group as less distinct, the more voluntary ethnicity becomes to its members.

On the other hand, many people whose families have been in the United States for several generations do not emphasize the national origin of their ancestors and do not view themselves as hyphenated Americans. The degree of identification with the original ethnic group varies from person to person and could be a matter of individual choice. Nonethnic identification is probably more likely among whites, especially when there has been intermarriage across several different ethnic groups. Since the Bureau of the Census did not ask citizens to identify themselves by an ethnic group until 1969, there are no significant data to show whether the trend is toward greater or lesser ethnic identification.

Ethnic Groups

Many definitions have been proposed for the term *ethnic group* over the past three decades. Gordon (1964) wrote that the ethnic identity of an American was based on national origin, religion, and race. More recent definitions have expanded the term to include sex and life-style (Pratte, 1979). For this discussion, however, ethnic group will be defined only as an individual's national origin or origins. Many authors identify Jewish Americans as an ethnic group, in part because many members of the Jewish faith emphasize their Jewishness, rather than their national origin, as the most meaningful basis of their identity. Jews from Germany, Spain, and India may share more commonalities because of religion than they share with non-Jewish Germans, Spaniards, or Indians. In this text, religious differences are examined separately from ethnicity, and thus Jewish Americans will be discussed in the chapter on religion.

A nation is a historically constituted stable community of people formed on the basis of a common language, territory, economic life, and psychological makeup or culture. Ethnic identity is determined by living in a nation or maintaining ancestral ties even after having emigrated from a country. The strongest support for the country of origin is usually based on continuing family ties in that country. However, family ties in the country of origin usually weaken after several generations. Without extensive tracing of the family lineage, most members of ethnic groups who have been in this country for a century could not identify relatives in their country of origin. Yet, support for the country of origin often continues to exist. For example, in the aftermath of the 1980 earthquake in Italy, Italian-Americans in all parts of the United States organized benefits to collect money for relief. When cuts are being made in foreign aid, ethnic groups have sometimes lobbied on behalf of their country of origin.

Many members of ethnic groups in the United States maintain some of the cultural uniqueness of their national origin. Often they also are viewed as members of a specific ethnic group by nonmembers. Some groups are forced into ethnic enclaves as a result of discrimination or socioeconomic factors and thus may tend to maintain their ethnic identity to a greater degree than those who do not live in the enclave. Other groups maintain their ethnic distinctiveness because of the advantage it provides.

Because of the unique nature of ethnic groups, both members and nonmembers have a tendency to focus on the traditional attitudes, behaviors, and customs of the group. However, the character of the ethnic group changes in differing degrees from its existence in the country of origin because of the group's experiences in the United States. Members within ethnic groups will have different attitudes and behaviors based on their experiences in the United States and the conditions in the country of origin at the time of emigration. Recent immigrants may have little in common with other ethnic group members whose ancestors immigrated a century or even twenty years before. At the same time, ethnic communities are undergoing constant change in population characteristics, locations, occupations, educational levels, and political and economic struggles. All of these aspects affect the nature of the group and its members.

Ethnic groups differ in cultural characteristics. The immigrants brought with them concepts of art, political styles, religious perspectives, and family styles (Greeley, 1974). Members are inherently ethnocentric; they regard their own cultural traits as natural, correct, and superior to those of other ethnic groups, who often are perceived as odd, amusing, inferior, or immoral (Yetman, 1985). The ethnic group allows for the maintenance of group cohesiveness; it helps sustain and enhance the ethnic identity of its members; and it establishes the social networks and communicative patterns that are important for the group's optimization of its position in society.

Some Americans can trace their roots to several nations. Marriage across ethnic groups gives children of such marriages a heritage of one or more ethnic groups. Many individuals, families, and groups in the United States have assimilated into the majority group and identify themselves as American only. Others maintain cultural ties with the nation from which their family emigrated; they often identify themselves as hyphenated Americans, such as Polish-Americans, Croatian-Americans, or Vietnamese-Americans. Ethnic groups that have recently immigrated here have not been assimilated and continue to manifest the culture and language of their nation of origin while learning to accommodate or assimilate the new culture. Oppressed minority groups, such as African-Americans, Mexican-Americans, Asian-Americans, and Native Americans, have historically been blocked from assimilation into the majority group and thus continue to identify strongly with their own ethnic groups.

The upper strata of oppressed ethnic groups naturally respond to existing injustices. They appeal to their "brothers and sisters" and begin to agitate about their lack of rights and power, claiming that their cause is the cause of the ethnic community as a whole. The broad masses within these ethnic groups do not always remain passive and unresponsive to these appeals. Sometimes they rally around the banner of these spokespersons because the harsh economic and political realities imposed on them by the dominant majority affect them even more than they do the upper strata of intellectuals and leaders. Thus, at different junctures, movements for democratic rights and economic justice are born among the different ethnic groups. These movements invariably entail a rise in the concern of the community with its original or indigenous culture, as this aspect of their lives also has been suppressed and excluded by the dominant majority.

This reaction was seen in the United States most recently in the civil rights movement of the 1960s as a result of African-Americans' recognition of their subordinate status in society. The call for black power followed years of civil rights struggle that led to the passage of the 1964 Civil Rights Act and the 1965 Voting Rights Act. Yet, changes were not apparent to most ethnic minorities. Although legislation guaranteed equality, many white Americans continued to fight desegregation of schools and other public facilities. Frustrations with the majority group led subordinate group members to identify strongly with other members of their ethnic group and to fight the discrimination and inequality with a unified voice.

Racial Groups

Are racial groups also ethnic groups? In the United States, many people use the two terms interchangeably. Race is a concept that was developed by physical anthropologists to assist them in describing the physical characteristics of people in the world. Racial groups include many ethnic groups, but ethnic groups may include members of one or more racial groups. How has such mixed usage of the terms developed in this country?

Race has been used by physical anthropologists during the last 200 years to describe groups of people by their physical attributes, including color of skin, texture of hair, shape of the nose, and other physical traits. These racial groups were classified into three major races—Caucasoid, Mongoloid, and Negroid—classifications that many of us learned in geography or history classes during our schooling. This classification system was further divided into a number of subgroups.

When people were isolated in geographical regions of the world, these distinctive racial groupings could be applied easily. However, racial groups have not remained isolated. Most countries now include members of all three major racial groups. In addition, reproduction among the racial groups has resulted in offspring of mixed racial heritages, perhaps even new racial groups. Within the major racial groupings, there has been reproduction across the subgroups. For example, the Caucasoid group includes the following subgroups: Alpines from central Europe, Nordics from northern Europe, and Mediterraneans from southern Europe. After persons from these three groups immigrated to the United States, intermarriage became more common than it would have if they had occupied distinct geographical areas in Europe. The children of such marriages have mixed racial ancestry from two different ethnic groups in most cases. Many African-Americans represent a mixture of two major racial groups, the Caucasoid and Negroid.

The usefulness of the term *race* to describe a group of people is very limited. In fact, the group of scientists who developed a 1950 UNESCO statement on race recommended that the term be dropped altogether (Montagu, 1972). Yet, racial classifications continue to be used to identify blacks, whites, Asians, and Native Americans. Knowing the race of a group provides little or no help in understanding the culture of that group. The UNESCO statement indicated that "national, religious, geographic, linguistic and cultural groups do not necessarily coincide with racial groups; and the cultural traits of such groups have not demonstrated genetic connection with racial traits" (p. 8).

Throughout U.S. history, racial identification has been used by policymakers and much of the population to classify groups of people as inferior or superior to another racial group. Some theorists (e.g., Ogbu, 1988, and Berreman, 1985) suggest that race as used in the United States is equivalent to caste in other countries. Both are "invidious distinctions imposed unalterably at birth upon whole categories of people to justify the unequal social distribution of power, livelihood, security, privilege, esteem, freedom—in short, life chances" (Barreman, 1985, p. 37).

Because the institutions of government in the United States were established by northern Europeans, power was also controlled by some members of that group, and thus, those individuals viewed themselves as the superior racial and ethnic group. At one time, slaves were viewed as so inferior to the dominant power group that they were counted by the government as three-tenths of a person. This phenomenon of racial consciousness in the United States was repeated on the West Coast in the late nineteenth century when Chinese immigrants of the Mongoloid racial group were charged an additional tax for their braids. Even the large influx of southern and eastern Europeans in the late nineteenth and early twentieth centuries led the dominant group to label the immigrants as inferior because they came from the Alpine and Mediterranean races. This feeling of the superiority of the Nordic race over all others became a popular and emotional issue of the American people during this period. It later led to the deadly Holocaust under German Nazism in World War II.

This American racist ideology was detailed in 1916 in *The Passing of the Great Race* by Madison Grant. Northern and western Europeans of the Nordic race were described as "the political and military genius of the world" (Higham, 1975, p. 221). Protecting the purity of the Nordic race became such an emotional and popular issue of the majority of U.S. citizens that laws were passed to severely limit immigration into this country from any region except northern European countries. Miscegenation laws legally prevented the marriage of whites to members of other races in many states until the Supreme Court declared the laws unconstitutional in 1967. The immigration quota system passed by Congress in 1921 remained in effect until it was repealed in 1965. The fact that race became a supreme value in state and federal law set the stage for the continued popular confusion between racial and ethnic identification today.

Once race identification was codified, it was acceptable, even necessary, to identify oneself by race. Federal forms and reports often classify the population based on a mixture of racial and language identification: white, black, Hispanic, Asian or Pacific Islander, and American Indian or Eskimo. The problem with identifying the U.S. population by such characteristics is that it tells little about the people in these groups. Although whites are numerically dominant, this classification includes many different ethnic groups. Moreover, the ethnic identification or actual racial heritage of African-Americans is not recognized by most observers. And the Hispanic grouping includes different racial groups and mixtures of racial groups as well as at least four distinct ethnic groups in this country: Mexican-Americans, Puerto Ricans, Cuban-Americans, and Central Americans.

Although ideas about racial superiority have found no support within the scientific community, many people continue to believe in the inferiority of nonwhite races. This belief can be observed in cases of mixed racial heritage. Individuals of black and white parentage are usually classified by observers as black, not white; those of Japanese-American and white heritage usually are classified as nonwhite. In some areas of the country, state laws specify that a small percentage of nonwhite heritage requires that one be classified as a minority group member, regardless of physical characteristics.

Race is no longer a function of biological or genetic differences among groups. It is a social category that is dependent on society's perception that differences exist and that these differences are important. Racial designations have become arbitrary and artificial, serving to isolate and separate groups of people in society (Yetman, 1985). In their study of racial formation in the United States, Omi and Winant (1986) discovered that

> historically, a variety of previously racially undefined groups have required
> categorization to situate them within the prevailing racial order. Throughout the
> nineteenth century, many state and federal legal arrangements recognized only three

racial categories: "white," Negro," and "Indian." In California, the influx of Chinese and the debates surrounding the legal status of Mexicans provoked a brief judicial crisis of racial definition. California attempted to resolve this dilemma by assigning Mexicans and Chinese to categories within the already existing framework of "legally defined" racial groups. In the wake of the Treaty of Guadalupe Hidalgo (1848), Mexicans were defined as a "white" population and accorded the political-legal status of "free white persons." By contrast, the California Supreme Court ruled in People v. Hall (1854) that Chinese should be considered "Indian" and denied the political rights accorded to whites. (p. 75)

African-Americans range in skin color along a continuum from white to black. Thus, it is not the color of their skin that defines them. It is based, in part, on sharing a common national origin that can be traced to numerous African tribes and European and Native American nations. African-Americans have become an ethnic group because they share a common history, language, economic life, and culture that have developed over four centuries of living in the United States.

Because individuals appear to be African-American is not an indication that they identify themselves as African-Americans. Some members will identify themselves as blacks. Others will identify themselves as a member of another specific ethnic group, for example, Puerto Rican or Nigerian-American or West Indian. Africans who are recent immigrants will probably identify themselves ethnically by the nation or tribe of origin. In the same way, Polish-Americans may be classified as white, but many will identify themselves as Polish-Americans rather than white.

To understand the cultural underpinnings of groups of people in the United States, ethnic and racial identity is often very important. Race has historically been important in this country only because racial identity singled out people as inferior to the Nordic race and thus made them eligible for discriminatory treatment. "Particular meanings, stereotypes and myths can change, but the presence of a system of racial meanings and stereotypes, of racial ideology, seems to be a permanent feature of U.S. culture" (Omi & Winant, 1986, p. 63).

Minority Groups

Minorities and *minority groups* are terms often used in discussions about ethnic groups and their relationships to the majority or dominant group in the United States and other countries. What determines whether an ethnic group is a minority group in a country? Although the term *minority* usually refers to a numerical minority, it is used in the ethnic context to connote a subordinate power position in society. Minority groups do not share in the benefits provided to the dominant majority group. Those minority groups without social, economic, or political power are sometimes referred to as oppressed groups. Numerical superiority does not guarantee majority status, as exemplified by the situation in South Africa, where thirteen million blacks are in a subordinate position to three million ruling whites.

Members of minority groups experience a wide range of discriminatory treatment and frequently are relegated to positions relatively low in the status structure of a society. Any ethnic group that does not have sufficient power to fulfill it political, economic, social, or cultural needs is in a subordinate position and can be regarded as an oppressed minority group (Teper, 1977). Minority status is also evident when an ethnic group must be constantly vigilant to see that its needs are met by society. Members of an oppressed group cannot be assured of receiving the same societal benefits as members of the majority group.

Ogbu (1988) has found that "subordinate minorities usually react to their subordination and exploitation by forming ambivalent or oppositional identities as well as oppositional cultural frames of reference" (p. 176). They do not view the attitudes and behaviors of the dominant group as appropriate for them. Many members of the minority group develop attitudes and behaviors that are clearly opposed to those of the dominant group. Minority group members who cross the boundaries into the dominant group "may experience both internal opposition or identity crisis and external opposition or peer and community pressures" (Ogbu, 1988, p. 176).

This opposition becomes very important in schooling because many subordinate groups (especially African-Americans, Mexican-Americans, and Native Americans) equate schooling with accepting the culture of the dominant group and giving up their own cultural identity. They believe "that in order for a minority person to succeed, academically, in school, he or she must learn to think and act white" (Ogbu, 1988, p. 177). In many cases, minority students resist assimilation by developing strategies of resistence, including poor academic achievement (Fordham, 1988; Gibson, 1988; Ogbu, 1988).

In the United States, minority status more often than ethnic identity has come to be identified with races other than white. Institutions in this country, for the most part, were developed and continued to be controlled by members of the majority group. Because members of this majority group are white, it is easy to identify those persons who are not members. Minority members usually have unique physical or cultural characteristics that make them easily identifiable. They have been, and in most cases continue to be, victims of racism and negative stereotypes, and they are usually disproportionately represented in the lower classes of society.

Native American peoples, African-Americans, and Mexican-Americans have long histories of oppression in the United States. Asian-American, Puerto Rican, and southern and eastern European ethnic groups have more recent histories of subordination, but most of the European groups have now become accepted as part of the majority. Immigrants from the Middle East, Central America, and Southeast Asia are the latest ethnic groups that suffer from an oppressed minority status.

INTERETHNIC RELATIONS

An area that has received a lot of media coverage is interethnic relations in the United States. This attention extends into the schools. Fights between students from different ethnic backgrounds are often described as ethnic or racial in origin, rather than personal. Educators express concern about developing and maintaining positive interethnic relations among students, teachers, and the communities. An examination of

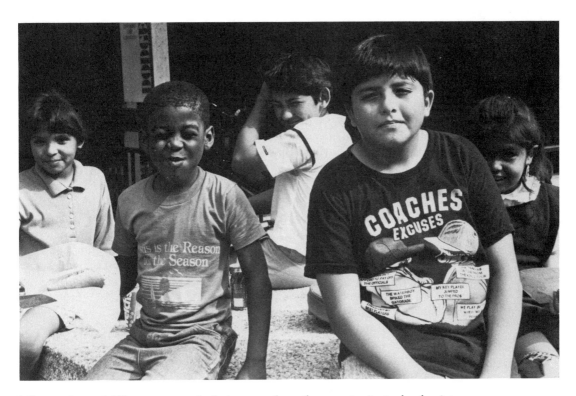

When students of different races and ethnic groups have the opportunity to develop interpersonal relationships, racial and ethnic relations are also likely to be improved.

(Photo by Willard Loftis).

factors that affect interethnic relations may help the professional educator understand the reasons for conflict between groups and the different perceptions of contact and conflict held by participants in interethnic communication.

Prejudice and Discrimination

Two causes of ineffective interethnic relations are prejudice and discrimination. Both stem from a combination of several factors: (1) a lack of understanding of the history, experiences, values, and perceptions of ethnic groups other than one's own; (2) stereotyping the members of an ethnic group without consideration of individual differences within the group; (3) judging other ethnic groups according to the standards and values of one's own group; (4) assigning negative attributes to members of other ethnic groups; and (5) evaluating the qualities and experiences of other groups as inferior to one's own. In other words, prejudice and discrimination are extreme forms of ethnocentrism.

"Prejudice is a negative attitude toward an entire category of people" (Schaefer, 1988, p. 55). This aversion to members of certain ethnic groups manifests itself in feelings of anger, fear, hatred, and distrust about members of the out-group. These attitudes are often translated into fear of walking in the neighborhood of the out-group, fear of being mugged by members of the out-group, distrust of any merchant from the out-group, anger at any advantages that members of the out-group may be perceived as receiving, and fear of a member of the out-group moving next door. "The forms of prejudice may range from a relatively unconscious aversion to members of the out-group to a comprehensive, well-articulated, and coherent ideology, such as the idology of racism" (Yetman, 1985, p. 11). Such an ideology undergirds the activities of the Nazis, Ku Klux Klan, and other white racist groups that currently exist in our society.

Since World War II, overt individual prejudice and discrimination have decreased dramatically. In the early 1940s, segregation of and discrimination against blacks were supported by the majority of whites. Today, most whites support policies against racial discrimination and prejudice. However, their support of government intervention to guarantee equality for minorities is not nearly as strong (Schuman, Steech, & Bobo, 1985). Moreover, during the 1980s, it became more acceptable to openly express one's prejudice, as evidenced by cross burnings and racist themes at fraternity parties on a number of college campuses. One wonders whether racial attitudes have really changed in the past fifty years or whether the prejudice against ethnic and racial groups other than one's own has just been less public.

Whereas prejudice focuses on attitudes, discrimination focuses on behavior. Discrimination "involves behavior that excludes all members of a group from certain rights, opportunities, or privileges" (Schaefer, 1988, p. 55). Prejudice is the arbitrary denial of the privileges and rewards of society to those whose qualifications are equal to the dominant group. Although prejudice may not directly hurt members of the out-group, it can be easily translated into discriminating behavior that harms members of the out-group.

Discrimination occurs at two levels: individual and institutional. Individual discrimination is attributed to or influenced by prejudice. Individuals discriminate against a member of the out-group for at least two reasons. Either they have strong prejudicial, or bigoted, feelings about the ethnic group, or they feel that societal pressures demand that they discriminate even though they may not be prejudiced. Realtors, personnel managers, receptionists, and membership chairpersons all work directly with individuals. Their own personal attitudes about members of certin ethnic groups can influence whether a house is sold, a job is offered, an appointment is made, or a membership is extended to a member of the out-group. The action of these individuals can prevent the member of the out-group from gaining the experiences and economic advantage that these activities offer.

An individual has less control in the other form of discrimination. Institutional discrimination cannot be attributed to prejudicial attitudes:

> Institutional discrimination refers to the effects of inequalities that are rooted in the system-wide operation of a society and have little relation to racially related attitudinal factors or the majority group's racial or ethnic prejudices. It involves "policies or practices which appear to be neutral in their effect on minority in-

dividuals or groups but which have the effect of disproportionately impacting upon them in harmful or negative ways" (Task Force on the Administration of Military Justice in the Armed Forces, 1972, p. 19). (Yetman, 1985, p. 17–18)

We face a dilemma because we have grown up in a society that has inherently discriminated against minority groups since the first explorers arrived. Throughout our lives, we have participated in a number of societal institutions, including schools, Social Security, transportation, and housing patterns. We have either benefited or not benefited adequately from some of those institutions. However, we often do not realize the extent that members of other ethnic groups receive the benefits and privileges of these institutions. Because we feel that we have never been discriminated against, we should not be led to believe that others do not suffer from discrimination.

Many individuals might argue that institutional discrimination no longer exists because today's laws require equal access to the benefits of society. Omi and Winant (1986) suggest that

> with the exception of some on the far right, the racial reaction which has developed in the last two decades claims to favor racial equality. Its vision is that of a "color-blind" society where racial considerations are never entertained in the selection of leaders, in hiring decisions, and the distribution of goods and services in general. As the right sees it, racial problems today center on the new forms of racial "injustice" which originated in the "great transformation." This new injustice confers group rights on racial minority groups, thus granting a new form of privilege—that of preferential treatment.
>
> The culprit behind this new form of "racism" is seen as the state itself. In attempting to eliminate racial discrimination, the state went too far. It legitimated group rights, established affirmative action mandates, and spent money on a range of social programs, which, according to the right, debilitated, rather than uplifted, its target populations. In this scenario, the victims of racial discrimination have dramatically shifted from racial minorities to whites, particularly white males. (p. 114)

The problem is that the criteria for access are often applied arbitrarily and unfairly. A disproportionately high number of minorities do not possess the qualifications for skilled jobs or college entrance or have the economic resources to purchase a home in the suburbs. As businesses and industries move from the city to the suburbs, access to employment by minorities who live in the inner city is limited. The crucial issue is not the equal treatment of those with equal qualifications, but the accessibility of minority group members to the qualifications and jobs themselves.

The consequences are the same in individual and institutional discrimination. Members of certain ethnic groups do not receive the same benefits from society as the majority group. Individuals are harmed by circumstances beyond their control because of their membership in a specific ethnic group. The role of teachers and other professional educators requires that they not discriminate against any student because of the student's ethnic background. This consideration must be paramount in assigning students to special education classes and in giving and interpreting standardized tests. Classroom interactions, classroom resources, extracurricular activites, and counseling practices must be evaluated to ensure that discrimination against students from various ethnic groups is not occurring.

Racism

Racism is a mixed form of discrimination and prejudice directed at ethnic groups that are racially different from the dominant group members. Traditionally, racism referred to the conscious or unconscious belief that members of racial groups other than one's own were innately inferior. Thus, in the early part of this century, eastern and southern Europeans were viewed by some as racially and intellectually inferior to the original northern and western European settlers. In this sense, racism is a form of prejudice. Often this prejudice was transferred by individuals and government policy into discrimination against immigrants in the form of literacy examination requirements to enter the country and strict immigration policies. Individual discrimination also prevailed in the availability of housing and jobs. It was often difficult for these immigrants to find acceptable work until they had relinquished their accents, their names, and other remnants of the old country.

Since the 1950s, the term *racism* has focused on prejudice and discrimination against people of color, especially African-Americans, Mexican-Americans, Puerto Ricans, Asian-Americans, and Native Americans. *White racism* is another term sometimes used in literature to describe this phenomenon. It refers to the belief that white people are inherently superior to people of color in significant ways and that in no significant ways are people of color superior to whites (Schuman, 1975).

Many whites may no longer believe that blacks are genetically inferior to whites, but many believe in another ideology. This "dominant white ideology is that of free will; anyone can 'better himself [herself]' if he [she] is not too lazy to make the effort" (Yetman, 1985, p. 15). Such an ideology refuses to acknowledge the impact of the oppressive social and economic conditions on subordinate group members. It places the responsibility for the disadvantage on the group itself. This emphasis implies that members of the minority group must certainly be inferior to whites, or they would be doing as well as whites. A comment often heard from whites is that their own ancestors were poor when they immigrated to this country, but that they worked hard to provide their families with all of the resources that moved them into the middle class, where they could enjoy the privileges and rewards of society. Some believe that if subordinate group members would work just as hard, they would also receive the same benefits. These individuals reject the existence of external impingements and disabilities that make it much more difficult for people of color to shed their minority status than it was for their own European ancestors. They ignore the fact that some people of color have adapted the cultural values and standards of the dominant group to a greater degree than many white ethnic groups. Yet discriminatory policies and practices prevent them from sharing equally in society's benefits with whites. In addition, the opportunities to gain qualifications with which people of color could compete equally with whites have been severely restricted throughout most of our history.

The most crucial factor in understanding racism is that the majority group has power over the minority group. This power has been used to prevent people of color from securing the prestige, power, and privilege held by whites. Racism is also practiced by some whites and their institutions to maintain a dominant-subordinate relationship with nonwhite groups. Professional educators must prevent such practices from occurring in their classrooms or schools.

Intergroup Conflicts

The reader should begin to realize why intergroup conflicts are likely to occur in the nation's schools. The fact that some groups receive more rewards from society than other groups can be observed by the members of oppressed groups. This resentment often causes tension between ethnic groups that can lead to conflict. It is not easier to accept a subordinate status just because most individuals of the dominant group are not prejudiced or do not discriminate. Whites often find this attitude frustrating because individually they may not deserve the criticism and blame laid on them by the oppressed groups. However, it is essential to understand the cause of the criticism, namely, the overt prejudice and discrimination faced by these groups. Historically, the oppressed groups have had to adjust to the dominant standards. Many minority members adopt the cultural patterns of the dominant group—a process called acculturation. However, no matter how much of the dominant culture has been adopted by minority groups, members of those groups assimilate into the dominant group only to the extent that the dominant group allows. African-Americans provide a classic example of this phenomenon.

Interethnic conflict is certainly not new in the United States, although the intensity of such conflicts has been mild compared to that in many other nations. Revolts were organized by slaves to overcome their oppressed role in society. Native American and European conflicts were common in the attempt to subjugate the native peoples.

What are the reasons for continued interethnic conflict as we enter the twenty-first century? Discriminatory practices have protected the superior status of the dominant group for centuries. When other ethnic groups try to share more equitably in the rewards and privileges of society, the dominant group must concede some of its advantages. Most recently, this concern about giving up some of the advantages of the oppressor has been reflected in reactions to affirmative action programs. When an African-American is offered a job over a white applicant, many whites state that affirmative action policies prevented them from getting the job; seldom do they state that the one selected was as well or better qualified for the position. As long as one ethnic group has an institutional advantage over other ethnic groups, some interethnic conflict is likely to occur.

Another reason for interethnic conflict is competition for economic resources. As economic conditions become tighter, fewer jobs are available. Discriminatory practices in the past have forced people of color into positions with the least seniority; as jobs are cut back, disproportionately high numbers are then laid off. The tension between ethnic groups increases as members of specific groups determine that they disproportionately suffer the hardships resulting from economic depression. Conflict sometimes occurs between oppressed groups when they are forced to share limited societal resources, such as low-income housing and access to bilingual education programs. Conflict as a result of inequitable distribution of economic rewards is likely to continue as long as members of ethnic groups can observe and feel those inequities (Appleton, 1983).

During the past fifty years, a number of educational strategies have been developed to reduce and overcome interethnic conflicts. These strategies have focused on training teachers to be effective in intergroup or human relations; attempting to change the prejudicial attitudes of teachers; fighting institutional discrimination through affirmative action and civil rights legislation; encouraging changes in textbooks and other resources to more accurately reflect the multiethnic nature of society; and attempting to remove discriminatory behavior from classroom interactions and classroom practices. All these strategies are important to combat prejudice and discrimination in the educational settings. Alone or in combination, however, the strategies do not appear to be enough. This fact is not to diminish the need for professional educators to further develop the strategies. It is not a sign of failure, but it is a recognition that prejudice, discrimination, and racism are diseases that infect all of society, not only the schools and professional educators.

ETHNIC IDENTITY

Students in a classroom are likely to come from several different ethnic groups, although physical differences are not always identifiable. Two white students who appear to be from similar backgrounds may actually identify strongly with their German or Polish background. The two families may live next door to each other in a similar houses, but the insides of the houses may be furnished or decorated differently. The churches that they attend will probably differ, as well as their ideas about raising children and maintaining the family. Their political ideologies are likely to differ markedly. Yet, students often are viewed as coming from the same cultural background if they have similar racial characteristics, even though their families may be African-American, Nigerian-American, Puerto Rican, or Jamaican-American. The educator must beware of assuming that all students who look alike come from the same ethnic background. Factors other than physical characteristics must be used to determine a student's ethnicity.

The degree of ethnic identity differs greatly from student to student, family to family, and community to community. Some students will identify with an ethnic group by participating in ethnic traditions, customs, clubs, organizations, and social cliques. The primary relationships of these students probably will be within the ethnic group, and their values and life-styles may be determined by the ethnic ethos. Often these students live in ethnic enclaves.

Some students superficially identify with an ethnic group. These students probably participate in some ethnic traditions, customs, clubs, or organizations, but they do not share in the fullest sense the ethos of that ethnic group. They may live in

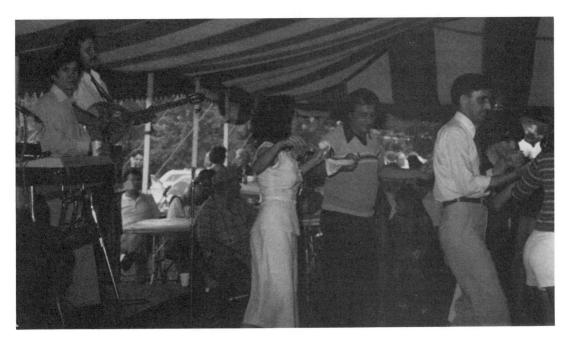

Many Americans maintain ties with their national origin or ethnic group. They often participate in traditional ethnic events, such as this Greek festival.

an ethnic enclave, but they are more likely to live in a community where identity with one's national origin is not important or valued.

Other students may have mixed ancestry, allowing them to identify with two or more national origins. Identification with one ethnic group more than others may occur, or students may view their ethnicity as just American. Some students may not see their ethnic identity as very important in understanding who they are. However, observers may continue to respond to them based on their identifiable ethnicity. Sometimes, the ethnic group itself makes it very difficult for an individual to withdraw from the ethnic group and assimilate into the majority group.

Some Americans grow up in ethnic enclaves and not in multiethnic communities. Chinatown, Little Italy, Harlem, and Little Saigon are examples of ethnic enclaves in the nation's cities. The suburbs also include pockets of families from the same ethnic background in addition to members of the dominant group. Throughout the country, there are small towns and surrounding farmland where the population comes from the same ethnic background, all the residents perhaps being African-American, German-American, Danish-American, Anglo-American, or Mexican-American. These individuals may be culturally encapsulated, so that most of their primary relationships and many of their secondary relationships are with members of their own ethnic group. They may not have the opportunity to interact with members of other ethnic groups or to recognize or share the richness of a second culture that exists in another ethnic setting. They may never learn how to live with people who speak a different language or dialect, eat different types of foods, and value things that their own ethnic group does not value. They often learn to fear or denigrate individuals from different ethnic groups primarily because their ways are seemingly strange and thus perceived as wrong or bad.

Unlike their white counterparts, most people of color usually are forced out of their ethnic encapsulation to achieve social and economic mobility. Many secondary relationships are with members of other ethnic groups because they often work with or for members of the dominant group. However, members of the dominant group rarely have the opportunity to develop even secondary relationships with members of other ethnic groups, particularly minority members. Dominant group members could spend their lives not knowing or participating in the culture of another ethnic group.

Ethnic enclaves help preserve a strong ethnic identity among their inhabitants. The group's value systems, traditions, language, and identity can be supported, and sometimes required, by the other members of the ethnic group. Some ethnic groups believe that solidarity is essential to the preservation of the ethnic group itself. For them the ethnic enclave is one means to ensure that the ethnic group does not become extinct.

With few exceptions, however, the ethnic enclave itself does not increase in size. Families move away because of job opportunities and economic rewards available outside of the community itself. Children who move away to attend college often do not return to reside. Yet some families continue to maintain a strong identity with the ethnic group even after they have moved away. Children of parents who have moved out of the ethnic enclave are less likely to maintain such strong identity with the ethnic group because many of the primary relationships are with members of other ethnic groups. Many whites become assimilated into the majority group. Others participate in some ethnic activities, although their acceptance and practice of the ethnic ethos may decrease significantly as they move geographically and emotionally away from the ethnic enclave. Second- and third-generation ethnics living in the suburbs often rediscover their ethnic ties and identity. Although their primary relationships may not be restricted totally to other members of the ethnic group, they tend to organize or join ethnic social clubs and organizations or revitalize their identification with their national origin.

One should be able to determine the importance of ethnicity in one's life. An individual inherits by birth certain ancestral ties that extend to one or more nations. Continued identification with that national origin can be preserved, recognized, or ignored by the individual.

An individual's degree of ethnic identity is influenced early in that person's life by whether or not the family members recognize or promote ethnicity as an important force in determining who they are. Sometimes, the choice about how ethnic one will be is imposed; this is particularly true for members of oppressed ethnic minority groups. When the ethnic group believes that strong and loyal ethnic identity is necessary to maintain the group solidarity, the pressure of other members of the group may make it difficult not to have a strong ethnic identity. For many members of the group, this ethnic identity provides them with the security of belonging and knowing who they are. The ethnic identity becomes the primary source of identification, and they feel no need to identify themselves differently. In fact, they may find it emotionally very difficult to sever their primary identification with that group.

Minorities often are classified as members of an ethnic group by objective characteristics. Because of prejudice and discrimination against minorities in this country, any minority individual faces the discriminatory practices used against all other members of that same group. Not all individuals view their ethnic origins as important in understanding who they are. Their membership in other microcultures may have a much greater impact on their identity than the nations from which their ancestors came. Many individuals from oppressed groups have been acculturated and share the same cultural characteristics with dominant group individuals. However, denied full access into the economic, political, and social spheres of the dominant group, they cannot assimilate. In the process of acculturation, some of these individuals reject the traditional culture of the ethnic group and are in a transitional stage between the ethnic minority group and the assimilated majority. The majority of these individuals probably function biculturally, participating as appropriate in either the oppressed group or the dominant group. Others reject the culture of the ethnic group to assimilate into the culture of the dominant group. If the dominant group denies assimilation, some of these individuals become suspended between two cultural groups, belonging to neither and developing problems with self-identity.

Educators must be aware of intragroup differences. We must beware of stereotyping all persons from the same ethnic group; many differences exist within all groups. The degree of ethnic identity differs greatly among individuals whom we classify as members of an ethnic group. Members of the same ethnic group differ greatly in their own historical experiences gathered from the old country as well as from this country. For example, families who emigrated from Vietnam in the early 1970s were predominantly from the wealthy and professional middle classes. They differ greatly in their social and economic backgrounds from Vietnamese who emigrated from peasant and rural backgrounds in the late 1970s. To expect the same cultural patterns for individuals from both groups might lead to ineffective instructional planning for them. For some students, membership in their ethnic group is very important in their self-identity. Knowing what students and their families expect within an ethnic context can be very helpful in preparing effective instructional strategies.

Identifying the degree of assimilation into the majority culture by students may be helpful in developing instructional strategies. Such information may help the educator understand the students' values, particularly what the students' expectations for school may be. It also allows the teacher to more accurately determine the learning styles of the students so that the teaching style can be effectively adapted to individual differences. The only way to know the importance of ethnicity in the lives of students is to objectively listen and observe them. Familiarity and participation with the community from which students come will also help the educator know the importance of microculture membership to students and their families.

Finally, the educator must remember that students from oppressed groups face societal constraints and restrictions that seldom affect dominant students. Such recognition is essential in the development of instructional programs and schools that effectively serve diverse populations that as yet do not share equally in the benefits that education offers.

EDUCATIONAL IMPLICATIONS

Educators must understand how ethnicity has affected the lives of students. Students from the dominant group have not suffered discrimination based on their ethnic backgrounds, whereas most minority students have. The impact of oppression on students must be recognized. Students know when a teacher or counselor does not respect and value the students' ethnic background. As educators, we cannot afford to reject or neglect students because their ethnic backgrounds are different from our own. We are responsible for making sure all students learn to think, read, write, and compute so that they can function effectively in society.

At this time, we are not very effective in teaching basic skills to all students, particularly minority students. Oakes (1988) reports that the following discrepancies in mathematics and science achievement still exist:

☐ Blacks and Hispanics consistently perform below the levels of whites on measures of end–of–high school achievement in mathematics and science.

☐ Minority low achievement in mathematics and science is undoubtedly more profound than test scores imply, considering the disproportionate number of poor, black, and Hispanic dropouts not represented in measures of high school achievement.

☐ Black and Hispanic high school graduates are less likely than whites to enter college.

☐ Blacks and Hispanics are underrepresented as college majors in science, mathematics, and engineering.

☐ Non-Asian minorities . . . are significantly underrepresented in science-, mathematics-, and technology-related careers. In 1984, for example, blacks, Hispanics, and American Indians (20 percent of the total population) constituted less than seven percent of this sector of the workforce. (pp. 107–108)

The lack of equitable achievement by minorities in these and other basic skills areas probably begins very early in a student's schooling, when disproportionate numbers are placed in low-level groups, where low achievement is expected. Upon entry into junior and senior high school, fewer minorities than whites seek or are placed in advanced, more rigorous academic classes. The mathematics and science courses taken vary considerably by race and class, leading to the unequal outcomes in achievement (Oakes, 1988).

There are at least two theories that educators should consider in developing strategies to better serve minority students. The cultural discontinuity theory attributes the differences in outcomes between students of oppressed groups and students of dominant groups to the differences between the culture and language of the school and those of the students. The school reflects the culture and values of the dominant society and usually ignores or denigrates the culture and values of the ethnic groups from which students come. For example, many schools have set aside the month of February to celebrate black history. This in itself may be a helpful strategy for learning about a specific ethnic group; however, it often substitutes for integrating the contributions and experiences of African-Americans throughout the curriculum during the whole school year. Other groups are studied only by students' participating in a traditional ethnic event or in tasting ethnic foods. The advantage in these cases goes to the students of the dominant group. The curriculum economically reflects their culture, and their views require little or no adjusting.

The structural inequalities theory "emphasizes the status of a particular minority or social class group within the socioeconomic structure of the host society and the group's relationship with the dominant majority" (Gibson, 1988, p. 30). The low achievement of minority students in schools reflects the social stratification system that operates in society, and most schools are designed to maintain that status quo. Thus, students from subordinate groups are tracked into low-ability groups and vocational programs.

Students are not always inactive participants in the stratification that occurs. Researchers are finding that many working-class boys and minority students develop resistance or oppositional patterns to handle their subordination within schools (Ogbu, 1988; Solomon, 1988; Willis, 1977). This opposition often takes the form of breaking school rules and norms, belittling academic achievement, and valuing manual over mental work. These students equate schooling with accepting the culture of the dominant group and thinking and acting white—characteristics that could have one expelled from the minority or class peer group. In many cases, especially for African-Americans, "students embrace education, the achievement ideology, and develop high educational aspirations. In the meantime, however, their counter-school activities do not allow them to achieve these ends" (Solomon, 1988, p. 260). While middle-class African-American students perform academically better than their working-class peers, they do not do as well as white students, in part because of this oppositional process.

Not all minority students adopt an oppositional form, and not all minority groups are equally affected. Asian-American students have high achievement records in mathematics and science and attend college at a rate disproportionately higher than other groups. One explanation might be that Asian-American adults are over-represented in professional occupations, which should indicate an income above that of most other minority groups. Oakes (1988) attributes their high levels of achievement and participation in mathematics and science to the economic advantages in the home backgrounds of many of these students. Generally, the cultural group values math and science skills, and families provide experiences that encourage their development. Whether these high achievement levels will be maintained by the more recent refugees from Southeast Asia has yet to be determined.

Recent immigrants also appear not to develop the oppositional forms of the long-established minority groups. Gibson (1988) found that they are more willing to accept school norms and succeed academically, in part because they compare the conditions of living in the United States with those in the country that they have just left. At the same time, many families are not willing to surrender their ethnic culture totally to become assimilated. In her study of Sikh immigrants in a California high school, Gibson (1988) found that families developed a strategy of accommodation and acculturation without assimilation. A high degree of academic success has also been found for Cuban, Central American, and Vietnamese refugees.

In responding equitably to ethnic differences, the educator should be able to (1) encourage students to build and maintain a positive self-concept, (2) use the ethnic backgrounds of students to teach effectively, (3) help students overcome their ethnic prejudices, (4) expand the knowledge and appreciation of the historical, economic, political, and social experiences of ethnic and national groups, and (5) assist students in understanding that the world's knowledge and culture have been and continue to be created from the contributions of all ethnic groups and nations. Schools need to provide environments in which students can learn to participate in the dominant society while maintaining distinct ethnic identities if they choose. Respect for and support of ethnic differences will be essential in this effort. We can help accomplish this goal by accurately reflecting ethnicity in the curriculum and positively using it to teach and interact with students. There are at least two curriculum approaches to incorporating broad ethnic content in the school curriculum: ethnic studies and multiethnic curriculum. Ethnic differences must also be examined in the interactions of students and teachers as well as in student assessment.

Curriculum Approaches

One approach to incorporating ethnic content is through ethnic studies. Ethnic studies are an extension or special segment of the curriculum that focuses on the history and contemporary conditions of one or more ethnic groups. A broader goal of ethnic studies is to "help students develop the ability to make reflective decisions on issues related to ethnicity and to take personal and public action to help solve the racial and ethnic problems in our national and world societies" (Banks, 1984, p. 20).

An advantage of ethnic studies courses is that they allow for in-depth exposure to the social, economic, and political history of a specific group. These courses are designed to correct the distortions and omissions about an ethnic group that prevail in textbooks. Events that have been neglected in textbooks are addressed, myths are dispelled, and history is viewed from the perspective of the ethnic group as well as the dominant group. Prospective teachers and other professional school personnel who have not been exposed to an examination of an ethnic group different from their own should take such a course or undertake individual study.

Traditionally, ethnic studies have been offered as separate courses that students elect from many offerings in the curriculum. Seldom have ethnic studies been required courses for all students. Too often the majority of students who choose these courses are students from the ethnic group or groups being studied. Although the information and experiences offered in these courses are very important to students with the same ethnic background, they are just as important for all students, regardless of their ethnic background.

The second approach to incorporating ethnic content affects the total curriculum of a school. A multiethnic curriculum permeates all subject areas at all levels of education, from preschool through adult education. All courses should reflect accurate and positive references to ethnic diversity. The amount of specific content about ethnic groups would vary according to the course taught, but an awareness and a recognition of the multiethnic nature of the nation can be reflected in classroom experiences. No matter how assimilated students in a classroom are, it is the teacher's responsibility to expose them to the ethnic diversity of this nation and the world.

Bulletin boards, resource books, and films that show ethnic diversity should constantly reinforce these realities, although teachers should not depend entirely on these resources for instructional content about ethnic groups. Too often, minorities are studied only during a unit on African-American history or Native Americans. Too often, minorities are not seen on bulletin boards or included in the reading lists when students study biographies, the basic food groups, labor unions, or the environment. If ethnic groups are included only during a unit or a week focusing on a particular group, students do not learn to view them as an integral part of society. They are viewed as separate, distinct, and inferior to the dominant group. A multiethnic curriculum prevents the distortion of history and contemporary conditions. Without it, the perspective of the dominant group becomes the only valid and correct curriculum to which students continually are exposed.

It is the educator's responsibility to ensure that ethnic groups become an integral part of the total curriculum. This mandate does not require the teacher to discuss every ethnic group. It does require that the classroom resources and instruction not focus completely on the dominant group. It requires that perspectives of ethnic groups and the dominant group be examined in discussions of historical and current events. For example, one should consider the perspective of Native Americans as well as the majority group in a presentation and discussion of early and contemporary conflicts.

Multiethnic education should include learning experiences that will help students examine their own stereotypes about and prejudice against ethnic groups. When students use derogatory terms for ethnic group members or tell ethnic jokes, teachers should use the opportunity to discuss attitudes about those groups. Students should not be allowed to express their hostility to other group members in a classroom that is multicultural.

Development of a multiethnic curriculum will require the educator to evaluate textbooks and classroom resources for ethnic content and biases. Although there have been advances in eliminating ethnic biases and adding information about ethnic groups in newer textbooks, many older textbooks are still used in classrooms across the nation. With many textbook revisions, ethnic content has been added to what already existed, rather than carefully integrating the material throughout the text. Biased books should not prevent the teacher from providing multiethnic instruction. Supplementary materials can fill the gap in this area. The biases and omissions in the texts can be used for discussions of biases and experiences of ethnic groups. However, none of these instructional activities will occur unless the educator is aware of and values ethnic differences and their importance in the curriculum.

Interaction Between Students and Teachers

The content of most courses reflects the ethnic awareness of the teacher. In addition to the course content and available resources, an understanding of ethnicity is an advantage in developing effective teaching strategies for individual students. It can assist the teacher in developing instructional strategies that build on students' ethnic experiences to help them learn concepts. Examples that demonstrate a concept can be personalized to the ethnic experiences and backgrounds of students. This technique helps students recognize that their ethnic identity is valued in the classroom; it also encourages all students in the classroom to respect the ethnic diversity that exists there.

Educational research shows that minority students, particularly recent non-European immigrants and students of color, sometimes are treated significantly differently from white students by their teachers. Because many white students share the same ethnic and middle-class culture with the teacher, they also share the same cultural cues that foster success in the classroom. Students who ask appropriate questions at appropriate times or who smile and seek attention from the teacher at times when the teacher is open to such gestures are likely to receive encouragement and reinforcement from the teacher. On the other hand, students who interrupt the class or who seek attention from the teacher when the teacher is not open to providing the necessary attention do not receive the necessary reinforcement. When students are from the same ethnic background as the teacher, many of these verbal and nonverbal cues are natural to both students and teacher. When the students and teacher are from different ethnic backgrounds, the verbal and nonverbal cues may be incongruent, to the detriment of the students (Brophy & Good, 1974).

Miscommunications with teachers are more likely to be initiated by students from oppressed groups than by dominant students. In response to the different treatment of students as a result, students begin to establish ethnic boundaries within the classroom. McDermott and Gospodinoff (1983) suggest that "under these conditions, ethnic solidarity becomes a refuge from the negative relationships offered to the children in the classrooms. In this way, the experience of belonging to a group was transformed into an experience of having enemies" (p. 229).

This situation is exacerbated as minority students see that students from the dominant group receive more opportunities to participate in instructional interactions and receive more praise and encouragement. Minority students receive fewer opportunities to participate, and the opportunities usually are of a less substantive nature. They also may be criticized or disciplined more frequently than white students.

Teachers tend to be more directive and authoritarian toward students of color and more open and democratic with white students (Gay, 1977). Unless teachers can critically examine their treatment of different students in the classroom, they will not know whether they treat students inequitably because of ethnic differences. Once that step has been taken, changes can be initiated to ensure that ethnicity is not a factor for automatically relating differently to students. Teachers may have to become more proactive in initiating interactions and providing encouragement, praise, and reinforcement to students from ethnic backgrounds different from their own.

How can teachers analyze their own classroom interactions and teaching styles? There are at least two types of data that should be collected: (1) how much talking is done by the teacher and individual students and (2) the nature of the interactions (e.g., giving praise, criticizing, asking questions, or initiating discussion). A number of instruments have been developed by researchers to assist in this process, and there are several possibilities for collecting the data. If equipment is available, teachers can videotape or audiotape a class and then systematically record the interactions as they view or listen to the tape later. An outside observer could be asked to record the interaction on an instrument while sitting in the classroom. Among other instruments, the reader might use Flander's Interaction Analysis or the Spaulding Teacher Activity Rating Schedule (STARS)—easily used rating instruments in which the type of interaction is recorded every few seconds (Guerin & Maier, 1983). An analysis of the data will show teachers how much of the class time they spend interacting with students and the nature of the interaction. The data could be used to show whether there are differences in interactions based on sex, ethnicity, or other characteristics of students. Such an analysis would be an excellent starting point for teachers who would like to ensure that they do not discriminate against students from different ethnic groups.

Every effort must be made to ensure that ethnic prejudices are not reflected in these interactions. To promote positive interactions between students from different ethnic backgrounds and between teacher and students, skills in intergroup or human relations are helpful to teachers.

Another area that teachers should investigate and change to better meet the needs of an ethnically diverse student population is that of teaching and learning styles. Both ethnicity and socioeconomic status appear to be important factors in learning style differences. Both teaching and learning styles can be categorized as either field-independent or field-sensitive. Field-independent teachers encourage independent student achievement and competition among students. Field-sensitive teachers are more interpersonally oriented and prefer situations that allow them to use personal, conversational techniques. Similarly, field-sensitive students perform better in social situations, such as group work; field-independent students work well on independent projects.

Generally, individuals from the dominant group are more likely to be field-independent than minority group members. This is not true in all cases, of course. Japanese-Americans and Chinese-Americans also tend to be more field-independent than field-sensitive. As individuals from minority groups become more assimilated, they are more likely to move closer to a field-independent learning style.

Ability to learn is not affected by where an individual falls along this continuum. However, learning styles are important in determining instructional strategies that will help, rather than hinder, students' ability to learn. Often the teacher's style differs from the learning style of some students, causing a classroom situation that may not be conducive to helping students reach their potential. Ramirez and Castaneda (1974) showed that teachers can learn to organize learning environments conducive to each cognitive style so that all students can benefit equally from teaching. They describe the ideal classroom for this bicognitive development as follows:

> [It is] one that allows children to work on individual projects and on group projects that afford close contact with the teacher and classmates. A program of study is developed for each student so that he or she has opportunity to work with both field-sensitive and field-independent peers. In this environment it would be possible for both field-sensitive and field-independent children to act as tutors. Classroom walls would be decorated with both field-sensitive and field-independent materials. (p. 145)

Teachers can identify their own teaching styles as well as the learning styles of most of their students. Understanding one's teaching style through this process is another positive step toward developing effective classroom strategies to meet the needs of all students.

Finally, the climate of the school must be supportive of ethnic diversity. Student governance should reflect ethnic diversity in selection of special programs, dances, and awards ceremonies. If equity is not being achieved in all aspects of schooling, educators need to carefully evaluate their practices to determine whether they are discriminatory. Most of us become so encapsulated in our own ethnic groups that we do not objectively view or accept our interactions with members of other groups as discriminatory. It is imperative that educators become more aware of such practices and have the skills to overcome discrimination against ethnic groups in schools.

Student Assessment

Throughout U.S. history, a racist ideology of the genetic superiority of certain ethnic groups has existed. This ideology has been reflected in national policies, such as voting rights and immigration. In both of these cases, literacy exams have been used to control the access of certain ethnic groups to entering the country or to basic civil rights. Similar practices are now manifested in the nation's schools.

Schools today conduct widespread testing of students for entrance into programs for the gifted, advanced courses, special education programs, colleges and universities, and professional schools. These standardized tests have limited the access of oppressed group members to more rigorous study at all educational levels. While these students are often prevented from entering professional schools, disproportionately large numbers of them are tested into special education programs for the mentally retarded, learning disabled, and emotionally disturbed.

Tests are trumpeted as measures of competence to graduate from high school, to enter upper-division college courses, to earn a baccalaureate degree, and to become certified to teach in the nation's classrooms. Many proponents of testing suggest that the tests alone can determine whether students know and perform at levels acceptable by society. Such tests are promoted as measures of quality in the nation's schools. Overwhelmingly, promoters suggest that anyone who cannot pass the appropriate test certainly cannot be qualified to move on to further study. In fact, however, such testing limits the access of many individuals to practice the career of their choice (Smith, 1985).

Individuals were first tested en masse by the army during World War I for the purpose of identifying potential officers. "Organizers of this testing effort . . . stressed the hereditary significance of intelligence, insisted they were discovering 'native' intelligence, and interpreted test results in a racist framework" (Weinberg, 1983, p. 60). A principal architect of this early testing effort and fervent supporter of heredity as the major determinant of intelligence, Princeton psychologist Carl C. Brigham had changed his mind by the 1930s. In a private memorandum, he wrote that belief in native intelligence was "one of the most serious fallacies in the history of science" and that IQ scores were "a composite including schooling, family background, familiarity with English, and everything else, relevant and irrelevant" (Weinberg, 1983, p. 65).

Nevertheless, educators and others continued to administer tests for the purpose of identifying native intelligence and thus sorting people appropriately for education and jobs for which they were most suited. Even more disturbing, some researchers continued to promulgate the ideology that intelligence is inherited and that there are genetic differences between racial groups. In the argument of heredity versus environment, proponents of the heredity of IQ most often based their evidence on studies of twins who had been separated and raised in somewhat different environments. Even though Cyril Burt, the preeminent researcher in this area, has since been acknowledged as a fraud because he deliberately distorted his data, proponents continue to insist that IQ is primarily attributable to genetic inheritance.

However, Burt never suggested that there were genetic differences in IQ between the races. This issue was brought to the forefront again by A.R. Jensen in a 1969 article. He contended that poor and ethnic minority children were seriously deficient in conceptual learning, such as problem solving and an ability to handle abstract ideas. Numerous geneticists refuted Jensen's racial hypothesis, indicating that there still is no convincing evidence that there are genetic differences in intelligence between the races (Weinberg, 1983).

Why is it, then, that students from oppressed groups continue to score lower on standardized tests than dominant group members? For one thing, these minority groups have suffered socioeconomic and cultural disadvantages for generations that have prevented them from competing equally with advantaged cultural groups. The second reason could be controlled by knowledgeable and sensitive educators. Most testing in schools is based on an Anglo-conformity model of appraisal. Psychologist Jane Mercer (1978) writes:

In making inferences about children's "intelligence" or "aptitudes," present procedures presume that America is a culturally homogeneous society in which all children are being socialized into essentially the same Anglo tradition. . . . [Existing tests] are to be used for diagnosis, prognosis, and prescription in education so that all children can be socialized to the existing social structure, i.e., the Anglo core culture. . . . [In the Anglo-oriented view,] the greater the sociocultural distance between the individual and the dominant core culture, the lower his or her score will be. Thus, persons more culturally distant from the Anglo core culture will score lower and will be considered "subnormal," ineligible for job placement, and inadmissible to college and graduate school. (p. 15)

As educators, we must be careful not to label poor and minority children as intellectually inferior because they score poorly on standardized tests. These scores too often influence the teacher's expectations for the academic performance of students in the classroom. It is essential that we maintain high expectations for all students, regardless of ethnic background and test scores. Standardized test scores can help determine how assimilated into the majority culture one may be, but it provides little evidence of how intelligent one is. There are many other factors that can be used to provide information about intelligence, for example, ability to think and respond appropriately in different situations.

Finally, in developing tests and using the results of standardized tests, the educator must recognize the inherent cultural bias that favors dominant students. Few tests have been developed from the bias of a minority group. One is the Black Intelligence Test of Bicultural Homogeneity (BITCH) (Williams, 1973), which is based on urban African-American culture. It includes language and terms familiar to this microculture. African-Americans consistently score better on this test than members of the dominant group. However, this and similar tests are rarely used to determine intelligence of individuals or groups. Test bias is a serious educational issue with devastating results to many minorities. A report of the National Alliance of Black School Educators (1984) stated:

Testing the intellect of African American children with alien cultural content is a scientific error and is, in our opinion, professional malpractice. Testing in order to *rank* children by intellect, to *rank* them by cognitive or behavioral style, or to *rank* them with "non-biased" assessment procedures is malpractice, in our opinion, unless such practices can be demonstrated by valid research to result in significant and meaningful changes in achievement for our children. (p. 28)

Educators must be aware that these cultural biases exist, and they must continually remind themselves not to rely on test scores as the only indication of students' intelligence. Educators are capable of making more valid decisions about ability based on numerous other objective factors about students. If decisions about the capabilities of minority students match exactly the standardized scores, the educator should reevaluate his or her own responses and interactions with these students. This is an area that none of us can afford to neglect.

SUMMARY

Almost from the beginning of European settlement, the population was multiethnic, with individuals representing many European nations, later to be joined by Africans and then Asians. The primary reasons for immigration were internal economic impoverishment and political repression in the countries of origin and the demands of a vigorous U.S. economy that required an expanded labor force. The conditions encountered by different ethnic groups, the reasons they came, and their expectations about life here differed greatly and have led ethnic groups to view themselves as distinct from others.

Ethnicity is a sense of peoplehood based on national origin. Although no longer useful in describing groups of people, the term *race* continues to be used in this country to classify groups of people as inferior or superior. Its popular usage is based on society's perception that racial differences are important—a belief not upheld by scientific study. The term *minority group* is useful in understanding relationships between groups. Oppressed minority groups lack social, economic, or political power in society. Members of these oppressed groups experience discriminatory treatment and often are relegated to relatively low-status positions in society.

Prejudice is "a negative attitude toward an entire category of people" (Schaefer, 1988, p. 55). Discrimination focuses on behavior that treats individuals differently because of their membership in a minority group. When discrimination is institutionalized, inequalities are inherent in policies and practices that benefit dominant group members while appearing to be neutral in their effect on different groups.

In a classroom, students are likely to come from several different ethnic groups, although physical differences are not always identifiable. Not all people view their ethnic origins as important in understanding who they are. Their membership in other microcultures may have a greater impact on their identity than the nations from which their ancestors came. Educators must beware of stereotyping all persons from the same ethnic group; many differences exist within the same group.

Two approaches to incorporating ethnic content in the curriculum are ethnic studies and multiethnic education. Ethnic studies are an extension or special segment of the curriculum that focuses on the in-depth study of the history and contemporary conditions of one or more ethnic groups. Often, ethnic studies are offered as separate courses. Multiethnic education is broader in scope in that it requires ethnic content to permeate the total curriculum; thus, all courses taught reflect the multiethnic nature of society.

Understanding ethnicity is an advantage in developing effective teaching strategies for individual students. Instructional strategies that build on students' ethnic experiences can be used to help students learn concepts. Educators need to periodically assess their interactions with students to determine whether they are picking up the verbal and nonverbal cues of all students appropriately. They also need to check whether students are being treated inequitably because of ethnic differences. Teachers should also assess their teaching styles, as well as the learning styles of students, so that they can develop teaching strategies that will assist students from different ethnic backgrounds in learning the material being taught.

Educators must examine how they are administering and using standardized tests in the classroom. Too often, testing programs have been used for the purpose of identifying native intelligence and thus sorting people for education and jobs. If disproportionately large numbers of minority students are scoring poorly on such tests and being placed in special classes as a result, the program must be reviewed. Many factors can be used to provide information about intelligence and ability, for example, the ability to think and respond appropriately in different situations.

QUESTIONS FOR REVIEW

1. Why is membership in an ethnic group more important to some individuals than to others?

2. Describe factors that cause subordinate group members to view ethnicity differently than dominant group members.

3. Describe differences and similarities in the immigration patterns of Africans, Asians, Central Americans, Europeans, and South Americans during the past four centuries.

4. Distinguish between prejudice and discrimination and describe their impact on subordinate group members in this country.

5. Why is race no longer used by most anthropologists to describe groups of people? Why does it remain so important in the social, political, and economic patterns of the United States?

6. What characteristics might an educator look for to determine a student's ethnic background and the importance it plays in that student's life?

7. List five ways in which an educator should be able to use ethnicity in the classroom.

8. Contrast ethnic studies and multiethnic education, and give the advantages of each.

9. How should the learning styles of students affect the instructional strategies of the teacher?

10. Why is the use of standardized tests so controversial today?

REFERENCES

Appleton, N. (1983). *Cultural pluralism in education.* New York: Longman.

Banks, J. A. (1984). *Teaching strategies for ethnic studies* (3rd ed.). Boston: Allyn and Bacon.

Berreman, G. D. (1985). Race, caste, and other invidious distinctions in social stratification. In N. R. Yetman (Ed.), *Majority and minority: The dynamics of race and ethnicity in American life* (4th ed.) (pp. 21–39). Boston: Allyn and Bacon.

Brophy, J. E., & Good, T. L. (1974). *Teacher-student relationships: Causes and consequences.* New York: Holt, Rinehart & Winston.

Fordham, S. (1988, February). Racelessness as a factor in black students' school success: Pragmatic strategy or Pyrrhic victory. *Harvard Educational Review, 58*(1), 54–84.

Gans, H. J. (1985). Symbolic ethnicity: The future of ethnic groups and cultures in America. In N. R. Yetman (Ed.), *Majority and minority: They dynamics of race and ethnicity in American life* (4th ed.) (pp. 429–442). Boston: Allyn and Bacon.

Gay, G. (1977). Curriculum for multicultural education. In F. H. Klassen & D. M. Gollnick (Eds.), *Pluralism and the American teacher: Issues and case studies.* Washington, DC: American Association of Colleges for Teacher Education.

Gibson, M. A. (1988). *Accommodation without assimilation: Sikh immigrants in an American high school.* Ithaca, NY: Cornell University Press.

Gordon, M. M. (1964). *Assimilation in American life: The role of race, religion, and national origins.* New York: Oxford University Press.

Greeley, A. M. (1974). *Ethnicity in the United States: A preliminary reconnaissance.* New York: Wiley.

Guerin, G. R., & Maier, A. S. (1983). *Informal assessment in education.* Palo Alto, CA: Mayfield.

Higham, J. (1975). Toward racism: The history of an idea. In N. R. Yetman & C. H. Steele (Eds.), *Majority and minority: The dynamics of racial and ethnic relations* (2nd ed.) (pp. 207–222). Boston: Allyn and Bacon.

McDermott, R. P., & Gospodinoff, K. (1983). Social contexts for ethnic borders and school failure. In H. T. Trueba, G. P. Guthrie, & K. Hu-Pei (Eds.), *Culture and the bilingual classroom: Studies in classroom ethnography* (pp. 212–230). Rowley, MA: Newbury House.

Mercer, J. R. (1978). Test "validity," "bias," and "fairness": An analysis from the perspective of the sociology of knowledge. *Interchange, 9,* 4, 5, 14–15.

Montagu, A. (1972). *Statement on race: An annotated elaboration and exposition of the four statements on race issues by the United Nations Educational, Scientific, and Cultural Organization.* New York: Oxford University Press.

National Alliance of Black School Educators. (1984). *Saving the African American child.* Washington, DC: Author.

Oakes, J. (1988). Tracking in mathematics and science education: A structural contribution to unequal schooling. In L. Weis (Ed.), *Class, race, and gender in American education* (pp. 106–125). Albany, NY: State University of New York Press.

Ogbu, J. (1988). Class stratification, racial stratification, and schooling. In L. Weis (Ed.), *Class, race, and gender in American education.* Albany, NY: State University of New York Press.

Omi, M., & Winant, H. (1986). *Racial formation in the United States: From the 1960s to the 1980s.* New York: Routledge & Kegan Paul.

Pratte, R. (1979). *Pluralism in education: Conflict, clarity, and commitment.* Springfield, IL: Thomas.

Ramirez, M., & Castaneda, A. (1974). *Cultural democracy, bicognitive development and education.* New York: Academic Press.

Schaefer, R. T. (1988). *Racial and ethnic groups* (3rd ed.). Boston: Little, Brown.

Schuman, H. (1975). Free will and determinism in public beliefs about race. In N. R. Yetman & C. H. Steele (Eds.), *Majority and minority: The dynamics of racial and ethnic relations* (2nd ed.) (pp. 375–380). Boston: Allyn and Bacon.

Schuman, H., Steeh, C., & Bobo, L. (1985). *Racial attitudes in America: Trends and interpretations.* Cambridge, MA: Harvard University Press.

Smith, P. (1985). The impact of competency tests on teacher education: Ethical and legal issues in selecting and certifying teachers. In M. Haberman (Ed.), *Research in teacher education.* To be published.

Solomon, R. P. (1988). Black cultural forms in schools: A cross national comparison. In L. Weis (Ed.), *Class, race, and gender in American education* (pp. 249–265). Albany, NY: State University of New York Press.

Task Force on the Administration of Military Justice in the Armed Forces. (1972). *Report.* Washington, DC: U.S. Government Printing Office.

Teper, S. (1977). *Ethnicity, race, and human development: A report on the state of our knowledge.* Chicago: Institute on Pluralism and Group Identity.

Weinberg, M. (1983). *The search for quality integrated education: Policy and research on minority students in school and college.* Westport, CT: Greenwood.

Williams, R. L. (1973). *Black intelligence test of cultural homogeneity (BITCH).* St. Louis: Williams & Associates.

Willis, P. E. (1977). *Learning to labour: How working class kids get working class jobs.* Farnborough, England: Saxon House.

Yancey, W. L., Ericksen, E. P., & Juliani, R. N. (1985). Emergent ethnicity: A review and reformulation. In N. R. Yetman (Ed.), *Majority and minority: The dynamics of racial and ethnic relations* (4th ed.) (pp. 185–194). Boston: Allyn and Bacon.

Yetman, N. R. (Ed.). (1985). *Majority and minority: The dynamics of racial and ethnic relations* (4th ed.). Boston: Allyn and Bacon.

SUGGESTED READINGS

Banks, J. A. (1983). *Teaching strategies for ethnic studies* (3rd ed.). Boston: Allyn and Bacon.

An excellent resource book for all teachers, particularly teachers of social studies at all levels. Includes key concepts for multiethnic studies, recommendations for organizing and planning the ethnic studies program, and historical overviews, annotated bibliographies, and instructional activities for a variety of American ethnic groups.

Cortes, C. E. (1976). *Understanding you and them: Tips for teaching about ethnicity.* Boulder, CO: Social Science Education Consortium.

A handbook for teachers at all levels. Includes an overview of how ethnicity should be treated in the curriculum, specific activities for ethnic studies, resources available, and instruments available for evaluating the outcomes of ethnic studies.

Hale, J. (1982). *Black children: Their roots, culture, and learning styles*. Provo, UT: Brigham Young University Press.

> *Conceptual framework for examining the development of African-American children. Includes curriculum recommendations with implications for early childhood education.*

King, E. W. (1980). *Teaching ethnic awareness: Methods and materials for the elementary school*. Santa Monica, CA: Goodyear.

> *Instructional strategies and classroom activities for teaching ethnic awareness to elementary students. Provides background information on why it is important to understand concepts and theories about multiethnic education.*

Longstreet, W. S. (1978). *Aspects of ethnicity: Understanding differences in pluralistic classrooms*. New York: Teachers College Press.

> *Profiles for five aspects of ethnicity: verbal communication, nonverbal communication, orientation modes, social value patterns, and intellectual modes. Includes recommendations for teachers.*

NCSS Task Force on Ethnic Studies Curriculum Guidelines. (1976). *Curriculum guidelines for multiethnic education*. Arlington, VA: National Council for the Social Studies.

> *Detailed guidelines for use by elementary and secondary schools in evaluating their commitment to multiethnic education, as shown in the curriculum and school climate. Includes a rationale and specific guidelines.*

Ramirez, M., III, & Castaneda, A. (1974). *Cultural democracy, bicognitive development and education*. New York: Academic Press.

> *An excellent resource for understanding and identifying the learning styles of students and the teaching styles of educators. Includes strategies for teaching students to function effectively in different learning styles as well as discussion of cultural democracy and bicognitive development.*

Weinberg, M. (1983). *The search for quality integrated education: Policy and research on minority students in school and college*. Westport, CT: Greenwood.

> *A critical examination of the research on the schooling of poor and minority children. Provides a historical background and legal framework, as well as discussions of race and intelligence, discriminatory educational processes, and desegregation.*

CHAPTER 4
Gender

We do not have the chance to choose whether we are going to be born female or male; our sex is determined before we are born, and it is one of the first characteristics noticed at birth. There are no questions asked about a baby's ethnicity, religion, or socioeconomic status, because the newborn will automatically be assigned the same microcultures as its parents. Society will react to these ascribed characteristics in unequal ways, but similarly to the way it has reacted to the parents. However, the sex of the baby will elicit different responses from both society and the family.

Parents tend to perceive male and female newborn infants differently, although there are no differences in other physical characteristics at birth. In a comparison of thirty newborns of the same length, weight, and Apgar scores (i.e., rating of the infant's color, muscle tone, reflexes, irritability, and heart and respiratory rates), researchers found that parents described girls and boys differently. Girls were more likely to be described as little, beautiful, pretty, and cute, whereas boys were described as big, strong, and hardy (Rubin, Provenzano, & Luria, 1974). Traditionally, baby gifts came wrapped in pink or blue paper to designate the sex of the newborn, and the name tags in the hospital nursery often are coded blue and pink. In many households, toys and clothes differ based on sex. More importantly, many parents and other individuals begin to treat their children differently based on their sex (Safilios-Rothschild, 1979).

What difference does our sex make to us and to our students? Other than different sex organs and reproductive capabilities, there really are not many biological differences between males and females, as we will see later in this chapter. Nevertheless, the popular, and sometimes "scientific," beliefs about differences between the sexes have not always matched reality.

For years, women were thought to be intellectually inferior to men and thus generally incapable of most professional and administrative work. Their nature made it imperative that men give orders and women take orders in the workplace. Because their strength was not comparable to that of men, women were also unable to obtain many manual or working-class jobs except for the most menial and lowest paid. Until recently, most women were expected to be homemakers, performing services for the family without remuneration.

Even though there is now clear evidence that women and men do not differ in intelligence, the percentage of men in the best-paying and most demanding professional jobs is disproportionately higher than the percentage of women in those jobs (see Figure 2–2). Because of technological advances, brute strength is usually no longer a requirement for most manual jobs, but the percentage of women in those jobs still falls far behind the percentage of men. Even today, many men and women believe that there are biological differences that prevent equality of the sexes.

In response to the patriarchical arrangements that keep women subordinate to men within the home and our capitalist system, strong women's movements have developed at different periods in our history. A number of the women and men in the antislavery movements prior to the Civil War raised concerns about women's issues, including divorce, property rights, the right to speak in public, abuse by husbands, work with little or no pay, and suffrage. A result was the Seneca Falls

Convention in 1848, where women first organized to fight against their oppression. In this effort, there were some male supporters, including Frederick Douglass. However, there were many women who were not supportive of equality and continued to accept their subordinate role. During this period, feminists were actively involved in fighting together with blacks and white abolitionists against slavery and for human and civil rights for all.

During the remainder of the nineteenth century, some changes became institutionalized. Most of these were in terms of protective legislation for women and children, not equal rights. Protective legislation made some manual jobs inaccessible to women because of the danger involved and limited the number of hours that could be worked and the time at which one could work. Unfortunately, feminists segregated their fight for equal rights from the struggles of other oppressed groups and refused to take a stand against Jim Crow laws and other violations of the civil rights of African- and Asian-Americans. The national and regional women's groups also pitted themselves against black men in the fight for the right to vote, which was granted to black men with the passage of the Fifteenth Amendment in 1870. The right to vote was not granted to women until 1919, after another vigorous struggle by suffragettes at the beginning of this century.

The most significant changes in the status of women were initiated in the 1960s, when feminists were able to gain the support of more women and men than at any previous time in history. As in the previous century, this movement developed out of the struggle for civil rights by African-Americans. In an attempt to defeat the Civil Rights Bill in Congress, a southern congressman inserted the words "or sex" to Title VII, declaring that discrimination based on "race, color, national origin, or sex" was prohibited. This legislation, which was approved in 1964, was the first time that equal rights had been extended to women. Still, the one-sentence Equal Rights Amendment (ERA), "Equality of rights under the law shall not be denied or abridged by the United States or by any state on account of sex," was defeated again in 1983, even though two-thirds of the U.S. population supported it.

The women's movements that were initiated in the nineteenth century were, and continue to be, dominated by middle-class white women. They have, for the most part, limited the struggle to women's issues rather than broader civil rights for all oppressed groups. This focus has prevented the wide-spread involvement in the movement of both men and women who are African-Americans, Asian-Americans, Hispanic Americans, and Native Americans. Support from the working class has also been limited. The lack of concern for general civil rights, resulting in the exclusion of other oppressed groups in a broader struggle, has been a major drawback of the women's movement since the Civil War.

Why do equal rights for women continue to be unmet? There are different views about the equality of the sexes. Feminists are supportive of equality in jobs, pay, schooling, responsibilities in the home, and the nation's laws. They believe that women and men should have a choice about working in the home or outside of the home, having children, and determining their sexual preference. Women should not have to be subordinate to men at home, in the workplace, or in society. The physical and mental violence that has resulted from such subordination should not be tolerated by society. The availability of child care and shared male and female responsibilities in the home are promoted.

On the other hand, there is a vocal group of antifeminists that includes both men and women who have fought against the Equal Rights Amendment and other equality issues. This group is led by political conservatives, especially those from a fundamentalist religious background. They believe that the primary responsibilities of a woman are to be a good wife and mother, and employment outside of the home is viewed as interfering with these expected roles. Homemaking is the career that should be pursued. The male is to be the primary breadwinner in the family, and a woman's dependency on the husband or father is expected. They believe that feminism and equal rights will lead to the disintegration of the nuclear family unit. Homosexuality and abortion are abhorred. These men and women were able to organize politically to defeat the ERA.

Regardless of one's identification with feminism, "most human beings live in single-sex worlds, women in a female world and men in a male world, and the two are different from one another in a myriad of ways, both subjectively and objectively" (Bernard, 1981, p. 3). Differences can be observed in sex segregation at social gatherings; concentrations in different occupations; dress and sex-specific grooming; and types of relationships, both between and within the sexes, such as dating behavior, sex-specific leisure activities, and stereotyped perceptions by members of each sex about themselves and the other sex (Safilios-Rothschild, 1979). "All human languages make a definite distinction between the sexes, and all societies use sex as the basis for assigning people to different adult roles" (Stockard & Johnson, 1980, p. 3). In the United States, men and women disproportionately enter different occupations and have different activities and opportunities in the economic world. "At school, at church, at work, at play, boys and girls and men and women are governed by different norms, rules of behavior and expectations; they are subject to different eligibility rules for rewards and different vulnerability to punishments" (Bernard, 1981, p. 4). In all known cultures, men's work is assigned higher prestige in society than women's work, regardless of the nature of the work. Male activities and roles are always recognized as predominantly important and given more authority and value than those undertaken by women (Rosaldo & Lamphere, 1974). In U.S. society, this inferior status is reflected in the inequities that exist in the prestige of different jobs held by men and women, the difference in wages earned by men and women, and the differential prestige and economic rewards for housework and child rearing compared to nonhousehold work. Of course, the range of social and economic differences within one sex is as great as it is between the sexes. There is no doubt that some women are economically and socially better off than many men. Nevertheless, women as a group have not been allowed a status equal to men in economic, social, and political spheres. In addition, differences between men and women are influenced by class, ethnicity, race, religion, and age.

Men are also greatly affected by society's view of gender expectations. The masculine characteristics that are rewarded in our society are independence, assertiveness, leadership ability, self-reliance, and emotional stability (Bornstein, 1982). However, Filene (1986) observes that "in reality, few men truly extinguished the need to be comforted, the fear of loneliness, the anxiety of being inept or wrong or unloved. But they had learned to hide those vulnerabilities behind tight lips and dry eyes—the masculine armor" (p. 213). Some men have established their own male liberation groups to promote choices beyond the traditional male roles. While occupation is still very important in a man's identification of who he is, the desire to be more involved in child rearing is gaining support.

Unlike the women's movement, which became social action, male liberation remains a personal, not political, matter. When a group holds power and privilege in society, it is difficult to relinquish it. "Men cannot be liberated from conventional male roles until institutions permit part-time and flexible work schedules as well as abundant, inexpensive child-care facilities. And men will not liberate themselves until they resolve the culturally entrenched definitions of control achievement and self-esteem" (Filene, 1986, p. 221).

Are there biological differences that prevent male- and female-assigned roles from being interchanged? Although women alone can bear offspring, does that also mean that only they can rear a child? Do biological differences suggest that we do different types of work?

DIFFERENCES BETWEEN MALES AND FEMALES

Most of us can easily identify physical differences between men and women by appearance alone. Girls tend to have lighter skeletons and different shoulder and pelvic proportions. During puberty, the proportion of fat to total body weight increases in girls and decreases in boys. The differences in physical structure contribute to a female's diminished strength, lower endurance for heavy labor, greater difficulty in running or overarm throwing, and better ability to float. Of course, environment and culture greatly influence the extent of these physical differences for both males and females. Thus, the feminine characteristics listed here can be altered with good nutrition, physical activity, practice, and different behavioral expectations (Barfield, 1976).

Other than sex organs, there are few observable differences between the sexes at birth. Boys tend to be slightly longer and heavier than girls. Girls have a lower percentage of their total body weight in muscle, and their lungs and heart are proportionally smaller. Although the proportion of different hormones in the body differs by sex, boys and girls have similar hormonal levels and similar physical development during the first eight years (Barfield, 1976). The onset of puberty marks the difference in hormonal levels that controls the physical development of the two sexes.

There are a number of other documented physical differences between the sexes. Males are more susceptible to physical disorders, disease, and early death. They seem to be more prone to speech defects (such as stuttering and language disorders), reading disabilities, limited vision, and hearing loss and deafness. Men exhibit peptic ulcers and skin disorders more often than women, whereas women are more likely to suffer from manic and depressive emotional psychoses (Barfield, 1976). Men are more likely than women to die from bronchitis, emphysema, asthma, cardiovascular disease, cirrhosis of the liver, hypertension, pneumonia, and influenza (Goldberg, 1976). More women attempt suicide, but more men succeed (Barfield, 1976). Some of these differences may be the result of different cultural expectations rather than a result of different physical makeup. For example, sex differences in incidence of cardiovascular disease may decrease as more women enter jobs associated with stress. Childless single and married women working in demanding careers suffer the lowest incidence of stress-related disease of all men and women in studies by researchers at the University of North Carolina. On the other hand, the highest incidence of heart disease occurs in women who are mothers and work in clerical positions (Radl, 1983). Because of different expectations and behaviors of the sexes in the past, it is difficult to determine how many of the differences mentioned here are actually a result of physical differences between females and males.

It is commonly thought that women are more sociable than men and that men have a higher achievement motivation (or that men are more aggressive). Within our culture, males and females are often assigned different psychological traits. In an exhaustive review of the literature on sex differences, Maccoby and Jacklin (1974) did find some psychological differences between the sexes, but not nearly as many as people attribute to the two sexes:

☐ On perception: (a) Infants of both sexes have similar responses to visual and auditory stimuli; (b) they both quickly develop more sustained interest in social events; and (c) research in other perceptual areas is inconclusive.

☐ On learning: (a) Both sexes respond to conditioning in similar ways; and (b) there is no difference between the sexes in the complex problem-solving strategies.

☐ On intelligence: (a) Beginning at ten years of age, girls excel at verbal tasks; (b) beginning in early adolescence, boys excel at mathematical tasks; and (c) between ten and twelve years of age, boys begin to excel on visual-spatial tasks.

☐ On achievement motivation: (a) Before college, there are no differences between the sexes; and (b) beginning in college, males have a higher internal locus of control (i.e., a stronger belief that they can control their own destiny).

☐ On sociability and affiliation: There are no differences between the sexes.

☐ On aggression and dominance: (a) Beginning at two years of age, boys are more verbally and physically aggressive; and (b) male readiness to aggress overtly and covertly is greater.

☐ On activity level: There are no differences between the sexes.

Thus, the only psychological differences are in the areas of verbal, mathematical, and visual-spatial tasks; aggression; and internal locus of control. Although there may be great psychological differences between individuals, there are few group differences between females and males.

Gender Differences

The sex differences discussed in the previous section describe the physical and psychological differences between the sexes, but that does not explain the many female and male characteristics attributed to both sexes in our society.

Gender is a term that better describes these differences as masculinity and femininity—the thoughts, feelings, and behavior that are identified as being either male or female. Although there are few physical and psychological differences between the sexes, their culturally determined behavior can differ greatly. Society reinforces these culturally determined differences. Many parents and teachers respond with disgust when these differences are abridged (e.g., when a boy shows feminine traits, or acts like a "sissy").

All of us identify ourselves as either female or male. This gender identity is the sum of our feelings about our sexual status; it reflects our conviction that biologically and behaviorally, we are either male or female (Swerdloff, 1975). Most people take their gender identity for granted and do not question it because it agrees with their biological identity. When it is established in the first few years of life, it is difficult to change gender identity.

One's recognition of the appropriate sex and gender identity occurs unconsciously early in life. It becomes a basic anchor in the personality and forms a core part of one's self-identity (Stockard & Johnson, 1980). By the age of two years, children realize that they are either a boy or girl and begin to learn their expected behaviors. By the time they are five or six years old, they have already learned their gender and stereotypical behavior (Bernard, 1981).

Although researchers are unsure how gender identity develops, the most important factor is the assignment of gender to an individual at birth by the doctor, parents, family, and friends. Biology does not necessarily determine whether an individual feels female or male. Instead, the "communications of the parents and others in the child's environment have a virtually irreversible effect on the child's gender identity" (Stockard & Johnson, 1980, p. 132). Children are trained for their masculine and feminine roles in society. Parents have different attitudes and treatment for the sexes, as demonstrated by their different reactions to boys and girls, their different methods of rearing each, and the importance they place on goals, depending on the sex of the child. The sex typing by parents is reflected in the personality attributes, intellectual performance, and occupational choices of their children.

The fact that gender identity is learned becomes clearer when males and females from other cultures are observed. During her field work in New Guinea, Margaret Mead (1935) observed three variations of male and female personalities. Both male and female Arapesh were cooperative, unaggressive, and responsive to the needs and demands of others. In contrast, the Mundugumor males and females were ruthless

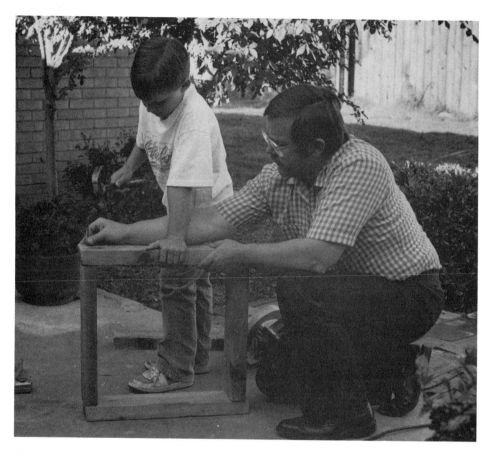

From an early age, most children adhere to the gender behavior and identity expected by society. (Photo by Sheryl Zelhart).

and aggressive, with few signs of a maternal cherishing aspect of personality. The Arapesh ideal was the mild, responsive man married to the mild, responsive woman; the Mundugumor ideal was the violent, aggressive man married to the violent, aggressive woman. In the third tribe, the Tchambuli, Mead found a genuine reversal of the sex attitudes of our own culture. The Tchambuli woman was dominant, impersonal, and the managing partner, while the man was less responsible and the emotionally dependent person. Mead's observations suggest that there is no basis for regarding aspects of behavior as inherently either male or female.

Gender should no longer be viewed in the traditional bipolar fashion as if masculine and feminine traits never coexist in an individual. Barfield (1976) summarizes this view: "An individual is not more or less masculine, or more or less feminine, but rather more or less aggressive, sexual, nurturant, ambitious, verbal, spatial, and so on" (p. 109).

SOCIALIZATION

Children are born with biological characteristics that are either male or female, but their gender is determined primarily by parents and others with whom they interact. In addition to family influence on gender identity, children learn appropriate sex behavior from reading, watching television, and playing with peers and toys (Safilios-Rothschild, 1979). The process of learning to behave in accordance with socially prescribed roles and expectations is called *socialization.* It is the process by which a child develops social skills and a sense of self.

During socialization, children internalize the social norms considered appropriate for their sex. They develop sex-appropriate behavior, personality characteristics, emotional responses, attitudes, and beliefs. These characteristics become so much a part of our self-identification that we forget they are learned and not innate characteristics. Individuals who demonstrate characteristics inappropriate to their sex are often chastised by society. Women are supposed to be feminine and men masculine, with society tolerating little crossover. Generally, females are allowed more flexibility in their gender identification than males in that the female with masculine traits is more acceptable in society then the male with feminine traits.

In most cases, children have been socialized differently depending on their sex. The socialization of boys has been oriented toward achievement and self-reliance, that of girls toward nurturance and responsibility. "Sex-typed socialization taught men to value work over home, while teaching women the opposite" (Filene, 1986, p. 220). Traditionally, it was believed that girls naturally learned their roles as wife and mother. The knowledge required to carry out these roles was not as highly valued by society as the knowledge required to achieve manhood. Especially in the middle class, girls learned to share and boys learned to compete (Filene, 1986).

Appropriate sex behavior is reinforced throughout the life cycle by social processes of approval and disapproval, reward and punishment. Studies show that there are substantive differences in the ways parents treat children of different sexes. Because mothers have primary responsibility for raising most children, the mother-child relationship in the early years is important in determining the male or female personality. The mother provides a girl an easily accessible model from the beginning. It is easy and natural for a girl to know and learn appropriate behavior by being with her mother much of the time during the preschool years. However, boys are not as likely to have readily available male models or masculine activities. At some point, the boy must break from his mother and establish his maleness separately from her (Rosaldo & Lamphere, 1974).

Socialization does not end with parents and friends. When the child enters school, the socialization process continues. In fact, achievement studies show that schooling is most effective when the values of school and family are similar. Generally, schools convey the same standards for sex roles as most parents in our society. The attitudes and values about appropriate sex roles are embedded in the curriculum of most schools. Elementary schools appear to imitate the mothering role with a predominance of female teachers and an emphasis on obedience and conformity. In classrooms, boys and girls tend to receive different feedback for their work, similar to the patterns used at home.

Sex/Gender Roles

Anthropologists have found that there are some universal practices related to sex roles. First, in all societies, men have clear control of political and military apparatus; in no known society do women have such control. Second, no society fosters achievement and self-reliance in females more than in males. Third, boys tend to seek dominance more than girls do and are significantly more physically and verbally aggressive. It is still unclear, however, whether these characteristics are near-universal sex role characteristics or a function of a near-universal cultural practice (Lee, 1976). There is no evidence that women could not control political and military apparatus or that achievement and self-reliance could not be fostered in them to the same degree as in men. The fact that these universal practices exist is the result of a historical development rather than the superiority of the male (de Beauvoir, 1974).

In every society, there are characteristic tasks, manners, and responsibilities associated with either women or men. Traditionally, women have had the primary responsibility for child rearing; men have had the responsibility for hunting (i.e., bringing home the paycheck in contemporary society) and warring (Rosaldo & Lamphere, 1974). Although the great strength and endurance of the male at one time may have been necessary in the division of labor to carry out numerous responsibilities, technology has rendered such physical strength unnecessary for most jobs that exist today. At the same time, child rearing does not have to be the total responsibility of the woman; men can learn to be as nurturing as women.

Today, men are still likely to have the primary responsibility for earning the income to support the family, although both the wife and husband work in 40 percent of all families and in 60 percent of middle-income families (Filene, 1986). Many women continue to fulfill the roles of mother and wife; the husband fulfills the roles of wage earner, father, and husband. However, these male and female roles are expanding and changing. Almost half of the nation's work force is female, and 90 percent of all women will work outside the home at some time. Today, a growing number of women are divorced, widowed, or otherwise alone and thus unable to depend on a male wage earner. They are forced economically to fulfill that role alone. Although both men and women now work in a variety of careers and share many roles and activities that were formerly sex-typed, many adults still retain their traditional sex roles as well.

Traditional feminine roles have less status than masculine roles. This female inferiority often leads to ambivalence, especially in the adolescent girl. There is growing evidence that "women who lack a sense of social and sexual entitlement, who hold traditional notions of what it means to be female—self-sacrificing and relatively passive—and who undervalue themselves are disproportionately likely to find themselves with an unwanted pregnancy and to maintain it through to motherhood" (Fine, 1988, p. 48). Teenagers from low-income families are particularly susceptible to fulfilling their female role through child bearing, no matter what their racial or ethnic backgrounds. In some cases, having a baby is the passage from childhood to adulthood. As a result, the children of teenage mothers will be disproportionately poor. The educational and occupational achievements of the mothers are often halted or delayed.

In a study of women teachers in an urban area, Weiler found that their choice of teaching as a career was based, in part, on the use of their nurturing and caring qualities. Because of their subordinate status, they found reasons not to pursue the math, science, or other professional careers that they had envisioned when they started college. The realities of racism and sexism influenced their final career decision. Weiler (1988) concludes:

> It is the internalization of a male hegemony that leads women to devalue their own worth and to assume that the career of a man is more important than their own, or that they are somehow "incapable" of doing math or science. Thus even when choices are freely made, they are choices made within a kind of logic of existing social structures and ideology. And this logic is learned very early and is reinforced through many institutions. Thus we see in these stories [of women teachers] the valuing of female nurturance, and at the same time women's sense of inadequacy; an acceptance that men are the *real people* and that girls and women are there to support them. (p. 89)

The sex role expectations are also reflected in schools. Girls and young women are expected to be well behaved and do well. Males are expected to be less well behaved and not to achieve academically as well as females prior to puberty. Many working-class males develop patterns of resistance to school and its authority figures because it is feminine and emphasizes mental rather than manual work (Willis, 1977).

Most people define the appropriate behaviors of males and females through their own ethnic and religious orientations. Males are not supposed to exhibit female characteristics and vice versa. In addition, individuals who choose homosexuality over heterosexuality are often not accepted as *real men* or *real women*, even though they may exhibit the same degree of masculinity or feminity as heterosexuals. Gay men share with heterosexual men a dominant position in relation to women, but are subordinate in relation to heterosexual men. As a result of the isolation and discrimination forces on homosexuals, gay cultural forms have developed. These include gay newspapers, magazines, churches, health clinics, and social clubs. Equality has yet to be extended to many females and males who openly define their sexual preference against the national norm.

Nevertheless, we are living in an era of changing norms, in which old, unequal roles are being rejected by many. These changes are resulting in many new uncertainties in which the norms of the appropriate sex role are no longer so distinct. As new norms develop, more flexible roles, personalities, and behaviors are evolving for both females and males.

Gender Stereotypes

Although gender roles tend to be gradually changing, they continue to be projected stereotypically in the socialization process. Masculine and feminine roles are learned early in childhood, not only from the parents but also from television and books to which many children are exposed. *Stereotypes* are exaggerated generalities that often are dangerous oversimplifications (Westoff, 1979). More specifically, Bornstein (1982) states that

> a *sex role stereotype* is the assumption that the male half of our population has in common another set of abilities, interests, values, and roles. Sex role stereotyping reflects oversimplified attitudes about males and females. It completely ignores individual differences. For example, the belief that all or most boys are good in math and science is a sex role stereotype. The belief that all or most girls are quiet and passive is another sex role stereotype. (p. 1)

Stereotyping narrowly defines the male and female roles and defines them for the two sexes as quite distinct from one another.

Stereotyping leads children to generalize that all persons within a group behave in the same way. Both males and females are often assigned traditional and rigid roles and characteristics in stereotypical presentations. Men and women become automatically associated with the characteristics and roles with which they are constantly endowed by the mass media and classroom materials. Careers are not the only areas in which sex stereotyping occurs. Male and female intellectual abilities, personality characteristics, physical appearance, social status, and domestic roles have also been sex stereotyped. Persons who differ from the stereotype of their group, especially gay men and women, are ostracized by the dominant group. Such role stereotyping denies individuals the wide range of human potential that is possible.

Television is one of the great perpetuators of sex role stereotyping. Studies show that by three years of age, children have already developed tastes in television programs related to age, sex, and race. By the time of high school graduation, the average child will have spent eleven thousand hours in the classroom and fifteen thousand hours in front of the television. Few children are exempt from this practice, since 97 percent of all homes in this country have one or more television sets (Bonk & Gardner, 1978). The influence of television is powerful, as observed in the following study:

> Quite simply, any steady diet of television will have a powerful influence on children. Its effect is, at least in part, the inevitable, natural consequence of observing behavior in others. Modeling—in which a child learns from witnessing the actions of other persons—is a cornerstone in social development. Television, by its very nature, brainwashes children in that it shapes the way they view the world and the kind of people they will be. We cannot rid ourselves of its influence. (Miles, 1975, p. 16)

The stereotypical roles portrayed on television do not reflect the available options being pursued by many males and females in today's society. The ideals and ideas of dominant America are incorporated into program development as symbolic representations of American society. They are not literal portrayals, yet these representations announce to viewers what is valued and approved in society. In recent years, some television shows have expanded female roles beyond that of a mother, nurse, teacher, or secretary. Women are sometimes seen as lawyers, police officers, and tough administrators. On a few shows, men are portrayed as nurturing fathers, usually when there is no mother available to handle those responsibilities. There is even a show on public television with a gay man as the central character. Overall, most shows still project men as strong and independent, while working women care for the children and are responsible for the house.

The written media is another area in which women and men continue to be stereotypically portrayed. Most newspapers have women's pages that include articles on fashion, food, and social events—pages specifically written for what is believed to be the interests of women alone. Many magazines are directed at predominantly male or female audiences.

Whereas the average adult spends about one hour daily reading newspapers, magazines, and books (Stockard & Johnson, 1980), children spend much of their reading time with school textbooks and assigned readings. How do the sexes fare in the resources used in classrooms across the nation? Studies show that both children and adults in textbooks are assigned rigid traits and roles based on sex stereotypes.

Many girls seen in textbooks play with dolls, give tea parties, work in the kitchen, and are frightened of animals and loud noises; they need to ask advice of others and seek assistance to solve problems. In illustrations, girls often are spectators, usually watching boys actively participate. In contrast, boys in textbooks are involved in important activities that prepare them for the careers to be pursued as adults. They save girls and mothers from danger. If there is a problem to solve, they are ingenious and creative enough to find the answer. Boys in textbooks are almost always active; they are swimming, running, riding a bicycle, winning a ball game, or solving mysteries (Gollnick, Sadker, & Sadker, 1982). In elementary readers, chances are four to one against a girl's possessing a boy's traits. Chances are even greater against a boy's being portrayed with a girl's traits (Women on Words and Images, 1975).

Adults also suffer from sex role stereotyping in textbooks. Overwhelmingly, women are portrayed as mothers who do not work outside the home. The few textbook women who work are usually single. The few working mothers are shown hurrying home from work to care for children and the house, while working fathers take children on trips or to a ball game. Textbook occupations for women are very limited. Textbook women most often work in service occupations, such as a cafeteria worker, cashier, cleaning woman, dressmaker, librarian, school crossing guard, nurse, teacher, or telephone operator. Occasionally, there is a female physician. Men are found working in about six times as many different occupations as women. In a major study of elementary readers, for example, men had positions in 147 different occupations, whereas women had jobs in only 26 (Women on Words and Images, 1975). Minority women are the most neglected in textbooks. In a study of the five most widely used primary and intermediate basal readers, King (1989) found that female minority representation in stories ranged from 7 to 15 percent. African-American characters were found the most often. Least often seen were only two Asian-American characters.

Although males appear to be blessed with more desirable characteristics, they also suffer from such stereotyping. For the most part, females are allowed more flexible roles. Many males do not fit the confining stereotype of textbooks, in which they are expected to be strong, brave, and intelligent at all times. Some boys (and men, too) show emotions in real life, but they almost never do in textbooks. Any sign of weakness may prevent them from becoming a "real man" because they lack the necessary characteristics. Although men change diapers, wash dishes, clean the house, and cook meals, they seldom do those chores in textbooks. Men are seldom shown in nurturing roles in the home or as a career. Some men today choose nonstereotyped careers, such as nursing or preschool teaching, but these careers do not exist in textbooks. Men are limited to rigid attributes, emotions, and responsibilities in textbooks, making them victims of sex stereotyping, too (Gollnick et al., 1982).

The sex stereotypes portrayed in the mass media do not accurately reflect the nation in which we live. The stereotypical household with a full-time working father, stay-at-home mother, and one or more school-age children at home was typical in 1950 of 70 percent of all U.S. households. Today, however, only 4 percent of all households fit the stereotype (Hodgkinson, 1986). About 30 percent of the families in this country are headed by a female, and one of every fifteen American children lives in a single-parent family. The greatest change in the stereotypical family has been the wife entering the labor force. By 1982, the two-income family had become the norm rather than the exception; over 50 percent of all wives were working, and 53 percent of these working wives had children under eighteen years old (U.S. Bureau of the Census, 1988). The 1950 nontraditional family became the traditional family of 1980, but the 1950 family is the one continually portrayed in the mass media and classroom materials. The fact that one type of household has been portrayed as more favorable is not the concern here. The major concern is the reflection of reality in our society—the recognition and portrayal of the variety of households that in fact do exist. Of course, it is not only the type of household that is stereotyped. In contemporary society, the male and female traditional roles are practiced interchangeably in a growing number of families. Both men and women work in nontraditional careers and share many of the formerly sex-typed roles. Even the portrayal of the woman who stays at home is stereotyped; the reality and difficulty of juggling the care of children and a husband, cleaning, cooking, shopping, doing laundry, repairing a leaky faucet, entertaining, and bookkeeping are seldom presented.

For many women, the role of wife, mother, and homemaker is very satisfying. Many men are quite satisfied to be the wage earner and to have their wives be primarily responsible for child rearing and homemaking. The problem occurs when either or both partners find these traditional sex-typed roles unrewarding (D. Sadker, 1975). Some men enjoy, or at least do not mind, sharing equally in the joys and frustrations of raising children and managing a house. Many women must work to supplement the family income in order to live reasonably comfortably and sometimes just to meet the essential needs of the family. A growing percentage of women are heads of households and must take on all of the roles of wage earner, mother, and homemaker at the same time.

Women are seriously hurt by sex-stereotyped roles because the roles assigned to women have less prestige in society. In pursuing a career, many women have learned both feminine and masculine characteristics to compete successfully in a masculine world. Feminine jobs, such as nursing, secretarial work, teaching, and cleaning, may

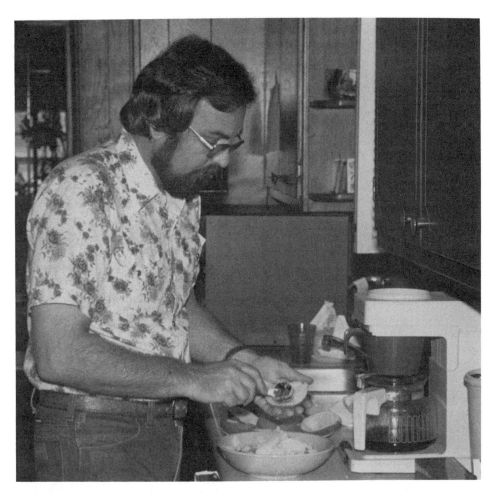

Today, many men take on household roles that were previously assigned almost completely to women.

better fit the stereotype of appropriate jobs for women, but they are low-status and low-paying jobs. Unfortunately, a disproportionately large number of women in the labor force continue to perform jobs that are similar to the traditional roles of homemaker, wife, and mother.

While females suffer from economic limitations and low self-esteem as a result of learning the stereotypical role, males are not exempt. They are often caught in roles that are dangerous to their health, frustrating, and unfulfilling. Total responsibility for the financial support of a family is a very demanding role—one that sometimes leads to heart attacks, hypertension, and other stress-related diseases. The *male mystique* in the United States implies that a man must be a successful earner first and a person second (R. Gordon, 1980). For example, the self-concept of a man suffers greatly when he is unemployed, because he is not fulfilling society's first expectation of him.

As a part of this mystique, males must always be proving that they are full-fledged males. In *The Hazards of Being Male*, Goldberg (1976) states:

> The "blessings" of being a young male in our culture are extremely mixed. From early boyhood on, his emotions are suppressed by others and therefore repressed by himself. In countless ways he is constantly being conditioned not to express his feelings and needs openly. Though he too has needs for dependency, he learns that it is unmasculine to act in a dependent way. It is also unmasculine to be frightened ("scared"), to want to be held, stroked, and kissed, to cry, etc. While all of these expressions of self are acceptable in a girl they are incompatible with the boy's sought after image of being tough and in control. (p. 183)

Young men are often expected to prove their masculinity through macho behavior. They face peer pressure to take risks to prove themselves worthy of being male. Thus, many race cars, brag of sexual prowess, and fight for honor. These behavioral and emotional constraints extend to adulthood, usually as internalized patterns that lead to the stigmatization of men who choose to work in traditionally feminine jobs—as nurses, librarians, or preschool teachers. Their hobbies are limited to sports, machines, hunting, and other masculine interests. Men who pursue traditionally feminine careers and hobbies are often ridiculed unless they have already proved their masculinity. These constraints prevent males from developing their nurturing traits in a way that would allow them to be as competent at child rearing as many women are.

Consciousness-raising activities to help men and women understand and evaluate the stereotyped roles for which they have been socialized have been extremely helpful in opening options for both groups. In many communities, one no longer has to have only feminine or masculine characteristics, behavior, or job options; it is becoming easier to have both. It is probably more accurate to describe individuals as more or less aggressive and more or less dependent rather than as feminine or masculine. More couples are sharing the role of wage earner—a traditionally sex-typed role for men. It is possible that in the future, a growing number of men will share more equally in the responsibilities of child rearing and homemaking. Optimistically, both men and women will be able to choose roles with which they are comfortable rather than having to accept a sex role determined by society.

SEX DISCRIMINATION

Throughout history, women have been assigned a subordinate role to men. A century ago, most women could not attend college, had no control of either their property or children, could not initiate a divorce, and were forbidden to smoke or drink. Because these outrageous inequities no longer exist and there are now laws to protect the rights of women, many people believe that men and women are treated equally in society. However, society continues to hold deep-rooted assumptions about how men and women should think, look, and behave. These societal expectations lead to discriminatory behavior based on sex alone.

"Sex discrimination is the denial of opportunity, privilege, role, or reward on the basis of sex" (Bornstein, 1980, p. 1). Often this discrimination is practiced by individuals in personal situations of marriage and family life as well as in their occupational roles of manager, realtor, secretary, or legislator. Socialization patterns within the family are discriminatory when children are taught self-differentiated behaviors. For example, girls are taught to be more obedient, neat, passive, and dependent, while boys are allowed to be more disobedient, aggressive, independent, exploring, and creative. These sex-differentiated behaviors prepare each for sex-specific jobs and severely limit the options available to an individual. Aggressive and independent individuals (usually men) are likely to manage those who are obedient and dependent (usually women).

Many of us discriminate on the basis of sex without realizing it. Because we are raised in a sexist society, we think our behavior is natural and acceptable, even when it is discriminatory. Women often do not realize the extent to which they do not participate equally in society—a sign that they internalize their distinct roles well during the socialization process. Most parents do not directly plan to harm their daughters by teaching them to be feminine. They do not realize that such characteristics may prevent their daughters from achieving societal benefits comparable to men. Too often, girls are encouraged to gain such societal rewards through marriage rather than by their own individual achievement and independence.

Many individuals outside the family also practice sex discrimination. The kindergarten teacher who scolds the boy for playing in the girls' corner is discriminating. The personnel director who hires only women for secretarial positions and only men as managers is overtly discriminating on the basis of sex. Such behavior prevents men from entering female occupations and vice versa. Educators have the opportunity to help all students break out of group stereotypes and to provide opportunities to explore and pursue a wide variety of options in fulfilling their potential individuals.

Sex discrimination not only is practiced by individuals, but also has been institutionalized in policies, laws, rules, and precedents in society. These institutional arrangements benefit one sex over the other. What are the results of individual and institutional sex discrimination?

When physical strength determined who performed certain tasks, men conducted the hunt for food, which required them to leave the home, while women raised food close to the home. With industrialization, this pattern of men working away from home and women working close to home was translated into labor market activity for men and non-labor market activity for women. Men began to work specific hours and receive pay for that work. By contrast, women worked irregular and unspecified working periods in the home and received no wages for their work (Kreps & Leaper, 1976). The value of a woman's work was never rewarded by money paid directly to her. It certainly was not as valued as the work of men, who contributed in labor market production. In our society, individuals who provide services for which they are paid have a higher status than those who are not paid for their work, such as homemakers.

Kreps and Leaper (1976) predicted that in the future, women will spend only about a decade less than men in the labor market. Unlike men, most working women maintain dual careers. In addition to their labor market activities, they generally have the responsibility for the home, including child care and housekeeping chores. Studies of family time allocation have found that few husbands increase their participation in work at home when the wife enters the labor force. The typical husband helps out with about 20 percent of the homemaking and child-rearing activities, regardless of whether the wife also works outside the home (Filene, 1986). Women who work outside the home usually have little reduction in their work at home. Instead, they reduce their amount of free time or the amount of time spent in homemaking activities.

Teenage pregnancy complicates even further women's participation in the labor force. "Young women with poor basic skills are three times more likely to become teen parents than women with average or above-average basic skills" (Fine, 1988, p. 48). Further, the children of these single teenage mothers are more likely than other children to be poor for long periods of their childhood. Many of these mothers must depend on welfare and/or work in low-paying jobs. This issue has been exacerbated by discrimination against pregnant teenagers in many of the nation's high schools.

Does the amount of education influence a person's participation in the labor market? Regardless of their education, men are expected to work in the labor market. For women, however, the acquisition of more education does not increase the likelihood of working after completing school. At the same time, the amount of education obtained by women does little to close the gap between the earnings of men and women. The more education received, the greater expected earnings for both sexes, but women with four years of college earn only slightly more than men who have only finished elementary school.

The difference in income between men and women generally increases with age. The difference shown in Figure 4–1 is not impacted by women who do not work. It reflects the income of male and female workers who work full-time. Why do these differences exist and continue to increase throughout life?

These discrepancies in income are due in part to the types of jobs held by the two groups. Women first entered the labor market in jobs that were similar to those performed in the home, such as sewing, teaching, nursing, and doing household services. Therefore, the stereotypes about the capabilities and roles of women in the domestic setting were transferred to the labor market. Jobs were defined according to their sex appropriateness. Women workers continue to be heavily concentrated in a few occupations. These jobs are accompanied by neither high prestige nor high income. Women continue to be extremely underrepresented as managers and as skilled workers.

It has been difficult for women to enter administrative and skilled jobs. There are fewer entry-level positions for these jobs than for the less prestigious ones. The available openings are often for jobs where there are short or nonexistent promotion ladders, few opportunities for training, low wages, few chances for stability, and

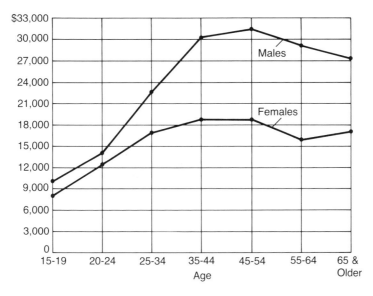

Figure 4–1   Median annual income of year-round, full-time workers over fifteen years old by sex and education: 1986.

poor working conditions. Clerical and sales jobs are examples of such jobs, but even the more professional jobs of teaching and nursing offer little opportunity for career advancement. "Efforts to train women for and place them in higher paying, traditionally male jobs, especially skilled trades, electronics, and coal mining, continue to face heavy resistance from private industry, organized labor, and often the government" (Shell, 1980, p. 14).

When men enter traditionally female fields, they often do not hold the same positions as women in the field. Less than 14 percent of all elementary teachers are men, but 53 percent of all high school teachers are men (U.S. Bureau of the Census, 1988). Male social workers are more often community organizers rather than group workers or caseworkers. Although the percentage of men participating in traditionally female jobs has increased over the years, they have become overrepresented in the higher-status, administrative levels of these occupations. For example, over 73 percent of all public school teachers are women, whereas over 82 percent of the principals are men (U.S. Bureau of the Census, 1988).

Sex segregation and wage discrimination also affect women in blue-collar and white-collar jobs. The majority of women enter the labor force at the lowest entry level of these categories, with unstable employment opportunities and low wages. Much of the discrimination against women in the labor force results from decisions of employers concerning promotions and wage increases. In addition, many of the occupations in which women are concentrated have not been organized by unions that might help change poor working conditions and low wages.

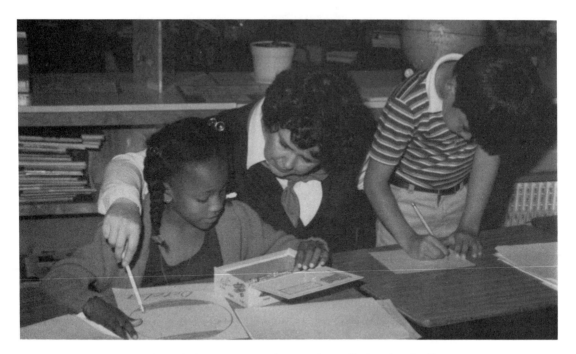

Women still work disproportionately in traditionally female jobs. For example, they make up over 82 percent of all elementary school teachers in this country.

Gradually, more women are entering traditionally male occupations, as barriers against their entry are broken. In 1950, for example, only 6.5 percent of all physicians and osteopaths were women; by 1986, 17.6 percent were women. The percentage of lawyers and judges has increased from 4.1 percent to 18.1 percent, but only 6 percent of all engineering jobs were held by women as late as 1986 (U.S. Bureau of the Census, 1988). Although more women are entering the traditionally male-dominated fields, they continue to face discrimination in wages earned. In 1955, women working full time earned 65 cents for every dollar earned by men; in 1988, they were still earning only 65 cents for every dollar earned by men. Such discrimination greatly affects the quality of life for women.

"Sexism is the degree to which an individual's beliefs or behaviors are prejudiced on the basis of sex" (Bornstein, 1980, p. 1). It is another term used to describe prejudice and discrimination against women at both the individual and institutional levels. It assumes that "human sexes have a distinctive make-up that determines their respective lives, usually involving the idea that one sex is superior and has the right to rule the other; a policy of enforcing such asserted right; a system of government and society based upon it" (Frazier & M. Sadker, 1973, p. 2).

Homophobia is another area of discrimination of which educators should be aware. Heterosexuality is the valued sexual preference that is promoted by the dominant power group in this country. It is so highly valued that laws and social practices have developed to try to prevent any other sexual preference. Until recently, laws in most states forbid sexual liaisons between members of the same sex; some states still have laws against sodomy. In many areas of the country where overt discrimination against homosexuals remains, gay men and women may not be able to find housing or jobs. Often they are not admitted to "straight" clubs and are vulnerable to attacks by straights on city streets. The National Gay and Lesbian Task Force collects data on reports of harassment and violence against gays, and such incidents have increased dramatically over the past few years.

Prior to the 1970s, most lesbians and gay men hid their homosexuality from their families, landlords, and the people with whom they worked because of the fear of rejection and retaliation. Following the 1969 Stonewall Inn riot in Greenwich Village, in which gays fought back against police, it became easier for many of them to openly admit their homosexuality. They, like other oppressed groups, extended the fight for civil rights to include their own struggle. As a result, "more than half of the states repealed sodomy laws, the Civil Rights Commission lifted its ban on hiring homosexuals, and the 1980 Democratic Party platform endorsed gay rights" (Filene, 1986, p. 218). In addition, the American Psychological Association dropped homosexuality from its list of mental disorders. Nevertheless, discrimination and prejudice against gay men and women remain, as evidenced by policies to prevent their organizing clubs on some college campuses. In addition, derogatory terms (e.g., sissy, faggot, and dyke) are used by many adults and students in schools. Much work is still required to overcome prejudices and discrimination based solely on sexual preference.

Professional educators have the responsibility of eradicating sexism in the classroom and school. The role of teachers and other professional educators requires that they not limit the potential of any student because of gender or sexual preference. Classroom interactions, resources, extracurricular activities, and counseling practices must be evaluated to ensure that students are not being discriminated against because of their gender.

GENDER IDENTITY

There is no choice about sex identity. We are either male or female because of biological distinctions in the reproductive organs. However, gender identity allows for flexibility in that an individual can have feminine and masculine characteristics. In fact, a person may learn both masculine and feminine traits and use different behaviors in appropriate situations. Thus, some men are aggressive in their work setting and yet are nurturing to their children in the family setting. Even in the work situation, some men are finding that feminine characteristics are desirable in employee relations and other aspects of the work world.

This adoption of both feminine and masculine traits as a part of one's gender identity leads to the development of an *androgynous* personality. This development moves away from the bipolar description of femininity and masculinity that requires rigid assignment of males and females to one or the other. Ideally, an androgynous individual would be able to choose from the full range of experiences along the continua shown below:

Dependent--Independent
Nurturant---Impersonal
Cooperative---Competitive
Emotional--Emotionless
Verbal--Spatial
Passive---Aggressive

With the interchanging of male and female roles as women stay in the labor force longer today, both groups are moving away from the rigid sex-specific roles and characteristics that were traditionally assigned to them. Androgynous individuals will not be forced into predetermined roles in life because of their sex. They will have the option to plan and pattern their lives as they choose.

The place where students are located along feminine-masculine continuum will vary as a result of past socialization practices and familial experiences. For instance, daughters of working mothers perceive significantly fewer differences between men and women, have higher educational aspirations, and are more likely to pursue careers than girls in families in which the mother does not work (Stewart, 1976). Increasingly, parents are encouraging their daughters to be explorers as well as mothers in play situations, and they are encouraging their sons to play with dolls as well as trucks. Still, many parents strongly believe that children should learn sex-specific roles and characteristics and are rigid in their enforcement of such appropriate behaviors.

The degree to which a student adheres to the traditional versus androgynous gender identity may be influenced by the family's ethnicity, socioeconomic level, or religion. Although the evidence is not conclusive, many studies indicate that working-class children are more aware of distinct sex roles than are middle-class children (Safilios-Rothschild, 1979). In addition, middle-class women are more likely to attend college immediately after high school than are women from working-class families. In an ethnographic study of high school women in a business work study program, Valli (1988) found that

> COOP [cooperative education program] students dissatisfied with the minimal challenge of office jobs did not, like middle-class young women, decide to pursue higher education. Even though many of them were clearly capable of college success, their working-class backgrounds exerted a strong influence on their life plans. Instead of college they projected part-time or temporary futures in beauty shops, travel agencies, nursery schools, and shopping malls. Nor did they, like working-class boys, have culturally-defined monetary reasons for staying in dissatisfying work environments. (p. 101)

Black and white working-class women value commonsense knowledge that they have gained through their lived experiences. "Their ways of knowing are embedded in community, family, and work relationships and cannot be judged by dominant academic standards" (Luttrell, 1989, p. 33). Although these women believe that both men and women have common sense, more value is placed on that of men. Working-class men gain their knowledge collectively in the workplace, while the women learn theirs individually as mothers and homemakers. It is accepted that individuals with accumulated academic knowledge seldom have the common sense that is required for working-class life. Still, many working-class women pursue additional education, most often in community colleges, to increase their ability to find better employment. After this, education is not sought until the women are older and have children. However, such academic achievement puts a strain on the working-class family, where men's knowledge has been more valued (Luttrell, 1989).

Membership in a specific ethnic group also influences the socialization patterns of males and females, but the degree to which the traditional sex roles are accepted will depend on the degree to which the family maintains the traditional patterns and on the particular experiences of the ethnic group in this country. Puerto Rican, Mexican-American, Appalachian, and Native American families that adhere to traditional religious and cultural patterns are more likely to encourage adherence to rigid sex roles than families that have adopted bicultural patterns. For example, labor market opportunities for Appalachian women who had moved into an urban area were found to be more influenced by their roles as Appalachian women than any other factor, including talent. These women "possess a strong cultural heritage emphasizing their identification with place [i.e., the mountains], their emotional strength, and their ability to manage family and other social relations with particular ability and energy. . . . Such an environment contributes to the image of the strong, independent woman" (Borman, Mueninghoff, & Piazza, 1988, p. 234). Because the Appalachian heritage does not easily fit into middle-class schools, students become alienated. In this culture, a female's transition from childhood to adulthood is noted by having a baby, which often leads to dropping out of school and going on welfare; later she might return to school to gain the skills necessary for employment. Most young women who break this pattern and choose academic achievement, completion of high school, and possible college attendance have adopted middle-class values and developed friendships outside the ethnic community. In many cases, they sacrificed their ethnic heritage in order to seek well-paying jobs and professional careers (Borman et al., 1988).

On the other hand, women in African-American families historically have worked outside the home and are less likely to hold strict traditional views about their roles. They have learned to be both the homemaker and wage earner. They are more likely than African-American men to complete high school and college. At the same time, African-American women who are poor and working class attain less schooling than any other ethnic group except Hispanic and Native American. Unlike many middle-class white women, "middle-class black women do not necessarily perceive marriage as a route to upward mobility or out of poverty" (Mickelson, 1989, p. 56).

It is dangerous to assume that students will hold certain views or behave in sex-typed ways because of their ethnicity or socioeconomic level. Individual families within those two microcultures vary greatly in their support of sex-typed roles for men and women and their subsequent behavior along a continuum of gender identity.

Religions, however, generally recognize and include masculine and feminine principles as part of their doctrine. Regardless of the specific religion, the religious rituals usually reflect and reinforce systems of male dominance:

> Because religion defines the ultimate meaning of the universe for a people, the impact may be deep and often emotional rather than intellectual. When male dominance is embodied within religion, it enters the arena that a society considers sacred. This may make it even less open to question and more resistant to change than other social areas. (Stockard & Johnson, 1980, p. 8)

Nevertheless, some of the more liberal religious groups support the move toward an androgynous personality for both sexes, while the more fundamentalist groups support a strict adherence to sex-differentiated roles.

The classroom teacher is likely to find students at different points along the gender identity continuum, both in their beliefs about female and male roles and in their actual behavior. The interaction of ethnicity, class, and religion is very important in determining one's gender role. Eduators should be aware that families and students will vary in the degree of adherence to traditional sex-typed roles. Without such an understanding, it may be difficult to open up options to all students, regardless of their sex.

EDUCATIONAL IMPLICATIONS

Education is seen by many people as a key to upward mobility and success in adulthood. The occupational roles that individuals pursue in adulthood are greatly influenced by their education in elementary and secondary schools. By the time students reach the secondary level, they have chosen, or been helped to choose, either a college preparatory program, a general education program, or a specific vocational training program. Males and females often select different secondary programs, especially in the vocational areas. When college students select a major, disproportionate numbers of males select technical and business majors over females selecting those fields of study. These early choices can make a great difference in later job satisfaction and rewards.

Educational experiences and outcomes continue to differ for males and females at all levels of experience:

☐ At ages nine, fourteen, and seventeen, girls perform higher on assessments of reading achievement, but by ages twenty-one to twenty-five, males perform at the same level as females in reading and literary proficiency (Mullis, 1987).

☐ By age nine, boys score higher than girls on mathematics achievement tests that require high-level thinking (Fennema & Carpenter, 1981).

☐ On all subsections of the SAT and ACT, males score higher than females (Dauber, 1987).

☐ Females receive 36 percent of the National Merit Scholarships (PEER, 1987).

☐ Males score higher on admission tests for graduate and professional schools [i.e., the Graduate Record Examination (GRE), the Medical College Admissions Test (MCAT), and the Graduate Management Admissions Test (GMAT)] (Brody, 1987).

Many persons believe that if the experiences of boys and girls are changed in school, they will achieve greater equality as adults. However, there is not common agreement even among feminists on how to accomplish this goal. Historians Tyack and Hansot (1988) found that

> some feminists believe that schools should consciously strive to create a gender-blind pedagogical order that will enlarge aspiration for both girls and boys and promote greater equality of opportunity by eliminating differential treatment of the sexes. Other feminists argue that male-defined values and practices permeate schools and that affirming and strengthening feminine qualities and ethical principles—making schools gender-sensitive rather than seemingly gender-neutral—is a worthier goal. Meanwhile, traditionalists, equally passionate, believe that schools should reflect and strengthen the separate spheres of men and women. (p. 34)

Programs designed to end sex stratification focus on education rather than on other societal institutions, probably because it is easier to effect change in schools than in many other institutions. Teachers, counselors, teachers' aides, coaches, and principals all have roles in eradicating the inequities that result from sexism. Schools have utilized two approaches in this process: women's studies and nonsexist education. In addition, laws have been passed at the federal level that influence education in this arena.

Women's Studies

Women's studies programs are similar to ethnic studies programs in their attempt to record and analyze the historical and contemporary experiences of a group that has usually been ignored in the general education courses taken by the majority of students. Courses in women's studies include concepts of consciousness-raising and views of women as a separate group with unique needs and disadvantages in schools and other institutions. They examine the culture, status, development, and achievement of women as a group (Sexton, 1976).

Women's studies have evolved in secondary and higher education as units in history, sociology, and literature courses; as separate courses; and as well-developed programs from which students can choose a major or minor field of study. Similar to the ethnic studies programs, the experiences and contributions of women and related concepts have been the focus.

For all students, women's studies often provide a perspective that is foreign. Historical, economic, and sociological events are viewed from the perspective of a group that has been in a position subordinate to men throughout history. Until students participate in such courses, they usually do not realize that 51 percent of the population has received so little coverage in most textbooks and courses. These programs allow students to increase both their awareness and knowledge base about women's history and contributions. Sometimes women are taught skills for competing successfully in a man's world or for managing a career and a family. In addition, many women's studies programs assist in developing a positive female self-image within a society that has viewed them as inferior to men. Psychological and career assistance to women is a part of some programs.

Although the content of women's studies is desperately needed to fill the gaps of current educational programs, it usually is a program set aside from the regular or general academic offerings. Instead of being required, it is usually an elective course. Thus, the majority of students may never integrate the information and concepts of women's studies into their academic work. The treatment of women as a separate entity also subtly suggests that the study of women is secondary to the important study of the world—a world that is reflected in textbooks and courses as one of males from a male perspective. All students need to learn about a world in which there are both male and female participants.

Nonsexist Education

Women's studies programs are a part of nonsexist education, but they become an integral part of the total education program in nonsexist programs rather than a separate luxury. Teachers may be required to use specific textbooks and materials within the classroom, but in general, teachers have control of the curriculum taught in their classrooms. Even with sexist materials, alert teachers can point out the discrepancies that exist between the sexes, discuss how and why such inequities are portrayed, and supplement the materials with information that provides a more balanced view of the roles and contributions of both men and women. Required readings can include those written by women as well as by men. At minimum, nonstereotypical male and female examples can appear on bulletin boards and in teacher-prepared materials.

All students should be exposed to the contributions of women as well as men throughout history. For example, history courses that focus primarily on wars and political power will almost totally focus on men; history courses that focus on the family and the arts will more equitably include both sexes. Science courses that discuss all of the great scientists often forget to discuss the societal limitations that prevented women from being scientists. (Women scientists and writers often had to use male names or give their work to men for publication.) Students are being cheated of a wealth of information about the majority of the world's population when women are not included as an integral part of the curriculum. The teacher controls the information and concepts taught to students. Thus, it is the teacher's responsibility to present a view of the world that includes other women and men and their wide ranges of perspectives.

Educators also should incorporate factual information on homosexuality. The contributions of gays to society should not be ignored. Homophobic name-calling by students could be used to provide facts and correct myths about homosexuality. "If adults criticize other forms of name-calling, but ignore antigay remarks, children are quick to conclude that homophobia is acceptable because gay men and lesbians deserve to be oppressed" (L. Gordon, 1983, p. 25).

It is also the responsibility of the teacher to provide all students the opportunities to reach their potentials. If girls constantly see boys as more active, smarter, more aggressive, and exerting more control over their lives, female students are being cheated. Boys who are always expected to behave in stereotypically masculine ways also suffer. Students are bombarded by subtle influences in schools that reinforce the notion that boys are more important than girls. This unplanned, unofficial learning, the *hidden curriculum,* has an impact on how students feel about themselves and others. Sexism is often projected in the following ways: in the messages that children receive in the illustrations, language, and content of texts, films, and other instructional materials; in the interaction of school authorities with male and female students; in the different roles of the two sexes in school rituals; and in the presence of influential role models (Bornstein, 1982).

An area over which all educators have control is their interactions with students. Consistently, researchers find that educators react differently to boys and girls in the classroom, on the athletic field, in the hall, and in the counseling office. Research studies have shown that low-achieving boys receive the most negative feedback from teachers; high-achieving boys receive the most positive feedback; and girls receive less feedback of either a negative or positive quality. Teachers ask "males more questions, give them more precise feedback, criticize them more, and give them more time to respond" (Sadker, Sadker, & Steindam, 1989, p. 46).

In mathematics classes, researchers have found differences in the interaction of teachers with boys and girls. Because most girls and boys have been socialized differently, some teaching strategies have been found more effective for girls than boys, and vice versa. Generally, the percentage of class time spent on mathematics did not differ, nor did the mathematics activities in which students participated. But teacher interactions with the two groups did differ in most cases. Teachers initiated more interactions with boys than with girls concerning classroom behavior. They more often worked individually with boys on classroom management, directions, and procedures. More social interactions were initiated with boys than with girls. In response to low-level mathematics questions, more called-out responses were received and accepted from boys. Teachers engaged boys in significantly more low-level and high-level interactions related directly to mathematics. At the same time, the researchers found that "the more that teachers asked high-level mathematics questions and interacted about mathematics at a high cognitive level with girls, the more girls learned about a higher cognitive level of mathematics" (Fennema & Peterson, 1987, p. 118). Girls were more likely to learn in cooperative mathematics activities; boys, on the other hand, learned better in competitive activities. Girls were influenced positively by the teacher's praise of a correct answer. Boys achieved better when the teacher corrected a wrong answer, but girls achieved better when the teacher prompted them for the correct answer. The differences between the achievement of girls and boys in mathematics classes appears to be related to the difference between dependence and independence (Fennema & Peterson, 1987). To help both girls and boys achieve well in mathematics will require different teaching strategies for boys than for girls.

When asked if they discriminate in the way they react to boys and girls in the classroom, most teachers respond "no." Once they critically examine their interactions, however, most teachers find that they do respond differently. The most important factor in overcoming sex biases in the classroom is the recognition that subtle and unintentional biases exist. Once these are recognized, the teacher can begin to make changes in the classroom and in the lives of the students in that classroom.

Nonsexist education is reflected in the school setting when students are not sorted, grouped, or tracked by gender in any aspect of the school program or environment. The teacher can develop a curriculum that does not give preferential treatment to boys over girls; that shows both sexes in aggressive, nurturing, independent, exciting, and emotional roles; that encourages all students to explore traditional and nontraditional roles; and that assists them in developing positive self-images about their sexuality. One's actions and reactions to students can make a difference.

Title IX

One law—Title IX of the 1972 Education Amendments—addresses the differential, stereotyped, and discriminatory treatment of students based on their sex. Title IX states that "no person shall, on the basis of sex, be excluded from participation in, be denied the benefits of, or be subjected to discrimination under any education program or activity receiving federal financial assistance." It protects students and employees in virtually all 16,000 public school systems and 2,700 postsecondary institutions in the United States. The law prevents sex discrimination in (1) the admission of students, particularly to postsecondary and vocational education institutions; (2) the treatment of students; and (3) the employment of all personnel.

What does Title IX require of teachers, counselors, principals, and other educators in kindergarten through twelfth-grade settings? The law clearly makes it illegal to treat students differently or separately on the basis of sex. It requires that all programs, activities, and opportunities offered by a school district be equally available to males and females. All courses must be open to all students. Boys must be allowed to enroll in home economics classes and girls allowed in industrial arts and agriculture courses. Regarding the counseling of students, Title IX prohibits biased course or career guidance; the use of biased achievement, ability, or interest tests; and the use of college and career materials that are biased in content, language, or illustration. Schools cannot assist any business or individual in employing students if the request is for a student of a particular sex. There can be no discrimination in the type or amount of financial assistance or eligibility for such assistance. Health and insurance benefits available to students cannot be discriminated against or excluded from any educational program or activity.

Membership in clubs and other activities based on sex alone is prohibited in schools, with the exceptions of YWCA, YMCA, Girl Scouts, Boy Scouts, Camp Fire Girls, Boys' State, Girls' State, Key clubs, and other voluntary and tax-exempt youth service organizations that have been traditionally limited to members nineteen years of age or younger of one sex. Rules of behavior and punishments for violation of those rules must be the same for all students. Honors and awards may not designate the sex of the student as a criterion for the award.

Probably the most controversial program covered by Title IX has been the area of athletics. Provisions for girls to participate in intramural, club, or interscholastic sports must be included in the school's athletic program. The sports offered by a school must be coeducational with two major exceptions: (1) when selection for teams is based on competitive skill and (2) when the activity is a contact sport. In these two situations, separate teams are permitted but are not required. Although the law does not require equal funding for girls' and boys' athletic programs, equal opportunity in athletics must be provided.

The law alone will not change the basic assumptions and attitudes people hold about appropriate female and male roles, occupations, and behaviors; but the law will equalize the rights, opportunities, and treatment of students within the school setting. Experience has shown that once discriminatory practices are eliminated and discriminatory behavior is altered, even unwillingly, changes in prejudiced attitudes often follow (Kearse, 1980). Equal treatment of students from kindergarten through college will more adequately encourage all students to explore available career options.

SUMMARY

Our culture determines in large part how parents will treat boys and girls. Although girls and boys are members of all other microcultures, the culture at large has different expectations of them based solely on their sex. Culture establishes the norms of acceptable sex-typed behavior. The sexes compose two distinct microcultural groups that are influenced greatly by a person's membership in other microcultures, such as ethnicity, religion, socioeconomic status, and age.

Anthropologists have observed many cultural differences in sexual behavior and in the division of labor between the sexes. However, research indicates that the biological differences between males and females have little influence on their behavior and roles in a culture. Instead, the differences within a society are primarily culturally determined rather than biologically determined.

The only psychological differences between males and females are in the areas of verbal, mathematical, and visual-spatial tasks; aggression; and internal locus of control. Although there may be great psychological differences between individuals, there are few group differences between females and males.

Socialization is the process of learning to behave in accordance with socially prescribed roles and expectations. It is during this period that children learn to be male or female. Male and female roles in our society are usually defined as quite distinct from one another and are often portrayed stereotypically by the media and reinforced in many families. Consciousness-raising activities over the past decade have helped men and women understand and evaluate the stereotyped roles for which they have been socialized, opening new options for both groups.

Sex discrimination has kept women in less prestigious and lower-paying jobs. Even the amount of education obtained by a woman does little to close the gap between the earnings of men and women—now at 65 cents earned by a woman for every dollar earned by a man. Such discrimination greatly affects the quality of life for women.

Although one has no choice about sex identity, gender identity allows for flexibility in that an individual can have either feminine or masculine characteristics or a combination of the two. The adoption of both feminine and masculine traits as part of one's gender identity leads to the development of an androgynous personality. The degree to which an individual adheres to the traditional versus androgynous gender identity will vary as a result of past socialization patterns and may be influenced by the family's ethnicity, socioeconomic level, or religion.

Women's studies and nonsexist education represent educational approaches to combating sexism in schools and society. Women's studies programs attempt to record and analyze the historical and contemporary experiences of women and usually are offered as separate courses. On the other hand, nonsexist education attempts to make the total school curriculum less sexist by incorporating content that reflects female as well as male perspectives. Nonsexist education also incorporates positive and supportive interactions of teachers with students. Educators are asked to be aware of behavior that discriminates against one of the sexes.

The federal government provides support for aspects of nonsexist education through Title IX of the 1972 Education Amendments. This law protects against the differential, stereotyped, and discriminatory treatment of students based on their sex.

QUESTIONS FOR REVIEW

1. What are the psychological differences between males and females?

2. In what ways are differences between the sexes culturally rather than biologically determined?

3. How does socialization into stereotyped roles harm females and males in our changing society?

4. Explain how sex discrimination has disproportionately impacted on women.

5. Define an androgynous personality, and explain why androgynous gender identity is not universally supported.

6. Contrast women's studies and nonsexist education, and explain the advantages of both.

7. How can teachers learn whether they are discriminating against students based on their gender?

8. How does homophobia manifest itself in schools? What can educators do toward eliminating the prejudice and discrimination that occur?

9. What impact has Title IX had on schooling over the past twenty years?

REFERENCES

Barfield, A. (1976). Biological influences on sex differences in behavior. In M. S. Teitelbaum (Ed.), *Sex differences; Social and biological perspectives* (pp. 62–121). Garden City, NY: Anchor Press.

Bernard, J. (1981). *The female world.* New York: Free Press.

Bonk, K., & Gardner, J. E. (1978). Sexism's universal curriculum. In The National Project on Women in Education, *Taking sexism out of education.* Washington, DC: U.S. Department of Health, Education and Welfare.

Borman, K. M., Mueninghoff, E., & Piazza, S. (1988). Urban Appalachian girls and young women: Bowing to no one. In L. Weis (Ed.), *Class, race, and gender in American Education* (pp. 230–248). Albany, NY: State University New York Press.

Bornstein, R. (1980). *Sexism in education.* Washington, DC: U.S. Department of Education, Women's Educational Equity Act Program.

Brody, L. (1987). *Gender differences in standardized examinations used for selecting applicants to graduate and professional schools.* Paper presented at the annual meeting of the American Educational Research Association, Washington, DC.

Dauber, S. (1987). *Sex differences on the SAT-M, SAT-V, TWSE, and ACT among college-bound high school students.* Paper presented at the annual meeting of the American Educational Research Association, Washington, DC.

de Beauvoir, S. (1974). *The second sex.* New York: Vintage Books.

Fennema, E., & Carpenter, J. (1981). The second national assessment and sex-related differences in mathematics. *Mathematic Teacher, 74*(7), 554–559.

Fennema, E., & Peterson, P. L. (1987). Effective teaching for girls and boys: The same or different. In D. C. Berliner and B. V. Rosenshine (Eds.), *Talks to teachers* (pp. 111–125). New York: Random House.

Filene, P. G. (1986). *Him/her/self* (2nd ed.). Baltimore: The Johns Hopkins University Press.

Fine, M. (1988, February). Sexuality, schooling, and adolescent females: The missing discourse of desire. *Harvard Educational Review, 58*(1), 29–53.

Frazier, N., & Sadker, M. (1973). *Sexism in school and society.* New York: Harper & Row.

Goldberg, H. (1976). *The hazards of being male: Surviving the myth of masculine privilege.* New York: Nash.

Gollnick, D. M., Sadker, M., & Sadker, D. (1982). Beyond the Dick and Jane syndrome: Confronting sex bias in instructional materials. In M. Sadker & D. Sadker (Eds.), *Sex equity handbook for schools* (pp. 60–95). New York: Longman.

Gordon, L. (1983). What do we say when we hear "faggot"? *Interracial Books for Children Bulletin, 14*(3, 4), 25–27.

Gordon, R. (1980). Ties that bind: The price of pursuing the male mystique. *Peer Report.*

Hodgkinson, H. (1986). *The schools we need for the kids we've got.* Paper presented at the 1987 annual meeting of the American Association of Colleges for Teacher Education, Washinton, DC.

Kearse, E. E. T. (1980). Affirmative action required to sever deep roots of sexism. *Jobs Watch, 1*(2), 1–2, 9, 23.

King, Y. M. (1989, March). *Equity in basal readers.* Paper presented at the annual meeting of the American Educational Research Association, San Francisco.

Kreps, J. M., & Leaper, R. J. (1976). Home work, market work, and the allocation of time. In J. M. Kreps (Ed.), *Women and the American economy: A look to the 1980s* (pp. 61–81). Englewood Cliffs, NJ: Prentice-Hall.

Lee, P. C. (1976). Introduction. In P. C. Lee & R. S. Stewart (Eds.), *Sex differences: Cultural and developmental dimensions* (pp. 1–5). New York: Urizen Books.

Luttrell, W. (1989, January). Working-class women's way of knowing. Effects of gender, race, and class. *Sociology of Education, 62*(1), 33–46.

Maccoby, E. E., & Jacklin, C. N. (1974). *The psychology of sex differences.* Stanford, CA: Stanford University Press.

Mead, M. (1935). *Sex and temperament in three primitive societies.* New York: Morrow.

Mickelson, R. A (1989, January). Why does Jane read and write so well? The anomaly of women's achievement. *Sociology of Education, 62*(1), 47–63.

Miles, B. (1975). *Channeling children: Sex stereotyping on prime time TV.* Princeton, NJ: Women on Words and Images.

Mullis, I. (1987). *Trends in performance for women taking the NAEP reading and writing assessments.* Paper presented at the annual meeting of the American Educational Research Association, Washington, DC.

PEER (Project on Equal Educational Rights). (1987, May 29). Equal education alert 7.

Radl, S. R. (1983). *The invisible women: Target of the religious new right.* New York: Dell.

Rosaldo, M. Z., & Lamphere, L. (Eds.). (1974). *Woman, culture, and society.* Stanford, CA: Stanford University Press.

Rubin, J. Z., Provenzano, F. J., & Luria, Z. (1974). The eye of the beholder: Parents' views on sex of newborns. *American Journal of Orthopsychiatry, 44*(4), 512–519.

Sadker, D. (1975, Winter). The feminist movement: Not for women only. *Journal of Teacher Education, 26*(4), 313–315.

Sadker, M., Sadker, D., & Steindam, S. (1989, March). Gender equity and educational reform. *Educational Leadership, 46*(6), 44–47.

Safilios-Rothschild, C. (1979). *Sex role socialization and sex discrimination: A synthesis and critique of the literature.* Washington, DC: National Institute of Education.

Sexton, P. C. (1976). *Women in education.* Bloomington, IN: Phi Delta Kappa.

Shell, R. W. (1980, January–February). Sex discrimination: Perpetuating a track system leading nowhere. *Jobs Watch, 1*(2), 1, 14.

Stewart, V. (1976). Social influences on sex differences in behavior. In M. S. Teitelbaum (Ed.), *Sex differences: Social and biological perspectives* (pp. 138–174) Garden City, NY: Anchor Press.

Stockard, J., & Johnson, M. M. (1980). *Sex roles: Sex inequality and sex role development.* Englewood Cliffs, NJ: Prentice-Hall.

Swerdloff, P. (1975). *Men and women.* New York: Time-Life Books.

Tyack, D., & Hansot, E. (1988, April). Silence and policy talk: Historical puzzles about gender and education. *Educational Researcher, 17*(3), 33–41.

U.S. Bureau of the Census. (1988). *Statistical Abstract of the United States.* Washinton, DC: Government Printing Office.

Valli, L. (1988). Gender identity and the technology of office education. In L. Weis (Ed.), *Class, race, and gender in American education* (pp. 87–105). Albany, NY: State University of New York Press.

Weiler, K. (1988). *Women teaching for change: Gender, class, and power.* South Hadley, MA: Bergin & Garvey.

Westoff, L. A. (1979). *Women–in search of equality.* Princeton, NJ: Educational Testing Service.

Willis, P. E. (1977). *Learning to labour: How working class kids get working class jobs.* Farnborough, England: Saxon House.

Women on Words and Images. (1975). *Dick and Jane as victims: Sex stereotyping in children's readers.* Princeton, NJ: Author.

SUGGESTED READINGS

Gates, B., Klaw, S., & Steinberg, A. (1979). *Changing learning, and changing lives.* Old Westbury, NJ: Feminist Press.

> *Curriculum that was created from the life experiences of working-class girls. Themes of race, class, and gender are critically analyzed.*

Guttentag, M., & Bray, H. (1976). *Undoing sex stereotypes: Research and resources for education.* New York: McGraw-Hill.

> *A documentation of a field survey and intervention program for changing sex role stereotyping in children. Provides a variety of curricular resources and lesson plans that can be used at elementary and secondary levels.*

Klein, S. S. (Ed.). (1985). *Handbook for achieving sex equity through education.* Baltimore: The Johns Hopkins University Press.

> *A comprehensive, scholarly, yet practical approach to the achievement of sex equity in schools. Addresses a variety of issues ranging from the need for institutional change in the visual arts curriculum to the kinds of programs required to meet the special needs of minority, gifted, rural, and adult women. Includes specific strategies for mathematics and science, reading and communication, social studies, visual arts, physical education and athletics, and career and vocational education.*

McRobbie, A., & McCabe, T. (Eds). (1981). *Feminism for girls.* Boston: Routlege & Kegan Paul.

> *An examination of the transmission of images and vlaues through the media and textbooks. Addresses the depiction of girls in literature, the nature of secretarial work, and the overt and hidden meanings of a popular girls magazine.*

Sadker, M., & Sadker, D. (1982). *Sex equity handbook for schools.* New York: Longman.

An excellent resource for prospective teachers. Includes chapters that address sex differences, sexism in education, sex bias in classroom interactions, sex bias in instructional materials, and sex equity in school organizations. Sample lessons and classroom activities are provided.

Schniedewind, N., & Davidson, E. (1983). *Open minds to equality: Learning activities to promote race, sex, class, and age equality.* Englewood Cliffs, NJ: Prentice-Hall.

A feminist curriculum for public schools.

Skolnick, J., Langbort, C., & Day,L. (1982). *How to encourage girls in math and science: Strategies for parents and educators.* Englewood Cliffs, NJ: Prentice-Hall.

Practical strategies for teachers to use in helping girls develop math and science skills and an interest in related careers. Includes descriptions and examples of sex role socialization and specific strategies and activites for kindergarten through eighth-grade students.

Sprung, B. (1975). *Non-sexist education for young children: A practical guide.* New York: Citation.

Guide for teachers on how to avoid sexist language and counteract social influences such as television and books. Describes how to create nonsexist environments that assist both boys and girls in nurturing and active roles. Includes five units of study for early childhood programs.

CHAPTER 5
Exceptionality

A significant segment of the population in the United States is made up of exceptional individuals. Twenty-five million or more individuals from every ethnic and socioeconomic group fall into one or more of the categories of exceptionality. Nearly every day, educators come into contact with exceptional children and adults. They may be students in our classes, our professional colleagues, our friends and neighbors, or individuals we meet in our everyday experiences.

Exceptional individuals include both handicapped and gifted individuals. Some, particularly the handicapped, have been rejected by society. Because of their unique social and personal needs and special interests, many exceptional individuals become a part of a microculture composed of individuals with similar exceptionalities. For some, this cultural identity is by ascription; they have been labeled and forced into enclaves by virtue of the residential institutions they have been sent to. Others live in the same communities by their own choosing. This chapter will provide an examination of the exceptional individual's relationship to society. It will address the struggle for equal rights and the ways the treatment of the handicapped often parallels that of oppressed ethnic minorities.

Exceptional children include both the handicapped and the gifted and talented. Definitions for exceptional children vary slightly from one writer to another, but Heward and Orlansky's (1988) is typical of most:

> The term *exceptional children* includes both children who experience difficulties in learning and children whose performance is so superior that special education is necessary if they are to fulfill their potential. Thus *exceptional* children is an inclusive term that refers to children with physical disabilities and children with learning and/or behavior problems, as well as children who are intellectually gifted. (p. 3)

This definition is specific to school-age children who are usually referred, tested to determine eligibility, and then placed in special education programs. Included in the process is the labeling of the child. At one end of the continuum are the gifted and talented children. At the other end are the handicapped (some of whom may also be gifted). The handicapped are categorized with labels such as mentally retarded, learning disabled, speech impaired, visually impaired, hearing impaired, emotionally disturbed (or behavior disordered), and physically and health impaired.

LABELING

The categorizing and labeling process has its share of critics. Opponents characterize the practice as demeaning and stigmatizing to the handicapped, with the effects often carried through adulthood. Earlier classifications and labels, such as moron, imbecile, and idiot, have become so derogatory that they are no longer used in a professional context. Some individuals, including many of the learning disabled and mildly retarded, were never considered handicapped prior to entering school. The school setting, however, intensifies their academic and cognitive deficits. Many, when they return to their homes and communities, do not seem to function as handicapped individuals. Instead, they participate in activities with their neighborhood peers until they return to school the following day, where they attend special classes (sometimes segregated) and resume their role in the academic and social structure of the school as handicapped children. The problem is so pervasive that it has led to the designation of "the six-hour retarded child." These are children who spend six hours a day as retarded children in our nation's schools. During the remaining eighteen hours a day away from the school setting, they are not considered retarded by the people they interact with (President's Committee on Mental Retardation, 1969). Heward and Orlansky (1988) suggest that the demands of the school seem to "cause" the mental retardation.

The labels carry with them connotations and stigmas of varying degrees. Some conditions are socially more acceptable than others. Visual impairment carries with it public empathy and sometimes sympathy. The public has for years given generously to causes for the blind, as evidenced by the financially well-endorsed Seeing Eye Institute, which produces the well-known guide dogs. The blind are the only handicapped group permitted to claim an additional personal income tax deduction by reason of their disability. Yet, the general public looks upon blindness as one of the worse afflictions imposed on humankind.

On the other hand, mental retardation, and to some extent emotional disturbance, are often linked to lower socioeconomic status. Both labels are among the lowest socially acceptable handicaps and perhaps the most stigmatizing.

Learning disabilities, the newest category of exceptionality, is one of the more socially acceptable conditions. While mental retardation is often identified with lower socioeconomic groups, learning disabilities tend to be more middle class in their identity. Whether these perceptions are accurate or not, middle-class parents more readily accept learning disabilities than mental retardation as a cause of their child's learning deficits. What has been observed is a reclassification of many children from mentally retarded to learning disabled (Ortiz & Yates, 1983).

While the labeling controversy persists, even its critics often concede its necessity. Federal funding for special education is predicated on the identification of individuals in specific handicapping conditions. These funds, which totaled over $1 billion in 1987 (Jordan & Zantal-Wierner, 1988), are so significant that many special education programs would all but collapse without them, leaving school districts in severe financial distress. Consequently, the labeling process continues, sometimes even into adulthood, where university students may have to be identified as learning disabled to receive necessary accommodations to their learning needs. Others are placed in jobs by vocational rehabilitation counselors, with labels more indicative of their learning problems than their work skills. This, in turn, tends to stigmatize, enhancing the likelihood of social isolation.

HISTORICAL ANTECEDENTS

The plight of the handicapped has in many instances closely paralleled that of oppressed ethnic groups. The history of the treatment of the handicapped has not shown society eager to meet its responsibilities. Prior to 1800, with a few exceptions, the mentally retarded, for example, were not considered a major social problem in any society. The more severely retarded were simply killed, or they died early of natural causes (Drew, Logan, & Hardman, 1988).

The treatment and care of the mentally and physically handicapped have typically been a function of the socioeconomic conditions of the times. In addition to attitudes of fear and disgrace brought on by superstition, early nomadic tribes viewed the handicapped as nonproductive and a burden, draining available resources. As civilization progressed from a less nomadic existence, the handicapped were still often viewed as nonproductive and expendable.

They were frequently shunted away to institutions designated as hospitals, asylums, and colonies. Many institutions were deliberately built great distances from the population centers, where the residents could be segregated and more easily contained. For decades, American society did not have to deal with its conscience with respect to its more severely handicapped. We simply sent them far away and forgot about them. Most Americans did not know of the cruel and inhumane treatment that existed in many facilities, and they did not really want to know. The mildly handicapped were generally able to be absorbed into society, sometimes seeming to disappear, sometimes contributing meaningfully to an agrarian society, often not even being identified as handicapped.

As society became more industrialized and educational reforms required school attendance, the academic problems of the handicapped became increasingly more visible. Special schools and special classes were designated to meet the needs of these children. Thus, society segregated these individuals, often in the guise of acting in their best interests.

The earlier attempts to provide for the educational needs of the handicapped often fell short. Personnel lacked training, and school districts accepted students on a selective basis. For the most part, only the more mildly handicapped were considered acceptable for the educational process. The moderately and severely handicapped were simply denied educational services. Parents were forced to pay for private services, keep the children at home, or institutionalize them.

Society's treatment of some handicapped groups, such as the mentally retarded, has frequently been questionable with respect to their civil rights. Krishef (1972) indicates that one-fourth of all states surveyed reported prohibitions against marriage between retarded individuals. Another third of the states either reported that no information was available or did not respond. Krishef further reports that twenty-four states permitted sterilization of the retarded, while only two states prohibited sterilization of the retarded. The Congressional Record reports fifteen states as having statutes authorizing compulsory sterilization of mentally ill or mentally retarded individuals.

Edgerton (1967) found that forty-four out of forty-eight retarded individuals released from a state institution had undergone eugenic sterilization. During the time of their institutionalization, sterilization was considered a prerequisite to release. Form letters sent to parents or guardians to gain consent for the procedure implied that sterilization could permit parole and would be in the individual's best interest. Follow-up interviews of the subjects indicated strong negative feelings regarding the sterilization that had been imposed on them. They viewed sterilization as an indelible mark of their institutionalization. Some felt deprived of the children they wanted, and there was a fear on the part of many that the secret they kept of their forced sterilization would be discovered by their partners.

The issue of marriage prohibitions and eugenic sterilization for the retarded raises serious social and ethical issues. The nonhandicapped segment of society, charged with the care and education of the handicapped, apparently views as its right and responsibility those matters dealing with sexual behavior, marriage, and procreation. In a similar way, educators determine the means of communication for the blind individual, either an oral/aural approach or a manual/total communication approach. Such decisions have profound implications, as they not only determine how these individuals will communicate, but to a great extent with whom they will be able to communicate. Too often, society seeks to dehumanize the handicapped by ignoring their personal wishes, making their critical decisions for them, and treating them as children throughout their lives.

DISPROPORTIONATE PLACEMENTS IN SPECIAL EDUCATION

In 1968, Dunn, in his seminal article, "Special Education for the Mildly Retarded: Is Much of It Justifiable?" pointed out the phenomenal increase of classes for the mentally retarded. Perhaps the most profound revelation was that 60 to 80 percent of the pupils taught in classes for the retarded were minority group children from low socioeconomic backgrounds. Questioning the proliferation of the classes for the mentally retarded, Dunn asserted that the extensive placement of these minorities in classes for the mentally retarded raised serious educational and civil rights issues.

In a classic study, Mercer (1973) documented the disproportionate placement of minorities in the Riverside, California, public school classes for the mentally retarded. While Mexican-American students there constituted only 11 percent of the general school population sampled, they made up 45.3 percent of the students in classes for the mildly retarded. Black children were placed in the same classes at a rate three times greater than their numbers in the school population at large. Whites, on the other hand, constituted 81 percent of the general school population but only 32.1 percent of the special education classes for the mentally retarded.

P. C. Chinn and Hughes (1987) analyzed the 1978–1984 U.S. Office of Civil Rights Surveys of Elementary and Secondary Schools. These surveys provided data regarding student enrollment and placement in special education classes. While Hispanics are no longer overrepresented in classes for the mildly mentally retarded in the national data, blacks continue to be. They are also overrepresented in classes for the moderately retarded and the seriously emotionally disturbed (SED). American Indians are overrepresented in classes for the moderately mentally retarded and learning disabled. Hispanics, blacks, and American Indians are all significantly underrepresented in classes for the gifted and talented. P. C. Chinn and Hughes emphasized that the national data obscure some state data, where minority groups may be over- or underrepresented in certain categories.

The issues of ethnicity, social class, and sex appear to be intricately intertwined with the issues of exceptionality. It is apparent that significant numbers of children from American Indian, black, and Hispanic families, many of whom come from lower socioeconomic backgrounds, are systematically excluded from classes for the gifted and talented. Large numbers of blacks, twice their numbers in the general school population, are placed in classes for the mildly mentally retarded. The extent of disproportionate placement of blacks in classes for the seriously emotionally disturbed is not as great as in classes for the mildly retarded, but enough to question the reasons for placement.

Other disturbing statistics include the fact that males are placed in classes for the seriously emotionally disturbed at a rate $3\frac{1}{2}$ times greater than for females (Office of Civil Rights, 1988), and children of lower socioeconomic backgrounds are also overrepresented in SED classes (Kauffman, 1981).

There are no simple solutions to the problems of disproportionate placement in special education classes. What is clear is that there are direct relationships to ethnicity, class, and sex. Laws related to special education have increased the law suits for alleged inappropriate placement, and school districts have responded by exercising more caution when making placements; yet, the problem persists.

What is known is that when a referral (usually from classroom teachers) is made for special education, the likelihood of placement is high. As many as 75 percent to 90 percent of special education referrals result in placement. High and Udall (1983) suggest that teacher attitudes toward culturally diverse students affect their referral rates.

Teachers, most of whom are white middle class, often have values that are incongruent with that of ethnic minority and lower socioeconomic students. Behaviors that may be considered within acceptable ranges in a child's home or community may be viewed as unacceptably aggressive by educators. These teachers may be prone to make referrals to special education in order to have the students removed from their classrooms (P. C. Chinn & Harris, 1990).

Differences in cognitive style may also result in perceiving children as less competent, particularly if the teacher is field-independent and the student is field-sensitive. Kitano and Kirby (1986) suggest that gifted children from culturally diverse backgrounds may go unnoticed because they express their talents in ways different from children in the majority culture.

Males are also placed in classes for the mildly retarded, moderately retarded, speech impaired, seriously emotionally disturbed, and learning disabled at higher percentages than females. They are placed in classes for the mildly retarded at $1\frac{1}{2}$ times, for the speech impaired at $1\frac{3}{4}$ times, for the seriously emotionally disturbed at $3\frac{1}{2}$ times, and for the learning disabled at $2\frac{1}{2}$ times the rate of placement for females. Males may indeed be more prone to some disabilities. However, the circumstances operating in the classroom with males may be similar to the situation with ethnic minorities and children from lower-class backgrounds. The majority of our teachers, particularly in the elementary school years, are female. They are socialized differently from males. In some instances, the teacher tolerance level for assertive or aggressive male students may preclude effective teacher-pupil relationships and may precipitate special education referrals.

The disproportionate placement of blacks and other minority groups has also been attributed to the assessement process. Special education placement is at least partially predicated on test scores. No test is culture-free, and some are inherently biased against children from culturally and linguistically different groups. Lack of skill or sensitivity on the part of test administrators has also been blamed for incorrect assessment results. *Larry P. v. Riles* (1972) was a major court case that found that some African-American children placed in special education classes for the retarded were victims of inappropriate assessment. The findings of the court have changed the entire placement process in California and have impacted on practices throughout the country.

The Office of Civil Rights (OCR) findings of disproportionate placement of blacks in classes for the moderately retarded is particularly distressing. The majority of the children in these classes have known central nervous system damage. Consequently, there are few challenges to the referral, assessment, or placement practices. Prior to the collection of data regarding special education placement and ethnicity, it was often assumed that moderate and severe mental retardation had no respect for ethnicity or social class. The OCR findings refute such an assumption. Blacks are placed in these classes at a rate 1½ times their representation in the general population. P. C. Chinn and Hughes (1987) state that

> the existence of poverty among some minority groups is a reality which cannot be logically disputed. The extent to which poverty and its concomitant problems contribute directly or indirectly to learning and behavior problems is difficult to determine. However, it is generally recognized that poverty, at least in extreme forms, may preclude adequate pre- and postnatal care, nutrition, and other environmental advantages. Absence of these favorable environmental conditions may place a child at greater risk. (p. 45)

In addition, there is a positive correlation between poverty and teenage pregnancies along with unwed motherhood (Berger, 1983). These situations, in turn, are directly related to children born preterm, which places the fetus and infant at risk. Children born at risk are in greater likelihood of sustaining physical insult or injury, sometimes permanent.

LITIGATION AND THE HANDICAPPED

In the last two decades, the U.S. Congress has passed two major pieces of legislation that will forever change the rights of handicapped individuals in the United States. Not unlike the treatment of ethnic minorities, many handicapped individuals throughout the country were disenfranchised of a meaningful education from the time educational services were first provided.

Section 504 was enacted through the legislative vehicle of Public Law 93–112, the Vocational Rehabilitation Act Amendments of 1973. This legislation is a counterpart to the Civil Rights Acts of 1964. It does for the handicapped essentially what the earlier legislation did for ethnic minorities. It is the basic civil rights provision with respect to prohibiting discrimination against America's handicapped. Though brief in its actual language, it has far-reaching implications. The statute states:

> No otherwise qualified handicapped individual in the United States . . . shall, solely by reason of his handicap, be excluded from the participation in, be denied benefits of, or be subjected to discrimination under any program or activity receiving Federal financial assistance.

In essence, Section 504 prohibits exclusion from programs soley on the basis of one's handicap. This means that a coach cannot bar a handicapped student from trying out for a team sport because he or she is learning handicapped. Nor can the band director stop another handicapped student for trying out for the school marching band. If, however, the first student cannot learn or remember the plays, or the second student cannot follow the marching formations, then the handicapped student can be cut from the team or the band in the same manner as a nonhandicapped student.

For years, handicapped students were routinely excluded from teacher education programs. Programs, schools, or colleges of education have admissions criteria to determine a student's eligibility to enter a teacher education program. Prior to the advent of Section 504, many of these programs required students to pass physical examinations that included hearing and vision tests. These tests effectively eliminated any hearing-impaired or visually impaired student from consideration for admission into teacher education. As in athletics, any student who cannot learn essential skills or perform essential teaching tasks can be eliminated from the program. But if barriers have been artificially created to exclude handicapped students, federal funds can be withheld, not only from the guilty program, but from the entire institution.

Public Law 94–142, the Education for All Handicapped Children Act, was passed by the U.S. Congress and signed into law by President Gerald Ford on November 29, 1975. The thrust of PL 94–142 is fivefold: (1) to provide a free and appropriate education for all handicapped children; (2) to ensure that school systems provide safeguards to protect the rights of handicapped children and their parents; (3) to educate handicapped children with nonhandicapped children to the maximum extent possible in the least restrictive environment; (4) to require that an Individualized Education Program (IEP) be developed and implemented for each handicapped child; and (5) to ensure that parents of handicapped children play an active role in the process used to make any educational decision about their handicapped children. States complying with the requirements of PL 94–142 receive federal funds to assist in providing services (Heward & Orlansky, 1988). While PL 94–142 applies to all handicapped children, ages three to twenty-one inclusive, who require special education or related services, Section 504 applies to all handicapped Americans, regardless of age.

PL 94–142 guarantees the right of a free and appropriate education. It provides for due process safeguards to ensure the educational rights of handicapped children. The heightened sensitivity of many educators to the rights as well as the capabilities of handicapped students have been coupled with the threat of litigation for noncompliance of the law. Consequently, more than ever, handicapped children and adults are becoming an integral part of the nation's educational system and are finding their rightful place in society.

While the progress that has been made in recent years is indeed encouraging, society's attitudes toward the handicapped has not always kept pace with their legal rights. As long as individuals are motivated more by fear of litigation than by a moral-ethical response, we cannot consider our efforts in this arena a success.

NORMALIZATION AND MAINSTREAMING

Much effort is directed today toward the concept of normalization. Normalization means "making available to the mentally retarded patterns and conditions of everyday life which are as close as possible to the norms and patterns of mainstream society" (Nirje, 1969, p. 181). Normalization was expanded and advocated in the United States by Wolfensberger (1972). He has subsequently suggested a rethinking of the term *normalization* and introduced the concept of "social role valorization"—giving value to the mentally retarded. He suggested that the "most explicit and highest goal of normalization must be the creation, support, and defense of valued social roles for people who are at risk of social devaluation" (Wolfensberger, 1983, p. 234).

Drew et al. (1988) suggest that normalization and social valorization have brought about an emphasis on deinstitutionalization, whereby individuals from large residential facilities for the retarded are returned to the community and home environments. They add that the concept is not limited to the movement away from institutions to a less restrictive environment, but also pertains to those individuals living in the community for whom a more "normal" life-style may be an appropriate goal.

The principles of normalization as they were first introduced were developed with the mentally retarded as the target group. In more recent years, the concept has broadened, so that all categories of handicapped individuals are now targeted. Berdine and Blackhurst (1985) follow the same principles and use almost the exact wording, substituting "handicapped people" for "the mentally retarded," urging that they, too, have the opportunity to live as close as possible to that of mainstream society.

Mainstreaming seemed to undergo a natural evolutionary process from the concept of normalization. While PL 94–142 mandates educating handicapped children in the "least restrictive environment," nowhere in the statute is the word *mainstream* used. However, "least restrictive environment" means that handicapped children are to be educated with nonhandicapped children whenever possible, in as normal an environment as possible. While the concept of least restrictive environment does not necessarily mean integration into regular education classes, the term *mainstreaming*, through common usage, refers to the practice of integrating handicapped children into regular education classes for all or a portion of the day. A goal in special education, therefore, is to mainstream as many handicapped children as is feasible.

Initially, mainstreaming was reserved for students with milder handicaps. A more current movement seeks to provide the moderately and severely handicapped with similar opportunities (Stainback & Stainback, 1985). While resistance to mainstreaming the mildly retarded is far less intense than it once was, resistance from some educators toward the more severely handicapped is still quite intense. The arguments against integrating severely handicapped children have often been centered on the presumed inability of normal children to accept their handicapped peers. In reality, some of the reservations may be more a reflection of educators who themselves are unable or unwilling to accept the dignity and worth of the severely handicapped.

The legal mandates do not eliminate the special schools or classes, but they do offer a new philosophical view. Instead of the physical isolation of the handicapped, an effort to allow the handicapped a more appropriate place in the educational setting is being promoted. There are still many handicapped children who apparently will not benefit appreciably from an integrated setting and are best educated in a special setting. As attitudes become more congruent with the laws, the handicapped may have more of an option in the decision to be a part of the mainstream or to form their own cultural groups.

EXCEPTIONALITY AND SOCIETY

Even in modern times, the treatment and understanding of any type of deviance have been limited. Society has begun to accept its basic responsibilities for the handicapped by providing for their education and care, but the social equality for the handicapped has yet to become a reality.

Society's view of the handicapped can perhaps be illustrated by the way the media portray the handicapped population. In general, when the media wish to emphasize the handicapped, they are portrayed as (1) children, usually severely mentally retarded with obvious physical stigmata, or (2) crippled persons, either in a wheelchair or on crutches. Thus, society has a mind-set on who the handicapped are. They are children or childlike, and they are severely handicapped mentally or physically or both.

Because society often views the handicapped as children, they are denied the right to feel and want like normal individuals. Teachers and other professional workers can often be observed talking about handicapped individuals in their presence, as if they are unable to feel any embarrassment. Their desire to love and be loved is often ignored, and they are often viewed as asexual, without the right to want someone else. Gliedman and Roth (1980) make the following statement:

> The able-bodied person sees that handicapped people rarely hold good jobs, become culture heroes, or are visible members of the community and concludes that this is "proof" that they cannot hold their own in society. In fact, society systematically discriminates against many perfectly capable blind men and women, cripples, adults with reading disabilities, epileptics, and so on. In other instances—and again the parallel with white racism is exact—beliefs about the incompatibility of handicap with adult roles may be not more than a vague notion that "anyone that bad off" cannot possibly lead an adult life, and not more respectable than the view that a handicapped person is mentally or spiritually inferior because he is physially dif-

ferent or that "people like that" have no business being out on the streets with "us regular folks." Like race prejudice, a belief in the social incapacity of the handicapped disguises ignorance or bigotry behind what we "see" to be an obvious biological fact. For, like Tycho Brahe (Danish astronomer) watching the sun "move" around the earth, we do not see our belief. We see a handicapped person. (pp. 22–23)

Gliedman and Roth (1980) suggest that with respect to discrimination, the handicapped are in some ways better off than blacks in that there is no overt discrimination, no organized brutality, no lynch mob "justice," and no rallies by supremist groups. However, in some ways the handicapped are worse off. Blacks and other groups have developed ethnic pride. Blacks started with "black is beautiful," and the Asians followed with "yellow is beautiful," the American Indians with "red is beautiful," and the Mexican-Americans with "brown is beautiful." In contrast, it is unlikely that one has ever heard a "cerebral palsy is beautiful" cry. Society opposes racism with the view that blacks are not self-evidently inferior, but at the same time takes for granted the self-evidently inferior status of the handicapped.

Stereotypes of the handicapped deny them a place in normal society. The handicap dominates our perception of the person's social nature. It creates a mind-set, and all perceptions are clouded by our view of deviance. The handicapped are viewed as vocationally limited and socially inept.

The handicapped are tolerated and even accepted as long as they maintain the roles ascribed to them. They are often denied basic rights and dignity as human beings. They are placed under the perpetual tutelage of those more knowledgeable and more capable than they. They are expected to subordinate their own interests and desires to the goals of a program decreed for them by the professionals who provide services to them.

Racists may be required by law to allow the African-American child in the public schools. They may have to work with an ethnic minority member. But they do not have to allow their children to play with the African-American child after school. The racist does not have to like the ethnic co-worker or invite this person home to socialize. Likewise, the general public may be required by law to provide educational and other services for the handicapped. The general public is prohibited by law against certain aspects of discrimination against the handicapped. No one, however, can require the person on the street to like the handicapped and to accept them as social equals. Many do not accept the handicapped. Just as racism leads to discrimination or prejudice against other races because of the belief in one's racial superiority, *handicappism* leads to stereotyping of and discrimination against the handicapped because of attitudes of superiority of some nonhandicapped individuals.

EXCEPTIONAL MICROCULTURES

Because of insensitivity, apathy, or prejudice, many of those responsible for implementing and upholding the laws that protect the handicapped fail to do so. The failure to provide adequate educational and vocational opportunities for the handicapped may preclude the possibility of social and economic equality. These social and economic limitations are often translated into rejection by nonhandicapped peers and ultimately into social isolation.

Not unlike many ethnic minority groups who are rejected by mainstream society, the handicapped often find comfort and security in each other, and in some instances they may form their own enclaves and social organizational structures. Throughout the country, one can find microcultures of groups such as the deaf, blind, and mentally retarded. In some instances, they congregate in similar jobs, in the same neighborhoods, and at various social settings and activities. For example, near Frankfort Avenue in Lousville, Kentucky, there are three major institutions providing services for the blind. The American Printing House for the Blind, the Kentucky School for the Blind, and the Kentucky Industries for the Blind are all within close proximity to each other. The American Printing House for the Blind, the leading publisher of materials for the visually impaired, employs a number of blind individuals. The Kentucky School for the blind is a residential school for the visually handicapped, and it also employs a small number of visually impaired individuals, including teachers. Finally, the Kentucky Industries for the Blind operates as a sheltered workship for the blind. With the relatively large number of blind persons employed by these three institutions, it is understandable that there are large numbers of blind individuals in the surrounding residential area. Living in this area allows them to live close enough to their work to minimize the many transportation problems related to their visual limitations. It also provides a sense of emotional security for the many who, in earlier years, attended the School for the Blind and lived on its campus and thus became a part of the neighborhood. The neighborhood community can also provide social and emotional security and feelings of acceptance. A few years ago, a mailing was sent from the Kentucky School for the Blind to its alumni. Ninety percent of the mailings had the same zip code as the school.

The Gifted

The gifted and talented usually do not experience the same type of discrimination and social rejection that many of the handicapped do. Yet, like the handicapped, they may suffer isolation from mainstream society and seek others with equal abilities, who may provide a feeling of acceptance as well as intellectual or emotional stimulation. Rejection of the gifted and talented may differ from that of the handicapped, because the roots may stem from a lack of understanding or jealousy rather than from the stigma that may relate to certain handicapping conditions.

Unfortunately, many gifted and talented students are not properly identified and as a result are not properly provided for in their educational programs. Unchallenged and bored with the routine of school, a few of these gifted children may resort to negative forms of behavior that jeopardize acceptance by classmates and teachers. This rejection may lead to social isolation that in turn may contribute to the development of alliances with other gifted and talented individuals who can provide understanding and acceptance and who have similar interests. Some gifted and talented individuals may not be rejected by others, but nevertheless seek others with similar talents and interests to provide the necessary or desired stimulation. The existence of Mensa, an organization whose membership prerequisites include high scores on

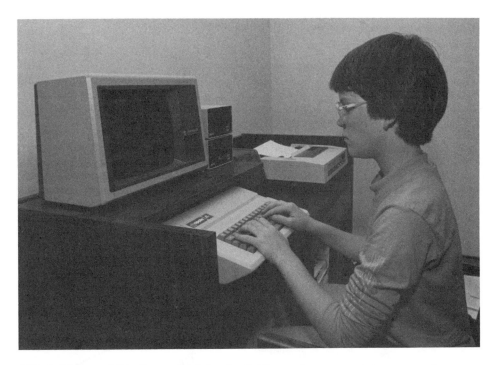

Gifted children exhibit diverse, high-level activities, such as computer programming.

(Photo by Sheryl Zelhart.)

intelligence tests, attests to the apparent need of some gifted individuals to be with others of their own kind.

The Mentally Retarded

It has been estimated that approximately 3 percent of the general population is mentally retarded. Translating this percentage into actual numbers suggests that there are 6.5 million or more retarded individuals living in the United States (Drew et al., 1988).

Many of the mildly retarded live independently or in community-based and community-supported group homes. The group homes provide a family-like atmosphere, and the homes are supervised by houseparents. Most of the moderately retarded who do not live in institutions tend to live at home. Many severely and profoundly retarded and some moderately retarded are institutionalized and are thus forced into their own cultural group or enclave, isolated from the rest of society.

Because of their intellectual limitations, frequent poverty, and minority status (through no fault of their own), the mentally retarded are often discriminated against and rejected. Because of their alienation from society, the mentally retarded may seek their own cultural identity.

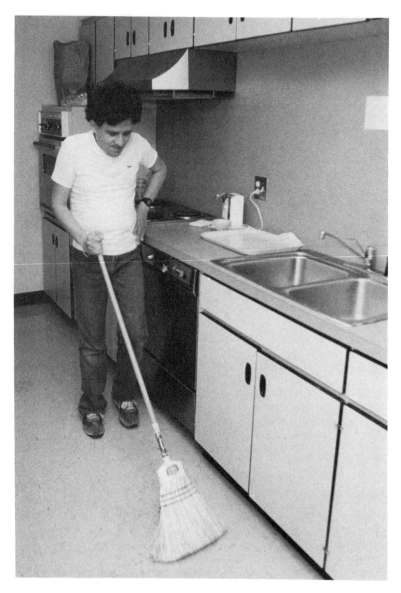

Group homes provide residents with an opportunity to learn skills for independent living.

(Photo by Sheryl Zelhart.)

The Deaf and Blind

Deaf or blind communities may exist when sensory-impaired individuals live in the same neighborhood, work together, socialize, and marry one another. In other cases, the microcultural group of sensory-impaired persons may consist of individuals from different communities. Because they do not feel part of the mainstream society and because they share many commonalities, such as language (sign language or braille), and may have similar interests, these handicapped individuals find comfort, satisfaction, and security in one another.

Of the various handicapping conditions, the visually impaired and the hearing impaired are among those most likely to form their own cultural groups. Both have a number of overriding factors that contribute to the need for individuals in these groups to seek out one another and to form cultural groups. The blind have limited mobility. Living in cultural enclaves allows them easier access to one another. They share the same forms of communication—oral language, braille, and talking books. Social and cultural interests created partly by their physical limitations can often be shared. The hearing impaired have communication limitations within the hearing world. Their unique means of communication provide them with an emotional as well as functional bond. Religious programs and churches for the deaf have been formed to provide services in total communication (including manual communication) and social activities.

The Physically and Health Impaired

Individuals with physical and health impairments often have conditions that interfere with their mobility. These limitations may have an impact on school, work, and social interactions.

Advances in biomedical science have in some instances reduced or even eliminated some of these conditions. On the other hand, advances in medical science have also contributed to the existence of these conditions. Infants and children who previously would not have survived the physical trauma resulting from severe disease or accidents are often spared the loss of life through advanced medical techniques. They are, however, sometimes left with permanent physical impairments, such as cerebral palsy, or are forced to endure a life as a paraplegic with limited wheelchair mobility.

The range and variety of conditions related to physical and health impairment are numerous, and it would serve no useful purpose in this chapter to attempt to list them. However, it is important to note the impact of physical disability on the individual, family, and society. Contemporary American society places great emphasis on physical beauty and attractiveness. Individuals who deviate significantly from physical norms are subject to possible rejection, even if their physical deviations do not interfere with functioning.

Society tends to place behavioral expectations on both men and women. Boys and men have specific masculine roles they are expected to assume. Boys are expected to be athletic. Physical impairments, however, may preclude athletic involvement. Unable to fulfill this role, the young paraplegic male may develop devalued feelings of self-worth or a feeling that he is less than a man. Feminine roles are also assigned, and physically handicapped women who are unable to assume these roles may suffer from feelings of inadequacy.

Individuals with physical handicaps may or may not become a part of a microcultural group related to the handicapping condition. Some function vocationally and socially as part of the mainstream society. With normal cognitive functioning and normal communication patterns, normal social interaction is possible but may be a function of the degree of impairment and the individual's emotional adjustment to the handicap. Some physically handicapped individuals may function in the mainstream world and also maintain social contacts with others with similar handicaps. Social clubs for physically handicapped individuals have been formed to provide experiences commensurate with functional abilities as well as a social climate that provides acceptance and security. Athletic leagues for competition in sports, such as wheelchair basketball, have been formed. Many marathon events (e.g., the Long Beach, California, marathon) now include competition for wheelchair entries.

The Emotionally Disturbed and Delinquent

Emotional disturbance and delinquency significantly affect the adequate functioning of the individual's family as a unit, as well as social contacts beyond the family. The behavior exhibited by these individuals is often negative and excessive, and the response to this behavior is typically rejection. Because the behavior may grossly affect the well-being of society, the individual and family are often held accountable for these actions, even if these actions are, in reality, beyond their willful control.

There is an apparent relationship between emotional disturbance and environmental factors. Graubard (1973) found that problems of aggression are reported in higher frequency among members of the lower class than among members of the middle or upper class. While some emotional problems in children stem from early negative interactions between parents and children, there are no solid research findings that would allow the blame for children's behavioral problems to be attributed primarily to their parents (Jacob, 1975). It has become increasingly evident that influences are transactional and interactional, and children affect their parents as much as their parents affect them.

It is clear that adverse environmental conditions contribute greatly to emotional disturbance. Where individuals are subjected to extreme stress, there is a greater likelihood for the development of emotional problems. Extreme poverty, for example, may subject an individual to constant stress, and the inability to cope with the stress results in emotional disturbances. Problems with delinquency, particularly in childhood and adolescence, may be related to lower socioeconomic circumstances, including being on public welfare, living in low-rent housing, and being a member of a minority group that tends to be caught in the low-income poverty cycle. Extreme stress caused by environmental deprivation can contribute to delinquent behaviors. However, it would be wrong to assume that children and adolescents faced with poverty-related stress are necessarily predisposed to delinquent behavior.

It has been speculated that some delinquent children are rebelling against social standards that are different from those of their own minority or disadvantaged group. In other instances, the resentment and negative behaviors may be directed against their own social and economic system, such as the maladjustment problems observed among individuals in middle and higher socioeconomic groups.

Some individuals who have no viable means to attain their goals may develop social alienation and maladjustment. Individuals from low-income groups, for example, are often confronted with the problem of wanting the material comforts of the middle and upper classes but not having a legitimate means to achieve these desires. Frustrated and disillusioned with their attempts to achieve through socially acceptable means, they may begin to seek less legitimate means that seem to bring more satisfying results.

The delinquent often forms or becomes part of a gang. The gang members form their own cultural group with their own values, morals, and standards. This may involve substance abuse with alcohol or other drugs. Those who are incarcerated in correctional institutions become a part of a larger microcultural group that also develops its own standards, values, and way of life.

NEEDS OF EXCEPTIONAL CHILDREN

There are many variables affecting the learning, cognition, and adjustment of handicapped individuals. Educators and others who work with the handicapped can do much to ensure that these variables impact in a positive manner.

The range and variety of experiences imposed on or withheld from persons with handicaps may result in undue limitations (Chinn & Chinn, 1979). Too often, parents and teachers assume that a child's visual limitation precludes the ability to appreciate the typical everyday experiences of sighted children. Blind children may not be able to see the animals in a zoo, but they can smell and hear them. They may not be able to enjoy the scenes along a bus route, but they can feel the stop-and-go movements, hear the traffic and people, and smell their fellow travelers. The deaf child may not be able to hear the sounds at the symphony or the crowd's roar at a football game. Both events, however, offer the possibility of extraordinary sensory experiences that the child needs exposure to. The child with cerebral palsy needs experiences such as going to restaurants, even if there is difficulty using eating utensils in a socially acceptable manner.

Well-adjusted individuals with a sensory handicap usually attain a balance of control with their environment (Chinn & Chinn, 1979). Individuals who depend completely on other members of the family and friends may develop an attitude of helplessness and a loss of self-identity. Handicapped individuals who completely dominate and control their environment with unreasonable demands sometimes fail to make an acceptable adjustment and may become selfish and self-centered.

It is critical to remember that exceptional children are children. Their exceptionality, although having an influence on their lives, is secondary to their needs as children. They are more like than unlike normal children. They therefore have the same basic needs as normal children. P. C. Chinn, Winn, and Walters (1978) identify three of those needs: communication, acceptance, and the freedom to grow.

Communication

Exceptional children are far more perceptive than many adults give them credit for being. They are sensitive to nonverbal communication and hidden messages that my be concealed in half-truths. They, more than anyone, need to deal with their exceptionality, whether it is a handicap or a gift. They need to know what their exceptionality is all about so that they can deal with it. They need to know how it will impact on their lives in order to make appropriate adjustments to make the best of their lives and reach their full potential. They need straight, honest communication tempered with sensitivity.

Acceptance

The society in which we live often fails to provide the exceptional child with a positive and receptive environment. Even the educational setting can be hostile and lacking in acceptance. The teacher can facilitate the acceptance of a child in a classroom by exhibiting an open and positive attitude. Students tend to reflect the attitude of the teacher. If the teacher is hostile, the students will quickly pick up these cues. If the attitude is positive, the students are likely to respond and provide a receptive environment for their handicapped classmates.

> J.B., a first-grade student who suffered from a hearing loss, was fitted with a hearing aid. When he came to school with the hearing aid, the students in the class immediately began whispering about the "thing" J.B. had in his ear. After observing the class behavior, the teacher assisted J.B. in a "show and tell" preparation for the next day. With the teacher's assistance and assurances, J.B. proudly demonstrated his hearing aid to the class. By the end of the demonstration, J.B. was the envy of the class, and any further discussion of the hearing aid was of a positive nature.

Freedom to Grow

Handicapped students need acceptance and understanding. Acceptance implies a freedom for the exceptional child to grow. There are times when it may seem easier to do things for a child rather than to take the time to teach the child.

> S.B. was a nine-year-old blind, orthopedically handicapped girl who attended a state residential school for the blind. She wore leg braces but had a reasonable amount of mobility with crutches. To save time and effort, fellow students or staff members transported her between the cottage where she lived and the classroom building in a wagon. One day her teacher decided she needed to be more independent in her travel to and from her cottage. To S.B.'s surprise, the teacher informed her after school that she would not ride back in the wagon but that he was walking her back. Angered, she denounced him as cruel and hateful in front of the entire class. She complained bitterly the full thirty minutes of their walk back to the cottage. After a

few days the complaining subsided and the travel time was curtailed. Within a few weeks S.B. was traveling on her own in ten minutes or less with newfound self-respect. (P. C. Chinn, Winn, & Walters, 1978, p. 36)

At other times, it may be tempting for teachers and parents to make extra concessions for the exceptional child. Often these exceptions preclude the emotional growth of the child and may later cause serious interpersonal problems.

> J.W. was a seven-year-old blind boy at the same state institute for the blind attended by S.B. He was a favorite of the staff members because he had such a pleasant personality and appeared to be so well adjusted. On a Sunday afternoon in the fall, he was assisting a staff member in making block prints for Christmas. The conversation turned to Christmas and J.W.'s wish for a transistor radio. This incident took place in 1960 when transistor radios were new on the market and very expensive. Since J.W. had already made his request to his parents, the staff member was confident that the parents would not deny this blind child his wish. To the surprise of the staff, J.W. returned after the holidays without a radio. He very philosophically explained to the staff that the radios were so expensive that if his parents granted his wish it would be at the expense of the other children in the family. Weeks later when J.W. returned from his birthday weekend at home, he entered his cottage with a transistor radio in hand, but in tears. He informed the staff that he and his younger brother Ralph had been fighting in the car on the way back and both had received a spanking. When a staff member went out to greet J.W.'s parents, his younger brother Ralph was still crying from the insult to his rear end. (P. C. Chinn et al., 1978, p. 36)

J.W.'s father was a laborer with a modest income. While their child's handicap created a number of adjustment problems for everyone, they had resolved to treat him as an equal in the family. As such he shared all of the family privileges. He also suffered the same consequences for inappropriate behavior. This attitude on the part of the parents was probably a primary factor in J.W.'s excellent adjustment to his handicap.

EDUCATIONAL IMPLICATIONS

The educational implications for working with exceptional individuals are numerous, and entire chapters could be devoted to each exceptionality. Educators should remember that exceptional children, both handicapped and gifted, are more like than unlike normal children. Their basic needs are the same as all children's. Abraham Maslow's theory on self-actualization is familiar to most students in education. To be self-actualized, or to meet one's full potential, Maslow (1954) theorized that one's basic needs must be fulfilled. That is, to reach self-actualization, one's physiological needs, safety needs, belongingness or love needs, and esteem needs must first be met. Although many handicapped individuals may never match the accomplishments of their normal peers, they can become proficient at whatever they are capable of doing. Educators can assist them by helping to ensure that their basic needs are met, allowing them to strive toward self-actualization.

Teachers must be constantly cognizant of the unique needs of their exceptional children. The exceptional adult may choose to become a part of, or may be forced by society to become a part of, a microcultural group. The interactions between educators and the exceptional child may not change what will eventually take place. Even if exceptional adults are a part of a microcultural group, they also will interact with the mainstream society on a regular basis. The efforts on the part of the educator to meet the needs of the child may ultimately affect the exceptional adult's interaction with society.

Teachers of children with physical and other health impairments may find it advantageous to check their student records carefully to determine potential problem situations with these students in the classroom. If the child has particular health problems that may surface in the classroom, the child's teachers need to be prepared for such situations so that they will know precisely what to do should the child have, for example, an epileptic seizure. The parents will most likely be able to provide precise instructions, and the school nurse could also provide additional recommendations. If the children are old enough to understand, they themselves can be a valuable source of information. Ask them what kind of adaptations, special equipment, or teaching procedures work best for them. Teachers should not be afraid of their own uncertainties. They should feel free to ask the student when they won't or don't want help. Teachers should treat their handicapped students as normally as feasible, neither overprotecting them nor giving or doing more for them than is needed or deserved. Allowing them to assume responsibility for themselves will do much to facilitate their personal growth.

SUMMARY

The concerns related to the disproportionate placement of ethnic minorities, males, and students from low-income families in special education programs have been addressed to focus on a long-standing educational problem. The issues raised are not intended to negate the fact that there are retarded as well as seriously emotionally disturbed and other handicapped children from both majority and minority groups. Rather, they are raised to call attention to problems in referral and assessment as well as the problems associated with poverty.

Handicapped adults often become a part of a microculture for the handicapped by ascription or by individual choice. They do not choose to be handicapped, and their situation often precludes full acceptance or integration into the world of those who are perceived to be physically, socially, or mentally normal. Their adjustment to their environment may be in part a function of the way they are perceived, treated, and accepted by educators. Consequently, teachers and other educators may have a greater influence on handicapped children than they themselves realize.

Public Law 94–142 and Section 504 of Public Law 93–112 guarantee all exceptional children the right to a free and appropriate education and freedom from discrimination resulting from their handicap. In spite of these mandates, equality still eludes millions of the handicapped in this country. Insensitivity, apathy, and prejudice contribute to the problems of the handicapped. Because of prejudice, institutionalization, or a desire to meet their own needs, some exceptional individuals form their own microcultures and some their own enclaves, where they live and socialize with one another. The laws can force services for the handicapped, but only time and effort can change public attitudes.

QUESTIONS FOR REVIEW

1. What are some of the objections to labeling handicapped children?
2. In what ways has the treatment of handicapped individuals paralleled that of oppressed minorities?
3. In what ways have ethnic minority children been disproportionately placed in special classes for the handicapped and gifted?
4. What are some of the variables contributing to the disproportionate placement of minorities in special education?
5. What are the major implications of Public Law 94–142 and Section 504 of Public Law 93–112?
6. Explain the concepts of normalization, social role valorization, and mainstreaming.
7. What are some of the negative ways that handicapped individuals are portrayed by the media and viewed by some members of society?
8. What are some of the ways in which exceptional individuals form their own microcultures?
9. What are some of the needs of exceptional children?

REFERENCES

Berdine, W. H., & Blackhurst, A. D. (1985). *An introduction to special education.* Boston: Little, Brown.

Berger, K. S. (1983). *The developing person through the life span.* New York: Worth.

Chinn, P. C., & Harris, K. C. (1990). Variables affecting the disproportionate placement of ethnic minority children in special education programs. *Multicultural Leader, 3,*(1)*,* 1–3.

Chinn, P. C., & Hughes, S. (1987). Representation of minority students in special education classes. *Remedial and Special Education, 8,*(4), 41–46.

Chinn, P. C., Winn, J., & Walters, R. H. (1978). *Two-way talking with parents of exceptional children: A process of positive communication.* St. Louis: Mosby.

Chinn, P. L., & Chinn, P. C. (1979). The child with learning problems. In P. L. Chinn, *Child health maintenance: Concepts in family-centered care* (2nd ed.) (pp. 784–801). St. Louis: Mosby.

Drew, C. J., Logan, D. R., & Hardman, M. L. (1988). *Mental retardation: A life cycle approach* (4th ed.). Columbus, OH: Merrill Publishing.

Dunn, L. (1968). Special education for the mildly retarded: Is much of it justifiable? *Exceptional Children, 7*, 5–24.

Edgerton, R. B. (1967). *The cloak of competence*. Berkeley: University of California.

Gliedman, J., & Roth, W. (1980). *The unexpected minority*. New York: Harcourt Brace Jovanovich.

Graubard, D. S. (1973). Children with behavioral disabilities. In L. M. Dunn (Ed.), *Exceptional children in the schools* (2nd ed.). New York: Holt, Rinehart & Winston.

Heward, W. L., & Orlansky, M. D. (1988). *Exceptional Children* (3rd ed.). Columbus, OH: Merrill Publishing.

High, M. H., & Udall, A. I. (1983). Teacher ratings of students in relation to ethnicity of students and school ethnic balance. *Journal of Education and the Gifted, 6*, 154–166.

Jacob, T. (1975). *The relationship between academic achievement and the demographic characteristics of hearing impaired children and youth*. Washington, DC: Gallaudet College.

Jordan, J. B., & Zantal-Wiener, K. (Eds.). (1988). *1987 special education year book*. Reston, VA: The Council for Exceptional Children.

Kauffman, J. M. (1981). *Characteristics of children's behavior disorders* (2nd ed.). Columbus, OH: Merrill Publishing.

Kitano, M. K., & Kirby, D. F. (1986). *Gifted education: A comprehensive view*. Boston: Little, Brown.

Krishef, C. H. (1972). State laws on marriage and sterilization of the mentally retarded. *Mental Retardation, 10*(3), 136–38.

Larry P. v. Riles, Civil No. C-71-2270,343F. Supp. 1306 (N.D. Cal., 1972).

Maslow, A. (1954). *Motivation and personality*. New York: Harper.

Mercer, J. (1973). *Labeling the mentally retarded*. Los Angeles: University of California Press.

Nirje, B. (1969). The normalization principle and its human management implications. In R. B. Kugel & W. Wolfensberger (Eds.), *Changing patterns in residential services for the mentally retarded* (pp. 227–254). Washington, DC: President's Committee on Mental Retardation.

Office of Civil Rights. (1988). *1986 elementary and secondary schools civil rights survey*. Washington, DC: Department of Education.

Ortiz, A., & Yates, J. R. (1983). Incidence of exceptionality among Hispanics: Implications for manpower planning. *National Association of Bilingual Education Journal, 7*(3), 41–53.

President's Committee on Mental Retardation. (1969). *The six hour retarded child*. Washington, DC: U.S. Department of Health, Education and Welfare.

Stainback, S., & Stainback, W. (1985). *Integration of students with severe handicaps into regular schools*. Reston, VA: Council for Exceptional Children.

U. S. Bureau of the Census. (1983). *Statistical abstract of the United States, 1984* (104th ed.). Washington, DC: Government Printing Office.

Wolfensberger, W. (1972). *Normalization: The principle of normalization in human services.* Toronto: National Institute on Mental Retardation.

Wolfensberger, W. (1983). Social role valorization: Proposed new form for the principle of normalization. *Mental Retardation, 21*(6), 234–239.

SUGGESTED READINGS

Drew, C. J., Logan, D. R., & Hardman, M. L. (1988). *Mental retardation: A life cycle approach* (4th ed.). St. Louis: Times Mirror/Mosby College.

An excellent developmental approach to mental retardation. Includes a sensitive view of mental retardation and its impact on the family. A chapter on legislative and legal issues related to the mentally retarded is also included.

Edgerton, R. B. (1967). *The cloak of competence: Stigma in the lives of the mentally retarded.* Berkeley: University of California Press.

A detailed follow-up of the lives of individuals released from Pacific State Hospital in California. Includes detailed portraits of selected subjects and concerns of these individuals living outside the institution. Considered a classic in the field of mental retardation.

Gliedman, J., & Roth, W. (1980). *The unexpected minority.* New York: Harcourt Brace Jovanovich.

An examination of how social rather than biological aspects of disability doom handicapped children and adults to stunted and useless lives. Demonstrates how discrimination against the handicapped is the result of stereotypes and misconceptions that distort the attitudes of both professionals and society at large.

Heward, W. L., & Orlansky, M. D. (1988). *Exceptional children* (3rd ed.). Columbus, OH: Merrill Publishing.

One of the few survey texts to include a chapter on culturally diverse exceptional children. An overview of all exceptionalities that will provide a good basic understanding of the gifted and talented as well as the various handicapping conditions.

CHAPTER 6
Religion

Congress shall make no law respecting an establishment of religion, or prohibiting the free exercise thereof; or abridging the freedom of speech, or of the press; or the right of the people peaceably to assemble, and to petition the Government for a redress of grievances. (First Amendment to the United States Constitution, 1791)

In the United States, close to 143 million individuals are affiliated with a religious group. In an average week, 42 percent of the adults attend a church or synagogue. Religion is clearly an important aspect of the lives of many individuals. Some individuals have little, if anything, to do with religion, but for others, including many children in American classrooms, their religion influences the way they think, perceive, and behave. The forces of religious groups are far from dormant. They can influence the election of school board members as well as the curriculum and textbooks used in the schools. Principals, teachers, and superintendents have been hired and fired through the influence of religious groups. This chapter will provide an overview of religion in the United States and its influence in the educational system.

The pluralistic nature of the school in which one teaches will be determined in great part by the geographical region of the United States. In most schools, there are boys and girls, exceptional students, students of different ages, and students from different socioeconomic levels. Because of various immigration and migration patterns throughout history, ethnic and religious groups have settled in different parts of the country. Although few areas remain totally homogeneous, a school community may be dominated by families that strongly identify with a particular ethnic group. More often, families identify strongly with the religious orientation of one or more denominations in the community. The perspective of a particular religious doctrine often influences what a family expects from the school and thus from the teacher. In an area where the religious perspectives and school expectations differ greatly, educators face numerous challenges. A look at the religious composition of schools in various sections of the country will provide a sense of the diversity one might face throughout a career in education.

A consolidated rural high school in the South may be attended primarily by students whose families are conservative Southern Baptist or Pentecostal. The church serves as the center of most community activities, and many families spend several nights a week at church or serving the church. Sex education is not allowed in the public school curriculum. Teachers may face harsh criticism if they teach about evolution or life-styles that conflict with those acceptable in that community. Textbooks and assigned readings are often scrutinized to ensure that the content does not stray far from the beliefs of this fundamentalist community.

At a middle school in northeastern Indiana, most students are from the same European background, but they dress and behave differently. Some of the students are from a local Old Order Amish community with strict codes for the dress of its members, while the majority of the other students are Mennonites. The former are very respectful and well behaved, but some are ridiculed by non-Amish students. After completing the eighth grade, the Amish students will no longer be part of the school system because their families withdraw them to work full-time on their farms.

Students from Catholic, Jewish, Protestant, and Buddhist families attend a suburban school on the West Coast. Some of the students in the school are from families that have no religious affiliation. Although the religious backgrounds of the students differ, they seem to share many of the same values. The school projects a generally liberal curriculum that includes sex education, ethnic studies, and religion courses.

Except for the students' celebration of various religious holidays, religion seems to have little impact on the students or the school.

At an inner-city school in an East Coast city, the religious backgrounds of students vary greatly. Some students attend Catholic services; others attend Baptist churches or storefront Pentecostal churches; some belong to a cult that has been established in the community; and others have no religious affiliation. Thus, some students are constantly involved in religious activities during their nonschool time. The school reflects little of these diverse religious perspectives in the curriculum or school environment.

Moving to the state of Utah, the educator will find a school in a moderate-size community dominated by members of the Church of Jesus Christ of Latter-Day Saints (Mormons). Many Mormon families serve their ward several nights every week and socialize almost solely with other Mormon families. Mormon beliefs do not allow smoking or drinking of alcohol, coffee, or tea. In that Utah community, most major institutions and businesses are controlled by this religious group. Religion itself is not taught as part of the school curriculum, but the perspective of the dominant religious group in this community is reflected in school and curriculum practices. Many students leave during school hours to receive religious instruction at a Mormon seminary adjacent to the school. Most of the elected officials are members of the Mormon church; thus, state and local laws affecting education reflect a Mormon influence.

People differ greatly in their beliefs about the role that religious perspective should play in determining school curriculum and environment. Like all other institutions in this country, schools have a historical background of rural, white, Protestant domination. Such domination has determined the holidays, usually Christian holidays, that are celebrated by schools. Moreover, the Protestant majority has determined the moral teachings that have been integrated into our public schools.

While the First Amendment affirms the principle of separation of church and state, it is one of the most controversial parts of the Constitution, as various individuals and groups tend to interpret it to meet their own needs and interests. For some, religious emphasis is appropriate in the public schools as long as it is congruent with their own religious persuasion. These same individuals, however, may be quick to cite the constitutional safeguards for separation of church and state if other groups attempt the infusion of their religious dogmas.

In most communities in this country, schools close in observance of Christmas and sometimes Easter (although Easter break may now be referred to as spring break). The Christian residents in these communities may realize that others in the community may not observe these Christian holidays, but they may also expect everyone to recognize their right to close the schools during their religious holy days. These individuals, however, may vigorously resist any attempts by other religious groups to close the schools in observance of their special religious days.

Equity and propriety are often in the eye of the beholder, and one's religious orientation may strongly influence one's perception of what constitutes objectivity, fairness, and legality.

Parents and churches disagree about the separation of church and state as required in the First Amendment. Since the removal of prayer from the schools by a 1963 Supreme Court decision, parent groups have continued to fight (sometimes successfully) to restore prayer in the schools through state and federal legislation. Parent groups have fought on religious grounds to prevent the teaching of sex education and evolution. Coming from different religious backgrounds, parents have fought verbally and physically over what books their children should read in literature courses and what curriculum should be used in social studies and science classes. Members of more liberal Protestant, Catholic, and Jewish denominations often argue that they want their children exposed to the perspectives of different religious and ethnic groups. Members of the more conservative, especially fundamentalist, groups argue that they do not want their children exposed to what they consider immoral perspectives and language inherent in such instructional materials.

Of all the microcultures examined in this book, religion may be the most problematic for educators. In one school, the religious beliefs of students appear to have little influence on what is taught in a classroom; in fact, the teacher is expected to expose students to many different perspectives. In another school, the teacher may be attacked for asking students to read *The Catcher in the Rye.*

Educators themselves vary in their beliefs about the role of religious perspective in education. If one shares the same religion or religious perspectives as the community, there will probably be little conflict between one's own beliefs and the beliefs reflected in the school. If the educator is from a religious background different from that prevalent in the community or has a perspective about the role of religion that differs from that of the community, misunderstanding and conflicts may arise that prevent effective instruction. If an educator does not understand the role of religion in the lives of the students, it may be difficult to develop appropriate instructional strategies. In some cases, it would be difficult to retain one's job.

This chapter will examine religion and its impact on a student's life, the various religions existing in the United States, the degree to which an individual identifies with a particular religious doctrine, and the educational implications of religion.

RELIGION AS A WAY OF LIFE

Religious pluralism has its foundation in the U.S. Constitution, as there were no ties between the government and a state or favored church. Although the separation of church and state is an integral part of our heritage, the two usually support each other. In many churches, the U.S. flag stands next to the church flag, and patriotism is an important part of religious loyalty. On the other hand, God has been mentioned in all inaugural addresses except Washington's second address (Bellah, 1974), and it is not an uncommon practice for politicians and preachers to refer to the United States as the promised land. The secular ideas of the American dream also pervade many religions in this country. In fact, religions often reflect the dominant values of our society (Greeley, 1982).

What does religion mean? Definitions range from general to specific. Yinger (1970) provides a general definition under which every individual could practice religion: "a system of beliefs and practices by means of which a group of people struggle with . . . the ultimate problems of human life" (p. 7). For this discussion, we will use a more specific definition, placing some parameters around the term as follows: "A religion is a unified system of beliefs and practices relative to sacred things, that is to say, things set apart and forbidden—beliefs and practices which unite into one single moral community called a church, all those who adhere to them" (Durkheim, 1969, p. 46).

Stark and Glock (1969) outline five dimensions of religion on which religious groups place different emphasis:

1. Belief: a certain theological outlook whose tenets the religious will acknowledge

2. Religious practice: worship and devotion that people follow to carry out their religious commitment

3. Experience: the feelings, perceptions, and sensations that ensure some contact with ultimate reality (i.e., a supernatural agency)

4. Knowledge: information about the basic tenets of one's faith, scriptures, and traditions

5. Consequences: the effects of religious belief, practice, experience, and knowledge on the person's daily life

What is expected of religious persons in these five dimensions will depend on the particular religious group to which they belong. A Southern Baptist will be expected to make a public profession of faith; a member of a charismatic church group may receive the Holy Spirit, as revealed in the ability to speak in tongues; and a member of the United Church of Christ may experience God through quiet prayer.

For most individuals, religion serves as a looking glass in which "humanity beholds its own image, its ideal portrait of itself, its highest intentions, its destiny" (Raschke, Kirk, & Taylor, 1977, p. 7). Western religions tend to emphasize individual control over life—an emphasis that prompts believers to blame the disadvantaged for their disadvantage (Stark & Glock, 1974). Many religions are particularistic in that members believe that their own religion is uniquely true and legitimate and all others are false (Wilson, 1978). Other religions accept the validity of various religions that have grown out of different historical experiences. The values and life-styles of families are affected by their religious beliefs (Greeley, 1982).

Nine out of ten Americans regard their religious beliefs as very, or at least fairly, important to them (Gallup Report, 1989). Although less than half of the population attends church weekly, most identify with a religious perspective that is reflected in their daily living (Gallup Report, 1987). Religion appears to have an influence in patterns of sex roles, marriage, divorce, birthrates, child training, sexual activity, friendships, and political attitudes. It may affect one's dress, social activities, and dietary habits, including alcohol consumption and smoking.

If the religious group is tightly knit, a member may have little chance to interact on a personal level with anyone other than another member of the same religion, especially if a religious school is maintained. Tight control over criteria for membership in the group and little contact with nongroup members are often key factors in maintaining the integrity of religious sects. The Hutterites and, to a great extent, the Amish have been able to survive in this way. Mormons, a much larger group, were able to grow with little outside interference once they were established in Salt Lake City. Even in suburban areas, friendship patterns are largely based on religious preference (Mueller, 1974).

Churches and their religious programs serve as a strong socialization mechanism in the transmission of values from one generation to another. Rituals, parables, and stories reinforce these values, and Sunday schools serve as primary agents for transmitting these values. Religious institutions are also responsible for reinterpreting social failure in spiritual terms, compensating for the lack of value realization, and functioning as an agent of social control by reward and punishment (Wilson, 1978).

All but 2 percent of the parents in this country believe that their children should have religious training for character building and as a means of keeping the family together (Gallup Poll, 1984). Children become aware of their religious identity as Protestant, Catholic, or Jew by five years of age, although they tend to equate religion with national and racial identities. By nine years of age, they are able to distinguish between religion and irreligion, and they can identify denominations by their practices. As one might expect, children of religious parents are more likely to be religious than children of nonreligious parents (Greeley, 1982).

In the United States, almost as many adults (40 percent) attend church or synagogue regularly as did their counterparts in 1939 (41 percent). Although not equal to the all-time high of 49 percent in 1955 and 1958, attendance from 1969 to 1986 deviated from only one or two pecentage points throughout that period (Gallup Report, 1987). Church and synogogue attendance patterns are listed in Table 6–1.

Weekly attendance at church or synagogue is apparently a function of one's microculture. In 1988, 18 percent more women (46 percent) attended weekly services than men (38 percent). Blacks (47 percent) attended more regularly than Hispanics (41 percent) or whites (41 percent). College graduates attended to a greater extent than nongraduates, and 20 percent more individuals sixty-five and older attended than those in the eighteen to twenty-four age-group. Southerners (45 percent) had a 9 percent higher attendance rate than Westerners (36 percent) (Gallup Report, 1989).

Thus, religious behavior is learned as a normal part of the socialization pattern. Religion and religious differences are important in our study of this pluralistic nation because it is a way of life for many people, as described by Wilson (1978):

> Religion is much more than a voluntary association of people with a common hobby or pastime. A denomination, sect, or church is also a community of people who intermarry, worship together as a family, choose their friends along religious lines, and socialize their children according to the teachings of their faith. Each faith, even each denomination, is a separate subcommunity as well as a voluntary association. It

Table 6-1 Church/Synagogue Attendance Among U.S.
Adults (Percentage Attending in Average Week)

Year	Percentage	Year	Percentage
1986	40	1968	43
1985	42	1967	43
1984	40	1966	44
1983	40	1965	44
1982	41	1964	45
1981	41	1963	46
1980	40	1962	46
1979	40	1961	47
1978	41	1960	47
1977	41	1959	47
1976	42	1958	49[a]
1975	40	1957	47
1974	40	1956	46
1973	40	1955	49[a]
1972	40	1954	46
1971	40	1950	39
1970	42	1940	37[b]
1969	42	1939	41

[a]High points.
[b]Low points.
From Gallup Report (1987), Religion in America, *259, 38.*

is a way of life, with social clubs, athletic leagues, insurance companies, professional societies, publishing houses, veterans groups, and even movie-rating committees. (p. 278)

RELIGIOUS PLURALISM IN AMERICA

Four decades ago, few Americans would have envisioned their country led by a Catholic president or foreseen an African-American minister elected as the majority whip in the U.S. House of Representatives. In very recent years, we have seen Jesse Jackson, an African-American minister, make a strong and serious bid for the Democratic party's presidential nomination. In the same election year, 1988, Pat Robertson, a popular tele-evangelist, was a serious candidate for the Republican nomination and received strong support financially and otherwise.

Table 6-2 Religious Preference 1986

| | **Major Faiths** | | | |
	Protestant	Catholic	Jewish	No Religious Preference
National	58%	27%	2%	9%
18–24 years	47	33	2	14
25–29 years	52	29	2	13
30–49 years	57	27	2	11
50–64 years	65	26	2	4
65 and older	69	23	2	4
Men	55	28	2	11
Women	61	26	2	7
East	39	45	5	10
Midwest	61	27	1	9
South	77	15	1	6
West	51	24	1	14
Whites	56	30	2	9
Blacks	81	7	a	10
Hispanics	19	70	1	8
College graduates	57	24	5	11
College incomplete	54	29	2	11
High school graduates	57	30	2	8
Not high school graduates	65	23	a	8
Republicans	66	22	1	8
Democrats	57	30	3	7
Independents	52	29	2	13
Household income:				
$40,000 and over	54	29	3	10
$25,000–$39,000	55	31	2	9
$15,000–$24,000	61	26	2	9
Under $15,000	62	24	1	9

[a]Less than 1%.

From Gallup Report (April 1987), Religion in America, 259, 20.

In recent years, we have observed thousands of young people, many white, led by a Korean minister and leader of the Unification church; we have seen African-Americans leaving traditional black Protestant churches and joining the ranks of the Black Muslims; and we have seen college students embracing Zen Buddhism.

Today, the electronic church (tele-evangelism) reaches the homes of millions of Americans, influences their lives and their voting patterns, and has helped to elect or defeat politicians and change the face of America for years to come. Thus, as Roof and McKinney (1985) suggest, religious groups are mediating structures that link families and individuals to the larger social order.

Americans tend to identify not only with major groups, such as Protestants, Catholics, or Jews, but also with smaller groups or denominations within these major religious microcultures. For example, former president Jimmy Carter, a Southern Baptist, identified himself as a "born again" Christian. Others may identify themselves as charismatic Catholics. It is important to note that within each major group, there is considerable heterogeneity. Conservative Protestants, for example, differ in many respects from their liberal counterparts. It is not unusual today to find conservative Protestants joining forces with conservative Catholics and Jews over moral or political issues, such as the prochoice/right to life debate.

Of the U.S. population, 90 percent identify themselves as belonging to one of three major faiths—Protestant, Catholic, or Jewish (see Table 6–2). Until early in this century, however, Protestantism was by far the dominant religious force in the country. Most of our institutions continue to bear the mark of the white Protestants who established them. After the great immigrations from southern and eastern Europe, Catholic Ireland, and Asia, however, pluralism described the religious diversity of the nation. Protestants as a group are still in the majority, with 58 percent of the population; 27 percent of the population identify themselves as Catholic, 2 percent as Jewish, 4 percent as others, and 9 percent as no religion (Gallup Report, 1987).

The fact that Americans place themselves in one of these three major faiths is misleading in understanding the great diversity of religious beliefs in this country. These three categories describe three historical religious groups that share the same Old Testament heritage, but they do not attest to the diversity of beliefs and interpretations of the Bible. Wilson (1978) states that there are 280 different religious bodies in the United States. Catholics compose the largest single denomination. Protestants as a group are the largest in numbers, followed by Catholics and Jews (Jacquet, 1987) (see Table 6–3).

A number of denominational differences have their origin in ethnic differences. The English established the Anglican (Episcopalian) and Puritan (later Congregational) churches here; the Germans established some of the Lutheran, Anabaptist, and Evangelical churches; the Dutch, the Reformed churches; the Spanish, French, Italians, Poles, and others, the Roman Catholic church; and the Ukrainians, Armenians, Greeks, and others, the Eastern Orthodox church. Over time, many of these separate ethnic denominations have united or expanded their membership to include other ethnic groups, although they may still be dominated by the original ethnic group. On the other hand, a different pattern has developed for black Americans because they often were not included in the expansion of membership. For example, 8 percent of all African-Americans are Methodist, and 54 percent are Baptists (Gallup Report, 1987). Most of those churches attended by blacks are for the most part racially segregated. Although many blacks attend integrated churches, the majority attend African-American churches.

Most denominations have remained in their traditional regional strongholds, with Catholics in the Northeast, liberal and moderate Protestants in the Northeast and

Table 6–3 Number of U.S. Churches and Members, by Religious Groups

	Number of Churches	Number of Members
Buddhist	100	100,000
Eastern Churches	1,659	4,025,698
Jews[a]	3,416	5,834,635
Old Catholic, Polish National Catholic, Armenian Churches	428	1,024,330
Protestants[b]	314,713	79,095,746
Roman Catholic	24,251	52,654,908
Miscellaneous[c]	1,124	191,046
Totals	345,961	142,926,363

[a]Including Orthodox, Conservative, and Reform branches.

[b]Some bodies included here are, strictly speaking, not Protestant in the usual sense, including, for example, Latter-Day Saint groups and Jehovah's Witnesses.

[c]This is a grouping of bodies officially non-Christian, including those such as Spiritualists, Ethical Culture Movement, and Unitarian-Universalists.

From Yearbook of American and Canadian Churches, 1987, *edited by Constant H. Jacquet. Copyright © 1987 by the National Council of the Churches of Christ in the U.S.A. Used by permission of the publisher, Abingdon Press.*

Midwest, and conservative Protestants in the South. Some groups, however, have expanded their base considerably. Episcopalians, Presbyterians, and members of the United Church of Christ are no longer as concentrated in the Northeast as they once were; some numerical base shifts have been made into the Sun Belt. Conservative Protestants, such as the Southern Baptists, are growing in all regions, including the Northeast and the West. Twenty-nine percent of Mormons are now in regions other than the West. Those without a religious preference are well represented in all regions, but continue to have the largest concentrations in the West (Roof & McKinney, 1985). The Jewish population tends to be located in metropolitan areas throughout the country, with the largest concentration in the mid-Atlantic region (Gallup Report, 1987).

Although religious pluralism has fostered the rapid accommodation of many American religious movements toward a mainstream of acceptability and respectability by society, groups such as the Jehovah's Witnesses and Seventh-Day Adventists have maintained their independence. Those smaller groups that maintain their distinctiveness historically have been victims of harassment by members of mainstream religious groups. Christian Scientists, Jehovah's Witnesses, Children of God, and the Unification Church are minority groups that have been subjected to such treatment in the past (Appel, 1983). Conflict among the three major faiths has also been intense at different periods in our history. Anti-Semitic and anti-Catholic sentiments are still perpetuated in some households and institutions in this country. Although religious pluralism in our past has often led to conflict, the hope of the future is that it will lead to a better understanding and respect for religious differences. In this section, we will examine in greater detail the three major faiths and then briefly discuss others that the educator may find in various communities.

Protestantism

Traditionally, Protestantism has stressed individualism, activism, and pragmatism for its members (Wilson, 1978). Many sects that separated from the Catholic church after the Reformation are now recognized as established Protestant denominations. There is no one doctrine or one church that is representative of Protestantism.

The history of Protestantism in this country is integrally mixed with the development of capitalism and the expansion of the West. Most of the better-known Protestant groups began as transplants of nonconformist European groups, including the Pilgrims and Puritans, Baptists and Quakers, Presbyterians, Mennonites, Marovians, and many Lutherans (Moseley, 1981). Jews and Catholics from England and Ireland were also among the early settlers, but they were clearly outnumbered by the Protestant groups.

Throughout the nineteenth and early twentieth centuries, Protestant groups maintained separate social communities based on common tradition and identity. The church served as the chief locus of social life in small towns and rural communities, bound by a common religious belief and national origin (Moseley, 1981). As these separate groups accommodated to Americanization, English replaced the immigrant language, and ethnic differences blurred. As these distinctions among religions diminished, doctrinal and liturgical distinctions were often accentuated. Although Protestantism has become characteristically American, remnants of ethnic identity remain in many Lutheran churches and the German sects of Mennonites, Marovians, and Brethrens. Segmentation remains with the Protestant denominations, but segregated from them, the black church has been the major institution over nearly two centuries that has allowed blacks the opportunity for self-expression. Over two hundred different sects and denominations that currently flourish in this country grew from these various sectional divisions.

The Dominant Protestant Influence.   The western Europeans who immigrated into this country in large numbers brought with them their various forms of Protestantism. Consequently, the political and social systems in the country still reflect the heavy influence of Protestantism. Although Protestants are no longer as dominant a force as they once were, they still claim 58 percent of the population (Gallup Report, 1987). Even that majority is divided along racial lines of black and white churches and denominations.

Has the political structure reflected the religious diversity that has developed over the past century? Table 6–4 shows the trends in the House of Representatives by denomination. In 1986, Protestants led to the group with 64.2 percent, which is 6.2

Table 6-4 Religious Affiliation of Members of the U.S. House of Representatives

Roman Catholic		141	(26.7%)
Jewish		37	(7%)
Eastern Orthodox		7	(1.3%)
Protestant (including Mormon and Unitarian)		339	(64.2%)
Methodist	74		
Episcopalian	60		
Presbyterian	57		
Baptist	54		
Lutheran	37		
Protestant (denomination not identified)	23		
United Church of Christ	16		
Mormon	11		
Unitarian	10		
Church of Christ	5		
Disciples of Christ	3		
Bible Church	2		
Christian Science	2		
No Affiliation		4	(0.76%)

Extracted from "Where Congress Go to Church," Christianity Today, 30, *44, December 12, 1986.*

percent higher than the 58 percent of the general population that indicated that they were Protestants (Gallup Report, 1987). Roman Catholics followed with 26.7 percent, which is almost identical to the Gallup poll's findings of 27 percent of the general population. Jewish congressional members made up 7 percent of the congressional seats, which was 5 percent higher than that of the general population. Those with no affiliation held less than 1 percent, considerably less than the general population's 9 percent. Eastern Orthodox congressional members held 1.3 percent of the House seats.

It is interesting to note, however, that the Protestant breakdown differs considerably from that revealed in the Gallup poll that year. Episcopalians, who made up only 2 percent of the general population in 1986, made up 11.4 precent of Congress. Presbyterians also made up 2 percent of the general population, but 10.8 percent of Congress; Methodists, 9 percent of the general population, but 14 percent of Congress; and Baptists, 20 percent of the general population, but only 10.2 percent of Congress. The two groups with the highest disproportionate representation are considered among the more liberal to moderate and higher socioeconomic Protestant groups. The Methodists, who are also overrepresented, are generally considered moderates and in the middle socioeconomic Protestant group. The Baptists (particulary Southern Baptists), who are significantly underrepresented, are considered in the conservative group and likely the lowest socioeconomic group of the four denominations mentioned here.

Members of liberal churches and Jews may be disproportionately overrepresented because historically, they have felt a responsibility for public issues. Another factor is probably related to the social class of members of these various denominations. Because holding political office can be quite costly, religious groups whose members are typically upper middle class are overrepresented in political offices (Carroll, 1979). In the past decade, evangelical churches also have actively entered the political arena, taking advantage of the fact that they are large, identifiable forces in society. In the elections since 1975, coalitions of these evangelical groups have pursued campaigns to elect persons with ultraconservative political views and free-enterprise economic principles.

The figures indicate that the political leadership reflects greater religious diversity than existed in the past. Is this an indication that Protestants, specifically, white Protestants, are willingly sharing the power that was almost totally theirs in the past? Carroll (1979) questions the current active political involvement of the evangelical groups and suggests that it may be an attempt to hold on to past control:

> Are such political and economic developments among evangelicals likely to be rather short-lived nativist attempts to hold back the tide of pluralism; that is, are they attempts by conservative white Anglo-Saxon Protestants to preserve their traditionally favored status in the face of increasingly invisible and vocal ethnic diversity? Or do the evangelicals constitute a genuine new force in American society that is likely to persist? It is clearly too early to tell, although we suspect the former is more probable. Religiocultural imperialism, such as Protestants of all varieties have exercised in the United States, dies hard, but it is unlikely to remain strong indefinitely in an increasingly pluralistic society. (p. 11)

Thus, Protestantism maintains not only the major religious influence on society, but also the dominant control of political leadership. Because Protestants continue to represent the majority of the population, such influence is to be expected. However, pluralism increasingly forces the sharing of power and resources among diverse groups of people in society.

Similarities Among Diversity. As one visits various Protestant services and listens to the different doctrines espoused by members, one often wonders how such a diverse conglomeration can be classified into one faith. This great diversity is reflected in the following examples:

> Incense lamps swing solemnly on silent chains. Smoke curls slowly through the pastel shafts of light penetrating the stained glass windows. A solemn acolyte approaches the alter carrying a huge, jewel-studded cross. Two other boys walk at his sides, each holding a three-foot-high golden candle. The priest, resplendent in intricately embroidered robes, raises a golden chalice and consecrates the dark wine within it. A choir chants softly.

A medieval service in a venerable English abbey? No. It is 1977, and we are witnessing high mass in an Episcopal cathedral.

The scene shifts. Business-suited evangelist Billy Graham addresses fifty thousand worshippers in a baseball stadium hired for the occasion. Six hundred giant billboards announce his coming. Special sound and lighting effects amplify God's message. The Reverend warns of a "divine computer" that compiles everyone's record of sins with terrifying efficiency. Each of us, he stresses, must find God before the final printout.

The scene shifts again. We are in the Amish country of Pennsylvania. Men in somber black suits and broad-brimmed hats, women in old-fashioned bonnets and long black dresses, are leaving their neat farms for the all-day Sabbath service. They ride in horse-drawn buggies. The Bible doesn't mention cars or telephones or trains or planes, so the Amish do without them.

Now we are in a Quaker meeting house. There are no stained-glass windows. There is no altar, no organ, no steeple, no ordained minister. The Friends (as the Quakers call themselves) meet in silent meditation and wait for a spiritual message to move one of them to speak. If no one gets a message during the worship hour, everyone will get up and go home. Not a word will have been spoken.

In the Appalachian log church or Indiana tent meeting, hands clap and feet stomp to the rhythms of tambourines and electric guitars. Here and there, someone falls to the ground in a trance—"saved" by coming to Jesus Christ.

In thousands of churches, millions of worshippers spend an hour each Sunday in quiet prayer, listening to the message of their minister, and reading the words of the Bible. ("Protestantism—World Religions," 1977, p. 22)

Let us look first at some commonalities among what appear to be very different beliefs and practices. Probably the most binding factor is that Protestants share a common faith that emanates from the Reformation, when there was a separation from the Catholic tradition. They reject the authority of the pope and believe that they individually communicate with God. Other similarities have little to do with religious doctrine, but are based instead on a shared American experience and its accompanying values.

To understand the differences that exist in Protestantism and that are often reflected in the classroom, the faith can be divided into two broad categories—liberal and conservative. Liberal Protestants make up approximately 9 percent of the population (Roof & McKinney, 1985). They attempt to rethink Christianity in forms that are meaningful for a world dominated by science and rapid change. They stress the right of individuals to determine for themselves what is true in religion. They believe in the authority of Christian experience and religious life rather than dogmatic church pronouncements of the Bible. Many liberal Protestants reject the traditional emphasis on the supernatural events of Jesus' recorded life, and they stress human dignity. They are most likely to support and participate in social action programs because of their belief that what individuals become depends greatly on an environment over which they have little control. The mainline, traditional denominations are included in this group. The United Church of Christ (a merger of Congregational with Evangelical and Reformed churches) and Episcopalian churches are examples, although the degree of liberalism depends on the individual congregation. Methodists and Disciples of Christ represent more moderate denominations within this category. They make up approximately 24 percent of the population (Roof & McKinney, 1985).

In the 1970s and 1980s several Protestant churches identified as liberal or moderate experienced staggering membership losses. In the 1970–1980 period, the United Presbyterian church lost 19 percent of its members; Disciples, 17 percent; Episcopalians, 15 percent; United Church of Christ, 11 percent; and United Methodists, 9 percent. The declines were rather abrupt, affecting all groups at about the same time. The losses were more the result of decreasing numbers of new members rather than increasing dropout rates. Younger adults were conspicuously absent among new members, raising speculation about a lost generation in these churches. In the liberal churches, the average age is noticeably high. Forty-two percent of the Disciples of Christ, 41 percent of the United Methodists, and 43 percent of the United Church of Christ are fifty-five years of age or older. By comparison, none of the conservative Protestant groups has more than 40 percent of its membership over fifty-five years of age. Some (e.g., Assemblies of God) have less than a third over that age. It is apparent that in comparison to their conservative counterparts, liberal Protestant groups are less successful in attracting and holding onto young members (Roof & McKinney, 1985).

Conservative religious groups generally believe that the Bible is inerrant, that the supernatural is distinct from the natural, that salvation is essential, and that Jesus will return in bodily form during the Second Coming. They emphasize personal morality rather than social ethics (Woodward, Barnes & Lisle, 1977). The conservative branch can be divided further into the fundamentalists, who are literalistic and inflexible, and the evangelicals, who are somewhat less literalistic and not so inflexible. Billy Graham's ministry would fit more appropriately into the second category. Evangelicalism is somewhat described as "the religion you get when you 'get' religion" (Woodward et al., 1977).

Conservative churches include the Churches of Christ and Southern Baptists. Assembly of God, other Pentecostal groups, and Church of the Nazarene also represent fundamentalist denominations. Some sects of the more liberal denominations have reacted to liberalism and established themselves as conservative groups, such as Wesleyan Methodist and Orthodox Presbyterian. Conservative Protestants make up approximately 15 percent of the population (Roof & McKinney, 1985).

Although the fundamentalist groups strictly and literally interpret the Bible, the different groups do not necessarily interpret it or practice their faith in the same way. The various sects and denominations are unrelenting in their belief that they are the one *true* church. Some groups, such as the Pentecostals, believe that their lives have been dramatically changed by infusion of the Holy Spirit—a spiritual baptism that results in the individual being about to speak in other tongues (Marty, 1975). Although the Pentecostals historically have come and gone in storefront ghetto churches and rural areas across the country, the Pentecostal church has been adopted as a charismatic sect by branches of many of the mainstream churches during the last decade (Briggs, 1977).

Some fundamentalist groups, such as the Mormons and Jehovah's Witnesses, do not even classify themselves as Protestants, although they are classified as such by nonmembers. These two groups and the Seventh-Day Adventists stand out from many other groups because the practice of their religion thoroughly pervades their way of life. Members of these groups proselytize as a part of their commitment to their beliefs. The *Watchtower*, a publication, is distributed door-to-door by Jehovah's Witnesses, and Mormon missionaries often work door-to-door. Members are unrelenting in their beliefs and in their commitment to prepare themselves for future fulfillment in the establishment of a latter-day sainthood and a life in heaven (Mormons), or in life after the Armageddon (Jehovah's Witnesses), or in the millennium after Christ's Second Coming (Adventists). The conservative groups have in recent years experienced rapid growth, often exceeding population growth rates. By 1967, Southern Baptists were the largest Protestant denomination. By 1985, Southern Baptists had 36,898 churches and a membership well in excess of fourteen million (Jacquet, 1987). In addition to increased church membership, church school enrollments, missionary support, book publications, and the establishment of private Christian schools attested to the movement toward and growth of conservatism (Roof & McKinney, 1985).

An examination of the responses of various Protestants to some basic doctrinal questions from a University of California survey conducted in the 1970s will show how great church differences are. In response to a question that asked if it is "absolutely necessary to believe in Jesus to be saved," 97 percent of the Southern Baptists and 38 percent of the Congregationalists responded affirmatively. Thirty-two percent of the Episcopalians and 80 percent of the Missouri Synod Lutherans "believe every word of the Bible is literally true." Finally, 99 percent of the Southern Baptists said they "believe in a real live devil" compared to 22 percent of the Congregationalists ("Protestantism—World Religions," 1977).

These differences in beliefs among Protestants themselves have resulted in many court cases to determine what can or cannot be taught to or asked of students in the public schools. Fundamentalism versus liberalism came to the forefront in the 1925 Scopes Trial, in which a biology teacher was convicted for teaching Darwin's theory of evolution. Although the teacher's conviction was later reversed, the argument continues today as fundamentalists push for state legislation preventing the teaching of evolution or instituting the teaching of creationism. Jehovah's Witnesses have been taken to court because their children have refused to salute the flag. The Amish have fought in courts to remove their children from public schools after they have completed the eighth grade. Finally, some of these religious groups continue to fight against the 1963 Supreme Court decision that disallowed prayer in school.

Thus, Protestants represent a pluralistic group that includes over two hundred different sects and denominations. Their beliefs range from very liberal to very fundamentalist. Members of the traditional churches can be located along the continuum from very fundamentalist to very liberal, with many of the liberal churches having sects that are fundamentalist and sometimes charismatic. The educator is expected to respect students and their beliefs no matter where they fall along this continuum or how they differ from the educator's own beliefs.

Catholicism

In 1985, the Roman Catholic Church was the largest U.S. denomination, with over fifty-two million members (Jacquet, 1987). Approximately 27 percent of the U.S. population identified themselves as Catholic (Gallup Report, 1987). Unlike the Protestant faith, which includes denominational pluralism, the Catholic faith is one denomination under papal authority. In this country, the Catholic faith has developed from Catholicism practiced by many different ethnic groups in the "old" countries. Although the doctrine and pattern of worship are uniform among churches, the individual parishes differ according to the race, ethnic background, and social class of their members (Salisbury, 1964).

Generally, a larger percentage of Catholics than non-Catholics have always attended church. In 1988, for example, the attendance figure for Catholics was 48 percent, compared to 45 percent for Protestants and 20 percent for Jews (Gallup Report, 1989). The religion has not spread significantly beyond the ethnic boundaries of the Catholic immigrations during the past two centuries. Over the past three decades, Catholics have increased in numbers from 22 percent of the population to 27 percent. This has been accomplished primarily through a high birthrate and through immigration. In recent years, Catholics have made spectacular gains in education, occupational status, and income. In 1986, Catholics (16 percent) compared favorably to Protestants (17 percent) with respect to college graduates and exceeded Protestants in household income (Gallup Report, 1987).

The movement toward conservatism has not been limited to Protestants. Some Catholics have objected to changes in liturgy and other areas of modernization instituted by Vatican II.

By becoming a uniquely American church, members of the Catholic church have not rejected the belief that they belong to the one universal church. Instead, they have accepted the fact that American society is intrinsically pluralistic and that their religion is one of the three major faiths that exists side by side with Protestantism and Judaism.

Judaism

Judaism is one of the oldest religions known to humanity and provides the historical roots of both Catholicism and Protestantism. Among the three major faiths in this country, Judaism represents only about 2 percent of the population. It has become one of the three major faiths primarily as a result of Jews from many different countries amalgamating under the identification of Jewish American.

Jewish immigrants were among the early settlers in this country, arriving here in small numbers with the 1654 New Amsterdam settlers. Those first American Jews were largely Sephardic Jews (i.e., Spanish and Portuguese Jews), who were gradually joined by other Jews from central Europe and Poland. Their numbers were small. By 1825, there were only about five thousand American Jews living along the East Coast. They established synagogues and auxiliary institutions to maintain their religion. In other areas of American life, they were rapidly acculturated and soon found that they also had to adapt their religious institutions and patterns in a way that was uniquely American (Herberg, 1960).

The remainder of the nineteenth century, however, changed the ethnic composition of the American Jewish population. Between 1820 and 1870, their ranks increased from five thousand to over two hundred thousand as a result of the many Germans immigrating to the United States. In a pattern similar to Catholic immigrations, the German immigrants did not immediately fuse with the native Jews. In fact, they initially identified themselves primarily as Germans rather than Jews. With their Protestant counterparts, these German immigrants moved with the advancing frontier rather than remaining in the cities along the coast. When there were enough German Jews settled together, they established Jewish institutions and movements that coexisted with those of their German neighbors. By the last quarter of the century, the roots of Reform and Conservative Judaism had emerged from the adaptation of the religion to American ways. They followed closely the Protestant-American pattern of decentralization and voluntarism (Herberg, 1960).

The final major change in the composition of the Jewish population in this country occurred between 1870 and 1924. Those 5½ decades brought nearly 2.5 million eastern European Jews, who settled in a few large cities. In addition to representing many nationalities with different languages, these Yiddish-speaking immigrants were strangers to the native Jews as well as to other Americans. World events, especially the increased persecution of Jews abroad, soon helped to unite the ethnically separate Jews in this country. Ethnic differences subsided as religion became the most salient feature of their self-identification (Herberg, 1960).

"The emergence of the third generation changed the entire picture of American Jewry and Judaism in America" (Herberg, 1960, p. 186). Ethnic and religious identity merged. The life-style evolved into the microculture of the American middle class. Education, including higher education, played an important role in the Jewish community by advancing young people from the working class into white-collar and professional positions. Religious practices and patterns were modified in ways that made them characteristically American. "The central place of the sermon, congregational singing, mixed choirs, organs, responsive readings, abbreviated services, the concluding benediction, and many other commonly accepted features obviously reflected the influence of familiar Protestant practice" (Herberg, 1960, p. 191). The three denominations, or divisions, of Jewish thought and practice—Orthodox, Conservative, and Reform—continued to meet the needs of the Jewish population.

Compared to Protestants and Catholics, the Jewish population has declined, partly a result of intermarriage and low birthrates. Yet, as a group, they remain a distinctive, identifiable religious minority whose social standing and influence are disproportionate to their numbers.

Jews in this country and throughout the world have been the target of prejudice and discrimination, sometimes leading to attempted annihilation of the population. The Jewish Holocaust, which resulted in the brutal deaths of millions of European Jews, was systematically conducted by one of the most economically and technically advanced nations. The civilized world cannot complacently sit back and ignore the

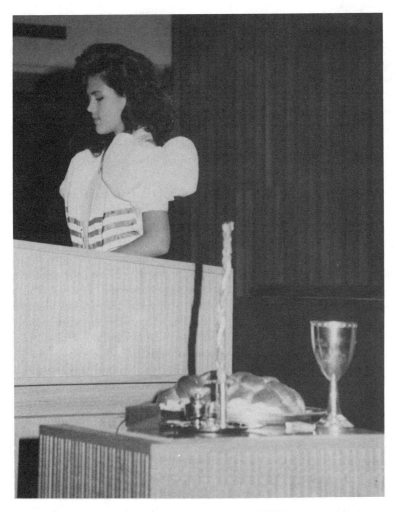

A thirteen-year-old Jewish female observes her Bat Mitzvah by reading from the Torah in Hebrew. The event marks her entry into religious adulthood.

fact that in spite of overwhelming evidence of what was being done by the Nazis, nothing was done to stop one of the greatest atrocities ever committed against humankind. As we approach the twenty-first century, other attempts at genocide persist. It is the responsibility of educators to help their students understand that even today, other holocausts are taking place.

Anti-Semitism is rooted in Jewish-Gentile conflicts that have existed for centuries. Discrimination has occurred in both occupational and social life. Jews have often been denied high-level corporate management positions and have been barred from membership in social clubs. There is evidence "that overall, religious people tend to be more anti-Semitic than nonreligious people" (Wilson, 1978, p. 316). The form and degree of anti-Semitism vary with world and national events; when non-Jews believe that events are the result of Jewish action, prejudices resurface in work and deed. Current events in the Middle East that involve Israel often initiate these reactions.

The conservative movement has involved American Judaism as well. Orthodox Judaism has seen a resurgence, growing more rapidly than either Reformed or Conservative groups in the 1970s. Growing numbers of Jews have turned to the more traditional faith, rejecting what some consider lax observance and permissiveness among the non-Orthodox groups. This is an apparent reversal from the earlier movement away from Orthodoxy toward the more liberal groups (Roof & McKinney, 1985).

About 75 percent of the nation's Jews live in five metropolitan communities (Herberg, 1960), and one-third live in New York City (Marty, 1979). Although Jews strongly identify with their religion, the Jewish practice of religion is relatively low regarding synagogue attendance and home religious observance (Carroll, 1979). Nevertheless, the American synagogue is the strongest agency in the Jewish community. Although they may not attend services as regularly (20 percent) as their Catholic and Protestant counterparts, a large percentage (44 percent) of Jews retain affiliation with the synagogue (Gallup Report, 1987). Many feel that Jewish identity does not require attendance at the synagogue; attending religious services and studying Jewish texts hold little interest for much of the Jewish population (Sklare, 1974). Attendance on High Holidays, however, is always at a maximum. The synagogue in America serves not only as a place of religious worship, but also as a primary base for Jewish identity and survival (Carroll, 1979).

Judaism, like the other two major faiths, has become an integral part of American society. "The American Jew . . . establishes his Jewishness not apart from, not in spite of, his Americanness, but precisely through and by virtue of it" (Herberg, 1960, p. 198). American Judaism emphasizes Jewishness as peoplehood and nationality more than as religion.

Other Religions

In addition to the three major faiths in this country, 4 percent of the population in 1986 indicated that they preferred another religion, and 8 percent responded "none" when asked about a religious preference (Gallup Report, 1987). What are the other religions that an educator might encounter in a community? They range from Christian religions that do not fall into the discrete categories of Protestantism or Catholicism to Islam, Eastern religions, and religions based on current psychological thinking.

One of the Christian religions that does not fall into the two major groupings is the Eastern Orthodox church. With four million members in the United States, Eastern Orthodoxy probably claims about one-fourth of all Christians worldwide. One of the reasons that the Eastern Orthodox church is less known in this country may be that its members, from Syria, Greece, Armenia, Russia, and the Ukraine, only immigrated during the last century. Although they split with the Roman Catholic church in 1054 over theological, practical, jurisdictional, cultural, and political differences, to many outsiders they appear very similar to the pre–Vatican II Catholic church. As the name suggests, Eastern Orthodoxy is steeped in tradition, as is apparent in its Divine Liturgy—a highly formal service of worship (Marty, 1975).

At least two other religions have a Christian heritage but seem to fall through the cracks of discrete categorization because of their beliefs. The Christian Scientists are one of these groups, with probably less than half a million members. Like some of the fundamentalist Protestant groups and others described in this section, their beliefs are so different from conventional religious beliefs that they attract public attention. They exist "to dispel illusion and bring people into harmony with mind, with God as All—away from what others call disease, sin, evil, matter, and death" (Marty, 1975, p. 205). Although they do not proselytize, they maintain reading rooms in business and shopping centers of many communities. *The Christian Science Monitor* is a highly respected general newspaper.

The second group that defies categorization is the Unitarian Universalists—a church that connotes liberalism to most people. Their membership has included several U.S. presidents (William Howard Taft, Thomas Jefferson, John Adams, and John Quincy Adams) and several New England writers (Henry Wadsworth Longfellow, James Russell Lowell, and William Cullen Bryant), helping to make the church an influence beyond that expected of a relatively small group. Unitarians are often found in suburbs, small towns, and college communities; many of the members could be described as political liberals. While many members have the highest respect for Jesus Christ, the church is "most open to the wisdom of non-Christian religions and may draw many of its readings from scriptures of Buddhism, Hinduism and religious philosophies" (Marty, 1975, p. 217). An expression of this openness, Unitarianism houses both Christian and non-Christian wings. The denomination follows no imposing standards of dogma or membership. Thus, their worship services appear extremely simple and are often experimental (Marty, 1975).

Islam now has more than two million followers in the United States. Some are immigrants from every area of the world, including the Mideast and Africa, or the children of these immigrants (Jacquet, 1987). This religion, however, is not solely an immigrant religion. As early as the 1930s, black Americans in Detroit were establishing the Nation of Islam (better known as the Black Muslims) as an alternative expression of black religion for blacks who populated the city's ghettos. Mosques now exist in cities across the country, and members are drawn from various religious and class lines. The religion addresses cultural identity, the acceptability and respectability of blackness, and economic self-help (Haddad, Haines & Findley, 1984). The past emphasis on racial awareness, the fight against white oppression, and hostility toward whites placed the church in a leadership role of the black power movement during the 1960s. Many have been drawn by the simple egalitarian teachings of Islam, which provides for self-identity and a clear purpose in life (Jacquet, 1987). The religion stresses self-determination for blacks, and members have been able to develop a successful economic program in the tradition of American capitalism. Until recently, membership had been limited to nonwhites.

Conversion to Islam usually requires a change in one's self-identity, and membership demands a high level of commitment (Haddad et al., 1984). "The individual

Muslims themselves are their own best currency of proselytism; they are clean, confident, prosperous, and respected" (Lincoln, 1974, p. 168). The strict dietary habits and other rules of living sometimes come into conflict with the public schools. Educators should be aware of the importance of such rules to believers in the Islamic religion.

The recent influx of Indochinese, Chinese, Koreans, and other groups has increased the religious pluralism in this country. These groups have brought with them, in addition to their religions, other aspects of their culture. The Laotians and Cambodians are primarily Buddhists, as are the Vietnamese. Some of the Vietnamese, however, are Taoists and Roman Catholics, and some, like the majority of the Korean immigrants, adhere to the teachings of Confucianism, which is more a philosophy than a religion. Most Koreans are likely to be Buddhists. However, a large minority are Protestants, and a smaller but still significant group are Roman Catholics. The majority of Hong Kong immigrants are Buddhists, with some Taoists. Many of these immigrants are also likely to adhere to the teachings of Confucius. Many of the recent immigrants from India and Pakistan have brought their Hindu and Moslem beliefs with them. The increasing religious diversity in this country is evident in the 1988 completion of the largest Buddhist temple/monastery in the Western Hemisphere, located in Hacienda Heights, a Los Angeles suburb.

Young people in many communities practice religions based on an Eastern religious tradition. This grouping includes the Hare Krishna, the Divine Light Mission, and the Unification Church. Members of some of these groups are very visible to the public. The Hare Krishna can be seen dancing with tambourines on sidewalks in larger cities, and members of the Unification Church may approach travelers in airports for donations. "The basic intent of each group is to help the individual become a part of a group seeking meaning and purpose for life" (Johnson, 1979, p. 99). Members of these religious movements are often well educated, young, and from different backgrounds. Many were involved with protest movements in the 1960s and sought a new religious consciousness. "In nearly all cases the life being shaped is disciplined, committed to the group, and devoted to discovering a dynamic inner self. The groups also demand that some expression of the religious feelings be demonstrated or shared with society at large" (Johnson, 1979, p. 99).

These various religions are practiced by a small minority of the population, but their presence in a community is often exaggerated beyond that warranted by their numbers. This notoriety often stems from the fact that their doctrine and practices are viewed as heretical by members of the major faiths, yet orthodox by the believers. In addition, members of the majority faiths, especially parents, fear the attraction of some of these groups because young people may desert the majority ranks.

INDIVIDUAL RELIGIOUS IDENTITY

Most Americans are born into their religion and baptized in the church of their parents, later joining that same church. Within the context of the religious freedom espoused in this country, however, individuals are always free to change their religion or to choose no religion. The greatest pressure to retain membership in the religious group in which one was born usually comes from the family and other members of that same religious group. Often it is more difficult for individuals to break away from their religious origins than to make breaks from any of the other microcultures of which they are members. Parents whose children have joined groups such as Hare Krishna or the Unification Church sometimes feel that their children (usually young adults) have been brainwashed by members of these religious cults, and some of these parents pay experts to remove their children from these religious groups and "deprogram" them. Families have been known to disown their children who marry outside of the faith. Thus, individual freedom of choice may be extremely limited by religious group membership.

Herberg's (1960) study of the three major faiths suggests that Americans are more likely to identify themselves by their membership in a religious microculture than by membership in any other subculture:

> To find a place in American society increasingly means to place oneself in one or another of these religious communities. And although this process of self-identification and social location is not in itself intrinsically religious, the mere fact that in order to be "something" one must be a Protestant, a Catholic, or a Jew means that one begins to think of oneself as religiously identified and affiliated. (p. 56)

When one's ethnic identity is very important to an individual, it is often combined with a religious identification. Irish Catholic, Russian Jew, and Norwegian Lutheran are examples of dual identification, and understanding the individual's relationship to both microcultures is important in understanding who the individual is.

The region of the United States in which one lives also affects the strength of identification with a specific religious group. In much of Georgia, many people will have the same or similar views; religious diversity is limited. On the other hand, religious diversity in New York is common. "At a party one is careful not to be critical of other religious groups, because the other partner to a conversation may be a member of one, an alumnus of another, and married to a member of a third" (Marty, 1979, p. 88). In many areas of the country, any deviation from the common religious beliefs and practices is considered heretical, making it very difficult for the nonadherent to be accepted by most members of the community. In other areas, the traditionally religious individual may not be accepted as a part of a community that is religiously liberal. Educators, as well as students, are usually expected to believe and behave according to the mores of the community—mores that are often determined by the prevailing religious doctrine and the degree of religious diversity.

Most communities have some degree of religious diversity, although the degree of difference may vary greatly, depending on the community. Often, students whose beliefs are different from those of the majority in the community are ostracized in school and social settings. Jews, atheists, Jehovah's Witnesses, and Pentecostals are among those groups whose members are sometimes shunned, suffering discrimination for their beliefs. Educators must be careful that their own religious beliefs and memberships do not interfere with their ability to provide equal educational opportunity to all students, regardless of their religious identification.

Religion Switching

Changing from one religious faith to another has been a common practice in this country. One-third of all Americans do not belong to the religious group to which they were born. Forty percent of Protestants today have changed religious affiliation at some time in their life (Roof & McKinney, 1985).

Switching from conservative to liberal Protestant churches has often accompanied upward mobility. Theologically liberal and higher-status churches have been in keeping with advances in education and occupation. Thus, the liberal churches have typically benefited from upward mobility, and Episcopalian, Presbyterian, and Congregationalist churches gained memberships at the expense of the moderate and conservative denominations. Today, however, this type of movement is seen to a lesser extent (Roof & McKinney, 1985).

Those shifting to the liberal churches have tended to be older, more educated, holding higher-status occupations, and, as might be expected, more liberal on moral issues. As a group, they tend to be less active in their new churches than the members of the conservative churches they have left (Roof & McKinney, 1985).

A second group of individuals involved in changing churches includes those who have switched to more conservative churches. As a group, they tend to be young and of lower socioeconomic status. While liberal churches have tended to have larger net gains, the conservatives have been able to attract or maintain members who are generally more loyal and active. The losers in the switching behavior of American churchgoers have been the larger, moderate denominations, such as the Methodists and Lutherans (Roof & McKinney, 1985).

A third group is switching to nonaffiliation. For every person who is raised with no religious affiliation and who later becomes involved in organized religion, over three people leave churches and become nonaffiliated with religious bodies. While all religious groups lose to nonaffiliation, moderate groups within the three major religious bodies are the major losers. The individuals involved in switching to nonaffiliation are predominantly males who are well educated (Roof & McKinney, 1985). The movement to nonaffiliation or unchurched, as it is sometimes designated, may be due in part to increasing social acceptance of nonparticipation in organized religion. Whereas those who did not belong to or did not attend church may have at one time been considered immoral or amoral, society appears to be increasingly more accepting, or at least tolerant, of the individual's right to determine the degree, if any, of religious participation. (It might be noted here that there was a time when some school districts required church attendance of their teachers.)

In some respects, the religious institutions (even those with a net loss) may gain from this switching behavior. Choices relating to churches or religious bodies become based more on genuine preference. Consequently, religious groups may tend to become more homogeneous, with clearer social and religious identities.

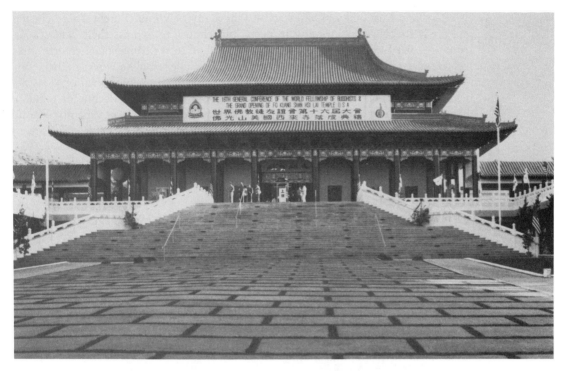

The Fo Kuang Shan Hsi Lai Temple opened in Hacienda Heights, California, in 1988. This Los Angeles County temple is the largest Buddhist temple in North America.

DECLINING MEMBERSHIPS

While church attendance has remained fairly constant, all three of the major religious communities have experienced membership declines in recent years. In 1974, 76 percent of adults in the United States identified themselves as church or synagogue members. By 1978, the figure had dropped to 68 percent, and by 1988, it had dropped to a low of 65 percent (Gallup Report, 1989; Roof & McKinney, 1985). Approximately 80 percent of Catholics and 73 percent of Protestants are church members, and 45 percent of Jews are members of a synagogue. In reality, many who say they are church members are effectively unchurched because of their lack of attendance or involvement. Using a more rigorous criteria, a major study in 1978 identified 41 percent of the adult population as unchurched because of lack of involvement in religious institutions. That same year, the Gallup poll found that 68 percent claimed church membership, a 9 percent discrepancy with the previously cited study (Gallup Report, 1989; Roof & McKinney, 1985). It is likely that if the more stringent criteria were applied today, a little over half of the adult population would qualify as active church members.

Roof and McKinney (1985) suggest that many of the unchurched are believers and are quite religious in many respects, but choose to express their beliefs apart from organized institutions. As a group, they tend to welcome social change, hold less to conservative values, and are less rooted in stable social networks in their communities (Roof & McKinney, 1985). About 35 percent of the population does not belong to a church or synagogue (Gallup Report, 1989). The decline of religious membership in recent years about equals the increase of those indicating no religious affiliation. This decrease in members may suggest a growing secular constituency that may be more irreligious than antireligious and which Roof and McKinney (1985) suggest is a force of growing cultural importance in a pluralistic society.

EDUCATIONAL IMPLICATIONS

Religious groups place different emphases on the need for education and have different expectations of what children should be taught. The Amish usually want to remove their children from formal schooling after they complete the eighth grade. The Hutterites do not want their children to attend school with non-Hutterite students, although the teacher is usually not a member of the religious community. Catholics, Lutherans, Episcopalians, Hutterites, and Seventh-Day Adventists have established their own schools to provide both a common education (i.e., the general, nonreligious skills and knowledge) and a religious education.

Public schools should be free of religious doctrine and perspective, but many people believe that schools without such a perspective do not provide a desirable value orientation for students. There is a constant debate about the public school's responsibility in fostering student morality and social responsibility. A major point of disagreement focuses on who should determine the morals that will provide the context of the education program in a school. Because religious diversity is so great in this country, that task is nearly impossible. Therefore, most public schools incorporate commonly accepted American values that transcend most religions. In response, some students are sent to schools operated by a religious body; other students attend religion classes after school or on Saturdays; and many students receive their religious training at Sunday school.

Although the U.S. Constitution requires the separation of state and religion, this does not signify that public schools and religion have always been completely separated. Until the 1962 and 1963 Supreme Court decisions determined that these practices were unconstitutional, some schools included religious worship and prayer in their daily educational practices. Although schools should be secular, they are influenced greatly by the predominant values of the community. Whether evolution, sex education, and values clarification are part of instruction in a school is determined in great part by the religious beliefs of a community. Educators must be cognizant of this influence before introducing certain readings and ideas that stray far from what the community is willing to accept within their belief and value structure.

Influence of the Religious Right

By the late 1970s, the ideologies of a conservative and increasingly influential group referred to as the Religious Right were clashing head-on with the ideologies of secular humanism. The battle was waged on two fronts: the family and the school. Controversies centered on the family and gender roles and issues such as abortion, the Equal Rights Amendment, and gay rights. The conservatives supported a return to traditional roles for men and women and opposed equal protection for women and homosexuals, such as the hiring of homosexuals as public school educators (Roof & McKinney, 1985).

The New Christian Right, referred to at times as evangelicals, became a potent force in the 1970s and 1980s partly because of the effective television ministries (dubbed the electronic church) of individuals such as Jerry Falwell, Pat Robertson, Jim Bakker, and Jimmy Swaggert. With their ability to reach millions in their own homes, these religious leaders have encouraged political involvement and have mounted efforts on issues such as school prayer, abortion, pornography, and national defense. The Religious Right has provided strong support or opposition for political candidates based on their voting records or position on issues (Roof & McKinney, 1985). In 1980 and 1984, they were a strong factor in the election of Ronald Reagan. In 1988, they supported Pat Robertson's candidacy and then supported Bush over the Democratic candidate they branded as a liberal.

Their efforts have altered the course of American history and will impact on the judicial systems in this country for decades. Ronald Reagan succeeded in appointing conservative justices to the Supreme Court. In 1990, the remaining liberal justices are of advanced age and one or more are likely to be replaced by more a conservative appointment by a conservative President elected in part by conservative constituents.

They have put pressure on the American educational system to return the schools to what they once were, to once again include the study of creation according to the Book of Genesis in addition to the previously mentioned school prayer. They have allied themselves with political conservatives, and together they work diligently to impose their convictions and values onto the schools. Today's educators cannot ignore the influence of these groups, which in some communities is very powerful.

Nationally, our adherence to the principle of separation of church and state has obviously been schizophrenic at best. Oaths are typically made on Bibles and often end with the phrase, "so help me God." Our coins and currency state, "In God we trust." We have military chaplains and congressional chaplains, and we hold congressional prayer breakfasts. This has been interpreted by some to mean that the separation of church and state simply means that there will be no state church (Welch, Medeiros, & Tate, 1981).

Complete separation of church and state, as defined by strict constitutionalists, would have a profound effect on our socioreligious life. It is likely that the American public wants some degree of separation of these two institutions, but it is equally likely that it would be outraged if total separation were imposed. Total separation would mean no direct or indirect aid to religious groups, no tax-free status, no tax deductions for contributions to religious groups, no national Christmas tree, no government-paid chaplains, no religious holidays, no blue laws, and so on. The list of religious activities, rights, and privileges that could be eliminated seems almost endless (Klein, 1983).

Among the controversial issues that surround the efforts of the New Right and fundamentalist religious groups are school prayer, tuition tax credits, and censorship.

School Prayer

In spite of the 1962 and 1963 Supreme Court decisions regarding school prayer, the conservative groups have persisted in their efforts to revive school prayer in the schools. The present law is in essence a voluntary prayer law. The law in no way precludes private prayer in school. The Supreme Court decisions do not prevent teachers or students from praying privately in school. Any teacher or student can offer his or her own private prayer of thanks before the noon meal or meditate or pray between classes and before and after school. Public group prayer is forbidden by law. Advocates of school prayer sometimes advance their efforts under the term "voluntary" prayer. The interpretation of what constitutes voluntary school prayer has become one of the main issues in the prayer controversy. Some of the proponents of school prayer advocate mandated school prayer, with individuals voluntarily choosing to participate or not participate. It is likely that if such laws were ever enacted, there would be considerable social pressure to participate that would be particularly difficult for younger children to resist (Welch et al., 1981).

Tuition Tax Credits

Tuition tax credits have been a major controversy within education. Proponents of tuition tax credits support income tax credits for parents who enroll their children in private schools. Many of those who support these tax credits believe that since the children in private schools reduce the number of students in public education and thereby reduce public education costs, their parents are entitled to some tax relief. Proponents further support the tax credits as a matter of social equity, encouraging greater pluralism, diversity, and competition in the American education system. The decision to send children to private schools is usually precipitated by parental desires to provide an education coupled with a religious environment, to provide an education superior to that available in the public schools, or, in some cases, to segregate their children from other children in the public schools.

Opponents to tuition tax credits see such legislation as a weakening of the public education system and an encouragement for some parents to abandon public education for their children for the exclusiveness of the private education sector. It was attacked by two U.S. senators as "segregation sanctioning—rip-off for the rich, creating a dual system of education: public schools for the poor, the handicapped and disadvantaged and private schools for the rest" ("Senate Scuttles," 1984, p. 13).

In 1983, the Supreme Court, in *Mueller v. Allen*, upheld Minnesota's allowance of income tax deductions for the cost of tuition and related education expenses. The

Minnesota law provides for income tax deductions regardless of whether a child attends public or private school—parochial or secular. Minnesota was able to convince the Court that the purpose of the law was to ensure a well-educated citizenry and to relieve the burden on public schools. The Court applied a three-part test that it often used to determine the unconstitutional establishment of religion. The Court determined that (1) the purpose of the tax law was not to aid religion; (2) the law did not have the primary effect of aiding religion; (3) the law did not promote excessive entanglement between church and state (Lines, 1983). With the Mueller decision, it is highly likely that other groups will attempt to emulate Minnesota's success through both federal and state tax laws.

Censorship

The discussion of censorship is included in this section because the censorship movement tends to be heavily influenced by many individuals from fundamentalist and conservative religious groups. Censorship of textbooks, library books, and other learning materials in education has become another major battleground in education for the New Right and other fundamentalist groups. Jenkinson (1979) estimates that there are no less than two hundred groups involved in public school censorship.

The impact of censorship in the public schools cannot be underestimated. It is a serious matter. Censorship, or attempts at censorship, have resulted in violence, where involved parties have been beaten and even shot. It has resulted in the dismissal or resignation of administrators and teachers. It has split communities and in the past thirty years has created nearly as much controversy as the desegregation of schools. Few can doubt the sincerity of censors and their proponents. Most, if not all, are absolutely certain that the cause they support is just and morally right and that for the sake of all, they are obligated to continue their fight.

At the other end of the continuum, opponents to the censors also tend to share a conviction that they are the ones that are in the right and that censors infringe on academic freedom, seeking to destroy meaningful education. Opponents to the censors feel that their antagonists thrive on hard times, when schools come under fire because of declining Scholastic Aptitude Test (SAT) scores, rising illiteracy rates, escalating costs of education, and increasing concern about violence and vandalism in the schools (Jenkinson, 1979). Other factors that prompt the activities of censors are the removal of school prayer, teaching methods that are branded as secular humanism, and programs such as values clarification, drug education, and sex education. Books written specifically for teenagers about subjects that are objectionable to some parents and in language others consider too realistic are often a source of concern. The emergence of African-American literature, sometimes written in the black vernacular, is sometimes the source of irritation or concern (Jenkinson, 1979).

Targets for the censors are those books and materials that are identified as disrespectful of authority and religion, destructive of social and cultural values, obscene, pornographic, unpatriotic, or in violation of individual and familial rights of privacy. Books written by homosexuals are frequently attacked.

Among the materials attacked by censors are materials that are considered non-racist or nonsexist. Magazines such as *Time, Newsweek,* and *U.S. News and World Report* are sometimes attacked because they publish stories about war, crime, death, violence, and sex. In a conservative community, a teacher can anticipate a negative reaction to the teaching of evolution without presenting the views on creationism.

In 1977, a survey of a selected number of secondary school teachers was conducted by the National Council of Teachers of English. One aspect of the survey requested the titles of books that were the focus of objections by would-be censors. A total of 145 titles were reported. Here is a list of the ten books receiving the most complaints, with *The Catcher in the Rye* receiving more than twice as many complaints as the two Steinbeck books tied for second place. The number of objections or complaints is listed in parentheses (Burgess, 1979).

1. *The Catcher in the Rye* (25)
2. *Of Mice and Men* (12)
3. *The Grapes of Wrath* (12)
4. *Go Ask Alice* (10)
5. *One Flew Over the Cuckoo's Nest* (8)
6. *Lord of the Flies* (7)
7. *My Darling, My Hamburger* (6)
8. *One Day in the Life of Ivan Denisovich* (6)
9. *Flowers for Algernon* (5)
10. *Love Story* (5)

In addition, certain dictionaries with words and definitions described as offensive have been forced off adoption lists. Curricula such as MACOS (Man—A Course of Study), a social studies course published by the National Science Foundation, a federal agency, have felt the full force of the censors' attack. The censors attacked the curriculum as containing topics such as wife swapping and cannibalism. Its defenders accused the censors of fostering misunderstanding by taking materials out of context. The battles over censorship continue, with both sides certain that they are right.

One can understand the concern of parents who are often influenced by censors. They believe that unless they choose sides and act, their children will be taught with materials that are anti-God, antifamily, anti-authority, anticountry, antimorality, and anti–law and order.

The failure to communicate effectively with parents has been cited as a major contributing source of alienation between educators and parents (Jenkinson, 1979; Kamhi, 1981). Failure to communicate the objectives of new curricula and to explain how these programs enrich the educational experience may cause suspicion and distrust. Many administrators and librarians indicate that communication with parents is more crisis oriented than continuous. Information about programs, policies, and procedures tends to be offered in response to inquiries or challenges rather than as part of an ongoing public relations effort.

A small Ohio community faced with parental challenges and rumors about a "dirty" book assigned to their children set up an evening course for parents entitled, "Books Our Children Read." In the class, parents read and discussed the book in question and others like it. As a result, the teachers learned something from the parents, and the parents, in turn, learned to respect and trust the teachers (Berkley, 1979).

Secular humanism has been one of the direct targets of the censors, particularly those affiliated with fundamentalist religious groups. The emphasis in secular humanism is a respect for human beings, rather than a belief in the supernatural. Its objectives include the full development of every human being, the universal use of the scientific method, affirmation of the dignity of humans, personal freedom combined with social responsibility, and fulfillment through the development of ethical and creative living (Welch et al., 1981).

The groups opposed to secular humanism cite two Supreme Court cases as evidence that secular humanism is a religion: *Torcaso v. Watkins* and *United States v. Seeger*. These cases were not heard by the Court to determine whether or not secular humanism is a religion. Nevertheless, the wording in the Court findings have been frequently used to support the postion that the Supreme Court recognizes secular humanism as a religion (Jenkinson, 1979).

However, secular humanism is not an organized religion like Roman Catholicism, Protestantism, and Judaism. It does not have rituals, a church, or professed doctrines. Its existence is in the minds of individuals who align themselves with these perspectives. The specific beliefs and manifestations of beliefs vary from one believer to another.

Teachers new to the profession or new to a community should never underestimate the determination of those involved in the censorship movement. Teachers would be well advised to make certain that they are fully aware of the climate within the community before introducing new, innovative, or controversial materials, teaching strategies, and books. Experienced colleagues and supervisors can usually serve as barometers as to how students, parents, and the community will react to the new materials or teaching techniques. With this type of information, the new teacher can proceed with a more realistic anticipation of the reception that can be expected.

Classroom Implications

Although religion and public schooling are to remain separate, religion can be taught in schools as a legitimate discipline for objective study. A comparative religion course is part of the curriculum offered in many secondary schools. In this approach, the students are not forced to practice a religion as part of their educational program. They can, however, study one or more religions.

As part of the curriculum, students should learn that the United States (and indeed the world) is rich in religious diversity. Educators portray their respect for religious differences by their interactions with students from different religious backgrounds. Understanding the importance of religion to many students and their families is an advantage in developing effective teaching strategies for individual students. Instructional activities can build on students' religious experiences to help them learn concepts. This technique helps students recognize that their religious identity is valued in the classroom and encourages them to respect the religious diversity that exists.

At the same time, educators should avoid stereotyping all students from one denomination or church. There is diversity within every religious group and domination. In each group, there is likely to be differences in attitudes and beliefs. For example, Southern Baptists may appear to be conservative to outsiders. However, among Southern Baptists, some would be considered part of a liberal or moderate group, whereas others may be identified as conservative. Some Southern Baptist churches may hold services so formal in nature that they might even be described as resembling an Episcopalian service.

It is the responsibility of educators to be aware of the religious diversity and the influence of religion in the community in which they work. They must also understand the influence of religion on the school's curriculum and climate in order to teach effectively. Finally, educators must periodically reexamine their own interactions with students to ensure that they are not discriminating against students because of differences in religious beliefs. It is imperative that educators recognize the influence of membership in a religious microculture in order to help students develop their potential.

SUMMARY

One's religion has considerable impact on how one functions on a day-to-day basis. Education may be greatly influenced by religious groups. Some private schools are established on religious principles, and in those schools, religion is an integral part of the curriculum. Even in public schools, attempts by religious groups are made regularly to influence the system. The degree of religious influence in the schools varies from one community to another. Educators should not underestimate the influence and strategies of conservative religious groups and would be well advised to know their community before introducing controversial materials.

QUESTIONS FOR REVIEW

1. Discuss how the religious atmosphere of a community can influence curriculum and instructional methodology.

2. To what extent does religion influence American life with respect to its importance to the individual and church or synagogue attendance?

3. What is the relationship of religion to public office?

4. What are the present trends with respect to membership in conservative, moderate, and liberal religious groups? What are the implications of these trends for the political and legal directions of the country?

5. What do present laws permit with respect to school prayer? How does the Religious Right want to change these laws?

6. Discuss censorship in the schools, including the targets of the censors.

7. How have Protestantism, Catholicism, and Judaism influenced American culture?

REFERENCES

Appel, W. (1983). *Cults in America: Programmed for paradise*. New York: Holt, Rinehart & Winston.

Bellah, R. N. (1974). Civil religion in America. In P. H. McNamara (Ed.), *Religion American style*. New York: Harper & Row.

Berkley, J. (1979). Teach the parents well: An anti-censorship experiment in adult education. In J. E. Davis (Ed.), *Dealing with censorship*. Urbana, IL: National Council of Teachers of English.

Briggs, K. A. (1977). Charismatic Christians. In H. L. Marx, Jr. (Ed.), *Religions in America*. New York: Wilson.

Burgess, L. (1979). A brief report of the 1977 NCTE censorship survey. In J. E. Davis (Ed.), *Dealing with censorship*. Urbana, IL: National Council of Teachers of English.

Carroll, J. W. (1979). Continuity and change: The shape of religious life in the United States—1950 to the present. In J. W. Carroll, D. W. Johnson, & M. E. Marty (Eds.), *Religion in America: 1950 to the present*. New York: Harper & Row.

Durkheim, E. (1969). The social foundations of religion. In R. Robertson (Ed.), *Sociology of religion*. Baltimore: Penguin Books.

Gallup Poll. (1984). *Religion in America*. Princeton, NJ: Gallup International.

Gallup Report. (1985). *Religion in America, 236*, 27.

Gallup Report. (1987, April). *Religion in America, 259*.

Gallup Report. (1989, September). *Religion in America*,

Greeley, A. M. (1982). *Religion: A secular theory*. New York: Free Press.

Haddad, Y. Y., Haines, B., & Findley, E. (1984). *The Islamic impact*. Syracuse, NY: Syracuse University Press.

Herberg, W. (1960). *Protestant—Catholic—Jew: An essay in American religious sociology*. New York: Anchor Press.

Jacquet, C. H., Jr. (Ed.). (1987). *Yearbook of American and Canadian churches, 1987*. Nashville: Abingdon Press.

Jenkinson, E. B. (1979). *Censors in the classroom*. Carbondale, IL: Southern Illinois University Press.

Johnson, D. W. (1979). Trends and issues shaping the religious future. In J. W. Carroll, D. W. Johnson, & M. E. Marty (Eds.), *Religion in America: 1950 to the present*. New York: Harper & Row.

Kamhi, M. M. (1981, December). Censorship vs. selection: Choosing the books our children shall read. *Educational Leadership, 211–213.*

Klein, J. P. (1983). Separation of church and state: The endless struggle. *Contemporary Education, 54*(3), 166–170.

Lincoln, C. E. (1974). *The Black church since Frazier.* New York: Schocken Books.

Lines, P. M. (1983, August 24). Impact of Mueller: New options for policymakers. *Education Week.*

Marty, M. E. (1979). Interpreting American pluralism: In J. W. Carroll, D. W. Johnson, & M. E. Marty (Eds.), *Religion in America: 1950 to the present.* New York: Harper & Row.

Marty, M. E. (Ed.). (1975). *Our faiths.* Royal Oak, MI: Cathedral Publications.

Mueller, S. A. (1974). The new triple melting pot: Herbert revisited. In P. H. McNamara (Ed.), *Religion American style.* New York: Harper & Row.

Protestantism—world religions. Pt. 6. (1977, April 7). *Senior Scholastic, 109,* 22–24.

Raschke, C. A., Kirk, J. A., & Taylor, M. C. (1977). *Religion and the human image.* Englewood Cliffs, NJ: Prentice-Hall.

Roof, W. C., & McKinney, W. (1985, July). Denominational America and the new religious pluralism. *Annals of the American Academy of Political and Social Science, 480,* 24–38.

Salisbury, W. S. (1964). *Religion in American culture: A sociological interpretation.* Homewood, IL: Dorsey.

Senate Scuttles. (1984). *Religion and Public Education, 11*(1), 13.

Sklare, M. (1974). The American synagogue. In P. H. McNamara (Ed.), *Religion American style.* New York: Harper & Row.

Stark, R., & Glock, C. Y. (1969). Dimensions of religious commitment. In R. Robertson (Ed.), *Sociology of religion.* Baltimore: Penguin Books.

Stark, R., & Glock, C. Y. (1974). Prejudice and the churches. In P. H. McNamara (Ed.), *Religion American style.* New York: Harper & Row.

Welch, D., Medeiros, D. C., & Tate, G. A. (1981, December). Education and the New Right. *Educational Leadership, 203–207.*

Wilson, J. (1978). *Religion in American society: The effective presence.* Englewood Cliffs, NJ: Prentice-Hall.

Woodward, K. L., Barnes, J., & Lisle, L. (1977). Born again! In H. L. Marx, Jr. (Ed.), *Religions in America.* New York: Wilson.

Yinger, J. M. (1970). *The scientific study of religion.* New York: Macmillan.

SUGGESTED READINGS

Anderson, C. H. (1970). *White Protestant Americans: From national origins to religious group.* Englewood Cliffs, NJ: Prentice-Hall.

> *A description of white Protestants in the United States. Includes a historical overview of white Protestant immigrations.*

Frazier, E. F. (1974). *The Negro church in America;* and Lincoln, C. E. (1974). *The black church since Frazier.* New York: Schocken Books.

> *Two essays on the historical and contemporary development of black churches in the United States.*

Herberg, W. (1960). *Protestant—Catholic—Jew: An essay in American religious sociology.* New York: Anchor Press.

> *A sociological study of the three major faiths in the United States. Describes Americans as "melting" into one of those three groups rather than a one-model American. Includes a brief history of each group. Considered a classic by some.*

Jenkinson, E. B. (1979). *Censors in the classroom.* Carbondale, IL: Southern Illinois University Press.

> *An examination of censorship in the public schools. Describes some of the major censorship battles that have taken place in this country, who some of the censors are, and the targets of censors.*

Marty, M. E. (Ed.). (1975). *Our faiths.* Royal Oak, MI: Cathedral Publications.

> *A description of the historical and contemporary experiences and beliefs of eight major Christian churches and nine additional groups outside of the mainstream.*

McNamara, P. H. (Ed.). (1974). *Religion American style.* New York: Harper & Row.

> *An anthology of readings on the relationship of religion and society.*

Podell, J. (Ed.) (1987). *Religion in American Life.* New York: Wilson.

> *Contains a number of interesting and provocative articles and essays regarding religion in the United States. Includes Roof and McKinney's excellent article related to religious pluralism in the country.*

Wilson, J. (1978). *Religion in American society: The effective presence.* Englewood Cliffs, NJ: Prentice-Hall.

> *Comprehensive coverage of recent literature in the sociology of religion. Describes the essence and growth of religion, religion and social integration, religious diversity and social conflict, and secularization.*

CHAPTER 7
Language

Some students come to school barely speaking English, some are bilingual, some speak a nonstandard dialect, and some use sign language. As the scene changes from school to school, the languages and dialects spoken also change. The scene, however, is indicative of the multilingual nature of the United States as a result of our multicultural heritage.

Students exhibit cultural similarities and differences related to language as well as to sex, class, ethnicity, religion, exceptionalities, and age. Because they speak one or more languages, as well as dialects of these languages, they are a part of another microcultural group. Of course, not all African-American children speak black English, nor do all Hispanics speak Spanish. Within most microcultures, members will vary greatly in the language or dialect used.

Unfortunately, society often attaches a stigma to bilingual students that characterizes them as "low-income, low-status persons who are educationally at risk" (Hakuta, 1986, p. 7). Rather than valuing and promoting the use of two or more languages, we expect students to replace their native language with English as soon as possible. Movements to establish English-only policies and practices bestow "official blessing upon state residents who speak English, and a repudiation of those residents who do not" (Spencer, 1988, p. 142). Individuals who have limited English proficiency frequently suffer institutional discrimination as a result of the limited acceptance of languages other than English.

Language is the means by which we communicate. It makes our behavior human. It can incite anger, elicit love, arouse bravery, and trigger cowardice (Thomson, 1975). It binds groups of people together. Language and dialect serve as a focal point for cultural identity. Individuals who share the same language or dialect often share the same common feelings, beliefs, and behaviors. It provides a common bond for individuals with the same linguistic heritage. Individuals traveling abroad are often pleased to find other travelers seeking their language or their particular dialect. The dialect or language used in the right situation can provide an individual with immediate acceptance or credibility (Chinn, 1985).

However, language is much more than just a means of communication. It is used to socialize children into their linguistic and cultural communities, developing patterns that distinguish one community from another. In an ethnographic study of the use of language in three culturally different communities in the Piedmont area of North Carolina, Heath (1983) discovered the following:

1. Patterns of language use in any community are in accord with and mutually reinforce other cultural patterns, such as space and time orderings, problem-solving techniques, group loyalties, and preferred patterns of recreation.

2. Factors involved in preparing children for school-oriented, mainstream success are deeper than differences in formal structures of language, amount of parent-child interaction, and the like. The language socialization process in all its complexity is more powerful than such single-factor explanations in accounting for academic success.

3. The patterns of interactions between oral and written uses of language are varied and complex, and the traditional oral-literate dichotomy does not capture the

> ways other cultural patterns in each community affect the uses of oral and writ-
> ten language. In the communities [in the study] occasions for writing and reading
> of extended prose occur far less frequently than occasions for extended oral dis-
> course around written materials. (p. 344)

Thus, the interaction of language and culture is complex but central to the socialization of children into acceptable cultural patterns.

Exactly how a language is learned is not known, but almost all children have
the ability to learn one or more native languages. In part through imitating older
persons, the children gradually learn. They learn to select almost instinctively the
right word, the right response, and the right gesture to fit the situation. By age five,
children have learned the syntax of their native language, and they know that words
in different arrangements mean different things (Neisser, 1983). The average adult
has fifty thousand words at his or her disposal, and in addition, can communicate
through numerous vocal sounds and gestures.

Native speakers of a language unconsciously know and obey the rules and customs
of their language community. Society and language interact constantly. To make
a wrong choice in word selection may come across as rude, crude, or ignorant.
Children who are learning a new language or who are unfamiliar with colloquialisms
may make wrong choices or even be surprised at the use of certain words when such
use is incongruent with their perceptions of what is proper. An Australian student
in a southwestern school was shocked when a girl in his class responded to his query
of what she had been doing with, "Oh, just piddling around." Her response was meant
to convey the message that she had been passing her time in idle activities. However,
from his frame of reference, the Australian student understood her to say that she
had been urinating. It is important for classroom teachers to recognize that students
who are new to a language may not always be able to make appropriate word selec-
tions or comprehend the meaning of particular dialects or colloquialisms.

The subtle and complex nature of the interaction between language and culture
sometimes makes it difficult for the student whose first language is not English to
fully master the English language as it is used in schools and institutions. Instruction,
practice, and exposure do assist in the mastery of vocabulary and grammar. However, total immersion in the new linguistic community may make it easier to master
the finer points of language usage and the associated subtleties that allow for alternative and appropriate ways of saying things at the appropriate times.

Thomson (1975) cites the example of Fiorello La Guardia, mayor of New York
City in the 1930s, to illustrate the different communication styles of different ethnic
groups. La Guardia, of mixed Jewish and Italian ancestry, was fluent in both Yiddish
and Italian, as well as the New York dialect of English. When speaking to Italian
audiences, La Guardia used the broad and sweeping gestures characteristic of the people of southern Italy. When speaking Yiddish to Jewish audiences, he utilized the
forearm chop identified with many eastern European Jews. When speaking English,
he used softer, less emphatic gestures more typical of English-speaking individuals.
The example of La Guardia not only suggests different communication styles among
different ethnic groups, but also suggests that individuals adjust their communica-

tion style, whenever possible, to suit the needs of the intended audience.

At an early age, a child acquires the delicate muscle controls necessary for pronouncing the words of the native language or for signing naturally if the child is deaf. As the child grows older, it becomes increasingly more difficult to make the vocal muscles behave in new, unaccustomed ways necessary to master a foreign language. For example, the Filipino is unaccustomed to the sounds associated with the letter *f*, which makes it difficult, if not impossible, for a Filipino to pronounce the word *four* properly. Perhaps even more difficult to learn are the vocabulary and structure of the new language.

All this tends to inhibit people from learning new languages and as such encourages them to maintain the one into which they were born. Although the United States is primarily an English-speaking country, there are many other languages spoken. Spanish, Italian, and sign language are the most commonly used languages other than English. Among the English-speaking, there are numerous dialects—from the Hawaiian pidgin to the southern drawl of Atlanta to the Appalachian white dialect to the Brooklyn dialect of New York. Each is distinctive, and each is an effective means of communication for those who share its linguistic style.

In the United States, it has been estimated that there are approximately five million school children whose native language is not English (Brown, Rosen, Hill, & Olivas, 1980). This figure does not include the millions of English-speaking children whose dialects are sometimes labeled as nonstandard. If adults were added to the totals of non-English-speaking and nonstandard-English-speaking individuals, the numbers would be in the tens of millions.

The multilingual nature of American society reflects the rich cultural heritage of its people. Such language diversity is an asset to the nation, especially in its interaction with other nations in the areas of commerce, defense, education, science, and technology. There is an advantage to being bilingual or multilingual that is often overlooked because of our ethnocentrism. In many other nations, children are expected to become fluent in two or more languages and numerous dialects.

THE NATURE OF LANGUAGE

> There is no such thing linguistically speaking as a good language or a bad language, a superior language or an inferior language. Each language is appropriate for its time, place and circumstances. All languages are complete in this respect. (Gonzalez, 1974, p. 565)

Each language does not necessarily have a word for every concept. A language may or may not have need to express certain concepts. The Aztecs had no word for horse or orange, since neither was known to them before the advent of the Spanish in Mexico. Likewise, there were originally no words in English for taco or piñata because these terms did not exist in the English culture. Borrowing and incorporating words into a language do not corrupt the language, but merely reflect the changing needs of languages (Gonzalez, 1974).

Different languages are equally good, since each is equally adequate for a given time and place (Gonzalez, 1974). Nevertheless, individuals from particular regions of the country often tend to downgrade the linguistic styles of other regions. For example, Easterners, citing the use of slow, extended vowels and the term "y'all," may be critical of the speech of Southerners. Southerners, on the other hand, may be critical of the speech and language patterns of people from Brooklyn, who seem to speak through their nose and use phrases such as "youse guys." The eastern dialect of English is appropriate in the East, the southern dialect appropriate in the South, and black English appropriate in many African-American communities (Gonzalez, 1974).

The needs and aspirations of a group change constantly, and these changes are reflected in language. For example, a third-generation Japanese-American who is born and raised in Maryland learns Japanese from both his grandparents and parents. Because of particular pride in his cultural and linguistic heritage, he continues to use his Japanese, teaching and speaking the language to his American-born Japanese wife and children. On his first trip to Japan, he has no difficulty in conversing with the people, but notices smiles, grins, and giggles when he speaks. When he asks if he has said anything humorous, the people politely explain that he is speaking as if he were someone out of the 1800s. His grandparents had immigrated to the United States in the 1800s and had maintained the language of that period. The language in Japan, however, had changed sufficiently to make his language patterns stand out as archaic.

In some areas, language changes are so gradual that they go unnoticed. In other circumstances, changes are more easily noted. There are expressions and words that tend to be identified with a particular period. Sometimes the language is related to particular microcultures for certain periods. For example, words and phrases such as "chilling," "hyped," and "def" may be a part of our language for a time, only to be replaced by other expressions.

All languages are systems of vocal sounds and/or nonverbal systems by which group members communicate with one another. Some languages do not have a written system. Sign language is a system of communication that is used primarily by the deaf to talk to each other. However, the fact that the language is not written or is not oral does not make it inferior to French, German, or English.

LANGUAGE DIFFERENCES

There are over three thousand known languages in the world, with one thousand in Africa alone. Language differences ultimately reflect basic behavioral differences between groups of people. Physical and social separation inevitably leads to language differences. The constant movement and settlement patterns of people, as well as natural barriers, such as mountains and rivers, isolated many of the early settlers in the United States. The lack of communication across communities in the early years of the country further contributed to the isolation. Thus, as language changes took place, different dialects of the same language developed in different communities (Wolfram & Christian, 1979).

Social variables also contribute to language differences. Both class and ethnicity reflect differences in language. The greater the social distance between groups, the greater the tendency toward language differences. Upwardly mobile individuals often adopt the language patterns of the dominant society, since it may at times facilitate social acceptance.

Sign Language

Not all language is oral. Deaf individuals are not able to hear the sounds that make up oral languages and have developed their own language for communication. American Sign Language (ASL) is a natural language that has been developed and used by deaf persons. Just in the past thirty years have linguists come to recognize ASL as a language with complex grammar and well-regulated syntax. A growing number of colleges and universities will accept fluency in ASL to meet a second-language requirement.

Just like oral languages, different sign languages have developed in different countries. ASL is used by 90 percent of the deaf adults in Canada and the United States (Neisser, 1983).

Deaf children are able to pick up the syntax and rhythms of signing as spontaneously as hearing children pick up their oral languages. They learn to think in it and translate other sign languages and lip reading into it. Both hearing and deaf children who are born into deaf families usually learn ASL from birth. However, 90 percent of the deaf children have hearing parents and do not have the opportunity to learn ASL until they attend a school for the deaf, where they learn it from their peers.

Although ASL is the only sign language that is recognized as a language, signed English is often used by the deaf to communicate with the hearing. Rather than having its own language patterns like ASL, it translates the English oral or written word into sign. Few hearing individuals know ASL because they rarely observe it. The deaf use it to communicate with each other.

The use of sign language is one of the components of the deaf microculture that sets its users apart from the hearing. In part because of the residential school experiences of many of the deaf, a distinct cultural community has developed. As a cultural community, they are "highly endogamous, with in-group marriages estimated at between 86 and 90 percent of all marriages involving deaf individuals" (Reagan, 1988, p. 2). Although ASL is the major language of the deaf community, many individuals are bilingual in English and ASL.

Bilingualism

In its short history, the United States has probably been host to more bilingual people than any other country in the world. One of the most fascinating aspects of bilingualism in the United States is its extreme instability, for it is a transitional stage toward monolingualism in English. Each new wave of immigrants has brought with it its own language and then witnessed the erosion of that language in the face of the implicitly acknowledged public language, English. (Hakuta, 1986, p. 166)

Language diversity in the United States has been maintained primarily because of continuing immigration from non-English-speaking countries. However, the incessant move toward monolingualism is a very rapid process (Hakuta, 1986). Schools have assisted in this process. Prior to World War I, native languages were used in many schools where a large number of ethnic group members were trying to preserve their language. In this country, the maintenance of native languages other than English now depends on the efforts of members of the language group through churches and other community activities. Now, even our bilingual education programs are designed to move students quickly into English-only instruction.

A major reason for learning English quickly is economic. The acquisition of a second language is important when it serves one's own social and economic needs. If immigrants have available only the most menial jobs in society, the need to learn English is minimal (Spencer, 1988).

During the civil rights movement of the 1960s, language-minority groups, especially Hispanics, began to celebrate their native language tradition. Other ethnic groups decried the loss of their native languages over a few generations and blamed the school's Americanization process for the loss. The passage of federal legislation for bilingual education resulted. Many of those early advocates, however, hoped that the bilingual programs would help maintain and promote the native language while teaching English skills.

What constitutes bilingualism? It implies the ability to use two different languages. There are differences of opinion about the degree of fluency required. Whereas some maintain that a bilingual individual must have nativelike fluency in both languages, others suggest that measured competency in two languages constitutes bilingualism (Bacca & Cervantes, 1989).

Hakuta (1986) has identified two types of bilingualism: subtractive bilingualism and additive bilingualism. Subtractive bilingualism occurs when the second language replaces the first. Additive bilingualism occurs when the two languages are of equal value and one does not dominate the other. The latter has the more positive effect on academic achievement.

Accents

An accent generally refers to how an individual pronounces words. Since the Japanese do not have the sound of an *l* in their language, many tend to pronounce English words that begin with the letter *l* as if they began with the letter *r*. Thus, the word *light* may be pronounced as if it were *right*, and *long* as if it were *rong*. Note that an accent differs from the standard language only in pronunciation. A dialect, however, may contain changes both in pronunciation and in grammatical patterns of the language system. For example, in Hawaiian pidgin English, "Don't do that" may evolve into "No make like dat." Teachers should be aware that persons who speak with an accent often speak standard English, but at this level of their linguistic development are unable to speak without an accent.

DIALECT DIFFERENCES

There is no agreement on the number of dialects of English spoken in this country. Shuy (1967) has identified approximately nine major dialect areas in the United States, such as western-southern, eastern-southern, northern, New England, and New York City. However, social, ethnic, age, and sex considerations complicate any attempt to isolate areas completely.

Idiolects

An idiolect is an individual's own version of what he or she perceives to be a particular dialect or language. No two individuals will have precisely the same understanding or perception of the content and structure of a language. When a set of idiolects develops with a variance that is sufficiently small enough to constitute a tightly clustered mode, it may be considered a dialect or a language (Goodenough, 1981).

Dialects

In the United States, English is the primary language. However, numerous English dialects are used throughout the country. Dialects are any given variety of language shared by groups of speakers. These varieties typically correspond to other differences between groups, such as ethnicity, religion, geographical location, social class, or age. People who share common characteristics often share the same language (Wolfram & Christian, 1979). All people speak a dialect of their language. Everyone belongs to some group that can be distinguished from other groups and as such speaks the dialect of that group.

Wolfram and Christian (1979) suggest that a nontechnical but popular use of the term *dialect* carries a negative connotation. It is sometimes used to refer to a particular variety of English that may have a social or geographical basis and that differs from what is considered standard English. Black English, Hawaiian pidgin English, and rural Appalachian English are often referred to as dialects in this manner.

Certain languages are sometimes improperly referred to as dialects. Examples are the labeling of African languages as African dialects or the languages of the various American Indians as Indian dialects. This improper practice would be synonymous to labeling French and German as dialects spoken in the different countries in Europe.

Dialects differ from one another in a variety of ways. Differences in vowels are a primary means of distinguishing regional differences, whereas consonant differences tend to distinguish social dialects. However, regional and social dialects cannot be divorced from one another because an individual's dialect may be a blend of both. In northern dialects, for example, the *i* in words such as *time, pie,* and *side* is pronounced with a long-*i* sound that Christian and Wolfram (1979) describe as a rapid production of two vowel sounds, one sounding more like *ah* and the other like *ee*. The second sound glides off the first so that *time* becomes *taem*, *pie* becomes *pae*, and *side* becomes *saed*. Southern and southern-related dialects may eliminate the gliding *e*, resulting in *tam* for *time*, *pa* for *pie*, and *sad* for *side*.

In the social dialects, consonants tend to distinguish one dialect from another. Common examples of consonant pronunciation differences are in the *th* sound and in the consonants *r* and *l*. In words such as *these, them,* and *those,* the beginning *th* sound may be replaced with a *d,* resulting in *dese, dem,* and *dose.* In words such as *think, thank,* and *throw,* the *th* may be replaced with a *t,* resulting in *tink, tank,* and *trow.* Christian and Wolfram (1979) suggest that middle-class groups may substitute the *d* for *th* to some extent in casual speech, whereas working-class groups make the substitution more often.

In some groups, particularly the black working class, the *th* in the middle or end of the word is not spoken. The *th* in *author* or *tooth* may be replaced with an *f,* as in *aufor* and *toof.* In words such as *smooth,* a *v* may be substituted for the *th,* resulting in *smoov.* In regional and socially related dialects, *r* and *l* may be lost, as in *ca* for *car* and *sef* for *self.*

Among the various dialects, differences in various aspects of grammatical usage can also be found. Christian and Wolfram (1979) suggest that nonstandard grammar tends to carry with it a greater social stigma than nonstandard pronunciation.

A common example of grammatical differences in dialect is in the absence of suffixes from verbs where they are usually present in standard dialects. For example, the *-ed* suffix to denote past tense is sometimes omitted, as in, "Yesterday we play a long time." Other examples of grammatical differences include the omission of the *s* used in the present tense to denote agreement with certain subjects. "She have a car" may be used instead of "She has a car." The omission of the suffix has been observed in certain American Indian communities, as well as among members of the African-American working class. In the dialect of some African-American working-class groups, the omission of the *s* in the plural form of certain words and phrases, as in "two boy" rather than "two boys," has been observed. Also often omitted in these dialect groups is the possessive *s,* as in "my friend car" instead of "my friend's car."

Variations in language patterns among groups are significant when compared by age, socioeconomic status, sex, ethnic group, and geographical region (Christian & Wolfram, 1979). For example, individuals in the forty- to sixty-year-old age-group tend to use language patterns different from those of teenage groups. Teenagers tend to adopt certain language patterns that are characteristic of their age-group. Slang words, particular pronunciation of some words, and certain grammatical contractions are often related to the teenage and younger groups. As the individual grows older, social pressures may encourage the dropping of those speech patterns. Although a teenager may refer to a good idea as "bumping," few fifty-year-old Madison Avenue executives would choose to use such an expression in a board meeting.

Social factors play a role in the choice of language patterns. The more formal the situation, the more formal the speech patterns. The selection of appropriate speech patterns appears to come naturally and spontaneously. Individuals are usually able to "read their environment" and to select from their large repertoire the language or speech pattern that is appropriate for the situation.

Christian and Wolfram (1979) also indicate that while the evidence is not conclusive, the range between high and low pitch used in African-American communities is greater than that which is found in white communities. Such differences would, of course, be the result of learned behavior. African-American males may tend to speak with a raspiness in their voice. American women, it has been suggested, may typically have a greater pitch distribution over a sentence than do men.

Other differences in dialects exist as well. Since educators are likely to find dialect differences in the classroom, additional reading in this area may be appropriate. The Suggested Readings at the end of this chapter include some helpful resources.

Bidialectalism

Certain situations, both social and professional, may dictate adjustments in dialect. Some individuals may have the ability to speak in two or more dialects, making them bidialectal. In possessing the skills to speak in more than one dialect, an individual may have some distinct advantages and may be able to function and gain acceptance in a greater number of cultural contexts. A large-city executive from an agrarian background may quickly abandon his three-piece suit and put on his jeans and boots when visiting his parent's home. When speaking with the hometown folks, he may put aside the standard English necessary in his business dealings and return to the hometown dialect that proves he is still the old country boy they have always known.

Likewise, an African-American school psychologist who speaks standard English both at home and at work may elect to include some degree of black English in her conference with African-American parents at the school. The vernacular may be used to develop rapport and credibility with the parents. This strategy may allow the psychologist to show the parents that she is African-American more than just in appearance and that she understands the problems of black children and parents. She may choose, however, not to use as much of the dialect as the parents in order to maintain her credibility as a professional. On the other hand, in a conference with white parents, the same psychologist may choose to be scrupulously careful to speak only standard English if she feels that this is necessary for effective communication.

Children tend to learn adaptive behaviors rapidly, a fact that is often demonstrated in the school. Children who fear peer rejection as a result of speaking standard English may choose to use their dialect even at the expense of criticism by the teacher. Others may choose to speak with the best standard English they possess in dealing with the teacher but use the dialect or language of the group when outside the classroom.

Educators must be aware of the child's need for peer acceptance and balance this need with realistic educational expectations. Pressuring a child to speak standard English at all times and punishing him or her for any use of dialects may be detrimental to the overall well-being of the child.

Standard English

Although standard English is often referred to in the literature, no single dialect can really be identified as such. In reality, however, the speech of a certain group of people in each community tends to be identified as standard. Wolfram and Christian

(1979) suggest that norms vary with communities and that there are actually two norms, informal standard and formal standard. The language that is considered proper in a community is the informal standard. Its norms tend to vary from community to community. Formal standard is the acceptable written language that is typically found in grammar books.

Since no particular dialect is inherently and universally standard, the determination of what is and what is not standard is usually made by people or groups of people who are in positions of power and status to make such a judgment. Teachers and employers are among those who are in such a position. These are the individuals who decide what is and what is not acceptable in the school and in their workplace. Thus, people seeking success in school and in the job market often tend to use the standard language as identified and used by those individuals in positions of power. Moreover, certain individuals may be highly respected in the community. Just as hairstyles are often influenced by people who are respected and admired, the language of those who are admired also serves as a model. Generally speaking, standard American English is a composite of the language spoken by the educated professional middle class. With the wide variations of dialects, there are actually a number of dialects of standard American English (Wolfram & Christian, 1979).

Perspectives on Black English

Black English, sometimes referred to as Ebonics or vernacular black English, is one of the better-known and more controversial dialects spoken in the United States. Black English is the primary dialect spoken by African-Americans who live in low-income communities. As Tolliver-Weddington (1979, p. 364) states, "Ebonics is spoken by a wide variation of black Americans (both educated and uneducated) and there is a wide variation in consistency and form."

Black English has long been a center of controversy. Most linguists and the majority of African-Americans consider it a legitimate system of communication. Others, however, consider it a substandard dialect and as such a poor form of English that should be prohibited in the schools and eliminated from students' speech as much as possible.

As stated previously, there is no one correct way to speak English; that is, no dialect is any better or more effective as a way to communicate than any other. Since black English is related to a specific ethnic group, attacks against it are sensitive issues, and controversy is inevitable. Among the critics of black English are some prominent African-Americans who feel strongly that linguistic assimilation into the mainstream is essential for success. However, the refusal of some to recognize black English as a legitimate form of communication is sometimes interpreted as Anglocentric arrogance, which furthers the controversy.

The widespread use of black English as a form of communication cannot be denied. It is the primary form of communication for the majority of one of the largest ethnic groups in the United States.

Although the terms *black English, vernacular black English,* and *Ebonics* are used interchangeably, *Ebonics* is the term preferred and adopted by some African-American behavioral scientists and researchers. It is more inclusive than the other terms, since it refers to both linguistic and related features of the language (Tolliver-Weddington, 1979). However, for the purpose of this text, the term *black English* will be used.

Woffard (1979) estimates that approximately 80 percent of Americans of African ancestry use black English consistently. Another 19 percent of African-Americans use language that, with the exception of slight differences in vocal quality and pronunciation, is indistinguishable from standard English. The remaining 1 percent use other dialects.

Covington (1975) suggests that teachers coming from cultural backgrounds different from those of students tend to misunderstand the language behavior and goals of the pupils. The available literature, she contends, may be written from a narrow perspective, which may cause negative attitudes toward African-American children and their language. Covington (1975) maintains that the use of black English does not necessarily interfere with school achievement, as some writers propose. Rather, teacher perceptions of the student language may be related to achievement. Teacher bias against African-American children, particularly those from low-income background, has been documented. Such bias is not limited to white teachers, since it has been found among African-American teachers as well. The teacher is essential to quality education; thus, the most important changes will occur only as teachers change.

NONVERBAL COMMUNICATION

Although most individuals think of communication as being verbal in nature, nonverbal communication can be just as important in the total communication process. Because it is so closely interwoven into the overall fabric of verbal communication, nonverbal communication often appears to be inseparable from it. Birdwhistell (1970) suggests that communication uses the channels of all the sensory modalities. That is, in the communication process, we employ gestures, postures, facial expressions, and different levels of voice volume and intonation that reveal our thoughts, feelings, intentions, and personalities. In essence, nonverbal communication includes all forms of communication that are neither spoken nor written.

Leubitz (1973) identifies four functions of nonverbal communication:

1. Nonverbal communication relays messages. A person's attitude, personality, manner, or dress may communicate.

2. Nonverbal communication can augment verbal communication. When upset, an individual may say, "I feel terrible about the way things have turned out." At the same time, the individual may be crying. The spoken words are reinforced by the nonverbal act of crying.

3. Nonverbal communication can contradict verbal communication. A wife finds her husband nervously pacing the floor and puffing on his cigarette when she returns home from the office. When asked if he had a bad day, he snaps back, "No! Everything is just fine."

4. Nonverbal communication can replace verbal communication. When verbal communication is not possible for some reason, such as trying to keep the noise level down or trying to communicate with someone who speaks a different language, communication can be transmitted by gestures, motions, and facial expressions.

The importance of nonverbal communication is illustrated by the amount of meaning it carries in a normal conversation. Knapp (1972) suggests that in a typical conversation between two people, less than 35 percent of the social meaning is actually transmitted by words, whereas more than 65 percent of the social meaning is conveyed through nonverbal channels. Chinn, Winn, and Walters (1978) stress that the total meaning of communication includes not only the surface message as stated (content), but also the undercurrent (emotions or feelings associated with that content). They suggest that the listener should watch for congruence between the verbal message and that which is sent nonverbally, such as by body language.

There are a number of physical features that relate directly to nonverbal communication. These features themselves communicate messages, sometimes inaccurately, although much depends on the perceptions of the observer. When first introduced to an individual, people instinctively form some type of impression before any words are actually spoken. These first impressions are often communicated by features such as body build, height, weight, skin color, and other noticeable physical characteristics.

Often the impressions are functions of the observer's cultural backgrounds. Research has supported the contention that definite prejudices are based on body characteristics. For example, physical attractiveness plays a part in the ability to persuade other people. Attractive people tend to be judged as more likable; and taller men tend to be given higher status (Knapp, 1972) and viewed as smarter in school (Wilson, 1968). The study of nonverbal behavior is usually divided into three major areas: proxemics, kinesics, and paralanguage.

Proxemics

Proxemics is the language of social space. It is concerned with the spatial distance between people. Cultural variables affect proxemics. The normal conversational distance between white Americans, for example, is about twenty-one inches. A distance much greater than this may make the individuals feel too far apart for normal conversation and a normal voice level. Individuals of other cultural groups, such as Arabs, Latin Americans, and southern Europeans, are accustomed to standing considerably closer when they talk. In contrast to these contact cultures, Asians, Indians, Pakistanis, and northern Europeans have been identified as noncontact cultures (Watson, 1970).

Baxter (1970) found that in the natural positioning of people, African-Americans tended to stand farthest apart. Whites maintained an intermediate distance, and Mexican-Americans stood the closest together. When a person from a cultural group that tends to stand close in conversation speaks with a white American, the white American often backs up while the other individual continually moves in closer.

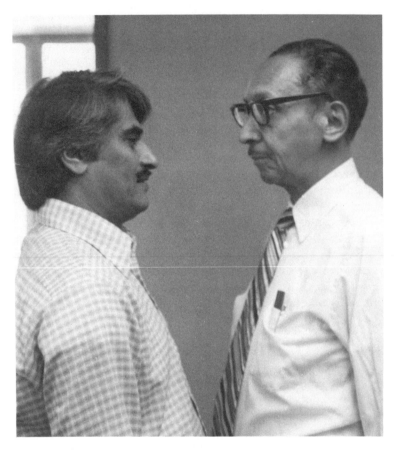

The individual on the left is maintaining a speaking distance considerably closer than that normal for white Americans. The person on the right shows some discomfort because the closeness is unnatural for him.

Several studies have shown that greater distance is maintained when one of the individuals is from a group that has marginal status in society (Wolfgang, 1979).

Among some cultural groups, physical contact is a common means of greeting. The English and French are separated by only twenty-one miles of water, yet there are vast differences in the way they greet their friends. A Frenchman may greet his male friends by kissing them on both cheeks. An Englishman, who typically avoids body contact, may avoid even a handshake.

At times, individuals protect their space by deliberately placing a barrier between themselves and those to whom they are speaking. A desk is an effective barrier. Moreover, a large chair behind the desk, in contrast to a smaller office chair on the other side, reinforces the individual's superior position.

Kinesics

Kinesics is the study of body language. It includes facial expressions, posture, gestures, and any other body movements that might carry some type of message. Body movements and gestures carry feelings and attitudes between people. The body language of students may tell the teacher whether what is being communicated is accepted or rejected. A student leaning forward in his or her seat may indicate receptiveness, whereas a student slouched in his or her seat with arms crossed could indicate rejection or boredom (Bull, 1983). However, the teacher should be careful not to assume that the student's body language means the same thing to the student and the teacher. These responses are culturally determined and must be interpreted within the student's cultural context rather than the teacher's.

At times, some body movement (or language) may convey information when there is no intention of doing so. Gestures such as the nervous drumming of fingers on a desk top are often unconscious and unintentional.

Paralanguage

Nonverbal communication is not necessarily nonvocal. Often what is being said depends on the manner in which it is said. For example, the single word *yes* can carry a message of defiance, resignation, acknowledgment, interest, agreement, or enthusiasm (Barnlund, 1968).

Paralanguage includes all production of sound that is vocal but nonverbal. It includes voice quality, ways of verbal expression, and sounds that are not verbal, such as laughing and crying. It is what is communicated through sounds that are not contained in the words themselves (Swenson, 1973).

There are two categories of paralanguage: vocalizations and vocal qualities. Vocalizations are sound and noises that are not words. Vocalizations are broken into three types: (1) vocal characterizers, which include sounds such as laughing, crying, sighing, and coughing; (2) vocal qualifiers, which include characteristics of sounds such as intensity (loud or soft) and pitch (high or low); and (3) vocal segregates, which are sounds other than words, such as "uh-huh," "mmmm," and "shhh." Among African-Americans, "um-huh-um-huh-um-huh-um-huh-um" may be used to express surprise, admiration, or total frustration, depending on the context in which it is used. "Uh-uh-uh-uh-h-h-h" and "um-m-m-m-m-m-uh" are similar expressions (Williams, 1975).

Vocal qualities include resonance, tempo, articulation control, and rhythm control. These different characterizations of voice can be manipulated as one speaks to communicate various messages. Anger, for example, tends to be expressed by a faster rate of speech, louder volume, and higher pitch. Sadness, for example, tends to be expressed through slower speech, lower volume, and lower pitch (Swenson, 1973).

Vocal cues provide listeners with remarkable amounts of information. Vocal cues alone can enable listeners to distinguish between male and female speakers, African-American and white speakers, and older and younger speakers, as well as distinguishing educational level and area of residence within a certain dialect region. A speaker's social class and status can often be determined based on the vocal characteristics of the individual.

In any discussion of nonverbal behavior, there are inherent dangers. As examples are given, the reader must realize that these are gross generalizations, and it should not be assumed that any given behavior can immediately be interpreted in a certain way. Hall (1977) cautions that nonverbal communications are often a prominent part of the context in which verbal messages are set. Although context never has a specific meaning, communication is always dependent on context. Hall (1977) further states the following: "Most people are lucky to have one subcultural system under control— the one that reflects their own sex, class, generation, and geographic region within a country. Because of its complexity, efforts to isolate out "bits" of nonverbal communication and generalize from them in isolation are doomed to failure" (p. 82).

EDUCATIONAL IMPLICATIONS

Language is an integral part of life and an integral part of our social system. The diversity and richness of our language systems in this country are a reflection of the richness and diversity of American culture. The ability of American educators to recognize and appreciate the value of different language groups will to some extent determine the effectiveness of our educational system.

All children bring to school the language systems of their culture. It is the obligation of each educator to ensure the rights of each child to learn in the language of the home until the child is able to function well enough in English. This may imply the use of English as a Second Language (ESL) or bilingual programs for limited-English-proficient children. Equally important is the responsibility to understand cultural and linguistic differences and to recognize the value of these differences while working toward enhancing the student's linguistic skills in the dominant language. While it is important to appreciate and respect the child's native language or dialect, it is also important that the teacher communicate the importance and advantages of speaking standard English in certain vocational and social situations.

Language and Educational Assessment

There are few issues in education that are as controversial as the assessment of culturally diverse children. The problem of disproportionate numbers of ethnic minority children in special education classes for the handicapped has resulted from such assessment. The characteristics of language have a direct relationship to the assessment of linguistically different children. Many of the educational and intelligence tests used to assess ethnic and linguistic minority children use norms for children primarily from white, middle-class backgrounds. Thus, such tests are often considered biased against the minority student.

Most intelligence tests rely heavily on language. Yet, there may be little attempt to determine a child's level of proficiency in the language or dialect in which a test is administered. For example, a Hispanic child may be able to perform a task that is called for in an intelligence test, but may not be able to understand the directions given in English. Even if a Spanish translation were available, it may not be in a dialect with which the child is familiar. Gonzalez (1974) suggests that using an unfamiliar Spanish dialect would be tantamount to administering the test in Chinese or Russian. The same may be true for Asians, African-Americans, or Native Americans who are being tested. The refusal to acknowledge the importance of the value of linguistic differences has resulted in inadequate services and in the inappropriate placement of children through highly questionable assessment procedures.

In 1970, the class action suit *Diana v. the California State Board of Education* was filed in a federal court on behalf of nine Mexican-American children from Spanish-speaking homes. The nine children had been placed in classes for the mentally retarded. Their diagnoses were based on IQ tests that relied heavily on verbal English, thereby ignoring the children's native language skills. The court determined

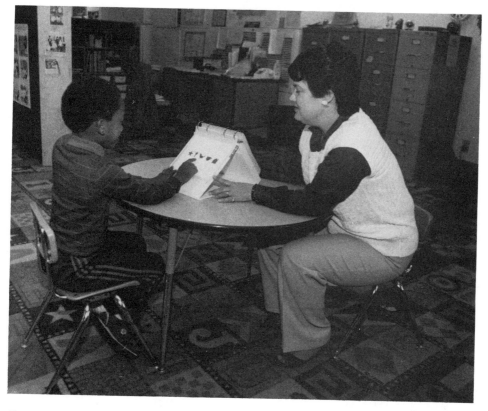

Tests such as the Kaufman ABC have been developed to reduce bias when used with culturally diverse children.

(Photo by Sheryl Zelhart).

that there was inherent cultural bias in the tests that discriminated against the plaintiffs. The case was eventually settled out of court with stipulated improvements in testing procedures and reevaluation of Mexican-American children already placed in classes for the retarded.

Guadalupe Organization, Inc., v. Tempe Elementary School District No. 3 et al. (1972) was a suit filed in Arizona that resulted from the disproportionately high placement of Yaquii Indian and Mexican-American children in classes for the mentally retarded. Placement had been based on the results of IQ tests given in English rather than in the children's native language. The out-of-court settlement required reevaluation of the students in these classes and testing in the primary language.

Dialects and Education

The issue of requiring a standard American English dialect in the schools is both sensitive and controversial. Since there is a close relationship between ethnic minority groups and dialects that are often considered nonstandard, this issue also has civil rights implications.

To require that standard English be spoken in the schools is considered discriminatory by some who think that such a requirement places an additional educational burden on the nonstandard-English-speaking students. As such, the insistence on standard English may hinder the acquisition of other educational skills, making it difficult for these students to succeed. It is argued that such practice denies the nonstandard-English-speaking students the same educational opportunities as others and thus morally, if not legally, denies them their civil rights.

Others argue that the school has the responsibility to teach each student standard English to better cope with the demands of society. There is little doubt that the inability to speak standard English can be a decided disadvantage to an individual in certain situations, such as seeking employment.

Dialect differences in the school may cause problems beyond the interference with the acquisition of skills (Wolfram & Christian, 1979). A second problem tends to be more subtle and involves the attitude of teachers and other school personnel toward students with nonstandard dialects. Too often, educators as well as other individuals make erroneous assumptions about nonstandard dialects, believing at times that the inability to speak a standard dialect reflects lower intelligence.

In a university classroom experiment, segments of two tape recordings in the area of language and culture were played. Neither speaker was identified; however, both are nationally prominent individuals in the field of linguistics. Both hold earned doctoral degrees, and both are from ethnic minority backgrounds. One individual speaks in standard English with no ethnic accent whatsoever. The other individual speaks in a combination of standard English and a slight black dialect. His speech patterns leave little doubt by his listeners that he is black.

After the two tape segments were played, the students were asked to indicate which of the two speakers in their opinion was the more intelligent. The class, which consisted of a number of African-American students, was unanimous in selecting the individual who spoke with the standard English dialect.

This simple classroom experiment suggests that most people have distinct pre-conceived notions about nonstandard-English-speaking individuals. If teachers and other school personnel react in this manner to students, the consequences could be serious. Students may be treated as if they were less intelligent than they are, and they may respond in a self-fulfilling prophecy in which they function at a level lower than they are capable of. In cases where children are tracked in schools, they may be placed in groups below their actual ability level. This problem surfaces in the form of disproportionately low numbers of African-American and Hispanic children being placed in classes for the gifted and talented (Office of Civil Rights, 1984). School administrators have cited the inability to appropriately identify these gifted and talented ethnic minority children as one of their biggest challenges. Teachers who have negative attitudes toward children with nonstandard dialects may be less prone to recognize potential giftedness and may be less inclined to refer these children for possible assessment and placement.

There are several alternatives for handling dialect in the educational setting. The first would be to accommodate all dialects, based on the assumption that they are all equal. The second would be to insist that only a standard dialect be allowed in the schools. This alternative would allow for the position that functional ability in such a dialect is necessary for success in personal as well as vocational pursuits.

A third alternative is a position between the two extremes, and it is the alternative most often followed. Native dialects are accepted for certain uses, but standard English is encouraged and insisted on in other circumstances. Students in such a school setting may be required to read and write in standard English, since this is the primary written language they will encounter in this nation. They would not be required to eliminate their natural dialect in speaking. Such a compromise allows the student to use two or more dialects in the school. It tends to acknowledge the legitimacy of all dialects while recognizing the social and vocational implications of being able to function in standard English.

The issue that seems to be at stake with some individuals who support the right to use nonstandard dialects is the recognition of the legitimacy of the particular dialect. Few, if any, will deny the social and vocational implications of dialects. Some parents may prefer to develop or have their children develop a standard dialect. However, the arrogant posture of some school officials in recognizing standard dialects as the only legitimate form of communication is offensive to many and may preclude rational solutions to this sensitive issue.

Bilingual Education

The language diversity that exists in the United States is naturally extended into the schools. In large urban and metropolitan school districts, there may be nearly one hundred different native languages spoken. Some students are bilingual in English and their native language. Others enter school speaking no English. Still others (3.6 million students) have limited English proficiency skills. Further, it is projected that the number of students with limited English proficiency will continue to increase by as much as 35 percent by the end of this century (Council for Chief State School

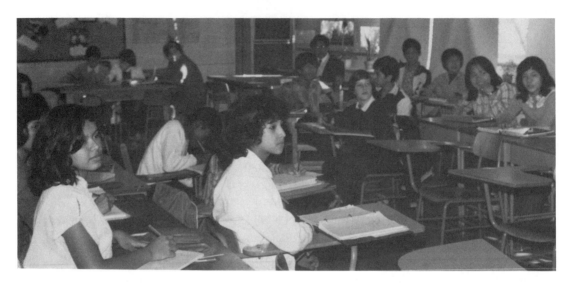

A bilingual education class in a metropolitan area often contains students from Hispanic and Southeast Asian backgrounds.

Officers, 1988). The challenge to provide an effective education for these students is met, in part, through the provision of bilingual education.

In 1974, a class action suit on behalf of eighteen hundred Chinese children was brought before the Supreme Court. The plaintiffs claimed that the San Francisco Board of Education failed to provide programs designed to meet the linguistic needs of those non-English-speaking children. The failure, they claimed, was in violation of Title VI of the Civil Rights Act of 1964 and the Equal Protection Clause of the Fourteenth Amendment. They argued that if the children could not understand the language used for instruction, they were deprived of an education equal to that of other children and were, in essence, doomed to failure.

The school board defended its policy by stating that the children received the same education afforded other children in the district. The position the board assumed was that a child's ability to comprehend English when entering school was not the responsibility of the school but rather the responsibility of the child and the family. In a unanimous decision, the Supreme Court stated the following: "Under state imposed standards, there was no equality of treatment merely by providing students with the same facilities, textbooks, teachers, and curriculum; for students who do not understand English are effectively foreclosed from any meaningful education" (*Lau v. Nichols*, 1974). Although the court did not mandate bilingual education for non-English-speaking or limited-English-speaking students, it did stipulate that special language programs were necessary if schools were to provide equal educational opportunity for such students. Hence, the Lau decision gave considerable impetus to the development of bilingual education.

In 1975 the Education for All Handicapped Children Act required each state to avoid the use of racially or culturally discriminating testing and evaluation procedures in the placement of handicapped children. It also required that placement tests be administered in the child's native language. In addition, communication with parents regarding such matters as permission to test the child, development of individualized education programs, and hearings and appeals must be in their native language.

Throughout the 1970s, the federal government and the state courts sought to shape the direction of bilingual education programs and mandate appropriate testing procedures for students with limited English proficiency (LEP). The Lau Remedies were developed by the U.S. Office of Education to help schools implement bilingual education programs. These guidelines prescribed transitional bilingual education and rejected English as a Second Language (ESL) as an appropriate methodology for elementary students. With a change of the federal administration in 1981, a shift to local policy decisions began to lessen federal controls. Emphasis was placed on the transition from the native language to English as fast as possible and the methodology for accomplishing the transition became the choice of the local school district. Thus, ESL programs began to operate alongside bilingual programs in many areas. While the future level of federal involvement in bilingual education is uncertain, there is little doubt among educators that some form of bilingual education is needed.

The definition of bilingual education that is generally agreed upon is "the use of two languages as media of instruction" (Baca & Cervantes, 1989, p. 24). Bilingual education has been supported, in part, by federal funds provided by the Bilingual Education Act of 1968 and reauthorized in 1974, 1978, and 1984. Hernández (1989) reports that

> federal policy encourages the establishment of programs using bilingual educational practices, techniques, and methods or of alternative instructional programs in school districts in which bilingual programs are not feasible (p. 83).

Thus, federal legislation defines bilingual education broader than does Baca and Cervantes. Methods other than the use of two languages are allowed and even encouraged. However, the Bilingual Education Act accounts for less than 10 percent of the total services provided to limited-English-proficient students (Secada, 1987).

Children who speak little or no English cannot understand English-speaking children or lessons that are presented in English. Not only are these children faced with having to learn new subject matter, but they must also learn a new language and often a new culture. It is likely that many of these children will not be able to keep up with the schoolwork and will drop out of school unless there is appropriate intervention. Approximately 45 percent of Mexican-American children drop out of school before the twelfth grade, and the attrition rate of Native American students is as high as 55 percent. Although language differences may not be the sole contributor to the academic problems of these children, they are considered by many to be a major factor (Garcia, 1976).

The primary goal of bilingual education is not to teach English or a second language per se, but to teach children concepts, knowledge, and skills in the language that they know best and to reinforce this information through the use of English (Baca & Cervantes, 1984). Two different philosophies currently shape programs in bilingual education: the transitional approach and the maintenance approach.

Transitional programs emphasize bilingual education as a means of moving from the culture and language most commonly used for communication in the home to the mainstream of American language and culture. It is an assimilationist approach in which the LEP student is expected to learn to function effectively in English as soon as possible. The native language of the home is used only to help the student make the transition to the English language. The native language is gradually phased out as the student becomes more proficient in English.

In contrast, maintenance bilingual programs provide a pluralistic orientation. The goal is for the LEP student to function effectively in both the native language and English. The student actually becomes bilingual and bicultural in the process, with neither language surfacing as the dominant one. The student's native language and culture are taught concurrently with English and the dominant culture.

Bilingual education can be justified as (1) the best way to attain maximum cognitive development for LEP students, (2) a means for achieving equal educational opportunity and/or results, (3) a means of easing the transition into the dominant language and culture, (4) an approach to educational reform, (5) a means of promoting positive interethnic relations, and (6) a wise economic investment to help linguistic minority students become maximally productive in adult life for the benefit of our society and themselves (Baca & Cervantes, 1984).

Whereas most bilingual educators favor maintenance programs, the majority of the programs in existence are transitional. Lack of trained personnel is one reason frequently cited for the predominance of transitional programs. Bilingual educators, however, strongly support the use of bicultural programs even within the transitional framework. A bicultural emphasis provides students with a recognition of the value and worth of their family's culture and enhances the development or maintenance of a positive self-image.

Bilingual education is not without controversy. It is an issue that stirs the emotions of many people as advocates or opponents. After analyzing letters to the editors of newspapers and testimony before Congress, Hakuta (1986) summarized the charges against bilingual education as follows:

> That there is no historical precedent for bilingual education; that most existing programs follow the maintenance model; that there is no popular support for bilingual education; that young children learn a second language in a very short period of time, so not much time is lost if they are placed in English-only classes; that education in the native language takes away valuable time that would otherwise be spent in English; that bilingual education is not effective; and that the number of eligible students is far smaller than originally estimated. [However,] there is research evidence that bears on all these points, evidence with which all too few of those who voice their opinions are familiar. (p. 210)

In a telephone survey, Hakuta and his students sampled the attitudes toward bilingual education in New Haven, Connecticut. Seventy percent of the respondents had favorable attitudes. They were also able to identify three distinguishing characteristics of those individuals who were against bilingual education. "First, men were more likely than women to oppose bilingual education. Second, men and women aged fifty or older tended to be more opposed. And third, men and women who had grown up using a non-English language at home were more opposed" (Hakuta, 1986, p. 212).

The opposition to bilingual education is due, in part, to the open acknowledgment of the legitimacy of non-English languages (Hakuta, 1986). Some people believe that it threatens the dominance of English as the national language. As a result, local and state laws to support two languages for official business often become emotional issues in a community.

Parents of LEP students also vary in their support for bilingual and ESL programs. Recent immigrants usually place high priority on their children's learning English in school. Less importance is given to studying the native language in schools. In a study of Punjabis and Mexican-American students in a California high school, Gibson (1988) concluded as follows:

> Immigrant minorities are less likely than involuntary minorities to favor bilingual education as an integral part of the regular instructional program of the public schools. . . . Those who equate an all-English curriculum with forced assimilation and Anglo conformity, favor bilingual-bicultural education. These same groups tend also to be those that feel most exploited by the dominant group and that view majority-group teachers with suspicion. (194–195).

Even this observation should not be generalized to all subordinate and new immigrant group members. Ethnic groups differ in their support for bilingual education, and individual families within the group may have different opinions about what is best for their children. Educators must be attuned to the beliefs of the community as they decide what strategies will be most effective in serving LEP students.

Advocates of bilingual education see the advantages in being bilingual. Although bilingual education programs have primarily been established to develop English skills for LEP students, some offer opportunities for English-speaking students to develop proficiency in other languages. In its position statement on bilingual education, the American Association of Colleges for Teacher Education (1985) states:

> It is desirable for native English-speaking children to participate in bilingual instruction programs, too. . . . Two advantages of dual language proficiency in this case include the learning that there are other equally valid ways of expressing ideas, and the development of respect for students who speak a different language at home, in the country, and the world. (p. 5)

In addition, bilingualism provides an individual with job market advantages. As our country becomes less parochial, there are more business and other contacts with individuals from other countries, providing decided advantages to bilingual individuals. Nevertheless, the controversy will continue as the dialogue develops about how pluralistic the nation should be.

English as a Second Language

English as a Second Language (ESL) is a program often confused with bilingual education. In this country, the learning of English is an integral part of every bilingual program. But the teaching of English as a second language in and by itself does not constitute a bilingual program. Both bilingual education and ESL programs promote English proficiency for limited English Proficiency (LEP) students. The approach to instruction distinguishes the two programs. Bilingual education accepts and develops native language and culture in the instructional process. Bilingual education may use the native language as well as English as the medium of instruction. ESL instruction, however, relies exclusively on English for teaching and learning. ESL programs are used extensively in this country as a primary medium to assimilate LEP children into the linguistic mainstream as quickly as possible. Hence, some educators place less emphasis on the maintenance of home language and culture than on English language acquisition, and they view ESL programs as a viable means for achieving their goals.

Sign Language and Education

Historically, most deaf students have been segregated from hearing students for their schooling experiences. Most states support one or more residential schools for the deaf. However, PL 94-142 (the Education for All Handicapped Children Act) calls for exceptional students to be mainstreamed into regular classrooms rather than being segregated in their own schools or classrooms. Because the residential schools have traditionally served as the place where American Sign Language (ASL) is learned and where the deaf culture is developed, there is concern among the deaf that the movement to mainstream them into regular classrooms may seriously hamper the transmittal of the culture (Reagan, 1988).

The major controversy in deaf education is between the use of an oral approach and the use of a manual approach. In the oral approach, students learn how to speak. Signing is used in the manual approach, but it is usually not ASL and is combined with speaking English. During the nineteenth century, sign language was used as a means of instruction. At the turn of the century, the oral approach took precedence and students were not permitted to sign in or out of the classroom. During the civil rights movements of the 1960s, the oral approach began to be replaced again by a manual approach (Neisser, 1983). Approximately one-third of the deaf programs in the United States still use the oral approach (Kannapell & Adams, 1984).

With the shift to mainstream deaf students into regular classrooms, more teachers will have deaf students in their classes. It will be important to become aware of the silence in which these students live and to develop strategies to make them an integral part of the class. Strategies could include helping all of the students learn about deafness and manual ways to communicate with each other. The culture of the deaf should be valued and extended into the classroom as much as possible. Paternalistic treatment should be avoided.

Nonverbal Communication in the Classroom

Cultural differences in appropriate nonverbal communications between students and teachers can be very frustrating to both. To begin to overcome such differences, the teacher must try to analyze particular nonverbal communications when students, especially those who are from a different cultural background, are not responding as the teacher expects. What the teachers perceive as inattention on the part of the student, or interruptions by the student at times considered inappropriate by the teacher, or even a tendency on the part of the student to look away from the teacher while being addressed may in fact be cases of miscommunication.

Too frequently, we jump to the conclusion that the student is not showing us respect when in fact the student is simply not following the informal rules of classroom etiquette. In most school settings, the students from subordinate groups are expected to become bicultural and adopt the nonverbal communication patterns of the dominant group while in school. A more positive approach to avoiding miscommunication would be for teachers also to learn to operate biculturally in the classroom.

Erickson (1979) suggests that teachers should reflect on what is occurring in the classroom when communications are not as expected. The first step is to "become more aware of what the nature of the trouble is" (p. 122). In the school setting, students should sometimes have access to teachers, counselors, or administrators who are from a culturally similar background. Teachers, meanwhile, could learn in a recipe fashion what the cultural cues of students mean and react appropriately. However, a more effective approach is to be able to analyze what is happening in the classroom and to respond based on what is known about the student and his or her cultural background.

SUMMARY

The Lau decision of 1974 ensures non-English-speaking children the right to an appropriate education that meets their linguistic needs. Even with a legal mandate, appropriate services may not always be delivered because of lack of tolerance or insensitivity to language or dialects other than that which is considered standard English. Because nonstandard dialects tend to have a negative stigma attached to them, some educators may refuse to view them as legitimate forms of communication. While they may indeed be legitimate forms of communication and may serve the speaker well in certain contexts, the use of nonstandard English dialects may preclude certain social and vocational opportunities.

Bilingual education has both its supporters and its detractors. Through proper educational programming, however, children with limited English proficiency can have the education to which they are entitled.

QUESTIONS FOR REVIEW

1. How is language a function of culture?

2. Explain why American Sign Language is considered a language parallel to English, German, Chinese, etc.

3. What are the advantages of being bilingual in the United States? How is bilingualism encouraged and discouraged within most educational settings?

4. What are dialects? What factors generally determine whether an individual becomes bidialectal?

5. Why is black English a controversial issue in education? How should it be handled in the classroom?

6. Why is it important to be sensitive to nonverbal communications between the teacher and student and among students?

7. Contrast maintenance and transitional bilingual education. Which do you think is more appropriate? Why?

8. When might English as a second language approach be the most appropriate strategy to use in a classroom?

9. What changes in your teaching methodology should you make when a deaf student is in your classroom? What changes should you make when you have a student or students whose native language is not English?

REFERENCES

American Association of Colleges for Teacher Education. (1985). *Educating a profession: Bilingual education*. Washington, DC: Author.

Baca, L. M., & Cervantes, H. T. (1989). *The bilingual special education interface*. Columbus, OH: Merrill Publishing.

Barnlund, D. C. (1968). *Interpersonal communication: Survey and studies*. Boston: Houghton Mifflin.

Baxter, J. (1970). Interpersonal spacing in natural setting. *Sociometry, 33*, 44.

Birdwhistell, R. L. (1970). *Kinesics and contexts: Essays on body motion communication*. Philadelphia: University of Pennsylvania Press.

Brown, G. H., Rosen, N. L., Hill, S. T., & Olivas, M. A. (1980). *The condition of education for Hispanic Americans*. Washington, DC: Government Printing Office.

Bull, P. (1983). *Body movement and interpersonal communication*. New York: Wiley.

Chinn, P. C. (1985). Language as a function of culture. *Social Education, 48*(5), 101–103.

Chinn, P. C., Winn, J., & Walters, R. H. (1978). *Two-way talking with parents of special children: A process of positive communication*. St. Louis: Mosby.

Christian, D., & Wolfram, W. (1979). *Dialogue on dialects*. Arlington, VA: Center for Applied Linguistics.

Council for Chief State School Officers. (1987, December). *Model interdepartmental state education agency strategies to meet the educational needs of limited English proficient students: Project summary*. Participant's Notebook for the conference on "Improving the Educational Achievement of Limited English Proficient Students."

Covington, J. (1975). Teachers' attitudes towards black English: Effects on achievement. In R. L. Williams (Ed.), *Ebonics: The language of black folks*. St. Louis: Institute of Black Studies.

Erickson, F. (1979). Talking down: Some cultural sources of miscommunication in interracial interviews. In A. Wolfgang (Ed.), *Nonverbal behavior: Applications and cultural implications* (pp. 99–158). New York: Academic Press.

Garcia, G. (1976). Learning in two languages. Bloomington, IN: Phi Delta Kappa Educational Foundation.

Gibson, M. A. (1988). *Accommodation without assimilation: Sikh immigrants in an American high school*. Ithaca, NY: Cornell University Press.

Gonzalez, G. (1974). Language, culture and exceptional children. *Exceptional Children 40*(8), 565–570.

Goodenough, W. H. (1981). *Culture, language and society*. Menlo Park, CA: Benjamin/Cummings.

Hakuta, K. (1986). *Mirror of language: The debate on bilingualism*. New York: Basic Books.

Hall, E. T. (1977). *Beyond culture*. Garden City, NY: Anchor Press.

Heath, S. B. (1983). *Ways with words: Language, life, and work in communities and classrooms*. New York: Cambridge University Press.

Hernández, H. (1989). *Multicultural education: A teacher's guide to content and process*. Columbus, OH: Merrill.

Kannapell, B., & Adams, P. (1984). *Orientation to deafness: A handbook and resource guide*. Washington, DC: Gallaudet College Press.

Knapp, L. (1972). *Nonverbal communication in human interaction*. New York: Holt, Rinehart & Winston.

Lau v. Nichols, 414, U.S., 563–572. (1974, January 21).

Leubitz, L. (1973). *Nonverbal communication: A guide for teachers*. Skokie, IL: National Textbook.

Neisser, A. (1983). *The other side of silence: Sign language and the deaf community in America*. New York: Knopf.

Office of Civil Rights. (1984). *1982 Elementary and secondary civil rights survey*. Washington, DC: Government Printing Office.

Reagan, T. (1988, Fall). Multiculturalism and the deaf: An educational manifesto. *Journal of Research and Development in Education, 22*(1), 1–6.

Secada, W. G. (1987). This is 1987, not 1980: A comment on a comment. *Review of Educational Research, 57*(3), 377–384.

Shuy, R. W. (1967). *Discovering American Dialects*. Champaign, IL: National Council of Teachers of English.

Spencer, D. (1988, May). Transitional bilingual education and the socialization of immigrants. *Harvard Educational Review, 58*(2), 133–153.

Swenson, C. H. (1973). *Introduction to interpersonal relationships*. Glenview, IL: Scott, Foresman.

Thomson, D. S. (1975). *Language*. New York: Time-Life Books.

Tolliver-Weddington, T. (1979). Introduction. *Journal of Black Studies, 9*(4), 364–366.

Watson, O. M. (1970). *Proxemic behavior: A cross cultural study*. The Hague: Mouton.

Williams, R. L. (Ed.). (1975). *Ebonics: The true language of black folks*. St. Louis: Institute of Black Studies.

Wilson, P. R. (1968). Perceptual distortion of height as a function of ascribed academic status. *Journal of Social Psychology, 74*, 97–102.

Woffard, J. (1979). Ebonics: A legitimate system of oral communication. *Journal of Black Studies, 9*(4), 367–382.

Wolfgang, A. (1979). The teacher and nonverbal behavior in the multicultural classroom. In A. Wolfgang (Ed.), *Nonverbal behavior: Applications and cultural implications* (pp. 159–174). New York: Academic Press.

Wolfram, W., & Christian, D. (1979). *Exploring dialects*. Arlington, VA: Center for Applied Linguistics.

SUGGESTED READINGS

Baca, L. M., & Cervantes, H. T. (1989). *The bilingual special education interface*. St. Louis: Merrill.

An excellent overview of bilingual special education. Contains basic but important information on general bilingual education, including litigation and legislation related to the rights of children with limited English proficiency.

Miller, P. W. (1981). *Nonverbal communication*. Washington, DC: National Education Association.

Short, easy-to-read monograph that emphasizes what research says to the teacher about nonverbal communications.

Ovando, C., & Collier, V. (1985). *Bilingual and ESL classrooms: Teaching in multicultural contexts*. New York: McGraw-Hill.

Overview of bilingual and ESL approaches to providing effective classroom experiences for the non-English-speaking and LEP students.

Tolliver-Weddington, T. (Ed.). (1979). *Journal of Black Studies, 9*(4).

A journal issue devoted entirely to black English. Includes some insightful research into the logic.

Williams, R. L. (Ed.) (1975). *Ebonics: The true language of black folks*. St. Louis: Institute of Black Studies.

An edited monograph that contains a number of excellent articles on black English.

Wolfram, W., & Christian, D. (1979). *Dialogue on dialects*. Arlington, VA: Center for Applied Linguistics.

Part of the Dialects and educational equity *series. Provides an informative and concise overview of dialects in a question-and-answer format.*

CHAPTER 8
Age

Each individual who lives long enough will become a part of every age microculture. Without choice, we must all go through the various stages in life and eventually join the ranks of the elderly. Like other microcultures, we feel, think, perceive, and behave in part because of the age-group to which we belong. In this chapter, we will examine each of the major age-groups: childhood, adolescence, young adulthood, middle age, and the aged. We will examine how ethnicity, gender, social status and other determinants of culture interface with these periods in an individual's life. We will examine how peer pressure affects behavior in some age-groups. Critical issues such as child abuse, adolescent substance abuse, and adolescent suicide will be examined. Finally, we will examine how an understanding of age-groups can affect the educational process.

> Mark McKenzie was a tenth-grader in an affluent school district in a southwestern suburban community. This community is essentially a new town. Twenty years ago, there were less than eight thousand residents in the town. Today, there are over seventy-five thousand. Most of the homes are in the $150,000 to $200,000 price range. Some homes sell in excess of $500,000. Crime in this community is almost nonexistent. At least a fourth of the students in high school drive their own cars. Several drive late-model Trans-Ams and Camaros, and a couple have Corvettes; one has a BMW convertible.
>
> Mark moved into this community with his family just two years ago. His family consists of a father, an engineer in a large high-tech company; a mother, a successful realtor; a brother in the eighth grade; and a sister in the sixth grade. Mark's parents are extremely fond of their children, but time commitments to their successful careers precludes extensive time and interactions with them. Mark has been promised a car for his next birthday.
>
> When Mark and his family moved from his previous home in the Midwest, he began to demonstrate occasional periods of depression. He had two extremely close friends he had grown up with and objected to the move vehemently. Since moving to his new home, Mark had made some casual friends, but none as close as his friends in his previous community.
>
> In the fall of Mark's sophomore year, he became more withdrawn. He attended no school social events and spent most of his nonschool hours in his room behind closed doors.
>
> In a conversation with two classmates the next spring, he stated that death brought people the ultimate peace and tranquility. He expressed the same sentiment in two poems written for his English class. His teacher considered the poetry good and passed off his expressions as a teenager's glamorization of death.

A month after writing the poems, Mark began giving away some of his prized possessions. A coin collection that he started five years ago and that he had always valued was given to his brother. He gave his stereo to his sister. When questioned by his parents, he would only reply that he had paid for these out of his own money and felt it was his prerogative to do what he wanted with them. "Besides," he stated, "I'm no longer interested in coins or music." Later, Mark gave his $300 guitar to his brother along with his baseball glove. Other personal items were given to his sister and a few to friends at school.

Shortly after giving away his possessions, Mark's depression seemed to dissipate and his behavior was such that it could be described as euphoric. His parents were pleased, and his father remarked that Mark finally got his act together. A week later, Mark's body was found in a wooded area less than half a mile from his home. He had died of a self-inflicted gunshot wound. Mark had become one of over six thousand teenagers who would end their own lives that year.

An understanding of the various childhood and adult groups is helpful in understanding and providing more appropriately for the needs of students. A student's classroom behavior may be a function of his or her relationship with parents, siblings, and significant others. As these individuals move through various age stages in their lives, their behavior may change as well as their relationship to the student. Consequently, the student's behavior may in part be influenced by the age changes of the significant people in his or her life.

How we behave is often a function of age. Although many adolescents behave differently from one another, the way they think, feel, and behave is at least partly because they are adolescents. At the same time, age does not stand alone in affecting the way a person behaves or functions. Ethnicity, socioeconomic status, religion, and gender interact with age to influence an individual's behavior and attitudes.

An African-American woman in her eighties, for example, may eat the type of food she does partly because her age and related health condition require eliminating certain foods from her diet. But her socioeconomic status may determine to some extent the foods she can afford to buy, and her ethnicity may determine some of her choices in foods. Her sex, language, handicap-nonhandicap status, and religious background may not influence eating habits to any significant degree. However, these other cultural variables, along with her age, may influence other types of behavior and functioning. From the time of birth through the last days of life, an individual's age may influence perceptions, attitudes, values, and behavior.

Although infancy as an age-group clearly determines certain behaviors, the discussion of age in this text will begin with early childhood and will end with the aged. Since educators become involved with children as early as three years of age, the discussion of age as a microculture will begin at this level.

CHILDHOOD

Childhood is viewed by individuals in many different ways. There is often a lack of agreement as to which years in a person's life should be included in infancy and which is early childhood. For the purpose of the text, childhood will be divided into three segments: early childhood, from three to five years of age; middle childhood, from six to eight years of age; and late childhood, from nine to eleven years of age.

Early Childhood

The period of early childhood (ages three to five years) is considered by some to be the age of discovery. This is a period when the child is primarily involved in developing a separate sense of self. The child assumes a more mature body structure and greater language facility that closely resemble those of adults. Erickson (1963) suggests that the major psychological thrust of this stage of life is the development and mastery of self as an independent human being, with a willingness to extend experiences beyond the family.

During infancy and the earliest years of childhood, children's companions are most likely to be parents, siblings, other close members of the family, and children in the immediate neighborhood. As the child's first social group, the family plays an integral part in the establishment of attitudes and socialization skills. The family, therefore, greatly influences how the child perceives and relates to other groups in the ensuing years.

The pervasive negativism of a toddler peaks between 2½ and 3 years of age and gradually diminishes during the early childhood years. In many instances, the standards and values of the family have been internalized and become evident in the child's actions. However, by the end of this period, the child may begin to question parental values as they are compared with those of peer groups and other influential adults. To the frustration of their parents, children at the later stages of early childhood may be less willing to abide by family codes of conduct (Whaley & Wong, 1987).

By the time children in this group reach four years of age, they become more involved in associative play. Their mental and physical maturity allows for participation in cooperative activities. They are ready for social patterns and receive satisfaction from playing with other children. About half of their playtime involves others (Kaluger & Kaluger, 1986).

During this period, sexual differences are evident in behavior. Boys tend to be more physically aggressive than girls. By the age of three, children become aware of physical and sexual differences, which may lead to curiosity and exploration. Curiosity is related to the eliminative function of the anatomy rather than the reproductive function (Whaley & Wong, 1987).

As previously stated, children's closest companions at this age are usually relatives and children in the neighborhood. However, with the increasing economic necessity for mothers to work, more school-age children are being placed in day-care settings. This type of situation increases the socialization process of these children and makes other children a part of their microcultural group. Socioeconomic status and

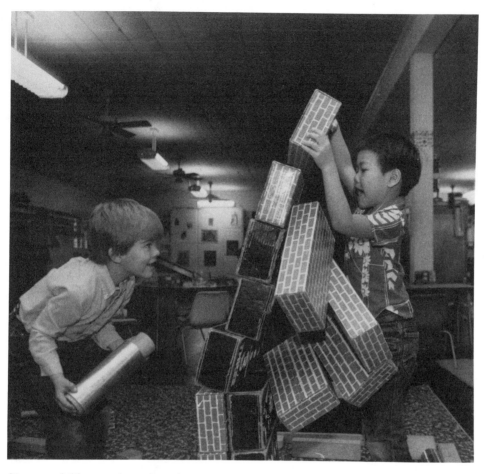

Younger children tend to select playmates more on qualities of age and size rather than sex or color.

(Photo by Sheryl Zelhart.)

ethnicity are again important determinants of who will be included in children's specific microcultures. Mothers from middle and upper socioeconomic groups may not need to work. Those who choose to can often be selective of the day-care setting to ensure an environment congruent with family values. Children from lower socioeconomic groups, however, may end up with a less than satisfactory day-care environment.

Ethnic identification is an important social development of this period. There is evidence that children as young as three years old respond to the different skin pigmentations of African- and Mexican-American children (Morland, 1972). By three or four years of age, white children tend to have positive associations with the color white and with white individuals. Black children have shown either no preference or preference for blacks in experimental studies. Minority group children tend to be more sensitive to racial cues and develop racial awareness earlier than their majority group peers (Katz, 1982). Different responses increase markedly from that time through the age of five years. Perception of differences at this age does not necessarily result in rejection. Younger white children may be unconcerned with ethnic identification and select playmates more on qualities of age and size rather than by sex or color. As they mature, however, they begin to respond to the prejudices of others, particularly those from the home environment. Meil and Kiester (1967) found that out of 237 white children studied in an elementary school, 79 percent preferred to play with other white children, 13 percent preferred to play with black children, 6 percent preferred to play with both, and 1 percent preferred to play with neither white children nor black children.

Comer and Poussaint (1975) indicate that ethnic identification may be different for black children than it is for white children. Whereas the average four-year-old black child is barely cognizant of racial differences, seven- and eight-year-olds understand these differences and may respond with anger and hostility if they have feelings of rejection or uncertainty related to race. This is a critical period in the lives of African-American children. They are exposed to the values, attitudes, and ways of the larger society, and these may or may not be congruent with those of their family. The children usually possess the maturity to sense the social conflicts in their parents, and this affects them as they formulate their own attitudes toward society. Comer and Poussaint (1975) suggest that black parents tend to teach their children attitudes that will enable them to handle the realities of being black in a white-dominant society. Similar development of attitudes is likely with other ethnic minority groups. The degree of awareness and intensity of feelings may be a function of the actual or perceived level of prejudice toward the particular group. Anselmo (1987) suggests that unless children have interracial families or child-care arrangements, information about race is provided by parents and others of the same racial background as the child. The evidence appears to refute the contention that children are "color-blind" with regard to racial differences.

Middle Childhood

Middle childhood (ages six to eight years) may bring about some of the most drastic changes in the life of children. For many children, it becomes the time when they leave the more confining atmosphere of their home to enter a school situation. Some children have nursery and kindergarten experiences before this time. However, this period marks the beginning of formal academic training for all children.

The middle childhood years mark a change in socialization focus. In the initial years of life, the primary influences on a child's social responses and reactions come from the family. By middle childhood, however, the influence from the school and peers predominate. The shift is neither sudden nor complete. For those attending day-care and preschool programs, the change begins earlier. The influence of the family remains significant throughout childhood, but the focus shifts from the immediate family to the school setting, where peers form a microcultural setting. The peers at this point become a dominant source of influence of life-style, dress habits, speech patterns, and standards of behavior and performance. Peer group standards become vitally important, and an effort is made to conform. Acceptance by the peer group becomes paramount, even above that of family acceptance. This is often a trying time for children, who must cope with peer group pressures that may be incongruent with the standards in their home. Success or failure in meeting peer group standards may be judged more harshly than previous judgments made in the home environment. The devastation that comes from not being accepted by the group may be the most severe that children have experienced. On the other hand, the feelings of success that come from achieving group approval are powerful and gratifying experiences.

This period may be a difficult time for an immigrant family. Children seeking peer acceptance may wish to become more acculturated than what is considered acceptable by parents seeking to maintain traditional cultural values. The conflicting values may emanate from the teachers as well as from peers. It is not uncommon to find children at this level resisting the language of the home as well as family values related to dress and behavior. During this period, children begin to identify with significant adults in their lives who serve as role models. This identification allows children to strengthen, direct, and control their own behavior in such a manner that it approximates the behavior of those they hold in esteem. Children often choose as role models individuals of the same sex who have similar physical traits, often their mother or father. Identification may also be with the parent of the opposite sex, or they may adopt other adult models with whom they can identify.

Children in their middle childhood tend to develop a code of behavior based on their perceptions of right and wrong, justice, and fairness. As they begin to try out their developing behaviors, they may find that it is contrary to that deemed acceptable by the family but congruent with the values of their peers. Clothing and hairstyles are typically influenced by the peer group. Small, close-knit groups of friends are formed, and nonmembers (both children and adults) are usually excluded. Group standards of loyalty and behavior are clearly delineated, any violations may be dealt with severely through criticism and even exclusion.

Children in this age-group begin to recognize socioeconomic differences. While the choice of friends may or may not be a function of socioeconomic levels, the type of playmates available may be. With the exception of the children transported away from their neighborhood schools, most children in their earlier years attend schools that are somewhat homogeneous in terms of socioeconomic level. Neighborhood playmates are even more homogeneous. During this period, however, an increasing awareness develops regarding the differences in material possessions found in different homes. The child begins to understand what is meant by rich and poor.

With one-fifth to one-fourth of our nation's children living below the poverty level, the effects of poverty are often manifested in the schools. In some areas of the country (e.g., southern California), the cost of living is so high that even some of those who technically live above the poverty level effectively live in poverty. Many of these children suffer from inadequate housing, nutrition, and medical care. Many of their homes have inadequate heat or cooling, which affects their sleep and physical well-being. Homes are often old and in neighborhoods where residents live in fear of their personal safety.

A recent study (Dolan, 1989) indicates that many of the nation's poor children are living in homes or areas where they are vulnerable to lead poisoning. Lead is found in the dust from the leaded paint in older homes, in automobile exhaust fumes, and in emissions from industry. One-fifth of the children examined were affected by lead poisoning, which often leads to irreversible neurological impairment manifested in learning disabilities, mental retardation, and behavioral problems.

Best friends are the ones who share secrets, private jokes, and adventures and come to your aid in times of need. In the course of best-friend relationships, there will be fights, threats, breakups, and reunions. These relationships, in which children experience the love and closeness of their peers, may serve as a foundation for heterosexual relationships of adulthood. In these relationships, neither child has authority over the other as in an adult-child relationship. To resolve their differences, the children often work out their own problems, with little or no assistance from their parents (Whaley & Wong, 1987).

Child Abuse.   Child abuse is a phenomenon that has been increasing in alarming proportions. The official reports of child abuse increased from 416,033 in 1976 to 614,291 in 1978, an increase of over 47 percent (Kaufman, 1983). Authorities believe that the actual number of child abuse cases far exceeds the officially reported cases, since many children are either too young or too afraid to report abuse themselves.

Child abuse appears to be more prevalent among lower socioeconomic groups, perhaps in part because of the frustrations and stress created by poverty. However, it is in no way restricted to this population and is found in all socioeconomic and ethnic groups.

Four criteria are often used in determining abusive behavior. They are willful malnutrition, sexual molestation, willfully inflicted trauma, and the isolation of a child in a dark area (e.g., in a closet). These behaviors involve a direct intent to bring injury or harm to the child either physically or psychologically. While at least one writer (Gelles, 1982) maintains that intent to harm must be accompanied by identifiable injuries to constitute child abuse, others regard abuse as deprivation of physical or emotional needs, either of which can be detrimental to the welfare of the child.

Thompson (1983) suggests that abusive behavior may take the form of interaction or lack of interaction between the parent (or significant others) and the child that are out of step with the family's cultural or social norms and that are harmful, detrimental, and counterproductive to a child's developmental, emotional, and physical maturity.

The causes of child abuse are numerous. Among the most prevalent are personality disorders, drinking, lack of parental maturity, an unwanted child, and drug use. Less prevalent but contributing to abuse are social structural conditions such as financial problems, work-related problems, and isolation from friends and relatives.

Late Childhood

Children in their late childhood (ages nine to eleven years) are usually quite adjusted to the change from family-oriented activites to peer-oriented activities. The peer group has considerable influence on attitudes, desires, and behavior—an influence that increases as children grow older. Children in this age-group are not prepared to abandon parental control (Whaley & Wong, 1987). Although they may complain about parental restrictions, they need and want the security of parental authority to assist them in coping with the ever-expanding problems of their environment.

Late childhood is a period of transition from the typical behavioral and social patterns of childhood to those of adolescence. Physical changes also take place at this time, and some children who mature early may experience changes more typically associated with the adolescent period.

The period is also characterized by the formation of cliques. The peer group provides a sense of belonging. The effects of exclusion from the peer group may be devastating. Children who fail to make entry into some group may enter adolescence without some of the necessary socialization skills and may be branded as misfits. Whaley and Wong (1987) suggest that younger children who are unable to secure full entry into the peer group tend to hang around the periphery of the group—watching, learning, and practicing skills, participating whenever they are allowed to or deemed worthy. Often, as children get older, full participation rights are granted.

Because children tend to have a strong need not to be different, group structure may be intolerant of those who are different. Handicapped children, children who are ethnically different, or children who do not conform to group standards may be excluded from membership.

While group identification and association are important to children's socialization process, there are some inherent problems. Peer pressure may induce behaviors that violate their personal standards. Smoking, drinking alcoholic beverages, experimenting with drugs, stealing, and engaging in sexual activity have often been initiated by peer group pressure. Not only do some of the behaviors involve risks of personal health and safety, but they also result in emotional trauma for both parents and children.

As already mentioned, three factors continually impact on children as microcultural groups are established. Sex, ethnicity, and socioeconomic status interface with other variables and often determine what the nature of the microcultural group will be. Among some children, religion, exceptionality, and language may determine the choice of friends and composition of their peer groups. In Utah, for example, the Mormon church exerts considerable influence over social as well as religious life. As such, peer groups or cliques may form in which religious background is an overriding element in determining membership. One clique may consist of children who are all of Mormon background, whereas another peer group may consist of all non-Mormon children.

Because some children attend special classes for exceptional children, there is a natural opportunity for groups to form outside the school situation in which exceptionality is the common ingredient of all members. In some instances, handicapped children may be treated somewhat like younger children in terms of peer group membership. This is more likely to be true of mentally retarded children than of children with other handicaps. If they are not totally excluded from peer group membership, they, like younger children, may remain on the periphery, watching and participating if they are allowed. However, unlike younger children who eventually gain entry as they get older, retarded children may remain on the periphery indefinitely, because advancement in chronological age may not be accompanied by advancement in social skills.

Language may also be a factor in either exclusion from or formation of peer groups among children. Children with limited English proficiency may be excluded from peer group participation. Other children may form cliques with Spanish or nonstandard English as a criteria for membership. In some instances, the peer group may influence members regarding language patterns. Children who talk in nonstandard English may work diligently toward developing standard English skills if this is valued by the peer group.

ADOLESCENCE

Adolescence is perhaps one of the most challenging times in the life of the individual and the family. It is a long transitional period (six years or so) during which the individual is "suspended" between childhood and adulthood. During adolescence, emancipation from the primary family unit is the central task of the individual. It is a difficult period for the young person, who is attempting to be free from the role of a child but is not fully equipped to assume the responsibilities of adulthood.

Adolescence is impossible to define in precise chronological terms. The literature suggests that the beginning age for this period is twelve or thirteen years. The end of adolescence is usually associated with the end of a high school education, about the age of eighteen years. In some instances, adolescence is treated synonymously with the teenage years, which span from thirteen to nineteen years of age.

In some cultures, entry into adulthood begins immediately after childhood. Adolescence as a stage of behavioral development does not exist (Whaley & Wong, 1987). However, in Western culture, an individual is seldom allowed or expected to make an immediate transition from childhood to adulthood. It is interesting to note that the anticipated state of extreme disequilibrium associated with adolescence and the period of "storm and stress" does not exist in some cultures in which adolescence does not exist. Cultural definitions of the role of the adolescent along with social attitudes have created a number of circumstances that cause this period of life to be what it is in our Western culture.

Whaley and Wong (1987) suggest that the ambiguity of society and parents regarding the attainment of adult status contributes to adolescents' confusion and ambiguity about themselves. For example, only in recent years were eighteen-year-olds allowed to vote, although they were eligible for military service. The age of adulthood varies from state to state, and the age for legal consumption of alcohol has varied from eighteen to twenty-one years of age.

There has been speculation that the behavioral turmoil associated with adolescence is related to the physiological changes that take place within the individual during this period. However, studies have provided little support for this contention. Rather, the changes that take place are gradual and fluctuate little on a day-to-day basis. These changes may contribute to the problems of the adolescent, but do not by themselves cause the problems.

The unique nature of the adolescent period has led to the designation of an adolescent culture. Coleman (1961) has identified five factors in American culture that have led to the development of a distinct adolescent culture:

1. The differences in skills, knowledge, and values result in communication problems between adolescents and their parents.
2. The parents and family no longer provide vocational training to the adolescents, as this is provided in the school and elsewhere.
3. Adolescents no longer are viewed as essential to contributing to the family income, and adolescents no longer or seldom enter the labor force at this time.
4. Adolescents are important consumers.
5. With compulsory school attendance, adolescents are in school longer, and those in school represent a larger and more pluralistic group.

In his field theory, Lewin (1939) has identified three factors in a younger person's life that create adolescent behavior considered typical in Western societies: (1) The greater mobility of adolescents (many have their own cars) expands their psychological field and enhances their ability for associations; (2) the marginal status between childhood and adulthood leads to conflicts in attitudes and values; and (3) there are physical and biological changes whereby the adolescents are neither children nor adults, requiring the development of a new body image several times during adolescence.

Peer Group

As in the middle and late childhood years, the peer group is an integral part of the adolescent's socialization process. In many respects, the adolescent peer group plays an even bigger role in the lives of individuals than does the childhood group. The peer group is a primary means in our society for adolescents to break from family influence and allegiance. Peer groups demand a sense of loyalty and solidarity. Membership in the group requires the willingness of individuals to lay aside personal goals, if necessary, for the good of the group. Group identification is marked by conformity in hair and clothing styles, behavior, language, and values. These characteristics of group membership exist in spite of strong inclinations toward individualization. The group is a vehicle for movement away from family control, and as such, contributes to the desire for individualization. While independence from the

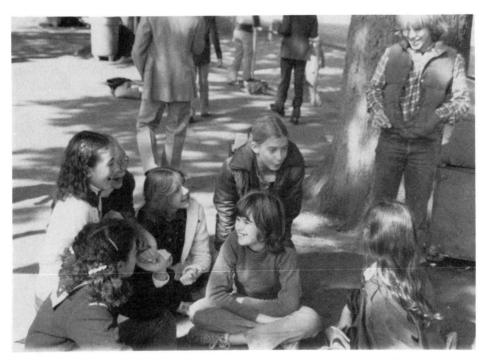

In childhood and adolescence, peers begin to be a dominant source of influence on social behavior.

primary family unit is one of the major objectives of the adolescent, it should be recognized that there are different types of independence. Newman and Newman (1986) suggest three types of independence: *Behavioral independence* may involve staying out beyond a curfew; *emotional independence* may be manifested by indifference to parents' anger; and *value independence* may be observed in values incongruent with those of parents.

Although there are a few who remain outside peer group participation, either by preference or rejection, the majority of individuals during the adolescent period find companionship and security within a group. Since most adolescents are insecure by nature, they readily conform to group values to gain approval and to ensure establishment in the group. The group fulfills the need for belonging and in many cases the need for esteem and status. The group offers adolescents acceptance and security. They can try out and experiment with a variety of roles with the support of those who face similar problems and who feel and behave the same way. They are able to stand together against those who they feel do not understand (Whaley & Wong, 1987).

Adolescents distribute themselves into a relatively predictable social hierarchy. The largest social division is the set, which may include individuals of both sexes.

Activities may relate to a particular sex, and this may cause separation into sexual groupings. Within the set are smaller, distinctive groups, or cliques, that consist of close friends with similar backgrounds, tastes, and interests. There are emotional attachments to one another in these groups, as opposed to the more casual relationships within the larger set. Membership is according to a specific standard. The cliques are usually made up of one sex, with girls more cliquish than boys (Whaley & Wong, 1987).

Relationship with Parents

As the adolescent shifts emotional ties from the family to peers, there may be a restructuring of the parent-adolescent relationship. Parents may be viewed more objectively. Parents may become more concerned about peer influence as they have increasingly less interaction with their child (Newman & Newman, 1986). These changes have the potential for turning the period of adolescence into one of dissonance and alienation from parents and other members of the family. However, one need only observe a few adolescent-family situations to realize that the degree of dissonance and alienation varies greatly.

The attitude of the parents may contribute to the alienation. Parents who expect problems with their children in the adolescent period sometimes fall into the trap of a self-fulfilling prophecy. Their expectation of alienation generates a hostile attitude on their part. This attitude is quickly sensed by the adolescents, and a vicious cycle is started. On the other hand, parents who have confidence in their children may promote a feeling of confidence and trust. These children often develop sufficient self-confidence to resist peer pressure when it is appropriate.

Alienation is disturbing to the families, to adult members of the community, and to the adolescents themselves. In their efforts to achieve autonomy, sexual functioning, and identity in order to become productive, self-sufficient individuals, some adolescents think that they must turn away from the family. There is considerable ambivalence, since young persons are usually unprepared to yield family support systems in the quest for independence. As adolescents assert their rights to assume adult behaviors, there is sometimes an inability to assume complementary adultlike responsibility. Recognizing this, parents are understandably reluctant to grant them adult privileges, which further adds to the alienation.

Many young people reach a higher level of education than their parents. Most parents support the intellectual and educational development of their children and often encourage their children to achieve a higher level than they did. Parents may find that their children sometimes develop the typical "intellectual" approach, viewing as worthy only the most vital aspects of life (as defined by them). They develop an attitude of superiority, looking down on anyone (including their parents) who in their opinion has a more mundane view of life. Often, neither parents nor children are able to comprehend the developing dynamics. Rejection and lack of communication develop. Problems can also develop if the parents are high achievers. There is both family and social pressure for the children to achieve in the same manner. If these standards cannot be met, alienation may result.

When family values are incongruent with those of adolescents' peer groups, the family standards may then be rejected to maintain peer group acceptance. Many adolescents therefore reject the validity and desirability of their family expectations. They view their family standards as wrong. If they do not meet the family standards, they do not consider themselves as failures, because it is not possible to fail if the standards are wrong in the first place.

Some ethnic minority adolescents can have unique problems. They may become alienated from society if they recognize the inequities of our social system as they relate to minority groups. They see how their parents have been unable to achieve, and they may become angry for their parents and for what they feel is in store for them. At times, parents assume a more passive acceptance of the social system or do not share in the same degree of frustration as their children. This difference in attitude or perception may alienate these children from their parents as well as from society.

Sexuality

During adolescence, physical development occurs to the point of sexual competence. This can be a difficult time for young persons, particularly if sexual development is either early or late. According to Gispert (1981), "Biologically, sexual maturation occurs at an earlier chronological age than in previous generations, while the sociological period of adolescence has been extended upward into the twenties by prolongation of studies, financial dependence of parents, and the trend toward marriage at a later age" (p. 32a).

A major psychological task facing adolescents is the integration of their perceptions of their developing bodies with their desire to develop their femininity or masculinity in the context of the expectations of their parents, peers, and society. There is no doubt that adolescents are, as a group, sexually active. National surveys suggest that 80 percent of adolescents have an accepting attitude toward sexual activity, and at least 60 percent are active sexually (Gispert & Falk, 1978). Zelnick and Kantner (1980) report that the proportion of fifteen- to nineteen-year-old females living in cities and surrounding suburbs reporting premarital sexual intercourse was 50 percent. The average age of first intercourse was 16.2 years. While the threat of the AIDS virus may now inhibit the sexual activity of some adolescents, it is apparent that this group is still sexually active.

Today's adolescents operate in a social environment that is considerably more liberal and permissive in sexual attitudes than that of their parents. Adolescents are continuously exposed to sexually oriented material in the media, with movies, television, and newspapers presenting the more permissive and liberal views. Peers may also encourage adoption of liberal views. On the other hand, parents may continue to hold the more conservative views of their generation.

When adolescents adopt liberal attitudes toward sexual behavior and their parents maintain conservative values, dissonance and alienation are inevitable. Unable or unwilling to turn to their parents and often lacking adequate sex education at school, adolescents may turn to their peers for support. Although they may be able to provide sympathetic understanding and support, the peers often are neither knowledgeable nor able to respond in an objective manner. The lack of appropriate information and knowledge may explain why half of all the illegitimate births in the United States involve adolescents.

Sex education and school clinics that provide information on sexuality and birth control can provide adolescents with the background to deal with their increased sexual awareness. They can, however, be a source of considerable controversy, and parents in some communities may resist these efforts or endeavors.

Adolescent Suicide

One of the most alarming developments in adolescent behavior is the dramatic increase in teenage suicides. Every day, an average of eighteen young Americans kill themselves, 5,000 to 6,500 a year. Every hour, fifty-seven children and adolescents try to take their own lives. There are well over a thousand attempts each day. Since 1955, there has been a 300 percent increase in adolescent suicides. Only accidents and homicides exceed suicide as a cause of adolescent deaths, and many of those deaths are suspected suicides (Gelman & Gangelhoff, 1983; Griffin & Felsenthal, 1983; Guetzloe, 1989).

While the United States once had a low rate of suicide among young people, the rate among young males is now among the highest in the world (Hendin, 1985). The statistics we have reported here are considered by researchers as inaccurate and understated (Guetzloe, 1989; Pfeffer, 1986). The number of reported suicides is probably less than half the actual number (Jobes, Berman, & Josselsen, 1986). This underreporting may be in part due to attempts to protect the family from the social and religious stigma associated with suicide. Consequently, many suicides are reported as accidental deaths (Hawton, 1986).

The increase in the adolescent suicide rate is due primarily to the increase in suicides among young males. By 1980, the ratio of male suicides to females was five to one. Most of the male victims are white (89 percent). While the suicide rate for males in other racial groups has also increased, it has remained lower than that of whites (Centers for Disease Control, 1986). The suicide rate for white males fifteen to nineteen years of age has been slightly over twice that of black counterparts. The rate of white females of the same age is higher than that of their black counterparts.

In 1983, a teenager in a Dallas suburb was killed in an accident. Within eight weeks, the accident victim's best friend took his own life, and two others did the same. In an eight-month period, there were sixteen suicide attempts by adolescents and young adults between the ages of thirteen and twenty-four in this community. The following year, four teenagers in a Houston suburb took their lives in a one-week period. Six killed themselves in a two-month period.

Numerous theories have been advanced for the adolescent suicide phenomenon. Among the reasons offered is the decline in religion, the breakup of the nuclear family, and the competitiveness in school (Gelman & Gangelhoff, 1983). The most common emotion felt by suicidal individuals is depression (Miller, 1975). Because of their youth and lack of experience in making accurate judgments, depressed adolescents are more prone to respond to the suggestion of suicide than an adult (Hyde & Forsyth, 1978). Adolescent depression is a function of a wide range of situations, perhaps involving failure, loss of a love object, or rejection. It can also be a function of bio-chemical imbalances in the brain (Hipple & Cimbolic, 1979). The loss of a parent through death, divorce, separation, or extended absence has been cited as a possible variable in adolescent suicides (Ray & Johnson, 1983). Less than 38 percent of this country's children live with both natural parents. Strong, stable support systems are unavailable to many children (Gelman & Gangelhoff, 1983). The loss of a parent may be viewed as parental rejection, which may lead to feelings of guilt in the adolescent (Ray & Johnson, 1983).

The Dallas suburb where the 1983 suicides took place has all the trappings of an ideal suburban community. Middle- to upper-level management and high-tech professionals occupy the community's many expensive homes, attracted by the community's good schools and low crime rate. Many of the community's teenagers have their own expensive cars. A closer look, however, provides some interesting statistics. Among its ninety thousand residents in 1983, there were about a thousand divorces a year. Of the residents, 82 percent had lived there less than ten years, 59 percent for four years or less. Almost everyone and everything there was new. There were few roots in the community.

Alienation in the family is cited as another major contributor to adolescent suicide. Where family ties are close, suicide rates are low; where families are not close, suicide rates are high (Cantor, 1976; Wenz, 1979). Adolescent suicide victims come from all socioeconomic backgrounds, but many are from middle- and upper-income homes. The parents in these homes are generally high-achieving individuals, and they expect similar behaviors from their children. Failure to conform to parental expectations may lead to alienation. There are, of course, many other causes of family alienation. Guetzloe (1989) lists the following risk factors that may be related to youth suicide: biological factors, psychiatric disorders, family problems, environmental and sociocultural factors, and factors related to learning and cognition.

No single variable or factor can be identified as the cause of adolescent suicide. However, adolescent suicide is an apparent response to the frustrations of life, and in the attempted suicides, it is a possible cry for help or a call to attention to the adolescent's profound problems. As Griffin and Felsenthal (1983) suggest, suicides are cries for help that have backfired, and which others can heed or help.

As previously discussed, the adolescent period is one of intense excitement as individuals assume more independent roles and adjust to physiological changes associated with this transition period. Distinct characteristics, such as peer group behavior, dress standards, and music preference, emerge. The adolescent's attitude, as well as that of parents and other important individuals, may determine whether or not the period becomes one of storm and stress or a positive transition into adulthood.

Substance Abuse

The use of harmful substances, primarily by children and adolescents has been one of the most problematic areas faced by parents, schools, and law enforcement agencies in the past two decades. It will inevitably continue to be a major problem in the 1990s. The problem is a national phenomenon, and many of the problems of adult substance abuse have their roots in adolescence.

Numerous problems related to substance abuse affect the community at large. Intravenous drug users are one of the high-risk groups of Acquired Immune Deficiency Syndrome (AIDS). The spread of the deadly virus among adolescents has by 1990 already exceeded expectations. In many cities, drug-related gang violence has led to the deaths of hundreds of adolescents. To support their habits, adolescents and adults have resorted to criminal activities.

Another major result of adolescent substance abuse has been the physical and mental effects on embryos and fetuses carried by adolescent drug and alcohol users. There is also increased risk of accidental deaths among infants when parents are involved in substance abuse. While some infant deaths are reported as accidents rather than being linked to drug use, they are often the result of negligence or violence related to the parents' (often adolescents themselves) substance use and reduced capacity to provide appropriate care (Cormerci, 1986).

In adolescence and early adulthood, over half the motor vehicle fatalities are associated with alcohol abuse. Many deaths are likely associated with other drug use (Cormerci, 1986).

The use of harmful substances among adolescents has reached alarming proportions. In 1985, the percentage of high school seniors admitting the use of such substances on a daily basis was 5 percent for alcohol, 20 percent for tobacco, 5 percent for marijuana, 0.4 percent for stimulants, and 0.4 percent for cocaine. The percentage of seniors reporting at least one-time use was 92 percent for alcohol, 69 percent for tobacco, 54 percent for marijuana, 26 percent for stimulants, and 17 percent for cocaine (Johnson, O'Malley, & Backman, 1986). Actual usage may be higher or lower in specific communities or schools.

These substances are used to produce altered states of consciousness. The adolescents that use them often seek relief, escape, or comfort from stress related to the prolonged and intense period of their life. The social institutions to which the adolescent must relate, including the family and particularly the educational system, may be perceived as unresponsive or openly hostile. Their inability to focus on long-range goals, their desire for immediate gratification, and their lack of appreciation for the consequences of their behavior may contribute to some adolescents' use of substances (Millman & Khuri, 1981). The use of "psycho-active drugs remains one of the few pleasurable options for many adolescents; it may be a predictable, reliable method to punctuate an otherwise unrewarding life" (p. 740).

The media, particularly television, in both commericials and programming, have tended to glamorize the use of substances such as alcohol. Children and adolescents who see entertainment and sports personalities promoting the use of beer, wine coolers, and so forth, tend to be influenced by what they think is "cool" behavior (Cohen, 1985). Some are obviously influenced by peers, using drugs to gain perceived acceptance. Others are sensation-hungry risk takers. After trying drugs for the first time, the adolescent may be drawn to repeated use by the dreamy state of altered consciousness, by the excitement, by heightened acuity, or by feelings of power and confidence. For some, the presumed benefits may come from visual hallucinatory experiences or a sexual sensation (Whaley & Wong, 1987).

There are two broad categories of adolescent drug users: the experimenters and the compulsive users. The experimenters make up the majority of adolescent drug users. A few progress from experimenters to compulsive users. While most experimenters will eventually abandon such use, the fear of progression to compulsive use is a serious concern of parents and authorities. Recreational users fall somewhere in between experimenters and compulsive users. For them, alcohol and marijuana are often the drugs of choice. Their use is primarily to achieve relaxation, and use is typically intermittent. However, for a few, the goal is intoxication, and these recreational users pose a threat to themselves and others (Whaley & Wong, 1987).

Whaley and Wong (1987) suggest that there are four groups of adolescents who are involved in substance abuse:

Social group:	These individuals are involved and motivated by social reasons. They are usually members of the same social group, and use tends to be intermittent.
Escapist group:	These individuals view the use of substances as a means to escape from feelings of anger and depression. Escape, however, is only temporary, and the problems remain unresolved.
Punitive group:	A small group of adolescents see the use of substances as a way of striking back at parents and others. If they are arrested, then others will also experience the suffering that they themselves feel.
Self-destructive group:	These individuals are particularly dangerous to themselves. Their behavior flirts with death, which sometimes becomes a reality either deliberately or accidentally.

The use of alcohol and drugs by adolescent males tends to exceed that of females. Sex ratios, however, vary with the type of substance. The use of amphetamines, for example, has been slightly higher among female high school seniors than among males. Sex differences in the use of tobacco has declined in recent years, as evidenced in the increasing rate of lung cancer among females. Racial differences in drug use tends to be small except for heroin use, which is two to three times more prevalent among blacks than among white adolescents. On the other hand, whites tend to be more involved in alcohol use than African-Americans. Rates of substance abuse tend to be higher in metropolitan areas (Spiegler & Harford, 1987).

The use of legal drugs usually precedes the use of those that are illegal. Three distinct stages of adolescent exposure and experience with drugs have been identified as (1) alcohol and tobacco use, (2) marijuana use, and (3) use of other illicit drugs (Spiegler & Harford, 1987).

The relationships between parents and their adolescents tend to have a bearing on the use of substances. For example, closeness to parents was found to have a positive correlation to moderate teenage drinking compared to heavy drinking. Drinking behavior was found to be less problematic among adolescents who reported similar interests and expectations as their parents. It has consistently been found that adolescents are more likely to drink and use drugs if their parents do (Fawzy, Coombs, & Gerber, 1983). Consequently, children of alcoholics are at high risk of developing alcoholism (Spiegler & Harford, 1987).

While it has been shown consistently that adolescents demonstrate drug use behaviors similar to those of their friends, peer influences are more important for certain substances than others. Use of both marijuana and alcohol is better predicted by the behavior of friends than is the use of other illicit drugs.

The problem of substance abuse is a national crisis and a national tragedy. It is a complex problem that deserves more attention of educators than the brief coverage here. The problem can and must be dealt with through the home, school, and law enforcement authorities as well as through social agencies and responsible media.

EARLY ADULTHOOD

To many, the early adult years, ages twenty to thirty-five or forty (Kaluger & Kaluger, 1986), represent the best years of their lives. To others, it is a time of important decision making coupled with stress and sometimes pain. Young adults are faced with some of the greatest decisions they will ever make in their lives. Some decisions are awesome because of the impact they may have for the remainder of an individual's life.

Decisions must be made regarding the possibility of education beyond high school. If the decision is to continue education, the type of training, as well as the place of training, must be decided. Vocational choices must be determined. Decisions are often made regarding marriage during this period. If the choice is to marry, the critical decision of choosing a mate must be made, as well as the decision of whether or not to have children.

Physical vitality, the excitement of courtship, marriage, the birth of children, and career satisfaction can bring considerable pleasure to individuals during this period of life. At the same time, unwise choices in education or vocation, along with frustration in courtship and failure in marriage, can bring frustration and grief.

During this time of life, individuals are at their physical and mental peak. They are stronger, more physically attractive, and more alert than they will ever be again in their lives. It is likely that many have the resilience to rebound from whatever failures and frustrations they will encounter at this time and that they will continue to enjoy this exciting period in their lives.

During early childhood, most individuals are faced with decisions about dating, marriage, and having children. However, these life experiences are not limited to the period of early adulthood. Dating, singleness, cohabitation, marriage, divorce, and childbearing can be experienced at any age from early adulthood through late adulthood. These issues are included in this section because initial decisions about them often are made during early adulthood.

Dating and Courtship

Whereas many different age-groups are involved in dating, it is an activity that primarily involves adolescents and young adults. Dating has several possible functions. It can serve as a recreational or social activity, be used to select a mate, or be a means to achieve status.

Today, more individuals than in the past view singleness as a viable and preferred option. Whereas part of this reflects a postponement of marriage, some will never marry (Glick, 1977). Changing role expectations, especially for women, greater occupational career opportunities for women, decreased emphasis on childbearing, and greater social opportunities for single persons contribute to this choice of life-style.

Cohabitation also has become an increasingly popular life-style among young individuals. In 1970, there were 523,000 reported unmarried couples cohabitating. In 1986, the number had increased to 2,220,000 (U.S. Bureau of the Census, 1987). Cohabitation allows individuals to share expenses, housing, and sexual and other personal relationships without a legally binding marriage arrangement. Couples may feel that such an arrangement allows for an easier dissolution of a relationship than does marriage.

Marriage and Divorce

Although there is no legal mandate that requires individuals to marry, the social pressures to do so are considerable. Influenced themselves by the social pressures and perhaps by their desire for grandchildren, parents may pressure their children to marry.

Mate selection is often influenced by an individual's cultural background. Although intermarriage across cultural boundaries has become increasingly more prevalent, a large percentage of individuals still marry within their own cultural group. Individuals tend to marry within their own racial or ethnic group, typically within their own language group, their own socioeconomic group, their own religious group, and their own age-group. Some handicapped individuals marry others with the same type of handicapping condition (e.g., blind individuals may select blind mates). However, there are exceptions, with an increasing number of individuals marrying across cultural lines.

With the increasing financial stress created by rising inflation and the assumption of additional expenses, such as a college education for children, dual careers have become a necessity in many families. In addition, changing social values tend to support the concept of women working for both their personal satisfaction and their financial satisfaction. Although these marriages are often characterized by role sharing and by self-fulfillment and self-expression for the woman, they are not without strains on family relationships. As women assume full-time careers, their husbands must often assume greater family responsibility than more traditional roles have prescribed. The effect of these additional responsibilities on the husband may be a function of his willingness to deviate from the traditional roles. When one partner is required to spend more time in career activities, the other must usually spend more time in home activities. There is a delicate balance between give-and-take in these relationships, and it must be worked out to minimize stress and feelings that one partner is being taken advantage of.

When a couple decides that their marriage is no longer viable and they are no longer committed toward keeping it as such, they may seek dissolution through divorce. The legal system, however, has traditionally made divorce difficult and expensive. For years, the courts required that guilt be assigned to one of the partners in a divorce and that punitive actions be assessed against the partner most responsible for the breakup. With the more recent trend toward no-fault divorces, the termination of marriages has been possible with minimal trauma for the parties involved (Hultsch & Deutsch, 1981).

The highest incidence of divorce is found in the age-group under twenty-five, the divorce rate being three times greater than the overall average. Women under the age of twenty are involved in half of the divorces reported annually (Kaluger & Kaluger, 1986). In 1970, the divorce rate in the United States was 3.5 per a population of one thousand. By 1976, the divorce rate reached a record high of five per one thousand (Hultsch & Deutsch, 1981). Apparently, the rate has now stabilized, as the rate in 1986 was identical to the rate ten years prior, five per one thousand (U.S. Bureau of the Census, 1987). Current estimates based on reported data indicate that about one in three marriages end in divorce. This compares to one in seven in 1920 and one in twelve in 1900 (Kaluger & Kaluger, 1986). These divorce trends do not necessarily indicate a movement away from the institution of marriage; 50 percent of divorced men under the age of thirty-five remarry within one year, and 50 percent of divorced women of the same age-group remarry within fourteen months. Within three years, 75 percent of divorced individuals remarry (Hultsch & Deutsch, 1981).

In a study by Wallerstein and Kelly (1980), women were three times more likely than men to precipitate divorce actions. Forty-three percent of the women stated they had been unhappy three-fourths of their married life. Twenty-seven percent of the men responded in the same manner. Women's complaints centered on affective, or emotional, failings related to their husband's personality, the quality of home life, the authority of the husband, and his values. Men's complaints centered on conflict and disagreements regarding their roles and those of their spouses. The authoritarian stance of the wife was also cited. Both men and women from higher-status groups complained more about the lack of emotional support and deficiencies in interpersonal relationships. Those from lower-status groups complained of the spouse's failings and lack of performance of tasks (Kelly, 1982).

Divorce is usually a stressful event for an individual. Not only is there loss of attachment, but there is also the loss of role functioning of either the husband or the wife. The individual may be faced with feelings of loneliness as well as lowered self-esteem. Adjustments must be made in finances, housing, child care, and household maintenance. Women tend to have greater difficulty adjusting to the process of separation, whereas men tend to have greater difficulty after a divorce (Stinnet & Walters, 1977). The stress related to divorce may be second only to death of a spouse in terms of the need to reorganize one's life.

Hetherington, Cox, and Cox (1979) found that divorced women feel overwhelmed by the quantity of tasks that they face. They lack the time and physical energy to meet the demands of household maintenance, financial tasks, child care, and occupational and social responsibilities. As more men are seeking and winning custody of their children, it is likely that some are experiencing similar difficulties. Both divorced men and divorced women indicate disorganization in family activities, such as eating on a regular basis.

Divorced individuals may demonstrate altered self-images and problems in emotional adjustment. Anxiety, anger, rejection, depression, and feelings of incompetence peak during the first year after a divorce and diminish after the second year. Women often experience economic stress, which can be attributed to the lack of financial experience and discrimination encountered in financial dealings. Women also report feelings of unattractiveness, helplessness, and loss of identity, their identity having been associated with their marital status. Men indicate a loss of structure in their lives.

Men often respond to their altered self-images with changes in life-style, such as in their dress style and the purchase of a sports car or motorcycle. Women, on the other hand, may respond with weight change, cosmetic surgery, or a change in hairstyle. These behaviors may be temporary, and they are often abandoned after a satisfying, intimate, heterosexual relationship develops, which improves the self-image.

Divorced individuals may initially have a negative attitude toward social activities. They may feel that the social world is one for couples and tends to exclude singles. Women may have a tendency to feel this even more strongly than men as a result of being locked into the world of their children (Hetherington et al., 1979). Divorced individuals may develop their own social or cultural groups that provide both a social outlet and a support system with understanding individuals experiencing similar problems and concerns.

While divorce has become increasingly more common, the high incidence rates provide little consolation for children. They usually suffer from the separation from one parent. They sometimes must deal with the mistaken notion that they were responsible for the breakup. They must suffer from the changes in the family financial structure, which almost invariably affects them. With a few exceptions, there are numerous "battle scars" and wounds that both parents endure during and after a divorce. The emotional drain on the parents may leave them less equipped to meet the needs of their children. Their patience may be limited, and children can easily feel picked on for behaviors that were previously ignored or unnoticed. Divorced parents may have problems relating to their children, and these problems may take the form of overindulgence, poor communication, or lack of consistent discipline. These problems often manifest themselves at school. On the other hand, some parents may lack the energy or the inclination to discipline their children properly. As the custodial parent seeks to develop new relationships, the children may spend more time with a sitter. It is not uncommon for children to foster hopes of a reconciliation between parents. As parents develop new relationships, children may see their hopes for reconciliation threatened.

Teachers who are aware that children in divorce situations are having adjustment problems should refer them on for appropriate intervention. Most children have a high level of resiliency and adaptability. With appropriate counseling for them and sometimes for their parents, the children's problems may be transitory. Teachers may assist parents by suggesting the names of competent child therapists and mental health clinics, which usually charge on a sliding scale, enabling any parent to secure necessary services.

MIDDLE AGE

The middle-aged group in American society now represents a significant portion of the total population. Approximately 25 percent of the population is between the ages of forty and sixty-four years. Middle age is typically viewed as a period of transition, and for some, a period of crisis or stress. Some theorists have compared the stress of middle age to the stress experienced in adolescence. According to Gould (1978): "Mid-life, then, is every bit as turbulent as adolescence, except now we can use all this striving to blend a healthier, happier life. For unlike adolescents, in midlife we know and can accept who we are" (p. 17).

Mid-life transition is usually a span of four to six years, culminating when individuals reach their early forties. The two basic tasks of this transition period are (1) the appraisal of earlier life structures and (2) the making of choices that will modify the earlier structures and provide a basis for living in middle adulthood. As individuals make new commitments or make recommitments to an earlier life structure, the transition phase is left behind, and full entry is made into middle adulthood.

Biological functioning peaks between the late teens and late twenties. By the beginning of middle age, most individuals have begun to notice various forms of physical decline. These are often characterized by loss of muscle tone and physical strength, decreased perceptual acuity, loss of teeth, slowing of central nervous system functioning, arthritis, periodontal (gum) disease, dermatological problems and other changes in pigmentation, and cardiac and other physiological dysfunctions. A number of changes in physical appearance, such as gray hair, baldness, wrinkles, and weight gain, accompany the physiological changes. Most of the physiological and appearance changes of middle age do not interfere with most routine daily functioning and are not likely to alter everyday life-styles significantly. However, these changes serve as reminders of advancing age and may have more psychological than physiological significance.

Although the mortality for this age-group may not be high compared to that of the aged, it is, of course, considerably higher than for young adults. Physical decline and occasional deaths of friends and associates in the same age cohort serve as reminders that death is inevitable. For young adults, life may seem endless. The concepts of retirement and death may seem abstract. However, to the middle aged, these concepts become realities, frightening realities for some. At mid-life, there tends to be a psychological shift in time perspective, as some individuals begin to view life from the perspective of time left to live as opposed to time since birth.

Career and Life Satisfaction

During middle age, many individuals reach the highest levels of their careers in both status and income. Many married women who have not been employed enter the labor market or return to work or school during this period (Siegler & Edelman, 1977). As previously indicated, the functions of middle age include appraising earlier structures. As individuals evaluate career choices and determine their level of satisfaction, they may conclude that they are not satisfied with their earlier choices and decide to change to a career that is more meaningful and satisfying.

The middle years are a time in which individuals are faced with transition. It is a difficult time for some who face retirement and advancing years unwillingly and reluctantly. It is a period in which individuals are able to reflect on the earlier decisions in life and measure comparative successes or failures. It is a time when children leave home and couples are able to commit a greater amount of time to their relationship and experience a higher level of marriage satisfaction.

THE AGED

All individuals who live in their mid-sixties will become members of the microculture of the aged, along with their membership in other microcultures. As with other minority groups, the aged are often discriminated against. But unlike discrimination against minority groups, the individuals who discriminate will also someday become a part of the aged group, and they themselves may become victims of discrimination. Butler and Lewis (1982) describe ageism as "a systematic stereotyping of and discrimination against people because they are old, just as racism and sexism accomplish this in relation to skin color and gender" (p. xvii). They further suggest that the elderly are stereotyped as senile, rigid in thought and manner, garrulous, and old-fashioned in morality and skills.

In our society, little value is placed on nonproduction. It is understandable, then, why some individuals may adopt an ageist attitude. American society also places much emphasis on physical beauty. The physical ideal is associated with youth, and the aging process only serves to remove an individual farther from the accepted norms related to physical beauty.

As the body changes because of the aging process, health problems may develop. Death itself is inevitable, and the older an individual becomes, the greater the likelihood of death. Because many of the aged live on a limited income, they often become victims of poverty. These realities of the aged, coupled with genuine philosophical and value differences with younger generations, may contribute to the attitudes of ageism. If ageists live long enough to become old, their attitudes may turn into self-hatred (Butler & Lewis, 1982).

Who Are the Aged?

The age of sixty-five years is often used as an arbitrary demarcation between middle and old age. This age has been used to determine retirement or services available for the elderly. The age of sixty-five itself has little relevance in describing various aspects of functioning, such as general health, mental capacity, psychological or physical endurance, or creativity. Gerontologists tend to designate the ages of sixty-five to seventy-four years as early old age, and seventy-five years and older as advanced old age. The use of age in years serves only as a convenience rather than as an accurate indicator of a person's physical and mental status (Butler & Lewis, 1982).

In 1986, there were an estimated 29.2 million people who were sixty-five years of age or older in the United States (U.S. Bureau of the Census, 1987). With the advent of modern medical technology and improved living conditions, average life expectancy in the United States is now 75.4 years (U.S. Bureau of the Census, 1987). This compares with an average life expectancy of 47 years in 1900, when only 4 percent of the population was sixty-five or older. Every day, while approximately 5,000 Americans reach the age of sixty-five, 3,400 individuals over the age of sixty-five die. This, however, provides a net increase of 1,600 a day into the ranks of the elderly. This translates into about 584,000 per year (Whitaker, 1981).

The aged constitute slightly more than 10 percent of the American population. As such, they constitute a statistical minority. The aged resemble other oppressed minority groups in that they suffer from prejudice, discrimination, and deprivation. On the other hand, they differ from other minority groups in that they are not born into their age-group.

There are three basic misconceptions that the rest of society tends to have regarding the aged:

1. Most elderly people are sick or infirm. The reality is that only 20 percent of persons over sixty-five years old are in this category, and only 10 percent are unable to engage in normal activity.

2. Most elderly people are senile. The fact is that less than 10 percent of the aged have incapacitating mental illness or senility.

3. Most elderly people cannot be productive. The reality is that as a group, the elderly are as productive as young workers, are less prone to job turnover, and have lower accident and absentee rates.

The aged are discriminated against in many areas that affect their well-being and life-style. For example, many employers discriminate against them in hiring and retention. In addition, many medical personnel admit that they prefer not to treat the elderly, and some younger people, because of their prejudices, appear to avoid the elderly (Palmore, 1978).

As a microculture, only some of the aged seem to have a sense of group identity. Some utilize chronological indices to determine the advent of old age, while the remainder generally use functional criteria, such as retirement or health conditions. Some are ashamed of old age and resist identification with the elderly. At the same time, some among the aged have adopted a militant posture, forming groups to protest and promote the rights of the elderly.

As a group, the aged make up a potent political force. As the federal and state governments move toward balancing their budgets, social and welfare programs have often been cut. With many of the elderly living on fixed incomes, they are rightfully fearful of cuts that impact directly on the quality of their lives. Consequently, as a group, they typically exercise their right to vote to a greater extent than other age-groups. The recognition of their voter influence was evident in the 1988 elections, where candidates openly courted the votes of this group, pledging to support their interests.

The aged are understandably concerned about voter issues related to the maintenance or enhancement of Social Security and health-care benefits. They are more likely than other groups to support "tax payer revolts" and resist any efforts toward revenue enhancement, which will affect their incomes. Since they are typically no longer involved in their education or that of their children, attempts to increase school revenues through taxes are often resisted. Efforts such as California's proposition 13, which rolled back property taxes but had a negative impact on education, have had wide support.

It has become increasingly more important to educators and their supporters that the aged, as well as other segments of the population, be appropriately sensitized to the importance of a well-educated society. In addition to the more altruistic reasons for supporting education, more pragmatic approaches may be appropriate, pointing out that a more educated citizenry detracts less from social/welfare programs and contributes more taxes to their support.

Interaction of Age with Ethnicity and Socioeconomic Status

In the United States, the life expectancy is lower for blacks than for whites. It can be assumed that the lower socioeconomic conditions accorded to African-Americans are prominent factors in this phenomenon. African-Americans make up nearly 12 percent of the general population but only about 8 percent of the older age-group. Poor health conditions for many of them contribute greatly to the disproportionately high mortality for this group. Butler and Lewis (1982) suggest that institutionalized racism falls most heavily on black men, and their average life expectancy in 1986 was 65.5 years of age, compared with 72 years of age for white men. With improved opportunities and living conditions for blacks, however, life expectancy of this group is on the rise, as evidenced by the increase of black elderly persons from 1.2 million in 1960 to 2.2 million in 1982 (U.S. Bureau of the Census, 1987).

At birth, the average life expectancy of a white person is more than 6½ years greater than that of a nonwhite. In addition, the nonwhite aged are more likely to be poor than their white counterparts. Butler and Lewis (1982) suggest that although there are more poor whites than poor blacks, the proportion of poor blacks is greater, and their poverty is more profound. Without the resources to provide for a quality retirement life, it is understandable why ethnic minorities as a group may tend to perceive old age less favorably than whites. However, within the traditional culture, older Native Americans do have the respect accorded them because of their cultural values, which identify wisdom and old age. Older Asian-Americans enjoy the deference paid to them by the young as part of their traditional Asian cultural values. However, individuals from these groups who are highly assimilated may respond to the aged in a manner more typical of the mainstream culture.

Socioeconomic status tends to be a major factor in the adjustment to old age. As with the earlier years in life, income influences longevity, health status, housing, and marital status for the aged. Elderly persons with a high income have a number of advantages associated with their greater financial resources. In earlier years, they were able to maintain better living conditions and better health care, which often translates into better health in the advanced years. Their financial resources enable them to maintain these higher living and health-care standards. This advantage, in turn, may result in extended quality leisure activities, such as travel, which makes the retirement years more pleasurable. It is understandable, therefore, why individuals from high socioeconomic backgrounds tend to view old age more favorably than those from low socioeconomic backgrounds.

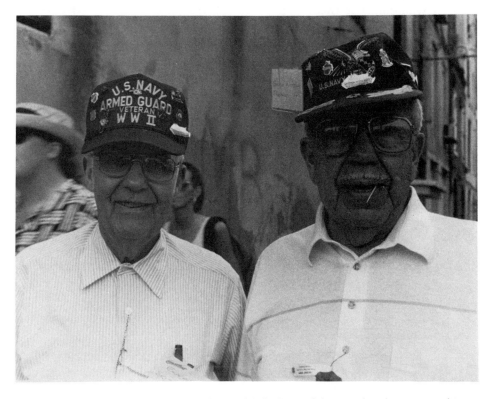

Many older people are able to travel and enjoy life far beyond the time that they stop working.

(Photo by Susan Tucker.)

Adjustment

Adjustment to old age is a function of a number of variables, such as sex, adequacy of support systems, socioeconomic status, ethnic background, and whether an individual faces old age alone or with a spouse. Old age usually brings with it retirement for the individual. A woman may find retirement less traumatic than a man; she typically has had to face numerous role adjustments in her life. As a mother, a woman may have had to leave the labor force—at least temporarily—to have children. The woman whose primary function during part of her life was that of mother had to change roles as her children grew and left home. Many men have had one primary role—the major breadwinner. Thus, for many men, retirement marks a dramatic change in life-style.

Widowers tend to face even greater adjustment problems than widows. Most women expect to become widows, whereas few men anticipate losing a spouse. Men are often unprepared to assume household responsibilities and find few men in similar situations to provide companionship and support. Widows, however, have a large potential group of other widows from whom to draw support. Older women may have better support systems than men; they may see their children and relatives more often than older men do (Itzin, 1970); they also tend to be more involved in community-level organizations and activities.

Palmore (1978) suggests that several trends will reduce prejudice against the elderly. Although a generation ago few gerontologists could be found, there are now thousands in the profession. Institutions for higher education are now offering numerous courses in gerontology, and centers for research and training in gerontology are opening around the United States. In addition, the federal government has now established the National Institute on Aging for Gerontological Research. These efforts in research and education will gradually undercut the roots of discrimination and prejudice against the elderly. Palmore (1978) suggests that we appear to be moving toward an age-irrelevant society in which age becomes irrelevant to a person's rights and opportunities.

As individuals mature in age, they will eventually move through a number of different age-groups, and as such, they will become members of different microcultures. As individuals join new age-group cultures they bring with them other aspects of culture, such as ethnicity, socioeconomic status, and sex. As these various cultures interface with one another and blend their individual unique qualities, they add to the rich pluralistic nature of American society.

EDUCATIONAL IMPLICATIONS

As with other microcultures, the various age-groups of the U.S. population contribute greatly to the pluralistic nature of this society. There are some basic educational considerations in the study of age-groups as a function of culture. American society in general has not always been viewed as particularly supportive or positive in its perception of all age-groups. The discussion on adolescence noted that this period is often viewed as a time of storm and stress, whereas in some cultures this period passes with few crises. In American society, the former view tends to prevail. In addition, advancing age is not viewed by the U.S. macroculture with the respect or reverence that is found in many other cultures. Ageism does exist and is regretfully as much a part of our social system as is racism and handicapism.

For these reasons, it is critically important that students be exposed to age as it relates to culture. Moreover, studying age and its relation to culture is important because students, if they live to full life expectancy, will become members of each age-group. Thus, unlike the study of different ethnic groups, students can learn to understand and appreciate microcultures of which they have been members, are presently members, or will eventually be members. By addressing the issues of various age-groups in the classroom, educators can assist students to better understand their siblings, parents, and other important persons in their lives. Knowledge can eliminate fear of the unknown as students begin to move into different age-groups at different times in their lives. It is important that issues related to age-groups be appropriately introduced into the curriculum. Students need to understand the concept of ageism. Just as the school assists students in understanding the problem of racism, the school should be responsible for helping students to understand the aged and to dispel the myths related to this group. Field trips to retirement homes or visits to the class by senior citizens may provide useful experiences. As students become aware of the nature and characteristics of each age-group, they will develop perceptions of each individual, regardless of age, as being an important and integral part of society.

It is critically important for educators to understand age as it relates to both students and their parents. Understanding the particular age-group characteristics and needs of the students can assist the educator to better understand and manage age-related behavior, such as reactions or responses to peer group pressure. Understanding the nature of parents, siblings, and other important individuals (e.g., grandparents) will assist the educator in parent-teacher relationships as well as in helping students to cope with their interaction with others.

For example, when the parents of a child in the third grade are in the process of separation and divorce, a teacher who understands the nature of such a traumatic event can better assist the student in school as well as help with some personal adjustment. As an elderly grandparent moves into the family setting, this event may impact on a child and affect classroom behavior.

The school is perhaps in the best position of any agency in the community to observe the effects of child abuse. The classroom teacher is an important agent in detecting and reporting abuse and in some states is required by law to do so. To do this, the teacher must be aware of the problem of abuse, the manifestations of abuse, and the proper authorities to whom abuse is reported. If the teacher's immediate supervisor is unresponsive to the reporting of a potential abuse problem, the teacher should then continue to seek help until it is provided by competent and concerned individuals in positions of authority.

The single most important factor in determining possible child abuse is the physical condition of the child. Telltale marks, bruises, and abrasions that cannot be adequately explained may provide reason to suspect abuse. Unusual changes in the child's behavior patterns, such as extreme fatigue, may be reason to suspect problems. The parents' behavior and their ability or lack of ability to explain the child's condition and the social features of the family may be reason to suspect abuse. While physical abuse or neglect may tend to have observable indicators, sexual abuse may occur with few if any obvious indicators. Adults may be unwilling to believe what a child is saying and may be hesitant to report alleged incidents. There is no typical profile of the victim, and the physical signs vary. Behavioral manifestations are usually exhibited by the victims but are often viewed as insignificant or attributed to typical childhood stress. Chronic depression, isolation from peers, apathy, and suicide attempts are some of the more serious behavioral manifestations of the problem (Sarles, 1980).

The majority of suicides are planned and not committed on impulse. The majority of suicide victims mention their intentions to someone. Of adolescents who commit suicide, 80 percent make open threats beforehand (Griffin & Felsenthal, 1983). There are often a number of warning signs that can alert teachers, other professionals, and parents. The following are some of the danger signals (Griffin & Felsenthal, 1983):

☐ Aggressive, hostile behavior

☐ Alcohol and drug abuse

☐ Passive behavior

☐ Changes in eating habits

☐ Changes in sleeping habits

☐ Fear of separation

☐ Abrupt changes in personality

☐ Sudden mood swings

☐ Decreased interest in schoolwork and decline in grades

☐ Inability to concentrate

☐ Hopelessness

☐ Obsession with death

☐ Giving away valued possessions

☐ Euphoria or increased activity after depression

If trouble is suspected by teachers or other school personnel, friendly, low-key questions or statements may provide an appropriate opening: "You seem down today"; "Seems like something is bothering you." If an affirmative response is given, a more direct and probing (but supportive) question may be asked. If there is any reason whatsoever to suspect a possible suicide attempt, teachers and other school staff should alert the appropriate school personnel. Teachers should recognize their limitations and avoid making judgments. The matter should be referred to the school psychologist, who should in turn alert a competent medical authority (i.e., a psychiatrist) and the child's parents. Assistance can also be obtained from local mental health clinics and suicide prevention centers. Prompt action may save a life.

Our coverage of adolescent substance abuse has been brief. But the importance of the problem is such that every educator should be aware of the problem and work toward providing children at an early age with appropriate drug education. No agency, group, or individual can wage an effective campaign against substance abuse alone. Only with a united effort can an effective battle be waged.

Hafen and Frandsen (1980) indicate that there are danger signs for drug or alcohol ingestion that may place the individual at life-threatening risk:

1. *Unconsciousness.* [The] individual cannot be awakened or if awakened lapses back into deep sleep.

2. *Breathing difficulties.* Breathing stops altogether, may be weak, or weak and strong in cycles. Skin may become bluish or purple indicating lack of oxygenated blood.

3. *Fever.* Any temperature above 100° F (38° C) is a danger sign when drugs are involved.

4. *Vomiting while not fully conscious.* In a stupor, semiconscious or unconscious state vomiting can cause serious breathing problems.

5. *Convulsions.* Twitching of face, trunk, arms or legs; muscle spasms or muscle rigidity may indicate impending convulsions. Violent jerking motions and spasms likely indicate a convulsion.

In the event that these signs are observed in the classroom, the school nurse should be summoned immediately. If none is available, then someone trained in CPR should be summoned. It would be advisable for a list of all personnel with CPR training to be made available for all teachers and staff.

As parents hurry children into adulthood, educators may also contribute to the hurrying process. Teachers, administrators, and support personnel should be cognizant of the fact that the children they teach and work with are children and not miniature adults. Children have but one opportunity to experience the wonders of childhood. In comparison to adulthood, childhood and adolescence are relatively short periods of time, and these young people should have every opportunity to enjoy these stages of their lives to the fullest extent possible.

SUMMARY

The study of age as a microculture is important to educators because it helps them to understand how the child or adolescent struggles to win peer acceptance and balance this effort with the need for parental approval. In some instances, the pressures from peers are not congruent with those that come from the home.

As each child develops into adolescence, we observe a growing need for independence. Adolescence for some is a time of storm and stress, while for others it passes with little or no trauma. Early adulthood is one of the most exciting times in life. It is a time for courtship, marriage, children, and career choices. It is a time when individuals reach their physical prime. Young adulthood can also be a threatening time, as choices made at this time often have a lifetime impact on the individual. While this is a time for many to marry, it is a time in which many also experience the frustrations of divorce.

Middle age is a time when some reach a mid-life transition. During this period, the individual appraises earlier life structures and makes decisions that affect those earlier structures and which provide a basis for living in middle adulthood. This is a period when the individual begins to notice various forms of physical decline, serving as a reminder that old age may be "around the corner."

With life expectancy increasing each year, those in the aged cohort increase in numbers daily. There is a net increase of over a half million into the ranks of the aged each year. Like the ethnic minorities and the handicapped, the aged face discrimination and prejudice in the form of ageism. Those who discriminate will someday become aged, perhaps to face the treatment that they themselves imposed on others.

QUESTIONS FOR REVIEW

1. What are the major characteristics of the childhood period?

2. Explain why child abuse is a problem, and cite the signs of child abuse.

3. When does ethnic identification begin in children, and how is it manifested?

4. How does peer group pressure influence children and adolescents?

5. What are the sources of alienation between adolescents and their families?

6. What is the extent of substance abuse among adolescents, and what are some of the underlying causes of substance use in this age-group?

7. What are the causes of adolescent suicide, and what are the warning signs?

8. Why is early adulthood an exciting yet threatening time in an individual's life?

9. What is mid-life transition?

10. How does old age relate to ethnicity and socioeconomic status?

11. What are the roots of ageism?

REFERENCES

Anselmo, S. (1987). *Early childhood development.* Columbus, OH: Merrill Publishing.

Butler, R. N., & Lewis, M. I. (1982). *Aging and mental health: Positive psychosocial and biomedical approaches* (3rd ed.). St. Louis: Mosby.

Cantor, P. (1976). Personality characteristics found among youthful female suicide attempters. *Journal of Abnormal Psychology, 85,* 324–329.

Centers for Disease Control (CDC). (1986, November). *Youth suicide in the United States, 1970–1980.* Atlanta, GA: Department of Health and Human Services.

Cohen, S. (1985). *Substance abuse problems* (Vol. 2). New York: Haworth Press.

Coleman, J. S. (1961). *The adolescent society.* Glencoe, IL: The Free Press.

Comer, J. P., & Poussaint, A. F. (1975). *Black child care: How to bring up a healthy black child in America.* New York: Simon & Schuster.

Cormerci, G. D. (1986). Foreclosing on life. *The Journal of Pediatrics, 109*(4), 723–725.

Dolan, M. (1989, June 2). Study finds perilous levels of lead in 20% of children. *Los Angeles Times,* pp. 1, 28–29.

Elkind, D. (1981). *The hurried child.* Reading, Mass.: Addison-Wesley.

Erickson, E. H. (1963). *Childhood and society* (2nd ed.). New York: Norton.

Fawzy, F. I., Coombs, R. H., & Gerber, B. (1983). Generational continuity in the use of substances: The impact of parental substance use on adolescent use. *Addictive Behaviors, 8,* 109–114.

Gelles, R. J. (1982). Problems in defining and labeling child abuse. In R. H. Starr, Jr. (Ed.)., *Child abuse prediction: Policy implication.* Cambridge, MA: Ballinger.

Gelman, D., & Gangelhoff, V. K. (1983, August). Teenage suicide in the sunbelt. *Newsweek, 15,* pp. 70–74.

Gispert, M. (1981, February). Sexual conflicts and concerns of adolescent girls. *Medical Aspects of Human Sexuality, 2,* 32a, 32e.

Gispert, M., & Falk, R. (1978). Adolescent sexual activity: Contraception and abortion. *American Journal of Obstetrics and Gynecology, 132,* 620–628.

Glick, P. C. (1977). Updating the life cycle of the family. *Journal of Marriage and Family, 39,* 5–15.

Gould, R. L. (1978). *Transformations: Growth and change in adult life.* New York: Simon & Schuster.

Griffin, M. E., & Felsenthal, C. (1983). *A cry for help.* Garden City, NY: Doubleday.

Guetzloe, E. C. (1989). *Youth suicide: What the educator should know.* Reston, VA: The Council for Exceptional Children.

Hafen, B. Q., & Frandsen, K. J. (1980). *Drug and alcohol emergencies.* Center City, MN: Hazelden Foundation.

Hawton, K. (1986). *Suicide and attempted suicide among children and adolescents.* Beverly Hills, CA: Sage.

Hendin, H. (1985). Suicide among the young: Psychodynamics and demography. In M. L. Peck, N. L. Farberew, & R. E. Litman (Eds.), *Youth suicide* (pp. 19–38). New York: Springer.

Hetherington, E. M., & Cox, M., & Cox, R. (1979). Stress and coping in divorce: A focus on women. In J. E. Gullahorn (Ed.), *Psychology and women in transition.* Washington, DC: Winston.

Hipple, J., & Cimbolic, P. (1979). *The counselor and suicidal crisis.* Springfield, IL: Thomas.

Hultsch, D. C., & Deutsch, F. (1981). *Adult development and aging.* New York: McGraw-Hill.

Hyde, M., & Forsyth, E. (1978). *Suicide.* New York: Franklin Watts.

Itzin, F. (1970). Social relations. In A. M. Hoffman (Ed.), *The daily needs and interests of older people*. Springfield, IL: Thomas.

Jobes, D. A., Berman, A. L., & Josselsen, A. R. (1986). The impact of psychological autopsies on Medical Examiners' Determination of Manner of Death. *Journal of Forensic Science, 31*(2), 177–189.

Johnson, L. D., O'Malley, P. M., & Bachman, J. G. (1986). *Drug use among American high school students and other young adults: National trends through 1985* [Publication No. (ABM) 86-1450]. Rockville, MD: National Institute on Drug Abuse.

Kaluger, G., & Kaluger, M. F. (1986). *Human development: The span of life* (3rd ed.). Columbus, OH: Merrill Publishing.

Katz, P. A. (1982). Development of children's racial awareness and intergroup attitudes. In L. G. Kutz (Ed.), *Current topics in early childhood education* (Vol. 4). Norwood, NJ: Ablex.

Kaufman, M. (1983). Physical abuse, neglect, and sexual abuse: Dimensions and framework. In N. B. Ebeling & D. A. Hill (Eds.), *Child abuse and neglect*. Boston: John Wright, PSG.

Kelly, J. B. (1982). Divorce: The adult perspective. In B. B. Wolman (Ed.), *Handbook of developmental psychology*. Englewood Cliffs, NJ: Prentice-Hall.

Lewin, K. (1939). Field theory and experiment in social psychology: Concepts and methods. *American Journal of Sociology, 44*, 868.

Meil, A., & Kiester, E. (1967). *The shortchanged children in suburbia*. New York: Institute of Human Relations Press, American Jewish Committee.

Miller, J. (1975). Suicide and adolescence. *Adolescence, 10*, 13–23.

Millman, R. B., & Khuri, E. T. (1981). Adolescence and substance abuse. In J. H. Lowinson & P. Ruiz (Eds.), *Substance abuse: Clinical problems and perspectives*. Baltimore: Williams & Wilkins.

Morland, J. K. (1972). Racial acceptance and preference of nursery school children in a southern city. In A. R. Brown (Ed.), *Prejudice in children*. Springfield, IL: Thomas.

Newman, B. M., & Newman, P. R. (1986). *Adolescent development*. Columbus, OH: Merrill.

Palmore, E. (1978). Are the aged a minority group? *Journal of the American Geriatrics Society, 26*, 214–216.

Pffeffer, R. (1986). *Suicidal child*. New York: The Guilford Press.

Ray, L. Y., & Johnson, N. (1983). Adolescent suicide. *The Personnel and Guidance Journal, 62*(3), 131–135.

Sarles, R. M. (1980). Incest. *Pediatric Review 2*(2), 51–54.

Siegler, I. C., & Edelman, C. D. (1977, April). *Age discrimination in employment: Implication for psychologists*. Paper presented at Western Psychological Association, San Francisco.

Spiegler, D. L., & Harford, T. C. (1987). Addictive behaviors among youth. In T. D. Nirenberg & S. A. Maistro (Eds.), *Developments in the assessment and treatment of addictive behaviors*. Norwood, NJ: Ablex.

Stinnet, N., & Walters, L. M. (1977). *Relationships in marriage and family*. New York: Macmillan.

Thompson, M. (1983). Organizing a human services network for primary and secondary prevention of the emotional and physical neglect and abuse of children. In J. E. Leavitt (Ed.), *Child abuse and neglect: Research and innovation*. Boston: Martinus Nijhoff.

U. S. Bureau of the Census. (1987). *Statistical abstract of the United States: 1988* (10th ed.). Washington, DC: Government Printing Office.

Wallerstein, J. S., & Kelly, J. B. (1980). *Surviving the breakup: How children and parents cope with divorce*. New York: Basic Books.

Wenz, F. (1979). Self-injury behavior, economic status, and the family anomie syndrome among adolescents. *Adolescence, 14*, 387–397.

Whaley, L. F., & Wong, D. L. (1987). *Nursing care of infants and children* (3rd ed.). St. Louis: Mosby.

Whitaker, J. D. (1981, April). Elderly women face years alone, often in poverty. *The Washington Post, 20*, pp. A1, A4, A5.

Zelnick, M., & Kantner, J. F. (1980). Sexual activity, contraceptive use and pregnancy among metropolitan-area teenagers: 1971–1979. *Family Planning Perspectives, 12*, 230–237.

SUGGESTED READINGS

Butler, R. N., & Lewis, M. I. (1982). *Aging and mental health: Positive psychosocial and biomedical approaches* (3rd ed.). St. Louis: Mosby.

This thorough and detailed treatment of the elderly provides insightful information of this growing segment of the population.

Guetzloe, E. D. (1989). *Youth suicide: What the educator should know*. Reston, VA: The Council for Exceptional Children.

A very good monograph written in two parts. Part I, "Toward an Understanding of Youth Suicide," provides information on trends, issues, statistics, risk factors, events precipitating suicide, treatment, and so forth. Part II, "Suicide Prevention in the School," has nine sections and includes school plans for intervention, assessment of suicide potential, working with parents, and counseling suicidal students.

Hultsch, D. C., & Deutsch, F. (1981). *Adult development and aging*. New York: McGraw-Hill.

This excellent treatment of various age groups provides some of the more recent research.

CHAPTER 9
Strategies for Multicultural Education

Educators are expected to assist students in reaching their academic, vocational, and social potentials. This task can be difficult and demanding when faced with a class-room of thirty students who have different educational needs and experiences. School records often indicate students' intellectual abilities as measured by standardized tests; physical problems; and psychological problems. More helpful than any of this information in providing successful educational experiences will be information regarding their cultural backgrounds. At the same time, there is sometimes a tendency to stereotype students' behavior and values based on racial and class characteristics that are easily identifiable. To use cultural information effectively in developing educational services, it is necessary to understand students' membership in various micro-cultures as described in earlier chapters of this book.

An educator should be able to understand and utilize students' cultural back-grounds in developing educational programs. However, the degree of identity with the various microcultures to which one belongs varies greatly from individual to in-dividual. The impact of one's membership in a specific microculture often has an even greater impact because of how others view it and its relationship to the dominant society. Educators must be careful not to stereotype students based on their member-ship in one of the many microcultures. Too often, teachers' expectations have been based on ethnic or class identity, with the result that equal education is not provided.

How can educators begin to use their knowledge about microcultural member-ships in the classroom? How do they begin to develop appropriate instructional strategies for thirty students in the classroom—thirty students who may have thirty different cultural backgrounds? It seems a lofty, almost insurmountable task to under-stand the cultural identities of the 30 to 150 students one may see daily. Often, educators meet only those parents who attend parent organization meetings or who schedule conferences with them. Sometimes, educators neither live, nor have ever lived, in the community in which their students live. This lack of firsthand knowl-edge about the community sometimes makes it difficult to understand the cultural differences and experiences of the residents of that community.

Multicultural education is a means for positively using cultural diversity in the total learning process. A critical element is the incorporation of issues and strategies related to membership in different microcultures, especially race, gender, and class. If we continuously address only one of these areas without referring to the interrela-tionships with the others, students will begin to think that they are totally separate elements of multicultural education. We cannot neglect one while trying to overcome the others. If we develop activities to fight racism, but continue to perpetuate sex-ism, we are not providing multicultural education. At the same time, we should not forget women of color and poor women when discussing women's issues. In the pre-ceding seven chapters, examples of educational strategies were outlined for the various microcultures. In all cases, membership in the other microcultures can—and should—be woven into these strategies. However, in this chapter, general recommendations for the delivery of multicultural education will be made.

Let us review the goals of multicultural education: (1) to promote the strength and value of cultural diversity; (2) to promote human rights and respect for those who are different from ourselves; (3) to acquire a knowledge of the historical and social realities of U.S. society in order to understand racism, sexism, and poverty; (4) to support alternative life choices for people; (5) to promote social justice and equality for all people; and (6) to promote equity in the distribution of power and income among groups.

TEXTBOOKS AND INSTRUCTIONAL MATERIALS

One can easily become overwhelmed by the total number of instructional materials available for use in the classroom. There are over five hundred thousand different materials available for classroom use. A recent edition of *Elementary/High School Textbooks in Print* listed over twenty thousand titles of textbooks alone, and the National Center for Educational Media listed over five hundred thousand unpublished titles. The textbook industry is big business. Over $1 billion a year is spent on elementary and high school books—more than is spent on all other hardcover and paperback books sold in the United States (Starr, 1989).

How important are instructional materials in the classroom? "Ninety percent of all classroom activity is regulated by textbooks" (Starr, 1989, p. 106). Much of the student's classroom time also is structured around printed material. How much control an educator has over the instructional materials to be used in the classroom often depends on the school district or state in which one teaches. There are now twenty-four states, including the two largest—Texas and California—where textbooks must be adopted by the state before they can be used in the classroom (Starr, 1989). In the other states, the teacher may have some role in selecting the textbook to be used in the classroom. Most often, however, texts are assigned to teachers. Although a few teachers serve on a school district committee or state committee to select textbooks for the area, most teachers have no role in the selection process.

Although it may seem that the teacher often does not have much control over the textbooks to be used in the classroom, it is an area in which the teacher can make many important decisions. In most cases, there is a great deal of latitude about the kind of supplementary materials to be used. In most cases, there is a choice about how dependent the curriculum is on the textbooks and materials that are assigned to the classroom. In many schools, students are expected to be at a certain level of academic competency by the time the school year ends. How the teacher ensures that students learn the necessary concepts depends on the teacher. As instructional decision makers, educators are in influential positions (Gollnick, Sadker, & Sadker, 1982).

Many teachers have come to rely heavily on the textbook. A textbook has often been used to determine the curriculum and subsequent instructional strategies. Remember the teacher who used to announce on the first day of school how far in the textbook students had to be by the last day of school? Even for teachers who do not rely heavily on the textbook to teach, it probably remains the most important educational tool in the classroom. Other than the teacher and the chalkboard, the textbook is probably the most standard item in all classrooms. How textbooks and

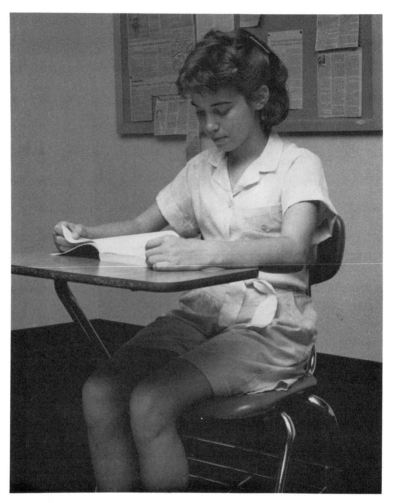

The textbook remains a standard item in the classroom. No matter how old textbooks are, the teacher can use them effectively to provide multicultural education.

(Photo by Sheryl Zelhart).

other instructional materials are used is extremely important in providing multicultural education.

One of the problems in depending on the textbook for classroom instruction is that many educators never question the validity of its contents. "Knowledge is often accepted as truth legitimizing a specific view of the world that is either questionable or patently false" (Giroux, 1988, p. 31). Too often, we read the information as if it were unquestionably accurate. Consequently, it is difficult to begin reading critically for multicultural content and sensitivity. A first step is to examine critically the materials used in the classroom. We must be able to recognize the biases that often exist in such materials and develop instructional strategies to counteract those biases. Sadker and Sadker (1978) have identified six forms of bias in classroom materials.

The first bias, *invisibility*, is the underrepresentation of certain microcultures in materials. This omission implies that these groups have less value, importance, and significance in our society (Sadker & Sadker, 1978). Invisibility in instructional materials occurs most frequently for women, minority groups, handicapped individuals, and older persons. After an analysis of the most widely used high school U.S. history text, for example, Trecker (1977) summarized the role of women as seen in these books as follows:

> Women arrived in 1619. They held the Seneca Falls Convention on women's rights in 1848. During the rest of the nineteenth century, they participated in reform movements, chiefly temperance, and were exploited in factories. In 1920 they were given the vote. They joined the armed forces during the Second World War and thereafter have enjoyed the good life in America. (p. 252)

A similar omission occurs for other groups that are subordinate to the dominant culture. It is a characteristic not only of history books but of texts in all subject areas.

Materials can be examined for invisibility simply by counting the number of times different groups are represented in the text, in illustrations, in various occupations, in biographies, or as main characters. This technique was used by researchers who analyzed 134 readers and found the following ratios regarding gender (Women on Words and Images, 1975):

Boy-centered stories to girl-centered stories	7:2
Male illustrations to female illustrations	2:1
Male occupations to female occupations	3:1
Male biographies to female biographies	2:1

Another study of science, math, reading, spelling, and social studies textbooks revealed that only 31 percent of all illustrations included girls and women and that the percentage of females decreased as the grade level increased. This same pattern was found for illustrations of people of color. The most invisible member of school texts was the minority female. She appeared only half as often as the minority male and made up only 7 percent of all girls and women in textbooks (Weitzman & Rizzo, 1974). Because children need strong positive role models for the development of their self-esteem, the omission of members of their own microcultures is serious. It often teaches members of those groups that they are less important and less significant in our society than are majority males.

A second bias, *stereotyping*, assigns traditional and rigid roles or attributes to a group. It denies the diversity, complexity, and variety of individuals (Sadker & Sadker, 1978). Stereotyping occurs across cultural groups. Probably the most common occurrence is in the area of vocational and career choices, especially for men, women, minority, and handicapped individuals. When Mexican-Americans are shown working only in fields as migrant workers and never in professional jobs, stereotyping is occurring. Such bias denies the reality of individual differences and prevents readers from understanding the complexity and diversity that occur within groups.

Selectivity and imbalance occurs when issues and situations are interpreted from only one perspective, almost always the perspective of the dominant group. The authors of textbooks collect hundreds of pages of notes from which they write the book. They must decide what is most important and should be included. The authors determine whether the emphasis in a history book will be on wars and political decisions or on families and the arts. As the authors select content, the contributions of one group of people may be highlighted, and those of another group may be partially or totally omitted. In a study of the portrayal of the labor movement in secondary school history textbooks, Anyon (1979) concludes that the textbook

> suggests a great deal about the society that produces and uses it. It reveals which groups have power and demonstrates that the views of these groups are expressed and legitimized in the school curriculum. It can also identify social groups that are not empowered by the economic and social patterns in our society and do not have their views, activities, and priorities represented in the school curriculum. The present analysis suggests that the United States working class is one such group; the poor may be another. Omissions, stereotypes, and distortions that remain in "updated" social studies textbook accounts of Native Americans, Blacks, and women reflect the relative powerlessness of these groups. (p. 382)

In Trecker's study (1977) of the most widely used history textbooks, she found that there was more information on the length of women's skirts than on the suffrage movement. Many issues, situations, and events described in textbooks are complex and can be viewed from a variety of perspectives. Often, only one perspective is presented. For example, the relationships between the U.S. government and the American Indians are usually examined only from the government's perspective in terms of treaties and protection. An American Indian perspective would also examine broken treaties and the appropriation of native lands. This is an example of bias through selectivity and imbalance.

Texts that focus primarily on the origins, heritage, and contributions of European settlers in this nation are not presenting a balanced perspective. With such emphasis on a specific microculture, women, persons of color, and handicapped individuals often do not learn about the contributions of members of their cultural groups to the development of our society. Such biases prevent all students—from both dominant and subordinate groups, male and female—from realizing the complexity of historical and contemporary situations and developments.

A fourth bias is *unreality*. Textbooks frequently present an unrealistic portrayal of our history and contemporary life experiences. Controversial topics are glossed over, and discussions of social movements, dissent, homosexuality, sex education, divorce, and death are avoided. "A recent survey of social studies textbooks found that the coverage of contemporary problems faced by the U.S. is so scant or disconnected that students find it difficult to understand the depth of passion these issues produced or their relevance to society today" (Woodward, Elliott, & Nagel, 1986,

p. 52). This unrealistic coverage denies children the information needed to recognize, understand, and perhaps someday conquer the problems that plague our society. When sensitive or unpleasant issues, such as racism, sexism, prejudice, discrimination, intergroup conflict, and classism, are not included in instructional materials, students are not provided guidance in handling such complex issues.

Contemporary problems faced by the handicapped or aged are often disguised or simply not included. American Indians, in discussions or illustrations, are often pictured in historical rather than a contemporary context. Most materials do not consider sex, race, and class biases that exist in employment practices and in salary schedules. The avoided issues include those that many students will have to face in the future. Obviously, the achievements and successes of the United States should be presented in textbooks. However, the problems and difficulties should be analyzed as well. No wonder students find that what is studied does not relate to their lives. "As a result, young Americans today display little interest and even less knowledge of social and political affairs" (Starr, 1989, p. 107).

Fragmentation and isolation refer to the way some publishers include certain microcultures in instructional materials. Issues, contributions, and information about various groups are separated from the regular text and discussed in a section or chapter of their own. This additive approach is easier to accomplish than trying to integrate the information throughout the text. The isolation of this information often has negative connotations or messages for students. This approach suggests that the experiences and contributions of these groups are merely an interesting diversion and not an integral part of historical and contemporary developments. There is nothing wrong with having some information separate from the regular text if it is not the only place students read about members of a specific microculture. The same phenomenon occurs when members of a specific microcultural group are illustrated interacting only among themselves and having little or no influence on society as a whole. Society is multicultural, and it is important that instructional materials and textbooks reflect this diversity as a part of the total text rather than discussing microcultures in a separate section.

Finally, *linguistic bias* is often seen in classroom materials, especially in the older editions that are often used. Examples include the use of masculine pronouns or only Anglo names throughout a textbook. Table 9-1 lists some nonsexist alternatives for some common words and phrases used in books. The lack of Spanish, Polish, Filipino, African, and other non-Anglo names in materials, as well as the lack of feminine pronouns or names will be evident to the sensitive teacher. When teachers are aware that linguistic bias blatantly omits female and many ethnic group references, they can develop strategies to correct the biases and to ensure that these groups are an integral part of the curriculum.

How do educators overcome the biases that exist in instructional materials, especially if they have been assigned a set of classroom materials that may be old and may not even include the positive changes of the past decade? They must become aware of the biases that often exist and then begin to critically examine the materials used in the classroom. Textbook analysis is neither a quick nor an easy task. How-

Table 9-1 Nonsexist Alternatives for Some Common Words and Phrases

Common Word/Phrase	Alternative
Mankind	Humanity, human beings, human race, people
Primitive man	Primitive people, primitive men and women
Man-made	Artificial, synthetic, manufactured
Congressman	Member of Congress, Representative
Businessman	Business executive, business manager
Fireman	Firefighter
Mailman	Mail carrier, letter carrier
Salesman	Sales representative, salesperson, salesclerk
Insurance man	Insurance agent
Statesman	Leader, public servant
Policeman	Police officer
Chairman	Presiding officer, chair, head, leader, coordinator, chairperson, moderator

From D. M. Gollnick, M. P. Sadker, & D. M. Sadker (1982), Beyond the Dick and Jane syndrome: Confronting sex bias in instructional materials. In M. P. Sadker & D. M. Sadker (eds.), Sex equity handbook for schools. New York: Longman, p. 72.

ever, there are evaluation instruments and studies that are helpful for examining classroom materials.

One does not have to depend totally on the text for instruction. When using the text, it is appropriate to point out omissions. Students can examine the author's perspective with the understanding that there may be other perspectives, and discussions can focus on some of these. For example, an examination of how several American Indian groups look at science would provide a perspective that contrasts with a traditional Western view of science. Students would begin to understand that environmentalism is not a new phenomenon.

If the textbook includes few or no women, older persons, or non-Anglos, students can talk about these omissions. Students can also be assigned to read other materials about the particular subject being studied that focus on the contributions of some of the omitted groups. Most schools have a library from which students can find materials to supplement classroom materials. In this way, the educator can ensure that students are presented a multicultural perspective.

In selecting instructional materials, one must do more than examine the content of the materials for the reflection of multiculturalism. One must also be concerned about the introduction of different perspectives as written by authors from a variety of microcultures. If students read only materials written by white men, they are being cheated out of other perspectives about the world and its events. By selecting such a narrow perspective, female students and students of color may have a difficult time identifying with the materials being used in the classroom.

This emphasis on the selection of multicultural materials is extremely important. It means exposing students to the multicultural nature of this country. All students—regardless of where they live or their religious or ethnic background—should know that other individuals come from different cultural backgrounds. Unless they help students understand the multicultural nature of American society, educators are not being honest about the world in which their students live.

CURRICULUM AND INSTRUCTION

In some school districts, teachers are provided at the beginning of the year with a curriculum guide that outlines the goals, objectives, and activities for their teaching assignments. In other schools, the textbook selected for the course serves as the curriculum guide for teachers. The teacher's guide that accompanies the textbook usually outlines activities and supplementary resources that can be used with the text. Other teachers are given instructions about the concepts to be taught throughout the year and the level that students are expected to attain when they finish the year. These teachers have the opportunity to select activities, supplementary materials, and textbooks that will assist in that process. How, then, does curriculum and instruction become multicultural? There are a number of concepts and components that should be included in a multicultural curriculum. Components of multicultural education that might be included are ethnic, minority, and women's studies; bilingual education; cultural awareness; human relations; and values clarification. Concepts include racism, sexism, handicappism, ageism, prejudice, discrimination, oppression, powerlessness, power, inequality, equality, and stereotyping.

Curriculum is more than the composite of courses that students are required to take—the so-called official curriculum. The school setting includes what researchers call a *hidden curriculum* as well. This hidden curriculum consists of the unstated norms, values, and beliefs about the social relations of school and classroom life that are transmitted to students (Giroux, 1988). Some observers of schools find that "students learn values and norms that would produce 'good' industrial workers. Students internalize values which stress a respect for authority, punctuality, cleanliness, docility, and conformity" (Giroux, 1988, p. 29).

Regardless of the level of formal schooling, multicultural education should permeate both the formal and hidden curriculum. It should be directed toward all students from both dominant and subordinate groups. It is important for students in a multicultural setting, as well as those in a more homogeneous setting, to develop a multicultural perspective.

Although communities are not always rich in ethnic diversity, there is always cultural diversity. Educators will need to determine the microcultures that exist in the community. Schools that are on or near Native American reservations will include students from the tribes in the area, as well as non–Native Americans. Urban schools typically include multiethnic populations and students from middle and lower socioeconomic levels; inner-city schools are likely to have a high proportion of poor students. Teachers in Appalachian-area schools will need to be aware of poor and middle-class families with fundamentalist backgrounds. Teachers who enter schools attended by students from different cultural backgrounds will need to adjust to that setting; otherwise, both students and teacher could suffer. However, the application of several principles can help the educator in developing multicultural curriculum and instruction.

Principle 1: Student Achievement

"Multicultural education must help students increase their academic achievement levels in all areas, including basic skills, through the use of teaching approaches and materials that are sensitive and relevant to the students' sociocultural backgrounds and experiences" (Suzuki, 1980, p. 34). If educators do not understand the community in which they teach, they may have a difficult time developing instructional strategies that can be related to the life experiences of the students in the classroom. Rural students often do not relate to riding a subway to work daily, and inner-city students seldom relate to a single-family house with a large yard. Because students do not relate these examples to their own life experiences does not mean that they should not learn about other life-styles based on different cultural backgrounds and experiences. It does mean that students' own cultural backgrounds and experiences should be used to teach basic academic concepts. For example, in one school, playing cards might be an appropriate aid in teaching some elementary math concepts; in another school, playing cards would be totally unacceptable. Instructional strategies must relate to the experiences of students. Gay (1977b) defines such teaching as *cultural context teaching* and suggests that teachers "carefully select illustrations, analogies, and allegories from the experiences of different ethnic [and cultural] groups to demonstrate or extricate the meanings of academic concepts and principles" (p. 54).

The cultural background of students in the classroom should guide teachers in developing strategies with which students can identify. An example of how a teacher was able to do this was described by a migrant student:

> I always am a little scared when I try a new school, yes; but I try to remember that I won't be there long, and if it's no good, I'm not stuck there like the kids who live there. . . . To me a good school is one where the teacher is friendly, and she wants to be on your side, and she'll ask you to tell the other kids of the things you can do, and all you've done—you know, about the crops and like that. There was one teacher like that, and I think it was up North, in New York it was. She said that so long as we were there in the class she was going to ask everyone to join us, that's what she said, and we could teach the other kids what we know and they could do the same with us. She showed the class where we traveled, on the map, and I told my daddy that I never before knew how far we went each year, and he said he couldn't understand why I didn't know because I did the traveling all right, with him, and so I should know. But when you look on the map, and hear the other kids say they've never been that far, and wish someday they could, then you think you've done something good, too—and they'll tell you in the recess that they've only seen where they live and we've been all over. (Coles, 1967, pp. 72–73)

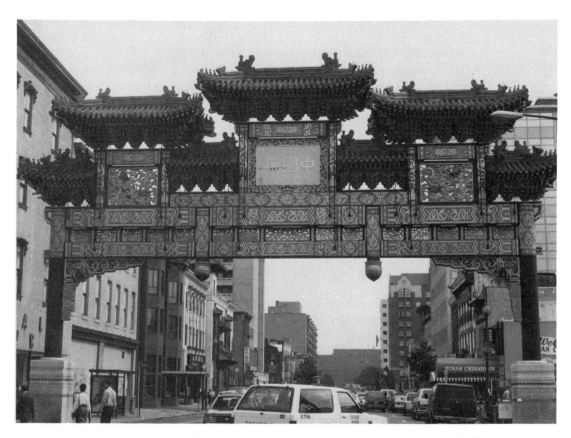

Some students live in easily identified ethnic communities like Chinatown. For others it will be difficult to determine their ethnic backgrounds from the community in which they live. Knowing the communities and the cultural backgrounds of the families of students in the classroom is an important aspect of multicultural education.

(Photo by Willard Loftis).

The teacher who is sensitive to experiences of students from different cultural backgrounds can make those students feel as much a part of the class as those from the dominant culture.

Principle 2: Voice

Attention to *voice* must be a part of multicultural instruction. What do we mean by voice in the classroom? It refers to the dialogue between persons, especially between teachers and students. Multicultural education calls for teaching that starts from the students' life experiences, not the experiences of the teacher, nor the experiences necessary to fit into the dominant school culture (Shor & Freire, 1987).

Through our microcultural memberships and their relationships with the dominant society, we learn multiple voices. Students can recognize the voices of their communities and that of the mass media as seen on television. Although students from subordinate groups often do not use the language of the school at home, they can mimic the teacher's voice in informal discussions with other students. Although many teachers grew up in a community where the dominant standard English was not the norm, they have learned it in their years of schooling. Some may be bidialectal or bilingual; others may have lost the native language or dialect.

Schools legitimize the voice of the dominant society—the standard English that is used primarily by the white, middle-class population. O'Connor (1988) suggests that

> in a group of similar thinking individuals of equal power, the accepted orientations of the community may parallel one's deep urges and encourage close ties between voice and consciousness. The wider and deeper the breach between the society and the individual's orientations, the more difficulty the individual will have in trying to appropriate the available terms for his or her use. Inclinations to express urges in a way that reflects preferred values will be delegitimized; he or she will need to develop a consciousness alienated from these choices, or disguise it. In some cases, the individual may lose the capacity for verbalization of his or her basic urges, experiencing what Freire (1970) calls a culture of silence. Attention to voice acknowledges this range of relationships between power relations and the process of representation. (p. 9)

In multicultural education, educators must be able to recognize the conflict between the voices of the official school and those of the students and learn how to use students' voices in developing effective curriculum and instructional strategies.

Success in school should not be dependent on one's adoption of the school's voice. "The organization of school discourse in a way that permits all cultural voices to search for skills and concepts to reconstruct their cultural principles in their own terms must come to serve as the basic formula for equal educational opportunity" (O'Connor, 1988, p. 20). One approach that teachers should consider is that of dialogic inquiry in the classroom. In this approach, instruction occurs as a dialogue between teacher and students. It requires that teachers know the subject being taught very well. Rather than depending on a textbook and lecture format, the teacher listens to students and directs them in the learning of the discipline through dialogue. Dialogic inquiry "is situated in the culture, language, politics, and themes of students" (Shor & Freire, 1987, p. 104). It incorporates content about the students' backgrounds as well as that of the dominant society. It requires discarding the traditional authoritarian classroom to establish a democratic one in which both teacher and students are active participants.

What should be the teacher's role when students bring to the classroom biased values and beliefs about other groups? It is important that the teacher be able to provide "a just structure to protect rights of all students" (O'Connor, 1988 p. 25). Although students have the right to hold biased beliefs, they must be challenged. As Friere (Shor & Freire, 1987) explains,

The educator has the right to disagree. It is precisely because the teacher is in dis-agreement with the young racist men or women that the educator challenges them. This is the question. Because I am a teacher, I am not obliged to give the illusion that I am in agreement with the students. . . . In the liberating perspective, the teacher has the right but also the duty to challenge the status quo, especially in the questions of domination by sex, race, or class. What the dialogical educator does not have is the right to impose on the others his or her position. But the liberating teacher can never stay silent on social questions, can never wash his or her hands of them. (pp. 174–175)

The dialogues developed through this approach could help students understand the perspectives brought to the classroom by other students from different cultural backgrounds. It will help them relate the subject matter to their real world and perhaps take an interest in really studying and learning it. Finally, "it is important that we help students to begin to consider how they are both created and limited by their particular life circumstances and to consider what alternative ways of working and living could be supported by other possible ways of defining one's work in the world" (Simon, 1989, p. 144).

Principle 3: Communications

In multicultural education, oral and nonverbal communication patterns between students and teachers are analyzed to increase the involvement of students in the learn-ing process. These communications between students and teachers can be problematic because of differences between the cultural backgrounds of students and teachers:

Just as cultures differ in the structure of their language, they also differ in the struc-ture of oral discourse. Moves made in teaching-learning discourse, who is to make them, and the sequence they should take will vary from culture to culture. These rules are not absolute laws governing behavior; in fact, they are closer to expecta-tions and norms by which participants make sense out of "the messiness of naturally occurring conversation" (Erickson, 1980). But when these patterns differ from cul-ture-of-teacher to culture-of-child, serious misunderstandings will occur as the two participants try to play out different patterns and assign different social meanings to the same utterance or gesture. (Ainsworth, 1984, p. 134)

These differences are likely to prevail in schools with large numbers of students from subordinate groups. The "silent Native American child" described by a number of writers provides such an example. Philips (1983) identified four types of classroom interaction used by teachers from the dominant culture in schools on the Warm Springs Indian Reservation:

1. The teacher interacts with all students by addressing them as a group or as a single student in the presence of the class; the students respond as a group or individually.

2. The teacher interacts with a subgroup of students rather than with the entire class.

3. A student interacts with the teacher while working independently, and there is no audience for the interaction.

4. Students interact in small groups that they run themselves.

Philips found that the students were reluctant to participate in the first two types of interaction, which are most commonly used in schools. In the last two types of interaction, the students were actively involved.

Teachers who are aware of these differences can redirect their instruction to primarily use the kinds of interaction that work most effectively with the student. At the same time, the teacher can begin to teach students how to interact effectively in the situations with which they are most uncomfortable. This approach will assist all students in responding appropriately in future classroom situations that are dominated by interactions with which they are not familiar. Further, Ainsworth (1984) suggests that "if teachers and students of many different cultural backgrounds in this multicultural nation are to avoid the embarrassment and anger caused by unwitting violation of sociolinguistic rules, both teachers and students must discover and make explicit these implicit rules" (p. 137). Refer to Chapter 7 for a detailed description of nonverbal communication patterns.

Principle 4: Learning and Teaching Styles

In multicultural education, the learning styles of students and the teaching style of the teacher are understood and used to develop effective instructional strategies. Knowing the cultural background of students should help the educator determine how to structure the classroom in order to provide the most effective instruction. Learning styles of students are often correlated with how assimilated they are into the dominant society. Students from subordinate groups are more likely to be field-sensitive than most students from the dominant group. Many Asian-American students are an exception; they are more likely to be field-independent. Most instruction in the past has been provided in a field-independent mode, which favors the students from the dominant group. Teachers are likely to become very frustrated when students don't work well independently or don't respond quickly enough to questions asked by the teacher. The following identifies the differences between these two types of students observed in classrooms.

Cognitive, or learning, styles refer to the ways in which individuals respond to a wide range of perceptual and intellectual tasks. Teaching style, meanwhile, affects the way the teacher presents information and responds to students in the classroom. When students are having problems learning, it may be more effective to examine our teaching styles than to focus on the students' IQs, emotional blocks, and personality conflicts (Dembo, 1977).

One example of differences in cognitive style is the impulsive/reflective dimension. Impulsive students respond rapidly to tasks; they are the first ones to raise their hands to answer the teacher's question and the first ones to complete a test. Reflective students, on the other hand, respond much slower, even though they usually have fewer errors than the impulsive responder. Knowing whether you tend to encourage more reflective or impulsive behavior can assist you in having a positive effect on student learning. If you tend to promote impulsive behavior, you will need to develop some strategies for fostering reflectiveness in students. At the same time, you should help reflective students learn to respond more impulsively in some situations, such as during timed tests.

One of the most widely investigated dimensions of learning style is that of field independence and field sensitivity. Field-sensitive individuals have a more global perspective of their surroundings; they are more sensitive to the social field. Field-independent individuals tend to be more analytical and can more comfortably focus

Table 9–2 Differences in Behavior Between Field-Independent and Field-Sensitive Students

Field-Independent Behaviors of Student	Field-Sensitive Behaviors of Students
Relationship to Peers	
• Prefers to work independently	• Likes to work with others to achieve a common goal
• Likes to compete and gain individual recognition	• Likes to assist others
• Is task oriented; is inattentive to social environment when working	• Is sensitive to feelings and opinions of others
Personal Relationship to Teacher	
• Rarely seeks physical contact with teacher	• Openly expresses positive feelings for teacher
• Is formal; restricts interactions with teacher to tasks at hand	• Asks questions about teacher's tastes and personal experiences; seeks to become like teacher
Instructional Relationship to Teacher	
• Likes to try new tasks without teacher's help	• Seeks guidance and demonstration from teacher
• Impatient to begin tasks; likes to finish first	• Seeks rewards that strengthen relationship with teacher
• Seeks nonsocial rewards	• Is highly motivated when working individually with teacher
Characteristics of Curriculum That Facilitate Learning	
• Details of concepts are emphasized; parts have meaning of their own	• Performance objectives and global aspects of curriculum are carefully explained
• Deals with math and science concepts	• Concepts are presented in humanized or story format
• Based on discovery approach	• Concepts are related to personal interests and experiences of children

Adapted from Ramirez, M., and Castañeda, A. (1974). Cultural democracy, bicognitive development and education. New York: Academic Press, Inc., pp. 169–170.

on impersonal, abstract aspects of stimuli in the environment. As you probably would expect, field-sensitive persons are more likely to choose careers in teaching or social work, while field-independent persons select mathematics and science.

Researchers have found that teachers and students can be mismatched in teaching and learning styles to the disadvantage of both. "Generally, field-independent teachers encourage independent student achievement and competition between individual students. In contrast, field-sensitive teachers are more interpersonally oriented and prefer situations that allow them to use personal, conversational techniques while interacting with students" (Dembo, 1977, p. 146). What are the differences in behavior between the two ends of this continuum? The following teacher behaviors (listed in Tables 9–2 and 9–3) can be observed in the classroom:

Table 9–3 Differences in Behavior Between Field-Independent and Field-Sensitive Styles

Field-Independent Teaching Styles	Field-Sensitive Teaching Styles
Personal Behaviors	
• Is formal in relationship with students; acts like authority figure	• Displays physical and verbal expressions of approval and warmth
• Centers attention on instructional objectives; gives social atmosphere secondary importance	• Uses personalized rewards that strengthen relationships with students
Instructional Behaviors	
• Encourages independent student achievement; emphasizes importance of individual effort	• Expresses confidence in student's ability to succeed; is sensitive to student's who are having difficulty and need help
• Encourages competition between students	• Gives guidance to students; makes purpose and main principles of lesson obvious; presents lesson clearly, with steps toward "solution" clearly delineated
• Adopts a consultant role; encourages students to seek help only when they experience difficulty	
• Encourages learning through trial and error	• Encourages learning through modeling; asks students to imitate
• Encourages task orientation; focuses student attention on assigned tasks	• Encourages cooperation and development of group feeling; encourages class to think and work as a unit
	• Holds informal class discussions; provides opportunities for students to see how concepts being learned are related to students' personal experiences

Field-Independent Teaching Styles	Field-Sensitive Teaching Styles
Curriculum-Related Behaviors	
• Focuses on details of curriculum materials	• Emphasizes global aspects of concepts; before beginning lesson, ensures that students understand the performance objectives; identifies generalizations and helps students apply them to particular instances
• Focuses on facts and principles; teaches students how to solve problems using short cuts and novel approaches	
• Emphasizes math and science abstractions; tends to use graphs, charts, and formulas in teaching, even when presenting social studies curriculum	• Personalizes curriculum; relates curriculum materials to interests and experiences of students as well as to teacher's own interests
• Emphasizes inductive learning and the discovery approach; starts with isolated parts and slowly puts them together to construct rules or generalizations	• Humanizes curriculum; attributes human characteristics to concepts and principles
	• Uses teaching materials to elicit expression of feelings from students; helps students apply concepts for labeling their personal experiences

Adapted from Ramirez, M., and Castañeda, A. (1974). Cultural democracy, bicognitive development and education. New York: Academic Press, Inc., pp. 177–178.

Teaching behaviors reflect the teacher's learning style. The teacher who is aware of his or her own teaching style can learn to organize instruction and classroom activities that are conducive to both cognitive styles. Ramirez and Castañeda (1974) found that these teachers were also able to teach students to become bicognitive. Bicognitive students are able to respond appropriately no matter what the situation— whether it is taking a standardized test or working in a group. Instruction that encourages field sensitivity includes group projects, close work with the teacher, and material in tune with the ethnic and social backgrounds of students. Field-independent instruction will focus on independent activities, minimal participation of the teacher, curriculum materials, charts and diagrams, and student work that emphasizes individual achievement.

The individual differences in learning and teaching styles develop from early and continuing socialization patterns. They are not indicative of general learning ability or memory. Members of the dominant cultural group in the United States tend to be more field-independent, while many subordinate group members are field-sensitive. To serve all students effectively, teachers might be aware of their own styles and be able to identify the learning styles of students in order to develop instructional strategies that are compatible with them. To be able to function bicognitively in the classroom and to teach students to operate bicognitively are goals that teachers should try to implement.

Principle 5: Formal Curriculum

Multicultural education must permeate the formal curriculum. This approach will probably require some major changes in the educational program. Educators should take affirmative steps to ensure that cultural diversity is integrated throughout the curriculum. The curriculum should promote students' in-depth exposure "to the variety and richness of American's multicultural history; such an education might help diffuse a latent racism and provide a solid foundation for social stability" (Pratte, 1979, p. 49).

With little effort, today's teacher can locate supplementary materials, information, and visual aids about most subordinate groups. This information should be included as part of the curriculum in every subject regardless of how culturally diverse the community is. It may be more difficult to find resources on microcultures where the membership is small or somewhat new to the United States, but it is not impossible. Although teachers cannot possibly address each of the hundreds of microcultures in this country, they should attempt to include the groups represented in the school community, whether or not all these groups are represented in the school. For instance, in western Pennsylvania, a teacher should include information about the Amish heritage in some aspect of the curriculum. This approach will help the Amish students feel a valued part of the school and will indicate to other students that cultural diversity is acceptable and natural in the community. In schools in the Southwest, teachers should be sensitive to Mexican-Americans and Native Americans and their unique experiences and contributions in that area. Knowledge of these groups should be integrated throughout the curriculum to a greater degree than in states where they make up less of the population. Thus, curricula for all subjects at all grade levels should include both dominant and subordinate microcultures.

Educators are cautioned against giving superficial attention to various microcultures. Multicultural education is not tasting ethnic food and learning ethnic dances. Even celebrating African-American history only during February is not multicultural education. It is much more complex and pervasive than setting aside an hour, a unit, or a month. It should influence the whole curriculum.

The amount of specific content about various microcultures will vary according to the course taught, but an awareness and a recognition of the culturally pluralistic nature of the nation can be reflected in all classroom experiences. No matter how assimilated or how ethnic students in a classroom are, it is the teacher's responsibility to expose them to cultural diversity.

An essential aspect of multicultural education is the critical examination of contemporary and historical issues. Most instructional content is presented from a dominant political perspective because that perspective pervades most textbooks and other resource materials adopted by school districts or states.

> Diverse perspectives can provide genuine alternatives to standardized knowledge. The presentation and critical discussion in classrooms of many interpretations of economics, labor, minority, and other social histories provides conceptual and behavioral options. This kind of classroom work fosters in students an awareness of the possibilities of social change and facilitates constructive activity. (Anyon, 1979, p. 386)

It is important for students to learn that individuals from other ethnic, religious, and socioeconomic groups may have different perspectives on the same issues and that these perspectives may be as valid as their own. On the other hand, perspectives and behaviors that degrade and harm members of other cultural groups are not considered valid by the authors of this text. The perspectives of the Ku Klux Klan and the Nazi party are examples of such invalid perspectives.

As an educator teaches about different values, life-styles, religions, and ethnic backgrounds, these differences must not be described as inferior to the educator's own. Students easily perceive such a superior attitude. Multiculturalism must not be viewed as a compensatory process. Multicultural education recognizes cultural differences as reflected in human relations, motivational incentives, and communication styles. Students should be helped to develop openness, flexibility, and receptivity to cultural diversity and alternative life-styles (Gay, 1977b). These educational experiences should encourage students to accept and prize diversity and should assist in reducing students' anxieties about encountering people who are culturally different (Gay, 1977b).

When one first begins to teach multiculturally, extra planning time will be needed to discover ways to make the curriculum and instruction multicultural. With experience, however, this process will become second nature to the effective teacher. In many schools, the teacher will expand the standard curriculum to reflect cultural diversity. When microcultures are introduced into the curriculum, they should be included in positive roles and not always in subordinate status roles.

Teaching multiculturally will require examining sensitive issues and topics. It will require looking at historical and contemporary events from the perspective of white men, African-American women, Puerto Ricans, Vietnamese, Central American refugees, Jewish Americans, and Southern Baptists. Reading books, poems, and articles by authors from various microcultural backgrounds will be helpful, as it will allow students to begin to understand the perspectives of other microcultural groups and how those perspectives differ from their own because of different experiences. Even without adding the literature of subordinate groups to the curriculum, teachers can help students understand the relationship of power and knowledge by comparing classical and contemporary writings in the subject being taught. This strategy can help students explore why some works are included in the curriculum while others are not (McLaren, 1988).

There are a number of resources for making the curriculum multicultural that include student and teacher activities. See the Suggested Readings at the end of the chapter for an annotated listing of selected resources. You may want to add one or more of these resources to a personal curriculum library for use in your own classroom.

Principle 6: Hidden Curriculum

Multicultural education must impact the hidden curriculum at all levels. Remember that the hidden curriculum includes the norms and values that undergird the formal curriculum. Although the hidden curriculum is not taught directly nor included in the objectives for the formal curriculum, it has a great impact on students and teachers alike. It includes the organizational structures of the classroom and school as well as the interactions of students and teachers.

Elements of the hidden curriculum are shaped by crowds, praise, and power (Jackson, 1968). As a member of a crowd, students must take turns, stand in line, wait to speak, wait for the teacher to provide individual help, face interruptions from others, and be distracted constantly by the needs of others. They must develop patience in order to be successful in the school setting. They must also learn to work alone within the crowd. Even though they share the classroom with many other students, they usually are not allowed to interact with classmates unless the teacher permits it. These same characteristics will be encountered in the work situations for which students are being prepared. They are not part of the formal curriculum, but central to the operation of most classrooms.

Praise can be equated with evaluation. Teachers evaluate students' academic performances by testing and responding to written and oral work. However, much more than academic performance is evaluated by teachers. Student behavior probably receives the most punishment, usually when classroom rules are not adequately obeyed. In a study of elementary classrooms, Jackson (1968) found that the hidden curriculum is reflected more in student difficulties than successes:

> Why do teachers scold students? Because, try as he [she] might, he [she] fails to grasp the intricacies of long division? Not usually. Rather, students are commonly scolded for coming into the room late or for making too much noise or for not listening to the teacher's directions or for pushing while in line. The teacher's wrath, in other words, is more frequently triggered by violations of institutional regulations and routines than by signs of his [her] students' intellectual deficiencies. (pp. 34–35)

Classroom research has found that teachers provide boys more negative attention than girls because boys tend to be more aggressive in the classroom. Girls are more often praised for being quiet, not interrupting, and writing neatly. Similarly, students who have been assigned a low-ability status often receive negative attention from the teacher because of not following the rules, rather than because they are not performing adequately on academic tasks.

In addition to evaluations based on academic performance and institutional rules, teachers often make evaluations based on personal qualities (Jackson, 1968). As was shown in the Rist study discussed in Chapter 2, students are sometimes grouped according to their clothes, family income, cleanliness, and personality rather than potential academic abilities.

The third aspect of the hidden curriculum is that of unequal power. In many ways this is a dilemma of childhood. By the time students enter kindergarten, they have been taught that power is in the hands of adults. The teacher and other school officials require that their rules be followed. In addition to the institutional rules, teachers may require that students give up their home languages or dialects in order to be successful academically or at least to receive the teacher's approval. Most often, students are required to adopt middle-class, white values to be successful.

How can the hidden curriculum reflect multicultural education? A first step is to recognize that it exists and that it provides lessons that are probably more important than the academic curriculum. Developing a more democratic classroom would help in overcoming the power inequities that exist. We should value students' curiosity and encourage it. Too often the requirements of the classroom place more value on following the rules (e.g., being quiet and handing in all assignments) than on learning. Trying hard is sometimes more important than being able to think critically. We should also evaluate our interactions with students to ensure that we are actually supporting learning rather than preventing it.

Principle 7: Critical Thinking

Multicultural education must teach students to think critically. What is critical thinking? Starr (1989) defines it as having "the freedom to ask questions and the tools to reason, liberating [one's] mind from unthinking prejudice, and promoting an appreciation for pluralistic democracy" (p. 107). Students should be supported in questioning the validity of the knowledge presented in textbooks and encouraged to explore other perspectives. "Children [and prospective teachers] who have been provoked to reach beyond themselves, to wonder, to imagine, to pose their own questions are the ones most likely to learn to learn" (Green, 1988, p. 14). However, critical thinking is not currently included in most classrooms. In a study of one thousand classrooms, Goodlad (1981) found that less than 1 percent of class time dealt with open-ended critical inquiry.

Starr (1989) discusses what critical thinking means in the classroom:

> In the critical thinking method, the teacher provides facts, then asks open-ended questions designed to get students to analyze. Instead of multiple-choice questions, the students write essays in which they argue a position logically, citing relevant evidence. Critical thinking also requires students to identify the assumptions underlying different positions and the values implicit in the assumptions. In the process, ethnocentric statements are consciously examined and stereotypes confronted. Sources of information are evaluated and propaganda techniques are made transparent. In science classes, critical thinking means performing experiments while not knowing what the result will be, and trying to explain the outcome. (p. 108)

Multicultural education must deal with the social and historical realities of American society and help students gain a better understanding of the causes of oppression and inequality, including racism and sexism (Suzuki, 1980). It is important that students be encouraged to investigate institutional racism and sexism and how societal institutions have served different populations in discriminatory ways. Even though we may overcome our own prejudices, and eliminate our own discriminatory practices against members of other cultural groups, the problem is not solved. It goes beyond what we individually control. The problem is societal and is imbedded in historical and contemporary contexts that we must help students understand.

For one, educators can help students examine their own biases and stereotypes related to different cultural groups. "Stereotypes caused by ignorance, hard times, and folk wisdom socialization can be countered by accurate information about the group(s) being stereotyped" (Garcia, 1984, p. 107). In this regard, the nonsexist, nonracist materials that have been developed over the past fifteen years are helpful.

We must beware of addressing cultural differences only in superficial ways that limit study to ethnic dances and food. These activities often only reinforce existing biases and prejudices rather than helping students understand the nature of cultural groups. Realistically addressing issues of oppression and equality are essential aspects of a curriculum that is multicultural.

Being able to think critically and to teach students to think critically is essential for a democratic society. These skills will help us realize the vision that Starr (1989) describes:

> It's a vision of active cooperation and mutually respectful disagreement, side by side. It's a vision of teachers being free to choose from a diversity of instructional materials and methods of evaluation, if and when they want. It's a vision of all points of view being given a sympathetic hearing, so that all students can have the courage of their own convictions. It's a vision of students feeling free to bring into the classroom issues that concern them in real life. It's a vision of learning together and growing together without being lost in the crowd. (p. 109)

Principle 8: Lived Realities

Multicultural education must start "where people are." Educators must know the community to understand the lived cultures of families in that community. Giroux (1988) suggests that

> a discourse be developed that is attentive to the histories, dreams, and experiences that such students bring to schools. . . . Searching out and illuminating the elements of self-production that characterize individuals who occupy diverse lived cultures is not merely a pedagogical technique for confirming the experiences of those students who are often silenced by the dominant culture of schooling; it is also part of a discourse that interrogates how power, dependence, and social inequality structure the ideologies and practices that enable and limit students around issues of class, race, and gender. (p. 106)

In a school in which a prayer is said every morning regardless of the Supreme Court's decision forbidding prayer in public schools, one should not teach evolution on the first day of class. In that school setting, one may not be able to teach sex education in the same way that it is taught in many urban and suburban schools. In another school, Islamic parents may be upset with the attire that their daughters are expected to wear in physical education classes, and they would not approve of coed physical education courses. Jewish students might wonder why the school celebrates Christian holidays and never Jewish holidays. Girls in some communities might question why they are restricted from participation in industrial arts courses and some vocational programs. In another part of the country, parents may be adamantly against their daughters' attending such courses. In 1974, parents in Kanawha County, West Virginia, bombed classrooms because they believed that the textbooks selected by the school district did not reflect their own values and, in fact, would corrupt their children. On the other hand, urban families in the same county strongly supported the inclusion of the broad range of perspectives offered in the textbooks.

It is essential that educators know their community as they develop curriculum and instruction for the classroom.

Because members of the community may revolt against the content and certain activities in the curriculum does not mean that the educator cannot teach multiculturally. It does suggest that the teacher must know the sentiments of the community before introducing concepts that may be foreign and unacceptable. Only then can the educator develop strategies for effectively introducing such concepts.

Principle 9: The Community Resource

Multicultural education must use the community as a resource. Multicultural teaching also will involve using the community as a resource in the classroom. If speakers are invited to talk with students, the teacher should be sure that they are not all from the same cultural background. Speakers should also be selected from different role groups.

In summary, teaching multiculturally means teaching about the real world—a world that includes individuals and groups with cultural backgrounds very different from one's own. As educators, we should understand that students receive cues about cultural differences not only in the classroom, but also from television, movies, advertising, and family discussions. We should be concerned about controlling or mediating many of these cues. Many misconceptions and distortions of individual and group differences are perpetuated through this social curriculum. It is our responsibility to help students understand the historical and contemporary experiences of their own and other groups. We live in an increasingly interdependent world and nation—a fact that requires us to learn to respect cultural differences and understand the differential power relationships that currently exist.

TEACHER BEHAVIOR

The heart of the educational process is in the interaction between teacher and student. It is through this action that the school system makes its major impact upon the child. The way the teacher interacts with the student is a major determinant of the quality of education the child receives. (U.S. Commission on Civil Rights, 1973, p. 3)

The development and use of multicultural materials and curricula are important and necessary steps toward providing multicultural education. Alone, however, these steps are not enough. A teacher's behavior in the classroom is a key factor in helping all students reach their potential, regardless of sex, ethnicity, age, religion, language, or exceptionality.

In addition, the teacher who is enthusiastic about multicultural education will be more likely to use multicultural materials and encourage students to develop more egalitarian views. In a project designed to promote sex equality in kindergarten and fifth- and ninth-grade classrooms, researchers found that teacher enthusiasm was a key factor in affecting attitudinal change of both boys and girls at all levels (Guttentag & Bray, 1976).

Other research studies have found that warmer and more enthusiastic teachers produce students with greater achievement gains. These teachers also solicit better affective responses from their students, which leads to classrooms with a more positive atmosphere. Warmth of the teacher seems to be especially important with disadvantaged students and students who are targets of prejudice and discrimination (Brophy, 1983). Many white students, on the other hand, are less affected by warmth and more affected by a teacher's teaching skills (St. John, 1971). Nevertheless, teachers will have to carefully assess the needs of individual students in the classroom in order to develop effective teaching strategies. One must beware of generalizing the research findings to all students. While democratic leadership style and teacher sincerity may be generally effective as teacher attributes, some lower-socioeconomic-level students may show better achievement from, and may actually prefer, authoritarian teaching (Brophy & Good, 1974).

"Recent teacher-effectiveness research has provided clear evidence that individual teachers do make a difference in student learning" (Good, 1983, p. 57). They can also make students feel either very special or incompetent and worthless. They can make the subject come alive, or they can be extremely dull. What are the qualities of teachers who make positive differences in the lives of their students? "When students are asked to describe successful teachers, one quality that comes up again and again is *fairness*—the ability to establish a democratic classroom where all students are treated equitably" (Sadker & Sadker, 1982, p. 97).

Teacher Expectations and Ability Grouping

Unfortunately, some teachers respond differently to students because of their microcultural memberships. Researchers have found different expectations and treatment of students based on their race, sex, and class. After reviewing research studies in this area, Brophy and Good (1974) observed that "in some school systems a student's career is somewhat determined as of the day he enters school simply on the basis of his clothing, appearance, and other factors related to the socioeconomic status of his family but not necessarily to his ability or potential" (p. 9).

Educators must beware of automatically expecting less academic achievement from minority and poor students than they expect from students from the dominant cultural group. Teachers' expectations are often based on generalizations that lower-class students and students from subordinate groups do not perform as well in school (Baron, Tom, & Cooper, 1985). When these generalizations are applied to all or most of the students from those groups, grave damage can be done, because students tend to meet the expectations of the teacher, no matter what their actual abilities are. Self-fulfilling prophecies about how well a student will perform in the classroom are often established early in the school year, and both students and the teacher unconsciously fulfill those prophecies. Educators need to develop strategies to overcome any negative expectations they may have for certain students and plan classroom instruction and activities that will help those student overcome such expectations.

Moreover, Garcia (1984) warns that you should not overcompensate for minority students either:

> Too often in the attempt to win over minorities, teachers have acquiesced to demands to "make it easy for the downtrodden." Or, teachers have recoiled with guilt when accused of being prejudiced because they gave low grades to minorities. Minorities need to be encouraged to excel in all areas of academic pursuits lest a self-fulfilling prophecy perpetuate lower academic expectations and outcomes for minorities. (p. 107)

Students from higher socioeconomic levels are often placed in higher academic tracks, and students from lower socioeconomic levels are placed in lower tracks, than their measured ability would predict. "One critical aspect of ability grouping is that membership in groups tends to remain quite stable over time, with the work of upper- and lower-ability groups becoming more sharply differentiated as time passes" (Good, 1987, p. 175). Teaching behavior for high-quality groups is much different than for low-ability groups; middle-ability groups usually receive treatment more similar to that of high-ability groups. Good (1987) describes the differences:

> The assignments extended to lows often are practice/review-oriented and, in a word, dull. Those extended to high-ability groups involve more abstraction and conceptualization and are more likely to involve students actively in constructing knowledge meaningfully. Students in low-ability groups are more likely encouraged to endure; students in high-ability groups, to think and to understand. (p. 175)

Teachers must be extremely careful that students are not placed at different academic levels based on their clothes, grooming, language, and behavior. To a large degree, students learn to behave in a manner expected of the group in which they are placed. Through tracking, educators have a great influence not only on directing a student's potential, but also on determining it by their initial expectations for that student. The sad reality is that tracking does not appear to work anyway.

Many educators think that grouping students makes the classroom more manageable. They also think that it is better for students because it meets their individual needs. In a study of twenty-five schools and hundreds of research studies, Oakes (1985) found that these assumptions are wrong. She concludes,

> Tracking seems to retard the academic progress of many students—those in average and low groups. Tracking seems to foster low self-esteem among these same students and promote school misbehavior and dropping out. Tracking also appears to lower the aspirations of students who are not in the top groups. And perhaps most important, in view of all the above, is that tracking separates students along socioeconomic lines, separating rich from poor, whites from nonwhites. The end result is that poor and minority children are found far more often than others in the bottom tracks. And once there, they are likely to suffer far more negative consequences of schooling than are their more fortunate peers. (p. 40)

The students who suffer the most from tracking practices are those from subordinate groups—the poor and minorities—who are disproportionately placed in the low-ability groups. Compared to students in other tracks, these students develop more negative feelings about their academic potential and future aspirations. Educational equality demands a different strategy. It should mean "that all students are provided with the same kinds of experience in schools—a common set of learnings, equally effective instruction, and equally encouraging educational settings" (Oakes, 1985, p. 135).

Cooperative Learning

When students and teachers are mutually involved in learning, trusting relationships are more likely to develop (Oakes, 1985). Cooperative learning is an instructional strategy that assists in developing these trusting relationships and in increasing academic achievement. In cooperative learning, students work together in small groups and are rewarded for their group performance. In the traditional classroom, on the other hand, the teacher often lectures or leads the discussion. Also, competitiveness is more frequently found in classrooms based on the values of the dominant culture, correlating more directly with field-independent learning and teaching styles. Cooperative activities are more supportive of field-sensitive learning and teaching styles. In some cooperative learning activities, competition is included, but it occurs between groups, rather than between individuals.

The research on cooperative learning activities indicates that there is often a positive effect on academic achievement. In addition, there is a positive effect on race relations, with students of different races being chosen as friends more often than occurs in traditional classroom settings. In addition, "minority students appear to gain academically as a result of participating in cooperative learning more than do white, middle-class students" (Wilkinson, 1988, p. 214). At the same time, white, middle-class students do not achieve less than in other situations; their achievement just does not increase as dramatically as does that of minority students.

Teacher Biases

Unknowingly, educators often transmit biased messages to students. For example, lining up students by sex to go to lunch reinforces the notion that boys and girls are distinct groups. Why not line them up by shoe colors or birth dates instead? What messages do students receive when girls are always asked to take attendance and boys are asked to move chairs; or when upper-middle-class students are usually asked to lead small-group work; or when retired people are never asked to speak to the class? Most educators do not consciously or intentionally stereotype students or discriminate against them; they usually try to treat all students fairly and equitably. However, we have learned our attitudes and behaviors in a society that has been ageist, handicappist, racist, sexist, and ethnocentric. Some biases have been internalized to such a degree that we do not realize that we are biased. When teachers are able to recognize the subtle and unintentional biases in their behavior, positive changes can be made in the classroom (Sadker & Sadker, 1982).

Classroom research has also found that teachers often treat boys and girls differently in the classroom. Boys receive more teacher disapproval and criticism than do girls. Boys tend to be more aggressive than girls, but these behavioral differences are not based on biological factors; instead, they are based on socialization patterns from birth. Traditionally, teachers have been part of the socialization process that teaches different male and female behavior based on sex. Although boys are often more aggressive, many of the differences observed in the way teachers treat the two sexes are based on their own beliefs about male and female behavior. Thus, boys are criticized in more harsh and angry tones, girls in more conversational tones (Brophy & Good, 1974). Teachers have more interaction with boys through discipline and instruction. They ask boys more direct and open-ended questions and are more likely to give boys extended directions so that they can learn to do things for themselves. In contrast, teachers are more likely to do things for girls, as shown by the following example:

> In one classroom, the children were making party baskets. When the time came to staple the paper handles in place, the teacher worked with each child individually. She showed the boys how to use the stapler by holding the handle in place while the child stapled it. On the girls' turns, however, if the child didn't spontaneously staple the handle herself, the teacher took the basket, stapled it, and handed it back (Serbin & O'Leary, 1975, p. 102).

Again, teachers must assess their interactions with boys and girls to determine whether they provide different types of praise, criticism, encouragement, and reinforcement based on the sex of the student. Only then can steps be taken to equalize treatment.

Teacher Attributes

Although there are many areas of teaching behavior that could be investigated here, the purpose is only to make teachers aware of the importance of their behavior in the provision of multicultural education. Good (1987) outlines six attributes of good teachers:

1. They view their main responsibility as teaching.
2. They know that diagnosis, remediation, and enrichment are key aspects of teaching.
3. They expect some difficulties in helping all students learn, but are prepared to provide the appropriate follow-up instruction that will be more successful.
4. They expect all students to meet at least the minimum specified objectives.
5. They expect to deal with individuals, not groups or stereotypes.
6. They build a stimulating classroom environment that makes learning enjoyable for all students, not just those in the high-ability group.

These six characteristics are essential in multicultural teaching. To provide the greatest assistance to all students, teachers cannot provide the same treatment to each student, since they should be working toward meeting individual needs and differences.

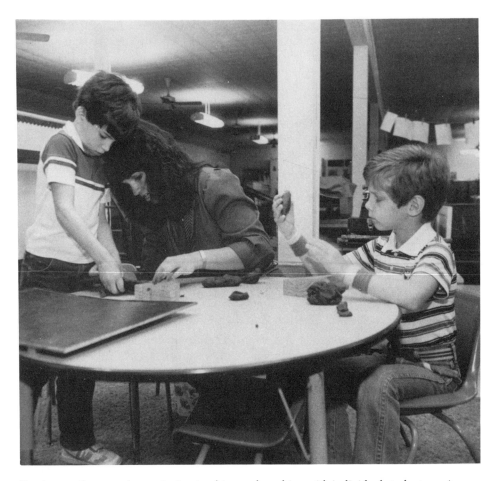

Teacher attributes such as enjoying teaching and working with individual students are important in the delivery of multicultural education.

However, teachers must be sure that they are not treating students differently based solely on the students' membership in certain microcultures.

The preceding suggestions were designed to help teachers become more aware of the importance of their behavior in providing equitable education. With the elimination of bias from the teaching process and the emergence of proactive teachers who seek to best meet the needs of individual students, the classroom can become a stimulating experience for most students, regardless of their cultural background and experiences. The area of teacher behavior is one in which the teacher has almost total control.

SCHOOL CLIMATE

Another area in which commitment to multicultural education can be evaluated is the general school climate. When visitors enter a school, they can usually feel the tension that exists when cross-cultural communications are poor. They can observe whether cultural diversity is a positive and appreciated factor at the school. If only minority students or only males are waiting to be seen by the assistant principal in charge of discipline, the visitors will wonder whether the school is providing effectively for the needs of all its students. If bulletin boards in classrooms show only white characters, visitors will question the appreciation of cultural diversity in the school. If the football team is made up primarily of minority players and the chess club of white players, they will wonder about the inclusion of students from a variety of cultural backgrounds in extracurricular activities. If school administrators are primarily men and most teachers are women, or if the teachers are white and the teacher aides are Hispanic, the visitors will envision discriminatory practices in hiring and promotional procedures. These are examples of a school climate that does not reflect a commitment to multicultural education.

Although all schools are multicultural, the cultural diversity that exists is not always positively reflected. A school that affirms multiculturalism will integrate the community in its total program. Not only will the educators know and understand the community, but the parents and community will know and participate in the school activities. As long as members of the community feel unwelcome in the school, they are not likely to initiate any involvement. The first step in multiculturalizing the school is the development of positive and supportive relations between the school and the community. Teachers can assist by asking community members to participate in class activities by talking about their jobs, hobbies, or experiences in a certain area. They can initiate contacts with families of students. They can participate in some community events. A sincere interest in the community, rather than disgust or patronage, will help to bridge the gap that often exists between the school and the community.

Staffing composition and patterns should reflect the cultural diversity of the country. At a minimum, they should reflect the diversity of the geographical area. Women, as well as men, should be school administrators; men, as well as women, should teach at preschool and primary levels. Minorities should be found in the administration and teaching ranks, not primarily in custodial and clerical positions.

Student government and extracurricular activities must include students from various microcultural groups. Except for female students, who do not participate in contact sports such as wrestling and football, there should be no segregation of students based on their membership in a certain microculture. In a school where multiculturalism is valued, students from various cultural backgrounds will hold leadership positions. Those roles will not automatically be delegated to students from the dominant cultural group of the school.

If the school climate is multicultural, it will be reflected in every aspect of the educational program. In addition to those areas already mentioned, assembly programs will reflect multiculturalism in their content, as well as in the choice of speakers. Bulletin boards and displays will reflect the cultural diversity of the nation, even if the community is not rich in cultural diversity. Cross-cultural communications among students and between students and teachers will be positive. Different languages and dialects used by students will be respected. Both girls and boys will be found in industrial arts, home economics, calculus, bookkeeping, and vocational classes. Minority students, as well as white students, will make up the college preparatory classes.

The school climate must be supportive of multicultural education. When respect for cultural differences is reflected in all aspects of the students' educational program, the goals of multicultural education will have been attained. Educators hold the key to attaining this climate.

PREPARATION FOR PROVIDING MULTICULTURAL EDUCATION

"A teacher in search of his/her own freedom may be the only kind of teacher who can arouse young persons to go in search of their own" (Green, 1988, p. 14). There are a number of actions that educators should undertake to prepare for the provision of multicultural education in the classroom. First, they should know their own cultural identity and the degree to which they identify with the various microcultures of which they are members. The degree of identification will probably change over time. Second, they should be able to accept the fact that they have prejudices that may affect the way they react to students in the classroom. When they recognize these biases, they can develop strategies to overcome or compensate for them in the classroom.

Educators need to learn about cultural groups other than their own. They might read about different cultural groups, attend ethnic movies or plays, participate in ethnic celebrations, visit different churches and ethnic communities, and interact with members of different groups. Teachers who enjoy reading novels should select authors from different cultural backgrounds. The perspective presented may be much different from one's own. Novels may help the reader to understand that other people's experiences may lead them to react to situations differently than the reader would. It is often an advantage to discuss one's reactions to such new experiences with someone else in order to clarify one's own feelings of prejudices or stereotypes.

Educators should make an effort to interact with persons who are culturally different from themselves. Long-term cultural experiences are probably the most effective means for overcoming fear and misconceptions about a group. One must remember, however, that there is much diversity within a group. One cannot generalize about an entire group based on the characteristics of a few persons. In direct cross-cultural contacts, one must learn to be open to the traditions and perspectives of the other culture in order to learn from the experience. Otherwise, one's own traditions, habits, and perspectives are likely to be projected as better rather than just different. If individuals can learn to understand, empathize with, and participate in a second culture, they will have had a valuable experience. If they learn to live multiculturally, they are indeed fortunate.

SUMMARY

Multicultural education is a means for positively using cultural diversity and equality in the total learning process. Goals of multicultural education are (1) to promote the strength and value of cultural diversity; (2) to promote human rights and respect for those who are different from oneself; (3) to acquire a knowledge of the historical and social realities of U.S. society in order to understand racism, sexism, and poverty; (4) to support alternative life choices for people; (5) to promote social justice and equality for all people; and (6) to promote equity in the distribution of power and income among groups.

Educators must become aware of biases that exist in most classroom materials and begin to integrate content about various ethnic, religious, gender, socioeconomic, and age groups. They should also supplement the curriculum with materials that will fill in the gaps left by regular classroom materials.

Multicultural education can help students increase their academic achievement levels in all areas, including basic skills, through the use of teaching approaches and materials that are sensitive and relevant to the students' sociocultural backgrounds and experiences. The voices of students and the community must be heard in order to deliver multicultural education. Oral and nonverbal communication patterns between students and teachers are analyzed and changed to increase the involvement of students in the learning process. In multicultural education, the learning styles of students and the teaching style of the teacher are understood and used to develop effective instructional strategies. Multicultural education must be integrated throughout the curriculum at all levels. It can help students to think critically, to deal with the social and historical realities of American society, and to gain a better understanding of the causes of oppression and inequality, including racism and sexism. Multicultural education must start "where people are." Finally, multicultural education should incorporate multicultural resources from the local community.

A teacher's behavior in the classroom is a key factor in helping all students reach their potential, regardless of sex, ethnicity, age, religion, language, or exceptionality. Educators should develop skills for individualizing instruction based on the needs of students. No longer can we afford to teach all students the same knowledge and skills in the same way. Individualizing the instruction is a way to help all students reach their potential and develop their unique talents. Teachers must make an effort to know all of their students and to build on their strengths and help them overcome their weaknesses. However, teachers must be sure that they are not treating students differently based solely on the students' membership in certain microcultures. We need to evaluate our own academic expectations of students, our practices of ability grouping, our own biases, and our attributes to ensure that we are helping all students have access to the same knowledge.

Educators will face a tremendous challenge in the next decade to use effectively the cultural diversity that students bring to the classroom. Every subject area can be taught in ways that reflect the reality of cultural differences in this nation and the world. Skills to function effectively in different cultural settings can also be taught.

For students to function effectively in a democratic society, they must learn about the inequities that currently exist. Otherwise, our society will never be able to overcome such inequities.

As educators, we must teach *all* children. The ultimate goal of multicultural education is to meet the individual learning needs of each student so that all students can progress to their fullest capacity. This goal has not been reached in the past, partly because educators have been unable to use effectively the cultural backgrounds of students in providing classroom instruction. As multicultural education reaches into all levels of schooling, the maximum development of all students, regardless of their cultural background, will be supported. Acceptance of the challenge to multiculturalize our schools is vital to the well-being of all citizens.

QUESTIONS FOR REVIEW

1. Define multicultural education, and describe how it is designed to help all students reach their potentials.

2. How is membership in microcultures related to multicultural education?

3. What is cultural context teaching? Give examples for the subject area that you plan to teach.

4. If the textbook that you have been assigned to use includes no information or examples pertaining to nondominant groups, what can you do to provide a balanced and realistic view of society?

5. Identify the principles for teaching multiculturally, and provide examples for implementing those principles in your own teaching.

6. Why have tracking systems developed in many schools? What are the characteristics used to track students? What is the danger in tracking students?

7. Identify teacher behaviors and attributes that should positively support the delivery of multicultural education.

8. In what situations would it be appropriate to use cooperative learning strategies?

9. What is your teaching style, and what strategies should you develop to work more effectively with students whose learning style is not compatible with your own?

10. What characteristics would you look for to determine if a school is committed to multicultural education?

REFERENCES

Ainsworth, N. (1984). The cultural shaping of oral discourse. *Theory into Practice, 23*, 132–137.

Anyon, J. (1979, August). Ideology and United States history textbooks. *Harvard Educational Review, 49*(3), 361–386.

Baron, R. M., Tom, D. Y. H., & Cooper, H. M. (1985). Social class, race and teacher expectations. In J. B. Dusek, V. C. Hall, & W. J. Meyer (Eds.), *Teacher expectancies* (pp. 251–270). Hillsdale, NJ: Lawrence Erlbaum Associates.

Brophy, J. E. (1983). Classroom organization and management. In D. C. Smith (Ed.), *Essential knowledge for beginning educators* (pp. 23–37). Washington, DC: American Association of Colleges for Teacher Education.

Brophy, J. E., & Good, T. L. (1974). *Teacher-student relationships: Causes and consequences.* New York: Holt, Rinehart & Winston.

Coles, R. (1967). *Migrants, sharecroppers, mountaineers.* Vol. 2 of *Children in Crisis.* Boston: Little, Brown.

Dembo, M. H. (1977). *Teaching for learning: Applying educational psychology in the classroom.* Santa Monica, CA: Goodyear.

Erickson, F. (1980). Timing and context in everyday discourse: Implications for the study of referential and social meaning. In R. Bauman & J. Sherzer (Eds.), *Language and speech in American society.* Austin, TX: Southwest Educational Development Laboratory.

Freire, P. (1970). *Pedagogy of the oppressed.* New York: Seabury.

Garcia, R. L. (1984). Countering classroom discrimination. *Theory into Practice, 23*, 104–109.

Gay, G. (1977a). Curriculum design for multicultural education. In C. Grant (Ed.), *Multicultural education: Commitments, issues, and applications* (pp. 94–104). Washington, DC: Association for Supervision and Curriculum Development.

Gay, G. (1977b). Curriculum for multicultural education. In F. H. Klassen & D. M. Gollnick (Eds.), *Pluralism and the American teacher: Issues and case studies* (pp. 31–62). Washington, DC: American Association of Colleges for Teacher Education.

Giroux, H. A. (1988). *Teachers as intellectuals.* Granby, MA: Bergin & Garvey.

Gollnick, D. M., Sadker, M. P., & Sadker, D. M. (1982). Beyond the Dick and Jane syndrome: Confronting sex bias in instructional materials. In M. P. Sadker & D. M. Sadker (Eds.), *Sex equity handbook for schools* (pp. 60–95). New York: Longman.

Good, T. L. (1983). Recent classroom research: Implications for teacher education. In D. C. Smith (Ed.), *Essential knowledge for beginning educators* (pp. 55–64). Washington, DC: American Association of Colleges for Teacher Education.

Good, T. L. (1987). Teacher expectations. In D. C. Berliner & B. V. Rosenshine (Eds.), *Talks to teachers* (pp. 159–200). New York: Random House.

Goodlad, J. I. (1981). *A place called school.* New York: McGraw-Hill.

Green, M. (1988). *The dialectic of freedom.* New York: Teachers College Press.

Guttentag, M., & Bray, H. (1976). *Undoing sex stereotypes: Research and resources for educators.* New York: McGraw-Hill.

Jackson, P. W. (1968). *Life in classrooms*. New York: Holt, Rinehart & Winston.

McLaren, P. L. (1988, May). Culture or canon? Critical pedagogy and the politics of literacy. *Harvard Educational Review, 58*(2), 213–234.

Oakes, J. (1985). *Keeping track: How schools structure inequality*. New Haven, CT: Yale University Press.

O'Connor, T. (1988, November). *Cultural voice and strategies for multicultural education*. Paper presented at the annual meeting of the American Educational Studies Association, Montreal, Canada.

Philips, S. U. (1983). *The invisible culture: Communication in classroom and community on the Warm Springs Indian reservation*. New York: Longman.

Pratte, R. (1979). *Pluralism in Education*. Springfield, IL: Thomas.

Ramirez, M., & Castañeda, A. (1974). *Cultural democracy, bicognitive development and education*. New York: Academic Press.

Sadker, M., & Sadker, D. (1978). The teacher educator's role. In S. McCune & M. Matthews (Eds.), *Implementing Title IX and attaining sex equality: A workshop package for postsecondary educators*. Washington, DC: U.S. Government Printing Office.

Sadker, M. P., & Sadker, D. M. (1982). Between teacher and student: Overcoming sex bias in classroom interaction. In M. P. Sadker & D. M. Sadker (Eds.), *Sex equity handbook for schools* (pp. 96–132). New York: Longman.

Serbin, L. A., & O'Leary, K. D. (1975, December). How nursery schools teach girls to shut up. *Psychology Today, 9*(7), 56–57, 102–103.

Shor, I., & Freire, P. (1987). *A pedagogy for liberation: Dialogues on transforming education*. South Hadley, MA: Bergin & Garvey.

Simon, R. I. (1989). Empowerment as a pedagogy of possibility. In H. Holtz, I. Marcus, J. Dougherty, J. Michaels, & R. Peduzzi (Eds.), *Education and the American dream: Conservatives, liberals and radicals debate the future of education* (pp. 134–149). Granby, MA: Bergin & Garvey.

Starr, J. (1989). The great textbook war. In H. Holtz, I. Marcus, J. Dougherty, J. Michaels, & R. Peduzzi (Eds.), *Education and the American dream: Conservatives, liberals and radicals debate the future of education* (pp. 96–109). Granby, MA: Bergin & Garvey.

St. John, N. (1971). Thirty-six teachers: Their characteristics and outcomes for black and white pupils. *American Educational Research Journal, 8,* 635–648.

Suzuki, B. H. (1980, April 23–25). *An Asian-American perspective on multicultural education: Implications for practice and policy*. Paper presented at the meeting of the National Association for Asian and Pacific American Education, Washington, DC. (ERIC Document Reproduction Service No. ED 205 633)

Trecker, J. L. (1977). Women in U.S. history high-school textbooks. In J. Pottker & A. Fishel (Eds.), *Sex bias in the schools: The research evidence* (pp. 146–161). Cranbury, NJ: Associated University Presses.

U.S. Commission on Civil Rights. (1973). *Teachers and students, Report 5, Mexican American education study: Differences in teacher interaction with Mexican American and Anglo students*. Washington, DC: Government Printing Office.

Weitzman, L. J., & Rizzo, D. (1974). *Biased textbooks: A research perspective*. Washington, DC: Resource Center on Sex Roles in Education.

Wilkinson, L. C. (1988). Grouping children for learning: Implications for kindergarten education. *Review of Research in Education, 15,* 203–223.

Women on Words and Images. (1975). *Dick and Jane as victims: Sex stereotyping in children's readers.* Princeton, NJ: Author.

Woodward, A., Elliott, D. L., & Nagel, K. C. (1986, January). Beyond textbooks in elementary social studies. *Social Education, 50*(1), 50–53.

SUGGESTED READINGS

Appleton, N. (1983). *Cultural pluralism in education.* New York: Longman.

An examination of goals for multicultural education and a conflict-sensitive curriculum. Includes goals for teacher and students. The list of teaching resources includes a comprehensive annotated list of helpful simulations.

Baker, G, C. (1983). *Planning and organizing for multicultural instruction.* Reading, MA: Addison-Wesley.

A multicultural approach to the curriculum that addresses philosophy and implementation. Includes excellent recommendations for the development of units in art, language arts, music, science, and social studies for the elementary classroom.

Banks, J. A. (1984). *Teaching strategies for ethnic studies* (3rd ed.). Boston: Allyn and Bacon.

An excellent resource of multiethnic concepts, teaching strategies, and resources for primary, intermediate, and high school levels. Includes strategies for the study of specific ethnic groups, including Native Americans, European-Americans, African-Americans, Mexican-Americans, Asian-Americans, Puerto Rican-Americans, Cuban-Americans, and Native Hawaiians. Also includes a useful chronology of key events related to ethnic groups in American history.

Bennett, C. I. (1986). *Comprehensive multicultural education: Theory and Practice.* Boston: Allyn and Bacon.

An overview of multicultural education that focuses on culture, individual differences, curriculum reform, and teaching concepts and strategies. Includes exercises that help readers clarify their thinking about the concepts presented and lesson plans for different components of multicultural education.

Bulletin. New York: Council on Interracial Books for Children.

A periodical published eight times a year. Includes thought-provoking, issue-oriented analyses of storybooks, textbooks, audiovisuals, and other learning materials. Includes surveys, teaching strategies, lesson plans and bibliographies, as well as regular departments that suggest useful resources and review children's books.

Codianni, A. V. (1981). *Toward educational equity for all: A planning guide for integrating multicultural/nonsexist education into the K-12 curriculum.* Manhattan, KA: Midwest Race and Sex Desegregation Centers.

An action document to assist schools in planning and implementing multicultural education throughout all subject areas from kindergarten to grade 12. Includes goals and outcomes for social studies, mathematics, language arts, and science.

Cortes, C., Metcalf, F., & Hawke, S. (1976). *Understanding you and them: Tips for teaching about ethnicity*. Boulder, CO: Social Science Education Consortium.

> *A multiethnic approach to classroom activities for all grades. Includes a helpful description of how to incorporate ethnicity in the curriculum and a discussion of evaluation instruments, including a list of references.*

DeCosta, S. B. (1984). Not all children are Anglo and middle class: A practical beginning for the elementary teacher. *Theory Into Practice, 23*(2), 155–162.

> *A focus on multicultural teaching in the elementary classroom. Includes suggested activities and resources that are available.*

Good, T. L. (1987). Teacher expectations. In D. C. Berliner & B. V. Rosenshine (Eds.), *Talks to teachers*. New York: Random House.

> *A presentation of research on teacher expectations. The most valuable sections of this chapter include practical skills for working with students who are failing and suggestions for improving performance of low achievers.*

Grant, C. A. (Ed.) (1977). *Multicultural education: Commitments, issues, and applications*. Washington, DC: Association for Supervision and Curriculum Development.

> *A multicultural approach to classroom activities for all grades. Includes background information on multicultural education and its implications for curriculum.*

Grant G. (Ed.). (1977). *In praise of diversity: Multicultural classroom applications*. Omaha: The University of Nebraska at Omaha, Teacher Corps, Center for Urban Education.

> *Fifty-one classroom activities for social studies, language arts, science, math, and art.*

Guidelines for selecting bias-free textbooks and storybooks. (1984). New York: Council on Interracial Books for Children.

> *Collection of criteria and checklists to identify stereotypes and other forms of bias against women, people of color, disabled people, and older people.*

Guttentag, M., & Bray, H. (1976). *Undoing sex stereotypes: Research and resources for educators*. New York: McGraw-Hill.

> *An excellent resource of suggestions for making the curriculum nonsexist at all levels. Includes a description of the research by the Nonsexist Intervention Project, on which the suggestions are based. Also includes bibliographies and list of resource organizations.*

Hansen-Krening, N. (1979). *Competency and creativity in language arts: A multiethnic focus*. Reading, MA: Addison-Wesley.

> *A multiethnic approach to language arts at the primary and intermediate levels. The lesson plans address sensory awareness, music, art, listening, speaking, writing, movement and nonverbal communications, creative dramatics, myths, legends, and folktales.*

Henslee, T., & Jones, P. (1977). *Nonsexist curricular materials for elementary schools*. Washington, DC: Office of Education, U.S. Department of Health, Education and Welfare.

> *Nonsexist activities and program suggestions for preschool and primary levels.*

Hernandez, H. (1989). *Multicultural education: A teacher's guide to content and process*. Columbus, OH: Merrill.

Practical guide for incorporating multicultural education in different aspects of class-room instruction and what teachers should know about students' homes, neighbor-hoods, and communities. Areas covered include the hidden curriculum, bilingualism, special/gifted education, instructional materials, and multicultural curriculum.

Kendall, F. E. (1983). *Diversity in the Classroom.* New York: Teachers College.

A resource book for preschool, primary-grade, and day-care teachers. Includes a resource unit and activities on affirming cultural diversity, as well as recommenda-tions for working with children and parents.

King, E. W. (1980). *Teaching ethnic awareness: Methods and materials for the elementary school.* Santa Monica, CA: Goodyear.

Multiethnic and nonsexist classroom activities for preschool and elementary levels. Includes an annotated listing of resources and curriculum materials.

Klassen, F. H., & Gollnick, D. M. (Eds.). (1977). *Pluralism and the American teacher: Issues and case studies.* Washington, DC: American Association of Colleges for Teacher Education.

A collection of papers presented at a conference on multiethnic education in teacher education. The chapters by Geneva Gay and James A. Banks are particularly helpful to educators at all levels. Includes an annotated listing of helpful resources for multi-culturalizing the curriculum.

McNeill, E., Allen, J., & Schmidt, V. (1975). *Cultural awareness for young children.* Dallas: The Learning Tree.

Multiethnic activities for preschool children. Based on activities developed and used at The Learning Tree, a multicultural preschool in Dallas.

Morris, L., Sather, G., & Schull, S. (Eds.). (1978). *Extracting learning styles from social/cultural diversity: A study of five American minorities.* Norman, OK: Southwest Teacher Corps Network.

A discussion of the uniqueness of Native American, Chicano, Afro-American, low-income white, and Asian-American cultures. Includes resultant learning styles and their implications for organizing classroom strategies.

NCSS Task Force on Ethnic Studies Curriculum Guidelines. (1976). *Curriculum guidelines for multiethnic education. Position Statement.* Arlington, VA: National Council for the Social Studies.

Guidelines describing the ideal characteristics of school environments consistent with ethnic pluralism. Includes a rationale for ethnic pluralism and a checklist for assessing specific school environments to determine the extent to which they reflect the idealized school described in the guidelines.

New Jersey Education Association. (1976). *Roots of America.* Washington, DC: National Educa-tion Association.

Multiethnic curriculum units for junior high social studies. Includes units on black Americans, Italian-Americans, Japanese-Americans, Jewish Americans, Mexican-Americans, Native Americans, Polish-Americans, and Puerto Ricans. Includes a bibliography and chronology for each ethnic group.

Northwest Regional Educational Laboratory & Washington Education Association. (1982). *The teacher, the classroom and multicultural education.* Portland, OR: Author.

> *A resource package of classroom activities for use in the elementary classroom. Includes a bibliography of resources.*

Pasternak, M. G. (1977). *Helping kids learn multi-cultural concepts: A handbook of strategies.* Nashville: Nashville Consortium Teacher Corps.

> *An excellent resource of teaching strategies and classroom activities developed and used by classroom teachers. Although the activities were developed for ten- to thirteen-year-old students, they could be adapted to any level. Includes annotated listings of basic multicultural resources and publishers.*

Perl, T. (1978). *Math equals: Biographies of women mathematicians and related activities.* Reading, MA: Addison-Wesley.

> *Classroom activities associated with the work of nine female mathematicians for all grade levels.*

Ramirez, M., & Castañeda, A. (1974). *Cultural democracy, bicognitive development and education.* New York: Academic Press.

> *An extremely helpful research report of the learning styles of Mexican-American children and teaching styles of their teachers. Describes an intervention strategy for training teachers to teach students to be bicognitive.*

Sadker, M. P., & Sadker, D. M. (Eds.). (1982). *Sex equity handbook for schools.* New York: Longman.

> *An overview of the critical areas of sex equity in schools and practical strategies for the elimination of sex bias in education. Includes lesson plans and units with a synopsis of relevant research and a narrative on the nature of sex bias in today's classrooms.*

Schniedewind, N., & Davidson, E. (1983). *Open minds to equality: A sourcebook of learning activities to promote race, sex, class, and age equity.* Englewood Cliffs NJ: Prentice-Hall.

> *Numerous activities for implementing multicultural education.*

Shor, I., & Freire, P. (1987). *A pedagogy for liberation: Dialogues on transforming education.* South Hadley, MA: Bergin & Garvey.

> *Conversations about teaching for liberation by two practitioners. Includes recommendations for dialogical teaching and developing critical thinking skills of students. Also addresses some of the problems teachers may face when using this approach, as well as giving recommendations for handling unruly behavior, silence, and discontent.*

Simms, R. L., & Contreras, G. (1980). *Racism and sexism: Responding to the challenge.* Washington, DC: National Council for the Social Studies.

> *An exploration of the responses of the social studies to racism and sexism. Includes a helpful resource list, including alternative publishers and projects that address these topics.*

Sleeter, C. E., & Grant, C. A. (1988). *Making choices for multicultural education: Five approaches to race, class, and gender.* Columbus, OH: Merrill.

> *An examination of five approaches to teaching multicultural education with a focus*

on the integration of race, class, and gender issues. Includes research activities and lesson plans that assist the reader in changing curriculum to implement the different approaches.

Strike, K. A., & Soltis, J. F. (1985). *The ethics of teaching.* New York: Teachers College, Columbia University.

Case studies and discussions about ethical situations that teachers may face in the nation's classrooms. Includes case studies and dialogues on a number of multicultural issues: the equal treatment of students, censorship, equality, grading policies, the Pledge of Allegiance, values clarification, social reproduction, equality of opportunity, separation of church and state, sex education, and teaching values.

Tiedt, P. L., & Tiedt, I. M. (1979). *Multicultural teaching: A handbook of activities, information, and resources.* Boston: Allyn and Bacon.

Multicultural activities, resources, and information for the elementary level. Although the activities are designed for use in bilingual classrooms, they are equally applicable to any classroom. Includes teaching strategies, book lists, important ethnic dates, and addresses of organizations.

Critical Incidents in Teaching

The critical incidents described in this section reflect real-life situations that have occurred in schools or classrooms or are parts of different incidents that have been combined to provide you with a problematic situation that could very well take place in your school. The purpose of this section is to provide you with an opportunity to examine your feelings, attitudes, and possible actions or reactions. In some respects, these exercises are not realistic for you as a potential problem solver; in many real situations, decisions must be made quickly, and you may not have even five minutes to ponder your options and decide on an appropriate action. However, these exercises in problem solving may facilitate and sharpen your skills to think critically, which may enhance your functioning in various school situations and help you to better meet the diverse needs of your students.

Sex/Gender Role Identification

Jane Irwin is the director of the Model Learning Center at a regional university located in the Southwest. The center is a kindergarten laboratory school located on the university campus to provide observation and practicum opportunities for students in the teacher education program. Ms. Irwin is affectionately referred to as Miss Janie by the children at the center. At the end of a lesson on health, the children are dismissed by Miss Janie for thirty minutes of free play in the classroom. Each child is free to select his or her activity of choice. The Model Learning Center is well equipped with a wide variety of play materials, and the children quickly move to their chosen activities. In the classroom are two undergraduate students in early childhood education who are in the center as part of their required practicum.

Some of the children choose puzzles, some a large playhouse, others an indoor slide, airplanes, dolls, and various other activities. One of the boys, Tim, moves over to an area where two of the girls are playing with dolls. Tim gently picks up a doll and begins combing its long blonde hair. Shocked by this behavior, one of the practicum students rushes over to Tim, helps him to his feet, takes the doll and comb out of his hands, places them on the floor and says, "Come with me" as she leads him by the hand to an area where two boys are playing with a model airplane and a helicopter. Picking up an airplane, she hands it to Tim and says, "Here, you play with this. Boys like airplanes, not dolls."

Miss Janie has observed the entire sequence of events as she sits at her desk watching her students and the university teacher education student.

Questions for Discussion

1. What should Miss Janie do with regard to the child who is now obediently playing with the airplane?
2. What should she do with regard to the class, since several children observed the incident?
3. What should she do with regard to the university student?

Religious Discrimination

Janice Furguson is a five-year-old Jewish girl living in a conservative Protestant community where there are few non-Christian families. She is the only Jewish child in her kindergarten class. She is an outgoing child, well liked by her classmates. While playing out in the playground with two of her classmates, one of them asks Janice what she expects to receive for Christmas. Janice answers by stating that her family does not observe Christmas. "Why not?" the other girls ask. "Because we're Jewish and we have Chanukah instead," Janice explains.

The next day, Janice, visibly upset, seeks out Mrs. Tedesco, her teacher, on the playground. "Mary Ellen said that her daddy told her that Jews were bad people because they killed Jesus. I don't think she wants to be my friend anymore."

Questions for Discussion

1. What can Mrs. Tedesco do for Janice to provide her with some immediate comfort?

2. What can or should Mrs. Tedesco do with regard to Mary Ellen?

3. Should Mrs. Tedesco do anything with regard to the class to stop a potential problem in bigotry from spreading? If so, what are some activities she can plan for her class?

Acceptance of Hearing-Impaired Student

Jeb Benson is a first-grade student in Ms. Storey's class. Unbeknownst to his classmates, Jeb, in the past two months, has been examined by an otologist, tested by an audiologist, and found to have a bilateral hearing loss of forty decibels. He has been fitted for a behind-the-ear hearing aid, and without either warning (except for Ms. Storey) or fanfare, has shown up in class with an unobtrusive but noticeable hearing aid in his right ear.

By the time Jeb sits down in his seat, several of his classmates have noticed his new hearing aid and are beginning to gossip about it. None know exactly what it is, and Jeb is acutely aware of the fact that his classmates are talking about him. He suddenly feels embarrassed and removes the hearing aid from his ear and places it in his pocket. From her desk, Ms. Storey observes all that is going on. She is determined to help Jeb feel comfortable wearing his hearing aid in her class.

Questions for Discussion

1. How can Ms. Storey facilitate Jeb's adjustment to his new hearing aid in the class?

2. What should she say to Jeb?

3. What, if anything, should she say to the class?

4. What activities could she devise to enhance acceptance and understanding of Jeb's problem?

Placement of a Child with Epilepsy

Mr. Potts is a sixth-grade teacher in a middle-class suburban school. After school, Mr. Potts finds a note in his box indicating that the principal and the special education resource room teacher would like to meet with him the next day before the students arrive.

At the meeting the next day, his principal, Dr. Levy, explains to him that a new student, Chris Erickson, will be placed in his class the following Monday morning. He is informed that Chris is slightly above average in academics and a personable young man. However, Dr. Levy wants Mr. Potts to know that Chris is an epileptic who occasionally has grand mal seizures. While the seizures are generally under control through medication, there is a good possibility that sometime during the school year Chris will have a seizure in the classroom.

At this time, Ms. Chang, the resource room teacher, describes the grand mal seizures. She explains that they are the most evident and serious type of epileptic seizure. They can be disturbing and frightening to anyone who has never seen one. Chris would have little or no warning that a seizure was about to occur. During a seizure, his muscles will stiffen and he will lose consciousness and fall to the floor. His whole body will shake violently, as his muscles alternately contract and relax. Saliva may be forced from his mouth, his legs and arms may jerk, and his bladder and bowels may empty. After a few minutes, the contractions will diminish, and Chris will either go to sleep or regain consciousness in a confused and drowsy state (Heward & Orlansky, 1988).

Stunned at this information, Mr. Potts sits in silence as Ms. Chang briefs him about what procedures to take if and when a seizure occurs in the classroom. She also explains to him that he should inform the other students that the seizure is painless to Chris and that it is not contagious.

Mr. Potts is aware that he has no option as to whether or not Chris will be in his class. Determined to make Chris' transition into his class as smooth as possible, and also determined that he will help his class adjust and prepare for the likely seizure, Mr. Potts begins to map out a plan of action.

Questions for Discussion

1. What can Mr. Potts do with regard to his class?
2. Should he talk to his class about Chris?
3. Should he explain what epilepsy is?
4. What should he say to Chris? What other actions can he take?

Student with a Health Problem

Michelle Adams is a third-grade teacher in a cattle and farming community of forty thousand in Colorado. Some of the residents in the community and students in the school come from lower socioeconomic backgrounds; others come from middle- and upper-class backgrounds. The students are primarily white, and several are descendants of early German settlers in the region. A few students are Hispanic, and some are children of migrant workers who work in the sugar beet fields. There are a handful of Asian students, mostly third- and fourth-generation Japanese-Americans.

On the day after Christmas vacation, Ms. Adams notes that one of her students, Terry, is constantly touching his teeth with his index finger. Walking over to his desk, she asks him what his problem is. "My teeth hurt," he replies. Asking him to open his mouth, she is shocked to see one of his teeth visibly eaten away with decay. "Do your parents know about this?" she asks the student. "Sure they do," he responds. "Then why don't you go to a dentist to have it taken care of?" she asks. "Cause we ain't got no money," he replies.

Questions for Discussion

1. Should Ms. Adams have pursued the questioning in front of the class?

2. What could she have done to minimize any embarrassment to Terry in front of his classmates?

3. Is the health and dental needs of a child the responsibility or concern of the teacher?

4. Should she contact Terry's parents? The principal? The school nurse?

Attempts to Censor

Mitchell Aoki is a second-year English teacher in a midwestern community of eighty thousand. He teaches sophomore and junior English classes. A fourth-generation Japanese-American, Aoki majored in English and religion and received his teaching credential from a private Southern Baptist university. His evaluations from his principal for his first year were considered excellent for a first-year teacher.

When his principal asks him to come to his office, Aoki is surprised when he is handed a letter from a parent. The letter reads:

> Suzanne came home crying in the heart. I don't know who this Mr. Aoki is, but he needs to know that it is important to respect the religious values of others even if he does not believe in our God. There will be retribution, for one cannot take the name of God in vain and not expect punishment for such blasphemy.

Stunned, Aoki asks the principal what the letter is all about? "That's what I was about to ask you," the principal replies.

"I never use profanity in front of the students. In fact, I don't use profanity at all," Aoki responds. "I don't know what this is all about. The letter implies that I'm a nonbeliever, a non-Christian. Maybe an atheist? I'm an active member of a Baptist Church. I even majored in religion."

"I know, Mitchell. That's why I'm trying to get to the bottom of this," the principal says.

Suddenly, it strikes Aoki. "It was the series of poems I read to the class last week. They were examples of poetry by some contemporary writers, and there was a passage in one where the author referred to someone as a 'God damned weasel.' I read that as a direct quote to a class of high school juniors and now I'm branded as a blasphemer! He's assuming that because of my ethnic background I'm religiously undesirable."

Questions for Discussion

1. Did Mitchell Aoki exercise poor judgment in reading a poem to the class that contained words offensive to the student and her father?

2. If he did nothing wrong, should he take precautions in the future to avoid similar reactions?

3. Should the student and father be contacted by Aoki? By the principal? By both? If so, what form should the contact take? A letter? A conference? An apology? An explanation? What type of explanation?

4. Are minority group teachers at greater risk of being perceived as nonmainstreamed in values, morals, and so on?

Differences in Socioeconomic Status

The middle school in a rural community of nine thousand residents has four school-sponsored dances a year. At the Valentines dance, a coat and tie affair, six of the eighth-grade boys showed up in rented tuxedos. They had planned this together, and their parents, among the more affluent in the community, thought it would be "cute" and paid for the rentals. The final dance of the year is scheduled for May, and it, too, is a coat and tie dance. This time, rumors are circulating around the school that "everyone" is renting a tux and the girls are getting new formal dresses. Three boys' parents are, according to the grapevine, renting a limousine for their sons and their dates. These self-imposed behaviors and dress standards are far in excess of anything previously observed at the middle school.

Several of the students, particularly those from lower socioeconomic backgrounds, have said that they will boycott the dance. They cannot afford the expensive attire, and they claim that the ones behind the dress-up movement have said that only the nerds or geeks would show up in anything less than a tux or a formal gown.

Questions for Discussion

1. Should the school administration intervene?

2. Should the parents be contacted?

3. Should the matter be discussed in the homerooms? In a school assembly?

4. Should the dance be canceled?

5. Should there be limits on how dressed up students can be? Could the school legally enforce limits?

6. Can and should there be any issue made on the hiring of limousine services for middle school students?

Religious Dietary Attitudes

Allison Beller is a fourth-grade teacher in a suburban school district. The community is primarily middle class. The children come from diverse ethnic and religious backgrounds. Part of her curriculum includes some basic lessons in cooking. Today's lesson involves the preparation of hamburgers. Beller is aware that one of the children is a vegetarian and that two others do not eat red meat. She has prepared burgers out of ground turkey for two and substituted what she felt was an appropriate alternative for the vegetarian child.

Beller is stunned, therefore, when the vegetarian child states before the class that eating hamburger is wrong and sinful. "My daddy says that hamburgers come from cows that are killed and it is wrong to kill cows or anything else. He says that if you eat the hamburgers, you are as bad as the people who killed the cow."

The other children in the class are also shocked at the accusation and sit in their places speechless.

Questions for Discussion

1. How should Ms. Beller respond to the accusation?
2. What should she say to the class?
3. Should she go on with the lesson?
4. Should she contact the child's parent? If so, what should she say and/or do?
5. Should she consult with the principal?
6. Should she discontinue the cooking lessons?

Observance of Religious Beliefs

Alexander Swanson ranks first in his senior class of 651 students with a 3.96 grade-point average. Dr. Diane Harris, the principal, is pleased to inform Alex that he will be the class valedictorian for the commencement in June. Alex is visibly pleased and shakes Dr. Harris' hand, thanking her as he leaves the office. As is her custom, Dr. Harris writes a letter to Alex's parents congratulating them on their son's achievements and informing them of his scheduled valedictory address on the first Saturday evening in June.

Three days later, when her secretary informs her that Mr. Swanson is on the phone, she expects to exchange pleasantries regarding Alex's accomplishments. Instead, Mr. Swanson informs her that it is quite impossible for Alex to make the valedictory address on graduation night because it will be the Sabbath, and their entire family will be attending their regular religious worship at that time. "Couldn't you make an exception this one time?" Dr. Harris asks.

"No, that is impossible," Mr. Swanson replies. "We would like you to change the graduation to Friday night instead," Mr. Swanson states.

"But that would be impossible," Dr. Harris explains. "The other high school has their commencement on Friday night, and the superintendent and many of the school board members attend both graduations. This was planned over a year ago."

"Then we are at an impasse, Dr. Harris. My son will not compromise his religious convictions," Swanson says firmly as he hangs up the telephone.

Questions for Discussion

1. What can Dr. Harris do?
2. Should the school district avoid scheduling Saturday commencements in the future?
3. Is there any way that Dr. Harris can provide Alex with the recognition he deserves without disrupting the commencement schedule or expecting him to compromise on his family's religious beliefs?

Student's Conflict Between Family and Peer Values

Wing Tek Lau is a sixth-grade student in a predominantly white and African-American southern community. He and his parents emigrated from Hong Kong four years ago. His uncle, an engineer at a locally based high-tech industry, had encouraged Wing Tek's father to immigrate to this country and open a Chinese restaurant. The restaurant is the only Chinese restaurant in the community, and it was an instant success. Mr. Lau and his family have enjoyed considerable acceptance in both his business and in his neighborhood. Wing Tek and his younger sister have also enjoyed academic success at school and appear to be well-liked by the other students.

One day when Mrs. Baca, Wing Tek's teacher, calls him by name, he announces before the class, "My American name is Kevin. Please, everybody call me Kevin from now on." Mrs. Baca and his classmates honor this request, and Wing Tek is "Kevin" from then on.

Three weeks later, Mr. and Mrs. Lau make an apppointment to see Mrs. Baca. When the teacher makes reference to "Kevin," Mrs. Lau says, "Who are you talking about? Who is Kevin? We came here to talk about our son, Wing Tek."

"But I thought his American name was Kevin. That's what he asked us to call him from now on," Mrs. Baca replies.

"That child," Mrs. Lau says in disgust, "is a disgrace to our family."

"We have heard his sister call him by that name, but she said it was just a joke," Mr. Lau adds. "We came to see you because we are having problems with him in our home," Mr. Lau states. "Wing Tek refuses to speak Chinese to us. He argues with us about going to his Chinese lessons on Saturday with the other Chinese students in the community. He says he does not want to eat Chinese food anymore. He says that he is an American now and wants pizza, hamburgers, and tacos. What are you people teaching these children in school? Is there no respect for family, no respect for our culture?"

Mrs. Baca, an acculturated Mexican-American who was raised in East Los Angeles, begins to put things together. Wing Tek, in his attempt to ensure his acceptance by his classmates, has chosen to acculturate to an extreme, to the point of rejecting his family heritage. He wants to be as "American" as anyone else in the class, perhaps more so. Like Wing Tek, Mrs. Baca had acculturated linguistically and in other ways, but had never given up her Hispanic values. She knows the internal turmoil Wing Tek is experiencing.

Questions for Discussion

1. Is Wing Tek wrong in his desire to acculturate?
2. Are Mr. and Mrs. Lau wrong in wanting their son to maintain traditional family values?
3. What can Mrs. Baca do to bring about a compromise?
4. Is there anything Mrs. Baca can do in the classroom to resolve the problem or to at least lessen the problem?

Placement of a Child with a Contagious Disease

At a special education student placement meeting, the first case involves a three-year-old male with a history of medical problems. The child is developmentally delayed and is not ambulatory. Further, the child is not toilet trained. He also lacks oral muscle control and drools constantly.

The medical report indicates that the student tests positive for cytomegalovirus (CMV). This is a herpes-like virus that is excreted in urine and saliva. CMV may result in mental retardation, severe hearing loss, microcephaly, and chronic liver disease when transmitted to newborns. A woman may have contracted CMV several years previously and been asymptomatic, but may transmit the virus in utero, during delivery, or via breast feeding. Eighty percent of all persons over age thirty-five show serologic evidence of previous infection. The majority of these infections are asymptomatic.

The school district's special education policy concerning CMV is checked by the placement committee, and it is discovered that there is *no* justification for excluding children who are known shedders of this virus. According to the "least restrictive environment" clause of PL 94-142, a special day class in a special school is the most appropriate placement.

Since the child is only three years old, he qualifies for only one of the seven preschool classes. The preschool program is run by an innovative instructional team consisting of five young female instructors (of childbearing age), one older female, one male teacher, and fourteen female assistants (of childbearing age). Three of the teachers are pregnant. The preschool staff members are a very strong, informal group. Further, four of the teachers have leadership roles on the school's steering committee.

The student placement meeting is concluded, and the parent is told that the child will be placed in one of the preschool classes and that transportation will begin in two weeks. Word leaks out that a child with CMV is about to enter the preschool program. A panic begins in the preschool department, and two teachers threaten to transfer if the child is put into their classroom.

Questions for Discussion

1. How should the administrator proceed?
2. How would you, as a teacher, react?
3. Where should the child be placed?
4. What would you do if the child was put in your class?

Racial Identification

Roosevelt High School annually celebrates Black History Month in February. The month-long study includes a convocation to celebrate African-American heritage. For ten years, students have organized and conducted this convocation in which the whole student body participates.

The students who have organized the event this year begin the convocation with the black national anthem. The African-American students, a few of the other students, and some of the faculty members stand for the singing of the anthem. Many of the African-American students become very angry at what they perceive to be a lack of respect by the students and faculty who refuse to stand.

In discussions that follow the convocation, some of the students and faculty who did not stand for the anthem argue that the only national anthem to which they should be expected to respond is their own national anthem. They say that it is unfair to be required to attend a convocation celebrating the heritage of one racial group when there is no convocation to celebrate their own racial or ethnic heritage.

Questions for Discussion

1. What may have been happening in the school that led to the tensions that surfaced during this convocation?
2. How may the African-American students perceive the refusal to stand by some of the students and faculty?
3. Do you think that the reasons for not standing during the anthem are valid? Why or why not?
4. If you are meeting with a class immediately after the convocation, how will you handle the tension between students?
5. What activities might be initiated within the school to reduce the interracial tensions that have developed?

Index